PRACTICAL
NEUROLOGY

FIFTH EDITION

PRACTICAL NEUROLOGY

FIFTH EDITION

José Biller, MD, FACP, FAAN, FANA, FAHA

Professor and Chairman

Department of Neurology

Loyola University Chicago

Maywood, Illinois

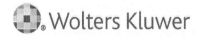. Wolters Kluwer

Philadelphia • Baltimore • New York • London
Buenos Aires • Hong Kong • Sydney • Tokyo

Acquisitions Editor: Kel McGowan
Product Development Editor: Andrea Vosburgh
Marketing Manager: Rachel Mante Leung
Senior Production Project Manager: Alicia Jackson
Design Coordinator: Elaine Kasmer
Manufacturing Coordinator: Beth Welsh
Prepress Vendor: S4Carlisle Publishing Services

5th edition

Library of Congress Cataloging-in-Publication Data
Names: Biller, José.
Title: Practical neurology / [edited by] José Biller, MD, FACP, FAAN, FAHA,
   professor and chairman, Department of Neurology, Loyola University
   Chicago, Stritch School of Medicine, Maywood, Illinois. Fifth edition.
Description: Fifth edition. | Philadelphia: Wolters Kluwer Heath, [2017] |
   Includes index.
Identifiers: LCCN 2016044459 | ISBN 9781496326959
Subjects: LCSH: Neurology.
Classification: LCC RC346.P685 2017 | DDC 616.8—dc23 LC record available at https://lccn.loc
   .gov/2016044459

LWW.com

This book is dedicated in memory of my parents Elena and Osías, and to my wife Rhonda, my children Sofía, Rebecca, Gabriel and Monique, my stepchildren Adam, Emily and Jon, and my grandchildren Selim, Ira, and Oz.

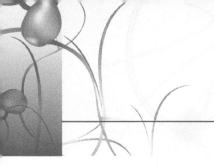

Contributors

Harold P. Adams, Jr., MD
Director
Department of Neurology
Comprehensive Stroke Center of Iowa Hospitals and Clinics
University of Iowa Hospitals and Clinics
Iowa City, Iowa

Joseph G. Akar, MD, PhD
Associate Professor of Medicine
Department of Medicine, Section of Cardiovascular Medicine
Yale University School of Medicine
New Haven, Connecticut

Sara Anderson-Kim, MS, RN, FNP-C, APN
Department of Otolaryngology—Head and Neck Surgery
Loyola University Medical Center
Maywood, Illinois

Alon Y. Avidan, MD, MPH
Professor of Neurology
Director
UCLA Sleep Disorders Center
UCLA Neurology Clinic
David Geffen School of Medicine
University of California Los Angeles
Los Angeles, California

Maria Baldwin, MD
Assistant Professor
Department of Neurology
VA Pittsburgh Healthcare System
University of Pittsburgh School of Medicine
Pittsburgh, Pennsylvania

Xabier Beristain, MD
Associate Professor of Neurology
Stritch School of Medicine
Loyola University Medical Center
Maywood, Illinois

José Biller, MD, FACP, FAAN, FANA, FAHA
Professor and Chairman
Department of Neurology
Loyola University Chicago
Stritch School of Medicine
Maywood, Illinois

Valérie Biousse, MD
Cyrus H. Stoner Professor of Ophthalmology
Professor of Ophthalmology and Neurology
Emory University School of Medicine
Atlanta, Georgia

Cynthia L. Bodkin, MD
Associate Professor in Clinical Neurology
Associate Professor in Physical Medical Rehabilitation
Indiana University School of Medicine
Indianapolis, Indiana

Troy Buck, MD
Assistant Professor of Anesthesiology
Department of Anesthesiology
Loyola University Chicago
Loyola University Medical Center
Maywood, Illinois

Marcello Cherchi, MD, PhD
Assistant Professor
Department of Neurology
Northwestern Feinberg School of Medicine
Chicago, Illinois

Melissa G. Chung, MD
Clinical Assistant Professor of Medicine
Division of Critical Care and Neurology
Department of Pediatrics
Nationwide Children's Hospital
The Ohio State University
Columbus, Ohio

Natalie L. Denburg, PhD
Associate Professor of Neurology and Neurosciences
Department of Neurology
University of Iowa Carver College of Medicine
Iowa City, Iowa

Kathleen B. Digre, MD
Professor of Neurology and Ophthalmology
Adjunct Professor of Obstetrics and Gynecology
University of Utah
Salt Lake City, Utah

Edward J. Dropcho, MD
Professor
Department of Neurology
Indiana University Medical Center
Indianapolis, Indiana

Andrew P. Duker, MD
Associate Professor of Neurology
Department of Neurology
James J. and Joan A. Gardner Family Center for Parkinson's Disease and Movement Disorders
University of Cincinnati
Cincinnati, Ohio

David W. Dunn, MD
Professor of Psychiatry and Neurology
Indiana University School of Medicine
Indianapolis, Indiana

Mark E. Dyken, MD, FAHA, FAASM, FANA
Professor of Neurology
Director
Sleep Disorders Center and Sleep Medicine and Clinical Neurophysiology Fellowship
Programs
Department of Neurology
University of Iowa Carver College of Medicine
Iowa City, Iowa

Nilüfer Ertekin-Taner, MD, PhD
Associate Professor of Neurology
Associate Professor of Neuroscience
Departments of Neurology and Neuroscience
Mayo Clinic
Jacksonville, Florida

Alberto J. Espay, MD, MSc, FAAN
Associate Professor of Neurology
Director and Endowed Chair
James J. and Joan A. Gardner Center for Parkinson's Disease and Movement Disorders
University of Cincinnati Academic Health Center
Cincinnati, Ohio

Eoin P. Flanagan, MBBCh
Assistant Professor of Neurology
Department of Neurology
Mayo Clinic
Rochester, Minnesota

Michael J. Frett, Jr., MD
Assistant Professor
Department of Anesthesiology
Loyola University Chicago
Stritch School of Medicine
Maywood, Illinois

Jeannette M. Gelauff, MD, PhD
Student
Department of Neurology
University Medical Center Groningen
Groningen, The Netherlands

Peter J. Goadsby, BMedSc, MBBS, MD, PhD, DSc, FRACP, FRCP, FMedSSci
Professor of Neurology
Director
NIHR-Wellcome Trust King's Clinical Research Facility
King's College
London, United Kingdom

Christopher G. Goetz, MD

Professor of Neurological Sciences
Professor of Pharmacology
Rush University Medical Center
Chicago, Illinois

Neill R. Graff-Radford, MBBCh, FRCP(UK)

David Eisenberg Professor of Neurology
Mayo Clinic
Jacksonville, Florida

Mark W. Green, MD

Director of Headache and Pain Medicine
Professor of Neurology, Anesthesiology, and Rehabilitation Medicine
Icahn School of Medicine at Mount Sinai
New York, New York

Michael W. Groff, MD

Director of Spinal Neurosurgery
Department of Neurological Surgery
Brigham and Women's Hospital
Boston, Massachusetts

Gregory Gruener, MD, MBA

Professor and Associate Chair
Department of Neurology
Loyola University Chicago
Stritch School of Medicine
Maywood, Illinois

Timothy C. Hain, MD

Professor Emeritus
Department of Physical Therapy and Human Movement Sciences
Northwestern University
Chicago, Illinois

Marcia J. Hay-McCutcheon, PhD, CCC-A

Associate Professor
Department of Communicative Disorders
The University of Alabama
Tuscaloosa, Alabama

Sara Hocker, MD

Assistant Professor of Neurology
Department of Neurology
Mayo Clinic
Rochester, Minnesota

Joseph R. Holtman, Jr., MD, PhD

Professor
Anesthesiology/Molecular Pharmacology and Therapeutics
Loyola University Chicago
Stritch School of Medicine
Maywood, Illinois

Holli A. Horak, MD
Associate Professor of Neurology
Department of Neurology
University of Arizona
Tucson, Arizona

Eric M. Horn, MD, PhD
Associate Professor
Department of Neurological Surgery
Indiana University School of Medicine
Goodman Campbell Brain and Spine
Indianapolis, Indiana

Tarik F. Ibrahim, MS, MD
(September 2, 1981 – July 30, 2016)
Neurosurgery Resident
Department of Neurological Surgery
Loyola University Medical Center
Maywood, Illinois

Kyoung Bin Im, MD, MS
Assistant Professor of Clinical Neurology and Psychiatry
University of Iowa Carver College of Medicine
University of Iowa Hospitals and Clinics
Iowa City, Iowa

Walter S. Jellish, MD, PhD
Professor and Chair
Department of Anesthesiology
Loyola University Chicago
Stritch School of Medicine
Maywood, Illinois

Robert G. Kaniecki, MD
Director
The Headache Center
Chief
Headache Division
Assistant Professor of Neurology
University of Pittsburgh School of Medicine
Pittsburgh, Pennsylvania

Aki Kawasaki, MD, PhD
Associate Professor
Faculty of Biology and Medicine
University of Lausanne
Department of Ophthalmology
Hopital Ophtalmique Jules Gonin
Lausanne, Switzerland

Bhupendra O. Khatri, MD
Director
Center for Neurological Disorders
Wheaton Franciscan Health Care
Milwaukee, Wisconsin

John C. Kincaid, MD

Professor of Neurology
Indiana University and Indiana University Health
Indianapolis, Indiana

Matthew L. Kircher, MD

Assistant Professor
Department of Otolaryngology—Head and Neck Surgery
Loyola University Chicago
Stritch School of Medicine
Maywood, Illinois

Athena Kostidis, MD

Clinical Assistant Professor of Neurology
Loyola University Medical Center
Maywood, Illinois

Sarah S. Kramer, MS, CCC-SLP

Speech and Language Pathology
Department of Speech Pathology
Loyola University Health System
Maywood, Illinois

Neeraj Kumar, MD

Department of Neurology
Mayo Clinic
Rochester, Minnesota

Krutika Kuppalli, MD

Assistant Professor
Division of Infectious Diseases
Department of Medicine
Loyola University Chicago
Stritch School of Medicine
Maywood, Illinois

John P. Leonetti, MD

Professor and Vice Chair
Department of Otolaryngology
Loyola University Chicago
Stritch School of Medicine
Maywood, Illinois

Betsy B. Love, MD

Clinical Associate Professor of Neurology
Loyola University Chicago
Stritch School of Medicine
Maywood, Illinois

Rimas V. Lukas, MD

Director of Medical Neuro-Oncology
Associate Professor
Department of Neurology
University of Chicago
Chicago, Illinois

Devin D. Mackay, MD
Assistant Professor of Clinical Neurology, Ophthalmology, and Neurosurgery
Indiana University School of Medicine
Indianapolis, Indiana

Raul N. Mandler, MD, FAAN, FANA
North Bethesda, Maryland

Omkar N. Markand, MD, FRCP(C), FACP, FAAN
Professor Emeritus of Neurology
Indiana University School of Medicine
Indianapolis, Indiana

Sam J. Marzo, MD
Professor and Chairman
Department of Otolaryngology—Head and Neck Surgery
Loyola University Chicago
Stritch School of Medicine
Maywood, Illinois

Nikolas Mata-Machado, MD
Instructor
Department of Neurology
Division of Child Neurology
Loyola University Chicago
Stritch School of Medicine
Maywood, Illinois

Matthew A. McCoyd, MD
Assistant Professor of Neurology
Loyola University Chicago
Stritch School of Medicine
Maywood, Illinois

Michael P. McQuillen, MD, MA
Former Chairman, Department of Neurology
The Medical College of Wisconsin and University of Kentucky College of Medicine
Professor of Neurology (retired)
Stanford University
Departmen of Neurology and Neurological Sciences
Palo Alto, California

Michael P. Merchut, MD, FAAN, FACP
Professor
Department of Neurology
Loyola University Chicago
Stritch School of Medicine
Maywood, Illinois

Richard T. Miyamoto, MD, MS (Otology)
Arilla Spence DeVault Professor Emeritus
Department of Otolaryngology—Head and Neck Surgery
Indiana University School of Medicine
Indianapolis, Indiana

Paul B. Nelson, MD
Professor
Department of Neurosurgery
Penn State Health College of Medicine
University Park, Pennsylvania

Nancy J. Newman, MD
LeoDelle Jolley Professor of Ophthalmology
Professor of Ophthalmology and Neurology
Instructor in Neurological Surgery
Director, Neuro-Ophthalmology
Emory University School of Medicine
Atlanta, Georgia

Russ P. Nockels, MD
Professor and Vice Chair
Department of Neurological Surgery
Loyola University Chicago
Stritch School of Medicine
Maywood, Illinois

Paul O'Keefe, MD
The John W. Clarke Professor and Chairman
Department of Medicine
Loyola University Chicago
Stritch School of Medicine
Maywood, Illinois

Emilio Oribe, MD, FACP
Affiliate Assistant Professor of Clinical Neurology
Weill Cornell Medical College of Cornell University
New York, New York

Javier Pagonabarraga, MD, PhD
Neurologist
Unit of Movement Disorders
Hospital Sant Pau
Barcelona, Spain

Robert M. Pascuzzi, MD
Professor of Neurology
Indiana University School of Medicine
Chairman
Neurology Department
Indiana University Health
Indianapolis, Indiana

Hema Patel, MD
Professor, Clinical Neurology
Department of Neurology, Section of Child Neurology
Riley Hospital for Children
Indiana University Medical Center
Indianapolis, Indiana

Marc C. Patterson, MD

Chair
Division of Child and Adolescent Neurology
Professor of Neurology, Pediatrics, and Medical Genetics
Mayo Clinic Children's Center
Mayo Clinic
Rochester, Minnesota

Valerie Purvin, MD

Professor
Departments of Ophthalmology and Neurology
Indiana Medical Center
Indianapolis, Indiana

Alejandro A. Rabinstein, MD

Professor of Neurology
Mayo Clinic
Rochester, Minnesota

Sarah L. Rahal, MD

Assistant Professor
Departments of Neurology and Pediatrics
Icahn School of Medicine at Mount Sinai
New York, New York

Adolfo Ramirez-Zamora, MD

Associate Professor of Neurology
Phyllis E. Drake Endowed Chair in Movement Disorders
Department of Neurology
Albany Medical College
Albany, New York

E. Steve Roach, MD

Wolfe Professor and Chief
Division of Child Neurology
The Ohio State University College of Medicine
Nationwide Children's Hospital
Columbus, Ohio

Christopher P. Robinson, DO, MS

Neurocritical Care Fellow
Department of Neurology
Mayo Clinic
Rochester, Minnesota

Robert L. Rodnitzky, MD

Professor and Chair Emeritus
Department of Neurology
University of Iowa College of Medicine
Iowa City, Iowa

Karen L. Roos, MD

John and Nancy Nelson Professor of Neurology
Professor of Neurological Surgery
Indiana University School of Medicine
Indianapolis, Indiana

Jordan Rosenblum, MD

Professor of Radiology and Neurology
Loyola University Chicago
Stritch School of Medicine
Maywood, Illinois

Mark A. Ross, MD

Professor of Neurology
Department of Neurology
Mayo Clinic Arizona
Scottsdale, Arizona

Sean Ruland, DO

Professor of Neurology
Department of Neurology
Loyola University Chicago
Stritch School of Medicine
Maywood, Illinois

Meridith Runke, MD

Assistant Professor for Clinical Neurology
Department of Neurology
Indiana University School of Medicine
Indianapolis, Indiana

Daniel E. Rusyniak, MD

Division Chief, Medical Toxicology
Medical Director, Indiana Poison Center
Professor of Emergency Medicine
Department of Emergency Medicine
Indiana University School of Medicine
Indianapolis, Indiana

Vicenta Salanova, MD, FAAN

Professor of Neurology
Director
Indiana University Epilepsy Program
Indiana University School of Medicine
Indianapolis, Indiana

Arash Salardini, MD

Assistant Professor, Behavioral Neurology
Yale University
New Haven, Connecticut

Peter A. Santucci, MD

Professor of Medicine
Section of Cardiac Electrophysiology
Loyola University Chicago
Stritch School of Medicine
Maywood, Illinois

Jeffrey L. Saver, MD
Professor of Neurology
David Geffen School of Medicine at UCLA
Director
Stroke Center
UCLA Ronald Reagan Medical Center
Los Angeles, California

Michael J. Schneck, MD, FAAN, FANA, FAHA
Professor of Neurology and Neurosurgery
Department of Neurology
Loyola University Chicago
Stritch School of Medicine
Maywood, Illinois

Eugene R. Schnitzler, MD
Professor of Neurology and Pediatrics
Loyola University Chicago
Stritch School of Medicine
Maywood, Illinois

Scott A. Shapiro, MD, FACS
Robert L. Campbell Professor of Neurosurgery
Indiana University School of Medicine
Indianapolis, Indiana

Jon Stone, MD
Consultant Neurologist and Honorary Reader in Neurology
Department of Clinical Neurosciences
University of Edinburgh
Edinburgh, United Kingdom

Rochelle Sweis, DO
Assistant Professor of Neurology
Department of Neurology
Loyola University Chicago
Stritch School of Medicine
Maywood, Illinois

Annya D. Tisher, MD
Clinical Fellow, Behavioral Neurology
Department of Neurology
Yale School of Medicine
New Haven, Connecticut

Laura M. Tormoehlen, MD
Assistant Professor of Clinical Neurology and Emergency Medicine
Neurology and Emergency Medicine
Indiana University School of Medicine
Indianapolis, Indiana

Daniel Tranel, PhD
Professor
Departments of Neurology and Psychology
University of Iowa
Iowa City, Iowa

Amy R. Tso, MD
Basic and Clinical Neuroscience
Institute of Psychiatry, Psychology and Neuroscience
King's College London
NIHR-Wellcome Trust King's Clinical Research Faculty
King's College Hospital
London, United Kingdom

Ergun Y. Uc, MD
Professor
Department of Neurology
University of Iowa and Iowa City VA Health Care System
Iowa City, Iowa

Michael W. Varner, MD
Professor
Department of Obstetrics and Gynecology
University of Utah Health Sciences Center
Salt Lake City, Utah

Eelco F. M. Wijdicks, MD, PhD
Professor of Neurology
Chairman of Neurocritical Care
Mayo Clinic
Rochester, Minnesota

David J. Wilber, MD, FACC, FAHA
George M. Eisenberg Professor of Cardiovascular Sciences
Director
Division of Cardiology
Cardiovascular Institute
Loyola University Chicago
Stritch School of Medicine
Maywood, Illinois

Torricia H. Yamada, PhD
Staff Neuropsychologist
Mental Health PSL
Minneapolis VAHCS
Minneapolis, Minnesota

Joseph Zachariah, MD
Neurointensive Care Fellow
Division of Critical Care Neurology
Mayo Clinic Hospital
Rochester, Minnesota

Phyllis C. Zee, MD, PhD
Benjamin and Virginia T. Boshes Professor in Neurology
Director
Northwestern Medicine Sleep Disorders Center
Director
Center for Circadian and Sleep Medicine
Northwestern University Feinberg School of Medicine
Chicago, Illinois

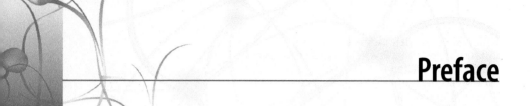

Preface

Welcome to the fifth edition of *Practical Neurology*. In addition to providing the necessary updates that incorporate the rapid advances of the science that informs the practice of clinical neurology, we have kept this new edition in the same accessible format of the prior editions, providing practical information. Its clarity of outline also allows this fifth edition to be scholarly by adding to the breadth of topics and presenting a wide range of neurologic conditions for review. The fifth edition of *Practical Neurology* is not intended to replace existing and more comprehensive reference and neurology textbooks. From the outset, we were determined to produce a textbook that covers the most important topics in a format that is complete, and effective for the neurologist in training, or the practicing neurologist needing an update.

In developing this "new and improved" text, we benefited greatly from the suggestions of users of previous editions and inputs from medical students, neurology residents, and neurology fellows. The first section (Chapters 1 to 39) of the book is directed at diagnosis. The second section (Chapters 40 to 63) addresses treatment. Many of the outstanding authors of chapters from previous editions are back again, but many new authors helped to achieve our more ambitious goals for this edition. To remain relevant, a number of new chapters were added: Approach to the Ataxic Patient (Chapter 29), Approach to the Patient with Functional Disorders in the Neurology Clinic (Chapter 33), Approach to the Patient with Suspected Brain Death (Chapter 34), Approach to Common Emergencies in Pediatric Neurology (Chapter 38), and Inherited Metabolic Neurologic Disorders (Chapter 49). The textbook is further enhanced by the addition of didactic videos for each chapter, concluding each chapter with a list of Key Points, and limiting references to those most relevant to the material presented. Our collective hope is that this clinically relevant, straightforward, and contemporary volume will meet the needs of a multidisciplinary readership.

My thanks are extended to all who have participated in this rewarding effort; and a heartfelt thanks to all the authors who worked diligently to bring this edition to fruition. Finally, I want to express my sincere appreciation to the many patients who participated in this textbook, as they volunteered to allow their own videos to be used to both educate and inform.

José Biller, MD, FACP, FAAN, FANA, FAHA

Acknowledgments

The success of this effort could not have been achieved without the support and professionalism of Andrea Vosburgh, Product Development Editor for Health Learning, Research and Practice at Wolters Kluwer. Organizing this book, and tracking all of the major logistical challenges, could not have been accomplished without the skills and dedication of Linda Turner, who kept me organized and helped to ensure that lines of communication were always clear.

Contents

Contributors   vi

Preface   xviii

Acknowledgments   xix

SECTION I. Diagnosis

1   Approach to the Patient with Acute Confusional State (Delirium/Encephalopathy)   1
Joseph Zachariah and Sara Hocker

2   Approach to the Patient with Dementia   15
Nilüfer Ertekin-Taner and Neill R. Graff-Radford

3   Approach to the Patient with Aphasia   29
Jeffrey L. Saver and José Biller

4   Approach to the Patient with Memory Impairment   40
Torricia H. Yamada, Natalie L. Denburg, and Daniel Tranel

5   Approach to the Comatose Patient   52
Michael P. Merchut

6   Approach to the Patient with Seizures   59
Vicenta Salanova and Meridith Runke

7   Approach to the Patient with Syncope   70
Peter A. Santucci, Joseph G. Akar, and David J. Wilber

8   Approach to the Patient with Gait Disturbance and Recurrent Falls   80
Xabier Beristain

9   Approach to the Patient with Sleep Disorders   93
Mark E. Dyken and Kyoung Bin Im

10   Approach to the Patient with Visual Loss   108
Devin D. Mackay, Valérie Biousse, and Nancy J. Newman

11   Approach to the Patient with Abnormal Pupils   121
Aki Kawasaki

12   Approach to the Patient with Diplopia   132
Devin D. Mackay and Valerie Purvin

13   Approach to the Patient with Facial Numbness   142
Arash Salardini and Betsy B. Love

14   Approach to the Patient with Facial Pain   153
Murray S. Flaster

15   Approach to the Patient with Facial Weakness   162
Sam J. Marzo and John P. Leonetti

16 Approach to the Patient with Dizziness and Vertigo 172
Timothy C. Hain and Marcello Cherchi

17 Approach to the Patient with Hearing Loss 190
Richard T. Miyamoto and Marcia J. Hay-McCutcheon

18 Approach to the Patient with Dysphagia 202
Alejandro A. Rabinstein

19 Approach to the Patient with Dysarthria 211
Sarah S. Kramer, Michael J. Schneck, and José Biller

20 Approach to the Patient with Acute Headache 218
Mark W. Green and Sarah L. Rahal

21 Approach to the Patient with Chronic and Recurrent Headache 227
Robert G. Kaniecki

22 Approach to the Patient with Neck Pain and/or Arm Pain 240
Scott A. Shapiro

23 Approach to the Patient with Low Back Pain, Lumbosacral
Radiculopathy, and Lumbar Stenosis 249
Eric M. Horn and Paul B. Nelson

24 Approach to the Patient with Upper Extremity Pain and Paresthesias
and Entrapment Neuropathies 258
Mark A. Ross

25 Approach to the Patient with Lower Extremity Pain, Paresthesias,
and Entrapment Neuropathies 272
Gregory Gruener

26 Approach to the Patient with Failed Back Syndrome 283
Tarik F. Ibrahim, Russ P. Nockels, and Michael W. Groff

27 Approach to the Patient with Acute Sensory Loss 291
Eoin P. Flanagan and Neeraj Kumar

28 Approach to the Hyperkinetic Patient 301
Javier Pagonabarraga and Christopher G. Goetz

29 Approach to the Ataxic Patient 318
Adolfo Ramirez-Zamora

30 Approach to the Hypokinetic Patient 328
Ergun Y. Uc and Robert L. Rodnitzky

31 Approach to the Patient with Acute Muscle Weakness 340
Holli A. Horak

32 Approach to the Patient with Neurogenic Orthostatic Hypotension,
Sexual and Urinary Dysfunction, and Other Autonomic Disorders 347
Emilio Oribe

33 Approach to the Patient with Functional Disorders
in the Neurology Clinic 368
Jeannette M. Gelauff and Jon Stone

34 Approach to the Patient with Suspected Brain Death 380
Christopher P. Robinson and Eelco F. M. Wijdicks

35 Neuroimaging of Common Neurologic Conditions 391
Jordan Rosenblum

36 Approach to the Selection of Electrodiagnostic, Cerebrospinal Fluid, and Other Ancillary Testing 406
Maria Baldwin and Matthew A. McCoyd

37 Approach to Common Office Problems of Pediatric Neurology 432
Eugene R. Schnitzler and Nikolas Mata-Machado

38 Approach to Common Emergencies in Pediatric Neurology 446
Melissa G. Chung and E. Steve Roach

39 Approach to Ethical Issues in Neurology 459
Bhupendra O. Khatri and Michael P. McQuillen

SECTION II. Treatment

40 Ischemic Cerebrovascular Disease 473
José Biller and Rochelle Sweis

41 Hemorrhagic Cerebrovascular Disease 494
Harold P. Adams, Jr.

42 Epilepsies in Children 510
Hema Patel and David W. Dunn

43 Epilepsy in Adults 530
Omkar N. Markand

44 Multiple Sclerosis 561
Matthew A. McCoyd

45 Movement Disorders 575
Andrew P. Duker and Alberto J. Espay

46 Dementia 588
Annya D. Tisher and Arash Salardini

47 Central Nervous System Infections 605
Karen L. Roos

48 Neurologic Complications in Acquired Immune Deficiency Syndrome 617
Krutika Kuppalli and Paul O'Keefe

49 Inherited Metabolic Neurologic Disorders 639
Marc C. Patterson

50 Spinal Cord Disorders 646
Athena Kostidis

51 Peripheral Neuropathy 663
John C. Kincaid

52 Myopathy 673
Holli A. Horak and Raul N. Mandler

53 Disorders of the Neuromuscular Junction 685
Robert M. Pascuzzi and Cynthia L. Bodkin

54 Therapy of Migraine, Tension-Type, and Cluster Headache 697
Amy R. Tso and Peter J. Goadsby

55 Chronic Pain 713
Troy Buck and Walter S. Jellish

56 Complex Regional Pain Syndrome 724
Joseph R. Holtman and Michael J. Frett, Jr.

57 Primary Central Nervous System Tumors 737
Edward J. Dropcho

58 Nervous System Complications of Cancer 750
Rimas V. Lukas

59 Neurotoxicology 763
Laura M. Tormoehlen and Daniel E. Rusyniak

60 Sleep Disorders 781
Phyllis C. Zee and Alon Y. Avidan

61 Dizziness and Vertigo 807
Matthew L. Kircher and Sara Anderson-Kim

62 Neurologic Diseases in Pregnancy 818
Kathleen B. Digre and Michael W. Varner

63 The ABCs of Neurologic Emergencies 839
José Biller, Rochelle Sweis, and Sean Ruland

Index 865

1

Approach to the Patient with Acute Confusional State (Delirium/Encephalopathy)

Joseph Zachariah and Sara Hocker

Acute confusional state is one of the most common reasons for neurologic consultation in a hospital setting. While there is no universally agreed-upon distinction between the terms, an acute confusional state is due to acute brain dysfunction and is typically referred to as either *encephalopathy* or *delirium*. Encephalopathy can be conceptualized as a global alteration in the content of consciousness and often the level of consciousness due to an underlying neurologic or systemic cause, which is usually acute to subacute in onset and reversible with treatment of the precipitating condition(s). Delirium is defined in the fifth revision of the *Diagnostic and Statistical Manual of Mental Disorders* (*DSM-5*) as a disturbance in attention, awareness, and cognition, developing over hours to days, fluctuating in severity throughout the day, and not attributable to any preexisting neurocognitive condition. The past decade has provided insight into the risk factors for and consequences of delirium, namely, long-term cognitive impairment and increased mortality. The terms *encephalopathy* and *delirium* are simply constructs for thinking about acute brain dysfunction and significant overlap exists. We will use the terms interchangeably or refer to *acute confusional state* for the remainder of this chapter.

The plethora of causes of acute confusional state can truly be daunting, and it requires both an experienced provider and an organized approach to identify the etiology or multiple etiologies in an individual patient. In most instances, acute confusional states are reversible as long as the etiology is recognized early. Early evaluation of the cause of acute confusional state is necessary to identify treatable causes where a delay in diagnosis may result in permanent morbidity or death. While a diagnosis of "encephalopathy" or "delirium" is useful for billing and coding purposes, it is not terribly informative to the medical team caring for the patient. Instead, identification of all potentially contributing factors can speed resolution of the confusional state by allowing the medical team to focus on modifiable factors.

PATHOPHYSIOLOGY

The pathophysiology of encephalopathy and delirium is poorly understood and varies with the etiology. For example, the pathophysiology of hepatic encephalopathy differs from that of the encephalopathy that results from administration of anticholinergic drugs. Still, the common pathophysiologic mechanism of all causes of acute confusional state is widespread dysfunction of the cortical and subcortical neurons. Alterations in the level of consciousness arise from disruptions to the reticular activating system (RAS) fibers due to bihemispheric injury, bithalamic injury, or the brainstem reticular formation. The RAS fibers are a network of neurons that connect the thalamus with the cortex and dorsal forebrain, which serve to regulate wakefulness and sleep–wake transitions. Focal populations of neurons may be affected or neuronal functioning may be diffusely disrupted. Other mechanisms include endothelial dysfunction, disrupted blood–brain barrier, alterations in cerebral blood flow and cerebral hypoperfusion, altered neurotransmitter and glucose composition, and excess of circulating inflammatory cytokines leading to microglial activation and mitochondria and astrocyte dysfunction.

The neurotransmitters acetylcholine and dopamine are known to play a central role in the regulation and communication of large numbers of neurons, and, thus, their alteration through medications can contribute to the development of an acute confusional state. As cholinergic neuronal pathways are widespread and critical in most executive brain functions, anticholinergic medications may induce hyperactivity and reduce attention through down-regulation of these pathways. Dopaminergic neurons are found primarily in the nigrostriatal, hypothalamic–pituitary and ventral tegmental areas, which then project diffusely to the frontal and temporal lobes. Dopamine agonists may contribute to an acute confusional state through upregulation of the dopamine pathways. Depletion of other monoamines including norepinephrine and serotonin also likely plays a role. Antidopaminergic agents (neuroleptics) are commonly used in management of delirium-related symptoms.

ETIOLOGIES

Innumerable etiologies of acute confusional state exist. A list of potential etiologies can be found in Table 1.1, and these can be separated into broad categories including structural

TABLE 1.1 Causes of Acute Confusional State

Structural

Traumatic contusions
Diffuse axonal injury
Intracranial hemorrhage (intraparenchymal, intraventricular, epidural, subdural, subarachnoid)
Cerebral infarction (arterial and venous)
Tumors (primary, metastatic, meningeal carcinomatosis)
Hydrocephalus
Paroxysmal sympathetic hyperactivity (autonomic storms)
Anoxic-ischemic brain injury
Central pontine myelinolysis

Metabolic

Electrolyte derangements (hyponatremia, hypernatremia, hypercalcemia)
Hyperosmolality, hypo-osmolality
Acid–base disorders (acidosis or alkalosis)
Hypercapnia
Hypoxia
Hypoglycemia or severe hyperglycemia
Uremia
Acute or chronic liver failure
Reye's syndrome
Pancreatic encephalopathy
Acute intermittent porphyria
Hypothyroidism or hyperthyroidism
Adrenal cortical insufficiency
Pituitary failure

Nutritional

Thiamine deficiency (Wernicke's encephalopathy)

Toxic

Acute alcohol intoxication/withdrawal
Opioid intoxication
Cocaine intoxication
Amphetamine intoxication
Phencyclidine intoxication
Sedative-hypnotic intoxication/withdrawal
Barbiturate intoxication/withdrawal
Benzodiazepine intoxication/withdrawal
Lithium intoxication
Carbon monoxide poisoning
Inhalant poisoning (i.e., amyl nitrite, toluene, nitrous oxide)
Malignant hyperthermia

TABLE 1.1 Causes of Acute Confusional State (*continued*)

NMS
Serotonin syndrome
Cefepime neurotoxicity
Metronidazole encephalopathy
Tacrolimus neurotoxicity
Infectious
Systemic infection
Sepsis
CNS infection (meningitis, encephalitis, or abscess)
Other
Nonconvulsive seizures, NCSE, or postictal state
Acute disseminated encephalomyelitis
Antibody-mediated encephalitis
Systemic lupus erythematosus
Paraneoplastic neurologic syndromes
PRES and the related hypertensive encephalopathy
Decompensated dementia
Post perfusion syndrome (due to disturbed microcirculation after cardiac surgery)
Hypothermia and hyperpyrexia
Sensory deprivation
Sleep deprivation

Abbreviations: CNS, central nervous system; NCSE, nonconvulsive status epilepticus; NMS, neuroleptic malignant syndrome; PRES, posterior reversible encephalopathy syndrome.

(trauma, vascular, neoplastic, anoxic-ischemic), metabolic, toxic, infectious, and other. This table is meant to be used as a guide and is by no means exhaustive.

A. Structural causes

Structural etiologies of altered mental status can be caused by trauma, anoxic-ischemic injury, hemorrhages, infarctions, neoplasms, and hydrocephalus. Trauma can result in hemorrhagic or nonhemorrhagic brain contusions or diffuse axonal injury, which produce varying degrees of encephalopathies. Patients with long-bone fractures from polytrauma can develop cerebral fat embolization manifesting as a transient encephalopathy with or without seizures and focal neurologic deficits lasting up to a month. While contusions and hemorrhages are easily identifiable on a noncontrast head computed tomography (CT), diffuse axonal injury and fat emboli are better visualized by magnetic resonance imaging (MRI) and should be considered when patients have persistent encephalopathy following trauma. Brain hemorrhages (intraparenchymal, subdural, epidural, or subarachnoid), infarctions, or tumors located in both cerebral hemispheres, the thalami, or brainstem can lead to an acute confusional state or varying degrees of stupor or coma. Lesions located in one cerebral hemisphere can be large enough to cause tissue shift and compression of the contralateral hemisphere, thereby producing an acute confusional state associated with focal neurologic deficits. In other cases, a lesion may be strategically located (i.e., in the frontal or temporal lobes) such that it produces acute confusion in the absence of significant edema. Carcinomatous meningitis, the diffuse infiltration of neoplastic cells into the meninges, may occur in the setting of leukemias, lymphomas, malignant melanoma, and lung or breast cancers. Patients with carcinomatous meningitis often present with headache, neck stiffness, and cranial nerve abnormalities because of direct infiltration of cancer cells. Severe hypoxemia or global reductions in cerebral blood flow can also cause irreversible injury because brain regions with high metabolic demand such as the basal ganglia and motor and occipital cortices suffer anoxic-ischemic injury.

B. Metabolic causes

"Metabolic encephalopathy" is one of the most common reasons for neurologic consultation in the hospital. Any acute organ dysfunction can produce an acute confusional state, and the severity varies depending on the degree of organ dysfunction and the rapidity over which it developed. For example, when renal failure develops very slowly over many months, the brain is often able to adapt, whereas when it develops suddenly over days to weeks, accumulation of toxins can lead to severe confusion or even coma. The exception is chronic liver failure, where patients may develop acute episodes of encephalopathy periodically without a corresponding acute decline in liver function. The most common causes of "metabolic encephalopathy" by far are liver or kidney dysfunction. Other causes include diabetic ketoacidosis and nonketotic hyperglycemic state, hyper- or hypothyroid states, or major electrolyte imbalances or acid–base derangements. Generally, encephalopathy resulting from metabolic derangements resolves with correction of the underlying organ injury, acid–base imbalance, and endocrine or electrolyte derangement. It is acceptable to rapidly correct the majority of these conditions (when possible); however, clinicians should exercise caution in the setting of an acute on chronic hyponatremia where rapid correction may precipitate a frequently irreversible osmotic demyelination syndrome otherwise known as *central pontine myelinolysis*.

C. Nutritional causes

Alcoholic patients are prone to several nutritional deficiencies, some of which may lead to a subacute or chronic cognitive decline. Thiamine deficiency, specifically, can produce an acute confusional state known as "Wernicke's encephalopathy" if patients are given glucose before thiamine repletion. Thiamine supplementation is therefore recommended before glucose administration in any patient with suspected or known chronic alcohol use as well as any patient with risk factors for nutritional deficiencies such as those with cancer, prior gastric bypass, inflammatory bowel disease, or eating disorders in order to avoid irreversible injury to the mamillary bodies. Wernicke's syndrome may variably result in a constellation of symptoms including acute encephalopathy, ophthalmoplegia, and ataxia. The full triad is rare.

D. Toxic causes

Toxic causes of encephalopathy include intoxication or withdrawal syndromes, drug–drug interactions, or drug toxicity in the setting of reduced renal or hepatic function. As discussed in the pathophysiology section, certain drugs have the potential at therapeutic levels to cause acute confusional states because of their alteration of neurotransmitter concentrations. While some drugs are more likely offenders than others, any drug is a potential culprit when it becomes supratherapeutic or when combined with the wrong drug.

When patients present for evaluation of acute encephalopathy, intoxication with a drug of abuse should be considered. When the encephalopathy develops after admission the patient may be withdrawing from a regularly used drug or alcohol. Urine and serum drug screens can detect most commonly used drugs of abuse; however, newer synthetic agents including bath salts and synthetic marijuana may not be detectable by conventional drug screens. Alcohol intoxication can be assessed through odor and serum alcohol levels but alcohol withdrawal symptoms are easily overlooked. Intoxication and withdrawal syndromes as well as certain drug interactions and toxicities may be life threatening and therefore require prompt recognition and timely intervention. Signs and symptoms of common culprits are listed in Table 1.2.

Neuroleptic malignant syndrome (NMS) and serotonin syndrome may develop during hospitalization of a patient on psychiatric medications. Both syndromes share common features including hyperpyrexia, rigidity, tachycardia, hypertension, and encephalopathy but important differences exist. Fentanyl and antiemetics are common precipitants of a serotonin syndrome in the hospital when they are initiated in patients receiving selective serotonin reuptake inhibitors.

Antineoplastic and immunosuppressive agents may potentiate a posterior reversible encephalopathy syndrome (PRES). PRES is a clinicoradiographic syndrome thought to be due to endothelial dysfunction and vasogenic edema preferentially affecting the posterior cerebral regions. The primary triggers include acute hypertension or blood pressure swings, sepsis, autoimmune conditions, cytotoxic medications (including antineoplastic and immunosuppressants), and pre-eclampsia or eclampsia. The majority of patients recover completely within 2 to 8 days. However, severe cases of PRES can lead to irreversible brain injury because of infarcts and hemorrhages in the areas of edema.

The most notable antibiotics causing severe encephalopathy are cefepime and metronidazole. In patients with renal impairment, serum and cerebrospinal fluid (CSF)

TABLE 1.2 Important Drug-Related Syndromes

Common intoxication syndromes	
Sedatives *Benzodiazepines, barbiturates, alcohol*	CNS depression, bradycardia, hypothermia, hypotension, apnea
Opioids *Oxycodone, heroin, morphine, methadone*	CNS depression, bradycardia, hypothermia, hypotension, apnea, miosis
Sympathomimetics/hallucinogenics *Cocaine, ephedrine, amphetamines* *Ecstasy, PCP, LSD, MDMA*	Agitation, hallucinations, diaphoresis, mydriasis, hyperthermia, hypertension, tachypnea, tremors, seizures
Anticholinergics *Scopolamine, antihistamines, atropine,* *Parkinson medications, antispasmodics*	Agitation, hallucinations, diaphoresis, mydriasis, hyperthermia, hypertension, tachypnea, tremors, seizures, dry skin/mucous membranes, urinary retention, decreased bowel sounds
Common withdrawal syndromes	
Sedatives	Agitation, tremors, seizures, autonomic dysfunction, tachycardia
Opioids	Agitation, mydriasis, nausea, vomiting, diarrhea, lacrimation, cramping, yawning, piloerection
Sympathomimetics	Psychomotor retardation, depression, excessive sleep
Anticholinergics	Diaphoresis, nausea, rebound anxiety, restlessness, palpitations, urinary urgency
Other	
Serotonin syndrome *Any combination of the following:* *MAOI, SSRI, TCA, fentanyl, MDMA, LSD,* *metoclopramide*	Encephalopathy, hypertension, tachycardia, hyperpyrexia, mydriasis, increased tone in the legs>arms, myoclonus/clonus, shivering, increased bowel sounds
NMS *Any combination of the following:* *Typical or atypical psychotics, Antiemetics,* *sudden withdrawal of* L-DOPA	Encephalopathy, hypertension, tachycardia, hyperpyrexia, rigidity, shivering
Cefepime neurotoxicity	Depressed consciousness, myoclonus

Abbreviations: CNS, central nervous system; NMS, neuroleptic malignant syndrome; PCP, phencyclidine; LSD, lysergic acid diethylamide; MDMA, 3,4-methylenedioxymethamphetamine; MAOI, monoamine oxidase inhibitor; SSRI, selective serotonin reuptake inhibitor; TCA, tricyclic antidepressant.

levels of cefepime can approach toxic thresholds to trigger seizures, confusion, myoclonus, and even coma. The pathophysiology of metronidazole-induced encephalopathy is less understood and is thought to occur as a result of modulation of neurotransmitters by the metabolites of metronidazole.

E. Infectious causes

Infections such as meningitis and encephalitis and opportunistic infections such as aspergillosis and toxoplasmosis in immunosuppressed individuals can undoubtedly result in acute confusional states by direct invasion of the brain and severe inflammation. These infections can variably lead to hemorrhages, arterial infarctions as a result of infectious vasculitis, venous ischemia from cerebral venous and dural sinus thrombosis, or abscess formation. Systemic infections, especially sepsis and septic shock, may also provoke robust cytokine storms that result in dysfunction of several cell types and disruption of neurotransmission and calcium homeostasis. Disruptions in blood–brain barrier expose the brain parenchyma to various circulating toxic infectious molecules or to inappropriately metabolized drugs due to concurrent liver or kidney injury. The severity of encephalopathy in sepsis is related to the severity of sepsis. It should be noted that septic encephalopathy can occur in the absence of overt organ injury.

1. Nonconvulsive seizures, nonconvulsive status epilepticus, or postictal state

Nonconvulsive seizures found in up to 8% of critically ill patients, nonconvulsive status epilepticus (NCSE), or postictal states can present as acute confusional states.

Nonconvulsive seizures or status epilepticus can be suspected in somnolent or lethargic patients found to have subtle twitching of the face or limbs or the patient may simply appear withdrawn and disengaged. The diagnosis is very challenging and can evade even the most experienced of clinicians.

F. Hypertensive encephalopathy

Sudden spikes of blood pressure due to any cause above the limit of cerebral autoregulation can result in endothelial injury, breakdown of the blood–brain barrier, and subsequent vasogenic edema. Hypertensive urgency and emergency are reversible when identified and managed early; however, delayed recognition can lead to hemorrhages, ischemia, and cerebral edema. It can also precipitate a syndrome of reversible encephalopathy and vasogenic edema, known as PRES (discussed earlier).

G. When no clear cause is identified "delirium"

Patients with any degree of underlying cognitive impairment can easily decompensate in the setting of an acute medical or neurologic insult, a condition known as "beclouded" or "decompensated" dementia. Patients with neurocognitive disorders are at higher risk for development of delirium and may take longer to recover from events such as anesthesia, sedatives, postoperative states, postictal states, and prolonged hospitalizations.

DIFFERENTIAL DIAGNOSIS OF ACUTE CONFUSIONAL STATE

The differential diagnosis of acute confusional state is shown in Table 1.3. Locked-in syndrome should be suspected in an otherwise unresponsive patient who is only able to blink and produce vertical gaze movements. Infarcts affecting the ventral pons disrupt corticospinal, corticopontine, and corticobulbar tracts but spare supranuclear eye movements and the RAS, thus preserving consciousness and vertical eye movements.

Transient global amnesia typically occurs in middle-aged or elderly persons and manifests clinically as an acute episode of amnesia for the present and recent past. Episodes are usually self-limited and last up to several hours. There is no consensus on the cause but hypotheses include a vascular etiology (either arterial or venous), a migrainous phenomenon or cortical spreading depression, seizures, or a psychogenic etiology.

Patients with psychiatric disease can develop acute mania, psychosis, catatonia, or dissociative fugue states. These should be differentiated from the acute confusional states discussed earlier as the management is very different. Catatonia presents as a motionless, apathetic state in which the patient is oblivious or does not react to external stimuli. Patients in this state make little or no eye contact and may be mute and rigid sometimes alternating with excitement, immobility, and waxy flexibility. Catatonia is treated with benzodiazepines, and in refractory cases, electroconvulsive therapy is indicated.

A. Case

A neurology consultation is placed for an elderly individual with progressive agitation and confusion after presenting with a mechanical fall fracturing several ribs and acute

TABLE 1.3 Differential Diagnosis of Acute Confusional State

Syndrome	Clinical Signs
Transient global amnesia	Alert, attentive, not oriented
Aphasia	Deficits within components of language: comprehension, fluency, repetition, writing and reading
Locked-in syndrome	Complete paralysis with the preservation of cognition, vertical gaze, and/or eye opening/closing
Psychiatric disorders	
Catatonia	Waxy flexibility, immobility, lethargic
Depression	Depressed mood with clear sensorium
Schizophrenia	Delusions with clear sensorium
Mania	Delusions, psychotic behavior, agitation, hyperactive

kidney injury. He was treated with oxycodone and fentanyl for pain, and subsequently with haloperidol and quetiapine for agitation. His confusion worsens and he begins to develop abnormal involuntary movements. Family recalls a previous admission related to another fall 2 years prior, which was also complicated by confusion and "twitching" and which took several weeks to resolve. Upon a detailed interview of family members, it is discovered that the patient has become slowly withdrawn over several years and occasionally demonstrates a unilateral resting tremor. On examination, he is inattentive, disoriented, and has prominent multifocal asterixis and myoclonus and there appears to be an underlying tremor (Video 1.1). No focal findings or meningeal signs were identified on examination.

B. **Diagnostic approach**

Determining the etiology of a patient's encephalopathy can be challenging. A systematic approach to an acutely altered patient will make the encounter less intimidating. A focused history, followed by an organized medical record review, careful clinical examination, and then prudent selection of diagnostic tests when necessary, including laboratory, imaging, and electrophysiologic studies, is recommended.

C. **Brief history**

The patient's history, arguably the most important step in elucidating the etiology of acute confusional state, is commonly sparse. The provider should interview members close to the patient including family members and first responders such as emergency medical staff and emergency room providers. Important questions apart from medical and psychiatric history, medication lists, and prior substance abuse include the following. How abruptly did the confusion begin? It is often enlightening to ask when the patient was last completely normal. Despite being consulted for acute confusion, in many instances this question will bring out a more subacute story of forgetfulness and lapses in judgment. Has the confusion been persistent or fluctuating? Has this happened before? Does the patient have access to drugs or medications of abuse? Has there been any exposure to sick contacts, carbon monoxide, or other potential neural toxins? Have there been any associated fevers or chills? A thorough 14-point review of systems is useful to ensure that all associated symptoms are identified as family members may not think to mention the recent initiation of an herbal supplement to help with their depression, for example, as they may not think it could be related to their presenting complaint.

CLINICAL MANIFESTATIONS

While the level of consciousness may be depressed in an acute confusional state, the hallmark of an acute confusional state is alteration of the content of consciousness and inattention. Attention refers to the ability to focus as well as to sustain and shift focus. Disorientation and deficits in memory, language, perception, and visuospatial ability are also prominent. Autonomic hyperactivity such as tachycardia, hypertension, and hyperhidrosis may accompany delirium; however, their presence should alert the provider to the possibility of acute brain injury (i.e., paroxysmal sympathetic hyperactivity), infection (encephalitis), or a toxidrome (serotonin syndrome or NMS). In delirious patients, agitation can predominate at night and drowsiness through the daytime, sometimes referred to as "sundowning." Hallucinations may occur as well as significant cognitive deficits. Patients with agitation, hallucination, and restlessness are easily seldom missed. This presentation is termed "hyperactive delirium" and accounts for less than 5% of episodes of delirium. The most common presentation is the so-called "hypoactive delirium," in which the patient appears withdrawn and lethargic.

The examination of an encephalopathic patient can be completed within a few minutes by an experienced provider. Certain causes of mental status changes can be discovered solely by thorough examination. The general examination includes an assessment of vital signs, respiratory pattern, and skin as outlined in Table 1.4. A hypersympathetic state manifesting as fever, tachycardia, hypertension, and tachypnea may indicate an early shock state, acute brain injury, or a toxidrome such as a serotonin syndrome or NMS. Hypothermia on the other hand may point toward sepsis, adrenal crisis, or a sedative, opiate, or alcohol overdose. Breath can have a fruity odor in a patient with diabetic ketoacidosis while alcohol intoxication and a garlic odor may indicate organophosphate toxicity. Skin examination may reveal dermatomal rashes or needle tract signs implicating varicella or drug abuse, respectively.

TABLE 1.4 Examination Findings in Encephalopathic Patients

Fever	Sepsis or other systemic infection
	Meningitis, encephalitis, brain abscess, or septic emboli
	Toxidrome
	Intracerebral hemorrhage
	Brain tumor
Hypothermia	Alcohol intoxication
	Opiate overdose
	Sedation
	Adrenal crisis
	Sepsis
	Environmental hypothermia
Hypertension	PRES/hypertensive encephalopathy
	Drug intoxication, i.e., stimulants
	Acute brain injury
	Toxidromes
Hypotension	Sedatives
	Shock
Tachycardia	Shock
	Toxidromes
	Acute brain injury
Bradycardia	Sedatives
	Increased intracranial pressure
	Organophosphate poisoning
Breath odor:	
Fruity	Ketoacidosis, alcohol intoxication
Garlic	Organophosphates
Tachypnea	Shock
	Metabolic acidosis
	Brainstem injury
Slow respirations	Sedatives
	Opiate overdose
	Brainstem injury
	Organophosphate poisoning
Ataxic breathing	Brainstem injury
Skin:	
Jaundice	Acute liver/biliary dysfunction
Needle tracks	Drug intoxication or withdrawal
Increased sweating	Toxidromes
	Hypoglycemia
	Organophosphate poisoning

Abbreviations: PRES, posterior reversible encephalopathy syndrome.

The mental status examination entails assessment of the level of consciousness, attention, orientation, memory, organization of thought, and mood. The level of consciousness can be described as alert, drowsy, somnolent, stuporous, and comatose. An alert individual is spontaneously awake. Drowsy patients require repeated verbal prompting to maintain alertness. A somnolent patient will transiently arouse to physical stimuli, commonly requiring tactile or even nociceptive stimulation, whereas a comatose patient will not arouse to any stimuli. This can be documented as spontaneous eye opening (alert), eye opening to voice (drowsy), eye opening to touch (somnolence), eye opening to pain (stupor), or no eye opening (coma). Attention refers to the ability to focus as well as to sustain and shift focus. Orientation testing should include orientation to patient's name, location including immediate location (i.e., hospital), city and state, time including day, date, month, year, and season, as well as purpose of hospitalization. Memory tests should be completed with remote history as well as immediate recall. Disordered thinking and emotional lability should also be noted if present.

A careful language examination can help to differentiate an acute aphasia from the tangential and mumbling speech of an encephalopathic or delirious patient. When alert, encephalopathic patients should be able to name simple objects, and repeat and follow simple commands although it may require significant redirection and repetition of the commands to complete this portion of the examination.

Examination of the cranial nerves can alert the provider to the presence of a structural brain lesion but some findings are easily explained by drugs. Mydriatic pupils are usually a result of sedative medications or overdose of anticholinergics but may also reflect a hypersympathetic state as is seen with in serotonin syndrome or NCSE. Miotic pupils on the other hand are most commonly reflective of opiate administration but can also result from sympathomimetic drugs of abuse or a pontine lesion. Bilaterally fixed pupils with absence of all other brainstem reflexes can reflect complete neuromuscular blockade or brain death. A unilaterally dilated pupil should raise concern in an encephalopathic patient as it reflects compression of the third nerve along its pathway, either as a result of a posterior communicating artery (PCOM) aneurysm, cavernous sinus syndrome, or herniation of the uncus of the temporal lobe. When it occurs in an alert patient it may still result from a PCOM aneurysm but is more likely to reflect administration of a topical mydriatic agent such as a scopolamine, antiemetic patch, or aerosolized respiratory medications. Oval pupils may reflect prior ocular surgery, midbrain disease, or increased intracranial pressure.

A forced gaze deviation or a gaze preference can be seen in unilateral hemispheric lesions. A destructive lesion such as an infarct affecting the frontal eye field will result in ipsilateral gaze deviation, whereas an irritative lesion such as an epileptic focus will produce a contralateral gaze deviation at the time of seizure occurrence. An irritative lesion can produce ipsilateral gaze deviation following a seizure. A downward gaze can reflect thalamic or dorsal midbrain injury, acute hydrocephalus, or raised intracranial pressure. Upward gaze is uncommon and poorly localizable. Skew deviation is a vertical misalignment of the eyes resulting from a cerebellar or brainstem injury. Ocular bobbing is rapid downward and slow upward correction that occurs spontaneously in the setting of pontine lesions. Slow downward followed by rapid upward correction is known as ocular dipping, which also localizes to the pons. Roving eyes are spontaneous slow horizontal movements of the eyes and are commonly observed in the setting of encephalopathy when the level of consciousness is depressed. The presence of roving eye movements is nonspecific and simply reflects the depression in the level of consciousness. Nystagmus noted in the primary resting position is frequently indicative of a toxidrome.

The corneal reflex arc may be interrupted by midbrain or pontine lesions. Note that patients who have had prolonged intensive care unit admissions can have scleral edema and patients who routinely use contact lenses will have a depressed corneal reflex.

Tone in a severely encephalopathic patient may be the most important part of the clinical examination. Increased tone throughout all limbs associated with fever can be indicative of a toxidrome such as neuroleptic malignant syndrome or malignant hyperthermia but may also occur as part of paroxysmal sympathetic hyperactivity (in the setting of acute brain injury) or in central nervous system (CNS) infections. When tone is disproportionately increased in the lower extremities when compared with the upper extremities, this suggests a possible serotonin syndrome and other signs should be sought (i.e., tremor-like movements, myoclonus, and increased bowel sounds). Unilateral hypotonia when accompanied by weakness is suggestive of a contralateral hemispheric infarction. Meningismus, Brudziński's, and Kernig's signs indicate meningeal irritation either by subarachnoid hemorrhage or by meningitis.

When possible, strength can be assessed by asking the patient to flex and extend individual muscle groups. However, when cooperation or level of consciousness is reduced, observation for amplitude, symmetry, and purpose of the movements is very informative. The presence of a restraint only unilaterally, for example, offers a clue to the presence of a hemiparesis. In a patient who is not moving spontaneously, motor response is assessed by administration of a painful stimulus to the nail bed of each extremity. The response may be described as localization, withdrawal/flexion, extension, or absent.

Many adventitious movements occur in encephalopathic patients and should be noted. Patients may have tremor-like movements, which may indicate shivering or low-amplitude clonic movements, myoclonus, spontaneous clonus, or asterixis. Fine motor twitching may suggest nonconvulsive seizures. Asterixis or negative myoclonus is the inability to sustain a motor contraction such as wrist extension or lip puckering. Myoclonus is a sudden involuntary twitch of a muscle. Both asterixis and myoclonus can accompany metabolic derangements such as renal or hepatic failure or may result from drug–drug interactions or drug toxicity such as gabapentin accumulation in the setting of renal disease.

ORGANIZED MEDICAL RECORD REVIEW

An organized review of the medical record often reveals laboratory or vital sign trends, medication combinations, newly initiated medications, previously documented examination changes, or previous hospitalizations with similar symptoms, among other pertinent information. The medical record should be examined in a systematic and organized manner such that important components are not overlooked. Clues to the etiology of encephalopathy can be attained by paying close attention to changes in vital signs or trends, such as a slow increase in the heart rate that may otherwise have gone unnoticed. Such a systematic review should include (1) vital sign review over the duration of the hospitalization, (2) laboratory review over the duration of the hospitalization, (3) review of the medication administration record, (4) review of prior neurologic examinations in the current hospitalization as well as in prior documented notes (to obtain a baseline), (5) and any prior neuroimaging.

In a consultation for altered mental status, the medication administration record may arguably be the most helpful in discovery of the etiology for encephalopathy. A careful review can result in identification of common deliriogenic medications such as anticholinergics in the elderly, high doses of fentanyl in the setting of chronic serotonin reuptake inhibitor use, or cefepime, which may be of concern in a patient with renal failure, to name a few. In addition to the administered medications, assessing for abruptly discontinued outpatient medications during ongoing hospitalization, namely benzodiazepines, may lead to identification of the cause of acute confusional state. Prior documented neurologic examinations may document a facial palsy that the patient's family had not noted, obviating the need for further evaluation of that finding and prior neuroimaging may explain a previously undocumented subtle hemiparesis.

DIAGNOSTIC TESTING

Tests that are potentially useful in aiding the evaluation of an encephalopathic patient include basic laboratory studies, toxicology studies, imaging, electroencephalography (EEG), and lumbar puncture (LP) for CSF analysis. These studies should be pursued in a judicious fashion rather than as a shotgun approach. Reflexively ordering an MRI, LP, and EEG on every encephalopathic patient does not require any training on the provider's part. A suggested diagnostic approach can be found in Figure 1.1.

General laboratory studies should include a complete chemistry panel including electrolytes, urea, creatinine, and blood glucose levels. Thyroid function studies, liver function studies, and ammonia levels may be indicated in some patients. In suspected individuals, a blood and urine toxicology screen should be obtained including an alcohol level. Patients with concomitant respiratory illness should have an arterial blood gas sampled to assess for hypercapnia or acidosis. In patients with fever, hypothermia, leukocytosis, subjective chills, or urinary symptoms, a urinalysis and blood cultures should be obtained. Take caution in attributing the cause for alterations of consciousness to mildly abnormal laboratory values. A mild case of urinary tract infection (UTI) or mild hypo- or hypernatremia should conclude the evaluation of encephalopathy only in rare cases such as elderly patients who have a history of acute confusional state associated with previous UTIs. Patients with serious electrolyte derangements, hypoglycemia, or hyperammonemia, on the other hand, may not require additional evaluation. Persistent encephalopathy upon correction of the suspected causal laboratory derangement, or in the presence of focal neurologic signs on examination should prompt further testing.

EEG has limited utility in the encephalopathic patient except to exclude nonconvulsive seizures or status epilepticus. Up to 8% of critically ill patients may suffer NCSE. Almost all patients with acute confusional state will have an abnormal EEG with either a posterior dominant rhythm frequency of less than 8 Hz or a relative decrease from an alpha wave of

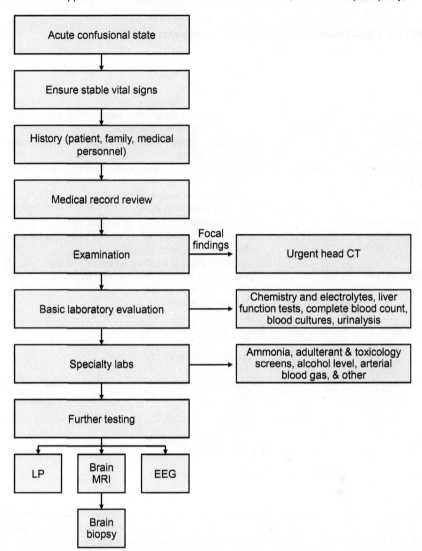

FIGURE 1.1 Approach to evaluation of acute confusional state. CT, computed tomography; EEG, electroencephalography; LP, lumbar puncture; MRI, magnetic resonance imaging.

10 to 12 Hz. As the encephalopathy worsens, the EEG background becomes disorganized, and high-voltage theta and delta activity appears with loss of EEG reactivity at frequencies less than 5 to 6 Hz. Triphasic waves, while classically associated with hepatic encephalopathy, are nonspecific and can be seen in any type of metabolic encephalopathy. Excessive beta activity is typically due to administration of benzodiazepines or anesthetic agents such as propofol. Table 1.5 outlines common EEG findings in encephalopathic patients and their clinical implications.

An LP for CSF analysis should be obtained in any patient with suspected meningitis and encephalitis, or in patients with suspected malignancy to assess for carcinomatous meningitis or paraneoplastic antibodies. Carcinomatous meningitis can occur in patients with lymphoma, leukemia, melanoma, and lung and breast cancers. CSF analysis is also warranted in most immunocompromised acutely encephalopathic patients to assess for opportunistic infections. When LP is performed, the minimum requirements for CSF analysis include cell count, glucose, protein, culture, and gram stain. A serum glucose obtained within the hour the LP is performed

TABLE 1.5 EEG Findings in Encephalopathic Patients

Triphasic waves	Nonspecific; may be seen in:
	Hepatic or renal disease
	Metabolic causes
	Anoxic-ischemic brain injury
	Hyperglycemic or hypoglycemic states
Periodic lateralizing epileptiform discharges	Implies the presence of a focal lesion
	That is ischemic stroke, intracerebral hemorrhage, or herpes simplex virus encephalitis
Generalized periodic epileptiform discharges	Implies severe diffuse cerebral dysfunction; may be seen in:
	CNS infections
	Severe metabolic encephalopathy
	Anoxic-ischemic brain injury
Diffuse slowing	Nonspecific; implies diffuse cerebral dysfunction
Burst suppression	Implies either profound or severe cortical injury; may be seen in:
	Anoxic-ischemic brain injury
	Anesthesia or use of anesthetic agents for sedation
Isoelectric (flat)	Implies absence of cortical function; may be seen in:
	Deep anesthesia
	Profound hypothermia
	Brain death
Alpha coma	May be seen in:
	Drug overdose
	Anoxic-ischemic brain injury
	Brainstem injury
Excess beta	May be seen with sedative/anesthetic administration:
	Benzodiazepines
	Barbiturates
	Propofol
Normal EEG	Locked-in syndrome
	Psychogenic causes

Abbreviations: CNS, central nervous system; EEG, electroencephalography.

allows for calculation of the CSF/serum ratio. Further testing is pursued if the initial tests are abnormal or depending on the clinical question. For example, if a paraneoplastic syndrome is suspected to be the cause of the patient's acute confusional state, a CSF paraneoplastic panel should be ordered even in the setting of a normal CSF cell count and chemistry.

A noncontrast head CT can identify the majority of structural causes of acute confusional state, including hemorrhage, tumors, infarction, hydrocephalus, and brain edema. An MRI is useful in the evaluation of acutely confused patients with suspected encephalitis, white matter processes (i.e., acute disseminated encephalomyelitis or PRES), brainstem infarctions, Wernicke's encephalopathy, multifocal lesions such as septic emboli or metastatic disease, or hypoxic-ischemic brain injury, where the CT may be normal.

Patients with acute confusional state but an otherwise normal physical examination and no fever, leukocytosis, or history of seizures, who meet diagnostic criteria for delirium, may not require any additional testing beyond a basic laboratory evaluation and medication review. A period of observation after initiation of reorientation, sleep enhancement, and other management strategies is recommended, with reconsideration of further testing (specifically neuroimaging) if the patient fails to improve over a specified period of time.

MANAGEMENT

Treatment strategies rely strongly on addressing the primary etiology of the acute encephalopathy. Once the etiology is discovered, successful correction of the encephalopathy depends on timely reversal of all contributing factors. For example, dialysis will eventually improve encephalopathy due to uremia; however, the rate of improvement will vary significantly and may be delayed in comparison with correction of the laboratory values. Lactulose administered for treatment of hepatic encephalopathy often readily improves the encephalopathy in most cases; however, delayed recognition and initiation of treatment may lead to permanent cognitive changes. In some instances, no specific contributing acute organ injury, infection, drug, or other etiology can be identified, and in these patients, if criteria for delirium are present, the management is focused on symptom control, maintenance of sleep–wake cycles, and frequent reorientation.

The yield of general nonpharmacologic approaches in the management of a patient with acute confusional state should not be underestimated. A comprehensive interdisciplinary approach includes prevention of aspiration, avoidance of skin breakdown by encouraging progressive mobility, and prevention of urinary retention or ileus. Prevention of sensory deprivation by means of visual or auditory assist devices, and gentle physical contact are several techniques that can easily be undertaken. Sleep enhancement can be requested in which disruptions are minimized (i.e., lab draws and nursing cares) during sleep hours. This helps promote a normal sleep–wake cycle. Familiarization of the patients with their environment by frequent reorientation, use of photographs of loved ones, or the physical presence of family members can aid in reducing behavioral disturbances. Bodily restraints should be used as a last resort in order to ensure patient and staff safety.

The pharmacologic management of behavioral dyscontrol related to acute confusional state primarily consists of antipsychotic agents. Haloperidol and chlorpromazine are typical antipsychotics historically used in the management of delirium. In an emergency where either the safety of the patient or care providers is at risk, haloperidol remains the drug of choice. More recently, atypical antipsychotics with their improved adverse effect profile such as quetiapine, olanzapine, and aripiprazole have been increasingly utilized. These newer agents have fewer extrapyramidal symptoms including akinesia, akathisia, acute dyskinesias or dystonic reactions, tardive dyskinesia, and parkinsonism. Aripiprazole is the agent of choice in patients with prolonged QTc on electrocardiogram. These medications may be administered on a scheduled as well as an as-needed basis but their use in the morning should be avoided if possible as they are frequently sedating. Benzodiazepines should be reserved for treatment of benzodiazepine withdrawal, alcohol withdrawal, catatonia, or for control of myoclonus or clonus in the setting of a toxidrome such as serotonin syndrome or neuroleptic malignant syndrome.

PROGNOSIS

The majority of acute confusional states are reversible with treatment of the underlying cause; however, many can result in permanent neurologic morbidity or mortality if diagnosis and treatment are delayed. For example, unrecognized PRES can lead to infarctions or hemorrhage. Untreated hyperammonemia can result in irreversible encephalopathy and delayed recognition of serotonin syndrome with sustained serotonergic overdrive can lead to fatal systemic complications from hyperthermia, rhabdomyolysis, and renal failure. Delirium related to prolonged hospitalization, recent operation, or sedation is also typically reversible; however, there is clearly an independent relationship between mortality and delirium in hospitalized patients. Furthermore, patients with delirium in the hospital may develop new long-term cognitive impairment.

COMMENTARY ON THE CASE

An underlying neurocognitive disorder with exposure to opiates in the setting of acute renal failure and a UTI likely resulted in this patient's acute encephalopathy. During routine laboratory testing, which also consisted of blood cultures and urinalysis, given his fever, a UTI was identified. He could be said to have decompensated dementia, delirium, or acute encephalopathy secondary to UTI, opiate administration, and acute kidney injury. All would apply. Opiates were discontinued, his infection was treated, and he was continued on an atypical antipsychotic (quetiapine), given his possible Parkinsonism. His confusion slowly resolved.

Key Points

- Any acute organ dysfunction can produce an acute confusional state and the severity varies depending on the degree of organ dysfunction and the rapidity over which it developed.
- Toxic causes of encephalopathy include intoxication or withdrawal syndromes, drug-drug interactions, or drug toxicity in the setting of reduced renal or hepatic function.
- Nonconvulsive seizures, status epilepticus, or postictal states can present as acute confusional states.
- Patients with underlying cognitive impairment can easily decompensate in the setting of an acute medical or neurologic insult, a condition known as "beclouded" or "decompensated" dementia.
- The differential diagnosis of acute confusional state includes locked-in syndrome, transient global amnesia, and psychiatric disease.
- Nonpharmacologic approaches to the management of acute confusional state include prevention of sensory deprivation, sleep enhancement, familiarization of the environment by frequent reorientation, use of photographs of loved ones, or the physical presence of family members.
- Haloperidol remains the drug of choice in an emergency where either the safety of the patient or care providers is at risk.
- The majority of acute confusional states are reversible with treatment of the underlying cause unless recognition is delayed.

Recommended Readings

Behrouz R, Godoy DA, Azarpazhooh MR, et al. Altered mental status in the neurocritical care unit. *J Crit Care*. 2015;30(6):1272–1277.

Brown TM. Drug-induced delirium. *Semin Clin Neuropsychiatry*. 2000;5(2):113–124.

Brummel NE, Vasilevskis EE, Han JH, et al. Implementing delirium screening in the ICU: secrets to success. *Crit Care Med*. 2013;41(9):2196–2208.

Cichoz-Lach H, Michalak A. Current pathogenetic aspects of hepatic encephalopathy and noncirrhotic hyperammonemic encephalopathy. *World J Gastroenterol*. 2013;19(1):26–34.

Dobbs MR. Toxic encephalopathy. *Semin Neurol*. 2011;31(2):184–193.

Ferenci P, Lockwood A, Mullen K, et al. Hepatic encephalopathy—definition, nomenclature, diagnosis, and quantification: final report of the working party at the 11th World Congresses of Gastroenterology, Vienna, 1998. *Hepatology*. 2002;35(3):716–721.

Fugate JE, Rabinstein AA. Posterior reversible encephalopathy syndrome: clinical and radiological manifestations, pathophysiology, and outstanding questions. *Lancet Neurol*. 2015;14(9):914–925.

Hocker SE, Wijdicks EF. Neurologic complications of sepsis. *Continuum (Minneap Minn)*. 2014;20(3, Neurology of Systemic Disease):598–613.

Lipowski ZJ. Delirium in the elderly patient. *N Engl J Med*. 1989;320:578–582.

Morandi A, Mccurley J, Vasilevskis EE, et al. Tools to detect delirium superimposed on dementia: a systematic review. *J Am Geriatr Soc*. 2012;60(11):2005–2013.

Seifter JL, Samuels MA. Uremic encephalopathy and other brain disorders associated with renal failure. *Semin Neurol*. 2011;31(2):139–143.

Sutter R, Kaplan PW. What to see when you are looking at confusion: a review of the neuroimaging of acute encephalopathy. *J Neurol Neurosurg Psychiatry*. 2015;86(4):446–459.

Towne AR, Waterhouse EJ, Boggs JG, et al. Prevalence of nonconvulsive status epilepticus in comatose patients. *Neurology*. 2000;54(2):340–345.

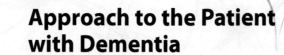

2 Approach to the Patient with Dementia

Nilüfer Ertekin-Taner and Neill R. Graff-Radford

In the *Diagnostic and Statistical Manual of Mental Disorders-V (DSM-V)* criteria, **dementia** is replaced by the term **Major Neurocognitive Disorder** and is defined as significant impairments in one or more cognitive domains such as amnesia, aphasia, apraxia, agnosia, topographical disorientation, executive dysfunction, dyscalculia, dysprosody, or agraphia. This impairment results in decline of social or occupational functioning in comparison with previous functioning and leads to loss of independence. The deficits should not occur exclusively during the course of delirium and should not be accounted for by another psychiatric condition, such as depression or schizophrenia. The *DSM-V* definition of **Major Neurocognitive Disorder** can be further specified as being due to Alzheimer's disease (AD), frontotemporal lobar degeneration (FTLD), Lewy body disease (LBD), vascular disease, traumatic brain injury, substance/medication use, HIV infection, prion disease, Parkinson's disease, Huntington's disease, another medical condition, multiple etiologies, or left as unspecified.

EPIDEMIOLOGY OF DEMENTIA

It is estimated that the worldwide prevalence of dementia in 2014 is 44 million patients, according to the World Alzheimer Report 2014. AD is the most common dementia etiology, accounting for 50% to 75% of the cases, followed by vascular dementia (VaD, 20% to 30%), frontotemporal dementia (FTD, 5% to 10%), and dementia with Lewy bodies (DLB). The number of people with dementia is expected to increase to 135 million in 2050, unless new therapies that delay its onset or progression are developed. An average 5-year delay in the age of dementia onset is expected to reduce its population prevalence by 50%. Thus, the public and socioeconomic impact of dementia is a significant worldwide problem.

RISK FACTORS AND ETIOLOGY

A. **Risk factors.** The following have been identified as risk factors for the development of dementia and/or AD in one or more studies: Nonmodifiable risk factors are increasing age, female sex, unfavorable perinatal conditions, early life development, and growth. Modifiable risk factors fall into vascular and psychosocial categories. The following are modifiable vascular risk factors for dementia: midlife hypertension, obesity, and hyperlipidemia; midlife and late-life diabetes mellitus, heart disease (peripheral atherosclerosis, heart failure, and atrial fibrillation), cerebrovascular disease, heavy alcohol intake, hyperhomocysteinemia due to low B_{12} and folate, and cigarette smoking. Declines in blood pressure, body mass index, and total cholesterol were shown to precede dementia. The following may be the socioeconomically modifiable risk factors for dementia: low education, poor social network, low mental or physical activity. The following have been proposed as potential protective factors for dementia, although their roles are yet to be proven in clinical trials: Statins, B group vitamins, "Mediterranean diet," nonsteroidal anti-inflammatory agents, antioxidants, omega-3 fatty acids, physical and mental exercise, and treating sleep disorders. Depression was also identified as a risk factor for dementia, although it is also possible that this is an early symptom. Regardless, depression and anxiety need to be recognized and treated in dementia.

B. **Etiology.** Table 2.1 lists many of the causes of dementia. Potentially reversible conditions were identified in 4% to 8% of dementia cases in different studies. Hydrocephalus, space-occupying lesions, psychiatric disease, medications, alcoholism, and substance abuse

TABLE 2.1 Causes of Dementia

Degenerative (See Tables 2.2 and 2.3)	Tumors
Vascular	Glioblastoma
Multiple infarction	Lymphoma
Single stroke	Metastatic tumor
Binswanger's disease	**Toxic/metabolic**
Vasculitis	*Vitamin B₂ deficiency*
Subarachnoid hemorrhage	*Thyroid deficiency*
Cerebral amyloid angiopathy	*System failure: liver, renal, cardiac, and respiratory*
Hereditary cerebral hemorrhage with angiopathy—	*Heavy metals*
Dutch type	*Toxins (e.g., glue sniffing)*
CADASIL	*Electrolyte abnormalities*
Subdural hematoma	*Hypoglycemia*
Infectious	*Parathyroid disease*
Meningitis (fungal, mycobacterial, and bacterial)	*Drugs*
Syphilis	*Alcohol*
AIDS dementia	**Traumatic**
Creutzfeldt–Jakob's disease	*Closed head injury*
Post-herpes simplex encephalitis	*Open head injury*
Lyme disease	Pugilistic brain injury
Whipple's disease	Anoxic brain injury
Progressive multifocal leukoencephalopathy	**Psychiatric**
Autoimmune/inflammatory	*Depression*
Systemic lupus erythematosus	*Personality disorder*
Sjögren's syndrome	*Anxiety disorder*
Multiple sclerosis	**Other**
Steroid responsive encephalopathy	*Symptomatic hydrocephalus*
Paraneoplastic	

Italics indicate the etiologic factor is at least partially reversible or treatable.

were the most frequent causes of nondegenerative and nonvascular dementia. Although treatment for the potentially reversible conditions may not lead to partial or full reversal of dementia, their identification and attempted treatment is crucial. Table 2.2 lists the degenerative causes of dementia by pathologic classification. It should be noted that in addition to causative Mendelian mutations, a genetic component is identified for most degenerative dementias, including AD, FTLD, and LBD. Genome-wide association studies identified risk loci for some of these conditions, which is expected to lead to the identification of new disease risk variants and genes. Table 2.3 includes the syndromic classification of degenerative dementias. It is important to acknowledge that the same underlying pathology may present as different clinical syndromes and different pathologies may present as the same clinical syndrome. Further, nearly half of the subjects with neuropathologic diagnosis of AD also have other pathologies such as LBD, vascular pathologies, and hippocampal sclerosis. Despite these complexities, the existing clinicopathologic correlations allowed for the development of diagnostic criteria for degenerative and VaDs, which is discussed in what follows.

CRITERIA FOR DIAGNOSIS

The following are the diagnostic guidelines for AD, VaD, DLB, and FTLD (the four most common causes of dementia in order). Also presented are the guidelines for diagnosis of mild cognitive impairment (MCI), which bridges the spectrum between dementia and normal cognition.

TABLE 2.2 Degenerative Dementias: Pathologic Classification

Amyloid/Tau
AD: Early-onset familial AD may have *APP, PSEN1,* or *PSEN2* mutations. Late-onset AD is the most common form.

Tau
Pick's disease
Corticobasal degeneration
Progressive supranuclear palsy
FTD with parkinsonism linked to chromosome 17 (tau mutations)
Tangle-only dementia
Argyrophilic grain disease

α-synuclein
LBD
Parkinson's disease dementia
Multisystem atrophy

Tau−/Ubiquitin+
TDP-43+
FTLD-TDP: May have *GRN, C9orf72, UBQLN2, VCP,* or *TDP43* mutations. Presents as FTD, ALS, or FTD+ALS.
UPS+
FTLD-UPS: May have *CHMP2B* mutations. Presents as FTD.
FUS/FET+
FTLD-FUS/FET: May have FUS mutations. Presents as ALS>>>FTD.
Neuronal intermediate filament inclusion disease
Basophilic inclusion body disease

Other
Huntington's disease
Dementia lacking distinctive histologic features
Progressive subcortical gliosis

The headers represent the primary neuropathologies for the syndromes listed underneath. Multiple neuropathologies can coexist.

Abbreviations: AD, Alzheimer's disease; FTD, frontotemporal dementia; FTLD-TDP, frontotemporal lobar degeneration transactive response DNA binding protein 43; FTLD-UPS, frontotemporal lobar degeneration ubiquitin proteasome system; LBD, Lewy body disease.

A. **Alzheimer's disease.** AD is characterized by both amyloid and tau pathology. The **National Institute of Neurological and Communicative Disorders and Stroke** and the **Alzheimer and Related Diseases Association** 1984 criteria for the diagnosis of AD have recently been modified to take into account (1) Patients with the pathophysiologic process of AD, which can be found in those with normal cognition, MCI, and AD. This pathophysiologic process, designated as AD-P, is thought to begin years before the diagnosis of clinical AD. (2) The diagnostic criteria for other diseases such as LBD and FTD. (3) MRI, positron emission tomography (PET) for imaging the amyloid beta protein (Aβ), ^{18}fluorodeoxyglucose (FDG) PET, and the cerebrospinal fluid (CSF) biomarkers Aβ42, total tau and phophotau. (4) Other clinical syndromes that do not present with amnesia but are related to AD pathology including posterior cortical atrophy and logopenic aphasia. (5) The dominantly inherited AD causing mutations in amyloid precursor protein, presenilin-1, and presenilin-2 (*APP, PSEN1, PSEN2,* respectively). (6) A change in age cutoffs noting persons under 40 and over 90 may have the same AD-P. (7) Many persons with possible AD in the past are now designated MCI.

TABLE 2.3 Degenerative Dementias: Syndromic Classification

MCI
Single domain
Amnestic
Nonamnestic
Multiple domain
Amnestic
Nonamnestic
AD
Typical
Primary and predominant memory impairment
Atypical
Posterior cortical atrophy
Logopenic aphasia
Corticobasal syndrome
FTD
Behavioral variant (bvFTD)
PPA
Progressive nonfluent aphasia
Semantic dementia and associative agnosia

Abbreviations: AD, Alzheimer's disease; bvFTD, behavioral variant frontotemporal dementia; MCI, mild cognitive impairment; PPA primary progressive aphasia.

In what follows, we present the 1984 criteria for probable and possible AD. Patients who meet the 1984 criteria for probable AD still meet criteria for probable AD. Additionally, we present the proposed new 2011 criteria for AD in Section **A.8** under Criteria for Diagnosis.

1. Criteria for the clinical diagnosis of probable AD.
    a. Dementia established by means of clinical examination and documented with the Mini-Mental State Examination, Blessed Dementia Rating Scale, or other similar examination and confirmed with neuropsychological tests.
    b. Deficits in two or more areas of cognition.
    c. Progressive worsening of memory and other cognitive function.
    d. No disturbance of consciousness.
    e. Onset between the ages of 40 and 90 years, most often after 65 years.
    f. Absence of systemic disorders or other brain diseases that in and of themselves could account for the progressive deficits in memory and cognition.
2. Supporting findings in the diagnosis of probable AD.
    a. Progressive deterioration of specific cognitive functions such as aphasia, apraxia (Video 2.1), or agnosia.
    b. Impaired activities of daily living and altered patterns of behavior.
    c. Family history of similar disorders, particularly if confirmed neuropathologically.
    d. Laboratory results as follows:
        (1) Normal results of lumbar puncture (LP) as evaluated with standard techniques.
        (2) Normal or nonspecific electroencephalography (EEG) changes (increased slow-wave activity).
        (3) Evidence of cerebral atrophy at computed tomography (CT) with progression documented by means of serial observation.
3. Other clinical features consistent with the diagnosis of probable AD, after exclusion of causes of dementia other than AD.
    a. Plateaus in the course of progression of the illness.
    b. Associated symptoms of depression; insomnia; incontinence; delusions; illusions; hallucinations; catastrophic verbal, emotional, or physical outbursts; sexual disorders; and weight loss.

    c. Other neurologic abnormalities for some patients, especially those with advanced disease, and including motor signs such as increased muscle tone, myoclonus, or gait disorder.

    d. Seizures in advanced disease.

    e. CT findings normal for age.

4. Features that make the diagnosis of probable AD uncertain or unlikely.

    a. Sudden, apoplectic onset.

    b. Focal neurologic findings such as hemiparesis, sensory loss, visual field deficits, and incoordination early in the course of the illness.

    c. Seizures or gait disturbance at the onset or early in the course of the illness.

5. Clinical diagnosis of possible AD.

    a. May be made on the basis of the dementia syndrome, in the absence of other neurologic, psychiatric, or systemic disorders sufficient to cause dementia and with variations in onset, presentation, or clinical course.

    b. May be made in the presence of a second systemic or brain disorder sufficient to produce dementia, which is not considered to be the principal cause of the dementia.

    c. Should be used in research studies when a single, gradually progressive, severe cognitive deficit is identified in the absence of any other identifiable cause.

6. **Criteria for the diagnosis of definite AD** are the clinical criteria for probable AD and histopathologic evidence obtained from a biopsy or autopsy.

7. **Classification of AD for research purposes** should specify features that differentiate subtypes of the disorder such as familial occurrence, onset before 65 years of age, presence of trisomy 21, and coexistence of other relevant conditions such as Parkinson's disease.

8. **Proposed new criteria for AD.** In 2011, National Institute on Aging and the Alzheimer's Association work group suggested new criteria for AD based on clinical and research evidence. All patients who met the 1984 criteria for probable AD described in A.1 would meet the current criteria. In addition, the following criteria are proposed:

    a. **Probable AD dementia with increased level of certainty.** This category includes patients with "probable AD dementia with documented decline" and "probable AD dementia in a carrier of a causative AD genetic mutation in *APP, PSEN1,* or *PSEN2* genes."

    b. **Possible AD dementia.** This category includes patients with an "atypical course" or "mixed etiology" and would not necessarily meet the 1984 criteria for possible AD. "Atypical course" is characterized by "sudden onset, insufficient historical detail or objective cognitive documentation of progressive decline." "Mixed etiology" includes subjects with concomitant cerebrovascular disease or features of DLB or "evidence for another neurologic disease or a non-neurologic medical comorbidity or medication use that could have a substantial effect on cognition."

    c. **Probable or possible AD dementia with evidence of the AD pathophysiologic process.** These criteria are proposed only for research purposes and incorporate the use of biomarkers, which are not yet advocated for routine diagnostic use. These biomarkers fall into the two categories of "brain amyloid β (Aβ) protein deposition," that is, low CSF Aβ42 and positive PET amyloid imaging; and "downstream neuronal degeneration or injury," that is, elevated CSF tau, decreased FDG uptake on PET in temporoparietal cortex, and disproportionate atrophy on structural MRI in medial, basal, and lateral temporal lobe, and medial parietal cortex. The biomarker profile will fall into clearly positive, clearly negative, and indeterminate categories.

B. **Vascular dementia.** There are different published diagnostic criteria for VaD: NINDS-AIREN (National Institute of Neurological Disorders and Stroke-Association Internationale pour la Recherche et L'Enseignement en Neurosciences), ADDTC (State of California Alzheimer's Disease Diagnostic and Treatment Centers), *DSM-IV,* and Hachinski Ischemia Scale. Their distinct features lead to differences in sensitivity and specificity. The first set of criteria discussed is the **NINDS-AIREN criteria for** VaD and is as follows:

1. The criteria for probable VaD include all of the following:

    a. Dementia defined similarly to *DSM-IV* criteria.

    b. Cerebrovascular disease defined by the presence of focal signs on neurologic examination, such as hemiparesis, lower facial weakness, Babinski's sign, sensory deficit, hemianopia, and dysarthria consistent with stroke (with or without history of stroke), and evidence of relevant cerebrovascular disease at brain imaging (CT or MRI), including multiple large-vessel infarcts or a single strategically situated infarct (angular gyrus, thalamus, basal forebrain, or posterior or anterior cerebral artery territories), as well as multiple basal ganglia and white matter lesions and white matter lacunes or extensive periventricular white matter lesions, or combinations thereof.

c. A relation between the two previous disorders manifested or inferred from the presence of one or more of the following: (1) onset of dementia within 3 months after a recognized stroke, (2) abrupt deterioration in cognitive functions, or (3) fluctuating, stepwise progression of cognitive deficits.

2. Clinical features consistent with the diagnosis of probable VaD include the following:
   a. Early presence of a gait disturbance.
   b. History of unsteadiness and frequent, unprovoked falls.
   c. Early urinary frequency, urgency, and other urinary symptoms not explained by urologic disease.
   d. Pseudobulbar palsy.
   e. Personality and mood changes, abulia, depression, emotional incontinence, or other subcortical deficits, including psychomotor retardation and abnormal executive functioning.

3. Features that make the diagnosis of VaD uncertain or unlikely include the following:
   a. Early onset of memory and other cognitive functions, such as language, motor skills, and perception in the absence of corresponding lesions at brain imaging.
   b. Absence of focal neurologic signs other than cognitive disturbance.
   c. Absence of cerebrovascular lesions on CT scans or MRIs.

4. **The term AD with cerebrovascular disease** should be reserved to classify the condition of patients fulfilling the clinical criteria for possible AD and who also have clinical or brain imaging evidence of relevant cerebrovascular disease.

5. The criteria for definite VaD are as follows:
   a. Probable VaD, according to core features.
   b. Cerebrovascular disease by histopathology.
   c. Absence of neurofibrillary tangles or neuritic plaques exceeding those expected for age.
   d. Absence of other clinical or pathologic disorders capable of producing dementia.

6. **Vascular dementia: ADDTC criteria** for VaD are as follows:
   a. The criteria for probable VaD include all of the following:
      (1) Dementia by *DSM-III-R* criteria.
      (2) Two or more strokes by history/examination and/or CT or T1-weighted MRI, or single stroke with clear temporal relationship to onset of dementia.
      (3) Presence of at least one infarct outside cerebellum by CT or T1-weighted MRI.
   b. The criteria for possible VaD include all of the following:
      (1) Dementia by *DSM-III-R* criteria.
      (2) Single stroke with temporal relationship to dementia or Binswanger defined as the following: (1) early-onset incontinence or gait disturbance not explained by peripheral cause, (2) vascular risk factors, and (3) extensive white matter changes on neuroimaging.
   c. The criteria for mixed dementia are as follows:
      (1) Evidence of AD or other disease on pathology examination plus probable, possible, or definite ischemic VaD.
      (2) One or more systemic or brain diseases contributing to patient's dementia in the presence of probable, possible, or definite ischemic VaD.
   d. The criteria for definite ischemic VaD are as follows:
      (1) Dementia.
      (2) Multiple infarcts outside the cerebellum on neuropathology exam.

7. Vascular dementia: **DSM-IV criteria** for VaD are as follows:
   a. Impaired memory.
   b. Presence of at least one of the following: aphasia, apraxia, agnosia, or impaired executive functioning.
   c. Symptoms impair work, social, or personal functioning.
   d. Symptoms do not occur solely during delirium.
   e. Cerebral vascular disease has probably caused the above deficits, as judged by laboratory data or by focal neurologic signs and symptoms.

8. Vascular dementia: Hachinski Ischemic Scale for VaD assigns points to each criterion. A total score >7 corresponds to multi-infarct dementia, whereas <4 is interpreted as AD. Each of the following criteria is shown with the associated number of points in parentheses.
   a. Abrupt onset (2)
   b. Stepwise progression (1)
   c. Fluctuating course (2)
   d. Nocturnal confusion (1)
   e. Relative preservation of personality (1)
   f. Depression (1)
   g. Somatic complaints (1)
   h. Emotional incontinence (1)
   i. History of hypertension (1)
   j. History of strokes (2)
   k. Associated atherosclerosis (1)
   l. Focal neurologic symptoms (2)
   m. Focal neurologic signs (2)

C. **DLB** is defined pathologically by the presence of cortical Lewy bodies composed mainly of α-synuclein and is part of a spectrum with Parkinson's disease, which has brainstem Lewy bodies. The McKeith criteria for the clinical diagnosis of DLB are as follows:
   1. Progressive cognitive decline interferes with normal social and occupational functioning
   2. Deficits on tests of attention, executive function, and visuospatial functioning are often prominent
   3. Prominent or persistent memory impairment may not be present early in the course of illness
   4. Two of the following core features are necessary for the diagnosis of **probable DLB,** and one is necessary for **possible DLB**:
      a. Fluctuating cognition or alertness
      b. Recurrent visual hallucinations
      c. Spontaneous features of parkinsonism
   5. **Suggestive features.** ≥1 suggestive feature + ≥1 core feature are sufficient for the diagnosis of probable DLB; ≥1 suggestive feature and no core features are sufficient for the diagnosis of possible DLB; probable DLB should not be diagnosed on the basis of suggestive features alone.
      a. REM sleep behavior disorder
      b. Severe neuroleptic sensitivity
      c. Low-dopamine transporter uptake in basal ganglia demonstrated by single photon emission computed tomography (SPECT) or PET imaging
   6. **Features supportive of the diagnosis** are repeated falls, syncope or transient loss of consciousness, severe autonomic dysfunction, tactile or olfactory hallucinations, systematized delusions, depression, relative preservation of mesial temporal lobe structures on CT/MRI, reduced occipital activity on SPECT/PET, low uptake meta-iodobenzylguanidine (MIBG) myocardial scintigraphy, prominent slow-wave activity on EEG with temporal lobe transient sharp waves.
   7. The following features suggest a disorder other than DLB:
      a. Cerebrovascular disease evidenced by focal neurologic signs or cerebral infarcts present on neuroimaging studies
      b. The presence of any other physical illness or brain disorder sufficient to account in part or in total for the clinical picture
      c. If parkinsonism appears only for the first time at a stage of severe dementia
   8. **Temporal sequence of symptoms.** DLB should be diagnosed when dementia occurs before or concurrently with parkinsonism (if it is present). The term Parkinson's disease dementia (PDD) should be used to describe dementia that occurs in the context of well-established Parkinson's disease.

D. **FTLD** involves focal atrophy of the frontal or temporal lobes or both, the distribution of atrophy determining the clinical presentation. The age at onset tends to be slightly younger (often before 65 years) than that for AD. Patients with clinical FTLD usually do not have Alzheimer's-type pathologic findings, but instead have other distinct pathology. According to recent consensus recommendations, there are five major neuropathologic classifications for FTLD based on the presence of abnormally accumulating protein as follows: FTLD-tau (includes Pick's disease and FTDP-17), FTLD-TDP (transactive response DNA binding protein 43; includes familial FTLD due to mutations in *GRN, C9orf72, UBQLN2, VCP, or TDP43*), FTLD-UPS (ubiquitin proteasome system; includes familial FTLD due to mutations in *CHMP2B*), FTLD-FUS/FET (fused in sarcoma; includes neuronal intermediate filament inclusion disease, basophilic inclusion body disease, familial FTLD due to *FUS* mutations), and FTLD-ni (no inclusions).

The two major phenotypes of FTLD are behavioral variant (bvFTD) and primary progressive aphasia (PPA). Three main variants of PPA are defined as nonfluent/agrammatic, semantic, and logopenic. International bvFTD Criteria Consortium (FTDC) published their first report on the comparison of 1998 Neary et al. criteria and their proposed criteria, which identified greater sensitivity. The proposed 2011 FTDC criteria for bvFTD need further evaluation, and are as follows: *Possible bvFTD* requires three of six clinically discriminating features (disinhibition, apathy/inertia, loss of sympathy/empathy, perseverative/compulsive behaviors, hyperorality, and dysexecutive neuropsychological profile). *Probable bvFTD* also includes functional disability and characteristic neuroimaging; and *bvFTD with Definite FTLD* requires histopathologic evidence of FTLD or a pathogenic mutation.

In comparison, the 1998 **Neary's criteria** for the clinical diagnosis of bvFTLD are as follows:

1. **In FTD,** character change and disordered social conduct are the dominant features initially and throughout the disease course. Instrumental functions of perception, spatial skills, praxis, and memory are intact or relatively well-preserved. Core criteria are as follows:
   a. Insidious onset and gradual progression.
   b. Early decline in social interpersonal conduct.
   c. Early impairment in regulation of personal conduct.
   d. Early emotional blunting.
   e. Early loss of insight.
2. Supportive diagnostic features of FTD are as follows:
   a. Decline in personal hygiene and grooming.
   b. Mental rigidity and inflexibility.
   c. Distractibility and impersistence.
   d. Hyperorality and dietary changes.
   e. Perseverative and stereotyped behavior.
   f. Utilization behavior.
   g. Speech and language features: aspontaneity and economy of speech; press of speech, stereotypy of speech, echolalia, perseveration, and mutism.
   h. Physical signs: primitive reflexes, incontinence, akinesia, rigidity, tremor, low and labile blood pressure.
   i. Investigations: Neuropsychology-significant impairment on frontal lobe tests in the absence of severe amnesia, aphasia, or perceptuospatial disorder; EEG-normal; imaging-predominant frontal or anterior temporal abnormality.

   Gorno-Tempini et al. have provided new classification and criteria for the PPA variants. It should be noted that while most PPA-nonfluent/agrammatic variant has FTLD-tau, most PPA-semantic variant has FTLD-TDP, and most PPA-logopenic variant has AD pathology, a definitive clinicopathologic correlation cannot be established. Thus, the following criteria represent clinical classifications.

   (1) Diagnosis of **PPA requires that the following criteria be met.**
      (a) Difficulty with language as the most prominent clinical feature.
      (b) Daily activities impaired primarily owing to language impairment.
      (c) Aphasia as the most prominent early deficit.
      (d) Deficit not accounted for by other disorders.
      (e) Deficit not accounted for by psychiatric diagnosis.
      (f) No prominent initial episodic memory, visual impairments.
      (g) No prominent initial behavioral disturbance.

(2) Clinical diagnosis of **PPA-nonfluent/agrammatic variant.**
    At least one of the following core features must be present:
  (a) Agrammatism in language production.
  (b) Effortful, halting speech with inconsistent speech sound errors and distortions (apraxia of speech). At least two of three of the following other features must be present:
    (1) Impaired comprehension of syntactically complex sentences.
    (2) Spared single-word comprehension.
    (3) Spared object knowledge.
(3) Imaging-supported **PPA-nonfluent/agrammatic variant diagnosis.**
    Both of the following criteria must be present:
  (a) Clinical diagnosis of nonfluent/agrammatic variant PPA.
  (b) Imaging must show one or more of the following results:
    (1) Predominant left posterior frontoinsular atrophy on MRI.
    (2) Predominant left posterior frontoinsular hypoperfusion or hypometabolism on SPECT or PET.
(4) **PPA-nonfluent/agrammatic variant with definite pathology.**
    Clinical diagnosis (criterion a below) and either criterion b or c must be present.
  (a) Clinical diagnosis of nonfluent/agrammatic variant PPA.
  (b) Histopathologic evidence of a specific neurodegenerative pathology (e.g., FTLD-tau, FTLD-TDP, AD, and others).
  (c) Presence of a known pathogenic mutation.
(5) Clinical diagnosis of **PPA-semantic variant.**
    Both of the following core features must be present:
  (a) Impaired confrontation naming.
  (b) Impaired single-word comprehension. At least three of the following other diagnostic features must be present.
    (1) Impaired object knowledge, particularly for low-frequency or low-familiarity items.
    (2) Surface dyslexia or dysgraphia.
    (3) Spared repetition.
    (4) Spared speech production (grammar and motor speech).
(6) Imaging-supported **PPA-semantic variant diagnosis.**
    Both of the following criteria must be present:
  (a) Clinical diagnosis of semantic variant PPA.
  (b) Imaging must show one or more of the following results:
    (1) Predominant anterior temporal lobe atrophy.
    (2) Predominant anterior temporal hypoperfusion or hypometabolism on SPECT or PET.
(7) **PPA-semantic variant with definite pathology.**
    Clinical diagnosis (criterion a below) and either criterion b or c must be present.
  (a) Clinical diagnosis of semantic variant PPA.
  (b) Histopathologic evidence of a specific neurodegenerative pathology (e.g., FTLD-tau, FTLD-TDP, AD, and others).
  (c) Presence of a known pathogenic mutation.
(8) Clinical diagnosis of **PPA-logopenic.**
    Both of the following core features must be present.
  (a) Impaired single-word retrieval in spontaneous speech and naming.
  (b) Impaired repetition of sentences and phrases. At least three of the following other features must be present:
    (1) Speech (phonologic) errors in spontaneous speech and naming.
    (2) Spared single-word comprehension and object knowledge.
    (3) Spared motor speech.
    (4) Absence of frank agrammatism.
(9) Imaging-supported **PPA-logopenic** diagnosis.
    Both criteria must be present.
  (a) Clinical diagnosis of logopenic variant PPA.

(b) Imaging must show at least one of the following results:
   (1) Predominant left posterior perisylvian or parietal atrophy on MRI.
   (2) Predominant left posterior perisylvian or parietal hypoperfusion or hypometabolism on SPECT or PET.

(10) PPA-logopenic with definite pathology.
   Clinical diagnosis (criterion a below) and either criterion b or c must be present.
   (a) Clinical diagnosis of **PPA-logopenic.**
   (b) Histopathologic evidence of a specific neurodegenerative pathology (e.g., AD, which is the most common pathology, FTLD-tau, FTLD-TDP, and others).
   (c) Presence of a known pathogenic mutation.

E. MCI is the transitional state between normal aging and dementia, and represents a condition with greater rate of progression to dementia than normal aging. Patients with amnestic MCI progress to AD at a rate of 10% to 15% per year. Initial criteria for MCI required the presence of memory impairment. Current criteria also recognize nonamnestic forms of MCI.

1. Criteria for MCI are as follows. Cognitive impairment that is not normal for aging, represents a decline, does not reach criteria for dementia, and does not impair activities of daily living.

2. Subtypes of MCI are as follows. Depending on the presence or absence of memory impairment and presence of one or more cognitive impairments, there are four types of MCI. Memory impairment present: amnestic MCI versus nonmemory cognitive impairment: nonamnestic MCI. Single domain (one domain impaired only) versus multiple domain. It is proposed that the expected outcome of single or multiple domain amnestic MCI is AD, of single or multiple domain nonamnestic MCI is less likely to be AD, although this is possible, and could be FTD or DLB.

3. New proposed research criteria for MCI. These criteria incorporate the use of biomarkers as described in A.8.c. When both Aβ and neuronal injury biomarkers are "positive" in a subject with MCI, it is suggested that these subjects have the highest likelihood of progressing to AD dementia; hence, the terminology of "MCI due to AD-High likelihood" is proposed. When only one set of biomarkers is positive, "MCI due to AD-Intermediate likelihood" and when both are negative, "MCI-Unlikely due to AD" is suggested. Additional work is needed for the validation of these criteria and standardization of biomarkers.

EVALUATION

A. History. It is essential that the history be obtained not only from the patient but also from an independent informant. In most cases the patient can be told, "I am now going to ask your spouse some questions, and if your spouse makes any errors, feel free to make corrections." Sometimes, the informant may not want to speak openly in front of the patient, so the clinician may want to arrange a separate interview, perhaps while the patient is undergoing another test or later by telephone.

1. **Patient difficulties.** Determine what difficulties the patient is having and what family members have noticed. Commonly, a patient with dementia may not know there is a memory difficulty or be able to give accurate details of the problem. Begin by asking the patient an open-ended question such as "What problems are you having?" This often does not elicit the desired responses. Even with specific questions such as "Are you having difficulty with your memory?" the clinician may not be told what the problems are. The informant may have to be asked specific questions, such as "What can't the patient do now that he (or she) could do before?" or "Does the patient sometimes ask the same question more than once in the same conversation?"

2. **Time course.** The time the family first noticed problems and the course the disease has taken over time are critical factors in the evaluation. A disease that is slowly progressive fits the profile of a degenerative disease such as AD. A disease that starts suddenly or follows a stepwise progression would be more in keeping with VaD. Rapidly progressive dementia (over a few months) suggests Creutzfeldt–Jakob's disease.

3. **Functioning of the patient.** Determine how well the patient has been functioning at work and at home, including performance of the basic activities of daily living. Patients with MCI are by definition able to function well. Patients with progressive nonfluent aphasia or semantic dementia usually are also able to function well. Ask what the patient does to keep busy. Does he or she read the newspaper, watch the news on television, keep the checkbook, do the shopping, prepare the meals, take part in a sport or hobby? Knowing this information helps in the planning of questions to ask during the mental status part of the examination.

4. **Issues of safety.** Ask whether the patient drives. If so, has the patient ever become lost while driving or had any accidents, near-accidents, or traffic violations? If the patient prepares meals, has he or she ever left the stove on? Does the patient keep weapons, and if so, has this posed any danger to the patient or to others?

5. **Etiologically directed history.** Include a history of vascular disease and risk factors, head injury, toxic exposure, symptoms of infection or exposure to diseases such as tuberculosis, psychiatric history such as depression, symptoms of depression (such as a change in weight, insomnia, crying, or anhedonia), medications, systemic illnesses, other past illnesses, and alcohol or tobacco use.

   The following questions may bring out symptoms of DLB: Does the patient have good days and bad days? What specifically cannot the patient do on bad days? Does the patient see things that are not there (visual hallucinations)? Does the patient act out dreams at night (rapid eye movement sleep behavior disorder)? Look for personality and behavioral changes in FTD with specific questions—for example, Does the patient drive recklessly, such as run stop signs or speed? Has the patient developed poor table manners such as eating excessively fast? Does the patient have rituals or do things repetitively?

6. **Family history.** Ask what the patient's parents died of and at what ages. Ask specifically whether there were memory problems in the later years. Then ask about the ages and health of the patient's siblings and children. Patients with late-onset AD commonly have a family history of disease. A strong family history for a younger patient suggests an autosomal dominant disease such as familial AD, familial FTLD, Huntington's disease, or spinocerebellar ataxia.

B. **Physical examination.**

1. Give a standardized short mental state test, such as the Folstein Mini-Mental State Examination or the Short Test of Mental Status. Asking about news events is a highly sensitive measure of recent memory. Be sure that the patient has been exposed to this information. Ask questions such as, Who is the president? What is his wife's name? Who was the last president? What is his wife's name? Note any evidence of aphasia, apraxia, or agnosia. Anomia with preservation of orientation suggests semantic dementia. Observe for lack of insight and disinhibited behaviors that occur in FTD.

2. Look for cardiovascular risk factors such as hypertension, arterial bruits, arrhythmia, and heart murmur.

3. Complete a full neurologic examination. Pay special attention to focal deficits such as visual field cuts, paresis, sensory loss, and ataxia. Posterior cortical atrophy, which most commonly has Alzheimer's-type pathology begins as progressive visual dysfunction similar to that of Balint's syndrome. Evaluate for any extrapyramidal difficulties, such as hypokinesia, increased muscle tone, a mask-like face, and micrographia. Determine whether the patient has any problem in walking. This is often best undertaken in the hallway rather than in the examining room. Note the patient's step size, speed of walking, arm swing, and ability to turn. The palmomental reflex and snout reflex are not particularly helpful because they are common among healthy elderly. The grasp reflex occurs late in the course of the disease.

C. **Laboratory studies.**

1. **Recommended in all cases** are complete blood count (CBC), chemistry panel, erythrocyte sedimentation rate, thyroid and liver function tests, folate and vitamin B12 levels, syphilis serologic testing, CT or MRI, and neuropsychological evaluation.

2. **Recommended selectively** are electroencephalography, LP, chest radiograph, HIV test, drug screen, SPECT or PET, heavy metal screen, copper, or ceruloplasmin.

3. **Electroencephalography** can be useful in diagnosing Creutzfeldt–Jakob's disease, differentiating depression or delirium from dementia, evaluating for encephalitis,

revealing seizures as causes of memory difficulties, and diagnosing nonconvulsive status epilepticus.

4. **LP** is recommended if the patient is suspected of having a paraneoplastic or limbic encephalopathy, cancer, CNS infection; hydrocephalus is seen at imaging; the patient is younger than 55 years; the dementia is acute or subacute; the patient is immunosuppressed; or vasculitis or connective tissue disease is suspected. In the setting where it is important to make a specific diagnosis, CSF amyloid β and tau protein levels jointly are reported to be 89% sensitive and 90% specific for AD. In the setting when Creutzfeldt–Jakob's disease is suspected often because the MRI diffusion image shows cortical ribboning or basal ganglia involvement, CSF 14-3-3 protein and CSF tau measurements plus the newer RT-QuIC (real-time quaking-induced conversion) are helpful.

5. **FDG (fluorodeoxyglucose)-PET** scan can be useful in differentiating FTD from AD. In one blinded study in which FDG-PET was used to evaluate those patients with and those without dementia, the sensitivity was only 38%, and the specificity was 88%. Also, biparietal hypometabolism supports the diagnosis of AD but is not specific.

6. **Amyloid PET scan.** There are now three FDA-approved isotopes for imaging brain $A\beta$ deposition. Many of the present studies evaluating $A\beta$ antibody to treat or prevent AD include only patients who have evidence of brain $A\beta$ deposits on amyloid PET scan. In this way, these drugs are accurately targeted, and those with non-AD dementias are excluded. When there is a disease-modifying treatment or disease preventative therapy, amyloid PET studies are expected to be used more often.

7. **Other diagnostic biomarkers.** The ε4 allele of the apolipoprotein E gene (apoE4) is a well-established risk factor for AD; however, the American Medical Association does not recommend apoE4 testing in the diagnosis of AD or if the patient's condition is presymptomatic. Mutations in the *PSEN1*, *PSEN2*, and *APP* genes can cause early-onset, autosomal dominant AD and are commercially available for testing. Genetic counseling is required before and after mutation testing. Structural imaging techniques including voxel-based morphometry, hippocampal volumetric measurement; functional imaging techniques including f-MRI, magnetic resonance spectroscopy, and amyloid PET imaging in the brain are emerging as imaging techniques with potential use for differentiating various dementia types and for preclinical diagnoses.

8. **Longitudinal biomarkers.** As mentioned earlier, these biomarkers are included in the new criteria for presymptomatic AD, MCI, and AD dementia, although additional research is needed for their validation and standardization. Longitudinal assessment of CSF amyloid β and tau protein, PET amyloid imaging, FDG-PET, and MRI volumetric studies lead to the hypothetical model of dynamic biomarker changes in AD, which posits the following order of changes: decrease in CSF amyloid β, increase in PET amyloid, increase in CSF tau and phospho-tau, decrease in MRI hippocampal volume and FDG-PET activity, cognitive impairment. Studies in asymptomatic carriers of early-onset familial AD mutation carriers suggest that changes in CSF biomarkers occur 15 to 20 years before symptom onset. Development of PET tracers to follow brain tau accumulation will be an important additional biomarker tool. These biomarkers will serve as valuable tools in tracking response to disease-modifying therapies once they become available.

DIFFERENTIAL DIAGNOSIS

Be aware of the possible causes of dementia listed in Table 2.1. The most important reversible causes include depression, medication, hydrocephalus, thyroid disease, vitamin B_{12} deficiency, fungal infection, neurosyphilis, subdural hematoma, and brain tumor.

ACKNOWLEDGMENT

This work was supported by National Institute of Aging grant P50 AG16574-02 and the State of Florida Alzheimer's Disease Initiative. NET is supported by National Institutes of Health grants R01 NS080820, U01 AG046139, RF1 AG051504, and R21 AG048101.

Key Points

- Neurodegenerative diseases constitute the most common etiology of dementia, but potentially reversible etiologies can also exist.
- AD is the most common dementia etiology, accounting for 50% to 75% of the cases, followed by VaD (20% to 30%), FTD (5% to 10%), and DLB.
- In addition to a thorough history and physical examination, blood tests for reversible causes of cognitive decline (including CBC, chemistry panel, vitamin B_{12} levels, thyroid, liver, kidney function tests), CT or MRI, and neuropsychological examination are needed for diagnosis, management, and counseling.
- Patients with atypical presentations, such as young age of onset, sudden onset, rapid progression, systemic illness, presence of noncognitive symptoms or signs, may require additional testing, such as EEG, LP, FDG-PET, or additional laboratory studies.
- AD typically presents as progressive worsening in memory, but atypical presentations with predominant involvement of other cognitive domains also exist.
- Clinical features that suggest DLB include fluctuations, hallucinations, parkinsonism, REM sleep behavior disorder, and neuroleptic sensitivity.
- FTD can present with predominant behavioral abnormalities or language impairment.
- Subjects with MCI have intact activities of daily living, but this condition can be a prodrome for dementia.

Recommended Readings

Albert MS, DeKosky ST, Dickson D, et al. The diagnosis of mild cognitive impairment due to Alzheimer's disease: recommendations from the National Institute on Aging-Alzheimer's Association workgroups on diagnostic guidelines for Alzheimer's disease. *Alzheimers Dement.* 2011;7(3):270–279.

American Psychiatric Association. *Diagnostic and Statistical Manual of Mental Disorders.* 4th ed. Washington, DC: American Psychiatric Association; 1994.

Becker P, Feussner JR, Mulrow CD, et al. The role of lumbar puncture in the evaluation of dementia: the Durham Veterans Administration/Duke University Study. *J Am Geriatr Soc.* 1985;33(6):392–396.

Boeve BF. Diagnosis and management of the non-Alzheimer dementias. In: Noseworthy JH, ed. *Neurological Therapeutics: Principles and Practice.* London, England: Martin Dunitz; 2003.

Boeve BF, Lang AE, Litvan I. Corticobasal degeneration and its relationship to progressive supranuclear palsy and frontotemporal dementia. *Ann Neurol.* 2003;54(suppl 5):S15–S19.

Cairns NJ, Bigio EH, Mackenzie IR, et al. Neuropathologic diagnostic and nosologic criteria for frontotemporal lobar degeneration: consensus of the Consortium for Frontotemporal Lobar Degeneration. *Acta Neuropathol (Berl).* 2007;114(1):5–22.

Corey-Bloom J, Thal LJ, Galasko D, et al. Diagnosis and evaluation of dementia. *Neurology.* 1995;45(2):211–218.

Ertekin-Taner N. Genetics of Alzheimer's disease: a centennial review. *Neurol Clin.* 2007;25(3):611–667.

Ertekin-Taner N. Genetics of Alzheimer's disease in the pre- and post-GWAS era. *Alzheimer's Res Ther.* 2010;2(1):3.

Folstein MF, Folstein SE, McHugh PR. "Mini-mental state": a practical method for grading the cognitive state of patients for the clinician. *J Psychiatr Res.* 1975;12(3):189–198.

Gorno-Tempini ML, Hillis AE, Weintraub S, et al. Classification of primary progressive aphasia and its variants. *Neurology.* 2011;76(11):1006–1014.

Graff-Radford NR, Godersky JC, Jones M. Variables predicting surgical outcome in symptomatic hydrocephalus in the elderly. *Neurology.* 1989;39(2):1601–1604.

Hardy J. Rogaeva E. Motor neuron disease and frontotemporal dementia: sometimes related, sometimes not. *Exp Neurol.* 2014;262(pt B):75–83.

Hejl A, Hogh P, Waldemar G. Potentially reversible conditions in 1000 consecutive memory clinic patients. *J Neurol Neurosurg Psychiatry.* 2002;73(4):390–394.

Jack CR Jr, Knopman DS, Jagust WJ, et al. Tracking pathophysiological processes in Alzheimer's disease: an updated hypothetical model of dynamic biomarkers. *Lancet Neurol.* 2013;12(2):207–216.

Kalaria RN, Maestre GE, Arizaga R, et al. Alzheimer's disease and vascular dementia in developing countries: prevalence, management, and risk factors. *Lancet Neurol.* 2008;7(9):812–826.

Knopman DS, Petersen RC, Cha RH, et al. Incidence and causes of nondegenerative nonvascular dementia: a population-based study. *Arch Neurol.* 2006;63(2):218–221.

Kokmen E, Naessens JM, Offord KP. A short test of mental status: description and preliminary results. *Mayo Clin Proc.* 1987;62(4):281–288.

McKeith IG, Dickson DW, Lowe J, et al. Diagnosis and management of dementia with Lewy bodies: third report of the DLB Consortium. *Neurology*. 2005;65(12):1863–1872.

McKhann G, Drachman D, Folstein M, et al. Clinical diagnosis of Alzheimer's disease: report of the NINCDS-ADRDA Work Group under the auspices of the Department of Health and Human Services Task Force on Alzheimer's disease. *Neurology*. 1984;34(7):939–944.

McKhann GM, Knopman DS, Chertkow H, et al. The diagnosis of dementia due to Alzheimer's disease: recommendations from the National Institute on Aging-Alzheimer's Association workgroups on diagnostic guidelines for Alzheimer's disease. *Alzheimers Dement*. 2011;7(3):263–269.

Morris JC, ed. *Handbook of Dementing Illnesses*. New York, NY: Marcel Dekker; 1994.

Mortimer JA. The epidemiology of Alzheimer's disease: beyond risk factors. In: Iqbal I, Mortimer J, Winblad B, Wisniewski H, eds. *Research Advances in Alzheimer's Disease and Associated Disorders*. New York, NY: John Wiley & Sons; 1995:3–11.

Neary D, Snowden J, Mann D. Frontotemporal dementia. *Lancet Neurol*. 2005;4(11):771–780.

Nordberg A. Towards early diagnosis in Alzheimer disease. *Nat Rev Neurol*. 2015;11(2):69–70.

Petersen RC. Mild cognitive impairment: current research and clinical implications. *Semin Neurol*. 2007;27(1):22–31.

Post SG, Whitehouse PJ, Binstock RH, et al. The clinical introduction of genetic testing for Alzheimer disease: an ethical perspective. *JAMA*. 1997;277(10):832–836.

Prince M, Albanese E, Guerchet M, et al. *World Alzheimer Report 2014: Dementia and Risk Reduction: An Analysis of Protective and Modifiable Factors*. London, England: Alzheimer's Disease International; 2014.

Qiu C, De Ronchi D, Fratiglioni L. The epidemiology of the dementias: an update. *Curr Opin Psychiatry*. 2007;20(4):380–385.

Rascovsky K, Hodges JR, Knopman D, et al. Sensitivity of revised diagnostic criteria for the behavioural variant of frontotemporal dementia. *Brain*. 2011;134(9):2456–2477.

Roman GC, Tatemichi TK, Erkinjuntti T, et al. Vascular dementia: diagnostic criteria for research studies: report of the NINDS-AIREN International Workshop. *Neurology*. 1993;43(2):250–260.

The Ronald and Nancy Reagan Research Institute of the Alzheimer's Association, the National Institute on Aging Working Group. Consensus report of the working group on: "molecular and biochemical markers of Alzheimer's disease." *Neurobiol Aging*. 1998;19(2):109–116.

Seprling RA, Aisen PS, Beckett LA, et al. Toward defining the preclinical stages of Alzheimer's disease: recommendations from the National Institute on Aging-Alzheimer's Association workgroups on diagnostic guidelines for Alzheimer's disease. *Alzheimers Dement*. 2011;7(3):280–292.

Thal LJ, Kantarci K, Reiman EM, et al. The role of biomarkers in clinical trials for Alzheimer disease. *Alzheimer Dis Assoc Disord*. 2006;20(1):6–15.

Whitwell JL, Jack CR Jr. Neuroimaging in dementia. *Neurol Clin*. 2007;25(3):843–857.

3 Approach to the Patient with Aphasia

Jeffrey L. Saver and José Biller

Aphasia is a loss or impairment of language processing caused by brain damage. Language disorders are common manifestations of cerebral injury. Reflecting the centrality of language function in human endeavor, the aphasias are a major source of disability.

PATHOPHYSIOLOGY

A. **Cerebral dominance.** The left hemisphere is dominant for language in approximately 99% of right handers and 60% of left handers.
B. **Neuroanatomy.** A specialized cortical–subcortical neural system surrounding the Sylvian fissure in the dominant hemisphere subserves language processing (Fig. 3.1). Circumscribed lesions in different components of this neurocognitive network produce distinctive syndromes of language impairment.

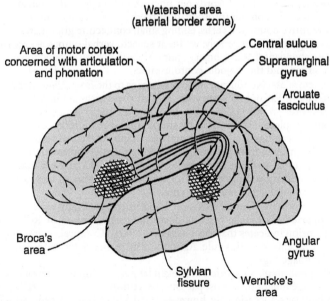

FIGURE 3.1 The neurocognitive network for language. The core perisylvian language cortices lie within the *dashed line* and include Broca's area in the inferior frontal gyrus, the supramarginal- and angular gyri in the parietal lobe, the subjacent arcuate fasciculus white matter tract, and Wernicke's area in the superior temporal gyrus. Extrasylvian sites that produce transcortical aphasias are found in surrounding cortices *(beyond dashed line)*. (Modified with permission from Mayeux R, Kandel ER. Disorders of language: the aphasias. In: Kandel ER, Schwartz JH, Jessell TM, eds. *Principles of Neural Science.* 3rd ed. New York, NY: Elsevier; 1991.)

ETIOLOGY

A. **Stroke.** Cerebrovascular disease is a frequent cause of aphasia. The perisylvian language zone is supplied by divisions of the middle cerebral artery (MCA), a branch of the internal carotid artery (ICA). The classic aphasic syndromes are most distinctly observed in ischemic stroke because vascular occlusions produce discrete, well-delineated brain lesions.

B. **Other focal lesions.** Any focal lesion affecting the language cortices will also produce aphasia, including primary and metastatic neoplasms and brain abscesses. **Primary progressive aphasia** (PPA) is a neurodegenerative syndrome characterized by slowly progressive, isolated language impairment in late life and focal atrophy of dominant frontotemporal cortices. Affected individuals frequently develop a generalized dementia after the first 2 years of illness. The three main variants of PPA and their anatomical correlate are as follows: (a) **nonfluent/agrammatic** (left posterior frontal and insular regions); (b) **semantic** (left anterior temporal); and (c) **logopenic** (left temporoparietal region). Among the causes of PPA are (1) tau-positive, ubiquitin/TDP 43-positive frontotemporal lobar degeneration and (2) a focal variant of Alzheimer's disease (AD) pathology.

C. **Diffuse lesions.** Diseases producing widespread neuronal dysfunction will disrupt language processing along with other cognitive and noncognitive neural functions. **Traumatic head injury** and **AD** are epidemiologically common causes of aphasic symptoms, although not of isolated aphasia.

CLINICAL MANIFESTATIONS

A. **Nonfluency versus fluency.** Fluency refers to the rate, quantity, and ease of speech production. In nonfluent speech, verbal output is meager (<50 words per minute), phrase length shortened (one to four words per phrase), production effortful, articulation often poor, and the melodic contour (prosody) disturbed. Nonfluent speakers often preferentially employ substantive nouns and verbs, eliding small connecting grammatical/functor words ("telegraphic speech"). Conversely, in fluent speech, verbal output is generous (and may even be more abundant than customary), phrase length normal, production easy, articulation usually preserved, and the melodic contour intact.

   1. **Anatomic correlate.** Nonfluency indicates damage to the frontal language regions anterior to the fissure of Rolando. Fluency signals that these areas are intact.

B. **Auditory comprehension impairment.** Impaired ability to understand spoken language ranges from complete mystification by simple one-word utterances to subtle failure to extract the full meanings of complex sentences. In informal conversation, aphasic patients often capitalize on clues from gestures, tone, and setting to supplement their understanding of the propositional content of a speaker's utterances. Examiners may underestimate the extent of auditory comprehension impairment if they fail to test formally a patient's comprehension deprived of nonverbal cues.

   1. **Anatomic correlate.** Comprehension impairment generally reflects damage to the temporoparietal language regions posterior to the fissure of Rolando. Preserved comprehension indicates that these areas are intact. (Comprehension of grammar is an important exception to this rule. Agrammatism is associated with damage to inferior frontal language regions.)

C. **Repetition impairment.** Repetition of spoken language is linguistically and anatomically a distinct language function. In most patients, repetition impairment parallels other deficits in spoken language. Occasionally, however, relatively isolated disordered repetition may be the dominant clinical feature (conduction aphasia). In other patients, repetition may be well preserved despite severe deficits in spontaneous speech (transcortical aphasias). Rarely, such patients exhibit echolalia, a powerful, mandatory tendency to repeat all heard phrases.

   1. **Anatomic correlate.** Impaired repetition indicates damage within the core perisylvian language zone. Preserved repetition signals that these areas are intact.

D. **Paraphasic errors.** Substitutions of incorrect words for intended words are paraphasias. Paraphasic errors are classified into three types.

   1. A **literal** or **phonemic paraphasia** occurs when only a part of the word is misspoken, as when "apple" becomes "tapple" or "apfle."

2. A **verbal** or **global paraphasia** occurs when an entire incorrect word is substituted for the intended word, as when "apple" becomes "orange" or "bicycle." A **semantic paraphasia** arises when the substituted word is from the same semantic field as the target word ("orange" for "apple"). Fluent output contaminated by many verbal paraphasias is **jargon speech.**

3. A **neologistic paraphasia** occurs when an entirely novel word not extant in the speaker's native lexicon is substituted for the intended word, as when "apple" becomes "brifun."

4. Anatomic correlate. Paraphasic errors may occur with lesions anywhere within the language system and do not carry strong anatomic implications. To some extent, phonemic paraphasias are more common with lesions in the frontal language fields and global paraphasias more common with lesions in temporoparietal areas.

E. Word-finding difficulty (anomia). Retrieval of target words from the lexicon is virtually always disturbed in aphasia. Patients may exhibit frequent hesitations in their spontaneous speech while they struggle with word finding. **Circumlocutions** transpire when patients "talk around" words they fail to retrieve, providing lengthy definitions or descriptions to convey the meanings of words they are unable to access.

1. Anatomic correlate. Word-finding difficulty occurs with lesions located throughout the language-dominant hemisphere and possesses little localizing value.

F. Reading and writing. In most cases of aphasia, reading impairment **(alexia)** and writing impairment **(agraphia)** parallel oral language comprehension and production deficits. Occasionally, however, isolated reading impairment, writing impairment, or both can occur in the setting of fully preserved oral language function.

1. Anatomic correlate. The anatomy of reading and writing incorporates both the core perisylvian language zones and additional function-specific sites. Reading requires primary and higher-level visual processing in the occipital and inferior parietal lobes. Writing depends on visual stores in the inferior parietal lobe and graphomotor output regions in the frontal lobe.

EVALUATION

A. History. Abrupt onset of language difficulty suggests a cerebrovascular lesion. Subacute onset may suggest tumor, abscess, or other more moderately progressive process. Slow onset suggests a degenerative disease, such as AD or frontotemporal lobar degeneration. Interviewing family members and other observers is crucial when the patient's language difficulty limits direct history-taking.

B. Physical examination.

1. Elementary neurologic signs. A detailed elementary neurologic examination allows identification of motor, sensory, or visual deficits that accompany the language disorder, aiding neuroanatomic localization. Important "neighborhood" signs are the presence or absence of hemiparesis, homonymous hemianopia or quadrantanopia, and apraxia.

2. Mental status examination. It is important to assess the patient's wakefulness and attentional function lest language errors resulting from inattentiveness be wrongly ascribed to intrinsic linguistic dysfunction. Nonverbal tests to evaluate memory, visuospatial, and executive functions should be used if severe language disturbance precludes routine verbal assessment.

3. Language examination. A careful language examination is critical in the evaluation of aphasia, profiling the patient's impaired and preserved language abilities and allowing a syndromic, localizing diagnosis (Video 3.1).

a. Spontaneous speech. The patient's spontaneous verbal output, in the course of conversation and in response to general questions, should be judged for fluency versus nonfluency and presence or absence of paraphasias. It is important to ask open-ended questions such as "Why are you in the hospital?" or "What do you do during a typical day at home?" because patients may mask major language derangements with yes/no answers and other brief replies to more structured interrogatories.

b. Repetition. The patient is asked to repeat complex sentences. If difficulty is evidenced, simpler verbal sequences from single-syllable words to multisyllabic words and short phrases are given to determine the level of impairment. At least one sentence rich in grammatical/functor words, such as "No ifs, ands, or buts," should be employed to test for isolated or more pronounced difficulty in grammatical repetition, as may be seen in Broca's and other anterior aphasias.

c. **Comprehension.** An initial judgment of auditory comprehension can be made in the course of obtaining the medical history and from spontaneous conversation. Tests that require no or minimal verbal responses are essential to the evaluation of auditory comprehension in individuals with severe disturbance of speech production and intubated patients.

(1) **Commands.** One simple bedside test is verbally to instruct the patient to carry out one-step and multistep commands, such as "Pick up a piece of paper, fold it in half, and place it on the table." Cautions to recall when interpreting results are (a) apraxia and other motor deficits may cause impairment not related to comprehension deficit and (b) midline motor acts on command, such as closing/opening eyes and standing up, draw on distinct anatomic systems and may be preserved even in the setting of severe aphasic comprehension disturbance.

(2) **Yes/no responses.** If the patient can reliably produce verbal or gestural yes/no responses, this output system may be used to assess auditory comprehension. Questions of graded difficulty should be employed for precise gauging of the degree of comprehension disturbance, using queries ranging from simple ("Is your name Smith?") to complex ("Do helicopters eat their young?").

(3) **Pointing.** This simple motor response also permits precise mapping of comprehension impairment by means of questions of graded difficulty. The examiner should employ both simple pointing commands ("Point to the chair, nose, door") and more lexically and syntactically complex pointing commands ("Point to the source of illumination in this room").

d. **Naming.** Difficulty with naming is almost invariable in all the aphasia syndromes. Consequently, naming tasks are sensitive, although not specific, means of testing for the presence or absence of aphasia.

(1) **Confrontation naming.** The patient is asked to name objects, parts of objects, body parts, and colors pointed out by the examiner. Common, high-frequency words ("tie," "watch") and uncommon, low-frequency words ("knot" of the tie, "watchband") should be tested.

(2) **Word-list generation.** Another type of naming test is to ask the patient to generate a list of items in a category (animals, cars) or words beginning with a given letter (F, A, S). Normal individuals produce 12 or more words per letter in 1 minute.

e. **Verbal automatisms.** Patients with profound disruptions of speech production should be requested to produce (a) overlearned verbal sequences, including the numbers from 1 to 10 and the days of the week; (b) overlearned verbal material, such as the pledge of allegiance; and (c) singing, such as "Happy Birthday to You." These utterances draw on subcortical and nondominant hemisphere areas and indicate residual capacities in impaired patients that may be capitalized on in rehabilitation.

f. **Reading.** Patients should be asked to read sentences aloud. Written sentences that are commands ("Close your eyes") allow simultaneous testing of reading aloud and reading comprehension.

g. **Writing.** In the order of difficulty, patients may be asked to write single letters, words, and short sentences. Obtaining a signature is insufficient because this overlearned sequence may be retained when all other graphomotor functions are lost.

C. **Laboratory studies.**

1. **Computed tomography.** Head computed tomography (CT) scan will delineate most focal structural lesions affecting the language regions of the brain. It may be normal in the first 24 hours following acute aphasia from new-onset ischemic stroke.

2. **Magnetic resonance imaging.** Brain magnetic resonance imaging (MRI) is somewhat more sensitive than CT at detecting morphologic abnormalities and is the preferred study if readily available. Imaging in the sagittal and coronal as well as axial planes allows precise mapping of lesions within known neural language regions.

SYNDROMIC DIAGNOSIS

Distinctive features of a patient's language disturbance may be employed to assign a syndromic diagnosis that has localizing value. Eight classical cortical aphasia syndromes are distinguished on the basis of fluency, comprehension, and repetition (Fig. 3.2). Approximately 60% of all aphasic patients exhibit one of these symptom clusters. Most of the remaining "atypical" aphasias will be found to harbor subcortical lesions. It is important to consider the time after onset when employing these syndromes for clinicoanatomic correlation. Soon after an acute insult, deafferentation, edema, hypoperfusion without infarction, and other mechanisms of diaschisis produce exaggerated clinical deficits. Later, neuroplasticity-mediated recovery of function reduces clinical deficits. The aphasia syndromes have maximal localizing value 3 weeks to 3 months after onset.

A. Perisylvian aphasias.

   1. Broca's aphasia. Patients with Broca's aphasia exhibit (a) nonfluent, dysarthric, effortful speech; (b) similarly disordered repetition; and (c) relatively intact comprehension, with mild difficulty in understanding syntax and relational grammar. Their verbal output is often "telegraphic," containing substantive nouns and verbs but omitting small, connecting, functor words. Most patients exhibit a faciobrachial hemiparesis. Patients often exhibit frustration over their language deficits and are at elevated risk for depression.

      a. Lesions producing Broca's aphasia lie in the posterior portion of the inferior frontal gyrus (Broca's area; Brodmann areas 44 and 45) and extend to involve surrounding motor, premotor, and underlying white matter territories. Lesions restricted solely to Broca's area produce mild, transient aphasia and more persistent dysarthria.

      b. Broca's area is supplied by the superior division of the MCA.

   2. Wernicke's aphasia. Patients with Wernicke's aphasia evince fluent, effortless, well-articulated output, almost always contaminated with paraphasias and neologisms. Repetition demonstrates a parallel impairment, with fluent but paraphasic output. The

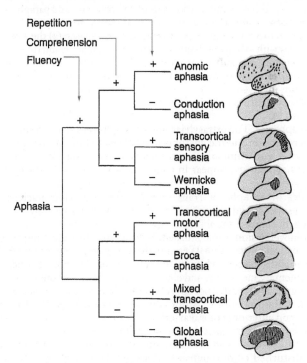

FIGURE 3.2 Algorithm for diagnosis and localization of the eight classical cortical aphasias.

leading feature of Wernicke's aphasia is a severe disturbance of auditory comprehension. Two types of behavioral responses to this comprehension deficit are observed. Most often in the acute phase, patients seem to be unaware of their inability to comprehend spoken language, calmly providing inappropriate and grossly paraphasic answers to observer's inquiries. Less frequently, patients are irritable and paranoid, perhaps because of their inability to understand what others say. A superior homonymous quadrantanopia is frequently present. However, the absence of more dramatic motor or sensory deficits, and the fluid production of speech, may mislead medical personnel into believing that the patient is confused or psychotic rather than aphasic, and may delay diagnosis while metabolic or psychiatric disturbances are sought.

    a. The core of lesions engendering Wernicke's aphasia map to the posterior third of the superior temporal gyrus (Wernicke's area; Brodmann area 22), an auditory association area. Lesion size may vary considerably, and damage often extends to the middle temporal gyrus and the inferior parietal lobe.

    b. Wernicke's area is supplied by the inferior division of the MCA.

3. Global aphasia. The most profound form of aphasia, called global aphasia, is characterized by drastically nonfluent output, severe disruption of comprehension, and little repetitive ability. Spontaneous speech is often absent initially, or marked by the production of a few stereotyped sounds. Patients neither read nor write. Hemiplegia is almost invariably present, and hemisensory loss and hemianopia are frequent.

    a. The typical insult involves the entire left perisylvian region, encompassing Broca's area in the inferior frontal lobe, Wernicke's area in the posterior temporal lobe, and all the interposed parietofrontal cortices. In rare cases, separate, discrete lesions of Broca's area and Wernicke's area produce global aphasia without hemiparesis.

    b. The perisylvian region lies within the territory of the MCA, and ICA and MCA occlusions are the most common causes of global aphasia.

4. Conduction aphasia. The hallmark of conduction aphasia is a disproportionate disruption of repetition. Comprehension of spoken language is relatively intact. Fluent spontaneous output is often marred by occasional hesitations and phonemic paraphasias, but is not as disturbed as repetition. Naming also tends to demonstrate mild paraphasic contamination. Motor and sensory disturbances are usually absent or mild.

    a. Two neural loci tend to give rise to conduction aphasia: (a) the supramarginal gyrus, sometimes with extension to the subinsular white matter, and (b) the primary auditory cortex, insula, and subjacent white matter. The arcuate fasciculus, a subcortical white matter tract connecting Wernicke's and Brodmann's areas, is often, but not invariably, involved.

    b. These regions are variably supplied by branches of the inferior or superior divisions of the MCA.

B. Extrasylvian aphasias. The extrasylvian aphasic syndromes share the clinical characteristic of preserved repetition and the anatomic trait of sparing of the core perisylvian language zone. They occur less commonly than the perisylvian aphasias. Many arise from watershed infarcts, but they may also appear in conjunction with tumors, abscesses, hemorrhages, and other lesions.

  1. Transcortical motor aphasia. Transcortical motor aphasia is characterized by discrepant spontaneous speech and repetition. Spontaneous output is severely disrupted, nonfluent, and halting. In contrast, the ability to repeat sentences verbatim is preserved, as is reading aloud. Comprehension is undisturbed. Naming may be mildly impaired.

    a. **Transcortical motor aphasia** results from damage at one of two foci: (a) prefrontal cortices and subjacent white matter anterior or superior to Broca's area or (b) the supplementary motor area and cingulate gyrus. These lesions disconnect Broca's area from limbic areas and other sources of the drive to communicate.

    b. Lesions anterosuperior to Broca's area lie in the vascular border zone between the middle and anterior cerebral arteries. The supplementary motor area and cingulate gyrus regions are irrigated by the anterior cerebral artery (ACA).

  2. Transcortical sensory aphasia. Patients with transcortical sensory aphasia exhibit severely disturbed comprehension of spoken language, but preserved repetition. Spontaneous speech is fluent, although often paraphasic. Echolalia—automatic repetition of overheard phrases—is common. Reading aloud may be fairly preserved, whereas reading comprehension is quite poor. Motor deficits are generally absent, but hemisensory deficits are common.

   a. Lesions may occur over a wide distribution posterior and superior to the posterior perisylvian region, including the middle temporal gyrus, the angular gyrus, and underlying white matter. These insults disconnect Wernicke's area from multiple posterior association cortices, preventing retroactivation by aural word forms of the widely distributed neural representations that convey their meanings.

   b. The lesions generally lie within the vascular watershed between the posterior cerebral artery (PCA) and MCA.

3. Mixed transcortical aphasia. This rare and remarkable condition is analogous to global aphasia, except for preserved ability to repeat. Spontaneous speech is minimal or absent. Patients are unable to comprehend spoken language, name, read, or write. Repetition of spoken language, however, is preserved. Patients are often echolalic. Mild hemiparesis and hemisensory loss affecting proximal greater than distal extremities may be observed.

   a. Lesions are an additive combination of those producing transcortical motor and sensory aphasias. Insults anterosuperior to Broca's area and posterosuperior to Wernicke's area cut off the perisylvian language zone from access to other cortices. **Isolation of the speech area** is a synonym for mixed transcortical aphasia.

   b. The lesions fall in the crescentic vascular border zone among the ACA, MCA, and PCA.

4. Anomic aphasia. These patients exhibit difficulty retrieving verbal tags in spontaneous speech and confrontation naming. The remainder of language functions is relatively intact. Auditory comprehension, repetition, reading, and writing are normal. Spontaneous speech is preponderantly fluent, although interrupted by occasional hesitations for word finding. In severe cases, output may be lengthy but empty, with recurrent circumlocutions.

   a. A wide variety of lesions, including both dominant and nondominant hemisphere loci, may produce anomic aphasia. Particularly common sources are insults to (a) the dominant inferior parietal lobe and (b) the dominant anterior temporal cortices. The latter insults have been associated with **category-specific naming deficits** in which naming in different semantic categories (e.g., living versus nonliving entities) is differentially impaired.

   b. The angular gyrus and anterior temporal cortices are supplied by different branches of the inferior division of the MCA.

C. Subcortical aphasia syndromes. Focal lesions confined to subcortical structures strongly interconnected with language cortices produce aphasia. Although the optimal classification system for the subcortical aphasias is a still contested and unsettled enterprise, two major profiles can be discerned according to neuroanatomic location of the lesions.

1. Striatal-capsular aphasia. The language deficit in striatal-capsular aphasia resembles that in anomic or transcortical motor aphasia. Patients may or may not be fluent but are almost invariably dysarthric. Mild to moderate anomia coexists with generally intact auditory comprehension, repetition, reading, and writing. Generation of complex syntactic sentences is impaired. Hemiparesis is common, hemisensory loss variable, and hemianopia infrequent. Lesions involve the left putamen, dorsolateral caudate, anterior limb of the internal capsule, and rostral periventricular white matter. This aphasia has been associated with both ischemic and hemorrhagic strokes.

2. Thalamic aphasia. The language deficit in thalamic aphasia resembles that in transcortical sensory aphasia. Output may be relatively fluent, auditory comprehension is deficient, and repetition is preserved. Impairments of naming, reading comprehension, and writing are also present. A contralateral emotional facial paresis (diminished facial movement in expressing spontaneous emotions but preserved facial movements to command) and contralateral hypokinesia are often the only elementary neurologic deficits. Lesions are situated in the left anterolateral thalamus. Thalamic aphasia has been associated with left thalamic infarction often involving the left tuberothalamic artery territory, and left thalamic hemorrhage.

D. Additional classical syndromes. Strategically placed lesions may produce dissociated impairments of reading, writing, and oral language function. Three syndromes with well-characterized localizing properties will be reviewed.

1. Alexia without agraphia (pure alexia). Alexia without agraphia, the first of the disconnection syndromes described by Joseph Jules Déjerine in 1892, presents as an acquired loss of

reading ability in a literate person, with preserved ability to write spontaneously. Reading is severely impaired, whereas spontaneous speech, repetition, and auditory comprehension are normal. Writing is preserved, but dramatically, after a delay, patients are unable to read phrases they themselves have written. Recognition of words spelled aloud and traced on the palm is normal. Only words presented visually pose difficulty. Patients frequently exhibit a slow, letter-by-letter reading strategy, painstakingly recognizing and stating aloud each letter in a word and then, from the string of spoken letters, determining the target word. A right homonymous hemianopia is common but not invariable. Disorders of color vision, including achromatopsia and color anomia, may be present.

The most common neuroanatomic substrate comprises simultaneous lesions of the left occipital lobe and the splenium of the corpus callosum, depriving the angular gyrus region critical for word recognition of visual input from either the left or right hemisphere. The smallest sufficient injury is a single lesion of the paraventricular white matter of the mesial occipitotemporal junction (the forceps major), interrupting interhemispheric and intrahemispheric visual tracts to the angular gyrus but sparing the corpus callosum and left occipital cortex. Etiologies include left PCA infarction, tumor, demyelinating disorders such as multiple sclerosis (MS) or acute disseminated encephalomyelitis (ADEM), toxoplasma or herpes encephalitis, and mitochondrial encephalomyopathy, lactic acidosis, and stroke-like episodes (MELAS).

2. **Alexia with agraphia.** Patients exhibit loss of literacy—inability to read or write—but relatively well-preserved oral language function. Speech is fluent, although anomia is often present, and auditory comprehension and repetition are intact. Hemisensory deficits are frequent, and hemiparesis and hemivisual disturbances are variable. A full-fledged Gerstmann's syndrome, including dyscalculia, dysgraphia, left–right confusion, and finger agnosia, may be present.

The underlying lesion classically involves the dominant inferior parietal lobule (angular and supramarginal gyri).

3. **Pure word deafness (auditory verbal agnosia).** Patients resemble Wernicke's aphasics. Comprehension and repetition of spoken language are impaired, whereas speech is fluent. Unlike in Wernicke's patients, however, paraphasias are rare and, more importantly, comprehension of written material is intact. Writing production is also normal. Although uncomprehending of word sounds, patients have intact hearing and are generally successful in identifying meaningful nonverbal sounds such as car horns or telephone rings.

Two types of lesions underlie pure word deafness, both disconnecting Wernicke's area from input from primary auditory cortices. Some patients harbor bilateral superior temporal lesions. A roughly equal number exhibit a single deep superior temporal lesion in the dominant hemisphere, blocking ipsilateral and crossing callosal auditory pathways.

E. **Aprosodia.** Meaning is conveyed not only through the propositional content of language, but also through prosody—the melody, rhythm, timbre, and inflection of the speaker. Prosody is frequently disturbed in nonfluent aphasia. However, patients may have normal propositional language yet exhibit disturbances of the production, comprehension, or repetition of prosody. Both cortical and subcortical dysfunctions can account for impaired prosody. In general, the nondominant hemisphere (most often the right) plays a greater role in production and comprehension of emotional prosody than does the dominant hemisphere.

DIFFERENTIAL DIAGNOSIS

Acquired speech impairments may result from disruption of lower-order neural and muscular mechanisms for implementing sound production rather than disturbances of central processing of language. It is important to distinguish these nonaphasic speech impairments from genuine aphasia, because they differ in their localizing significance and spectrum of etiologic causes.

A. **Dysarthria.** Dysarthria is abnormal articulation of spoken language. At least five types of nonaphasic dysarthria may be distinguished. (a) **Paretic dysarthria** is caused by weakness of articulatory muscles. Soft, low-pitched, nasal voicing is characteristic. Causes include myopathies, neuromuscular junction disorders such as myasthenia gravis, and lower motor neuron disease. (b) In **spastic dysarthria**, speech is typically strained, slow, and monotonic. Bilateral upper motor neuron lesions compromising the corticobulbar tracts are the cause.

(c) In **ataxic dysarthria**, jerky irregular speech rhythm and volume are noted, reflecting lesions to the cerebellum or its connections. MS is a common cause. (d) **Extrapyramidal dysarthrias** include hypokinetic dysarthria, which is seen in parkinsonism and choreic dysarthria, which is observed in Huntington's disease and other chorea syndromes. (e) In **aphemia (apraxia of speech),** small lesions within Broca's area (Brodmann areas 44 and 45) or the left frontal oral motor cortex near the face M_1 area produce dysarticulation without disturbing core language function.

Aphasic dysarthria—dysarticulation occurring as one manifestation of an aphasic language syndrome—is common with anterior aphasias such as Broca's syndrome. The nonaphasic dysarthrias may be distinguished from aphasic dysarthria by demonstrating preserved intrinsic language functions including naming, comprehension, and reading. Intact writing is most telling, showing normal productive language capacity when a nonoral output channel is employed.

B. **Mutism.** Aphasia—disordered language—can be securely diagnosed only on the basis of exemplars of disturbed output (or comprehension). Patients with acute-onset aphasia, especially Broca's or global aphasia, are often unable to speak for the first few hours or days. However, a wide variety of other insults can produce total cessation of verbal output (articulation and voice). The full differential diagnosis of mutism includes (a) psychiatric etiologies (schizophrenia, depression, catatonia, and psychogenic illness); (b) abulia/akinetic mutism (bilateral prefrontal, diencephalic, and midbrain lesions); (c) acute dominant supplementary motor area lesions; (d) pseudobulbar palsy; (e) locked-in syndrome from bilateral ventral pontine or midbrain lesions; (f) acute bilateral cerebellar lesions; (g) lower motor neuron lesions; and (h) laryngeal disorders.

C. **Thought disorders.** When an intact language apparatus is placed in service of an underlying thought disorder, bizarre utterances arise that superficially resemble the fluent aphasic output of patients with Wernicke's or conduction aphasia. Demographic features are helpful, recognizing that schizophrenia with psychotic speech of new onset tends to appear in individuals in their 20s and 30s, whereas fluent aphasias cluster in older individuals with vascular risk factors. Several features of the utterances also distinguish thought-disordered from fluent aphasic speech. (a) Paraphasias are common in aphasia but rare in schizophrenia. (b) The neologisms of aphasics are frequent and changing, whereas those of schizophrenics are infrequent and consistent. (c) Open-ended questions tend to prompt briefer responses in aphasics than in schizophrenics. (d) Bizarre and delusional themes appear only in schizophrenic discourse.

COURSE

Both undamaged language or perilesional regions of the left hemisphere, and language homologous regions of the right hemisphere or both, are thought to support post aphasia recovery. Some degree of spontaneous recovery of language function is invariable after a static brain injury. An initial accelerated period of improved function occurs over the first few days or weeks after insult and is attributable to resolution of edema, ischemic penumbra, and other causes of dysfunction at a distance from the site of permanent injury. The second, slower phase of recovery reflects utilization of parallel circuits, retraining, and structural neural plasticity. The bulk of this functional recovery takes place in the first 3 months after injury, and some may continue up to 1 year, rarely longer. Among the aphasia syndromes, the greatest recovery compared with baseline tends to occur in Broca's and conduction aphasias. Anomic aphasia is a common end stage into which other aphasia subtypes tend to evolve.

Factors favoring greater spontaneous improvement, as well as response to speech therapy, are young age, left-handedness or ambidexterity, higher education, smaller lesion size, no or few nonlanguage cognitive defects, absence of emotional difficulties such as depression and neglect, and strong family support. Patients with traumatic aphasia tend to recover more fully than patients with ischemic lesions.

REFERRAL

A. **Neurologist.** Most patients with aphasia should undergo neurologic consultation. The neurology specialist will confirm the presence of aphasia, clarify the type, aid in etiologic diagnosis, and provide the patient and family with an informed prognosis.

In selected cases, neurologists or physiatrists may consider pharmacotherapy of aphasia. Small case series have suggested that stimulants, cholinesterase inhibitors, dopamine agonists, and other neurotransmitter modulators may augment language therapy. Piracetam, donepezil, memantine, and galantamine have been found to be effective adjuncts to treatment of chronic poststroke aphasia in some studies. However, few well-validated randomized trials have been completed in this area, and more research is needed. Repetitive transcranial magnetic stimulation (rTMS) especially when combined with language therapy or other therapeutic approaches may promote language recovery, by releasing the perilesional fields from tonic inhibition.

B. Speech and language pathologist. All patients with aphasia should have an evaluation by a speech and language pathologist. The speech therapist will perform a formal diagnostic assessment, profiling the patient's language strengths and weaknesses with normed tests. A variety of standardized language assessment batteries, including the Boston Diagnostic Aphasia Examination, the Western Aphasia Battery, the Porch Index of Communicative Ability, and the Communication Abilities in Daily Living, may be drawn on to survey a patient's abilities. The therapist then employs the results to design and implement an individualized treatment program of aphasia therapy.

Systematic language rehabilitation programs improve patient outcome. Treatment is tailored to each individual's pattern of linguistic and cognitive competencies and deficits, exploiting spared brain systems to reestablish, circumvent, or compensate for lost language capacities. A variety of deficit-specific programs are available to supplement general language stimulation. For nonfluency, treatments include (a) melodic intonation therapy, (b) sign language and other gestural communication training, and (c) communication boards. Syntax training may benefit agrammatism. Specific word-retrieval therapies have been developed for anomia and comprehension training programs for auditory comprehension deficits.

Speech therapy programs generally last for 2 to 3 months, in 30- to 60-minute sessions conducted two to five times per week. Recent studies suggest that intense treatment (at least 2 hours a day, at least 4 days per week) during a short period may be more effective than a similar number of sessions spread out over a longer time period. Self- and family-administered home exercises provide additional stimulation. Computer-based training is expanding in scope and sophistication.

C. Neuropsychologist. Patients who have major nonlinguistic cognitive deficits in addition to aphasia, and whose diagnosis is unclear, should undergo neuropsychological evaluation. Formal neuropsychological evaluation with tests that minimize language requirements allow a more detailed profiling of memory, visuospatial reasoning, executive function, praxis, and concept formation than can be obtained by bedside mental status examination. Findings may aid the physician in making a diagnosis by suggesting the pattern of neural system involvement and the speech pathologist in prescribing therapy by identifying the extent to which different extralinguistic capacities can support various compensatory strategies.

D. Patient support groups. The National Aphasia Association (National Aphasia Association, 350 Seventh Avenue, Suite 902, New York, NY 10001, 1-800-922-4622, www.aphasia.org) is an excellent resource for patients and their families. The American Heart/Stroke Association and National Stroke Association also provide beneficial programs and information.

Key Points

- The left cerebral hemisphere is dominant for language in over 90% of all individuals.
- Assessing for aphasia involves evaluation of fluency, repetition, comprehension, reading, and writing.
- Aphasia after stroke affects approximately one out of five stroke patients.
- Aphasia has a negative impact on health-related quality of life.
- Aphasia is complicated by high rates of depression and social isolation.
- Alexia without agraphia is often due to a lesion in the left occipital lobe extending to the posterior corpus callosum disconnecting the right visual cortex from language areas in the left temporal lobe.

Recommended Readings

Alexander MP, Hillis AE. Aphasia. *Handb Clin Neurol*. 2008;88:287–309.

Allen L, Mehta S, McClure JA, et al. Therapeutic interventions for aphasia initiated more than six months post stroke: a review of the evidence. *Top Stroke Rehabil*. 2012;19(6):523–535.

Baker JM, Rorden C, Fridriksson J. Using transcranial direct-current stimulation to treat stroke patients with aphasia. *Stroke*. 2010;41:1229–1236.

Berthier ML, Pulvermüller F, Dávila G, et al. Drug therapy of post-stroke aphasia: a review of current evidence. *Neuropsychol Rev*. 2011;21:302–317.

Blair M, Marczinski CA, Davis-Faroque N, et al. A longitudinal study of language decline in Alzheimer's disease and frontotemporal dementia. *J Int Neuropsychol Soc*. 2007;13:237–245.

Bookheimer S. Functional MRI of language: new approaches to understanding the cortical organization of semantic processing. *Annu Rev Neurosci*. 2002;17:151–188.

Broca P. Remarks on the seat of the faculty of articulate speech, followed by the report of a case of aphemia (loss of speech). In: Rottenberg DA, Hochberg FH, eds. *Neurologic Classics in Modern Translation*. New York, NY: Hafner Press; 1977:136–149.

Catani M, Jones DK, Ffytche DH. Perisylvian language networks of the human brain. *Ann Neurol*. 2005;57:8–16.

Coslett HB, Brashear HR, Heilman KM. Pure word deafness after bilateral primary auditory cortex infarcts. *Neurology*. 1984;34(3):347–351.

Cuomo J, Flaster M, Biller J. Right brain: a reading specialist with alexia without agraphia: teacher Interrupted. *Neurology*. 2014;82:e5–e7.

Damasio H, Tranel D, Grabowski TJ, et al. Neural systems behind word and concept retrieval. *Cognition*. 2004;92:179–229.

Flamand-Roze C, Falissard B, Roze E, et al. Validation of a new language screening tool for patients with acute stroke: the Language Screening Test (LAST). *Stroke*. 2011;42:1224–1229.

Floel A, Cohen LG. Recover of function in humans: cortical stimulation and pharmacological treatment after stroke. *Neurobiol Dis*. 2010;37:243–251.

Gorno-Tempini ML, Hillis AE, Weintraub S, et al. Classification of primary progressive aphasia and its variants. *Neurology*. 2011;76:1006–1014.

Grossman M, Ash S. Primary progressive aphasia: a review. *Neurocase*. 2004;10:3–18.

Hillis AE. Aphasia: progress in the last quarter of a century. *Neurology*. 2007;69:200–213.

Kass JS, Arciniegas DB, Arora G, et al. Behavioral neurology and neuropsychiatry. *Continuum (Minneap Minn)*. 2015;21(3).

Kelly H, Brady MC, Enderby P. Speech and language therapy for aphasia following stroke. *Cochrane Database Syst Rev*. 2010;(5):CD000425.

LaPointe L, ed. *Aphasia and Related Neurogenic Language Disorders*. 4th ed. New York, NY: Thieme; 2011.

Martin PI, Naeser MA, Ho M, et al. Research into transcranial magnetic stimulation in the treatment of aphasia. *Curr Neurol Neurosci Rep*. 2009;9(6):451–458.

Mesulam MM. Primary progressive aphasia: a language-based dementia. *N Engl J Med*. 2003;349:1535–1542.

Nadeau SE, Crosson B. Subcortical aphasia. *Brain Lang*. 1997;58(3):355–402.

Oliverira-Souza R, Moll J, Caparelli-Dáquer EMA. Broca's aphemia: an illustrated account of its clinico-anatomic validity. *Arq Neuropsiquiatr*. 2007;65(4-B):1220–1223.

Ross ED. The aprosodias: functional-anatomic organization of the effective components of language in the right hemisphere. *Arch Neurol*. 1981;38(9):561–569.

Wildgruber D, Ackermann H, Kreifelts B, et al. Cerebral processing of linguistic and emotional prosody: fMRI studies. *Prog Brain Res*. 2006;156:249–268.

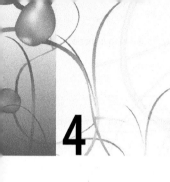

4

Approach to the Patient with Memory Impairment

Torricia H. Yamada, Natalie L. Denburg,
and Daniel Tranel

The term **amnesia** refers to conditions in which patients lose, partly or completely, the ability to learn new information or to retrieve information acquired previously. Amnesia (also referred to here as *memory impairment or memory dysfunction*) is common in neurologic diseases that affect the telencephalon or diencephalon and is a defining characteristic and frequently an early manifestation of some of the most frequently encountered neurologic diseases, including Alzheimer's disease (AD). As such, reports of memory impairment must be taken seriously.

Accurate diagnosis and effective management of memory disorders are important. A considerable clinical challenge is presented, however, by the facts that the most frequent neurologic diseases affect older adults and a certain degree of decline in memory is associated with normal aging. Hence, it can be difficult to differentiate reports of memory problems that may be normal manifestations of aging versus a signal of the presence of neurologic disease. Memory problems are common in nonneurologic conditions such as psychiatric disease, and this constitutes another reason for careful diagnosis. Such distinctions often require laboratory testing that can be conducted by neuropsychological assessments.

TYPES OF MEMORY AND MEMORY SYSTEMS IN THE BRAIN

There are several fundamental distinctions between different types of memory and the neural systems to which different types of memory are related (Table 4.1).

Working memory depends on the integrity of the frontal lobes. More specifically, recent functional imaging studies have linked working memory to the dorsolateral prefrontal sector of the frontal lobes. A laterality effect has also been noted wherein verbal working memory tasks depend on the left dorsolateral prefrontal sector, whereas spatial tasks depend on the right dorsolateral prefrontal sector.

A. Anterograde and retrograde memory.
   1. **Anterograde memory** refers to the capacity to learn new information—that is, to acquire new facts, skills, and other types of knowledge. It is closely dependent on neural structures in the mesial temporal lobe, especially the hippocampus and interconnected

TABLE 4.1 Subdivisions of Memory

Dichotomy	Characteristics
Retrograde	Retrieval of knowledge acquired previously, especially knowledge acquired before the onset of brain injury
Anterograde	Learning of new knowledge, especially learning of knowledge after the onset of brain injury
Verbal	Words, names, verbally coded facts; word-based material
Nonverbal	Faces, geographic routes, complex melodies; spatially based material
Declarative	Information that can be brought into consciousness, "declared," held in the "mind's eye"
Nondeclarative	Performance-based, motor output, habits and conditioning, automatic tendencies
Short term	Ephemeral (30–45 s), limited capacity (7 ± 2 words, numbers)
Long term	Permanent, unlimited capacity

structures, such as the amygdala, the entorhinal and perirhinal cortices, and other parts of the parahippocampal gyrus.

2. **Retrograde memory** refers to the retrieval of information that was acquired previously—that is, retrieval of facts, skills, and other knowledge learned in the recent or remote past. This type of memory is related to nonmesial sectors of the temporal lobe, including the polar region (Brodmann's area 38), the inferotemporal region (including Brodmann's areas 20, 21, and 36), and the occipitotemporal region (including Brodmann's area 37 and the ventral parts of areas 18 and 19). Autobiographical memory, a special form of retrograde memory that refers to knowledge about one's own past, is linked primarily to the anterior part of the nonmesial temporal lobes, especially in the right hemisphere.

B. Verbal and nonverbal memory. Knowledge can be divided into that which exists in **verbal** form, such as words (written or spoken) and names, and that which exists in **nonverbal** form, such as faces, geographic routes, and complex musical patterns. This distinction is important because it is generally believed that the memory systems in the two hemispheres of the human brain are specialized differently for verbal and nonverbal material (Table 4.2). Specifically, systems in the left hemisphere are dedicated primarily to verbal material, and systems in the right hemisphere are dedicated primarily to nonverbal material. This arrangement parallels the general arrangement of the human brain, in which the left hemisphere is specialized for language and the right hemisphere for visuospatial processing. This distinction applies to almost all right-handed persons and to approximately two-thirds of left-handed persons. (In the remaining minority of left-handers, the arrangement may be partially or completely reversed.)

C. Declarative and nondeclarative memory.

1. **Declarative memory** (also known as **explicit memory**) refers to knowledge that can be "declared" and brought to mind for conscious inspection, such as facts, words, names, and individual faces, which can be retrieved from memory, placed in the "mind's eye," and reported. The acquisition of declarative memories is intimately linked to the functioning of the hippocampus and other mesial temporal lobe structures.

2. **Nondeclarative memory** (also known as **implicit memory**) refers to various forms of memory that cannot be declared or brought into the mind's eye. Examples include sensorimotor skill learning, autonomic conditioning, and certain types of habits. Nondeclarative memory requires participation of the neostriatum, cerebellum, and sensorimotor cortices. A remarkable dissociation between declarative and nondeclarative learning and memory has been repeatedly found among patients with amnesia (including those with Korsakoff's syndrome, bilateral mesial temporal lobe lesions, medial thalamic lesions, and AD). Among such persons, sensorimotor skill learning and memory are often preserved, whereas declarative memory is profoundly impaired.

D. Short- and long-term memory.

1. The term **short-term memory** is used to designate a time span of memory that covers from 0 to approximately 45 seconds, a brief period during which a limited amount of information can be held without rehearsal. Also known as primary memory, it does not depend on the hippocampus or other temporal lobe memory systems but is linked closely to cerebral mechanisms required for attention and concentration, such as subcortical frontal structures.

TABLE 4.2 Hemispheric Specialization of Memory Systems

Left	Right
Verbal	Nonverbal
Words	Patterns
Names	Faces
Stories	Geographic routes
Lyrics	Complex melodies
Sequential, feature based	Holistic, gestalt based
Lexical retrieval	Unique personal knowledge

2. The term **long-term memory** refers to a large expanse of time that covers everything beyond short-term memory. Also known as secondary memory, it can be divided into **recent** (the past few weeks or months) and **remote** (years or decades ago). Unlike short-term memory, the capacity of long-term memory is enormous, and information can be retained in long-term memory almost indefinitely. The mesial temporal system, including the hippocampus, is required for the acquisition of knowledge into long-term memory. Other systems in the temporal lobe and elsewhere are required for the consolidation and retrieval of knowledge from long-term memory.

E. **Working memory** refers to a short time during which the brain can hold several pieces of information actively and perform operations on them. It is akin to short-term memory but implies a somewhat longer duration (several minutes) and more focus on the **operational** features of the mental process rather than simply the acquisition of information. It can be thought of as "online" processing and operating on knowledge that is being held in activated form.

CLINICAL MANIFESTATIONS

Although the etiology of cognitive impairment may differ, the *Diagnostic and Statistical Manual of Mental Disorders*, fifth edition (*DSM-5*), now generally classifies neurocognitive disorders as major neurocognitive disorder and mild neurocognitive disorder while retaining the term dementia as a way to describe neurodegenerative conditions (Video 4.1). Associated etiology medical codes for neurocognitive disorders include AD, frontotemporal lobar degeneration, Lewy body disease, vascular disease, traumatic brain injury, substance/medication induced, human immunodeficiency virus (HIV) infection, prion disease, Parkinson's disease, and Huntington's disease (in addition to categories that are unspecified or related to another medical condition). Several frequent neurologic conditions damage memory-related neural systems and lead to various profiles and severities of amnesia (Table 4.3).

Degenerative Diseases

A. Cortical dementia.
1. **AD** is characterized by two principal neuropathologic features—the neurofibrillary tangle and the neuritic plaque. Early in the course of the disease, the entorhinal cortex, which is a pivotal way station for input to and from the hippocampus, is disrupted by neurofibrillary tangles in cortical layers II and IV. The perforant pathway, which is the main route for entry into the hippocampal formation, is gradually and massively demyelinated. The hippocampus eventually is almost deafferentated from cortical input. AD also breaks down the efferent linkage of the hippocampus back to the cerebral cortex through destruction of the subiculum and entorhinal cortex. The hallmark behavioral sign of this destruction is amnesia—specifically, an anterograde (learning) defect that covers declarative knowledge but largely spares nondeclarative learning and retrieval.

TABLE 4.3 Causes of and Conditions Associated with Amnesia

Degenerative disease (e.g., Alzheimer's, Pick's, and Parkinson's)
Head injury
Cerebrovascular event (e.g., infarction and ruptured aneurysm)
Toxic conditions (e.g., alcoholism)
Anoxia, ischemia
Herpes simplex encephalitis (HSE)
Surgical ablation
Neoplasm
Normal pressure hydrocephalus
Transient global amnesia (TGA)
Functional amnesia

Early in the course of the disease, retrograde memory is relatively spared, but as the pathologic process extends to nonmesial temporal sectors, a defect in the retrograde compartment (retrieval impairment) appears and gradually worsens.

2. **Frontotemporal dementia** is characterized by symmetric atrophy of the frontal and temporal lobes. The earliest and most prominent cognitive symptoms involve personality and behavioral changes. Although reports of memory problems are common in frontotemporal dementia, they are never the sole or dominating feature. Severe amnesia is considered an exclusionary criterion. Memory functioning is described as selective (e.g., "she remembers what she wants to remember"). Knowledge regarding orientation and current autobiographical events remains largely preserved.

3. **Frontal lobe dementia** is another form of cortical dementia. It involves focal atrophy of the frontal lobes, which causes personality changes and other signs of executive dysfunction. This condition is similar to Pick's disease, except that there is no predominance of Pick bodies.

   a. **Pick's disease,** characterized by Pick bodies (cells containing degraded protein material), is an uncommon form of cortical dementia that often shows a striking predilection for one lobe of the brain, producing a state of circumscribed lobar atrophy. The disease is often concentrated in the frontal lobes, in which case personality alterations as well as compromised judgment and problem solving, rather than amnesia, are the prominent manifestations. However, the disease can affect one or the other temporal lobe and produce signs of a material-specific amnesia.

B. **Subcortical dementia.**

1. **Parkinson's disease** is focused in subcortical structures and influences memory in a manner different from cortical forms of dementia such as AD and Pick's disease. Disorders of nondeclarative memory (e.g., acquisition and retrieval of motor skills) are more prominent, and there may be minimal or no impairment in learning of declarative material. Patients with Parkinson's disease often have more problems in **recall** of newly acquired knowledge than in **storage.** When cuing strategies are provided, the patients have normal levels of retention. **Lewy body disease** is also a neurodegenerative condition characterized by Lewy bodies that share genetic and pathologic features of both Alzheimer's and Parkinson's disease. Core features can include, but are not limited to, fluctuating cognition, hallucinations, and parkinsonism.

2. **Huntington's disease** is also concentrated in subcortical structures and amnesia of patients with Huntington's disease resembles that of patients with Parkinson's disease. In particular, there is disproportionate involvement of nondeclarative memory. Patients with Huntington's disease also tend to have disruption of **working memory.**

3. **Progressive supranuclear palsy** is another primarily subcortical disease process that frequently produces problems with memory. In general, however, the associated amnesia is considerably less severe than that of AD. Laboratory assessment often shows relatively mild defects in learning and retrieval despite the patient's reports of forgetfulness.

C. **Other degenerative conditions.**

1. **Dementia related to HIV/acquired immune deficiency syndrome (AIDS)** is notable for varying degrees of memory impairment, with severity being roughly proportional to disease progression. Early in the course, memory defects may be the sole signs of cognitive dysfunction. The problems center on the acquisition of new material, particularly material of the declarative type. Memory defects in this disease appear to be attributable mainly to defective attention, concentration, and overall efficiency of cognitive functioning rather than to focal dysfunction of memory-related neural systems. Various investigators have found that the rate of percentage of CD4 lymphocyte cell loss is associated with and may represent a risk factor for cognitive dysfunction among persons with HIV/AIDS.

2. **Multiple sclerosis (MS)** patients have varying degrees of amnesia, although the severity can wax and wane considerably in concert with other neurologic symptoms. Many patients with MS have no memory defects during some periods of the disease. When present, the memory impairment most commonly manifests as defective recall of newly learned information. Encoding and working memory are normal or near-normal. Patients with MS often benefit from cuing. The amnesia of MS usually affects declarative material of both verbal and nonverbal types; defects in nondeclarative memory are rare.

3. **Head injury.** Several distinct types of amnesia are associated with head injury.
   a. **Posttraumatic amnesia** refers to the period of time following head trauma during which patients do not acquire new information in a normal and continuous manner despite being conscious. During this time, the patient may appear alert and attentive and may even deny having memory problems. It becomes apparent later that the patient was not forming ongoing records of new experiences. Information is not encoded, and no amount of cuing will uncover memories that would normally have been acquired during this period. The **duration** of posttraumatic amnesia is a reliable marker of the severity of head injury and constitutes one of the best predictors of outcome.
   b. **Retrograde amnesia** is the defective recall of experiences that occurred immediately before the head injury. Information from the time closest to the point of injury is most likely to be lost. The extent of retrograde amnesia typically "shrinks" as the patient recovers, and patients are typically left with only a small island of amnesia for the few minutes or hours immediately before the trauma.
   c. **Learning defects (anterograde amnesia)** can occur in moderate and severe head injuries when there is permanent damage to mesial temporal lobe structures, such as the hippocampus. The impairment is centered on declarative knowledge; nondeclarative learning is rarely affected. The defect may be unequal for verbal and nonverbal material if there is asymmetry of the structural injury.
4. **Cerebrovascular disease.**
   a. **Stroke** is a frequent cause of amnesia, and the nature and degree of memory disturbance are direct functions of which neural structures are damaged and to what extent. Amnesia is most likely to result from infarction that damages the mesial temporal region, the basal forebrain, or the medial diencephalon, especially the thalamus.
      (1) In the **mesial temporal lobe,** the parahippocampal gyrus and hippocampus proper can be damaged by infarction in territories supplied by branches of the middle cerebral or posterior cerebral arteries. (Strokes in the region of the anterolateral temporal lobe are uncommon.) Infarction of this type is almost always unilateral and almost always produces incomplete damage to mesial temporal memory structures; hence, the profile is one of a partial material-specific defect in anterograde memory for declarative knowledge.
      (2) The most severe memory impairment results from bilateral infarcts situated in the anterior part of the **thalamus** in the interpeduncular profundus territory. Unilateral lesions caused by lacunar infarction in anterior thalamic nuclei produce material-specific learning defects reminiscent of those observed with mesial temporal lobe lesions. Patients with thalamic damage, however, tend to have both anterograde and retrograde defects. In the retrograde compartment, a **temporal gradient** to the defect is common—that is, the farther back in time one goes, the less the severity of the amnesia.
   b. **Ruptured aneurysms** located either in the anterior communicating artery or in the anterior cerebral artery almost invariably cause infarction in the region of the basal forebrain—a set of bilateral paramidline gray nuclei that includes the septal nuclei, the diagonal band of Broca, and the substantia innominata. The amnesia associated with basal forebrain damage has several distinctive features. Patients have an inability to link correctly various aspects of memory episodes (when, where, what, and why). This problem affects both the anterograde and retrograde compartments. Confabulation is common among patients with basal forebrain amnesia. Cuing markedly improves recall and recognition of both anterograde and retrograde material.
   c. **Vascular dementia** (VaD) refers to conditions in which repeated infarction produces widespread cognitive impairment, including amnesia. The term is used most commonly to denote multiple small strokes (lacunar strokes) in the arterioles that feed subcortical structures; hence, the usual picture is "subcortical" dementia. The memory impairment in VaD generally affects encoding of new material (anterograde amnesia), and nondeclarative learning also may be defective. Retrograde memory tends to be spared.
5. **Toxic conditions.**
   a. **Alcoholism** can produce permanent damage to certain diencephalic structures, particularly the mammillary bodies and dorsomedial thalamic nucleus, which have

been linked to amnesic manifestations. This presentation is known as **alcoholic Korsakoff's syndrome** or **Wernicke–Korsakoff's syndrome.** The amnesic profile in patients with Korsakoff's syndrome is characterized by (1) anterograde amnesia for both verbal and nonverbal material with defects in both encoding and retrieval, (2) retrograde amnesia with a strong temporal gradient—that is, progressively milder defects as one goes farther back in time, and (3) sparing of nondeclarative memory. Confabulation is characteristic of patients with Korsakoff's syndrome, especially in the early days following detoxification.

b. **Other neurotoxins** such as metals, especially lead and mercury, solvents and fuels, and pesticides, can cause amnesia from acute or chronic exposure. The relation between exposure to these substances and cognitive dysfunction is poorly understood, but there is little doubt that memory impairment often does result from excessive exposure to these neurotoxins. The amnesia tends to manifest as a deficiency in new learning (anterograde amnesia) that covers various types of materials, including verbal, nonverbal, and nondeclarative. Defects of concentration, attention, and overall cognitive efficiency are frequent contributing factors. In most cases, the memory impairment occurs in the setting of more widespread cognitive dysfunction.

6. **Anoxia/ischemia,** which frequently occurs in the setting of cardiopulmonary arrest, often leads to the selective destruction of cellular groups within the hippocampal formation. The extent of damage is linked to the number of minutes of arrest. Brief periods of anoxia/ischemia can cause limited damage, and longer periods produce greater destruction. With a critical length of deprivation, the damage concentrates bilaterally in the CA1 ammonic fields of the hippocampus. The result is selective anterograde amnesia affecting declarative verbal and nonverbal material. The amnesia associated with anoxia/ischemia is reminiscent of the memory defect produced by early-stage AD.

7. **Herpes simplex encephalitis** (HSE) causes a severe necrotic process in the cortical structures associated with the limbic system, some neocortical structures in the vicinity of the limbic system, and several subcortical limbic structures. The parahippocampal gyrus—particularly the entorhinal cortex in its anterior sector and the polar limbic cortex (Brodmann's area 38)—is frequently damaged. HSE also may destroy neocortices of the anterolateral and anteroinferior regions of the temporal lobe (Brodmann's areas 20, 21, anterior 22, and parts of 36 and 37). The destruction may be bilateral, but with the advent of early diagnosis and treatment, circumscribed unilateral damage has become more common. The profile of amnesia caused by HSE is dictated by the nature of neural destruction. Damage confined to the mesial temporal region produces anterograde declarative memory impairment. When HSE-related pathologic changes extend to nonmesial temporal structures in anterolateral and anteroinferior sectors, the amnesia involves progressively greater portions of the retrograde compartment. The retrograde defect can be quite severe if nonmesial temporal structures are extensively damaged and, in the worst case, a patient can lose almost all capacity to remember declarative information from the past and are not able to learn new information **(global amnesia).**

8. **Surgical ablation** of intractable epilepsy, especially temporal lobectomy, can result in memory impairment. Even if the resection spares most of the hippocampus proper, the resection usually involves other anterior regions of the mesial temporal lobe, including the amygdala and entorhinal cortex, resulting in mild but significant memory defects. In the most common presentation, the patient has a material-specific learning defect (nonverbal if the resection is on the right, verbal if it is on the left) after temporal lobectomy. In addition, the amnesia affects only declarative knowledge. However, mild retrograde amnesia can also result if there is sufficient involvement of the anterolateral and anteroinferior temporal sectors. Generally speaking, patients whose seizures began at an early age are less affected by temporal lobectomy than are patients whose seizures began later.

9. **Neoplasms** can lead to amnesia, depending on their type and location. Impaired memory is a common symptom of brain tumors, especially those centered in the region of the third ventricle (in or near the thalamus) or in the region of the ventral frontal lobes (in or near the basal forebrain). The most common therapies for high-grade malignant brain tumors, including resection and radiation, often produce memory defects. Radiation necrosis, for example, can damage the lateral portions of the temporal lobes and lead to a focal retrograde amnesia.

10. **Normal pressure hydrocephalus** is a partially reversible condition in which gait disturbance, incontinence, and dementia, especially memory impairment, compose a hallmark triad of presenting features. Early in the course, memory impairment can be minimal, but most patients with normal pressure hydrocephalus go on to have marked memory defects. The typical situation is anterograde amnesia for declarative material; however, problems with attention and concentration can exacerbate the amnesia and make the patient appear even more impaired than he or she actually is.

11. **Transient global amnesia** (TGA) is a short-lasting neurologic condition in which the patient has prominent impairment of memory in the setting of otherwise normal cognition and no other neurologic defect. The duration of TGA is typically approximately 6 or 7 hours, after which the condition spontaneously remits, and the patient returns to an entirely normal memory status. The cause of TGA is unknown, although psychological stress, vascular factors, seizure, and migraine have all been proposed as causes. During the episode, the patient has severe impairment of anterograde memory for verbal and nonverbal material. Retrograde memory is impaired to a lesser degree. After recovery, patients are unable to remember events that transpired during the episode, and sometimes a short period of time immediately before the onset of TGA also is lost. Otherwise, there is no long-term consequence.

12. **Functional amnesia** can occur in the absence of any demonstrable brain injury, as a consequence of severe emotional trauma, hypnotic suggestion, or psychiatric illness. These presentations have been called *functional amnesia* to differentiate them from amnesia caused by "organic" factors, although at the molecular and cellular levels the mechanisms may not be distinguishable. A common form is **functional retrograde amnesia**, in which the patient loses most or all memory of the past (including self-identity), usually after a severe emotional or psychological trauma. Curiously, anterograde memory can be entirely normal, and the patient may even have "relearning" of the past. Spontaneous recovery is frequent, although most patients are never able to remember events that transpired during the episodes in which they had amnesia. Another interesting form is **posthypnotic amnesia**, the phenomenon whereby patients cannot remember events that transpired while they were under hypnosis.

EVALUATION

A. History.
1. Onset. Through careful history-taking, the clinician should determine as precisely as possible the timing of the **onset** of the problem. Memory defects that began years ago and have gradually worsened over time point to degenerative disease, such as AD. Reports of sudden memory impairment among younger patients, for whom psychological factors (e.g., severe stress and depression) can be identified as being temporally related to the problem, should raise the question of nonorganic etiologic factors.
2. Course. The history-taking should document carefully the **course** of the concern. Progressive deterioration in memory signals a degenerative process. Memory defects after head injury or cerebral anoxia, by contrast, tend to resolve gradually, and reports to the contrary raise the question of other (psychological) factors.
3. Nature. The clinician should explore the **nature** of the problem. With what types of information, and in what situations, is the patient having trouble? Patients may produce vague, poorly specified concerns (e.g., "My memory is bad" or "I'm forgetful"), and it is important to request specific examples to form an idea as to the actual nature of the problem. Patients tend to use the term "memory impairment" to cover a wide range of mental status abnormalities, and, again, elicitation of examples is informative. Patients who say they "can't remember" may actually have circumscribed impairment of word finding, proper name retrieval, or hearing or vision.
B. Bedside examination. Memory assessment is covered to some extent by almost all bedside or screening mental status examinations. If patients pass such examinations, do not report memory impairment, and are not described by spouses or caretakers as having memory difficulties, it is safe to assume that memory is broadly normal. If any of these conditions are not met, a more complete evaluation of memory is warranted. Referral for neuropsychological assessment provides the most direct access to such evaluation.

1. **Learning.** Can the patient learn the examiner's name? Three words? Three objects?
2. **Working memory.** Backward spelling, serial subtraction, and repeating numerical strings of digits backward are good probes of working memory.
3. **Delayed recall.** It is important to ask for the retrieval of newly acquired knowledge after a delay, for example, approximately 30 minutes. This may reveal a severe loss of information on the part of a patient who performed perfectly in an immediate recall procedure.
4. **Retrograde memory.** The patient should be asked to retrieve knowledge from the past. This should be corroborated by a spouse or other **collateral person**, because patients with memory defects may confabulate and otherwise mislead the examiner.
5. **Orientation.** The patient should be asked for information about time, place, and personal facts. Defects in orientation are often early clues to memory impairment.
6. **Attention.** Marked impairment of attention produces subsequent defects on most tests of memory. The diagnosis of amnesia, however, should be reserved for patients who have normal attention but still cannot perform normally on memory tests. Attentional impairment per se is a hallmark of other abnormalities, not necessarily of an amnesic condition.

C. **Laboratory studies** of memory are conducted in the context of neuropsychological assessment, which provides precise, standardized quantification of various memory capacities. Examples of some widely used procedures are as follows.

1. **Anterograde memory.** Most conventional neuropsychological tests of memory, including the *Wechsler Memory Scale*, fourth edition (*WMS-IV*), and other such instruments, assess **learning of declarative knowledge.** It should not be assumed that all aspects of memory are normal simply because the patient passes these procedures. For example, these tests do not measure nondeclarative memory, and they rarely provide adequate investigation of the retrograde compartment. Nonetheless, the *WMS-IV* and related procedures provide sensitive, standardized means of quantifying many aspects of memory.

   a. **Verbal.** In addition to several verbal memory procedures that comprise part of the *WMS-IV* (e.g., paragraph recall and paired-associate learning), there are several well-standardized list-learning procedures in which the patient attempts to learn and remember a list of words. The Rey Auditory–Verbal Learning Test, for example, requires the patient to learn a list of 15 words. Five successive trials are administered, and then a delayed recall procedure is performed after about 30 minutes. The patient's learning capacity, learning curve, and the degree of forgetting can be determined.

   b. **Nonverbal memory tests** typically involve administration of various designs, such as geometric figures, that the patient must remember (e.g., *WMS-IV* Visual Reproduction and the Benton Visual Retention Test). Face-learning procedures also provide good tests of nonverbal memory.

2. **Retrograde memory.** There are several standardized procedures for measuring retrograde memory, including the Remote Memory Battery, the Famous Events Test, and the Autobiographical Memory Questionnaire. These procedures probe recall and recognition of various historical facts, famous events and persons, and autobiographical knowledge. Corroboration of retrograde memory, particularly with regard to autobiographical information, is extremely important to determine the severity of retrograde memory defects.

3. **Nondeclarative memory.** A standard procedure for measuring nondeclarative learning is the Rotary Pursuit Task, which requires the patient to hold a stylus in one hand and attempt to maintain contact between the stylus and a small metal target while the target is rotating on a platter. Successive trials are administered and are followed by a delay trial. This procedure allows the measurement of acquisition and retention of the motor skill.

4. **Working memory.** The Digit Span Backward and Sequencing subtests from the *WAIS-IV*, as well as the Letter–Number Sequencing and Arithmetic subtests, provide a sensitive means of quantifying working memory. In Letter–Number Sequencing, the patient is read a combination of numbers and letters of varying lengths and is asked to repeat them by first stating the numbers in ascending order and then the letters in alphabetical order. In Arithmetic, patients must mentally solve math problems. The Trail-Making Test, which requires the patient to execute a psychomotor response while tracking dual

lines of information, is also a good probe of working memory. Another commonly used procedure is the Paced Auditory Serial Addition Test, in which the patient must add numbers in an unusual format under increasingly demanding time constraints. Finally, the Spatial Span subtest from a previous version of the *Wechsler Memory Scale* (*WMS-III*) is the visual–spatial analog of the aforementioned auditory–verbal subtest, Digit Span. Rather than recalling numbers in forward and backward order, spatial span requires the examinee to replicate, forward and backward, an increasingly long series of visually presented spatial locations.

5. **Long-term memory.** The ability to acquire new information, in addition to consolidate and store that information and retrieve it at a later time, is the real crux of memory. In a practical sense, it is not very helpful to have normal short-term memory if one cannot transfer the information into a more permanent storage area. Hence, delayed recall and recognition procedures, which yield information about the status of long-term memory, are very important in memory assessment and can also provide information regarding the etiology of memory impairments.

DIFFERENTIAL DIAGNOSIS

Different causes of amnesia have different implications for diagnosis and management. The following common differential diagnoses are particularly challenging.

A. **Normal aging.** A seemingly minor but practically difficult challenge is to differentiate true memory impairment from the influences of normal aging. Aging produces certain declines in memory, which can be misinterpreted by patients and clinicians alike as signs of neurologic disease. Many older adults who report "forgetfulness" turn out to have peer-equivalent performances on all manner of standard memory tests, and the diagnosis of amnesia is not applicable. Patients may be quick to interpret any episode of memory failure as a sign of AD, or they may adamantly deny memory dysfunction in the face of obvious real-world impairment. Consequently, careful quantification of the memory profile aids in the differential diagnosis.

B. **Psychiatric disease.** Many psychiatric diseases produce some degree of memory impairment. Accurate diagnosis is critical, because most memory defects caused by psychiatric disease are reversible, unlike most of amnesia that occurs in the setting of neurologic disease.

1. **Dementia related to depression (sometimes called pseudodementia)** is a condition that produces memory impairment and other cognitive defects resembling "dementia" but not caused by neurologic disease. Severe depression is the typical cause. Patients with pseudodementia often have memory impairment such as anterograde amnesia that is quite similar to that in the early stages of degenerative dementia. However, depressed patients respond to treatment with antidepressant medications and psychotherapy; when the affective disorder lifts, memory returns to normal.

2. **Depression** is a common cause of memory impairment among all age groups. Distinguishing features, however, help differentiate amnesia due to depression from amnesia caused by neurologic disease. Depressed patients tend to have problems in concentration and attention, and they may have defects in working memory and other short-term memory tasks. Long-term memory is less affected, and retrograde memory is normal. Apathetic, "don't know" responses are common among depressed patients, whereas patients with a neurologic disorder more often give incorrect, off-target responses. Depressed patients also tend to describe their memory problems in great detail, whereas patients with a neurologic disorder, such as those with suspected Alzheimer's dementia, generally discount memory problems. Patient history is informative and the clinician can usually find evidence of major stress, catastrophe, or other circumstances, and it is apparent that the onset of the memory problems coincided with the onset of the affective disorder.

3. **Schizophrenia** and **bipolar disorder** can also cause memory impairments among all age groups. Similar to depression, individuals diagnosed with schizophrenia or bipolar disorder often demonstrate difficulties with attention and concentration that affect learning or encoding (e.g., frontal lobe systems disruption). That is, it is difficult to have memory for an item not learned. Such individuals might have less difficulty retrieving

what they have learned and might also be able to cue up or recognize items more readily than an individual who might have a neurologic condition.

C. **Side effects of medications.** Many medications commonly prescribed for older adults produce adverse side effects on cognitive function, including memory. It is important to know what medications a patient has been taking and to account for the extent to which those medications may be causing memory impairment. The history often reveals that the onset of memory problems coincided with or soon followed the beginning of use of a particular medication. Memory defects caused by medication side effects also tend to be variable—for example, worse at certain times of the day. The main problems concern attention, concentration, and overall cognitive efficiency; memory defects are secondary.

DIAGNOSTIC APPROACH

The diagnostic approach to a patient with amnesia should include any procedures necessary for establishing both the most likely **cause** and the precise **nature** of the memory impairment. The most commonly used procedures are as follows.

A. **Neurologic examination** should establish whether a memory problem is present, the general degree of severity, and the history of the problem. It is not uncommon for patients with amnesia to underestimate or even deny the problem; information from a spouse or caretaker is a critical part of the history. Careful mental status testing can provide sufficient characterization of the amnesia profile.

B. **Neuroimaging procedures,** including magnetic resonance imaging (MRI) and computed tomography (CT), are almost always helpful in diagnosing the cause of amnesia. Functional imaging, such as positron emission tomography, may demonstrate abnormalities suggestive of AD (e.g., bilateral parietotemporal hypometabolism) earlier in the natural course of the disease than may MRI, CT, or clinical assessment.

C. **Neuropsychological assessment** provides detailed quantification of the nature and extent of memory impairment. Such testing should be considered for almost all patients with amnesia, although there may be instances in which the mental-status-testing portion of the neurologic examination provides sufficient information.

CRITERIA FOR DIAGNOSIS

The diagnosis of amnesia is appropriate whenever there are memory defects that exceed those expected given the patient's age and background. Some conditions, such as severe aphasia, make it difficult to assess memory in a meaningful way. Amnesia should not be diagnosed if the patient is in a severe confusional state, in which attentional impairment rather than memory dysfunction is the principal manifestation (e.g., delirium). Otherwise, amnesia can occur in isolation or coexist with almost any other form of impairment of mental status. It is customary to regard patients as having **amnesia** if there is considerable discrepancy between the level of intellectual function and one or more memory functions. There are many different subtypes of amnesia. Diagnosis of such subtypes usually requires fine-grained quantification, such as that provided in a neuropsychological laboratory.

REFERRAL

A. **Neuropsychological** evaluation is appropriate for almost all patients with manifestations of amnesia. The following situations that occur commonly in clinical practice particularly call for such a referral.

1. **Precise characterization of memory capacities.** For a patient who has sustained brain injury, neuropsychological assessment provides detailed information regarding the strengths and weaknesses of the patient's memory. In most instances, memory assessment should be performed as early as possible in the recovery period. This evaluation provides a baseline to which recovery can be compared. Follow-up assessments assist in monitoring recovery, determining the effects of therapy, and making long-range decisions regarding educational and vocational rehabilitation.

2. **Monitoring the status of patients who have undergone medical or surgical intervention.** Serial neuropsychological assessment of memory is used to track the course of patients

who are undergoing medical or surgical treatment for neurologic disease. Typical examples include drug treatment for patients with Parkinson's disease, seizure disorder, surgical intervention for patients with normal pressure hydrocephalus, or a brain tumor. Neuropsychological assessment provides a baseline memory profile with which changes can be compared and provides a sensitive means of monitoring changes in memory that occur in relation to particular treatment regimens.

3. **Differentiating neurologic and neuropsychiatric disease.** Neuropsychological assessment can provide evidence crucial to the distinction between amnesic conditions that are primarily or exclusively neurologic and those that are primarily or exclusively neuropsychiatric. A common diagnostic dilemma faced by neurologists and psychiatrists is differentiating "true dementia" (e.g., cognitive impairment caused by AD) and "pseudodementia" (e.g., cognitive impairment associated with depression).

4. **Medicolegal situations.** Cases in which "brain injury" and "memory impairment" are claimed as damages by plaintiffs who allegedly have sustained minor head injuries or have been exposed to toxic chemicals. In particular, there are many cases in which hard or objective signs of brain dysfunction (e.g., weakness, sensory loss and impaired balance) are absent, neuroimaging and electroencephalogram (EEG) findings are normal, and the entire case rests on claims of cognitive deficiencies, particularly memory dysfunction. Neuropsychological assessment is crucial to the evaluation of such claims.

5. **Conditions in which known or suspected neurologic disease is not detected with conventional neurodiagnostic procedures.** There are situations in which the findings of standard diagnostic procedures, including neurologic examination, neuroimaging, and EEG, are equivocal, even though the history indicates that brain disease and amnesia are likely. Examples include the early stages of degenerative dementia syndromes and early HIV-related dementia. Neuropsychological assessment in such cases provides the most sensitive means of evaluating memory.

6. **Monitoring changes in cognitive function over time.** In degenerative dementia in particular, equivocal findings in the initial diagnostic evaluation are not uncommon. In such cases, follow-up neuropsychological evaluation can provide important confirming or disconfirming evidence regarding the status of the patient's memory and possible progression of a disease process.

B. **Rehabilitation.** Another common application of neuropsychological assessment is the case in which a patient undergoes cognitive rehabilitation for amnesia. Neuropsychological data collected at the initial assessment can help determine how to orient the rehabilitation effort. Subsequent examinations can be used to measure progress during therapy.

Key Points

- There are several different types of memory that must be understood in order to identify neuroanatomical correlates. As examples, working memory involves the frontal lobe while anterograde and declarative memory involves the mesial temporal lobes.
- The etiology of memory impairments can differ, so it is important to always identify specific memory problems, as well as the onset and course of the memory impairments.
- Some common causes of memory impairment can be attributable to neurodegenerative diseases, such as cortical (e.g., AD) and subcortical disease (e.g., Parkinson's disease), as well as other neurodegenerative conditions (e.g., MS), head injury, cerebrovascular and psychiatric disease.
- A neuropsychological evaluation is especially useful to objectively quantify memory impairments and the nature of the impairments, including anterograde memory, verbal memory, nonverbal memory, retrograde memory, nondeclarative memory, working memory, and long-term memory.
- Neuropsychological evaluations are appropriate for almost all patients with memory complaints to characterize the memory impairments in addition to providing information about monitoring and outcomes, aid in differential diagnosis, and provide recommendations.

Recommended Readings

Adolphs R, Tranel D, Denburg NL. Impaired emotional declarative memory following unilateral amygdala damage. *Learn Mem*. 2000;7:180–186.

Alexander MP. Mild traumatic brain injury: pathophysiology, natural history, and clinical management. *Neurology*. 1995;45:1253–1260.

Attix DK, Welsh-Bohmer KA, eds. *Geriatric Neuropsychology: Assessment and Intervention*. New York, NY: Guilford Press; 2006.

Bachevalier J, Meunier M. Cerebral ischemia: are the memory deficits associated with hippocampal memory loss? *Hippocampus*. 1996;6:553–560.

Baddeley AD. Working memory. *Science*. 1992;255:566–569.

Cabeza R, Nyberg L. Imaging cognition: II: an empirical review of 275 PET and fMRI studies. *J Cogn Neurosci*. 2000;12:1–47.

Cohen NJ, Squire LR. Preserved learning and retention of pattern-analyzing skill in amnesia: dissociation of knowing how and knowing that. *Science*. 1980;210:207–210.

Corkin S. Lasting consequences of bilateral medial temporal lobectomy: clinical course and experimental findings in H.M. *Semin Neurol*. 1984;4:249–259.

Damasio AR. Time-locked multiregional retroactivation: a systems-level proposal for the neural substrates of recall and recognition. *Cognition*. 1989;33:25–62.

Hannula DE, Tranel D, Cohen N. The long and the short of it: relational memory impairments in amnesia, even at short lags. *J Neurosci*. 2006;26:8352–8359.

Heindel WC, Salmon DP, Shults CW, et al. Neuropsychological evidence for multiple implicit memory systems: a comparison of Alzheimer's, Huntington's and Parkinson's disease patients. *J Neurosci*. 1989;9:582–587.

Hyman BT, Kromer LJ, Van Hoesen GW. A direct demonstration of the perforant pathway terminal zone in Alzheimer's disease using the monoclonal antibody Alz-50. *Brain Res*. 1988;450:392–397.

Kroll NE, Markowitsch HJ, Knight RT, et al. Retrieval of old memories: the temporofrontal hypothesis. *Brain*. 1997;120:1377–1399.

Lezak MD, Howieson DB, Bigler ED, et al. *Neuropsychological Assessment*. 5th ed. New York, NY: Oxford University Press; 2012.

Markowitsch HJ. Which brain regions are critically involved in the retrieval of old episodic memory? *Brain Res Rev*. 1995;21:117–127.

Milner B, Squire LR, Kandel ER. Cognitive neuroscience and the study of memory. *Neuron*. 1998;20:445–468.

Ravdin LD, Katzen HL, eds. *Handbook on the Neuropsychology of Aging and Dementia*. New York, NY: Springer; 2013.

Silverman DH, Truong CT, Kim SK, et al. Prognostic value of regional cerebral metabolism in patients undergoing dementia evaluation: comparison to a quantifying parameter of subsequent cognitive performance and to prognostic assessment without PET. *Mol Genet Metab*. 2003;80(3):350–355.

Smith GE, Bondi MW. *Mild Cognitive Impairment and Dementia: Definitions, Diagnosis, and Treatment*. New York, NY: Oxford University Press; 2013.

Squire LR. Memory and the hippocampus: a synthesis from findings with rats, monkeys, and humans. *Psychol Rev*. 1992;99:195–231.

Tranel D, Damasio AR. The covert learning of affective valence does not require structures in hippocampal system or amygdala. *J Cogn Neurosci*. 1993;5:79–88.

Tranel D, Damasio AR, Damasio H, et al. Sensorimotor skill learning in amnesia: additional evidence for the neural basis of nondeclarative memory. *Learn Mem*. 1994;1:165–179.

Tranel D, Damasio H, Damasio AR. Amnesia caused by herpes simplex encephalitis, infarctions in basal forebrain, and anoxia/ischemia. In: Boller F, Grafman J, eds. *Handbook of Neuropsychology*. 2nd ed. Amsterdam, The Netherlands: Elsevier Science; 2000:85–110.

Van Hoesen GW. The parahippocampal gyrus. *Trends Neurosci*. 1982;5:345–350.

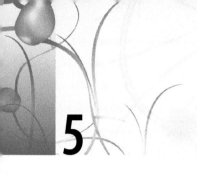

5   Approach to the Comatose Patient

Michael P. Merchut

Interpersonal communication and cognitive behavior require sufficient wakefulness, arousal, or alertness. Patients in the persistent vegetative state appear conscious or awake at times, but show little to no communicative or cognitive ability. **Coma** is the unconscious, sleep-like state of patients who are unresponsive to stimuli, where it is critical to find and treat any number of reversible causes.

Arousal is a function of the **ascending reticular activating system (ARAS)**, a complex pathway from dorsal pons to midbrain to intralaminar thalamic nuclei and basal forebrain, with diffuse cortical connections. Single structural lesions, such as an ischemic infarct or tumor, may produce coma by directly disrupting this pathway in the upper brainstem. However, a unilateral cerebral hemispheral lesion does not produce coma unless it creates enough edema and midline shift to adversely affect the ARAS bilaterally, typically at the thalamic level. Coma may also occur from extensive, severe, bilateral cortical lesions, such as multiple hemorrhages, or from metabolic processes suppressing cortical function in a global way, such as drug intoxication or hypoglycemia. If treated immediately, hypoglycemic coma may resolve completely, as may other toxi-metabolic etiologies. Certain causes of coma, such as fulminant encephalitis, are progressively fatal, and the patient never wakens. In other situations, such as anoxic encephalopathy, the patient may "wake up" after several days of coma, yet remain in a persistent vegetative state with poor or no cognitive recovery.

EVALUATION

A. History.
   1. Sudden onset of coma is suggestive of the following:
      a. Intracranial hemorrhage (prodromal severe headache may accompany spontaneous subarachnoid hemorrhage [SAH] or cerebral hemorrhage).
      b. Critical brainstem infarction or bilateral embolic cerebral infarcts.
      c. Significant cerebral hypoperfusion after cardiopulmonary arrest.
      d. Observed or unwitnessed head trauma.
   2. Confusion or delirium preceding coma is suggestive of a toxi-metabolic etiology (organ dysfunction or infection, electrolyte disorder, medicinal or drug toxicity).
   3. Important information to obtain immediately consists of the following:
      a. Current medications, especially any diabetic, epileptic, cardiac, or anticoagulant drugs.
      b. Any history of adverse or allergic medicinal reactions.
      c. Any history of recent head trauma, febrile or other illness, or previous neurologic symptoms.
      d. Any use of recreational drugs.
B. Physical examination.
   1. A rapid **general or systemic examination** may provide important clues for the etiology of coma.
      a. **Hypertension** to an extreme degree may point to causes other than an acute cerebral hemorrhage or infarction, including hypertensive encephalopathy, cocaine abuse, or eclampsia.
      b. **Hypotension** reflects hypovolemia, cardiogenic or septic shock.
      c. **Fever** accompanies systemic or central nervous system infections, as well as malignant hyperthermia, neuroleptic malignant syndrome, or serotonin syndrome.
      d. **Hypothermia** after cold exposure may even mimic brain death.

e. **Cutaneous bleeding** around the eyes or mastoid area accompanies skull fractures. More diffuse hematomas suggest a systemic bleeding disorder. Infective endocarditis may cause "splinter" nail bed or palmar/plantar hemorrhages, producing coma by means of cerebral infarcts or abscesses.

f. **Jaundice, ascites,** and hepatosplenomegaly may be noted in hepatic coma.

g. An **arrhythmia or heart murmur** may be clues for cardiogenic shock, cerebral cardioemboli, or infective endocarditis.

h. Once cervical spine stability is assured, the finding of **nuchal rigidity** suggests infective meningitis or SAH, but may disappear in deeper stages of coma.

i. **Papilledema** develops a few hours after severe elevation in intracranial pressure.

C. Although the **neurologic examination** in coma is limited, a level of deficit or focal lesion may be revealed and improvement or deterioration noted by serial observations. Developed initially for use in trauma patients, the **Glasgow Coma Scale** is an easy and reproducible scoring system for all medical personnel, as is the more recently developed **FOUR Score** (see Table 5.1), which is better in assessing brainstem reflexes and breathing patterns.

1. Motor responsiveness.
   a. Descriptive observations of any verbal and motor responses from the patient are more helpful than using brief terms (stuporous, obtunded) with variable meaning.
   b. Verbal responses include oriented conversation, disoriented communication, meaningless words or sounds, to unresponsiveness.
   c. Motor responses include spontaneous limb movements, limb movements on command, limb withdrawal to noxious stimuli, to unresponsiveness.
      (1) Decorticate posturing (upper limb flexion with lower limb extension, uni- or bilateral) localizes the deficit to the cerebral hemispheres or thalamus.

TABLE 5.1 Coma Scales

Glasgow Coma Scale	Full Outline of Unresponsiveness (FOUR)
Eye response	**Eye response**
4, eyes open spontaneously	4, eyelids open or opened, tracking, or blinking to command
3, eyes open to command	3, eyelids open but not tracking
2, eyes open to pain	2, eyelids closed but open to loud voice
1, no eye opening	1, eyelids closed but open to pain
	0, eyelids remain closed with pain
Motor response	
6, follows commands	**Motor response**
5, localizes pain	4, thumbs up, fist or peace sign
4, withdraws from pain (flexion)	3, localizing to pain
3, decorticate posturing to pain	2, flexion response to pain
2, decerebrate posturing to pain	1, extension response to pain
1, no motor response	0, no response to pain or generalized myoclonus status
Verbal response	**Brainstem reflexes**
5, oriented and converses	4, pupil and corneal reflexes present
4, disoriented and converses	3, one pupil wide and fixed
3, uses inappropriate words	2, pupil or corneal reflexes absent
2, incomprehensible sounds	1, pupil and corneal reflexes absent
1, no verbal response	0, absent pupil, corneal and cough reflex
	Respiration
	4, not intubated, regular breathing pattern
	3, not intubated, Cheyne–Stokes breathing pattern
	2, not intubated, irregular breathing
	1, breathes above ventilator rate
	0, breathes at ventilator rate or apnea

(2) Decerebrate posturing (upper and lower limb extension, uni- or bilateral) localizes the deficit to the midbrain (red nucleus).

(3) If required, noxious stimuli include rubbing the sternum, or applying firm but gentle pressure to the forehead or nail beds.

(4) Asymmetrical limb movements or hypertonia occur with structural brain lesions, whereas symmetrical motor responses are typical with toxi-metabolic conditions.

(5) Bilateral myoclonic jerks, asterixis, or tremulousness strongly suggest toxi-metabolic causes of coma.

(6) Asymmetrical or focal, rhythmical movements may be subtle clues when non-convulsive status epilepticus causes coma.

2. **Respiratory patterns** do not strictly correlate with the level of brain dysfunction as once thought and may be obscured if the patient is mechanically ventilated.

   a. Cheyne–Stokes' breathing is observed as periods of increasing, then decreasing, tidal volumes and respiratory rate, followed by seconds of apnea.

   (1) It occurs more commonly in elderly patients, with or without systemic medical problems or congestive heart failure.

   (2) It may occur from bilateral cerebral lesions or a unilateral lesion with brain shift.

   b. Persistent hyperventilation occurs more often from pulmonary causes like pneumonitis, and rarely from midbrain lesions.

   c. Arrhythmical, irregular respirations accompany dysfunction at the medulla, where critical cardiorespiratory centers are located.

3. **The pupils** are typically small but reactive to light in the elderly, as well as those in toxi-metabolic coma, even when other cranial nerve reflexes are absent.

   a. A unilaterally large pupil unreactive to light ("fixed or blown pupil") in an unresponsive patient represents dysfunction of third cranial nerve pupilloconstrictive fibers.

   (1) Most commonly found with ipsilateral temporal lobe compression of the third cranial nerve (uncal herniation) from hemorrhage or edema.

   (2) Rarely due to a ruptured intracranial aneurysm at the junction of the internal carotid-posterior communicating artery.

   (3) Asymmetrical pupils and decreased pupillary light reflexes are independent predictors of a structural lesion causing coma.

   b. Bilateral midposition to large, unreactive pupils may occur with midbrain lesions or terminal anoxic brain injury.

   c. Pinpoint, reactive pupils are caused by extensive pontine lesions interrupting the descending sympathetic pupillodilator fibers; however,

   (1) pinpoint pupils can also be caused in older patients by cholinergic eyedrops for glaucoma, and

   (2) narcotic overdose can also produce small pupils.

4. **Ocular reflexes,** which are cortically suppressible in an awake patient, indicate preserved brainstem function when found in a comatose patient.

   a. The oculocephalic ("doll's eyes") reflex occurs when the examiner passively turns the head to one side, eliciting a normal lateral conjugate rolling of the eyes to the opposite side.

   b. The oculovestibular ("cold caloric") reflex occurs after instillation of 50- to 200-cc ice water into one ear canal, with the head elevated 30 degrees, eliciting a slow, tonic deviation of both eyes toward the irrigated ear, after several seconds delay.

   (1) Ensure that the tympanic membrane is intact, so nonsterile water and debris cannot enter the middle ear.

   (2) Ensure there is no impacted cerumen in the ear canal, causing a false-negative test.

   (3) Lateral jerk nystagmus of the eyes toward the nonirrigated ear occurs in conscious patients, but not comatose patients where cortical function is depressed.

   c. Ocular reflexes

   (1) should not be checked in trauma patients until cervical spine stability is assured,

   (2) may be absent because of previous labyrinthine trauma, mastoiditis or toxicity from benzodiazepines or barbiturates, and

   (3) appear asymmetrical from a structural lesion affecting the brainstem, or from facial bone fractures restricting extraocular muscle function.

d. In coma,
   (1) the eyes are slightly divergent at rest,
   (2) conjugate lateral deviation of the eyes toward one side occurs from a lesion in the contralateral brainstem or ipsilateral cerebral hemisphere,
   (3) persistent, rhythmical nystagmus may be a subtle finding of nonconvulsive status epilepticus, and
   (4) "ocular bobbing" consists of repetitive downward jerks of the eyes, with slower updrift, because of pontine lesions with poor outcome.
e. Blinking
   (1) occurs spontaneously if the pontine ARAS is intact and
   (2) along with vertical eye movements may be the only motor functions (and means of communication) in a patient with the "locked-in syndrome" (see section Differential Diagnosis).

ETIOLOGY

A. **Toxi-metabolic coma** accounts for almost two-thirds of unresponsive emergency room patients.
   1. A confusional state or delirium occurs initially, followed by symmetrical motor or ocular reflex findings and preserved pupillary light reflex.
   2. Exceptionally, hemiparesis or aphasia may be due to hyperglycemic, hypoglycemic, hyponatremic, or dysosmolar states.
   3. Tremulousness, myoclonic jerks, and asterixis are typical.
   4. Drug intoxication or overdose may also lead to subsequent traumatic brain injury and structural lesions leading to coma.
B. **Structural causes of coma** account for about one-third of unresponsive emergency room patients.
   1. Asymmetrical motor or ocular reflex findings occur early.
   2. A unilaterally dilated pupil unresponsive to light indicates uncal herniation until proven otherwise.

DIFFERENTIAL DIAGNOSIS

A. Brain death.
   1. Irreversible, critical loss of brain and brainstem function.
      a. Comatose patient with absence of all brainstem reflexes, including spontaneous respiration (abnormal bedside apnea test: no observed breaths despite $pco_2 \geq 60$ mm, while on 100% oxygen).
      b. The cause of coma is known and sufficient to cause brain death, such as cardiopulmonary arrest.
   2. No improvement occurs during observation and treatment.
      a. Observation is at least 6 hours in adults, 12 hours to 2 days for children.
      b. Hypothermia, hypotensive shock, and drug intoxication have been ruled out or treated.
      c. Ancillary testing may help to confirm the clinical diagnosis (absent cerebral blood flow on radioisotope brain scan, or "flat-line" electroencephalogram [EEG]).
B. Persistent vegetative state (or "unresponsive wakefulness syndrome").
   1. After several days of coma, the patient appears intermittently awake, breathes spontaneously, and exhibits primitive reflexes or eye-roving behavior.
   2. Severe cerebral damage persists, however, and no meaningful communication or cortical responsiveness occurs.
   3. Patients showing some impersistent, subtle signs of awareness (visual pursuit, pain localization) are felt to be in a "minimally conscious state" (MCS).
C. "Locked-in syndrome."
   1. The patient may appear to be in a persistent vegetative state, and is unable to move the limbs and face, or gaze laterally ("de-efferented").
   2. Vertical gaze and eyeblinking are preserved, and serve as a means of proving that communication and cortical functions are preserved (the patient accurately blinks once for "yes," or twice for "no" in response to the examiner).

3. Caused by an extensive pontine infarction or profound neuromuscular paralysis, such as Guillain–Barré syndrome.

D. **Thalamic lesions.**
1. Bilateral lesions interrupting the projections of the intralaminar thalamic nuclei of the ARAS to the frontal lobes can produce an inattentive, unresponsive, but still wakeful state.
2. Paramedian thalamic syndrome (see Video 5.1).
   a. Lethargic patient with quadriparesis, impaired vertical gaze, and bilateral asterixis.
   b. Caused by bilateral infarction of the dorsal midbrain and thalamus.

E. **Nonconvulsive status epilepticus.**
1. Occasionally, continual or persistent generalized seizures may occur in the absence of obvious clinical convulsive activity.
2. Subtle clinical manifestations include rhythmical nystagmus, or twitching of an eyelid or part of the face or limb.
3. Obtain an emergent EEG recording and assess the response to IV benzodiazepine boluses.

F. **Psychiatric unresponsiveness.**
1. Occurs rarely, and remains a diagnosis of exclusion.
2. In the absence of drug overdose, brainstem reflexes and spontaneous breathing should be preserved, and no focal neurologic deficits are seen.
3. EEG brain wave frequencies are more similar to that of the awake state than the diffuse EEG slowing typical of toxi-metabolic coma.
4. Psychiatric patients may become comatose from other medical or neurologic disorders as well, or from therapeutic drug therapy (neuroleptic malignant or serotonin syndromes).

MANAGEMENT

A. Initial approach for a comatose patient.
1. Maintain **a**irway, **b**reathing, and **c**irculation, with intubation, ventilation, and fluid/pressor support as needed.
2. Urgently correct any hypothermia, which, if profound, can mimic brain death.
3. If trauma has occurred or is strongly suspected, establish stability of the cervical spine (computed tomography [CT] scan) before moving the head, as occurs with testing the oculocephalic (doll's eyes) reflex.
4. Rule out hypoglycemia, especially in diabetic patients, with an immediate fingerstick glucose reading (or empirical infusion of 50% dextrose if immediate testing is not available). Before any glucose infusion in malnourished patients, prevent Wernicke's encephalopathy with adequate thiamine supplementation, such as 500 mg IV (infused over 30 minutes) tid, followed by 250 mg IV daily for 5 days (see Chapter 63).
5. Check basic bloodwork (blood count, electrolytes, glucose, renal and liver functions, ammonia level, thyroid functions, protime, activated partial thromboplastin time, arterial blood gas, possibly carbon monoxide [CO] level if CO poisoning suspected) and urine drug screen.
6. The prognosis of coma following cardiac arrest improves with therapeutic hypothermia initiated within 6 hours, achieving a core temperature of 32° to 34°C for 24 hours, followed by slow rewarming.

B. Comatose patient with suspected hemorrhage.
1. After the initial approach above, perform a brain CT scan without contrast in a known or suspected trauma patient to rule out intracranial hemorrhage.
2. Nontraumatic SAH is suspected with prodromal headache and sudden loss of consciousness.
   a. Rule out SAH with a brain CT scan without contrast.
   b. Perform a lumbar puncture (LP) if SAH is still strongly suspected but not seen on brain CT scan.
   c. If SAH is found, request neurosurgical consultation and urgent conventional cerebral angiogram or CT angiogram.

C. Comatose patient with fever or septic syndrome.
1. After the initial approach above, examine the patient for any likely systemic focus of infection, such as abscess or peritonitis.

2. Panculture blood and urine, obtain chest X-ray.
3. Perform LP to exclude meningitis (in absence of focal neurologic findings, papilledema, bleeding disorder, or local infection over the lumbar spine) and begin initial broad-spectrum antibiotic coverage plus dexamethasone (see Chapter 63).
4. If LP is contraindicated, request emergent brain CT scan with and without contrast, and neurosurgery consultation.
5. Especially in the case of *Herpes simplex* encephalitis, a brain magnetic resonance imaging (MRI) scan may help reveal typical frontotemporal lesions.

D. Comatose patient with focal findings on neurologic examination.

1. After the initial approach above, exclude hemorrhage with a brain CT scan without contrast.
2. Investigate and treat intracranial hemorrhage or other cause of brain edema or shift.
3. If brain CT scan is normal, obtain brain MRI with and without contrast, including diffusion-weighted sequences, if patient is stable. MR or CT angiography may be urgently done when there is a strong suspicion of ischemic infarction, because acute interventions (mechanical thrombectomy, intravascular thrombolysis) may be helpful. Basilar artery thrombosis often presents with coma.
4. If brain CT and MRI scans are normal, perform EEG to exclude electrical status epilepticus or postictal state.

E. Comatose patient without focal findings on neurologic examination.

1. After the initial approach above, consider administration of IV naloxone or flumazenil, respectively, for possible narcotic or benzodiazepine overdose. Be ready to treat any drug withdrawal symptoms.
2. If no toxi-metabolic causes become obvious, obtain a brain CT scan or brain MRI scan if patient is stable.
3. If brain CT and MRI scans are normal, perform an EEG to exclude electrical status epilepticus or postictal state.

Key Points

- Coma from toxi-metabolic causes typically begins with confusion or delirium, followed by symmetrical motor or ocular reflex findings and preserved pupillary light reflex.
- Coma due to structural lesions usually presents early with asymmetrical motor or ocular reflex abnormalities, followed later by changes in attention or consciousness.
- The prognosis of coma following cardiac arrest improves with therapeutic hypothermia initiated within 6 hours.

Recommended Readings

Castaigne P, Lhermitte F, Buge A, et al. Paramedian thalamic and midbrain infarcts: clinical and neuro-pathological study. *Ann Neurol.* 1981;10:127–148.

Giacino JT, Ashwal S, Childs N, et al. The minimally conscious state: definition and diagnostic criteria. *Neurology.* 2002;58:349–353.

Hypothermia after Cardiac Arrest Study Group. Mild therapeutic hypothermia to improve the neurologic outcome after cardiac arrest. *N Engl J Med.* 2002;346(8):549–556.

Laureys S, Celesia GG, Cohadon F, et al. Unresponsive wakefulness syndrome: a new name for the vegetative state or apallic syndrome. *BMC Medicine.* 2010;8:68.

Merchut MP, Biller J. Assessment of acute loss of consciousness. In: Loftus CM, ed. *Neurosurgical Emergencies.* 2nd ed. New York, NY: Thieme Medical Publishers; 2008:3–10.

Plum F, Posner JB. *The Diagnosis of Stupor and Coma.* 3rd ed. Philadelphia, PA: FA Davis; 1982.

Thomson AD, Cook CC, Touquet R, et al. The Royal College of Physicians report on alcohol: guidelines for managing Wernicke's encephalopathy in the accident and emergency department. *Alcohol Alcohol.* 2002;37(6):513–521.

Tokuda Y, Nakazato N, Stein G. Pupillary evaluation for differential diagnosis of coma. *Postgrad Med J.* 2003;79(927):49–51.

Wallis WE, Donaldson I, Scott RS, et al. Hypoglycemia masquerading as cerebrovascular disease (hypoglycemic hemiplegia). *Ann Neurol.* 1985;18:510–512.

Wijdicks EFM. Altered arousal and coma. In: Wijdicks EFM. *Catastrophic Neurologic Disorders in the Emergency Department.* 2nd ed. Oxford, England: Oxford University Press; 2004:53–93.

Wijdicks EFM, Bamler WR, Maramattom BV, et al. Validation of a new coma scale: the FOUR score. *Ann Neurol.* 2005;58:585–593.

Young GB, Ropper AH, Bolton CF, eds. *Coma and Impaired Consciousness.* New York, NY: McGraw-Hill; 1998:307–392.

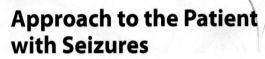

6 Approach to the Patient with Seizures

Vicenta Salanova and Meridith Runke

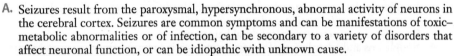

A. Seizures result from the paroxysmal, hypersynchronous, abnormal activity of neurons in the cerebral cortex. Seizures are common symptoms and can be manifestations of toxic–metabolic abnormalities or of infection, can be secondary to a variety of disorders that affect neuronal function, or can be idiopathic with unknown cause.
   1. **Nonrecurrent seizures**—for example, toxic–metabolic, hypoxia.
   2. **Recurrent seizures** or epilepsy—inherited, acquired, or structural cortical lesions.
B. The **international classification of epileptic seizures** consists of two main categories—partial seizures and generalized seizures.
   1. **Partial seizures** (focal) result from localized epileptogenic lesions, except in children with benign focal epilepsy, who have no structural lesions. Partial seizures are subdivided into
      a. **Simple partial seizures,** if there is preservation of consciousness.
      b. **Complex partial seizures,** if there is impairment of consciousness. A partial seizure typically begins as a simple partial seizure consisting of an aura reflecting the site of seizure origin (or ictal spread to the symptomatogenic area) and then evolves into a complex partial seizure. Both simple and complex partial seizures can evolve into secondarily generalized seizures.
   2. **Generalized seizures** can be convulsive or nonconvulsive and are subdivided into absence (typical and atypical absences), myoclonic, clonic, tonic, tonic–clonic, and atonic seizures.
C. There is also an **international classification of epilepsy** and epilepsy syndromes. This classification takes into account the age at onset, possible etiologic factors, inheritance, findings at neurologic examination, prognosis, and seizure type (partial or generalized).
   1. Localization-related epilepsy.
      a. **Idiopathic** (benign childhood rolandic and occipital epilepsy).
      b. **Symptomatic,** which is acquired and based mainly on the anatomic localization.
   2. Generalized epilepsy and syndromes.
      a. **Idiopathic** with **age-related** onset (e.g. benign neonatal familial convulsions, childhood and juvenile absence epilepsy, juvenile myoclonic epilepsy, epilepsy with grand mal seizures on awakening).
      b. **Symptomatic** (e.g., infantile spasms, Lennox–Gastaut syndrome). The international classification includes two other categories: (1) epileptic syndromes with both focal and generalized seizures (e.g. acquired epileptic aphasia) and (2) special syndromes (e.g. febrile convulsions). This chapter reviews the etiology, clinical manifestations, evaluation, and differential diagnoses of some of these types of seizures with emphasis on patients with partial seizures.

ETIOLOGY

A. Toxic–metabolic.
   1. Systemic illness. Hypoglycemia, nonketotic hyperglycemia, hypoxia, hypocalcemia (in patients with or without a history of hypoparathyroidism), hyponatremia (inappropriate antidiuretic hormone syndrome and water intoxication), hypomagnesemia, uremia and hepatic failure, sickle-cell anemia, thrombotic thrombocytopenic purpura, and Whipple's disease.

2. **Drugs and toxins.** Cocaine, amphetamines, phencyclidine, lidocaine, and lead poisoning. Others can lower the seizure threshold and increase the risk of seizures usually among patients with other predisposing factors (tricyclics, theophylline, phenothiazine, and penicillins).

3. **Withdrawal syndromes.** Alcohol, hypnotics.

4. **Pyridoxine deficiency.**

B. Acquired structural lesions.

1. **Infection.** Brain abscess, meningitis, encephalitis (e.g., herpes simplex encephalitis), postinfectious encephalomyelitis, cysticercosis, opportunistic infections in acquired immunodeficiency syndrome (AIDS), and neurosyphilis.

2. **Vascular.** Vasculitis (systemic lupus erythematosus, hypersensitivity, and infectious vasculitis), ischemic or hemorrhagic cerebrovascular disease, cerebral venous thrombosis, arteriovenous malformation, and cavernous angioma.

3. **Trauma.** Usually penetrating, subdural hematoma.

4. **Neoplasms** and other lesions. Primary or metastatic tumors, hamartomas, and cortical dysplasia.

5. **Mesial temporal sclerosis.** Usually postfebrile convulsions (Fig. 6.1).

6. **Other.** Alzheimer's disease, Creutzfeldt–Jakob disease, Paraneoplastic disorders limbic encephalitis, Rasmussen encephalitis, and, in rare instances, multiple sclerosis.

7. Autoimmune epilepsy with neural autoantibodies including voltage-gated potassium channel complex, glutamic acid decarboxylase, collapsing response-mediator protein, and anti-NMDAR (N-methyl-D-aspartate receptor) encephalitis.

C. Familial.

1. Primary generalized epilepsy.

2. Benign focal epilepsy of childhood.

3. Febrile convulsions.

4. Autosomal-dominant nocturnal frontal lobe epilepsy (ADNFLE).

5. Familial temporal lobe epilepsy (FTLE).

D. **Other genetic syndromes** associated with seizures (tuberous sclerosis complex, neurofibromatosis type 1), disorders of amino acid, lipid, and protein metabolism (e.g., phenylketonuria, maple syrup urine disease, porphyria).

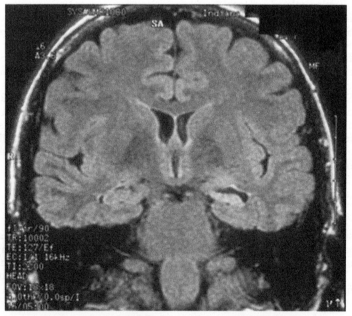

FIGURE 6.1 MRI showing left mesial temporal sclerosis. MRI, magnetic resonance imaging.

CLINICAL MANIFESTATIONS

A. **Metabolic–toxic and hypoxic insults.** Patients with seizures attributable to metabolic or toxic causes have generalized tonic–clonic seizures, but focal seizures and epilepsia partialis continua can occur with nonketotic hyperglycemia. Posthypoxic coma usually causes multifocal myoclonus; however, periodic lateralized epileptiform discharges (PLEDs) may be seen, at times associated with focal motor seizures.

B. **Meningitis and encephalitis** can cause either generalized or focal seizures with secondarily generalized seizures. Patients with herpes simplex encephalitis often have complex partial seizures typical of those of temporal lobe origin. The electroencephalogram (EEG) shows focal slowing in one or both temporal regions and PLEDs. Magnetic resonance imaging (MRI) shows hypodense lesions in one or both temporal lobes.

C. **Partial seizures** (functional–anatomic classification of epilepsy). Clinical features and EEG findings indicate focal origin.

1. **Temporal lobe seizures** are the most common partial seizures. In many of these patients, the seizures are refractory to medical treatment (Video 6.1).

   a. **Signs and symptoms.** The findings at neurologic examination are often normal, except for memory dysfunction, which can be seen in patients with bitemporal epilepsy. Most of these patients have an epigastric aura (nausea, an epigastric rising sensation, stomach upset, or even pain). Other auras consist of fear, complex visual or auditory hallucinations, déjà vu, and olfactory and gustatory sensations. The clinical manifestations are stereotypical, and most patients have one seizure type. Most patients exhibit staring, unresponsiveness, and oroalimentary and gestural automatism. Some patients also have contralateral arm dystonic posturing. Ictal or postictal language difficulties also have lateralizing value. Ictal speech occurs in patients with seizures arising from the nondominant temporal lobe. Patients with seizures originating from the dominant temporal lobe may exhibit ictal and postictal dysphasia.

   b. **Etiologic factors and pathologic features.** Mesial temporal sclerosis is the most common pathologic finding. There is a strong association between mesial temporal sclerosis and prolonged complex febrile seizures in patients younger than 5 years of age. There is usually a silent interval between the occurrence of febrile seizures and the onset of mesial temporal lobe epilepsy, which often begins toward the end of the first decade of life or soon after. Other pathologic findings include tumors, such as ganglioglioma, cortical dysplasia, and cavernous malformation. As many as 15% of patients with medically refractory temporal lobe epilepsy have evidence of a dual pathologic process. Mesial temporal sclerosis can occur with temporal lobe developmental lesions such as cortical dysplasia and subependymal heterotopia.

   c. **EEG findings** include epileptiform discharges over the anterior temporal region and often polymorphic slowing. About 30% to 40% of these patients have bitemporal independent interictal epileptiform discharges, usually with predominance on the side of ictal onset.

   d. **Imaging studies.** MRI volumetric studies usually show a smaller hippocampus and increased signal intensity on T2-weighted images that are indicative of hippocampal sclerosis. These changes can be seen in as many as 80% of patients with refractory temporal lobe epilepsy.

   e. **Secondarily generalized** tonic–clonic seizures and convulsive status epilepticus can occur; nonconvulsive complex partial status epilepticus is rare.

   f. Patients with temporal lobe seizures should be differentiated from patients with **FTLE**. The first series described FTLE as a benign disorder with late age of onset, excellent outcome, and normal finding on the MRI of the head. A second report, however, showed that some cases of FTLE were refractory to medical treatment, requiring surgical treatment. The most recent report concluded that FTLE is a clinically heterogeneous syndrome. The authors found hippocampal atrophy in 57% of their patients, including those with a benign course or remission of seizures. They concluded that the findings indicated the presence of a strong genetic component in the development of mesial temporal sclerosis in the families studied.

2. **Focal motor seizures.** These seizures originate in the vicinity of the rolandic motor cortex. Consciousness is preserved.

   a. **Signs and symptoms.** Examination may show contralateral mild hemiparesis or hyperreflexia. Seizures commonly begin with focal contralateral twitching of the face or hand and then spread to involve the rest of the extremity. When seizures originate in the nondominant hemisphere, patients are usually able to speak during the seizures. When seizures originate in the dominant hemisphere, patients may have ictal and postictal aphasia. Clonic eye movements, blinking, and conscious contraversion may also occur. Ictal focal motor manifestations, postictal hemiparesis, and postictal aphasia are contralateral to the side of seizure onset. Some patients have continuous focal motor activity (epilepsia partialis continua lasting weeks, months, or even years).

   b. **Imaging studies.** Focal structural lesions are common.

   c. **EEG** shows focal slowing and focal epileptiform discharges over the frontal lobe; however, some patients have no epileptiform discharges on scalp recordings or have bifrontal epileptiform abnormalities.

   d. Patients with focal motor seizures have to be differentiated from patients with benign rolandic epilepsy with centrotemporal spikes, which begins between the ages of 3 and 13 years. These children have normal findings at neurologic examination and imaging studies. They have nocturnal generalized seizures and partial seizures beginning in the face with preservation of consciousness, at times with speech arrest. The EEG shows centrotemporal, high-amplitude, broad, sharp waves and slow discharges, with a horizontal dipole, occurring predominantly during sleep. The prognosis is excellent.

3. **Supplementary motor seizures** originate in the supplementary motor cortex, which is located in the mesial frontal lobe anterior to the primary motor leg area.

   a. **Signs and symptoms.** Examination is usually normal. Almost one-half of these patients have a somatosensory aura consisting of tingling or numbness of the extremities, which can be contralateral or bilateral. These patients have unilateral or bilateral tonic posturing of the extremities at onset, vocalization, speech arrest, and laughter. Other manifestations include fencing posture, thrashing, kicking, and pelvic movements. Responsiveness is preserved unless the seizure evolves into a secondarily generalized tonic–clonic seizure. Supplementary motor seizures are common during sleep and are of short duration without postictal confusion or amnesia.

   b. **Imaging studies.** MRI of the head may show lesions in the supplementary motor area.

   c. The **EEG** may show epileptiform discharges over the vertex, but some patients may have no interictal epileptiform discharges on scalp recordings. Ictal recordings are often nonlateralized. A few patients may have no ictal EEG changes during scalp recordings.

4. **Complex partial seizures of frontal lobe origin**

   a. **Signs and symptoms.** The examination is usually normal. Patients may have a cephalic aura that is followed by staring or looking ahead, unconscious contraversion, and complex motor automatism such as bicycling, kicking, thrashing, running, and bouncing up and down. Vocalization and tonic posturing may occur toward the end of the seizure as manifestations of ictal spread to the supplementary motor area. Complex partial (nonconvulsive) status epilepticus, manifested by alteration of consciousness with automatic behavior often in a cyclical manner lasting hours to days, also may occur. Secondarily generalized tonic–clonic seizures and convulsive status epilepticus are believed to be more common in patients with frontal lobe seizures.

   b. **Imaging studies.** MRI may show lesions in the frontopolar, dorsolateral, orbitofrontal, and other frontal regions.

   c. The **EEG** may show focal slowing and interictal epileptiform discharges over one frontal lobe, lateralized to one hemisphere, or bilateral frontal epileptiform abnormalities.

   d. These patients with acquired frontal lobe epilepsy should be differentiated from those with **ADNFLE**. In ADNFLE, the seizures begin in childhood and usually persist through adult life. They occur in clusters during sleep and are characterized by vocalization, thrashing, hyperkinetic activity, or tonic stiffening. Patients have normal findings at neurologic examination and on imaging studies. An ictal EEG may show bifrontal epileptiform discharges. The seizures usually respond to carbamazepine monotherapy. These seizures are often misdiagnosed as parasomnia or familial dyskinesia.

5. **Occipital lobe seizures** are rare, but they may be difficult to differentiate from seizures originating from the posterior temporal lobe. These patients have to be differentiated from patients with benign occipital epilepsy, the onset of which is in childhood and has similar symptoms but no occipital lesions. The age at onset of benign occipital epilepsy ranges from 15 months to 17 years (with a peak between 5 and 7 years), and more than one-third of patients have family histories of epilepsy.

   a. Signs and symptoms. Occipital manifestations are common. Patients may have visual field defects, visual auras consisting of elementary visual hallucinations described as colored flashing lights, or ictal blindness. Other manifestations include contralateral eye deviation, a sensation of eye movement, nystagmoid eye movements, and blinking. After the occipital manifestations, many patients have typical temporal lobe automatism as well as focal motor seizure activity resulting from ictal spread to the temporal and frontal lobes. Because of these different spread patterns, many patients have more than one type of seizure. Almost two-thirds of patients have lateralizing clinical features, such as contralateral head deviation and visual field defects, contralateral to the epileptogenic zone.

   b. Imaging studies. On computed tomography (CT) scans and (magnetic resonance) MR images, many patients have occipital lesions ipsilateral to the epileptogenic zone.

   c. The **EEG** may show focal slowing and epileptiform discharges over one occipital lobe. However, most often the EEG shows posterior temporal epileptiform discharges. Some patients have bilateral posterior temporal–occipital epileptiform abnormalities.

6. **Parietal lobe seizures** are uncommon.

   a. Signs and symptoms. The examination may show contralateral impaired two-point discrimination, but more often the findings are normal. These patients have somatosensory aurae described as contralateral tingling or numbness and painful and thermal sensations. Other aurae consist of disturbances of body image, a sensation of movement in one extremity, or a feeling that one extremity is absent. Vertiginous sensations and visual illusions can occur, as can an aphasic aura. Some of these patients have seizures of multiple types as a result of ictal spread to the temporal and frontal lobes. Tonic posturing of extremities, focal motor clonic activity, head and eye deviations, and temporal lobe automatism are commonly observed.

   b. Imaging studies. MRI may show focal lesions in the parietal lobe.

   c. The **EEG** most often shows lateralized epileptiform discharges to one hemisphere rather than localized discharges.

D. Primary (idiopathic) generalized epilepsy. There is usually a family history of epilepsy. The first clinical manifestations indicate involvement of both cerebral hemispheres. This form of epilepsy can be **convulsive** or **nonconvulsive**.

1. **Childhood absence epilepsy** begins between the ages of 4 and 8 years. The findings at neurologic examination are normal.

   a. Signs and symptoms. There is a brief loss of consciousness, usually lasting 10 seconds or less and almost always lasting less than 30 seconds. There is no aura or postictal confusion. Blinking, brief facial twitching, or other clonic component, decreased postural tone, and automatism such as swallowing, lip smacking, and fumbling with clothes are common. Some patients also may have tonic–clonic seizures.

   b. The **EEG** shows the typical generalized, bilaterally synchronous 3-Hz spike–wave epileptiform discharges. Hyperventilation for 3 to 5 minutes often provokes an absence seizure with typical generalized, bifrontally dominant, regular, synchronous 3-Hz spike–wave complexes with abrupt onset and termination. In some patients, the epileptiform discharges may be maximum over the posterior head regions.

   c. The **prognosis** is favorable, and for many patients the seizures remit in adolescence. The prognosis is less favorable if tonic–clonic seizures occur.

   d. Absence status. Rare patients may have prolonged confusion that lasts hours or all day and is associated with continuous 3-Hz spike–wave discharges.

2. **Juvenile absence epilepsy** is less common than childhood absence epilepsy.

   a. The **clinical manifestations** are similar, but seizures begin during puberty or later. The absences tend to occur on awakening and are not as frequent as those in the childhood form. Myoclonic seizures also may occur.

   b. The **EEG** may show generalized 3-Hz spike–wave discharges or higher-frequency (4 to 5 Hz) discharges.

c. The **prognosis** is not as favorable as in the childhood form, and generalized tonic–clonic seizures are more frequent. Absence status is also more frequent than in the childhood form.

3. Juvenile myoclonic epilepsy. Age at onset is in the second decade. The findings at neurologic examination are normal. The diagnosis is often missed because of failure to recognize the myoclonic jerks.

   a. Signs and symptoms. These patients have awakening myoclonic and generalized tonic–clonic seizures. Absence seizures occur in 15% of patients. During brief myoclonic jerks, consciousness is preserved. Myoclonic seizures may precede the onset of generalized tonic–clonic seizures by a few years, or they may have simultaneous onset. The generalized tonic–clonic seizures usually follow a series of myoclonic seizures. Seizures may be precipitated by sleep deprivation or alcohol intake.

   b. The **EEG** shows generalized polyspike and wave discharges in most patients. Some patients are photosensitive and have photoparoxysmal responses. During the myoclonic jerks, the EEG shows abrupt onset of high-amplitude polyspike and wave complexes lasting from 2 to 10 seconds.

   c. Prognosis. Although these patients have an excellent response to valproic acid, the electroclinical trait persists for life, and most patients need lifelong treatment.

4. Generalized tonic–clonic seizures. A patient with primary generalized tonic–clonic seizures usually has a family history of epilepsy. The findings at neurologic examination are normal. Age at onset is usually during puberty.

   a. Signs and symptoms. There is no aura. A few patients may have a prodrome (nervousness, irritability) hours before the seizure. The seizure begins with brief tonic flexion of the axial muscles and muscular contraction of the extremities followed by a longer period of tonic extension of the axial muscles. The mouth is closed, and this may lead to tongue biting. Apnea can occur as a result of contraction of the respiratory muscles. The arms are semiflexed, and the legs are extended. After the tonic phase, there is diffuse tremor, and then there is a clonic phase. Autonomic changes usually occur at the end of the tonic phase. Heart rate and blood pressure can more than double during the tonic phase. There is also increased bladder pressure.

   b. **Complications** during a prolonged tonic–clonic seizure may include tongue biting, dislocation of shoulders, vertebral compression fractures, aspiration pneumonia, and even sudden death. The mechanism of sudden death is unclear; several factors, such as apnea, pulmonary edema, and cardiac arrhythmias, may be involved.

   c. The **EEG** shows generalized 4- to 5-Hz spike–wave activity, or multiple spike–wave complexes. More irregular spike–wave discharges can occur. The likelihood of recording the epileptiform discharges increases if the EEG is obtained 1 to 5 days after a seizure. Some patients have a photoparoxysmal response with bisynchronous, generalized irregular spike and spike–wave discharges. EEG ictal changes show generalized low-voltage fast activity (recruiting rhythm) followed by high-amplitude generalized polyspike or polyspike and wave discharges. During the clonic phase, high-amplitude polyspike or polyspike and wave discharges alternate with low-amplitude slowing. Postictally, there is low-amplitude slowing.

   d. **Generalized tonic–clonic status epilepticus** begins with recurrent, brief tonic–clonic seizures without full recovery of consciousness or with a prolonged generalized tonic–clonic seizure lasting 30 minutes.

E. Secondary (symptomatic) generalized epilepsy. These patients have multifocal cortical abnormalities, including infantile spasms (West's syndrome) and Lennox–Gastaut syndrome.

   1. West's syndrome. The onset is usually between 3 and 6 months of age and always before 1 year. Some infants have no identifiable etiologic factors (cryptogenic subgroup). Symptomatic West's syndrome is more common and can result from trauma, infection, Down's syndrome, tuberous sclerosis, phenylketonuria, and other disorders. These infants have frequent infantile spasms, developmental delay, and a characteristic EEG pattern (hypsarrhythmia).

   2. **Lennox–Gastaut syndrome** is one of the most severe epileptic syndromes. These children usually have developmental delay, neurologic deficits, and seizures of multiple types, which are often medically refractory (drop attacks, atypical absence, myoclonic,

tonic, and tonic–clonic seizures). The EEG shows generalized slow (<2.5 Hz) spike–wave discharges.

a. **Drop attacks** represent atonic seizures and are characterized by sudden loss of tone, at times preceded by a generalized clonic jerk. There is head drop, and often the child collapses. The ictal EEG shows an electrodecremental response.

b. **Atypical absences** usually last longer than typical absences and are commonly associated with motor findings and postictal confusion. They are more common during drowsiness and are not usually activated by hyperventilation. The EEG shows generalized slow spike–wave discharges and diffuse slowing of the background.

c. **Absence status** is common. Patients come to medical attention with prolonged absences (spike–wave stupor), blinking, and at times facial twitching with continuous generalized spike–wave discharges.

d. **Tonic seizures** are common in Lennox–Gastaut syndrome. The arms are elevated in a semiflexed position, and there is impairment of consciousness and autonomic changes.

EVALUATION

A. **History.**
1. The following should be documented: **age at onset** and **frequency** of seizures, **family history** of epilepsy, psychosocial history, possible etiologic factors such as history of head trauma, difficult birth, febrile seizures, meningitis, or encephalitis. **Precipitating factors** include medical illnesses that can lead to metabolic abnormalities and exposure to drugs or toxins.
2. The **presence and type of aura,** detailed description of the seizure by a family member, presence of automatism, ictal speech, dystonic or tonic posturing, postictal language difficulties, Todd's paralysis, or the presence of myoclonus can help to **differentiate focal from generalized seizures.**
3. **Response to antiepileptic drugs (AEDs)** and possible side effects.

B. **Physical examination.**
1. **Detailed examination,** including the skin, for signs of neurocutaneous lesions associated with seizures, such as neurofibromatosis type 1, tuberous sclerosis complex, and Sturge–Weber syndrome. Cranial bruits may be present in patients with arteriovenous malformations, and cervical bruits in patients with seizures resulting from cerebrovascular disease.
2. **Limb asymmetry** suggestive of injuries early in life. **Focal neurologic deficits,** such as subtle hemiparesis, hyperreflexia, decreased two-point discrimination, or visual field defects, may suggest the location of the epileptogenic lesion. **Memory deficits** can be elicited in some patients with bitemporal epilepsy.

C. **Laboratory studies** include complete blood cell count; a Venereal Disease Research Laboratory (VDRL) test; measurement of erythrocyte sedimentation rate and blood levels of glucose, calcium, sodium, and magnesium; liver and renal function tests; drug and toxicology screening if indicated by the history or examination findings; and human immunodeficiency virus testing for patients with risk factors. If the clinical manifestations suggest limbic encephalitis and autoimmune epilepsy is suspected, neural autoantibodies including voltage-gated potassium channel complex, glutamic acid decarboxylase, and NMDAR antibodies should be ordered.

D. **Cerebrospinal fluid examination** is performed if vasculitis or infection is suspected or if the serologic result is positive for syphilis.

E. The **EEG** is essential to confirm the diagnosis of epilepsy and to characterize the seizure type. It usually shows focal slowing and epileptiform abnormalities in patients with partial seizures or generalized epileptiform discharges in those with generalized seizures. Seizures are rarely recorded on routine EEGs. The exception is absence seizures, which can be precipitated by hyperventilation. Metabolic encephalopathy associated with seizures usually has diffuse slowing or periodic patterns, such as triphasic waves, in patients with hepatic or renal failure.
1. **Activation procedures,** such as photic stimulation, hyperventilation, and sleep, are performed.

2. Special electrodes. Earlobe, anterior temporal, or zygomatic electrodes are often used. Nasopharyngeal electrodes are traumatic and produce artifacts, and they should not be used. Sphenoidal electrodes are reserved for patients undergoing presurgical evaluation.

3. Video EEG recordings. In some patients with recurrent seizures and no interictal epileptiform discharges on serial EEGs, prolonged video EEG recording may be needed to confirm the diagnosis and to characterize the seizure type.

F. Imaging studies. When the history, neurologic examination, EEG findings, and seizure type suggest partial seizures, the procedure of choice is **MRI of the head.** Although the CT of the head may be helpful, some patients with partial seizures have lesions that do not appear on CT scans, such as hamartoma, cortical dysplasia, low-grade glioma, or cavernous malformation.

DIFFERENTIAL DIAGNOSIS

The **differential diagnosis** includes many neurologic, psychiatric, and medical disorders. The most common are psychogenic seizures and syncopal episodes.

A. **Syncope** is defined as a brief episode of loss of consciousness as a result of a transient decrease in cerebral blood flow. Episodes last a few seconds. Brief tonic–clonic movements and incontinence of urine and feces can occur (convulsive syncope). An EEG during the prodromal period (light-headedness) shows diffuse high-amplitude slowing, and when tonic or clonic activity occurs, the EEG result is isoelectric.

B. **Psychogenic seizures** are suspected when a patient has seizures precipitated by stress when others are present, no response to anticonvulsants, seizures of long duration up to 15 or 30 minutes or even hours, side-to-side head movements, pelvic thrusting, arrhythmic jerking, bilateral motor activity with preservation of consciousness, bizarre and aggressive behavior, and crying. There is no postictal confusion after generalized tonic–clonic jerking. However, some of these symptoms (bizarre complex automatism, pelvic thrusting, bilateral motor activity) can occur among patients with complex partial seizures of frontal lobe origin and supplementary motor seizures.

C. Panic attacks.

D. Cerebrovascular disorder. Transient global amnesia.

E. Migraine with brainstem aura.

F. Sleep disorder. Narcolepsy.

G. Movement disorder. Myoclonus, choreoathetosis, familial paroxysmal dystonia.

H. Paroxysmal vertigo.

I. Toxic–metabolic disorder. Alcohol withdrawal, hypoglycemia.

J. Daydreaming episodes.

DIAGNOSTIC APPROACH

A. The **history and examination** are central to determine the type of seizure (generalized or focal, psychogenic, related to syncope or metabolic causes, and so on), obtain descriptions of the aura (if present) and the seizure by a witness, and identify subtle neurologic deficits. It is helpful to ask a family member to mimic the seizure. After the initial evaluation, a presumptive etiologic diagnosis and a tentative seizure classification are often possible and should determine the extent of the evaluation.

B. **Laboratory evaluation** should include serum electrolytes, baseline renal and hepatic function tests to rule out metabolic causes, drug screening, and other tests as indicated by the history and examination findings.

C. If syncope is suspected, **electrocardiography** and **Holter monitoring** are performed as indicated by the history and examination findings. More extensive evaluation for cardiac causes of syncope may be needed.

D. **Sleep and awake EEGs** are obtained with activation procedures (hyperventilation and photic stimulation) and special electrodes. An ambulatory EEG may be helpful in the evaluation of patients with suspected seizures or pseudoseizures or suspected convulsive episodes of syncope.

E. **Prolonged video EEG** may be needed to confirm the diagnosis, characterize the seizure type, and exclude psychogenic seizures. Complex partial seizures of frontal lobe origin and supplementary motor seizures are often misdiagnosed as psychogenic seizures, and ictal recordings are often needed.

F. **Sleep studies** (multiple sleep latency test and polysomnography) may be needed in the evaluation of some patients with suspected sleep disorders.

G. **MRI** should be performed on patients with partial seizures and secondary (symptomatic) generalized epilepsy.

REFERRAL

A. For patients with recurrent seizures, an initial **neurologic consultation,** including an EEG to clarify the seizure type, allows the proper choice of anticonvulsants.

B. When the diagnosis remains unclear after the initial evaluation or there is lack of response to anticonvulsants, the patient should be referred to a **Comprehensive Epilepsy Center.** Evaluation at such centers includes prolonged video EEG with sphenoidal electrodes. It is important to emphasize that patients with poorly controlled epilepsy have a higher mortality rate than does the general population. Death is usually caused by accidents, status epilepticus, sudden unexplained death, cardiac arrhythmias, and suicide. However, when seizures are completely controlled after surgery, the mortality rate is not different from that of the age-matched general population.

1. **Because** the treatment and prognosis are based on the seizure type and epileptic syndrome, **ictal recordings** are invaluable and allow the proper choice of anticonvulsants.

2. Ictal recordings are the most effective way to diagnose psychogenic seizures, but patients with psychogenic seizures may also have epileptic seizures, and **all the habitual seizure types** should be recorded. To compound the problem, some patients with supplementary motor seizures and other simple partial seizures may have no ictal EEG changes on scalp recordings, or the EEG activity may be obscured by muscle artifacts. Inpatient prolonged video EEG recordings with reduction of AEDs may clarify the diagnosis by recording secondarily generalized seizures.

C. **Identification of surgical candidates and recent advances in the treatment of medically resistant partial epilepsy.** Approximately 3 million people in the USA have epilepsy and 30% to 40% of these patients are refractory to medical treatment. These patients should be referred to a comprehensive epilepsy program, for the diagnosis and treatment of their medically resistant epilepsy. Two randomized clinical trials for temporal lobe epilepsy demonstrated the benefits of surgical treatment; however, despite that, surgical treatment for epilepsy remains underutilized. Prolonged video EEG with surface electrodes and in some patients with intracranial electrodes, 3-Tesla head MRI, tests of focal functional deficits (fluorodeoxyglucose positron emission tomography scans), functional MRIs, to lateralize language, and neuropsychological testing and the intracarotid amobarbital procedure to assess language and memory are conducted at epilepsy centers to identify surgical candidates.

D. Patients with medically refractory temporal lobe epilepsy are the largest group of patients undergoing epilepsy surgery, and 70% to 80% of these patients become seizure free after surgery. A longitudinal study of a large number of patients who underwent temporal resection showed the lasting benefits of epilepsy surgery. The best surgical outcome was observed among patients with small lesions such as cavernous malformations, and mesial temporal sclerosis. Studies have also shown considerable improvement in the quality of life of patients who became seizure free after surgery.

E. **Neurostimulators in epilepsy.** Vagal nerve stimulation was approved for the treatment of patients with refractory partial epilepsy who are not candidates for surgical resection. In clinical trials, 30% to 40% of patients with medically refractory partial seizures had a reduction in seizures of at least 50%.

The SANTE trial (Stimulation of the Anterior Nucleus of the Thalamus for Epilepsy) reported the results of 110 patients who participated in a multicenter, double-blind, randomized controlled trial of bilateral stimulation of the anterior nuclei of the thalamus for localization-related epilepsy. The long-term efficacy and safety of deep thalamic stimulation (DBS) for drug-resistant partial epilepsy found that the median percent seizure reduction from baseline was 69% at 5 years of follow-up. There was also a significant improvement in the responder rates, seizure severity, quality of life, and reductions in most severe seizures. Based on the results of the SANTE trial, DBS for epilepsy was recently approved in Europe, but remains investigational in the United States.

The responsive neurostimulation (RNS) provided class I evidence that responsive cortical stimulation is effective in significantly reducing seizure frequency in adults who had failed two or more antiepileptic medication trials, and had one or two seizure foci. Based on the RNS trial responsive neurostimulation was recently approved in the United States for adults with medically refractory partial onset seizures who meet the above criteria.

Key Points

- Seizures result from paroxysmal, hypersynchronous, abnormal activity of neurons in the cerebral cortex, and can be manifestations of toxic–metabolic abnormalities or of infection or secondary to a variety of disorders that affect neuronal function, or idiopathic with unknown cause.
- The international classification of epileptic seizures consists of two main categories: partial seizures and generalized seizures.
- Partial seizures (focal) result from localized epileptogenic lesions, except in children with benign focal epilepsy who have no structural lesions.
- Temporal lobe seizures are the most common partial seizures, and most of these patients have an epigastric aura, staring, and oroalimentary and gestural automatisms. The head MRI often shows mesial temporal sclerosis.
- There are 3 million people with epilepsy in the United States and 30% to 40% of these patients have medically resistant epilepsy, and these patients should be referred to a comprehensive epilepsy program for evaluation and treatment.

Recommended Readings

Barbaro NM, Quigg M, Broshek DK, et al. A multicenter, prospective pilot study of gamma knife radio-surgery for mesial temporal lobe epilepsy: seizure response, adverse events, and verbal memory. *Ann Neurol.* 2009;65(2):167–175.

Bergey GK, Morrell MJ, Mizrahi EM, et al. Long-term treatment with responsive brain stimulation in adults with refractory partial seizures. *Neurology.* 2015;84:810–817.

Berkovic S, McIntosh A, Howell RA, et al. Familial temporal lobe epilepsy: a common disorder identified in twins. *Ann Neurol.* 1996;40:227–235.

Cendes F, Cook MJ, Watson C, et al. Frequency and characteristics of dual pathology in patients with lesional epilepsy. *Neurology.* 1995;45:2058–2064.

Engel J Jr, McDermott MP, Wiebe S, et al; Early Randomized Surgical Epilepsy Trial (ERSET) Study Group. Early surgical therapy for drug-resistant temporal lobe epilepsy: a randomized trial. *JAMA.* 2012;307(9):922–930.

Fisher R, Salanova V, Witt T, et al. Electrical stimulation of the anterior nucleus of the thalamus for treatment of refractory epilepsy. *Epilepsia.* 2010;51(5):899–908.

French JA, Williamson PD, Thadani VM, et al. Characteristics of medial temporal lobe epilepsy: I: results of history and physical examination. *Ann Neurol.* 1993;34:774–780.

Gloor P, Olivier A, Quesney LF, et al. The role of the limbic system in experiential phenomena of temporal lobe epilepsy. *Ann Neurol.* 1982;12:129–144.

Lüders H, Lesser R, eds. *Epilepsy: Electroclinical Syndromes.* London, England: Springer-Verlag; 1987.

Morrell MJ; RNS System in Epilepsy Study Group. Responsive cortical stimulation for the treatment of medically intractable partial epilepst. *Neurology.* 2011;77:1295–1304.

Morris HH III, Dinner DS, Lüders H, et al. Supplementary motor seizures: clinical and electrographic findings. *Neurology.* 1988;38:1075–1092.

Penfield W, Jasper H. *Epilepsy and the Functional Anatomy of the Human Brain.* Boston, MA: Little, Brown and Company; 1954.

Salanova V, Andermann F, Olivier A, et al. Occipital lobe epilepsy: electroclinical manifestations, electrocorticography, cortical stimulation and outcome in 42 patients treated between 1930 and 1991. *Brain.* 1992;115:1655–1680.

Salanova V, Andermann F, Rasmussen T, et al. Parietal lobe epilepsy: clinical manifestations and outcome in 82 patients treated surgically between 1929 and 1988. *Brain*. 1995;118:607–627.

Salanova V, Markand O, Worth R. Temporal lobe epilepsy surgery: outcome, complications, and late mortality rate in 215 patients. *Epilepsia*. 2002;43(2):170–174.

Salanova V, Morris HH, Van Ness P, et al. Frontal lobe seizures: electroclinical syndromes. *Epilepsia*. 1995;36:16–24.

Salanova V, Witt T, Worth R, et al. Long-term efficacy and safety of thalamic stimulation for drug resistant partial epilepsy. *Neurology*. 2015;84:1017–1025.

Salanova V, Worth R. Neurostimulators in epilepsy. *Curr Neurol Neurosci Rep*. 2007;7:315–319.

Scheffer I, Bhatia K, Lopez-Cendes I, et al. Autosomal dominant frontal lobe epilepsy: a distinctive clinical disorder. *Brain*. 1995;118:61–73.

Toledano M, Britton JW, McKeon A, et al. Utility of an immunotherapy trial in evaluating patients with presumed autoimmune epilepsy. *Neurology*. 2014;82:1578–1586.

Willie JT, Gross RE. Role of repeat ablation to treat seizure recurrence following stereotactic laser amygdalohippocampotomy. *Neurosurgery*. 2015;62(1):233–234.

Wyllie E, ed. *The Treatment of Epilepsy, Principles and Practice*. 4th ed. Philadelphia, PA: Lippincott Williams & Wilkins; 2006.

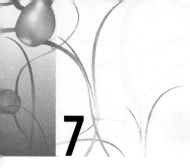

7

Approach to the Patient with Syncope

Peter A. Santucci, Joseph G. Akar, and David J. Wilber

Syncope is often used broadly to describe transient loss of consciousness (TLOC) and postural tone followed by spontaneous recovery. Though application of the term varies, modern usage commonly refers specifically to the subgroup of these related to transient global cerebral hypoperfusion (distinguishing syncope from TLOC from other causes such as seizure, trauma, or psychogenic causes). Though often of benign etiology, syncope can also be the manifestation of a dangerous underlying disorder or the precursor to sudden death. Even in benign forms, it can severely impact quality of life, not only by causing anxiety, but also by the potential restrictions on driving and work that may be necessary. In the United States, syncope accounts for approximately 1% of emergency department visits leading to over $2 billion of costs per year. More than a million individuals a year are evaluated for syncope and related injuries (e.g., falls, fractures), which not only creates a high cost burden on the healthcare system, but also is indicative of the significant impact on patient well-being and quality of life.

ETIOLOGY

Syncope is broadly defined as most commonly cardiovascular in etiology. Either a generalized or local cerebral impairment of blood/oxygen delivery can cause the loss of consciousness. Despite frequent referral for neurologic investigation after syncope, primary neurologic causes of TLOC are uncommon. However, neurally mediated cardiovascular causes resulting in impaired oxygen delivery (e.g., neurocardiogenic/vasovagal episodes) are the most common cause of syncope.

Even in cases where seizure-like motor activity is witnessed after the loss of consciousness, these may be a consequence of a cardiovascular etiology and an assessment for such is often warranted. Other causes of TLOC may present similarly and at times may be difficult to distinguish on initial evaluation.

Cardiovascular causes include decreased cardiac output secondary to abnormalities in heart rate (HR) and/or stroke volume, impairment of cerebral blood flow (CBF), and decreased blood pressure related to hypovolemia or decreased peripheral vascular resistance. Any medical condition causing one of these features may lead to the development of syncope. As shown in Table 7.1, the causes of syncope can be classified into broad categories: neurally mediated syncope, impaired orthostatic tolerance, cardiac arrhythmias, structural heart disease, and cerebrovascular steal syndromes. Based on pooled data from five studies, the incidence of the major causes of syncope is shown in Table 7.2.

Often multiple mechanisms can contribute to syncope. For example, medications, dehydration, or postprandial fluid shifts can exacerbate mild preexisting orthostatic intolerance, neurally mediated syncope, sinus node dysfunction, and impaired autoregulation of CBF. This is especially true in the elderly in whom syncope is commonly multifactorial.

Orthostatic intolerance can occur in several forms, including orthostatic hypotension, classic neurocardiogenic syncope, and postural orthostatic tachycardia syndrome (POTS). Some overlap can exist between these etiologies.

A. **Neurally mediated syncope,** also referred to as neurocardiogenic, reflex, or vasodepressor syncope, is common and results from the activation of a reflex that produces a significant vasodilatory (vasodepressor) and/or bradycardic (cardioinhibitory) response. Typically, it occurs after prolonged standing or sitting and may be reproduced on tilt-table testing. Long-term follow-up studies have shown that neurally mediated syncope carries a benign prognosis and a similar survival outcome to those patients with no history of syncope.

TABLE 7.1 Causes of Transient Loss of Consciousness

Syncopal

Neurally mediated
    Vasovagal syncope
    Carotid sinus syncope
    Situational syncope (cough, swallow, micturition, defecation, postprandial, and so on)
    Glossopharyngeal neuralgia
Orthostatic intolerance
    Orthostatic hypotension
        Volume depletion
        Medications
        Autonomic failure syndromes
        Primary autonomic failure (Parkinson's disease, MSA)
        Secondary autonomic failure (e.g., diabetes mellitus, amyloidosis)
        Alcohol or illicit drugs
        Postexercise
    POTS
Cardiac arrhythmias
    Bradyarrhythmias
        Sinus node dysfunction
        Atrioventricular conduction system disease
        Implantable device malfunction (pacemaker or defibrillator)
    Tachyarrhythmias
        Paroxysmal supraventricular and ventricular tachycardias
        Primary electrical abnormalities (long QT syndrome, Brugada's syndrome)
        Cardiomyopathies: Arrhythmogenic right ventricular dysplasia, hypertrophic,
            other cardiomyopathy
        Drug induced (e.g., torsades de pointes, bradycardia)
Structural cardiovascular disease
    Obstructive valvular disease, particularly aortic stenosis
    Hypertrophic obstructive cardiomyopathy
    Atrial myxoma
    Aortic dissection
    Pericardial tamponade
    Pulmonary embolism
Cerebrovascular
    Subclavian steal syndrome
    Stroke/TIA (uncommon)

Nonsyncopal

Seizure
Psychogenic
Metabolic and other conditions
    Electrolyte derangements
    Hypoglycemia
    Hypoxemia
    Anemia

Abbreviations: MSA, multiple system atrophy; POTS, postural orthostatic tachycardia syndrome, TIA, transient ischemic attack.

Table 7.1 shows various etiologies that can lead to neurally mediated syncope. Almost all of these etiologies can be diagnosed by a carefully taken history. Classic vasovagal syncope may be considered in this group and usually occurs in the setting of emotional or orthostatic stress, although it can also have an atypical presentation with no clear triggering events or premonitory signs. A careful history should also diagnose the etiology of several causes

TABLE 7.2 Incidence of Major Causes of Syncope and Transient Loss of Consciousness

Cause	%
Vasovagal	18
Situational	5
Orthostatic	8
Cardiac	18
Medication	3
Psychiatric	2
Neurologic	10
Carotid sinus	1
Unknown	34

of situational syncope (e.g., postprandial, postmicturition, postdefecation). Syncope due to carotid sinus hypersensitivity occurs in the setting of inadvertent mechanical pressure on the carotid sinus and can be reproduced by carotid sinus massage. Glossopharyngeal neuralgia may present with syncope associated with painful swallowing.

B. **Orthostatic hypotension/orthostatic intolerance syndromes** can cause inadequate cerebral perfusion leading to syncope upon rising from a sitting or supine to an upright position. The most common mechanism of hypotension is the loss of peripheral vascular tone because of failure of the autonomic nervous system to maintain peripheral vascular resistance. This can occur because of a primary dysfunction of the autonomic nervous system associated with several neurodegenerative conditions (multiple system atrophy) or because of diseases causing secondary autonomic nervous system failure (e.g., diabetes, amyloidosis). Multiple systems atrophy (MSA) encompasses a group of sporadic progressive neurologic disorders characterized clinically by autonomic dysfunction (i.e., orthostatic hypotension, impotence, urinary retention or incontinence, and so on), parkinsonism, and ataxia in any combination. Medications, alcohol, and drug toxicity should also be considered when evaluating orthostatic hypotension. Volume depletion (e.g., dehydration, hemorrhage, Addison's disease) may cause or exacerbate orthostatic syncope. Combinations of medications that contribute to orthostatic hypotension are a particularly common and overlooked cause.

POTS is a form of orthostatic intolerance in which the HR elevates (>30 bpm) in response to orthostatic stress in the absence of hypotension (blood pressure decrease <20 mm Hg). Although presyncope is more common, syncope also occurs in addition to a variety of other symptoms.

C. **Cardiac arrhythmias** often present with syncope because of a decrease in cardiac output. This can occur in bradycardia (e.g., sinus arrest, heart block) or tachycardia (e.g., nonsustained ventricular tachycardia/fibrillation). It is relatively uncommon for supraventricular tachycardias to cause syncope in the absence of other structural heart diseases or the Wolff–Parkinson–White syndrome (i.e., preexcited atrial fibrillation). Arrhythmic syncope may indicate a risk for sudden death and should be aggressively managed. In patients with congestive heart failure (CHF), syncope is associated with an increased risk of cardiovascular and total mortality.

D. **Structural heart disease** can cause syncope because of the inability to produce sufficient cardiac output to match demand. Obstructive valvular heart disease and hypertrophic cardiomyopathy are well-established etiologies. Primary pump failure due to myocardial dysfunction can also lead to syncope; however, associated ventricular arrhythmias are a more common cause. Other less common conditions include atrial myxoma and pericardial tamponade.

E. **Cerebrovascular and other vascular** causes of syncope are rare. These include acute aortic dissection and steal syndromes, such as subclavian steal, in which CBF is shunted away from the brain. Obstruction of CBF is a rare cause of true syncope. Most carotid artery distribution transient ischemic attacks (TIAs) cause unilateral visual impairment, weakness, or loss of sensation. Posterior circulation TIAs generally manifest as vertigo, diplopia, unilateral or bilateral hemianopia, ataxia or disequilibrium, but not loss of consciousness. Rare patients with TIA may have TLOC, but isolated syncopal episodes without accompanying neurologic symptoms should generally not be ascribed to a TIA.

F. **Psychogenic "syncope" (pseudosyncope)** is a form or TLOC mimicking syncope that occurs without any substantial changes in hemodynamics and is often associated with a prior significant psychologic event. Physical causes must be excluded. It and other causes are included in the differential diagnosis of TLOC, but are usually distinguished from true syncope.

G. **Syncope of unknown origin** is a diagnosis made after a careful history, physical examination, and selected laboratory tests have failed to elucidate a specific etiologic factor. Up to 40% of syncope may fall into this category. This diagnosis is clinically useful because it is associated with a prognosis considerably better than that of patients who have identifiable cardiac or neurologic causes of syncope. Although long-term follow-up studies have shown that patients with syncope and a history of cardiac or neurologic disease may have increased mortality rates, those patients with syncope of unknown causation have a distinctly better prognosis.

H. **TLOC from neurologic or other causes,** such as seizures or concussion, are distinct from syncope and are covered elsewhere (see Chapters 6, 37, 42, and 43).

EVALUATION

The evaluation of syncope should address these key questions:

- Was the loss of consciousness attributable to true syncope or to other causes? A careful history is crucial for making the diagnosis and excluding nonsyncopal etiologies. Table 7.3 lists some conditions that are commonly distinguished from syncope, some of which are associated with a TLOC.
- Which distinguishing features exist that may indicate the diagnosis? Table 7.4 lists features of vasovagal syncope, seizures, and cardiac syncope.
- Is heart disease present? This is an important question not only for diagnosis, but also for prognosis. Patients with syncope often have a fairly benign clinical course in the absence of heart disease. On the other hand, the presence of cardiac disease may carry a much more ominous prognosis.
- Is the patient at risk of sudden death? As syncope can be a manifestation of a life-threatening condition, a determination of patient risk should be made relatively early on.

Answering these questions can often largely be accomplished by an astute evaluation of the history and physical examination alone. Additional studies are used as needed to provide further insight or to guide therapy.

A. History.
The history is by far the most crucial component of the evaluation of syncope. In many cases, a good history alone can point to the diagnosis and afford a good evaluation of risk. Particular attention should be paid to the following points:

TABLE 7.3 Conditions to be Distinguished from Syncope

Disorders not associated with loss of consciousness
   Falls
   Drop attacks
Disorders associated with loss of consciousness
   Psychogenic (may or may not have loss of consciousness)
   Metabolic disorders
      Hypoglycemia
      Hypoxia
      Hyperventilation with hypocapnia
   Epilepsy
   Medication/pharmacologic (anesthetic/sedating including recreational drugs,
      alcohol)

TABLE 7.4 Typical Features of Vasovagal Syncope, Seizure, and Cardiac Syncope

	Vasovagal	Seizure	Cardiac
Feature onset	Subacute onset	Sudden onset or brief aura	Sudden onset
	Prodromal weakness, nausea	Auditory hallucinations or visual changes	None, chest pain, dyspnea, palpitations diaphoresis, and other cardiac symptoms may be present
Typical milieu or precipitating factor	Fatigue	Spontaneous onset	Often spontaneous onset
	Delayed prolonged standing or skipping meals	Triggered by flashing lights or monotonous sensory stimulation	During or following exertion
	Crowded enclosed confines pregnancy pain or trauma emotional situation		Known or suspected structural heart disease
Posture at time of onset	Standing or sitting	Standing, sitting, or supine	Standing, sitting, or supine
Appearance	Pallor	Normal or cyanotic stertorous respiration	Pallor transient loss of awareness
	Brief tonic–clonic motor activity possible	Stereotypic motor activity	Brief periods of tonic–clonic motor activity possible
	Occasional urinary incontinence	Urinary incontinence common	Urinary incontinence uncommon
Residual	Rapid recovery	Delayed recovery	Rapid or briefly delayed recovery
	Recurrence with resumption of upright posture possible	Postictal cognitive impairment	If prolonged hypoxia, evidence of central nervous system injury present system
		Todd's paralysis	Symptoms of cardiac dysfunction

1. Patient characteristics. In addition to the patient's current age and gender, the age of onset of syncope yields relevant clues in recurrent cases. A long-standing history of syncope from a young age in an otherwise healthy individual may suggest a neurocardiogenic etiology. Comorbidities are often relevant to the diagnosis. The most important prognostic factor in patients presenting with syncope is the presence of cardiac disease. Known comorbidities such as coronary artery disease, hypertension, congestive heart failure, hypertrophic obstructive cardiomyopathy, and valvular disorders require special emphasis. Symptoms associated with cardiac conditions such as palpitations, dyspnea, fluid retention, decreased exercise tolerance, lightheadedness, or chest pain require further evaluation.

2. Events leading to syncope. A patient's activity and posture before the episode should be noted. Syncope that occurs while supine may favor either an arrhythmic etiology or seizure, and largely excludes the etiologies dependent on orthostatic stress. Conversely, syncope occurring shortly after standing is typically because of orthostatic hypotension, while syncope during prolonged standing is most often neurocardiogenic. Vasovagal syncope is likely if the event was triggered by fear, pain, emotional distress, or blood draw.

Syncope occurring during or immediately after urination, defecation, coughing, or swallowing is a feature of situational syncope. Postprandial syncope is characterized by episodes that occur 15 to 90 minutes following meals. Syncope in the setting of neck manipulation such as extension, flexion, rotation, or compression (e.g., a tight shirt collar, necktie, or during shaving) may suggest carotid sinus hypersensitivity.

Syncope in the setting of exercise is particularly worrisome for a cardiac etiology. Syncope during physical exertion is a characteristic finding in aortic stenosis, atrioventricular (AV) block, or tachyarrhythmias, whereas loss of consciousness after exercise should arouse suspicion for hypertrophic cardiomyopathy or ventricular arrhythmia.

3. **Prodromal signs and symptoms** often provide clinically relevant information. Very brief prodromal symptoms lasting only seconds are a characteristic of cardiac causes, situational syncope, and orthostatic hypotension. Cardiac causes of syncope often do not have any prodromal symptoms or may present with dizziness and/or palpitations. On the other hand, vasovagal syncope typically has a more sustained warning period accompanied by symptoms of nausea, diaphoresis, and flushing. Focal neurologic symptoms such as vertigo, diplopia, ataxia, dysarthria, hemiparesis, and unilateral numbness are uncommon and may be indicative of a TIA as the cause of the loss of consciousness.

4. Events during the syncopal period. Though this typically requires the presence of a witness, obtaining as much detail as possible regarding the events during the syncopal episode may be highly valuable. The patient may be amnestic for events before, during, and after the episode. Often patients deny the loss of consciousness, even when it occurs. A detailed history confirming a true loss of consciousness and describing neuromuscular activity is extremely valuable. Although prolonged episodes of cerebral anoxia (more than 10 to 15 seconds) can induce brief involuntary motor activity, the presence of more sustained episodes of alternating tonic and clonic muscle action is strongly suggestive of a seizure. Urinary incontinence is more frequent among patients with seizures, although it can accompany syncope of any cause. Fecal incontinence is more specific for seizures.

5. Postsyncopal events. Details of events immediately following the loss of consciousness may provide important diagnostic clues. This history may also need to be obtained from witnesses. Prolonged duration of confusion, amnesia, or lethargy is more consistent with seizure activity rather than a cardiac or neurally mediated event. Similarly, the presence of focal neurologic symptoms or signs points to an inciting neurologic event such as a seizure with residual functional deficit (Todd's paralysis) or ischemic injury. Facial pallor points to syncope, facial plethora is more suggestive of seizure, and diffuse muscle soreness suggests seizure activity (see Chapters 5, 6, 42, and 43).

6. Family history. A family history of syncope, arrhythmias, or early sudden cardiac death may point to a genetic condition linked to ventricular arrhythmias, even in the absence of structural heart disease. Such a history should prompt more detailed cardiac investigation.

7. Comorbid conditions. In addition to the emphasis placed on obtaining a detailed history of any cardiovascular pathology, other comorbidities may be of relevance.

The history taker should address the possibility of neurologic disorders predisposing to seizures mimicking syncope. This includes primary or metastatic neoplasia, as well as a history of previous trauma, infection, and ischemic or hemorrhagic injury to the brain. Medical conditions such as diabetes mellitus, alcohol abuse, vitamin B_{12} deficiency, or other metabolic disorders are associated with peripheral or autonomic neuropathy and can cause orthostatic hypotension.

A gynecologic history should be elicited in appropriate patients to identify risk factors for pregnancy, particularly in ectopic locations. Pregnant patients are at increased risk of syncope because of orthostatic hypotension and vasovagal reactions. Moreover, a ruptured ectopic pregnancy occasionally manifests with syncope.

A history of anxiety disorders and depression is important to elucidate. Psychiatric illness should be suspected as a potential etiology, especially in patients with severe, atypical, repetitive, and drug-refractory episodes. Patients with psychogenic syncope may have reproducible symptoms on tilt-table testing despite a normal HR, blood pressure, and electroencephalography (EEG).

Finally, careful review of the patient's medication list is essential. Antihypertensive and other drugs can cause syncope by reducing cardiac output and lowering peripheral vascular resistance. As shown in Table 7.5, many antihypertensive and psychotropic medications can induce orthostatic hypotension. Numerous drugs can prolong the QT interval and may provoke ventricular arrhythmias that lead to syncope. Combinations of drugs can often be the culprit.

TABLE 7.5 Agents Causing or Exacerbating Orthostatic Hypotension

Angiotensin-converting enzyme inhibitors
Angiotensin receptor blockers
α-Blockers
β-Blockers
Calcium channel blockers
Diuretics
Nitrates
Sildenafil citrate
Phenothiazines
Opiates
Tricyclic antidepressants
Ethanol
Bromocriptine

B. Physical examination.
1. Vital signs should include an assessment of orthostatic hypotension, which is defined as a decrease of 20 mm Hg in systolic blood pressure or 10 mm Hg in diastolic blood pressure following standing from a supine position. It is important that the supine blood pressure be obtained after at least 5 minutes of recumbency and the standing blood pressure measured initially and again after the patient has been erect for at least 2 minutes.
2. Given the prognostic importance of cardiac disease, a detailed cardiovascular examination should be performed. Palpation of the carotid arteries may demonstrate weak and delayed carotid pulsation (pulsus parvus et tardus), which occurs with hemodynamically significant aortic stenosis, or biphasic carotid pulsation (pulsus bisferiens), which may be found in hypertrophic obstructive cardiomyopathy. Similarly, particular attention should be paid to the presence of systolic–crescendo–decrescendo murmurs, implying the presence of aortic stenosis or hypertrophic obstructive cardiomyopathy. Peripheral edema, elevated jugular venous pressure pulmonary crackles, hepatomegaly, and a third heart sound (S_3) signify heart failure. The presence of a carotid bruit signifies a high likelihood of diffuse atherosclerotic vascular disease involving the cerebral, coronary, and peripheral vasculature. A supraclavicular bruit and a diminished upper extremity arterial pulsation are evidence of subclavian steal syndrome.

   If carotid sinus supersensitivity is suspected, carotid massage can be performed in the absence of a bruit or known atheromatous disease. Carotid sinus hypersensitivity can be detected by means of monitoring changes in blood pressure and HR after 5 to 30 seconds of unilateral carotid artery massage. Responses are characterized as cardioinhibitory, vasodepressor, or mixed. Carotid sinus hypersensitivity is more common in older patients. Electrocardiographic and resuscitation equipment should be available.
3. A screening neurologic examination should be pursued to detect cognitive impairment, the presence of focal neurologic defects indicative of either acute neurologic injury or a preexisting substrate for a seizure disorder, peripheral neuropathy that would predispose to orthostatic hypotension, or a movement disorder that would cause nonsyncopal falls.
4. A digital rectal or stool examination should be considered if there is concern about gastrointestinal bleeding.
C. Laboratory and other studies.
1. Electrocardiography (ECG)
   a. ECG. The resting 12-lead ECG is an important test for both prognosis and triage. Although it is relatively uncommon for the ECG to directly demonstrate an arrhythmic cause for syncope, the presence of pathologic Q waves, left axis deviation, left bundle branch block, or left ventricular hypertrophy may point to underlying cardiac pathology. Severe sinus bradycardia or AV block may be diagnostic. Other ECG signs may suggest pulmonary embolism

      Repolarization abnormalities also may provide clues critical to determining the etiology of syncope. These include long QT intervals (long QT syndrome), epsilon waves with precordial T-wave inversions (arrhythmogenic right ventricular dysplasia/cardiomyopathy), and right bundle branch block with coved ST elevation in leads V1-V3 (Brugada's syndrome). Abnormally short QT intervals may also be relevant.

b. **Ambulatory electrocardiography.** Ambulatory electrocardiography has become a critical tool in the diagnosis of syncope. Because of the transient nature of arrhythmias causing syncope, routine 12-lead ECGs rarely capture the culprit arrhythmia, and extended monitoring is often required to make a definitive diagnosis. Several types of monitors could be used, depending on the frequency of the symptoms: 24-hour continuous recordings, patient-activated looping and nonlooping event monitors, and continuous 24-hour monitors that can be worn up to a period of 30 days or more.

Ambulatory monitoring has limited specificity because certain rhythm disturbances, such as brief pauses, premature atrial and ventricular contractions, and nonsustained ventricular tachycardia, can be detected even when they are not responsible for the syncope. Thus, it is important to correlate the findings of ambulatory monitoring with symptoms. If symptoms occur during monitoring and no ECG abnormalities are detected, a rhythm disturbance is effectively excluded as an etiologic factor.

c. **Implantable loop recorder (ILR).** Of increasing utility, subcutaneous ILRs for long-term monitoring have become an essential tool in the evaluation of syncope of unknown etiology. Newer-generation ILRs can be injected in the anterior chest in a brief procedure requiring only a local anesthetic, and have the energy to run for several years. These devices can unmask or exclude cardiac arrhythmias as the cause of infrequent episodes of recurrent syncope when all other evaluation has been inconclusive.

2. **Echocardiography** is one of the most widely used tests when evaluating patients for cardiac disease. Echocardiography can provide clues regarding the etiology of syncope such as valvular heart disease or atrial myxoma. More importantly echocardiography can confirm or exclude the presence of left ventricular dysfunction, which is associated with a risk of sudden cardiac death and which carries important prognostic implications.

3. **Blood laboratory testing.** Serum electrolyte abnormalities should be excluded. Elevated prolactin levels have been reported in some patients hours after generalized tonic–clonic seizures. The same is true for creatine kinase levels, although increased serum concentrations also can be caused by injury during a syncopal episode. Serum glucose levels are most valuable at the time of the event, particularly in evaluation of diabetic patients who have recently increased their insulin or oral hypoglycemic therapy or decreased their caloric intake. A complete blood count is occasionally helpful if blood loss or severe anemia is suspected.

Arterial blood gas analysis can be useful in evaluation of the occasional patient in whom pulmonary embolism is suspected because of the history, physical examination findings, or ECG results.

4. **Stress testing or coronary angiography** to assess for coronary ischemia is appropriate in some patients, particularly the elderly, those with exertional symptoms (syncope, chest pain, or dyspnea), cardiomyopathy, or ventricular arrhythmias.

5. **Electrophysiologic testing** is used to assess the integrity of the sinus node, cardiac conduction system, as well as the predisposition to ventricular and supraventricular arrhythmias. However, sensitivity is limited. The results are most often abnormal in patients with known heart disease or those with significant abnormalities on a routine ECG. Findings of greatest diagnostic value include inducible monomorphic ventricular tachycardia, markedly abnormal sinus node recovery times, inducible supraventricular tachycardia with hypotension, significant infra-His conduction disease, and pacing-induced infra-His block. Recent studies have shown that patients with underlying left ventricular dysfunction are at high risk of arrhythmic death and benefit from prophylactic defibrillator insertion even in the absence of syncope. Thus, patients with syncope and left ventricular dysfunction may not necessarily benefit from electrophysiologic testing to assess inducibility of ventricular arrhythmias.

6. **Tilt-table testing.** The utility of tilt-table testing for the diagnosis of neurocardiogenic syncope remains poorly defined. It is only a moderately sensitive and specific test. A positive result is reproducible only 70% of the time. The limited reproducibility of the test and the variable natural history of unexplained syncope reduce its utility. Abnormal response patterns to tilt-table testing include the vasovagal response, which consists of a decrease in blood pressure (vasodepressor) and bradycardia (cardioinhibitory), and

the dysautonomic response, which represents a failure of the autonomic system to compensate for an acute decrease in venous return that occurs with upright posture. Thus, the HR does not significantly change while the blood pressure declines. A third response to tilt-table testing is the POTS response in which there is a significant increase in HR in response to upright positioning.

7. **Radiographic studies/magnetic resonance imaging (MRI).** Routine head computed tomography (CT) and MRI of the brain have low yields but may be useful in the evaluation of patients who have sustained major head trauma, have a newly diagnosed seizure disorder, or have focal deficits on the neurologic examination (see Chapter 35). In addition, cardiac CT and MRI are becoming valuable means of detecting abnormal cardiac substrate that may not have been found by other means.

8. **EEG** is not required routinely, but should be performed when clinical evaluation points to seizure or in syncope of undetermined etiology when there is adequate suspicion (see Chapter 36).

9. **Device interrogation.** Patients with syncope in the presence of implanted pacemakers or implantable cardioverter defibrillators should have the devices checked by appropriate personnel. Not only should device malfunction be excluded as a cause of syncope, but modern devices store a plethora of diagnostic information that may be useful in diagnosis.

MANAGEMENT

The majority of syncope is of cardiovascular cause, and the diagnosis is often suggested after a complete history and physical examination. The goals of syncope management are twofold. One is prevention of further syncope and its potential effects including physical injury, driving risks, and work restrictions. Even more important is the prevention of sudden death in those at risk. Some patients with syncope from life-threatening cardiac disorders may appear healthy and be otherwise asymptomatic. For example, highly functional athletes, including at the professional level, may have malignant conditions (hypertrophic cardiomyopathy, genetic causes of ventricular arrhythmias, and so on) that lead to sudden cardiac death.

If the cause is unclear, evaluation of a resting 12-lead ECG should be performed in nearly all patients. Patients with symptoms or signs of cardiac disease, those with abrupt syncope without warning, and those with a concerning family history of sudden death receive more detailed cardiac evaluation, which often includes echocardiography, evaluation for coronary artery disease, and referral to a cardiologist or electrophysiologist. Further cardiac testing, including electrophysiologic studies and/or long-term cardiac monitoring, may be appropriate (see Video 7.1). Patients with unexplained syncope at high risk may be appropriate for preventive therapies, including the implantation of cardiac rhythm devices. Neurocardiogenic syncope can sometimes be difficult to manage because of the limitations of currently available therapies. Some orthostatically induced causes can also be challenging. Treatment should be in accordance with recent guidelines. When the symptoms are deemed not to be of cardiovascular etiology or are nonsyncopal (e.g., seizure, psychogenic, traumatic), the patient should be managed accordingly or referred to the appropriate specialist.

Key Points

- Syncope, even when broadly defined, is most commonly cardiovascular in etiology.
- Though most cases are of benign etiology, recurrent symptoms can severely impact quality of life and should be aggressively managed.
- Syncope can be the initial manifestation of serious cardiovascular conditions that may place the patient at risk of sudden death.
- With proper knowledge and questioning, the diagnosis is often suggested after a complete history and physical examination.
- The goals of syncope evaluation and management are twofold. One is the prevention of further syncope when feasible. However, the evaluation of risk and the prevention of sudden death are even more critically important.
- An assessment for heart disease is appropriate in many cases, particularly if the diagnosis is uncertain after the initial evaluation.

Recommended Readings

Brignole M. Diagnosis and treatment of syncope. *Heart.* 2007;93:130–136.

Brignole M, Albani P, Benditt D, et al. Guideline on management (diagnosis and treatment) of syncope. *Eur Heart J.* 2004;25:2054–2072.

Fenton AM, Hammill SC, Rea RF, et al. Vasovagal syncope. *Ann Intern Med.* 2000;9:714–725.

Grubb BP, Kosinski D. Dysautonomic and reflex syncope syndromes. *Cardiol Clin.* 1997;15:257–268.

Kapoor WN. Syncope. *N Engl J Med.* 2000;25:1856–1862.

Kenny RA, Brignole M, Dan G-A, et al. Syncope Unit: rationale and requirement—the European Heart Rhythm Association position statement endorsed by the Heart Rhythm Society [published online ahead of print June 24, 2015]. *Europace.* doi:10.1093/europace/euv115.

Middlekauff HR, Stevenson WG, Stevenson LW, et al. Syncope in advanced heart failure: high risk of sudden death regardless of origin of syncope. *J Am Coll Cardiol.* 1993;21:110–116.

Moss AJ, Zareba W, Hall J, et al. Prophylactic implantation of a defibrillator in patients with myocardial infarction and reduced ejection fraction. *N Engl J Med.* 2002;346:877–883.

Moya A, Sutton R, Ammirati F, et al; Task Force for the Diagnosis and Management of Syncope of the European Society of Cardiology (ESC), European Heart Rhythm Association (EHRA), Heart Failure Association (HFA), Heart Rhythm Society (HRS). Guidelines for the diagnosis and management of syncope (version 2009). *Eur Heart J.* 2009;30(21):2631–2671.

Olshansky B, Poole JE, Johnson G, et al. SCD-HeFT Investigators. Syncope predicts the outcome of cardiomyopathy patients: analysis of the SCD-HeFT study. *J Am Coll Cardiol.* 2008;51(13):1277–1282.

Saklani P, Krahn A, Klein G. Syncope. *Circulation.* 2013;127:1330–1339.

Sheldon RS, Grubb BP, Olshansky B, et al. 2015 Heart Rhythm Society expert consensus statement on the diagnosis and treatment of postural tachycardia syndrome, inappropriate sinus tachycardia, and vasovagal syncope. *Heart Rhythm.* 2015;12(6):e41–e63.

Soteriades ES, Evans JC, Larson MG, et al. Incidence and prognosis of syncope. *N Engl J Med.* 2002;347:878–885.

Zaidi A, Clough P, Cooper P, et al. Misdiagnosis of epilepsy: many seizure-like attacks have a cardiovascular cause. *J Am Coll Cardiol.* 2000;36:181–184.

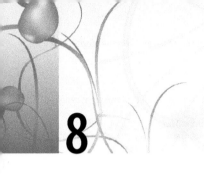

Approach to the Patient with Gait Disturbance and Recurrent Falls

8

Xabier Beristain

The act of walking is often perceived as a natural and simple activity, yet is a very complex motor skill. Therefore, any disruption of the anatomical structures involved in generating and maintaining a normal posture and gait would translate into a gait disorder. Gait and balance disorders are very common and a significant source of disability and diminished quality of life, with about 20% of older adults having difficulty walking or requiring an assistive device to ambulate. Arguably balance and gait examination is one of the most informative parts of the neurologic exam and able to provide a significant insight about the patient's functional status.

PATHOPHYSIOLOGY

A. **Locomotion** could be described as cyclic, patterned movements of the limbs with advancement in space and requiring controlled integration of posture and movement. Postural control is required to assure dynamic and static stability. For effective locomotion, appropriate locomotor patterns have to be generated and modified as needed on the basis of goals; inputs obtained from somatosensory, vestibular, and visual pathways; and changing environmental factors. These inputs are also combined with experience to adjust to the environmental conditions and anticipate any potential threatened stability. These anticipatory mechanisms may require tapping into the working memory and cognitive abilities that unfortunately can already be affected in patients with brain disorders.

B. **Anatomy and physiology.** The generation and control of locomotion are governed by a three-level network that also requires anticipatory postural adjustments mediated by the corticoreticulospinal system. The three levels include the spinal central pattern generator (CPG), the brainstem locomotor regions, basal ganglia output and its descending pathways, and control from the cerebral cortex (Fig. 8.1).

   1. **Spinal locomotor CPGs.** The spinal cord generates muscle activation patterns with reciprocal burst of activity in flexor and extensor muscles of the same limb. The rhythmic alternation of right and left limb movements is achieved through second-order interneurons in the Rexed lamina that project to the contralateral side. The activity of the CPG is modulated by sensory proprioception feedback and skin afferents. The centers for postural muscle synergies are likely localized rostrally, in the ventromedial reticular formation, as suggested by spinal cats that can walk but cannot maintain balance.

   2. **Brainstem locomotor regions** include three areas involved in locomotion: the **mesencephalic locomotor region (MLR)**, the **subthalamic locomotor region (SLR)**, and the **cerebellar locomotor region (CLR)**. The **MLR** is located mainly in the cuneiform nucleus, by the pedunculopontine nucleus (PPN), and receives inputs from the prefrontal cortices and the SLR. It is hypothesized that the excessive inhibitory effects exerted by the basal ganglia over the PPN/MLR maybe the pathophysiologic basis for gait disturbance in Parkinson's disease. Because the **SLR** is part of the lateral hypothalamus, it may contribute to emotional motor behaviors that would be mediated by the MLR. The **CLR** is located in the medial aspect of the cerebellar white matter. The CLR appears to exert its action on locomotor rhythm generation through the MLR. Muscle tone is influenced both by inhibitory and excitatory pathways at the brainstem level. The inhibitory system, mainly mediated by the PPN, regulates postural muscle tone, rhythm, and pattern of locomotion. The excitatory reticulospinal tract from the mesencephalic reticular formation, in addition to activating the CPG, increases postural tone. The vestibulospinal tract controls the overall level of muscle tone while

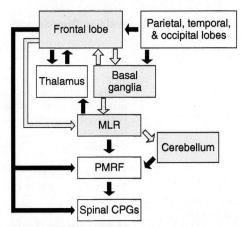

FIGURE 8.1 Summary of important areas involved in human locomotion. *Shaded areas* are hypothesized to be important in the development of HLGDs. CPGs, central patterns generators; HLGD, high-level gait disorder; MLR, mesencephalic reticular formation; PMRF, pontomedullary reticular formation. (From Nutt JG. Higher-level gait disorders: an open frontier. *Mov Disord.* 2013;28(11):1560–1565.)

the rubrospinal tract may regulate flexor muscle activity during locomotion such as when stepping over obstacles.

3. **Cortical locomotor areas.** The **premotor (PM)** and the **supplementary motor area (SMA)** are very important for gait initiation. PM cortex may be responsible for sensory-guided gait initiation, whereas the SMA may be also important for postural control. The temporoparietal cortex may integrate inputs from visual, vestibular, and proprioceptive pathways that would help to generate, in real-time, motor programs by the PM and SMA to adapt to a changing walking environment or situation.

ETIOLOGY

A. **Gait disturbances.** A gait disturbance could be understood as a gait pattern that deviates from the accepted "normal" gait; in that sense defective synchrony, fluency, smoothness and symmetry while walking, among other features, would represent an abnormal gait. A gait disturbance may be caused by disruption at any level of the neuraxis, and following the proposal by Nutt, Marsden, and Thompson gait disorders can be classified in a hierarchical anatomically based system. This classification divides gait disorders into low-level, middle-level, and high-level gait disorders (HLGDs) (Table 8.1). It should be taken into account that multiple factors are often at play to cause gait disturbance, particularly in the elderly.

B. **Causes of recurrent falls.** Errors in judgment and environmental hazards are responsible for one-third to one-half of the falls. About one-third of people older than 65 years may fall at least once a year, with one-fourth of them suffering a serious injury and about 5% of them having a fracture. Most of the patients with recurrent falls have neurologic disease, and the incidence of falls in hospitals and nursing facilities is almost three times the rates for community-dwelling older adults over 65 years of age. Common cause of recurrent falls include peripheral neuropathy, residual of stroke, diffuse cerebral ischemic disease, parkinsonian syndromes, dementing illnesses, effects of medication, orthostatism, vestibulopathy, and poor vision, among others.

CLINICAL MANIFESTATIONS

A. **Features of normal walking.** The gait cycle is defined as the time between successive heel–floor contacts with the same foot, and it consists of two steps that would be one stride (Fig. 8.2). The gait cycle can be divided into two phases: **stance phase** and **swing**

TABLE 8.1 Higher-, Middle-, and Lower-Level Gait Disorder and Their Anatomical Correlates

Levels	Anatomical Level	Balance and Gait Pattern
	Psychological/psychiatric	Variable: slow, buckling knees
Higher	Cortex	Different patterns: cautious, parkinsonian, ataxic,
Higher	Subcortical	spastic, magnetic, gait ignition failure, disequilibrium
Middle	Basal ganglia	Parkinsonian/dystonic/choreic
Middle	Thalamus	Astasia/ataxia
Middle	Cerebellum	Cerebellar ataxia
Middle	Brainstem	Ataxia/spasticity
Middle	Spinal cord	Spastic gait/tabetic gait
Lower	Peripheral nerve	Sensory ataxia/vestibular disequilibrium/visual
	Proprioception, vestibular, visual	disequilibrium
Lower	Neuromuscular junction	Waddling
Lower	Muscle	Waddling, steppage, Trendelenburg
	Skeleton	Antalgic/compensatory for deformities

phase. About 60% of the gait cycle is spent in the stance phase and 10% of that time is bipedal support. The stance phase is when the foot is on the ground; the swing phase is the time when the foot is in the air. The stance phase can be divided into initial double-limb support, single-limb stance, and second double-limb support. The swing phase is divided into initial swing, mid swing, and terminal swing. Gait parameters such as step length, cadence, and step height are shown in Table 8.2.

1. **Stride length (length of two successive steps) and cadence (steps per minute)** determine the velocity of walking. Gait velocity and step length are lower among women while cadence is higher in women. The most commonly affected gait parameters in older individuals are the reduction of walking speed and step length and increase in bipedal support. The magnitudes of arm swing, toe–floor clearance, and hip and knee rotations

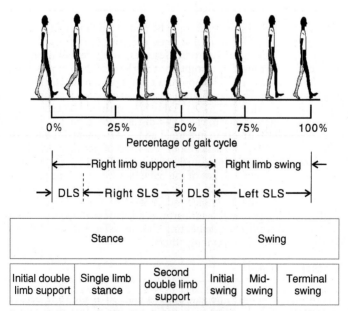

FIGURE 8.2 Phases of the normal gait cycle, expressed as percentage of total stride. DLS, double-limb support; SLS, single-limb support.

TABLE 8.2 Gait Parameters

Stance phase	When the foot is on the floor
Swing phase	When the foot is in the air
Stance time	The time when the foot is on the floor
Swing time	The time when the foot is in the air
Cadence	Number of steps per minute
Step length	Distance advanced by one foot compared to the position of the other
Stride length	The sum of two consecutive step lengths or the distance advanced by one foot compared to its prior position
Step time	Time between heel strike of one foot to heel strike of the other foot
Gait cycle	The time between two consecutive heel strikes of the same foot
Stride time	Time for a full gait cycle
Average gait velocity	Stride length divided by stride time

are proportional to stride length and velocity. Reduced gait velocity is a nonspecific sign of an underlying medical condition and is associated with reduced long-term survival.

2. **The total-body center of mass** oscillates vertically and horizontally during ambulation. The maximal vertical oscillation happens during the single-limb support, while the most lateral horizontal excursions of the center of gravity occur at the times of mid-single-limb support. These vertical and horizontal excursions of the center of mass are optimized to consume the least amount of energy. Therefore, most gait disorders are associated with increased energy expenditure during ambulation.

B. **Normal development of walking.** Most children walk independently by 15 months, and failure to walk by 18 months should be investigated as it could be indicative of an underlying central nervous system (CNS) pathology, neuromuscular disease, visual impairment, or vestibular disease. Maturation of gait and balance probably continues throughout childhood, but most of this maturation is accomplished by 3 or 4 years of age. By 5 years, the child should be able to walk, run, hop, skip, and jump.

C. **Abnormal patterns of walking.** Gait abnormalities can be classified in a hierarchical way as emerging from disturbances at different levels of the neuraxis and neuromuscular system. With this in mind, we may divide gait disorders as lower-, middle-, and higher-level gait disorders on the basis of the levels of motor control of locomotion. It should also be taken into account that the characteristics of an abnormal gait are usually a combination of the underlying pathologic process, compensatory mechanisms, and potential development of secondary musculoskeletal abnormalities.

1. **Lower-level gait disorders**

   The clinical characteristics of lowest- and middle-level gait disorders are predictable and consistent with the observed neurologic and neuromuscular deficits. The associated compensatory mechanisms are appropriate although limited by the underlying pathologic process and do not have a maladaptive counterproductive quality. Lower-level gait disorders are caused by disease of the muscles, peripheral nerves, skeletal pathology, peripheral vestibular system, and anterior visual pathway.

   a. **Steppage gait.** Steppage gait is seen in the context of weakness of foot dorsiflexion and could be uni- or bilateral. For the toes to clear the ground during the swing phase of gait and to avoid tripping, it will require an exaggerated knee and hip flexion on the affected leg; the step is high and short, and the foot commonly slaps the floor at the end of swing phase. Peroneal nerve injury, radicular compromise, and a demyelinating neuropathy are common causes of this gait pattern.

   b. **Waddling and Trendelenburg gaits.** The waddling gait pattern can be seen with bilateral hip girdle muscle weakness and in patients with bilateral orthopedic hip problems. Gait is wide based, short stepped, and associated to increased alternating lateral body sway and excessive hip drop. Increased arm abduction may also occur as well as exaggerated lumbar lordosis if there is superimposed weakness of the paraspinal muscles. Trendelenburg gait is characteristic of unilateral hip abductor weakness, and it is associated with ipsilateral lurching of the torso and hip drop on the contralateral side while standing on the leg of the affected side.

c. **Sensory ataxia.** The ataxic gait is characterized by wide base with variability in step length, and there is considerable stride-to-stride variability. This is associated with unsteadiness, and it is not specific for a particular location in the neuraxis: it can be seen in the context of proprioceptive deficits (i.e., sensory ataxia), cerebellar dysfunction (i.e., cerebellar ataxia), and pontine and thalamic pathology. The problem is more obvious when the eyes are closed (Romberg test). Abnormal postural sway can be present during stance with eyes open and closed.

d. **Visual disequilibrium.** Sensation of being off balance in the context of acute visual distortion such as when putting new prescription glasses on. This is typically associated with increased base of support, cautiousness, and tentative steps.

e. **Vestibular disequilibrium.** Acute vestibular dysfunction may cause vertigo, with potential nystagmus, instability, and a tendency to veer or fall toward the affected side. When the problem is chronic, the symptoms are usually less dramatic, but the gait tends to be still cautious and mildly wide based, and the patient has difficulty with Romberg maneuver and tandem walking. Patients are able to stand and walk without assistance despite their disequilibrium.

f. **Sensory disequilibrium.** It refers to feelings of unsteadiness when there is a conflict among inputs from visual, proprioceptive, and vestibular pathways. Acutely, this can be associated with falls but it may become chronic specially if there is significant loss of at least two of these sensory modalities or there is no adjustment of the CNS to the conflictive information from the different sensory modalities. In this setting, the gait is slow and cautious, with increased bipedal support.

2. **Middle-level gait disorders**

Middle-level gait disorders are caused by ascending or descending sensorimotor tract lesions, cerebellar dysfunction, bradykinesia, and hyperkinetic movement disorders.

a. **Spastic gait and scissoring.** Lesion of the corticospinal tracts causes spastic gaits that can be hemiparetic or paraparetic depending if the lesion is uni- or bilateral. In spastic gaits there is often a component of associated weakness. **Spastic hemiparetic** gaits are characterized by lower limb hyperextension with difficulty to flex hips and knees and excessive plantar flexion and inversion of the foot. Arm swing is reduced with flexor or dangling arm posture. The base of support is narrow and because of the hyperextension of the leg, to clear the ground while walking, will require a semicircular movement at the hip during the swing phase (circumduction; Video 8.1). Patients with little spasticity and appropriate proximal strength may clear the floor during the swing phase with increased hip flexion. **Spastic paraparesis** is more commonly seen in patients with spinal cord injuries and shares some features with hemiparetic gaits. In a sense, it could be imagined as walking on water up to the waist level. In addition, in many cases, arm swing and upper limb posture are relatively normal depending on the level of the pyramidal tract compromise. **Spastic diplegic gait** could be understood as a bilateral hemiparetic gait with some particular features; the knees and hips are significantly flexed and hips are also adducted during the gait cycle, causing the legs to cross each other in a pattern termed "scissoring." Compared to bilateral hemiparesis in adults, in spastic diplegia the upper extremities and bulbar musculature are usually much less affected than the lower extremities.

b. **Cerebellar ataxia** occurs typically in patients with bilateral damage to the cerebellum. Gait is wide based with significant stride-to-stride variability. Upper and lower limb movements are uncoordinated and abnormal postural sway during quiet stance is present. Different patterns of gait abnormality can be seen depending on what regions of the cerebellum are involved (i.e., lateral, intermediate, and medial functional zones). The medial zone (vermis) regulates extensor tone and dynamic balance control, and modulates the rhythmicity of flexor and extensor muscles. Therefore, a rostral vermian and paravermian lesion produces a predominantly trunkal and lower limb ataxia. This pattern of cerebellar degeneration is typically seen in chronic alcoholism and chronic thiamine deficiency. Caudal midline vestibulocerebellar damage produces disequilibrium and eye movement abnormalities. Patients tend to fall toward the side of the cerebellar or central vestibular lesion. Damage to the vestibular nuclei can produce a sensation that the environment is tilted and that the body is being pulled toward the side of the lesion. The intermediate cerebellar zone is important while performing precise goal-directed limb movements. The lateral cerebellum plays a significant role in adjusting to a new context or when strong visual guidance is required during ambulation but it seems to be less important in uninterrupted walking.

c. **Parkinsonian gait.** Short-stepped shuffling gaits are often referred to as parkinsonian gaits and are typically seen among patients with frontal lobe and basal ganglia dysfunctions. The typical gait in Parkinson's disease is narrow-based with short and slow steps and associated with stooped-over posture, stiff trunk, and diminished asymmetric arm swing. Turns are characteristically slow, requiring multiple steps, often more than four or five steps. Festination is the tendency to walk faster and faster with diminished step length, like trying to chase the center of gravity, and it is often seen in patients with freezing of gait (FoG). In cases of cerebrovascular disease with parkinsonian-like gait the base of support tends to be wider than in classic Parkinson's disease and arm swing has higher amplitude than the step length.

d. **Choreic gait** is characterized by superimposed abnormal hyperkinetic movements on top of the normal gait pattern, causing random extremity and trunk movements and postural shifts that can give the gait a bizarre, dance-like appearance ("chorea"). Choreic gait is often associated to increased risk of falling.

e. **Dystonic gait** is a pattern of walking in which extremity and trunkal movements and postural shifts are interrupted by tonic or phasic co-contractions of antagonistic muscles in a fairly stereotypic fashion. There is often some foot intorsion and the disorder can be task specific, making walking backward sometimes easier than walking forward. The abnormal postures and patterns observed while walking will depend on the extent of the dystonic disorder and give the gait a bizarre appearance.

3. **Higher-level gait disorders**

HLGDs are caused by impairment of the cortical–basal ganglia–thalamocortical pathways. Over the years multiple terms have been used to describe these walking difficulties, such as lower-body parkinsonism, gait apraxia, magnetic gait, or frontal lobe gait disorders to name a few. HLGD is not a single entity and it encompasses several potential gait patterns that are characterized by some of the following features:

a. Bizarre or inadequate postural synergy, limb and trunkal placement, and interactions with the environment (e.g., leaning backward when trying to get up from a chair).

b. Poor or absent rescue responses to postural perturbation.

c. Variable performance based on changes in the environment or emotional status.

d. Freezing or hesitation with seemingly insignificant environmental challenges (e.g., FoG while going through a doorway).

Bilateral lesions produce more significant disturbances of gait and it is often seen in parkinsonian syndromes and dementias as well as in extensive cerebrovascular disease. Unilateral lesions, on the other hand, cause a tendency to fall away from the lesion.

Some HLGD gait patterns:

1. **Cautious gait.** It is a gait pattern characterized by a widened base, slow speed, and diminished step length that resembles someone walking on ice. This is seen when an individual is walking in response to a real or perceived lack of balance and it is more commonly seen in elderly people. It is associated with slightly stooped posture, increased double-limb support, widened base, and reduced arm swing. This pattern can be seen in patients with cerebrovascular disease and neurodegenerative disorders but, unfortunately, this pattern of walking is nonspecific and provides with no significant clues to understand the underlying pathologic process.

2. **Fear of falling.** This is a maladaptive behavior in which perceived disequilibrium or previous falls have triggered an abnormal gait pattern. This is characterized by a tendency to grab or hold onto other people, walls, or furniture when trying to walk for fear of falling. This fearfulness is very often out of proportion to the actual walking abilities and it can be very limiting to the point that the patient may refuse to walk.

3. **FoG.** It is an episodic and brief spell of absence or significant reduction of forward progression while trying to walk to the point that feet may seem to be glued to the ground. Patients move their extremities relatively normally while seated or recumbent, but their feet appear to stick to the floor while walking. When the difficulty happens as the patient is trying to initiate gait it is called **start hesitation** or gait ignition failure; if it happens before getting to a target destination it is called **destination hesitation.** Environmental distractions and obstacles such as going through a doorway exacerbate or trigger FoG.

4. **Frontal and subcortical disequilibrium.** Disequilibrium due to acute unilateral frontal lobe lesions causes patients to fall away from the side of the lesion; lesion in the basal ganglia, ventrolateral thalamus, or dorsolateral midbrain causes a tendency to fall backward and laterally away from the lesion. However, when the lesions affect both frontal lobes or the subcortical structures just mentioned, the disequilibrium is more profound and sustained. This disequilibrium is characterized by poor synergy between postural and locomotor abilities and they are associated to inappropriate and very often counterproductive adjustments; patients may lean the wrong direction in such a way that stability and locomotion are compromised. This causes difficulty keeping balance while standing and potentially while sitting as well.

4. **Other gait disorders**

   a. **Antalgic gait.** Stance and gait are modified to reduce pain and decrease time in the stance phase on the affected limb is the norm. This is associated commonly to limping. The actual gait pattern would change depending on the location of the pain, for example, with hip pain it will be the so-called "abductor lurch" with shifting of the upper torso toward the painful hip during the single-limb stance on the painful hip and there is no hemipelvis drop like the one seen in Trendelenburg gait. In addition to pain, skeletal deformities are also associated to changes in stance and walking.

   b. **Functional/psychogenic gait.** Psychiatric disorders such as depression and schizophrenia may affect walking and balance; very often these patients walk slower and with diminished step length. Conversely, patients with psychogenic gait disorders tend to display bizarre and variable gait patterns that do not fit with known patterns of organic gait disorders. The most common patterns include excessive slowness, buckling of the knees, and acrobatic-like gait (i.e., **astasia–abasia**). Patients frequently lean, lurch, and gyrate in a manner that requires good balance and coordination. With distraction or suggestion patient's gait may improve even if this is more challenging than the original spontaneous gait observed (e.g., asking patient to walk on heels or toes; reciting months of the years backward while walking). Sudden onset of symptoms, a paroxysmal course, inconsistent and changing gait patterns, or acrobatic-like postures or gait while retaining the ability to perform quick steady normal turns should prompt considering a functional etiology. However, the clinician should exercise caution when making this diagnosis as some brain disorders may be associated to bizarre-appearing gaits.

EVALUATION

A. **History** is critical in determining the cause of the gait difficulties and it should be focused on the nature of the problem, timing, modifying factors, falls, and comorbidities that may have a negative impact on the ability to walk. This is important to establish the cause and potentially suggest the most appropriate workup and therapeutic approach in patients with gait difficulties.

   1. **Functional disability** is largely determined with a careful history. The frequency and circumstances of falls and the ability to perform various activities of daily living (dressing, bathing, climbing stairs, and getting in and out of bed and chairs) are important measures of disability.

   2. **Associated signs and symptoms** may suggest the cause such as rest tremor in Parkinson's disease, vertigo in vestibulopathies, urinary incontinence in patients with normal pressure hydrocephalus (NPH) or multiple system atrophy (MSA), paresthesia in patients with neuropathy or muscle wasting in patients with neuromuscular disease, for instance.

B. **Physical examination** is aimed at trying to anatomically localize the lesion and establish the degree of disability. This should include a full neurologic exam and a general physical

TABLE 8.3 Inspection and Examination of Gait and Posture

Balance while sitting	If balance while sitting is poor it would suggest profound imbalance or weakness
Standing up from a sitting position	Does the patient sequence the appropriate movements to stand up? Does the patient need to use hands to stand up from a chair?
Balance while standing	Can the patient stand without assistance? Does the patient need a wide base of support to stand? Does he/she sway with the eyes open?
Balancing on one foot	Is the patient able to stand on one foot for at least 10 sec? (healthy adults up to 80 yr may stand at least that long on one foot)
Gait initiation	How long does it take to start walking? Is the step length appropriate while starting to walk?
Gait parameters	Pay attention to step length and height, cadence, rhythmicity, and speed that should be over 1 m/sec
Base width	Distance between malleoli should be zero inches (unless anatomical deformities or obesity); more than that is abnormal but nonspecific
Arm swing	Amplitude, rhythmicity, and asymmetries should be noted. Abnormal in parkinsonian syndromes although not specific; it can be seen in orthopedic problems as well
Posture	Erect, stooped, hyperextended, tilted, twisted
FoG	Can be triggered by dual activities, turning or when going through doorways or narrow spaces
Romberg and enhanced Romberg test	Stand with feet together and see if patient sways both with eyes open and closed. If sway is worse with the eyes closed (positive Romberg) it would suggest vestibular or proprioceptive deficits. An enhanced Romberg test is a Romberg test done in tandem position
Tandem	Walking with one foot in front of the other
Turning	Number of steps needed to perform a 180 degrees turn while walking (1–2 steps is normal)
Dual task	Does the patient freeze up or stop walking when asked to perform a cognitive task?
Timed up and go	Walking from a chair, walk 3 m, turn and return to the chair (>14 sec may indicate risk of falling)
Pull test	The pull test evaluates the rescue response. To perform the test, the patient assumes a normal stance, and is instructed to hold his/her ground when briskly pulled backward at the shoulders by the examiner. The test is abnormal if the patient takes more than 1–2 steps to regain balance (the examiner must catch the patient, if necessary, to prevent a fall)

exam emphasizing the observation of gait parameters, posture, range of motion tandem walking, and the use of provocative tests such as the Romberg tests (Table 8.3). A detailed vestibular examination may be indicated in some patients (Table 8.4). Attention should be paid to localizing signs such as pyramidal signs, tremor, sensory changes, or dysmetria, for instance. The general examination should also look for physical signs of musculoskeletal problems, poor eyesight, cardiovascular diseases, and the possibility of orthostatism that could impact balance and walking.

C. **Laboratory studies** help to confirm the cause of the suspected gait disorder or to clarify the differential diagnosis inferred from the history and physical exam. The clinical suspicion should guide the clinician when deciding what studies are appropriate to answer the question at hand.

1. **Blood work** including a complete blood count, chemistry panel, and thyroid, renal, and liver function studies are frequently performed. Based on the clinical findings a vitamin B_{12} level is appropriate in cases of neuropathy, suspected subacute combined degeneration of the spinal cord, or elderly patients with cognitive difficulties and gait problems, for instance. Multiple other blood tests may be appropriate depending on the clinical suspicion. A lumbar puncture would be indicated in patients with suspected NPH to drain between 40 and 60 mL of cerebrospinal fluid (CSF) (i.e., Fisher's test) and establish if this would improve their ability to walk.

TABLE 8.4 Vestibular Evaluation

Nystagmus	Nystagmus is an involuntary, oscillatory, rhythmic eye movement with at least one slow phase Central nystagmus can be horizontal, vertical, or torsional Peripheral nystagmus is very often horizontal–torsional and it can be suppressed by visual fixation In benign paroxysmal positional vertigo of the posterior semicircular canal the nystagmus is typically vertical/rotatory
Hallpike's maneuver	The Hallpike's maneuver should be performed in patients with episodic vertigo especially if positional. With the patient sitting, the examiner turns the head to one side and rapidly places the patient in a supine position with the head overhanging the exam table. The patient is asked to keep the eyes open. The test is positive if a nystagmus and/or vertiginous symptoms similar to the ones described by the patients are triggered by the maneuver. The maneuver should be also performed with the head turned to the other side
Horizontal head impulse test (head thrust)	This test evaluates the vestibulo-ocular response (VOR) that it is necessary to maintain stable visual fixation while the head is moving The patient is asked to fixate on the examiner's nose, and the examiner quickly rotates the patient's head 20 degrees across the midline to the other side. A good technique is required as the most important factor of this maneuver is the acceleration (instructional videos can be found at http://novel.utah.edu/Newman-Toker/collection.php). When the head is rotated toward the side of a peripheral vestibular lesion, the eyes fail to be on target because of the impaired VOR and the head rotation is followed by a corrective saccade toward the examiner's nose. In patients presenting with an acute vestibular syndrome, a normal head–impulse response usually suggests a central lesion
Past pointing	With eyes open, the patient is to touch the fingers of the examiner. Then, with eyes closed, the patient tries to perform finger–nose–finger test. In case of labyrinth dysfunction it would be deviation to either the left or right in the direction of the affected labyrinth
Fukuda stepping test	Marching in place with eyes closed for 50–100 steps causes a deviation of more than 45 degrees in the direction of the affected labyrinth

2. **Imaging studies** such as brain MRI and head computed tomography (CT) scans are performed as needed, looking at the brain for enlarged ventricles, space-occupying lesions such as subdural fluid collection, old ischemic strokes, cerebral atrophy, and diffuse white matter changes. Evaluation of the spine may uncover evidence of space-occupying lesions, spinal stenosis, or spinal deformities that may cause walking difficulties. In cases of suspected degenerative parkinsonian syndromes a dopamine transporter scan may shed some light and show diminished uptake of the radioactive ligand in the striatum.
3. **Radiography** of the hips, spine, and extremities is performed as needed especially if orthopedic causes are suspected.
4. **Electromyography and nerve conduction studies** are helpful when suspecting a neuropathic or myopathic problem.
5. **Videonystagmography** and other vestibular and otologic tests may be helpful when a vestibular dysfunction is suspected as these tests may help distinguish central from peripheral vestibular disorders.
6. Comprehensive **gait and balance analysis** using instrumentation with optoelectronic systems, quantitative posturography, and shoe-integrated wireless sensor systems is possible but not widely available. Their role in the evaluation of most patients with gait difficulties is not well established at this point.

DIFFERENTIAL DIAGNOSIS

Differential diagnosis would depend on the gait patter observed and detailed history and physical exam. In older adults with fairly symmetric abnormal gait patterns it can be difficult to establish

TABLE 8.5 Differentiating the Neurologic Causes of Geriatric Gait Disturbances

Clinical Feature	Parkinson's Disease	White Matter Cerebrovascular Disease	NPH	PSP	MSA	Cervical Spondylosis
Asymmetric parkinsonism	++	+		+		
Pill-rolling rest tremor in the hands or rest tremor in the lower limbs	++					
Facial masking	++			++	++	
Reduced arm swing	++			++	++	
Good response to levodopa	++					
Postural instability and falls during the first year of symptoms		+	+	++	+	+
Prominent speech impairment during the first year of symptoms		+		++	++	
Stepwise progression		++				
Dementia in the first year or two of symptoms		++	+	++		
Subcortical white matter degeneration and microinfarcts		++				
Urinary dysfunction	+	+	++	+	++	+
Definite improvement after removal of 40–60 mL CSF by means of lumbar puncture			++			
Hydrocephalus (>0.3 Evans' ratio)			++			
Supranuclear downward gaze palsy				++		
Ataxia				+	++	
Early symptomatic orthostatic hypotension					++	
Spondylotic cervical spine and cord compression						++
Numb clumsy hands and Romberg's sign						++
Spastic lower limb movement						++

Abbreviations: +, suggestive; ++, highly suggestive; CSF, cerebrospinal fluid; NPH, normal pressure hydrocephalus; PSP, progressive supranuclear palsy.

the origin of the gait and balance problem because of a significant overlap of symptoms. Some of the conditions with fairly symmetric gait difficulties seen in older adults are shown in Table 8.5.

DIAGNOSTIC APPROACH

The **diagnostic approach** is based on trying to identify the primary cause or causes of gait disturbance and all contributing comorbidities. Most of the gait abnormalities seen in older patients are multifactorial and some of these comorbidities can be easily overlooked as individually their relative weight in causing gait difficulties might be low. However, multiple, and apparently minimal, problems can add up and significantly contribute to walking and balance difficulties. Some examples of comorbidities worth exploring include vitamin B_{12} deficiency, arthritic limbs, spinal deformities, neuropathy, deconditioning, hypothyroidism, depression, foot disorders, cardiopulmonary disease, orthostatic hypotension, visual impairment, vertigo, and medications (e.g., sedative-hypnotics, anticonvulsants, antipsychotics, and antiemetics). These contributing conditions are frequently more treatable than the primary neurologic illness.

CRITERIA FOR DIAGNOSIS

Criteria for diagnosis of gait **disorders** are heavily based on the medical and surgical history and findings on physical exam.

A. The diagnoses of neurodegenerative diseases (e.g., Parkinson's disease, MSA, and progressive supranuclear palsy [PSP]) are based largely or entirely on the history and physical examination.

B. The diagnoses of other central and peripheral causes of gait disturbance are corroborated with neuroimaging or electrophysiologic studies, as needed.

C. The diagnosis of **idiopathic** NPH is particularly challenging as the symptoms are not specific and the classic clinical triad of **gait disturbance**, **urinary incontinence**, and **cognitive dysfunction** may also occur in patients with vascular dementia, chronic subdural hematoma, and degenerative dementia. In addition, enlarged ventricles can be seen in patients with cerebral atrophy and dementia (i.e., "hydrocephalus ex-vacuo") that may already display some of those symptoms. Unfortunately, there is no ideal test to predict clinical response to CSF shunting.

   1. Unequivocal improvement in gait after removal of 40 to 60 mL of CSF through a lumbar puncture supports the diagnosis but does not occur in all patients as it has a low sensitivity, between 30% and 60%. Improvement after external lumbar CSF drainage for 3 days is more sensitive (over 80%) and specific, but has increased risk of complications.

   2. Improvement is achieved by approximately 50% of patients and sustained improvement by 30%. Complications occur in 20% of cases. Patients with an identifiable cause of hydrocephalus (e.g., aqueductal stenosis, Chiari's malformation, and previous meningitis or subarachnoid hemorrhage) are more likely to respond than are those with idiopathic hydrocephalus.

   3. Radiologic evidence of ventricular enlargement is necessary to establish the diagnosis of NPH. The **Evans' index** has been used to establish evidence of ventriculomegaly. The Evans' index is the ratio at the maximal frontal horn ventricular width divided by the inner diameter of the skull in axial cuts; a ratio >0.3 indicates ventriculomegaly. Unfortunately the index does not guarantee a beneficial response to ventriculoperitoneal shunting of CSF. As such the Evans' index has little role to play in the decision to shunt CSF in patients with suspected NPH.

D. **White matter brain lesions** have been linked to impaired balance, slower gait, and reduced mobility. White matter hyperintensities seen on T2-weighted MRI images in the frontal lobe and periventricular regions show the strongest relationships with balance and gait difficulties; in particular, bilateral symmetric periventricular white matter lesions in the frontal and occipito-parietal regions have been found to be sensitive (frontal) or specific (occipito-parietal) in discriminating individuals with increased difficulties with their mobility. These white matter lesions can be measures through MRI imaging by using the **Fazekas scale**. This scale quantifies the amount of white matter T2 hyperintensities, usually attributed to chronic small vessel ischemia, and gives them a grade, from 0 to 3, based on size and degree of confluence of white matter lesions. Moderate and severe white matter lesions according to the Fazekas scale have been, on average, independently associated with a deterioration of gait and balance.

REFERRAL

A. Neurologic consultation. All older adults should be asked about falls at least once a year. If there is an abnormal gait or recurrent falls they will require further evaluation by a clinician with appropriate skills and experience.

   1. A second opinion is advisable before shunting a patient with presumed NPH and before operating on a patient with presumed cervical spondylosis.

   2. Drug-resistant parkinsonism is strong evidence against the diagnosis of idiopathic Parkinson's disease.

B. **Physical therapy and vestibular rehabilitation** are considered cornerstones of management of gait and balance disorders. Vestibular rehabilitation is indicated when unsteadiness and vestibular dysfunction are involved and aimed at promoting vestibular adaptation and compensation. Prevention of falls should focus on physical conditioning and encourage regular physical activity. It should ideally be delivered through a multidimensional physical therapy activity program tailored to the patient's needs; it should include exercises to enhance strength, endurance, balance, and flexibility. A comprehensive safety evaluation of the patient's home by a physical therapist or visiting nurse is appropriate to establish potential fall hazards and suggest adaptations to the home environment. These adaptations may include the installation of handrails, raised toilet seats, grab bars in the shower, adequate lighting, and rubber floor mats among others. Elimination of throw rugs, clutter, and uneven surfaces would also decrease the risk of falls. The use of appropriately fitting shoes, with relatively firm slip-resistance soles and low heels is recommended and shoes with slippery soles, high heels, sleepers, and flip-flops should be avoided. Regarding mobility devices such as canes and walkers may improve balance and mobility if properly fit and should be prescribed after a complete evaluation by a physical therapist.

C. **Referral to a podiatrist, orthopedist, or rheumatologist** should be considered when skeletal or foot abnormalities contribute or cause significant walking difficulties.

Key Points

- Gait and balance disorders are common, especially among older adults, and a significant source of disability and limited quality of life.
- An active lifestyle is an important part of minimizing the risk of falls and balance difficulties as inactivity leads to deconditioning.
- Walking is a complex motor behavior that can be affected by lesions at multiple levels of the neuraxis and musculoskeletal system.
- A gait problem is the result of the primary gait difficulty and the associated compensatory mechanism.
- A gait pattern can help establish what structures of the neuraxis are affected and therefore localize the lesion; some gait disorders are very stereotypic and easy to identify (i.e., low- and mid-level gait disorders) while others are very variable and can be very challenging to diagnose and manage (i.e., HLGDs).
- Good proprioception, vision, and vestibular inputs are needed to maintain good balance; impairment of at least two of these inputs can seriously affect balance and this is the basis of the Romberg test.
- Central and peripheral vestibulopathies can cause balance difficulties but distinguishing both can be challenging at times; in peripheral vestibulopathy, all the signs are ipsilateral except for the fast component of the nystagmus. Lack of long-tract signs is not by itself indicative of a peripheral etiology. The head thrust test if performed properly can distinguish both (i.e., it is abnormal in peripheral vestibulopathies).
- Extensive white matter abnormalities seen on T2-weighted images and fluid attenuation inversion recovery (FLAIR)–weighted images on MRI, especially bilateral frontal or occipito-parietal periventricular ones, are associated with poor balance and walking difficulties.
- Defective cognition, in particular executive dysfunction, is linked to worsened performance while walking as shown in dual-task paradigms (e.g., more difficulty walking when asked to recite months of the year backward).
- There is significant overlap in the walking pattern of NPH and Parkinson's disease. However, a way to help distinguishing both is that Parkinson patients can be very responsive to external cueing while NPH patients are not.
- There is no good algorithm to clearly diagnose and treat patient with NPH; a robust response to removal of 40 to 60 mL of CSF is very encouraging but the sensitivity of this test is very low in predicting response to CSF drainage. Trying an external lumbar drain for a few days is more sensitive but more prone to complications.

Recommended Readings

Amboni M, Barone P, Hausdorff JM. Cognitive contributors to gait and fall: evidence and implications. *Mov Disord.* 2013;28(11):1520–1533.

American Geriatric Society, British Geriatric Society, American Academy of Orthopedic Surgeons Panel on Falls Prevention. Guideline for the prevention of falls in older persons. *J Am Geriatr Soc.* 2001;49(5):664–672.

Gallia GL, Rigamonti D, Williams MA. The diagnosis and treatment of idiopathic normal pressure hydrocephalus. *Nat Clin Pract Neurol.* 2006;2:375–381.

Ghosh S, Lippa C. Diagnosis and prognosis in idiopathic normal pressure hydrocephalus. *Am J Alzheimers Dis Other Demen.* 2014;29(7):583–589.

Kreisel SH, Blahak C, Bäzner H, et al. Deterioration of gait and balance over time: the effects of age-related white matter change—the LADIS study. *Cerebrovasc Dis.* 2013;35:544–553.

Lim MR, Huang RC, Wu A, et al. Evaluation of the elderly with an abnormal gait. *J Am Acad Orthop Surg.* 2007;15:107–117.

Maetzler W, Nieuwhof F, Hasmann SE, et al. Emerging therapies for gait disability and balance impairment: promises and pitfalls. *Mov Disord.* 2013;28(11):1576–1586.

Newman-Toker D. Symptoms and signs of neuro-otologic disorders. *Continuum (Minneap Minn).* 2012;18(5):1016–1040.

Nutt JG. Higher-level gait disorders: an open frontier. *Mov Disord.* 2013;28(11):1560–1565.

Nutt JG, Horak FB, Bloem BR. Milestones in gait, balance and falling. *Mov Disord.* 2011;26(6):1166–1174.

Nutt JG, Marsden CD, Thompson PD. Human walking and high level gait disorders, particularly in the elderly. *Neurology.* 1993;43:268–279.

Takakusaki K. Neurophysiology of gait: from the spinal cord to the frontal lobe. *Mov Disord.* 2013;28(11):1483–1491.

Zheng, JJ, Delbaere K, Close JCT, et al. Impact of white matter lesions on physical functioning and fall risk in older people: a systematic review. *Stroke.* 2011;42:2086–2090.

9 Approach to the Patient with Sleep Disorders

Mark E. Dyken and Kyoung Bin Im

This chapter focuses on primary sleep disorders described in the third edition of the *International Classification of Sleep Disorders (ICSD)*. The greatest difficulties in approaching patients with sleep disorders often relate to an incomplete sleep history, as only a few diagnoses require formal polysomnography (PSG). Nevertheless, the patient usually cannot recall a pathologic event that occurs during sleep, and as such, an attempt to substantiate the sleep history with a bed partner, family member, or close associate should be made.

GENERAL APPROACH

A. **The sleep history.** What is the sleeping environment and bedtime routine? When is bedtime (regular or irregular)? What is the sleep latency (the time to fall asleep "after the head hits the pillow")? What is the sleep quality? Is it restful or restless and, if restless, why? How many arousals occur per night and for what reasons? What is the final awakening time? Is assistance in waking necessary? How does the patient feel on waking? How many hours of sleep are needed for refreshment? Does the patient nap, and, if so, when, how often, how long, and how does the person feel after the nap (refreshed, unchanged, worse)? Does the patient experience excessive daytime sleepiness (EDS) or frank sleep attacks? A 2-week sleep diary, started before the initial clinic appointment, can diagnose disorders like inadequate sleep hygiene, a problem in 1% to 2% of adolescents and young adults and in up to 10% of the sleep-clinic population that presents with insomnia (Fig. 9.1).
   1. The degree of sleepiness can rate the severity of any sleep disorder through operational **definitions:** mild—sleepiness that impairs social or occupational performance during activities that require little attention (reading or watching television); moderate—sleepiness that impairs performance during activities that require some attention (meetings and concerts); and severe—sleepiness that impairs performance during activities that require active attention (conversing or driving).
   2. **Subjective measure scales,** like the Epworth sleepiness scale, can be used to qualify, quantify, and follow problems with sleepiness (Fig. 9.2). Chronically sleep-deprived persons can underestimate their sleepiness. Over time, they lose the reference point from which to make comparisons and forget what it feels like to be fully rested. In such cases, EDS can be reported as memory loss, slow mentation, and amnestic periods with automatic behavior.
B. **The wake history.** A history of insomnia and EDS can lead to, exacerbate, or result from a variety of medical and mental disorders and from drug or substance use/abuse.

TYPES OF SLEEP DISORDERS

A. **Insomnia.** The *ICSD* criteria demand a history of "persistent difficulty with sleep initiation, duration, consolidation, or quality that occurs despite adequate opportunity and circumstances for sleep, and results in some form of daytime impairment," evidenced by the patient, or the patient's parent or caregiver as at least one of the following: sleepiness, fatigue, malaise, impaired attention, concentration, or memory; social, vocational, or school dysfunction; mood disturbance; reduced motivation, energy, or initiative; and errors or accidents at work or driving. The *ICSD* formally differentiates chronic (complaints at least three times a week for at least 3 months) and short-term insomnias (significant complaints for less than 3 months).

	Mon. a.m.	Tues. a.m.	Wed. a.m.	Thurs. a.m.	Fri. a.m.	Sat. a.m.	Sun. a.m.
1. What time did you go to bed last night?							
2. How many minutes did it take you to fall asleep?							
3. How many times did you wake up?							
4. How many total minutes did the awakenings keep you awake?							
5. What time did you wake up?							
6. What time did you get out of bed?							
Please use Wakefulness key below to answer the following questions:	Mon. p.m.	Tues. p.m.	Wed. p.m.	Thurs. p.m.	Fri. p.m.	Sat. p.m.	Sun. p.m.
1. How awake were you in the morning?							
2. How awake were you in the afternoon?							
3. How awake were you in the evening?							
4. Did you nap today? When and for how long?							

*Level of Wakefulness key:

1 – Very sleepy
2 – Fairly sleepy
3 – Mix of sleepy and alert feelings
4 – Fairly alert
5 – Very alert

FIGURE 9.1 Example of a typical week-at-a-glance sleep diary.

An earlier edition of the *ICSD* defined clinical and pathophysiologic subtypes that might provide some utility when approaching any given patient with insomnia.

1. **Adjustment (acute) insomnia.** This term has been used to describe insomnia that immediately follows a clearly identifiable stressor and is expected to resolve when the stress ends or the patient adapts. Adjustment insomnia is often associated with anxiety and depression related to the specific stressor.
2. **Psychophysiologic insomnia.** This is a conditioned insomnia due to learned, sleep-preventing associations. It can represent persistent adjustment insomnia, where an external (or internal) stressor leads to a state of arousal "racing mind" in association with bedtime at home (patients often sleep better in the sleep lab; the "reverse first-night effect").
3. **Paradoxical insomnia.** Patients complain of severe insomnia with no objective evidence of disturbed sleep or daytime impairment. PSG studies show that these individuals overestimate their sleep latencies and underestimate their sleep times. Patient concerns are not alleviated when they are presented with these objective findings. High-frequency activity on electroencephalographic power-density measures may alter sleep perception in this patient population.

THE EPWORTH SLEEPINESS SCALE

Name: _____

Today's date: _____ Your age (years): _____

Your sex (male = M; female = F): _____

How likely are you to doze off or fall asleep in the following situations, in contrast to feeling just tired? This refers to your usual way of life in recent times. Even if you have not done some of these things recently try to work out how they would have affected you. Use the following scale to choose the *most appropriate number* for each situation:

0 = would *never* doze
1 = *slight* chance of dozing
2 = *moderate* chance of dozing
3 = *high* chance of dozing

Situation	Chance of dozing
Sitting and reading	_____
Watching TV	_____
Sitting, inactive in a public place (e.g.a theater or a meeting)	_____
As a passenger in a car for an hour without a break	_____
Lying down to rest in the afternoon when circumstances permit	_____
Sitting and talking to someone	_____
Sitting quietly after a lunch without alcohol	_____
In a car, while stopped for a few minutes in the traffic	_____

Thank you for your cooperation

FIGURE 9.2 The Epworth sleepiness scale. A score of 10 or greater suggests EDS. (From Johns MW. A new method for measuring daytime sleepiness: the Epworth sleepiness scale. *Sleep.* 1991;14:540–545, with permission.)

4. **Idiopathic insomnia.** This lifelong disorder is reported in 1% of young adults, beginning in infancy or early childhood. It has no known precipitators or major psychological concomitants, but may be associated with attention-deficit/hyperactivity disorder (ADHD) and dyslexia. A genetic abnormality in sleep/wake mechanisms is suspected. PSG often shows reduced body movements despite severely disturbed sleep.

5. **Insomnia due to (another) mental disorder.** In this diagnosis, insomnia is a symptom of a mental disorder, but its severity demands treatment as a distinct problem, which often improves the underlying mental disorder. Major depression is frequently associated with insomnia and reduced rapid eye movement (REM) sleep latency, but PSG is not needed for diagnosis.

6. **Inadequate sleep hygiene.** This presents as a primary or secondary diagnosis in over 30% of sleep-clinic patients. It involves two categories of habits inconsistent with good sleep: practices that produce increased arousal (e.g., caffeine and nicotine use) and practices that are inconsistent with the principles of sleep organization (variable bedtime and awakening times). Important factors can include engaging in mentally or physically stimulating activities too close to bedtime and failure to maintain a comfortable sleeping environment.

7. **Behavioral insomnia of childhood.** There are two types seen in up to 30% of children (possibly more frequent in boys) after 6 months of age. Sleep-onset association type occurs with dependency on a specific stimulation, object, or setting for sleep. Sleep-onset

associations are extremely prevalent and are only a disorder if highly problematic. Limit-setting type occurs with bedtime stalling, or refusal in toddlers and preschoolers. This problem is often due to poor practices of the caregiver.

8. Insomnia due to drug or substance. This is suppression or disruption of sleep during consumption or exposure to a drug, food, or toxin, or upon its discontinuation. The PSG in chronic alcohol withdrawal can reveal light and fragmented sleep that may persist for years.

9. Insomnia due to a medical condition. Disorders that cause discomfort (comfort is necessary for normal sleep) and neurodegenerative problems (with disruption of normal central sleep/wake mechanisms; poorly formed or absent sleep spindles are common) are representative of many possible etiologies. This diagnosis should only be considered when insomnia causes marked distress and warrants specific attention.

B. Sleep-related breathing disorders (SRBDs). In addition to the wake/sleep history, PSG is required in diagnosing SRBDs. PSG is the combined sleep monitoring of electroencephalography (EEG), electromyography (EMG), electrooculography (EOG), and physiologic measures that include airflow, respiratory effort, and oxygen saturation (Sao_2). PSG differentiates four sleep stages—non-REM (NREM) stages N1, N2, and N3, and REM (stage R). An obstructive apnea is a drop in airflow by $\geq 90\%$, in association with continued inspiratory effort, for ≥ 10 seconds in adults, or the duration of two baseline breaths in children. A central apnea is an absence of inspiratory effort for ≥ 10 seconds in adults, or, in children, for 20 seconds, or the duration of two baseline breaths in association with an arousal, awakening, or a $\geq 3\%$ Sao_2 reduction. A mixed apnea occurs when there is initially absent inspiratory effort, followed by resumption of inspiratory effort in the second part of the event. Hypopneas in adults occur with a ≥ 10-second period of reduced airflow of $\geq 30\%$, with an Sao_2 reduction of $\geq 3\%$ (or an associated arousal). In children, a hypopnea requires a $\geq 30\%$ fall in airflow for duration of two baseline breaths, in association with an arousal, awakening, or $\geq 3\%$ Sao_2 reduction. Severity of an SRBD is suggested by the apnea–hypopnea index (AHI)—the average number of apneas and hypopneas per hour of sleep.

1. Obstructive sleep apnea disorders. Obstructive sleep apnea (OSA) is associated with repeated episodes of upper airway obstruction. From 30 to 60 years of age, the prevalence ranges from 9% to 24% for men and 4% to 9% for women. Obstructions often result in oxygen desaturation, elevation in $PaCO_2$, and arousals, which disrupt sleep continuity and can lead to EDS. This syndrome often occurs among sleepy, middle-aged, overweight men with insomnia who snore. Premenopausal women are less commonly affected. This disorder has also been associated with systemic and pulmonary hypertension, nocturnal cardiac arrhythmia and angina, gastroesophageal reflux, nocturia, and an overall reduction in quality of life. Predisposing factors include familial tendencies, redundant pharyngeal tissue (e.g., adenotonsillar hypertrophy), craniofacial disorders (e.g., micrognathia, retrognathia, nasal obstruction), endocrinopathy (e.g., acromegaly, hypothyroidism with myxedema), and neurologic disease.

   a. OSA, adult

      (1) History. The patient or bed partner often reports restless, unrefreshing sleep and sleep maintenance insomnia with arousals associated with gasping, choking, or heroic snoring, possibly exacerbated by fatigue, alcohol, weight gain, or the supine sleeping position. Snoring may force the person to sleep alone and persist even when sitting. Although patients may not report daytime sleepiness, problems with fatigue, memory, and concentration are frequent. A family history of similar problems should be carefully sought.

      (2) Examination. The blood pressure, body mass index (BMI—weight in kilograms per square meter of height), and neck and waist circumference should be documented, as hypertension and obesity may relate to OSA. Of general concern (following western standards) are a BMI ≥ 30 kg/m^2, a neck circumference of >40 cm (15.7 inches), and a waist circumference (often measured at the iliac crest) >102 cm (40.2 inches) in men, and >88 cm (34.6 inches) in women. These are frequent signs in OSA that may predict comorbidities in the metabolic syndrome, heart disease, and stroke. Oral and nasopharyngeal patency and abnormalities of the tonsils, adenoids, tongue, soft and hard palate, uvula, nasal

septum, turbinates, and temporomandibular joint as well as fatty infiltration of soft tissues in the upper airways should be documented.

(3) **PSG.** Recurrent obstructions and respiratory effort-related arousals (RERAs) contribute to EDS. (However, the frequency of events correlates poorly with sleepiness severity.) Events generally appear worse in the supine position and during REM sleep. Tachy–brady cardiac arrhythmias and asystole may be documented. The diagnosis of OSA is considered with an obstructive AHI, or respiratory disturbance index (RDI; the obstructive AHI + the average number of RERAs/hour of sleep) ≥5, and when there is at least one symptom; EDS, insomnia, arousals with shortness of breath or choking, and witnessed loud snoring/apneas, or significant comorbidity; arterial hypertension, coronary artery disease, congestive heart failure (CHF), atrial fibrillation, stroke, mood disorders, or diabetes. The diagnosis is also given whenever the obstructive AHI or RDI is ≥15 (even in the absence of symptoms or comorbidities).

(4) **Differential diagnosis.** Loud snoring and RERAs, as part of the upper airway resistance syndrome (UARS), can lead to EDS without the standard PSG evidence of OSA (as RERAs are pathophysiologically similar to obstructions). During PSG, defining RERA requires esophageal balloon (or nasal pressure/inductance plethysmography) monitoring that reveals ≥10 second episodes of respectively increasing negative pressure, or flattening of nasal pressure waveforms (that correspond to increased respiratory effort), which terminate with arousal. In addition, isolated snoring, central sleep apnea (CSA), nonobstructive alveolar hypoventilation, narcolepsy, and restless legs syndrome (RLS) may manifest similarly to OSA in regard to disruptive sleep and EDS.

(5) **Other tests.** In severe cases, an interdisciplinary approach may necessitate electrocardiography, chest radiography, echocardiography, and pulmonary function tests (addressing pulmonary hypertension and right ventricular hypertrophy), cephalometric evaluations of the upper airways, and extensive cerebrovascular assessments.

b. **OSA, pediatric.** The prevalence of OSA is 2% in the general pediatric population, with girls and boys being affected equally, but with a higher prevalence in African American relative to White children. Some children may have OSA breathing patterns similar to adults; nevertheless, younger children may be prone to obstructive hypoventilation (long periods of persistent partial upper airway obstruction).

(1) **History.** Snoring and difficulty breathing are common, often with reports of associated neck hyperextension and diaphoresis. Cognitive and behavioral complications (ADHD) are frequent, with EDS being reported especially in older children.

(2) **Examination.** Although children can have OSA secondary to large tonsils and adenoids, obesity is becoming a more common etiology. Pectus excavatum may result from chronic paradoxical respirations. Patients with craniofacial abnormalities, Down syndrome, neuromuscular diseases, cerebral palsy, gastroesophageal reflux (with upper airway edema), mucopolysaccharidosis, sickle cell disease, or who are post cleft palate repair may be prone to OSA.

(3) **PSG.** Even relatively short obstructions may lead to severe hypoxemia as children have faster respiratory rates with lower functional residual capacities than adults. OSA in children is defined by an obstructive AHI ≥1.

(4) **Differential diagnosis.** In children, UARS, isolated snoring, CSA, nonobstructive alveolar hypoventilation, narcolepsy, and RLS may manifest similar to OSA in regard to disruptive sleep and EDS. In the pediatric PSG, RERAs are defined by a sequence of ≥2 breaths, characterized by increasing respiratory effort, flattening of the inspiratory portion of the nasal pressure waveform, snoring, or an elevation in the end-tidal Pco_2 leading to an arousal from sleep.

2. **CSA syndromes**
   a. **CSA with Cheyne–Stokes breathing (CSB).** PSG defines CSB as at least three consecutive cycles of a crescendo/decrescendo breathing with a central AHI of ≥5, and/or a cyclic crescendo/decrescendo pattern that lasts ≥10 consecutive minutes. CSB is most prominent in NREM sleep (usually absent or attenuated in REM).

It occurs predominately in men >60 years of age, with a prevalence up to 45% in CHF, and in 10% of strokes. CHF (a poor prognostic sign), stroke, and possibly renal failure are the most important precipitating factors.

b. **CSA due to a medical disorder without CSB.** A majority of the medical conditions with CSA are associated with brainstem lesions and cardiac or renal disorders.

c. **CSA due to high-altitude periodic breathing.** The only known predisposing factor to this disorder is when an individual has an increased hypoxic ventilatory responsiveness. This leads to hyperventilation on rapid ascent to altitudes >4,000 m and a hypocapnic alkalosis that, during sleep, inhibits ventilation (usually the first night), leading to central apneas in NREM sleep that alternate with hyperpneas in cycles of 12 to 34 seconds (often leading to shortness of breath, frequent arousals, and EDS). This is considered a normal, and transient, adaptive phase to higher altitudes.

d. **CSA due to medication or substance.** Regular use (>2 months) of long-acting opioids (methadone and time-release morphine and hydrocodone) can lead to CSA (often in association with obstruction, hypoventilation, and periodic breathing). The presumed etiology is from an effect on μ-receptors on the ventral surface of the medulla.

e. **Primary CSA.** This idiopathic disorder is more frequent in middle-aged to elderly males, associated with a low-normal waking $PaCO_2$ (<40 mm Hg), and high chemoresponsiveness (evidenced as central apneas) to the normal rise in $PaCO_2$ that occurs in sleep. Significant primary CSA with an AHI >5 can lead to arousals with shortness of breath, insomnia, and EDS.

f. **Primary CSA of infancy (apnea of prematurity <37 weeks conceptual age, apnea of infancy ≥37 weeks, ≤1 year conceptual age).** Central, mixed, obstructive apneas or hypopneas (most notably in active/REM sleep) associate with signs of physiologic compromise (hypoxemia, bradycardia, the need for resuscitative measures), but progressively decrease as the patient matures during the early weeks of life. The prevalence varies inversely with conceptual age (in 84% of infants <1,000 g, and <0.5% of full-term newborns), as it is related to developmental immaturity of brainstem respiratory centers. This has not been established as an independent risk factor for sudden infant death syndrome.

3. **Sleep-related hypoventilation disorders.** These syndromes often coexist with elements of OSA and CSA.

a. **PSG.** In adults, hypoventilation during sleep can be scored in either of the following situations: if there is an increase in the arterial Pco_2 (or surrogate; transcutaneous or end-tidal Pco_2) to a value >55 mm Hg for ≥10 minutes, or there is ≥10 mm Hg increase in arterial Pco_2 (or surrogate) during sleep (in comparison with an awake supine value) to a value exceeding 50 mm Hg for ≥10 minutes. In children, hypoventilation during sleep can be scored when >25% of the total sleep time as measured by either the arterial Pco_2 (or surrogate) is spent with a value >50 mm Hg.

(1) **Obesity hypoventilation syndrome.** These patients must hypoventilate (as defined by an arterial $PaCO_2$ [or surrogate] >45 mm Hg) while awake, and the hypoventilation must be primarily related to mass loading from obesity (as defined by a BMI >30 kg/m²; >95th percentile for age and sex for children). Prolonged periods of decreased tidal volume and sustained arterial oxygen desaturation (for several minutes) are usually seen, but not required for diagnosis. OSA is diagnosed as a separate entity in 80% to 90% of these patients. The serum bicarbonate level is routinely elevated secondary to renal compensation for the respiratory acidosis that follows chronic hypercapnia.

(2) **Congenital central alveolar hypoventilation syndrome (CCHS).** CCHS can lead to polycythemia, pulmonary hypertension, heart failure, and death. It is a rare congenital genetic disease (most cases due to de novo mutations in the *PHOX2B* gene) associated with failure of automatic central control of breathing, usually evident at birth, and requiring intubation. Most patients have a polyalanine point mutation and severity relates to a greater number of polyalanine repeats. Patients may progress to adequate waking breathing with normal daytime $PaCO_2$ levels, although some continue to show daytime hypoventilation, and others may need continuous ventilatory support. All will continue to require ventilatory support during sleep. Rarely individuals can present in adulthood, especially when

stressed with general anesthesia or respiratory illness. Although central apneas may occur, the PSG primarily shows hypoxemia and hypercapnia that associate with decreased tidal volume and respiratory rate, with hypoventilation generally appearing worse during slow wave (stage N3) sleep. CCHS is often associated with Hirschsprung's disease (approximately 16%), autonomic dysfunction, neural tumors, and dysphagia.

    (3) Sleep-related hypoventilation due to a medical disorder. This section includes a variety of disorders.

        (a) Lower airway obstruction occurs in disorders with obstruction or increased airflow resistance below the larynx, such as chronic obstructive pulmonary disease (COPD); chronic bronchitis and emphysema; bronchiectasis; cystic fibrosis; and α_1 antitrypsin deficiency. The greatest risk factor for COPD (the third leading cause of death in the United States) is cigarette smoking. Patients with COPD and significant sleep hypoxemia have increased pulmonary hypertension and mortality. Lower airway obstructive disease is evidenced by a forced expiratory volume exhaled in one second/forced vital capacity ratio <70% of predicted values.

        (b) Pulmonary parenchymal or vascular pathology can be documented using pulmonary function tests, radiography, echocardiography, pulmonary artery catheter measurements, and hemoglobin studies. Associated diseases include interstitial lung diseases, pulmonary hypertension, sickle cell anemia, and cystic fibrosis. Worse pulmonary function and a lower waking SaO_2 increases the risk for sleep hypoventilation/hypoxemia, and subsequent polycythemia and cardiac dysrhythmias. PSG findings are generally worse in REM sleep.

        (c) Neuromuscular and chest wall disorders can cause hypoventilation secondary to reduced contractility of the ventilatory musculature (intercostals, accessory muscles, and diaphragm), or due to anatomic distortion of the chest wall (which causes inefficient breathing). This often affects patients with obesity, amyotrophic lateral sclerosis, myasthenia gravis, muscular dystrophies, kyphoscoliosis, postpolio syndrome, and spinal cord injuries with diaphragmatic paralysis. The course of the breathing disturbance approximates the severity of the underlying condition, and can put the patient at risk for pulmonary hypertension, cor pulmonale, and cognitive dysfunction. Spirometry in patients with neuromuscular and chest wall disorders generally reveals a restrictive ventilatory dysfunction, with a forced vital capacity that is frequently <50% of predicted.

C. Central disorders of hypersomnolence. These disorders involve dysfunction of the normal central wake/sleep centers. The ascending reticular activating system (ARAS) of the brainstem promotes wakefulness through two pathways, leading to diffuse cortical projections. A ventral hypothalamic system excites the lateral nucleus (LN) and tuberomammillary nucleus of the hypothalamus, which relays to cholinergic basal forebrain cells, while a dorsal thalamic route stimulates nonspecific midline and intralaminar nuclei, while inhibiting the reticular nucleus of the thalamus. The central sleep-onset system has a hypothalamic "sleep switch" in the preoptic area of the hypothalamus (the ventrolateral and median preoptic nuclei). These nuclei have reciprocal inhibitory relays with multiple waking centers.

    1. Narcolepsy (types 1 and 2). Classically begins during puberty or young adulthood with EDS. Sleep attacks can occur while driving, engaged in active conversation, or eating. Once sleepiness stabilizes, it generally does not progress, but the other symptoms associated with narcolepsy may come and go. Cataplexy, often precipitated by strong positive emotion (usually mirth), involves attacks that range from brief sensations of weakness to essential paralysis. The spells are transient and do not produce cognitive impairment. Thirty-three percent to eighty percent of narcoleptics have the ancillary symptoms of hallucinations and sleep paralysis. Hypnagogic (at sleep onset) and hypnopompic (on awakening) hallucinations are generally frightening visual, auditory, or movement perceptions that essentially represent dreaming while awake. Sleep paralysis occurs during the transition from sleep to waking (or waking to sleep). The patient may experience brief paralysis (seconds to minutes) with the inability to speak. Other symptoms of narcolepsy can include insomnia, poor memory, depression, and automatic behaviors. Narcolepsy is associated with pathologic REM sleep mechanisms, clinically evidenced as EDS, cataplexy, sleep paralysis, and hypnagogic/hypnopompic hallucinations. In narcolepsy type 1 these symptoms are due to a deficiency of wake-promoting neuropeptides (orexins/ hypocretins) in the LN of the hypothalamus, as defined by cerebrospinal fluid (CSF) hypocretin (Hcrt)-1 concentration, measured by immunoreactivity, as either ≤110 pg/ mL or <1/3 of mean values obtained in normal subjects with the same standardized assay. Narcoleptics with cataplexy, and approximately 24% of narcoleptics without cataplexy, have low CSF Hcrt-1 concentrations and are given the formal diagnosis of narcolepsy type 1. Narcoleptics without cataplexy and with CSF Hcrt-1 levels >110 pg/mL or >1/3 of mean values obtained in normal subjects with the same standardized assay are given the formal diagnosis of narcolepsy type 2. Another clinical and pathophysiologic subtype is narcolepsy type 1 due to a medical condition, primarily central nervous system (CNS) disorders with lesions of the hypothalamus resulting from head trauma, tumors, or autoimmune and paraneoplastic disorders associated with anti-Ma2 or anti-aquaporin-4 antibodies.

a. **PSG and the multiple sleep latency test (MSLT).** The diagnosis of narcolepsy requires objective measurements, and includes documenting abnormalities of REM sleep utilizing PSG/MSLT. These evaluations should be preceded by at least 1 week of actigraphic recording with a sleep log to help rule out insufficient sleep, shift work, or another circadian sleep disorder that could appear similarly on PSG/MSLT. The patient must also discontinue any drug that affects their sleep for a minimum of 14 days (or five times the half-life of the drug and its metabolites) prior to the PSG/ MSLT. This should be confirmed with a urine drug screen. REM sleep is defined on PSG and MSLT as a "relatively low voltage, mixed frequency EEG" of alpha and theta waveforms, associated with "saw-tooth" waves, which occurs with an EOG that shows REMs and an EMG that documents atonia. In diagnosing narcolepsy, the MSLT should be performed approximately 2 hours after the patient awakens from the overnight PSG (which assures adequate sleep, with the goal of at least 7 hours of sleep, and a paucity of other sleep disorders, including SRBDs). The MSLT is a series of five 20-minute attempts at napping (during the patient's normal waking hours), which are separated by approximately 2-hour intervals. A mean sleep latency (the average time it takes the patient to fall asleep after the beginning of each individual nap period) ≤8 minutes and two or more naps during which REM sleep appears (a sleep-onset rapid eye movement period [SOREMP]) are classically associated with narcolepsy. A SOREMP (within 15 minutes of sleep onset) on the preceding PSG may replace one of the SOREMPs required for diagnosis on the MSLT.

b. **Split-screen, video-PSG studies.** As patients are infrequently examined during a cataplexy attack, the suspicion of cataplexy is usually based on the clinical history. Nevertheless, split-screen, video-PSG studies in individuals with frequent spells, performed during actual cataplectic events precipitated by emotional provocation, have shown REM sleep patterns during periods when patients were able to give appropriate responses to detailed questioning. Similar results have been documented during episodes of sleep paralysis and hypnagogic hallucinations.

c. **Genetics.** The risk of narcolepsy type 1 in first-degree relatives of affected patients is 1% to 2% (a 10-fold to 40-fold risk increase). Relatives of individuals with narcolepsy type 1 may be prone to partial narcolepsy symptoms suggesting narcolepsy type 2. The major histocompatibility complex of chromosome 6 contains genetic markers for narcolepsy. For nearly all patients with narcolepsy type 1 the mapping of specific human leukocyte class II antigens (DQ1 and DR2) reveals a subtype human leukocyte antigen allele DQB1*0602. The presence of the DQB1*0602 allele in approximately 45% of patients narcolepsy type 2 (and in 12% to 38% of controls) indicates that genetic testing alone is not sufficient for the diagnosis of narcolepsy.

d. **Orexins/hypocretins.** Narcolepsy type 1 is caused by a deficiency of LN hypothalamic hypocretin (orexin) wake-promoting neuropeptide signaling, and approximately 24% of narcoleptics without cataplexy have low CSF Hcrt-1 levels (8% have intermediate levels; >110 pg/mL, ≤200 pg mL).

2. **Idiopathic hypersomnia.** This is generally a lifelong disorder (remission rate of 14%) of EDS, which routinely begins in adolescence (mean age of onset 16.6 to 21.2 years),

and is associated with self-reported routine total sleep times ≥ 10 hours in at least 30% of patients. The use of 24-hour PSG monitoring has documented 24-hour sleep times (major sleep episode plus naps) ≥ 660 minutes. About 36% to 66% report sleep inertia (sleep drunkenness), defined as prolonged difficulty waking with automatic behaviors and confusion. About 46% to 78% of patients report long (often >1 hour) unrefreshing naps. There are no reports of cataplexy and no more than 1 SOREMP on PSG/MSLT studies, while the mean sleep latency averages 7.8 to 8.3 minutes. The autonomic concomitants implied by the frequency of associated headaches, orthostasis, perception of temperature dysregulation, and Raynaud's-type phenomena suggest hypothalamic dysfunction; nevertheless, relatively recent CSF studies have shown normal orexin/hypocretin and histamine levels.

3. **Kleine–Levin Syndrome (KLS).** The KLS is rare (prevalence of 1 to 2 cases per million; 500 cases reported) and begins during the second decade in 81%, with a male–female ratio of 2:1. It is characterized by baseline normalcy interrupted by relapsing-remitting episodes of hypersomnolence associated with cognitive, psychiatric, and behavioral disturbances. The first episode is often associated with an infection or alcohol use, and recurs every 1 to 12 months (median 3 months), typically resolving after a median of 14 years. During episodes the patient may sleep as long as 20 hours, are generally amnestic for waking confusion, hyperphagia (66%), hypersexuality (53% primarily men), infantile/depressed behaviors (53%; primarily women), and hallucinations/delusions (30%). Birth and developmental problems and Jewish heritage are risk factors for KLS. In addition, the frequency of HLA DQB1*02 was increased in one retrospective, multicenter study of 30 KLS patients. Brain MRI is normal, but functional brain imaging during episodes is frequently abnormal, variably showing hypometabolism in the thalamus, hypothalamus, mesial temporal lobe, and frontal lobe, with half of the patients showing persistent abnormalities when asymptomatic. Postmortem examinations have been performed in four cases with inconsistent findings that include perivascular lymphocytic infiltrations in the hypothalamus, thalamus, amygdala, grey matter of the temporal lobes, diencephalon, and mesencephalon, raising on occasion the suspicion of localized encephalitis. An autoimmune etiology is suggested by the combined clinical onset during adolescence that is often associated with infection and the HLA DQB1*02. Finally, menstrual-related KLS is a very rare clinical and pathophysiologic subtype (18 reported cases), where episodes occur exclusively just before or during menses. Response to estrogen and progesterone has suggested a reproductive disturbance in these cases.

4. **Hypersomnia due to a medical condition.** The conditions that can cause hypersomnia through direct effects on wake/sleep mechanisms include neurodegenerative disorders, brain trauma and tumors, encephalitis, genetic disease, and stroke. The diagnosis of narcolepsy type 1 due to medical condition is given when these conditions lead to cataplexy.
   a. **Hypersomnia secondary to Parkinson's disease.** In Parkinson's disease (PD), hypersomnia may result from degeneration of dopaminergic cells in the substantia nigra and cholinergic neurons in the basal forebrain.
   b. **Posttraumatic hypersomnia.** Hypersomnolence has been reported with a frequency of 28% in traumatic brain injury. This type of hypersomnia has been reported even in mild head injury (without loss of consciousness), and also during recovery from posttraumatic coma (where early PSG return of sleep spindles and normal sleep–wake cycling is a positive prognostic sign). In some cases this hypersomnolence may result from injury to the hypothalamic hypocretin/orexin neurons or other wake-promoting centers in the brain.
   c. **Genetic disorders associated with primary CNS somnolence.** Specific genetic disorders associated with hypersomnia include Norrie's disease, Niemann–Pick type C disease, myotonic dystrophy, Prader–Willi syndrome, fragile X syndrome, and Moebius syndrome. In Niemann–Pick disease type C, accumulation of unesterified cholesterol and sphingolipids in the hypothalamus, with a subsequent reduction in orexin/hypocretin, may be a cause of sleepiness. In myotonic dystrophy, hypothalamic (orexin/hypocretin) dysfunction, and loss of serotonin in the dorsal raphe nucleus, may account for hypersomnolence. Smith–Magenis syndrome is associated with reversal in the normal pattern of melatonin secretion (serum levels are high during the day, rather than at night).

    d. **Hypersomnias secondary to brain tumors, infections, or other CNS lesions.** Tumors, infections, strokes, sarcoidosis, or neurodegenerative lesions especially in the hypothalamus or rostral midbrain can produce EDS.

    e. **Hypersomnia secondary to endocrine disorders.** Hypersomnia secondary to endocrine disorder is typified by hypothyroidism. A significant reduction in slow wave activity can be induced by hypothyroidism.

    f. **Hypersomnia secondary to metabolic encephalopathy.** This includes encephalopathies related to hepatic, renal, adrenal, and pancreatic failure, toxin exposures, and some inherited childhood metabolic disorders.

    g. **Residual hypersomnia in patients with adequately treated OSA.** Residual sleepiness in this population may be caused by hypoxic injury to central monoamine waking systems.

  5. **Hypersomnia due to a medication or substance.** This includes use, abuse, and cessation of stimulants, and sedative-hypnotic drugs.

  6. **Hypersomnia associated with a psychiatric disorder.** These are related to psychiatric conditions that include adjustment, personality, schizoaffective, mood, and seasonal affective disorders. Subtypes include hypersomnia associated with a major depressive episode (atypical depression and bipolar type II disorder), and conversion disorder (or as an undifferentiated somatoform disorder).

  7. **Insufficient sleep syndrome.** This is due to voluntary, but unintentional, chronic sleep deprivation. Patients are preoccupied with etiologies they presume are responsible for their sleepiness (causes other than a reduced total sleep time), and their symptoms, which may include irritability, malaise, and reduced concentration.

D. Circadian rhythm sleep–wake disorders. A circadian rhythm sleep–wake disorder (CRSWD) occurs when there are incongruities between the sleep–wake schedule demanded by society and the intrinsic sleep–wake pattern of the patient (determined in large part by the circadian pacemaker—the suprachiasmatic nuclei of the anterior hypothalamus). When not extrinsic or self-imposed ("jet lag" or shift work), these problems are believed to result from abnormal intrinsic physiologic responses to environmental time cues (*Zeitgebers*) such as sunlight (which exerts its effects through retinal–hypothalamic pathways). The patient's state of sleepiness or arousal subsequently is out of synchrony with that of the general population. The result is alternating sleepiness and insomnia when the patient tries to follow a normal schedule.

  1. **History.** In many cases, a sleep log can be diagnostic. The accurate, 1- to 2-month documentation of all bedtimes, final awakening times, and nap times can help differentiate a circadian rhythm disorder from poor sleep hygiene. The log should be filled out during a vacation or "free" time so as to avoid societal constraints that prevent the patient from following their intrinsic sleep–wake pattern.

  2. **Other tests.** Actigraphy is a method for recording limb movement using a device (usually placed on the wrist) that records movement. Digitized data are downloaded to a computer, and computer algorithms are used to approximate wake and sleep periods over prolonged periods of time. The American Academy of Sleep Medicine (AASM) indicates actigraphy is reliable and valid for detecting sleep in healthy populations, and useful in the routine evaluation of CRSWDs, insomnia, and EDS. In addition, some sleep disorder centers can monitor hormonal rhythms [such as dim-light melatonin onset], and 24-hour body temperature fluctuations, which can lose normal circadian fluctuations and amplitudes in CRSWDs.

    a. **Delayed sleep–wake phase disorder.** This occurs with a prevalence rate up to 16%, and is primarily noted in adolescents and young adults, and individuals with evening-type personalities (as defined by the Horne–Ostberg questionnaire). There is an association with polymorphisms in the circadian clock gene *hPer3*, with a positive family history in 40%. Patients report chronically late bedtimes with late final awakening times (delayed over 2 hours relative to societal norms), which can be confirmed with a sleep logs and actigraphy (over at least 7 days). These individuals do not report sleepiness unless they attempt to follow the normal societal sleep–wake schedule.

    b. **Advanced sleep–wake phase disorder.** Persons with this syndrome go to sleep very early in relation to the setting of the sun, arise very early in relation to sunrise, and do not report excessive sleepiness during their "normal" waking hours. This tendency increases with age, and has a prevalence of 1% in middle-aged and older adults. Almost all patients are considered morning-type personalities. In younger patients genetic factors may be involved, possibly with an autosomal-dominant inheritance pattern, in association with a mutation in the circadian clock gene *hPer2*. This CRSWD is generally addressed only if it impairs the quality of the patient's work, social, or family life.

c. **Irregular sleep–wake rhythm disorder.** In this disorder there is no definitive sleep–wake rhythm. Patients subsequently have intermittent nocturnal insomnia and variable periods of daytime sleepiness, which generally result in three or more irregularly timed naps during a 24-hour period. The total sleep time during a 24-hour is normal, but the timing of sleep is not predictable. This disorder can be seen in the institutionalized elderly, in association with dementia, and in children with intellectual disabilities.

d. **Non-24-hour sleep–wake rhythm disorder.** Also known as hypernychthemeral syndrome, these patients have an inability to synchronize (entrain) the physiologic desire for a sleep–wake schedule that is greater than 24 hours with a normal 24-hour day. Subsequently these patients continually "phase delay" and on a day-to-day basis show a progressive 1- to 2-hour delay of bedtime and final awakening times. When they attempt to keep regular sleep–wake schedules (fixed bedtime and final awakening times), they experience recurrent periods without sleep problems (when their intrinsic schedules match society's), which are then followed by the gradual onset of periods associated with sleep-onset insomnia, difficulty waking in the morning, and daytime sleepiness (when their intrinsic schedules are out of synchrony with society's). These patients are often blind and the disorder has been reported with intellectual disability, schizophrenia, and rarely in the otherwise normal population. Upon diagnosis, imaging studies of the brain can be considered, as this disorder has been associated with suprasellar lesions.

e. **Shift work disorder.** In this disorder insomnia and EDS result when the patient works during the normal physiologic sleep period. The prevalence of shift work in industrialized countries is 20% and the estimated prevalence of insomnia/EDS because of shift work is 2% to 5%. This disorder may complicate gastrointestinal and cardiovascular disorders, cause social difficulties, or lead to drug dependency in attempts to improve sleep, and presents work-related safety concerns.

f. **Circadian sleep–wake disorder not otherwise specified.** Degenerative diseases (including Parkinson's and Alzheimer's disease), blindness, and hepatic encephalopathy can alter the function of the biologic clock and lead to insomnia and EDS. Sleep-related problems can then influence the severity of the underlying condition (e.g., "sun downing" and nocturnal wandering in dementia).

E. **Parasomnias.** These are undesired sleep-related physical events, associated with semipurposeful behaviors and elevated autonomic activity. Of the parasomnias, only the REM sleep behavior disorder (RBD) requires PSG for diagnosis.

1. **NREM-related parasomnias.** Confusional arousals, sleepwalking, and sleep terrors are closely related parasomnias formally referred to as disorders of arousal (from NREM sleep). They can occur in a familial pattern, are primarily noted in children, and generally begin in slow-wave (stage N3) sleep during the first third of the night. The spells are associated with general lack of environmental responsiveness, automatic actions, confusion, disorientation, and occasional injuries. After these events, from which the patient is generally unarousable, there is usually amnesia without dream recall.

a. **Confusional arousals.** These are prevalent in children (17.3% in children 3 to 13 years of age) and adults <35 years of age (2.9% to 4.2% in adults >15 years of age), with a lifetime prevalence of 18.5%. The childhood form usually appears around 2 years of age and diminishes in occurrence after 5 years age. Young children may sleepwalk when they become adolescents. Adolescents and adults can have the variants: severe morning sleep inertia and sleep-related abnormal sexual behaviors. Severe morning sleep inertia is a persistent problem that can lead to sleep-related injury (risk of motor vehicle accidents), violent behavior, poor work performance, and social problems. Sleep-related abnormal sexual behaviors can lead to assaultive behaviors followed by morning amnesia.

b. **Sleepwalking.** This occurs with a lifetime prevalence up to 18.3% (peaking by 8 to 12 years of age), and in up to 4% of adults (with associated violent behaviors occurring more frequently in men). The rate of familial sleepwalking is 60% when both parents are affected. Childhood sleepwalking can lead to injury, but usually resolves by puberty.

c. **Sleep terrors.** These occur with a prevalence rate up to 6.5% in children, and in 2.2% of adults. Adults may have associated bipolar, depressive, or anxiety disorders. The onset is usually between 4 and 12 years with resolution often during puberty. During the spell, the patient often appears frightened, with tachycardia, tachypnea, diaphoresis, and inconsolable screaming and crying that can last from a few seconds to 20 minutes.

2. **REM-related parasomnias.**

a. **RBD.** This disorder is associated with violent behavior during sleep that reflects dream enactment. Events begin during REM ("dreaming" or "paralyzed") sleep and are followed, after arousal, by reports of dream imagery compatible with the actions observed during the spell. This disorder generally appears after the age of 50 years, in elderly men, with a prevalence of 0.38% to 0.5% in the elderly and the general population. It is often associated with synucleinopathies (neurodegenerative disorders like PD and dementia with Lewy bodies (DLB), where there are neuronal lesions from aggregates of insoluble α-synuclein protein). A conversion rate (often after a delay of more than a decade) up 82% has been reported from idiopathic RBD to parkinsonism/dementia. RBD is reported in 46% of individuals with PD, 50% with DLB, and in >90% multiple system atrophy. The patients have histories of potentially harmful sleep-related body movements associated with dreaming. Patients frequently report sleep-related injuries, which include bruises, lacerations, dislocations, fractures, and subdural hemorrhage. The pathophysiology may be degeneration of REM-atonia pathways. The PSG shows that during REM sleep, muscle tone is generally elevated (REM without atonia). Periodic limb movements during sleep (PLMS) are seen in 75% of patients during NREM sleep. Behaviors appearing as dream enactment may be appreciated during REM sleep.

(1) **Clinical or pathophysiologic subtypes.** The parasomnia overlap disorder occurs when RBD occurs with a disorder of arousal, sleep-related eating disorder, sex-somnia, or rhythmic movement disorder (RMD). Status dissociatus is diagnosed when the PSG has no discernable sleep stages, but behaviors that resemble sleep and suggest dreaming and RBD. This can be seen in a broad range of underlying neurologic and medical conditions.

F. **Sleep-related movement disorders**

1. **RLS.** RLS is clinically diagnosed by symptoms that form the acronym URGE: an **U**rge to move the limbs (usually the legs), that is worse at **R**est, improves with movement (**G**oing), and is most evident in the **E**vening (often when attempting to go to sleep). In children there may be an association with ADHD. This symptom complex affects up to 10% of the general adult population, 30% of patients with rheumatoid arthritis, and up to 20% of patients with uremia (up to 62% of those on hemodialysis). It is reported almost twice as often in women, possibly related to the 11% to 20% prevalence recognized after the 20th week of pregnancy. There are early- and late-onset types of RLS. The early-onset form begins <45 years of age, is slowly progressive, and highly familial with 40% to 92% reporting affected family members. Linkage analyses have shown that a gene variant of *BTBD9* is estimated to confer a population attributable risk of 50% for RLS. The late-onset form typically, rapidly progresses and aggravating factors are common. Etiologic elements may relate to physiologic mechanisms associated with relative central dopamine and iron deficiencies (serum ferritin <18 to 50 μg/L, iron saturation <16% to 20%).

2. **Periodic limb movement disorder (PLMD).** PLMS are reported in 80% to 90% of patients with RLS, in up to 34% of patients >60 years of age, and in up to 15% of insomniacs. When PLMS are significantly elevated and they have an adverse effect on sleep or daytime functioning, the diagnosis of PLMD is made. Gene variants *BTBD9* and *MEIS1* (found in genome-wide studies of RLS) appear to influence the expression

of PLMS. PLMD can be exacerbated by tricyclic antidepressants, monoamine oxidase inhibitors, and hypnotics, and during withdrawal from benzodiazepines, barbiturates, and antiepileptic drugs. On PSG, the PLMS appear as elevated, predominantly 50 to 150 Hz, EMG activity from the tibialis anterior muscle, which persists for 0.5 to 5.0 seconds and coincides with episodes of repetitive, stereotypic extensions of the large toe with ankle, knee, and hip flexion. Consecutive movements have an intermovement interval ≥5 seconds and ≤90 seconds (generally 20 seconds to 40 seconds), and occur primarily in stage N2 sleep. PLMS are considered significant when the PLM index (the average number of PLMS per hour of sleep) is >5 in children and >15 in adults. New actigraphic monitors with high sampling rates can adequately detect PLMS, and promise to be a powerful research tool to study the known night-to-night variability of PLMS. There is controversy regarding whether autonomic arousals associated with PLMS (characterized by significant heart rate and blood pressure surges) provide a mechanism for possible increased risk for cardiovascular and cerebrovascular disease.

3. **Sleep-related RMD.** RMD primarily affects children. The movements are sleep related, stereotypical, repetitive movements of the head, neck, or large muscle groups and are often associated with rhythmic vocalization that includes head banging, body rocking, and leg banging (Video 9.1). Rhythmic body movements often begin in normal children between 8 and 18 months of age and rarely lead to injury. These movements generally resolve by 5 years of age, although persistence may be associated with stress, stimulus deprivation, or CNS lesions. Family members are generally concerned about the noise and sometimes violent nature of these behaviors. PSG studies have shown that rhythmic movements tend to arise from stage N1 or N2 sleep and occur with a frequency of 0.5 to 2 Hz. A series of movements generally lasts <15 minutes.

OTHER INVESTIGATIONAL TOOLS AND OPTIONS

A. **The maintenance of wakefulness test (MWT).** The MWT is a MSLT variant that is performed while the patient attempts to maintain wakefulness in an environment conducive to sleep (a warm, dark room, while lying in a semireclining position). The sleepiness documented utilizing an MWT may more accurately translate to a work situation when compared to the MSLT. The AASM Standards of Practice Committee recommends the MWT begin 2 hours after awakening from overnight sleep. It consists of four, 40-minute naps; each nap separated from the next by a 2-hour interval. A mean sleep latency <8 minutes is abnormal, whereas values between 8 and 40 minutes are of uncertain value. The use of an MWT has been approved in some occupations where sleepiness is hazardous, to justify a change in employment, and to support disability. No sleep is the strongest evidence for the ability to maintain wakefulness, but does not guarantee safety in regard to hypersomnolence.

B. **Brain imaging and EEG.** In some hypersomnias due to a medical condition, imaging of the brain and routine EEG may be of prognosticating value. In posttraumatic coma with hypersomnolence, radiographic evidence of hydrocephalus predicts poor treatment response. In Alzheimer's disease, clinical progression, secondary to degeneration of cholinergic neurons in the basal forebrain, often correlates with EEG loss of sleep spindles, slow waves, and REM sleep patterns. The use of extended PSG montages, which have extra channels, can allow more thorough assessment of variables such as the EEG (for nocturnal seizures) and EMG (for sleep-related movement and behavior disorders). Daytime provocative studies can be used to appropriately characterize phenomena such as cataplexy.

C. **Others.** Routine laboratory studies may be needed to rule out anemia, hypoxemia, infection, and metabolic and endocrinologic abnormalities. A Minnesota Multiphasic Personality Inventory with an interview by a neuropsychologist or psychiatrist familiar with sleep disorders can be helpful in cases in which an affective disorder is suspected. There is promise that for a number of intrinsic sleep disorders, such as narcolepsy, genetic testing may help to confirm the diagnosis.

D. **Referral to a sleep disorder center.** When sleep problems persist, greatly impair quality of life, or necessitate formal sleep studies for diagnosis or therapy (SRBDs and narcolepsy), referral to a reputable sleep disorder center should be considered.

SUMMARY

The general approach to the patient with a sleep disorder should always begin with the sleep history. The many specific questions necessary for diagnosing a variety of unique sleep disorders are neatly summarized in the *ICSD*s. The use of PSG is essential in diagnosing SRBDs, central disorders of hypersomnolence, and the RBD. The MSLT can delineate the types of pathologic sleepiness specific to narcolepsy and idiopathic hypersomnolence, whereas the MWT has been used to assess treatment efficacy and job suitability. In certain cases, basic metabolic panels, drug screens, genetic testing, and a variety of laboratory studies, including arterial blood gases (ABGs), complete blood counts, renal function tests, and CSF analyses, are of value. Occasionally, brain imaging, to address potential lesions affecting the ARAS and specific wake/sleep CNS centers, is important. An approach that properly combines clinical acumen with the appropriate diagnostic tools generally leads to a solid diagnosis, which allows successful therapeutic interventions.

Key Points

- It is imperative when approaching a patient with a suspected sleep disorder, to begin with a full sleep history for which the many specific questions necessary to diagnose any given disorder are clearly summarized in the *ICSD*s.
- The *ICSD*s define many sleep disorders, and only a few require PSG for diagnosis. These include the SRBDs and RBD (and in conjunction with an MSLT, the central disorders of hypersomnolence, as typified by narcolepsy types 1 and 2).
- In certain cases sleep diaries/actigraphy, properly timed urine drug screens, genetic testing, and CSF analyses (narcolepsy type 1), and waking ABGs and $PaCO_2$ monitoring (sleep-related hypoventilation/hypoxemia) can be invaluable.
- An approach combing clinical acumen (based on a solid sleep history) and when indicated, diagnostic tools (which can include sleep diaries/actigraphy, PSG/MSLT, drug screens, ABGs, genetic testing, and CSF analyses) generally lead to solid diagnosis and successful treatment of many sleep disorders.

Recommended Readings

American Academy of Sleep Medicine. *International Classification of Sleep Disorders: Diagnostic and Coding Manual.* 2nd ed. Westchester, IL: American Academy of Sleep Medicine; 2005.

American Academy of Sleep Medicine. *International Classification of Sleep Disorders.* 3rd ed. Darien, IL: American Academy of Sleep Medicine; 2014.

Arand D, Bonnet M, Hurwitz T, et al. The clinical use of the MSLT and MWT. *Sleep.* 2005;28(1):123–144.

Berry RB, Brooks R, Gamaldo CE, et al; for the American Academy of Sleep Medicine. *The AASM Manual for the Scoring of Sleep and Associated Events: Rules, Terminology and Technical Specifications, Version 2.0.* Darien, IL: American Academy of Sleep Medicine; 2012. www.aasmnet.org

Dyken ME. Cerebrovascular disease and sleep apnea. In: Lenfant C, Bradley TD, Floras JS, eds. *Sleep Apnea: Implications in Cardiovascular and Cerebrovascular Disease.* New York, NY: Marcel Dekker; 2000:285–306.

Dyken ME, Lin-Dyken DC, Poulton S, et al. Prospective polysomnographic analysis of obstructive sleep apnea in Down syndrome. *Arch Pediatr Adolesc Med.* 2003;157:655–660.

Dyken ME, Lin-Dyken DC, Seaba P, et al. Violent, sleep-related behavior leading to subdural hemorrhage: polysomnographically documented REM sleep behavior disorder with split-screen electroencephalographic-video analysis. *Arch Neurol.* 1995;52:318–321.

Dyken ME, Lin-Dyken DC, Yamada T. Diagnosing rhythmic movement disorder with video-polysomnography. *Pediatr Neurol.* 1997;16:37–41.

Dyken ME, Rodnitzky R. Periodic, aperiodic and rhythmic motor disorders of sleep. *Neurology.* 1992;42:68–74.

Dyken ME, Somers VK, Yamada T, et al. Investigating the relationship between stroke and obstructive sleep apnea. *Stroke.* 1996;27:401–407.

Dyken ME, Yamada T, Glenn CL, et al. Obstructive apnea associated with cerebral hypoxemia and death. *Neurology.* 2004;62:491–493.

Dyken ME, Yamada T, Lin-Dyken DC. Polysomnographic assessment of spells in sleep: nocturnal seizures versus parasomnias. *Semin Neurol.* 2001;21(4):377–390.

Dyken ME, Yamada T, Lin-Dyken DC, et al. Diagnosing narcolepsy through the simultaneous clinical and electrophysiologic analysis of cataplexy. *Arch Neurol.* 1996;53:456–460.

Iber C, Ancoli-Israel S, Chesson A, et al; for the American Academy of Sleep Medicine. *The AASM Manual for the Scoring of Sleep and Associated Events: Rules, Terminology and Technical Specifications.* 1st ed. Westchester, IL: American Academy of Sleep Medicine; 2007.

Kushida CA, Littner MR, Morgenthaler T, et al. Practice parameters for the indication for polysomnography and related procedures: an update for 2005. *Sleep.* 2005;28(4):499–521.

Littner M, Kushida CA, Anderson MW, et al. Practice parameters for the role of actigraphy in the study of sleep and circadian rhythms: an update for 2002. *Sleep.* 2003;26:337–341.

Littner MR, Kushida C, Wise M, et al. Practice parameters for clinical use of multiple sleep latency test and the maintenance of wakefulness test. *Sleep.* 2005;28(1):113–121.

Sleep-related breathing disorders in adults: recommendations for syndrome definition and measurement techniques in clinical research. *Sleep.* 1999;22(5):667–689.

Young T, Palta M, Dempsey J, et al. The occurrence of sleep-disordered breathing among middle-aged adults. *N Engl J Med.* 1993;328:1230–1235.

Young T, Peppard P, Palta M, et al. Population-based study of sleep-disordered breathing as a risk factor for hypertension. *Arch Intern Med.* 1997;157:1746–1752.

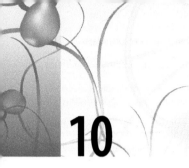

10 Approach to the Patient with Visual Loss

Devin D. Mackay, Valérie Biousse, and Nancy J. Newman

Visual loss is associated with many potential causes and localizations. The patient history can help narrow the diagnostic possibilities. Does the visual loss affect one eye or both eyes? Was the onset of visual loss abrupt or gradual? The potential causes of visual loss can be substantially narrowed on the basis of the temporal sequence of the patient's symptoms, age, gender, and the anatomic localization of the responsible lesion.

Patients often first seek evaluation from an ophthalmologist or optometrist with vision complaints. Commonly, if the ophthalmologic examination is normal or the suspected localization of the lesion involves the intracranial pathways of vision, the patient may be referred to a neurologist. Other patients in the inpatient or outpatient setting may first see a neurologist for their vision complaint. It is important that neurologists be able to perform a basic examination of the visual system, be able to distinguish optic neuropathies from other forms of visual loss, and be able to localize intracranial lesions of the visual pathways. Accurate localization of the visual abnormality facilitates the formation of an appropriate differential diagnosis and judicious use of confirmatory diagnostic testing.

HISTORY

The diagnosis of visual loss begins with a history from the patient of the details of their visual disturbance.

Is the vision disturbance binocular or monocular? The most helpful initial determination is whether the visual loss involves one or both eyes. It may be necessary to inquire if the patient checked by covering one eye at a time, especially in cases of transient visual loss. This is the first step in localization of the lesion, as visual loss involving only one eye localizes anterior to the optic chiasm and visual loss involving both eyes may be the result of an abnormality involving the optic chiasm or retrochiasmal visual pathways, or more rarely, bilateral anterior lesions.

Other helpful questions to narrow the differential diagnosis include, 'Is the vision disturbance transient or persistent, of abrupt or gradual onsent? Are there any other associated symptoms?' The remainder of the chapter addresses how the answers to these questions are often useful.

CLINICAL EXAMINATION OF THE VISUAL SYSTEM

A. **Visual acuity.** Distance visual acuity is best assessed using a distance Snellen chart (or equivalent) with the patient's corrective lenses in place. Alternatively, or if the vision complaint is primarily at near, near visual acuity can be measured using a handheld near acuity card. It is essential to measure near acuity with the patient's reading glasses on (in patients in their 40s or older), so presbyopia is not mistaken for dysfunction of the visual pathways. It is often helpful to start at the bottom of the chart/card and work up to the acuity line where the patient can correctly identify at least half of the characters. In Snellen notation, correct identification of 4/6 characters on the 20/20 line would be recorded as 20/20−2. A plus notation is used to denote when the patient correctly identifies one or more characters on the next smallest line, but less than half. If a patient cannot read any characters on the acuity chart, visual acuity can be tested by counting fingers. This is notated as "count fingers" acuity at the number of feet the fingers were held from the face, such as "count fingers at 2 feet." If the patient is unable to count fingers, the ability to see hand movements is tested (recorded as "hand motion"). If unable to see hand movements, light perception (LP) is tested by asking the patient whether they are able to see a bright light shone directly in the eye (recorded as "LP"). "No light perception" may be abbreviated as "NLP." Visual acuity is often normal in patients with a chiasmal or retrochiasmal visual field defect, but if abnormal, the acuity is the same in both eyes. Patients may have difficulty reading a part of the acuity line that extends into the abnormal visual field. Acquired visual acuity deficits not because of the need for eyeglasses (refractive error) imply a deficit of central vision. Optic neuropathies are typically characterized by a loss of visual acuity, defective color vision, a relative afferent pupillary defect (RAPD) (if unilateral or asymmetric), and may be accompanied by optic disc pallor or edema. A macular abnormality can cause loss of acuity and decreased color vision, but does not cause an RAPD.

B. **Color vision testing.** A book of Ishihara or Hardy–Rand–Rittler pseudoisochromatic color plates can be used to test color vision in each eye separately. These books are not available in many neurology offices, but pseudoisochromatic color vision tests can also be found in smartphone applications and internet-based resources, although their clinical validity has not yet been rigorously studied. Approximately 1% to 2% of men and 0.5% of women have a congenital red–green color deficiency. A bedside or office alternative to pseudoisochromatic color plates is the "red cap test" in which a red object (such as the cap of a bottle of dilating eye drops) is shown to each eye separately, and the patient is asked to compare the red in each eye, screening for **red desaturation**. In optic neuropathies, color vision deficiency often occurs early or out of proportion to visual acuity and can be a sensitive indicator of optic nerve dysfunction.

C. **Pupils.** The single most important and useful objective bedside test of anterior visual pathway function is the pupillary light response. With unilateral optic nerve damage, the pupillary reaction to light will be less brisk than the response in the unaffected eye, which is an **RAPD**. An RAPD is assessed by the "swinging flashlight test," in which a bright light is shown directly in one eye just long enough for the pupil to constrict, following which the light is quickly moved to the other eye, again just long enough to allow the pupil to constrict. The light is alternated between the two eyes with careful attention to the briskness of the pupillary response. A less brisk reaction or dilation of the pupil when light is shone in the affected eye denotes an RAPD (<u>Video 10.1</u>). As the term "relative" explicitly states, an RAPD refers to a defect in the pupillary reaction to light of one eye *relative* to the other, and therefore *bilateral* RAPDs cannot exist. If vision loss in one eye has resulted in complete blindness, the direct reaction to light in that eye will be absent, known as an **amaurotic pupil**.

D. **Confrontation visual fields** should be performed at a comfortable distance from the patient with the examiner's head at the same level as the patient's. The patient covers one eye with their hand and is instructed to fixate on the examiner's nose without looking at the examiner's fingers. The examiner positions their head such that their nose is in the center of the patient's visual field. The examiner presents one, two, or five fingers in each of the four quadrants of vision. Slowness to respond or an incorrect response in one quadrant or hemifield may be an early sign of homonymous visual field loss. If the patient is able to count fingers in each quadrant, fingers can be presented in any two adjacent quadrants simultaneously while asking the patient to compare the brightness and clarity of the fingers on each hand. Decreased brightness or clarity of one set of fingers may help increase the sensitivity of the examination and detection of a subtle hemianopia (suggestive of a chiasmal or retrochiasmal defect) or altitudinal visual field defect (may be seen with optic nerve or retinal disorders, such as anterior ischemic optic neuropathy [AION] or a branch retinal artery occlusion[BRAO]).

E. **Ophthalmoscopy** is typically performed with a handheld direct ophthalmoscope by most neurologists, which affords a magnified view of the posterior pole of the eye and facilitates a close view of the optic disc and retinal vessels. Recognition of abnormalities of the appearance of the optic disc is a key to the diagnosis of diseases affecting the anterior visual pathways. Pupillary dilation may be performed with 2.5% phenylephrine and 1% tropicamide. Details worth noting include the cup-to-disc ratio, appearance of the retinal vessels including spontaneous venous pulsations, the presence of hemorrhages or exudates, swelling or pallor of the optic discs, appearance of the macula, and the foveal light reflex.

F. **Visual field testing.**

1. **Static perimetry. Humphrey (Fig. 10.1A) and Octopus perimetry** uses static targets to test the central 24 to 30 degrees of the visual field. The test is performed in many

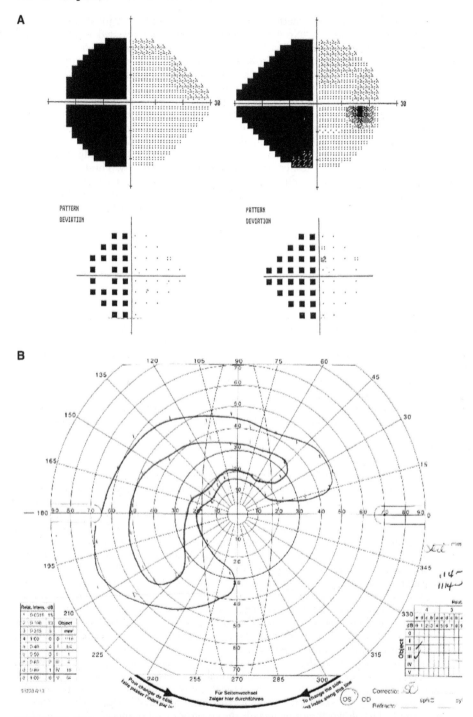

FIGURE 10.1 Visual fields. **A:** Humphrey visual fields showing a complete left HH. **B:** Goldmann visual field of the left eye showing a temporal and superior island of vision with vision loss centrally and inferonasally. The nasal field is to the right and the temporal field is to the left. HH, homonymous hemianopia. (See color plates.)

ophthalmology offices and is the most common form of perimetry performed. The test is sensitive, well validated, and capable of quantifying a visual field abnormality and following the defect over time.

2. **Kinetic perimetry.** Goldmann perimetry (Fig. 10.1B) uses moving lights of variable size and brightness to map the visual field using a kinetic technique. It is performed in an ophthalmologist's office, but technicians trained in this method are becoming increasingly difficult to find. It is technician-dependent, and has largely been supplanted by static perimetry. It is less sensitive than automated static perimetry, but can be useful in patients who perform automated perimetry poorly, have severe visual loss, or have a suspected visual field defect outside the central 30 degrees of vision.

3. **Tangent screen examination** is rarely used today. It can be performed on a black felt screen located 1 m from the patient. A light is shone on the screen by the examiner from behind the patient and the visual field can be mapped. It can be especially helpful in screening for nonorganic "tunnel" vision. Patients with organic visual loss experience enlargement of the visual field when farther away from the screen. However, patients with nonorganic visual loss may insist the visual field size remains the same even with increasing distance from the screen.

G. Neuroimaging.

1. **Computed tomography (CT)/magnetic resonance imaging (MRI).** Imaging studies are often an essential part of the evaluation of a patient with vision loss, and determination of what area to image and the most useful protocol depends on the localization determined by the history and examination. An MRI of the orbits with and without contrast is the preferred neuroimaging study for monocular vision loss suspected to localize to the optic nerve. In cases of possible optic neuritis, imaging should also include the brain to assess the risk of multiple sclerosis. For bitemporal vision loss, even if asymmetric, perform imaging of the optic chiasm and sella with contrast, as in an MRI of the sella/pituitary. An MRI of the brain, with and without contrast, is best for the evaluation of the retrochiasmal visual pathways. CT has the advantages of lower cost and faster image acquisition time, but exposes the patient to radiation and provides inadequate detail of soft tissues that may be affected with vision loss, such as the optic nerves and brain parenchyma. CT can still be very useful in patients who have a contraindication to MRI.

H. Electrophysiologic testing.

1. **Visual evoked potentials (VEPs).** This test can be helpful in selected clinical situations, particularly in cases of suspected prior optic neuritis or suspected nonorganic visual loss. In patients with normal visual acuity and no color visual loss, a prolonged P100 latency may be seen in patients with a previous history of optic neuritis, which reflects subtle incomplete recovery of myelination of the anterior visual pathway. In patients with suspected nonorganic visual loss, a normal VEP waveform and latency can confirm normally functioning intracranial visual pathways. However, patients can focus in the distance, past the VEP fixation target stimulus, and alter the test results. Therefore, a normal VEP in the setting of suspected nonorganic visual loss is very useful, while an abnormal VEP may be inconclusive.

2. **Electroretinography (ERG)** is a test of electrical potentials generated by retinal photoreceptor function. A full-field ERG generates one waveform from the pooled response of photoreceptors from each eye separately, while a multifocal ERG generates multiple waveforms from small groups of adjacent cells in the retina and can detect more localized disturbances of retinal function. ERG is most commonly used to detect conditions such as retinitis pigmentosa and retinal dystrophies. Much like VEPs, a normal result may be useful in supporting a diagnosis of nonorganic visual loss when other structural and functional visual pathway testing is normal.

ACUTE TRANSIENT MONOCULAR VISUAL LOSS

A. Clinical features. Acute transient monocular visual loss (TMVL) has a variety of potential causes. TMVL from a vascular cause (retinal transient ischemic attack) is often referred to as "amaurosis fugax." Patients may have difficulty distinguishing between truly monocular visual loss and a binocular homonymous hemifield defect, particularly if the visual loss event is short-lived or followed by a headache. The history is most likely to be reliable in patients who covered one eye during the event to determine whether one or both eyes were involved. Monocular visual loss may be reported as being sudden in onset, when in reality it was suddenly discovered when the unaffected normal eye was covered.

B. **Time course.** Distinction among the various causes of TMVL can be achieved to some degree with careful consideration of the time course of symptoms. TMVL occurring primarily with positional changes lasting several seconds is most suggestive of transient visual obscurations (TVOs) that occur with increased optic nerve head pressure in susceptible patients, such as those with papilledema (most common), an anomalous and crowded optic nerve head, or optic nerve head drusen. Visual loss over a period of minutes is more likely to be associated with a vascular cause. Common causes of true TMVL include retinal emboli (artery-to-artery emboli or cardiac emboli) and retinal/ocular hypoperfusion. Young patients with frequent TMVL and a negative workup may have vasospasm of a retinal artery. A loss of vision for minutes to hours involving a homonymous portion of the vision in both eyes may be a sign of cerebral transient ischemic attack or migraine.

C. **Approach to TMVL.**

Patients not yet examined by an eye care provider should undergo an eye examination with measurement of best-corrected acuity and intraocular pressure, dilated funduscopic examination, and visual field testing. Findings and testing that may be helpful in narrowing the diagnostic possibilities include:

1. Ophthalmoscopic evidence of asymmetric optic disc cupping (intermittent angle-closure glaucoma), optic disc anomalies (crowded, drusen, and so on), evidence of retinal embolism (hemorrhages, exudates, cholesterol emboli [Hollenhorst plaque], platelet, fibrin, or calcium emboli), and retinal hypotensive retinopathy (retinal hemorrhages with dilation of the veins).

2. An RAPD (Marcus Gunn pupil), visual field loss in both eyes, loss of visual acuity, and color vision deficiency all help localize a possible vision abnormality. TMVL with exercise or exposure to heat may occur in patients with a history of demyelinating or other forms of optic neuropathy (Uhthoff's phenomenon).

3. Proptosis is a sign of intraorbital disease and can be associated with intermittent visual loss due to vascular or optic nerve compression, especially with eye movement in certain directions (gaze-evoked amaurosis).

4. Cardiac murmurs or carotid bruits.

5. Laboratory studies that may be helpful in the evaluation of TMVL include:
   a. Complete blood count (CBC), including platelet count
   b. Erythrocyte sedimentation rate (ESR)—in all patients over age 50
   c. C-reactive protein (CRP)—in all patients over age 50.

6. Cervical vascular imaging is important as vascular TMVL may reveal ipsilateral carotid disease or aortic arch atheroma (depending on local availability, carotid Doppler ultrasound and/ or transcranial Doppler, MR angiography [MRA], or CT angiography may be performed).

7. Brain imaging (ideally brain MRI with diffusion-weighted imaging) is systematically obtained acutely, looking for concomitant acute cerebral ischemia (in which case a brain MRI and MRA of the head and neck are usually performed).

8. Cardiac evaluation typically includes a transthoracic echocardiogram with agitated saline bubble study or transesophageal echocardiogram with careful examination of the aortic arch, left atrial appendage, and interatrial septum looking for a patent foramen ovale, atrial septal defect, and/or atrial septal aneurysm.

9. In patients with a negative vascular and cardiac workup, evaluation for a hypercoagulable state should be considered.

PERSISTENT MONOCULAR VISUAL LOSS

Monocular visual loss can localize anywhere from the spectacles a patient is wearing (or not wearing) to the optic nerve. Vision loss involving the optic chiasm or retrochiasmal visual pathways involves both eyes. The neurologist must be familiar with the clinical findings that help distinguish an optic neuropathy from ophthalmic causes of visual loss. Optic neuropathies are characterized by a loss of central visual acuity, decreased color vision often out of proportion to acuity, an RAPD (when vision loss is unilateral or asymmetric), and often an abnormal optic disc appearance such as pallor or edema. Exceptions exist, such as AION, which often spares central visual acuity, or typical retrobulbar optic neuritis in which the funduscopic appearance is normal during the acute phase. Nevertheless, the presence of an RAPD is one of the most reliable indicators of unilateral or asymmetric optic nerve dysfunction.

A. Acute/subacute clinical syndromes involving the optic nerve.

1. Optic neuritis. Inflammation of the optic nerve occurs most often in younger patients and presents with monocular visual loss and is associated with pain with eye movements in >90% of cases. The visual loss is most often central or altitudinal, but may involve any portion of the visual field. Patients may report colors as dim or "washed out." Two-thirds of patients have a normal optic disc appearance acutely, while one-third have optic disc edema. Visual acuity can range from 20/20 to NLP, but most often is between 20/50 and 20/200. Visual recovery occurs over weeks and the prognosis for visual recovery is very good. Poor recovery of vision following an episode of suspected optic neuritis should prompt consideration of neuromyelitis optica, or a vascular event, such as ischemic optic neuropathy.

2. AION. AION typically presents in older patients with acute, monocular visual loss, which may worsen over several days. Acutely, all patients should have optic disc edema (Fig. 10.2A) and an RAPD (if unilateral and no prior contralateral optic nerve damage) (Video 10.1). There are two forms of AION:

   a. Nonarteritic AION (NAION). Approximately 90% of AION cases are nonarteritic and one of the most important risk factors is a structural predisposition from a small, nearly cupless, optic disc (Fig. 10.2B). This "disc at risk" is predisposed to an ischemic cascade in which ischemia leads to optic disc swelling, which causes compression of fibers in the already crowded optic nerve head, leading to a decrease in optic nerve head blood flow that further increases ischemic damage and swelling, and so on. NAION is typically painless and characteristically associated with an altitudinal, nasal quadrantic, or central scotoma visual field defect. Patients with a history of NAION are at increased risk for involvement of the second eye. While some providers offer a course of oral steroids in selected cases, no treatment has yet been proven effective in the treatment of NAION.

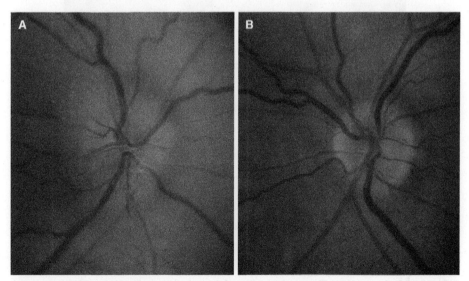

FIGURE 10.2 **A:** NAION showing acute optic disc edema in the right eye, with small peripapillary hemorrhages and exudates, as well as optic disc hyperemia. **B:** The optic disc in the patient's fellow eye is small and cupless, known as a "disc at risk" for NAION. NAION, nonarteritic anterior ischemic optic neuropathy. (See color plates.)

b. **Arteritic AION (AAION).** AAION tends to occur in older individuals than those with NAION, and giant cell arteritis (GCA) is the most common cause. Symptoms suggestive of GCA include a new headache, scalp tenderness, preceding episodes of TMVL, and jaw claudication. Polymyalgia rheumatica may also be present. AAION typically causes sudden, severe, permanent visual loss. Visual acuity is usually 20/200 or less and visual field defects range from an altitudinal visual field defect to a large central scotoma or even complete blindness. The optic disc is always swollen acutely, and is often also pale ("pallid edema"). ESR, CRP, and CBC should be checked emergently and if the clinical history and laboratory results are suggestive, intravenous high-dose corticosteroids should be started without delay. A temporal artery biopsy should be performed, but treatment of suspected GCA should not be delayed under any circumstances. The prognosis for visual recovery is poor. The risk of involvement of the second eye in GCA without adequate treatment is very high, and may occur within hours or days.

3. **Leber's hereditary optic neuropathy (LHON)** is a disorder of mitochondrial DNA, inherited through the maternal lineage. It presents as subacute, painless, monocular visual loss over days, and most commonly affects men in their teens to twenties (8:1 men to women). The second eye becomes similarly affected weeks to months after the first eye. During the acute phase, the optic disc may appear slightly swollen with a mildly hyperemic appearance (Fig. 10.3). After at least several weeks, the nerve fiber layer becomes atrophic, particularly in the region of the papillomacular bundle. Both optic discs become pale after nerve fibers are lost. Visual acuity typically ranges between 20/200 and 20/800 and there are dense central scotomas. Confirmation of the diagnosis is made with genetic testing screening for specific mutations in the mitochondrial DNA.

B. Chronic monocular visual loss from optic neuropathy

1. **Compressive optic neuropathies** are typically painless and may slowly progress over years, or may progress more quickly, depending on the nature of the compressing

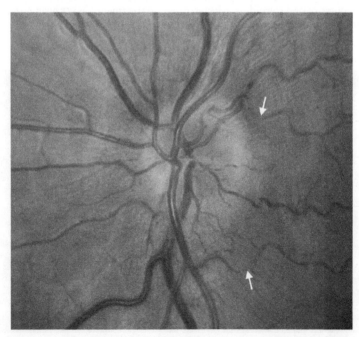

FIGURE 10.3 Acute LHON. There is thickening of the retinal nerve fiber layer (**RNFL**) surrounding the optic disc. The RNFL has a faintly white striated appearance and is oriented in a radial pattern from the optic disc. The thickened RNFL partially obscures some of the retinal vessels (*white arrows*). There is also hyperemia of the optic disc, with a "reddish" appearance. LHON, Leber's hereditary optic neuropathy. (See color plates.)

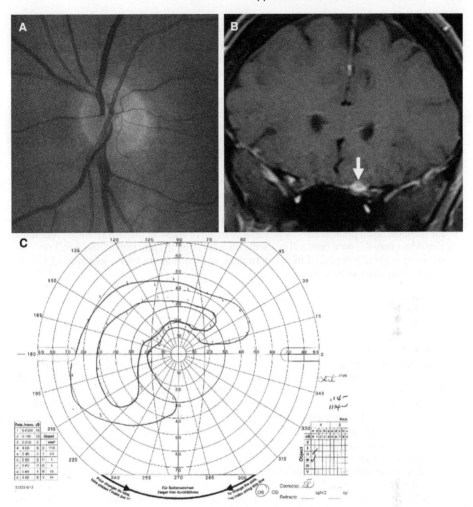

FIGURE 10.4 Planum sphenoidale meningioma causing a compressive optic neuropathy. **A:** Fundus photograph showing the patient's normal-appearing left optic disc. **B:** Coronal post-contrast T1-weighted MRI showing enhancement of a mass encasing and compressing the left optic nerve (*arrow*), which was missed on a prior MRI performed without contrast. **C:** Goldmann visual field of the patient's left eye showing a preserved island of vision superotemporally. (See color plates.)

lesion (Fig. 10.4). If the optic nerve is compressed by a mass within the orbit, there may be proptosis, limitation of extraocular motility, eye movement-induced transient visual loss (gaze-evoked amaurosis), conjunctival congestion, and chemosis. If optic nerve compression occurs within the optic canal or intracranially, proptosis occurs late, or may not occur at all. Clinically, there are features of optic neuropathy and the optic disc may appear normal (Fig. 10.4A), or exhibit optic disc edema, pallor, or both. Retino-choroidal collateral (shunt) vessels may develop on the optic disc in the setting of chronic disc swelling from optic nerve compression and impaired venous drainage.
2. **Other causes of optic neuropathy** include glaucoma (usually involves both eyes), dominant optic atrophy, toxic exposure (methanol, ethylene glycol, ethambutol), vitamin deficiency (vitamin B_{12}), damage from papilledema or trauma, and inflammatory, infectious, and infiltrative optic neuropathies.

SUDDEN BINOCULAR VISION LOSS

A. **Acute onset binocular visual loss** is most often because of chiasmal or retrochiasmal visual pathway lesions. Occasionally, acute binocular vision loss can be because of bilateral optic nerve dysfunction, such as ischemic optic neuropathy or optic neuritis (especially with neuromyelitis optica). On examination, one optic disc may be pale and atrophic, indicative of prior damage, and the other disc may show signs of acute damage, such as optic disc edema. This is characteristic of the **"Foster Kennedy syndrome"** in which a frontal tumor can cause an ipsilateral compressive optic neuropathy, as well as optic disc edema in the contralateral eye because of elevated intracranial pressure. A **"pseudo-Foster Kennedy syndrome"** can occur in conditions in which the optic disc edema is not because of papilledema. For example, prior AION in one eye may leave optic disc pallor, while acute AION in the fellow eye causes optic disc edema.

    TVOs occur in patients with increased tissue pressure at the optic nerve head, which may be associated with papilledema, optic nerve head drusen, or an otherwise anomalous optic disc. TVOs are experienced as transient blurring or dimming of the vision, lasting for seconds, often precipitated by postural changes or Valsalva maneuver. Rarely, binocular visual loss may follow a cerebral or cardiovascular angiography procedure. A full recovery of vision is usually expected in hours to days, and permanent vision loss related to toxic contrast exposure is very rare.

BINOCULAR VISUAL LOSS DUE TO OPTIC CHIASM DYSFUNCTION

A. Clinical features

  1. Bitemporal visual loss. Compression of the inferior portion of the optic chiasm, as in an expanding pituitary adenoma under the chiasm, results in superior bitemporal visual loss. Compression of the optic chiasm from above may occur with an aneurysm of the anterior cerebral artery or a craniopharyngioma and causes inferior bitemporal visual loss. Complete bitemporal defects are usually due to tumor compression of the chiasm, or may occur with a traumatic tear of the optic chiasm.

      Some patients may not notice their bitemporal visual loss and may instead experience other symptoms related to instability of the two preserved nasal visual fields. These symptoms may include intermittent diplopia, loss of objects, and vertical sliding of one hemifield relative to the other. This "slip" in the retinas causes one-half of the image to slip vertically and/or horizontally in relation to the other half because of the brain's difficulty in finding overlapping corresponding portions of intact visual field. These symptoms are known as **"hemifield slide"** phenomena.

  2. Junctional syndrome. If dysfunction of the optic chiasm occurs at the point where one optic nerve meets the chiasm, a **junctional** syndrome occurs in which vision loss occurs centrally in that eye, and superotemporally in the fellow eye. In its most severe form, complete vision loss in one eye is accompanied by complete temporal hemifield loss in the fellow eye.

  3. **Pituitary apoplexy.** An acute hemorrhage into a pituitary tumor or the pituitary gland **(pituitary apoplexy)** can cause the abrupt onset of unilateral or bilateral visual loss and may be accompanied by ocular motility disturbances related to dysfunction of cranial nerves III, IV, or VI. Headache, fever, and a stiff neck may be associated symptoms. Apoplexy may occur spontaneously or result from infarction following cardiac surgery or carotid endarterectomy. The diagnosis may be confirmed with an MRI or CT scan. Only rarely does pituitary apoplexy cause pure visual loss and is more often associated with some ocular motility disturbance. Pituitary apoplexy is a "don't miss" diagnosis among the various causes of sudden bilateral visual loss.

B. Clinical approach to nonacute binocular visual loss

  1. As with more acute visual loss, attempt to localize the deficit with the available history.

  2. On examination, visual acuity, color vision, and confrontation visual fields should all be assessed.

  3. Ophthalmoscopy may reveal important clues. For example, optic disc pallor is indicative of intracranial visual pathway injury, usually to the optic nerve, at least 4 to 6 weeks after

an acute event. Hemorrhages and optic disc edema can be acute or chronic. **Bowtie pallor**, in which there is pallor of the temporal and nasal optic disc, sparing the superior and inferior disc, occurs when the fibers that cross at the optic chiasm (nasal optic disc and papillomacular bundle/temporal optic disc) are atrophic because of damage of the optic chiasm or pregeniculate retrochiasmal visual pathways.

HOMONYMOUS HEMIANOPIA

Homonymous hemianopia (HH) is a term used to describe hemifield loss that is on the same side of the vertical meridian in both eyes (Fig. 10.5). A HH can be complete or incomplete depending on the extent of hemifield involvement, and congruous or incongruous (in incomplete hemianopias), depending on how similar the visual field is in one eye compared with the other. Associated signs, such as hemiparesis, hemisensory loss, aphasia, or parietal neglect, also give clues to the localization. In general, the more posterior the visual pathway lesion in the post-geniculate visual pathways, the more congruous the visual field defect between the two eyes.

A. **Localization.** HH localizes to the retrochiasmal visual pathways on the side of the brain opposite the visual field defect, which include the optic tract, the lateral geniculate nucleus (LGN), optic radiations (geniculocalcarine tract), and occipital cortex.

    1. **Optic tract.** A HH accompanied by an RAPD on the same side as the hemianopia is a sign of optic tract dysfunction.

    2. **LGN.** The LGN has a dual blood supply from the lateral choroidal artery (a branch of the posterior cerebral artery) and the anterior choroidal artery (a branch of the internal carotid artery). Occlusion of the lateral choroidal artery causes a homonymous

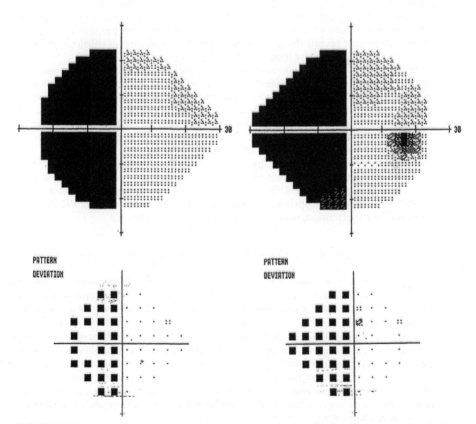

FIGURE 10.5 Homonymous hemianopia. Humphrey visual fields showing a complete left HH. HH, homonymous hemianopia.

sectoranopia around the horizontal meridian, and occlusion of the anterior choroidal artery causes a HH sparing the sector around the horizontal meridian. Mass lesions of the LGN more often produce a complete HH.

3. **Primary visual cortex.** Occipital lobe damage produces pure visual loss if the damage is confined to the calcarine cortex (primary visual cortex). Total loss of the calcarine cortex on one side will give a complete HH. Commonly, the macular region of calcarine cortex is "spared" to some extent because a large part of the visual cortex closest to the occipital pole subserves the inner 20 degrees of the visual field. Also, there may be a dual blood supply to the occipital pole, with anastomoses from branches of the middle and posterior cerebral arteries. Small occipital pole infarcts that cause visual loss within the central 20 degrees of the visual field can be difficult to detect by standard perimetry.

B. **Migraine aura.** One of the most common causes of episodic homonymous visual loss is the visual aura of migraine, which some patients may mistakenly believe is associated with visual loss in only one eye (the eye with the temporal visual field defect). Characteristic features include positive visual phenomena such as colored lights that flicker or shimmer in a zig-zag pattern surrounding an area of visual loss ("scintillating scotoma") that may expand over a period of minutes. Other descriptions include a "heat wave" like the appearance just above a road in the distance on a hot day, or a central visual image in both eyes "as if a flashbulb just went off." These visual events usually last from 5 to 60 minutes and are often followed by a headache. The headache is classically unilateral, but may be generalized. Some patients, especially older migraineurs, may have only the visual aura without a headache, called *acephalgic migraine*.

C. **Occipital lobe epilepsy.** Seizures with primarily visual manifestations without secondary generalization may be seen in patients with metastatic brain tumors, meningiomas, gliomas, and arteriovenous malformations affecting the occipital lobes. The seizures may produce homonymous flickering lights, flashes, and colors, but unlike migraine, there is no characteristic buildup and progression of visual symptoms from the center to the periphery. A head CT or brain MRI usually reveals the responsible lesion and an electroencephalogram (EEG) may show epileptiform activity localized to the occipital region.

D. **Degenerative diseases.** The Heidenhain variant of sporadic Creutzfeldt–Jakob disease (CJD) may present with a rapidly progressive HH as the condition affects the occipital lobes out of proportion to other brain regions. Rarely, patients with other neurodegenerative diseases, such as Alzheimer's disease (AD), may develop a HH. CJD can be distinguished from AD by the time course of symptom progression and characteristic MRI and EEG changes. Progressive multifocal leukoencephalopathy may present with a HH and demyelinating changes on MRI that characteristically spare the U-fibers.

E. **Posterior reversible encephalopathy syndrome (PRES)** can present with a HH in cases with asymmetric involvement of the occipital lobes, or cerebral blindness when there is bilateral involvement. PRES is likely related to cerebral edema from failure of the blood–brain barrier to appropriately compartmentalize intravascular fluid. PRES can be precipitated by hypertension, toxic medications, and various diseases.

VISION DISTURBANCES RELATED TO HIGHER COGNITIVE DYSFUNCTION

These visual disturbances are most commonly caused by embolic stroke, but may also be caused by primary or metastatic tumors, or other lesions. The unusual symptoms produced by lesions of the association visual areas in the brain, often with a lack of vision loss, frequently go unrecognized.

A. **Alexia without agraphia** is caused by damage to the connections between both visual cortices and the angular gyrus. This condition can be associated with a HH in the case of a left occipital infarct that also involves the splenium of the corpus callosum. Alexia without agraphia can also exist without a HH with lesions to the splenium of the corpus callosum (outflow from the right occipital lobe) and the connections of the left occipital lobe to the angular gyrus. In all cases, words "read" by the occipital lobes are not properly relayed to the appropriate language centers in the dominant hemisphere.

B. **Balint's syndrome** is characterized by visual disorientation, optic apraxia ("spasm of fixation"), optic ataxia (defect in visually guided hand movements), and simultanagnosia (inability to put together pieces of a visual scene) due to bilateral damage to the border zone between the middle and posterior cerebral artery territories in the high parietal lobes. Affected patients may have difficulty articulating their visual disturbance, but are not typically demented or aphasic.

C. **Bilateral inferior temporal lobe damage** with damage to the V4 area of the fusiform gyrus may cause **prosopagnosia** (the inability to recognize faces) and **central achromatopsia** (central color vision loss).

   1. **Prosopagnosia** is the inability to recognize individual faces, but patients may also have trouble recognizing their car, dog, or other items among similar items. They can identify classes of objects, but have difficulty singling out a specific individual within a general class or group without other clues. They may compensate by becoming increasingly adept at recognizing features of a person's voice or the way they walk to help identify them. There may be a homonymous superior quadrantic visual field defect or no associated visual loss. Patients may have a sudden deficit from bilateral inferior temporal lobe damage or a previously damaged inferior temporal lobe and then a second lesion to the other inferior temporal lobe. Less commonly, a patient may have prosopagnosia with a unilateral right inferior temporal lobe lesion.

   2. **Central achromatopsia** can involve one hemifield in both eyes (hemiachromatopsia) or the entire visual field. The degree of color loss may vary from profound achromatopsia to more subtle desaturation of colors. The responsible lesions are in the inferior temporal lobes.

D. **Anton syndrome** is caused by extensive bilateral damage to both the occipital and parietal lobes, causing visual loss and denial of blindness. Patients often confabulate elaborately in answering questions about their visual environment.

NONORGANIC VISUAL LOSS

Patients with nonorganic vision loss claim partial or total visual loss in one or both eyes despite normal eyes and intracranial visual pathways. The vision loss can be voluntary or involuntary. Severe vision loss in one eye, when related to an optic neuropathy, is always accompanied by an RAPD. The lack of an RAPD in the case of severe monocular vision loss may raise suspicion for nonorganic visual loss after other intraocular causes have been excluded by an ophthalmologist. Various examination techniques can be used to confirm nonorganic visual loss. An optokinetic flag or drum can screen for optokinetic nystagmus in each eye individually. The presence of an optokinetic response requires visual acuity of at least 20/400. A mirror can also be held in front of the patient's face and then tilted up and down and side to side. The eyes will usually move to orient the patient in space or follow the patient's own reflection. Moderate binocular nonorganic visual loss (e.g., acuity of 20/50 in both eyes) can be difficult to prove, as the lack of an RAPD and a normal optokinetic response offer no additional useful information. Electrophysiologic testing, such as a VEP or ERG, can be helpful. Patients can voluntarily alter these tests to give an abnormal response, so these tests are most helpful when the results are normal. Severe bilateral nonorganic visual loss can be inferred from failure of proprioception tests that appear to require vision, such as "bring the tips of your index fingers together" or "sign your name." Having the patient make several hand signals that are both shown and described followed by one in which the sign is shown, but not described, can sometimes uncover nonorganic visual loss.

A. Approach to the patient with suspected nonorganic visual loss.

   1. Observe the patient carefully, including how they entered the examination room, their response to visual cues, eye contact, and resistance to testing. Document each visual test performed and the patient's response, including behavior.

   2. Greater resistance to the examination may be seen in deliberate malingerers more often than naïve nonorganic patients who may be oblivious to obvious contradictions in their examination performance.

   3. Once the examination is complete, confronting the patient is rarely helpful. Suggesting that the vision is "better than the patient is aware" and is likely to improve can be helpful. Malingerers may accuse the examiner of not believing their symptoms or suggesting that they are simply "all in their head."

4. Radiographic (CT and MRI) and electrophysiologic studies (ERG and VEP) should be interpreted for the patient to be sure that no doubts regarding the etiology of vision loss remain. The patient should be told that there is no disease of the nervous system causing these symptoms. It may be useful to reassure them that "the structure and function of the eyes and the parts of the brain that control vision are working normally. In some people, the brain temporarily has trouble using the eyes and parts of the brain that control vision, even though they are normal."

5. It can be counterproductive to hope for a placebo effect by prescribing unnecessary eye drops or a medication, which undermines the assertion that there is no disease causing the symptoms. Artificial tears are reasonable to recommend to patients with signs or symptoms of dry eyes.

B. General rules in the evaluation of patients with vision loss

1. Perform a history and examination with localization of the vision loss in mind.

2. Perform imaging studies specific to the localization determined by your history and examination. For example, for monocular vision loss suspected to localize to the optic nerve, perform an MRI of the orbits with and without contrast. In cases of possible optic neuritis, imaging should also include the brain. For bitemporal vision loss, even if asymmetric, perform imaging of the optic chiasm and sella with contrast, as in an MRI of the sella/pituitary.

3. An evaluation by an ophthalmologist should always be performed in cases of monocular or binocular vision loss that do not clearly localize to the optic nerves or intracranial pathways of vision. The ophthalmology evaluation can include automated visual field testing, fundus photography, and optical coherence tomography that may not be available in most neurology clinics.

Key Points

- In patients with visual loss, the history and examination should first focus on localization, which helps with forming an appropriate differential diagnosis and directing additional testing.
- In the absence of a severe unilateral retina problem (which should be easily visible to an ophthalmologist), an RAPD indicates an optic neuropathy.
- MRI of the orbits with contrast and fat suppression techniques is the imaging modality of choice in patients with a suspected optic neuropathy.
- Patients with visual loss not obviously ascribable to a lesion of the intracranial pathways of vision should always be examined by an ophthalmologist.
- Patients with nonorganic vision loss may still have an organic cause of vision loss, with conscious or subconscious embellishment.

Recommended Readings

Atkins EJ, Newman NJ, Biousse V. Lesions of the optic nerve. *Handb Clin Neurol.* 2011;102:159–184.

Biousse V, Newman NJ. *Neuro-Ophthalmology Illustrated.* 2nd ed. New York, NY: Thieme; 2016.

Feske SK. Posterior reversible encephalopathy syndrome: a review. *Semin Neurol.* 2011;31(2):202–215.

Grzybowski A, Zülsdorff M, Wilhelm H, et al. Toxic optic neuropathies: an updated review. *Acta Ophthalmol.* 2015;93(5):402–410.

Miller NR. Neuro-ophthalmologic manifestations of nonorganic disease. In: Miller NR, Newman NJ, eds. *Walsh and Hoyt's Clinical Neuro-Ophthalmology.* Vol 1. 6th ed. Baltimore, MD: Lippincott Williams & Wilkins; 2004.

Newman NJ, Biousse V. Diagnostic approach to vision loss. *Continuum (Minneap Minn).* 2014;20(4):785–815.

Prasad S. Diagnostic neuroimaging in neuro-ophthalmic disorders. *Continuum (Minneap Minn).* 2014;20(4):1023–1062.

11 Approach to the Patient with Abnormal Pupils

Aki Kawasaki

The pupil size at any given moment is determined by the sum of active sympathetic and parasympathetic inputs to two iris muscles, the radial dilator and the sphincter. Ambient illumination and mental alertness are two important influences on the resting pupil size. An abrupt increase in light will trigger the pupil light reflex and conversely, sudden darkness will lead to reflex pupillary dilation.

The retina is the source of light information for the pupil light reflex. The axons of a special subset of retinal neurons, called the intrinsically photosensitive retinal ganglion cells, form a monosynaptic conduit from the retina to the paired pretectal olivary nuclei of the dorsal midbrain (retinotectal tract). This is the afferent limb of the **pupillary light reflex** and is carried in the optic nerve. Similar to the afferent visual signals, the axons carrying pupillomotor signals that derive from the nasal retina decussate at the optic chiasm.

The pretectal olivary nuclei integrate light information along with other supranuclear influences and then transmit to the Edinger–Westphal nuclei of the oculomotor nuclear complex. The projections are both ipsilateral and contralateral, forming a second decussation of the light reflex pathway at the pretectum (Fig. 11.1). The Edinger–Westphal nuclei are the origin of the oculo-parasympathetic pathway whose activation results in iris sphincter contraction for pupillary constriction and ciliary muscle contraction for accommodation.

Pupillary dilation is a reflex response to sudden arousal or darkness and is mediated by the sympathetic pathway (Fig. 11.2). The oculo-sympathetic pathway is a three-neuron pathway that originates in the hypothalamus and signals contraction of the iris dilator muscle.

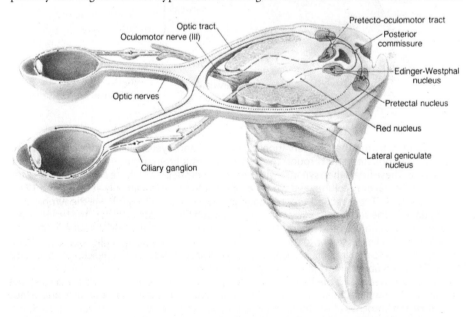

FIGURE 11.1 Diagram of the path of the pupillary light reflex. (From Miller NR, Newman NJ, Biousse V, et al, eds. In: *Walsh and Hoyt's Clinical Neuro-Ophthalmology: The Essentials.* 2nd ed. Philadelphia, PA: Wolters Kluwer Health/Lippincott Williams & Wilkins; 2008:316.)

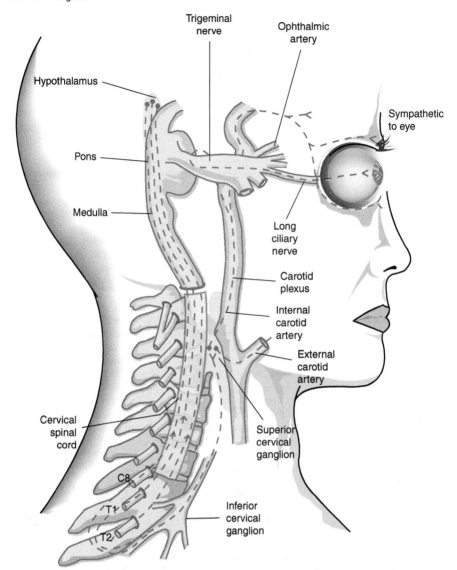

FIGURE 11.2 Sympathetic innervation of the pupil and eyelids. First-order hypothalamic (central) neurons descend through the brain stem (midbrain, pons, medulla) and cervical spinal cord. These fibers then synapse with preganglionic neurons whose cell bodies like in the intermediolateral gray column and whose axons exit the core ipsilaterally at C8; T1 and T2 via the ventral roots. These second-order (preganglionic) fibers travel rostrally via the sympathetic chain, traverse the superior mediastinum, pass through the stellate ganglion (the fusion of the inferior cervical ganglion and the first thoracic ganglion), and terminate in the superior cervical ganglion, which lies posterior to the angle of the mandible. The postganglionic axons ascend within the carotid plexus, which surrounds the internal carotid artery to reach the cavernous sinus. The pupil fibers briefly join the sixth nerve then follow branches of the first division of the trigeminal nerve and the long ciliary nerve to reach the iris dilator muscle. Fibers to the tarsal muscles (Müller's muscles) also travel within the carotid plexus to the cavernous sinus then may join branches of the third nerve before reaching the upper and lower eyelids. Sudomotor fibers, for example, for sweating to the lower face, follow the external carotid and then the facial arteries. (From Liu GT, Volpe NJ, Galetta SL, eds. *Neuro-Ophthalmology Diagnosis and Management.* 2nd ed. Philadelphia, PA: WB Saunders/Elsevier; 2010. Reprinted with permission.)

PUPILLARY EXAMINATION

Both the static and dynamic aspects of the pupils should be examined. This includes noting the resting pupil size in dim and bright illumination, comparing the speed and amplitude of pupillary movement to a light stimulus (and to darkness, if indicated) and comparing the pupil response between the two eyes.

A. **Hippus.** An awake patient sitting quietly in room light may show small, irregular, spontaneous oscillations of pupil size, known as *hippus*. It reflects fluctuations in the central modulating signals to the Edinger–Westphal subnuclei.

B. **Pupil size**

Baseline pupil size is dependent on many factors, and in particular the level of ambient light. Under dim light conditions, pupils are largest (7 to 9 mm) during the teenage years and then gradually decrease with increasing age. Asymmetry of pupil size, or anisocoria, of 0.4 mm or more is visible to the unaided eye. Depending on the pathology, the magnitude of anisocoria varies under different light conditions.

1. Anisocoria whose magnitude is greater under bright light suggests an inability of the larger pupil to constrict. This may be due to a defective iris, sphincter muscle failure, or impairment along the oculo-parasympathetic pathway.

2. Anisocoria that is more apparent in darkness implies a failure of dilation; thus, the smaller pupil is likely to be the faulty one.

C. **Testing the pupil light reflex**

Have the patient fixate on a distant target in a darkened room. Shine a bright focal light (a non-halogen penlight is not bright enough) directly onto one pupil for 3 seconds and note the speed and amplitude of constriction. Do this two or three times for a mental "average." Remember that a pupil that constricts poorly to direct light stimulation may be due to an optic neuropathy (defective afferent limb), interruption along the oculo-sympathetic pathway (defective efferent limb), or a damaged iris sphincter (defective mechanics). The latter two mechanisms result in anisocoria.

D. **Performing the alternating light test**

This is the standard clinical technique for identifying asymmetry of afferent pupillomotor input between the two eyes, referred to as the **relative afferent pupillary defect (RAPD)**.

1. **Technique.** Have the patient fixate a distant target in a dark room. Shine a bright focal light directly onto one pupil for 3 seconds, and then quickly swing the light onto the other pupil for 3 seconds. Repeat this for four or five alternations of light stimulation and watch the illuminated pupil (direct light response). The amplitude and velocity of pupillary constriction as well as the degree of redilation that occurs within the 3 seconds of light stimulation should be symmetric between the two eyes.

2. **A large RAPD** is present if the pupil of the "bad" eye simply dilates when the light is alternated back onto it after being on the "good" eye. In other words, the bad eye sees so little, if any, light that reflex dilation to darkness is instead initiated. Note that an RAPD is not a cause of anisocoria (Video 11.1).

3. **A small-to-moderate RAPD** is sometimes difficult to detect. The bad eye "sees" enough light to initiate pupillary constriction on direct stimulation but it is a less vigorous response compared to that of the good eye. The pupil of the bad eye also "escapes," that is, redilates sooner after the initial constriction (Video 11.2).

RELATIVE AFFERENT PUPILLARY DEFECT

The presence of an RAPD indicates unilateral or asymmetric injury to the afferent limb of the pupillary light reflex. In most instances, an RAPD is associated with optic nerve damage. Cataracts, corneal opacities, and vitreous lesions do not cause an RAPD, despite causing significant visual disturbance.

A. **Optic nerve lesions.**

1. An RAPD is a sensitive indicator of optic nerve dysfunction. A small RAPD often persists in patients with previous optic neuritis in whom vision has recovered.

2. The magnitude of RAPD is better correlated with the extent of visual field loss than with visual acuity. Patients with optic neuropathy and RAPD can have 20/20 acuity.

3. The extent of damage in bilateral optic nerve disorders is rarely symmetric. Therefore, an RAPD is generally found on the side with greater damage. An exception to the rule occurs in patients with Leber hereditary optic neuropathy or autosomal-dominant optic atrophy. These patients have visual loss because of optic nerve dysfunction and yet maintain relative preservation of the pupil light reflex. This visual–pupillary dissociation is presumably related to a greater resistance of intrinsically photosensitive retinal ganglion cells to neurodegeneration caused by mitochondrial dysfunction.

B. Retinal lesions. Less commonly, an RAPD results from severe retinal disorders associated with severe visual loss.

1. Large unilateral retinal lesions such as central retinal artery occlusion, large retinal detachment, or trauma produce an obvious RAPD. A dilated funduscopic examination usually confirms the diagnosis.

2. In the patient with poor acuity, a central scotoma and yet displays no-to-minimal RAPD, look for a macular lesion. Multifocal electroretinography may be indicated.

C. Optic chiasm. Lesions of the optic chiasm that produce bilateral but asymmetric visual dysfunction cause an RAPD in the eye with greater amount of visual field loss.

D. Optic tract lesions. In the patient with a homonymous hemianopsia due to an optic tract lesion, an RAPD may be present in the contralateral eye. A tract RAPD reflects the greater proportion of decussating axons compared to nondecussating axons at the optic chiasm.

E. Pretectal nucleus. A unilateral dorsal midbrain lesion such as stroke or tumor that damages the pretectal olivary nucleus on one side can produce a small RAPD in the contralateral eye. This is the rare occurrence of RAPD without associated visual loss.

MECHANICAL ANISOCORIA: "OPHTHALMOLOGIC" ANISOCORIA

Two iris muscles modulate pupil size and shape—the sphincter and the dilator. Damage to one or both iris muscles can distort the size, shape, and mobility of the pupil. Ocular pathologies such as trauma, infection, or surgery are common causes of a mechanical anisocoria. It is important to consider and identify ocular causes of anisocoria in order to avoid unnecessary neurologic evaluation.

A. History. Inquire about any previous infection, inflammation, trauma, or surgery involving the eyes, including laser procedures.

B. Examination

1. Marked irregularity of the pupillary margin, unusual distortion of pupillary shape, and a difference in iris color suggest that the iris structure and framework are damaged. Such findings are appreciated with direct observation (Fig. 11.3).

2. A slit lamp examination of the iris is needed to identify most other causes of mechanical anisocoria such as synechiae (adhesions), small sphincter tears, transillumination defects, and inflammation (Fig. 11.3). A dusting of iris pigment may form a ring on the lens of a patient who has had a blow to the eye.

UNILATERAL MYDRIASIS: NEUROLOGIC OR PHARMACOLOGIC?

Once mechanical causes of anisocoria are ruled out, it is important to confirm that the mydriatic pupil is the abnormal one. It should have a poor light reflex compared to the smaller pupil. The three most common nonocular conditions to cause unilateral mydriasis (a large, poorly reactive pupil) are oculomotor (third) nerve palsy, tonic pupil, and pharmacologically dilated pupil. The first two conditions represent an interruption somewhere along the oculo-para-sympathetic pathway. The preganglionic oculo-parasympathetic fibers originating in the Edinger–Westphal subnucleus travel with motor fibers of the oculomotor nerve and synapse in the ciliary ganglion of the orbit. The postganglionic parasympathetic fibers travel in the short ciliary nerves and innervate the iris sphincter, which mediates pupilloconstriction, and the ciliary muscle, which mediates accommodation. A tonic pupil results from damage to the postganglionic parasympathetic neurons and fibers to the eye. The neurotransmitter at the iris sphincter is acetylcholine.

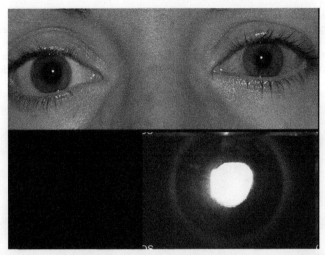

FIGURE 11.3 Patient with uveitis and anisocoria. The left pupil is ovoid in shape and has a weak response to light stimulation and near effort **(top)**. Slit lamp examination shows transillumination defects of the iris and irregular atrophy of the sphincter **(bottom)**. Inflammation-induced iris damage is the cause of this patient's anisocoria. (See color plates.)

A. Oculomotor (third cranial) nerve palsy

   Lesions that damage the preganglionic parasympathetic pupil fibers of the oculomotor nerve nearly always damage one or more motor fibers as well. With rare exception, a unilateral mydriasis that appears as an isolated finding (no ptosis, no diplopia) is not likely to be an oculomotor nerve palsy.

   1. Clinical features of unilateral mydriasis due to oculomotor nerve palsy
      a. Large poorly reactive pupil. The pupil on the side of the nerve palsy is the larger pupil and constricts poorly to both light stimulation and near (accommodative) effort.
      b. Responsiveness to pilocarpine. A mydriatic pupil from an oculomotor palsy will always constrict vigorously to topical full-strength (1% to 4%) pilocarpine. This is because pilocarpine acts directly on cholinergic receptors of the sphincter muscle. In about two-thirds of cases, such a pupil may also respond similarly well to dilute 0.125% pilocarpine, if cholinergic denervation supersensitivity of the sphincter has developed.
      c. Ipsilateral ptosis. The ptosis of an oculomotor nerve palsy may range from a slight, barely noticeable ptosis to complete ptosis.
      d. Ocular motility disturbance. A deficit of infraduction, supraduction, and/or adduction is nearly always present on the side of the larger pupil. **Caution:** Sometimes only one or two motor functions are disturbed, for example, an oculomotor nerve palsy with only ptosis and supraduction deficit. Cross-cover or red glass testing is important for detecting subtle ophthalmoplegia in patients with partial oculomotor nerve palsy.
   2. **Etiology of oculomotor nerve palsy** (see Chapter 12).
   3. Workup. **An acute and isolated oculomotor nerve palsy with pupillary involvement warrants emergent neuroimaging** to look for pituitary apoplexy, brainstem stroke, or expanding posterior communicating artery aneurysm. Remember that early compression by an aneurysm can cause a partial oculomotor palsy and no initial pupillary dysfunction. Investigation of other causes of an oculomotor nerve palsy should be directed by the clinical presentation.

B. Tonic pupil (Adie pupil)

   A tonic pupil is the most common neurologic cause of unilateral mydriasis in an otherwise healthy and alert patient. It is caused by injury to the ciliary ganglion in the orbit or to the postganglionic short ciliary nerves destined to the iris sphincter and ciliary muscle.

   1. **Symptoms** are anisocoria, photophobia, blurred near vision, and brow ache.

2. Clinical features (Fig. 11.4)
   a. **Large pupil.** An acute tonic pupil is a freshly denervated pupil. It is often very dilated and quite unreactive to light stimulation and near effort.
   b. **Sectoral palsy of the iris sphincter.** Parasympathetic denervation of the iris sphincter is often incomplete. The sphincter segments with preserved innervation are able to

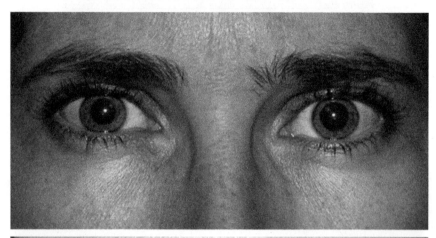

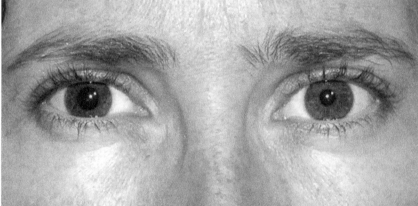

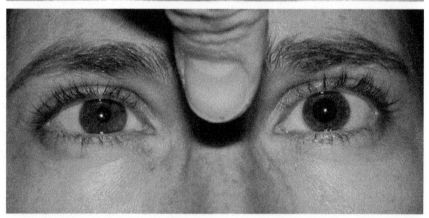

FIGURE 11.4 Patient with right tonic pupil. Pupils are dilated almost equally in very dim light (**top**). Under bright light, observed marked anisocoria is observed (**middle**). The right pupil shows a better constriction to near effort (LND) (**bottom**). LND, light-near dissociation. (See color plates.)

contract and tighten the pupillary margin like a pulled purse string. The denervated segments (palsied) are immobile and the adjacent pupillary margin remains flat. This clinical sign is present at all stages of tonic pupil. Slit lamp examination of the iris is required. Sectoral sphincter palsy is not observed in mydriasis because of third nerve palsy or pharmacologic manipulation.

c. **Poor light reaction.** The pupil light reflex of a tonic pupil is weak, sometimes appearing to be completely absent. This clinical sign is, like sectoral palsy, present at all stages of tonic pupil.

d. **Poor pupil near response and accommodation paresis.** Accommodation and pupillary constriction to near effort, like the pupil light reflex, are lost in the acute phase. Unlike the light reflex, these responses later recover (see **section B.4 under Unilateral Mydriasis: Neurologic or Pharmacologic?**).

e. **Light-near dissociation (LND).** Several weeks to months after denervation, the accommodative fibers in the short ciliary nerves resprout and often reinnervate (aberrantly) the iris sphincter. This restores the pupillary near response but not the light reflex. Thus, LND develops during the subacute stage of tonic pupil. Because of the aberrant reinnervation, the pupillary constriction to near effort is delayed and slow and sustained, and hence the term "tonic."

f. **Pupillary redilation** after pupilloconstriction to near effort (accommodation) is delayed and slow, owing to the tonicity of pupilloconstriction. Sometimes, patients complain of difficulty with vision after prolonged near work.

g. **Baseline pupil size.** An acute tonic pupil is large. After several months, the baseline pupil size starts to decrease. A chronic tonic pupil is often a miotic pupil that constricts poorly to light and dilates poorly in darkness. The near response is, however, more vigorous.

3. **Pharmacologic testing for cholinergic denervation supersensitivity.**

a. Place two drops of dilute pilocarpine (0.125% or less) in each eye. Wait 30 to 45 minutes.

b. Dilute pilocarpine usually has no effect on a normal eye. Constriction of the suspected pupil is a positive test for cholinergic supersensitivity and indicates cholinergic denervation of the iris sphincter (Fig. 11.5).

c. Mydriasis from oculomotor nerve palsy (preganglionic parasympathetic denervation) and tonic pupil (postganglionic parasympathetic denervation) may both demonstrate cholinergic denervation supersensitivity to dilute pilocarpine.

4. Pathophysiology

a. **Acute denervation.** Parasympathetic fibers carried in the oculomotor (third) nerve synapse at the ciliary ganglion in the orbit. Injury to the ciliary ganglion or the short ciliary nerves (carrying postganglionic parasympathetic fibers) denervates the ciliary muscle and the iris sphincter; thus, accommodation and pupilloconstriction are acutely abolished. Sectoral palsy of the iris is, however, often visible at the slit lamp.

b. **Aberrant reinnervation.** Sometime after the acute denervation injury, the accommodative fibers originally destined for the ciliary muscle resprout and reinnervate the ciliary muscle. Thus, accommodation (near vision) recovers. The resprouting accommodative fibers also send collateral branches to the iris sphincter (aberrant reinnervation) such that the pupillary near response recovers but with slow and tonic pupillary movements. The original pupilloconstrictor fibers tend not to regenerate; thus, the pupil light reflex remains poor or absent.

Agent	Mechanism of Action	Test Procedure	Positive Result	Example of Patient with Right Tonic Pupil
Pilocarpine 0.125% or less	Denervation supersensitivity of cholinergic receptors on the iris sphincter to weak cholinergic agonist	Put 2 drops of dilute (0.125%) pilocarpine in both eyes. Wait 45 minutes.	Larger (suspected) pupil becomes smaller pupil Or Suspected pupil constricts more than normal pupil	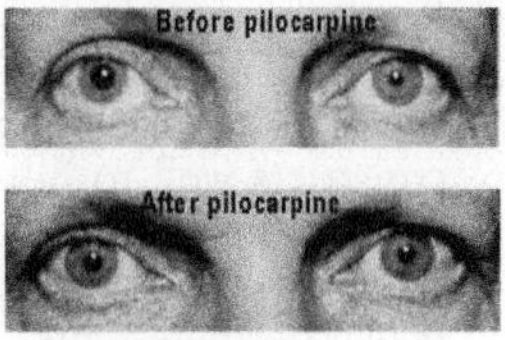

FIGURE 11.5 Pharmacologic testing for cholinergic denervation supersensitivity.

TABLE 11.1 Common Lesions along the Oculo-Parasympathetic Pathway that Cause a Large, Poorly Reactive Pupil

Preganglionic: Oculomotor Nerve Palsy	Postganglionic: Tonic Pupil
Brainstem (midbrain)—"fascicular"	Intraorbital
Ischemia	Viral ganglionitis
Hemorrhage	Trauma
Tumor	Ocular surgery
Arteriovenous malformation	Tumor
Interpeduncular fossa, subarachnoid space	Systemic autonomic neuropathy
Basilar artery aneurysm	Hereditary neuropathy (e.g., Charcot–Marie–Tooth disease, Riley–Day syndrome)
Basal infection (granulomatous meningitis, fungal meningitis)	Acquired peripheral neuropathy (diabetes, alcohol, toxins, amyloid, vasculitis)
Intraneural ischemia—"vasculopathic" (e.g., diabetes, hypertension)	Idiopathic (Adie's) tonic pupil
Cavernous sinus, superior orbital fissure	
Tumor (e.g., meningioma, pituitary adenoma)	
Inflammation (Tolosa–Hunt syndrome)	
Cavernous carotid aneurysm	
Thrombosis	
Fistula	

Brainstem "fascicular" oculomotor nerve palsy occasionally occurs as an isolated finding but is more commonly associated with other neurologic deficits (i.e., Weber's, Benedikt's, Claude's, and Nothnagel's syndromes). Vasculopathic oculomotor nerve palsy tends to spare the pupil. Compressive lesions typically involve the pupil.

5. **Etiology.** The most common form of an acute unilateral tonic pupil is Adie pupil, an idiopathic condition that typically affects women between the ages of 20 and 40 years (see Table 11.1). **An isolated unilateral tonic pupil in an otherwise healthy person does not require imaging studies.** Recent literature has emphasized that a unilateral tonic pupil can be an early manifestation of neurosyphilis. Workup of an isolated unilateral tonic pupil is serologic testing for syphilis and inflammatory disease. Unilateral tonic pupil in the context of other systemic or neurologic signs or bilateral tonic pupils suggests a systemic inflammatory condition, autonomic neuropathy, or even paraneoplastic condition, and the workup should be expanded accordingly.

6. **Management.** Management is aimed at symptom relief: reading glasses for accommodation loss, sunglasses for photosensitivity. In children, however, careful refractive correction may be recommended to avoid development of amblyopia in the eye with acute tonic pupil. Regular refraction should continue as the tonic pupil evolves.

C. **Pharmacologic mydriasis**

1. Parasympatholytic or anticholinergic ophthalmic agents include atropine, cyclopentolate, and tropicamide. Products containing atropine-like substances include scopolamine patch, certain insecticide, plants, and anticholinergic inhalants, for example, ipratropium, used to treat respiratory disease. An atropinized pupil is very large, in the order of 8 to 9 mm, and does not react to light or near stimulation. It is also unreactive to full-strength (1% to 4%) pilocarpine.

2. Sympathomimetics are adrenergic substances that cause mydriasis by excessive stimulation of the dilator muscle without paralysis of the sphincter muscle. Thus, a pharmacologic mydriasis from a sympathomimetic agent retains some degree of light reaction and constricts well to full-strength pilocarpine. Additional clues to sympathomimetic mydriasis are preserved near vision, conjunctival blanching, and eyelid retraction. Common topical sympathomimetic agents include epinephrine, phenylephrine, and ocular decongestants.

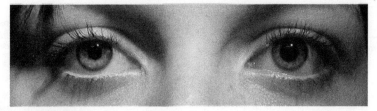

FIGURE 11.6 This patient has an anisocoria that, in the absence of significant ptosis, was initially thought to be physiologic in origin. Topical apraclonidine testing, however, confirmed a right Horner's syndrome. (See color plates.)

ANISOCORIA GREATER IN DARKNESS: NEUROLOGIC ANISOCORIA VERSUS PHYSIOLOGIC ANISOCORIA

A. Horner's syndrome (an oculo-sympathetic defect)
  1. Clinical characteristics
      a. **Ptosis.** Sympathetic denervation of the tarsal lid muscles leads to droopiness of the upper lid and elevation of lower lid (upper and lower lid ptosis). Together they create the impression of enophthalmos. Upper lid ptosis is generally mild and is absent in 12% of patients with Horner's syndrome (Fig. 11.6).
      b. **Anisocoria.** The anisocoria is not marked in room light, often 1.0 mm or less, but becomes more apparent in dim lighting. As the anisocoria stems from a failure of the smaller pupil to dilate, the light reflex is normal in patients with Horner's syndrome.
      c. **Pupillary dilation lag.** Turn the room light off abruptly and watch both pupils. The normal pupil dilates promptly within a few seconds. The Horner's pupil dilates slowly, taking 20 to 30 seconds to reach baseline size in darkness. Pupillary dilation lag is a very specific sign of an oculo-sympathetic defect but is demonstrable in only about half of patients with Horner's syndrome.
      d. **Ipsilateral facial anhidrosis** is variably present.
      e. **Heterochromia iridis** (different iris color) suggests congenital sympathetic denervation. Asymmetry of hair texture is also a sign of congenital Horner's syndrome.
  2. Pharmacologic diagnosis
      a. **Topical cocaine test.** Cocaine is an indirect sympathomimetic and, when placed on the normally innervated eye, causes pupillary dilation and lid retraction. A sympathetically denervated eye will not respond to topical cocaine and as such, the post-cocaine anisocoria is larger than the pre-cocaine anisocoria (Fig. 11.7).
      b. **Topical apraclonidine test.** Apraclonidine has weak alpha-1 agonist action, which can be used to look for adrenergic denervation supersensitivity. A sympathetically denervated pupil will dilate in response to apraclonidine, and a reversal of anisocoria following apraclonidine is diagnostic (Fig. 11.8). Apraclonidine is not used in infants.

Agent	Mechanism of Action	Test Procedure	Effect on Normal Eye	Effect on Horner Eye	Positive Result	Example of Patient with Right Horner Syndrome
Cocaine (4% or 10%)	Indirect sympathomimetic via inhibition of the reuptake of norepinephrine in postsynaptic junction	Put 2 drops of cocaine in both eyes Wait 45 minutes	Pupil dilation, lid retraction, conjunctival blanching	None	Postcocaine anisocoria of 1.0 mm or more (smaller pupil is the Horner's pupil)	Before cocaine 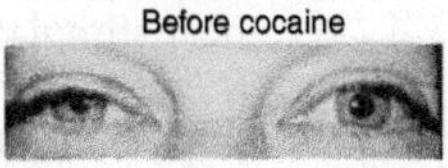 After cocaine 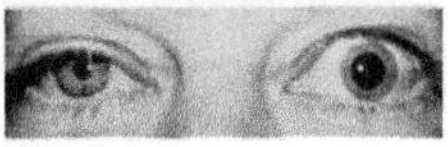

FIGURE 11.7 Pharmacologic testing for Horner's syndrome using topical cocaine.

Agent	Mechanism of Action	Test Procedure	Effect on Normal Eye	Effect on Horner Eye	Positive Result	Example of Patient with Left Horner Syndrome
Apraclonidine (0.5% or 1%)	Denervation sensitivity to weak agonist action at postsynaptic alpha 1 adrenergic receptors	Put 1 drop of apaclonidine in both eyes Wait 45 minutes	None	Pupil dilation, lid retraction, conjunctival blanching	Postapraclonidine reversal of anisocoria (larger pupil is Horner' pupil)	Before apraclonidine 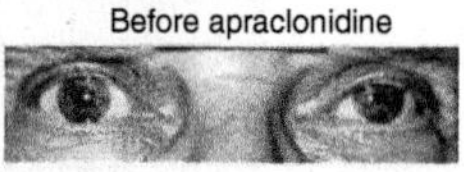 After apraclonidine 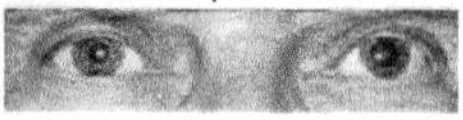

FIGURE 11.8 Pharmacologic testing for Horner's syndrome using topical apraclonidine.

3. Localization
   a. **Central Horner's syndrome** is usually accompanied by other symptoms or signs of brainstem dysfunction (e.g., Wallenberg's syndrome). Anhidrosis involves the whole ipsilateral face, neck, and body.
   b. **Preganglionic Horner's syndrome** causes ipsilateral anhidrosis of the face and neck. Weakness and wasting of the ipsilateral hand muscles suggest injury at the C8–T2 spinal rootlets or brachial plexus. Pain in the supraclavicular fossa suggests a superior sulcus lesion (Pancoast's syndrome). Past surgical procedures, use of central catheters, or trauma to the neck or chest may be a cause of oculo-sympathetic injury. Thyroid enlargement (goiter), cancer, and surgical resection may also cause preganglionic Horner's syndrome.
   c. **Postganglionic Horner's syndrome** is not associated with clinically appreciable facial anhidrosis. Pain in the jaw, ear, throat, or peritonsillar area suggests carotid pathology, particularly dissection. Associated ipsilateral trigeminal dysfunction (dysesthesia, numbness) or an ipsilateral sixth nerve palsy localizes the lesion to the parasellar–cavernous sinus region of the skull base.
4. Etiology of Horner's syndrome
   In general, a central Horner's syndrome is stroke related. Preganglionic lesions are notoriously neoplastic, and postganglionic lesions are mostly benign. **Note: A painful postganglionic Horner's syndrome should be evaluated for internal carotid artery dissection,** especially in the acute setting when the risk of stroke is high and anticoagulation may be warranted. Carotid dissection must be differentiated from cluster headaches, which can cause postganglionic Horner's syndrome in up to 22% of cases.
B. Aberrant regeneration of the oculomotor nerve
   1. Pathophysiology. When a structural lesion compresses or transects the oculomotor nerve, the fibers innervating the extraocular muscles can sprout misguided collaterals that aberrantly innervate the iris sphincter. Primary ischemic injury such as diabetic third nerve palsy does not cause aberrant regeneration.
   2. Clinical characteristics
      a. **Synchronous unilateral pupilloconstriction** during attempted adduction, supraduction, or infraduction of the globe. This occurs from coactivation of an extraocular muscle and the iris sphincter.
      b. Poor light reflex. Because the original parasympathetic fibers to the iris sphincter have been disrupted by the structural lesion, the pupil responds poorly to light and near stimulation.
      c. Reversed anisocoria. In some cases, the aberrantly innervated pupil is the larger pupil under bright light and the smaller pupil in darkness.
C. Physiologic anisocoria
   1. This disorder is also called benign or essential anisocoria.
   2. Incidence. Approximately 20% of the general population have pupillary inequality of 0.4 mm or more in dim lighting.
   3. Clinical characteristics
      a. The difference in pupil size is usually 1.0 mm or less and can vary in amplitude (even within a few minutes).

  b. The anisocoria is slightly greater in darkness than in bright light. Patients often notice their anisocoria "disappears" in the sunlight.

  c. Physiologic anisocoria occasionally will "reverse" sides—that is, the larger pupil can be on one side at first but on the other side later.

  d. All reflex pupillary movements are normal and symmetric (light reflex, near response, and dilation in dark). All responses to pharmacologic tests are symmetric.

 4. Workup: None.

LIGHT-NEAR DISSOCIATION

Under normal conditions, the amplitude of pupillary constriction to a light stimulus is greater than that to a near effort. Never test the near response with a bright light, because the two stimuli summate and create the false impression of LND. LND occurs under the following circumstances.

A. The most common cause of LND is optic neuropathy, which results in reduced afferent pupillomotor input.

B. A central lesion may interrupt the afferent signal from the eye (light reflex) but spare the afferent signal mediating the near response. Such a lesion is usually situated in the dorsal midbrain.

 1. Midbrain LND. This form of LND is a feature of the sylvian aqueduct syndrome or dorsal midbrain syndrome. Both pupils are typically midsize and show poor response to light stimulation. However, the pupil constriction with near effort is normal. Associated motility dysfunction includes bilateral lid retraction, supranuclear vertical gaze palsy, and convergence–retraction nystagmus.

 2. Argyll Robertson pupils. Both pupils are very small and often irregular in shape. They demonstrate an absence of the light response, a preserved near response, as well as poor dilation in darkness. Visual function is intact. Argyll Robertson pupils are distinguished from bilateral chronic tonic pupils (which have LND) by the briskness of the pupil constriction to near effort. In both cases, syphilis must be ruled out.

C. The light response and the near response are initially both damaged, but the near response is restored via aberrant regeneration of the short ciliary nerves. The classic example is a tonic (Adie) pupil.

Recommended Readings

Cooper-Knock J, Pepper I, Hodgson T, et al. Early diagnosis of Horner's syndrome using topical apraclonidine. *J Neuroophthalmol.* 2011;31:214–216

Davagnanam I, Fraser CL, Miszkiel K, et al. Adult Horner's syndrome: a combined clinical, pharmacological, and imaging algorithm. *Eye.* 2013;27:291–298.

Kardon RH, Bergamin O. Adie's pupil. In: Levin LA, Arnold AC, eds. *Neuro-Ophthalmology: The Practical Guide.* New York, NY: Thieme;2005:325–339.

Kardon RH, Denison CE, Brown CK, et al. Critical evaluation of the cocaine test in the diagnosis of Horner's syndrome. *Arch Ophthalmol.* 1990;108:384–387.

Kawasaki A. Disorders of pupillary function, accommodation and lacrimation. In: Miller NR, Newman NJ, Biousse V, Kerrison J, eds. *Walsh and Hoyt's Clinical Neuro-Ophthalmology.* 6th ed. Baltimore, MD: Lippincott Williams & Wilkins; 2005:739–805.

Kawasaki A. Diagnostic approach to pupillary abnormalities. *Continuum (Minneap Minn).* 2014;20:1008–1022.

LaMorgia C, Ross-Cisneros FN, Sadun AA, et al. Melanopsin retinal ganglion cells are resistant to neurodegeneration in mitochondrial optic neuropathies. *Brain.* 2010;133:2426–2438.

Thompson HS, Corbett JJ, Cox TA. How to measure the relative afferent pupillary defect. *Surv Ophthalmol.* 1981;26:39–42.

Thompson HS, Kardon RH. The Argyll Robertson pupil. *J Neuroophthalmol.* 2006;26:134–138.

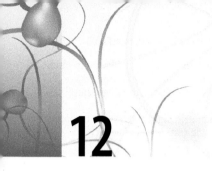

12 Approach to the Patient with Diplopia

Devin D. Mackay and Valerie Purvin

Normal binocular vision is accomplished by focusing slightly different views of the same object on the fovea of each eye. When the visual axes are misaligned, the images fall on non-corresponding areas of the two retinas, usually experienced as **diplopia.** Binocular diplopia is characterized by resolution with covering either eye and is a hallmark of ocular misalignment. Occasionally, patients interpret this as blurring rather than doubling of the image, but the "blur" is relieved by closing either eye. The absence of diplopia despite ocular misalignment and intact vision usually implies a very long-standing (often congenital) disorder.

MONOCULAR VERSUS BINOCULAR DIPLOPIA

By far, the most important question in the evaluation of diplopia is whether the double vision is monocular or binocular. Monocular diplopia is not due to ocular misalignment, but is an optical disorder, due to an uncorrected refractive error, corneal aberration (e.g., dry eyes) or lenticular change (cataract). Rare cases of monocular diplopia due to neurologic disease, termed "cerebral polyopia," can be identified by the presence of diplopia in both eyes, associated homonymous visual field loss, and other symptoms of disordered visual integration. Finally, unlike monocular diplopia due to ocular disease, cerebral diplopia does not resolve with pinhole. Patients with monocular diplopia should be referred to an ophthalmologist for further evaluation and treatment.

HISTORY

A. Description. After establishing that a patient's diplopia is binocular, and therefore due to ocular misalignment, the abnormality can often be further localized and the differential diagnosis narrowed with some specific questions. "Is the misalignment horizontal or vertical?" "Is it worse in any particular direction of gaze or head posture?" "Is it worse at distance or at near?" For example, diplopia associated with a sixth nerve palsy (NP) will be horizontal, worse at distance (as with driving), and worse with gaze in the direction of the palsy. "Is it constant or intermittent?" Diplopia that is not present immediately upon awakening, but worsens during the day is suggestive of myasthenia gravis. More prominence of diplopia with fatigue is nonspecific and frequently described by patients with an underlying phoria that intermittently escapes fusion. "Is there any history of strabismus or ocular misalignment as a child?" "Has the diplopia changed since onset?"

B. Associated symptoms. Patients should also be questioned regarding accompanying symptoms. "Is there eye or head pain?" The presence of pain with eye movement suggests an orbital condition, usually inflammatory. Diplopia associated with pain in the distribution of the first division of the trigeminal nerve (V_1) may localize to the cavernous sinus or superior orbital fissure. Unilateral or bilateral sixth NP associated with headache suggests increased intracranial pressure (ICP). Other symptoms of increased ICP include transient visual obscurations and pulsatile tinnitus. Patients over the age of 50 with diplopia should be questioned regarding symptoms of giant cell arteritis, including scalp tenderness, jaw claudication, proximal muscle stiffness, and constitutional symptoms. In individuals with painless, pupil-sparing diplopia, myasthenia gravis is always a consideration; ask about ptosis, dysphagia, dysarthria, difficulty holding the head up, fatigue with chewing, and limb weakness. Finally, patients should be questioned about other symptoms referable to a brainstem disorder such as dizziness, incoordination, ataxia, numbness, and weakness.

TERMINOLOGY

A. A **phoria**, also termed a **latent deviation**, is a tendency toward ocular misalignment that is only detectable when binocular vision is interrupted (i.e., when one eye is covered). A **tropia**, or **manifest deviation**, is an ocular misalignment that is present with both eyes viewing. Many normal individuals have some degree of underlying phoria that, under normal viewing conditions, is easily held in check by fusional vergence mechanisms. The fusional system is fairly delicate, however, and can be disrupted by a number of factors including advancing age, intercurrent illness, minor trauma, and medications that have central nervous system (CNS) depressant properties such as sedative/hypnotics, pain medications, and anticonvulsants. The vertical fusional system is less robust than the horizontal mechanism.

B. The prefix attached to either term indicates the direction of the manifest or latent deviation: an **eso**tropia is an inward deviation of the eye, **exo**tropia outward, **hyper**tropia upward, and **hypo**tropia downward. Common abbreviations used for charting include ET, XT, and HT, with the latter referring to a hyper deviation, by convention. **Ortho**phoria indicates that the eyes are aligned, even with one eye covered.

C. Ocular misalignment may be the same in all fields of gaze, termed **comitant**, or may vary depending on the position of gaze, termed **incomitant**. This distinction is important because misalignment due to weakness of an extraocular muscle is always worse in the direction of action of that muscle (incomitant). Nonparetic misalignment (e.g., congenital esotropia) is the same in all fields of gaze (comitant). The term **strabismus** is nonspecific, simply referring to any form of ocular misalignment or deviation. Eye movements tested with both eyes viewing are called **versions**, and eye movements tested with only one eye viewing are called **ductions**. Infraduction indicates a downward movement, supraduction an upward movement, abduction a movement away from the midline, and adduction a movement toward the midline. In vergence movements, the eyes are moving in opposite directions at the same time: **convergence** (inward movement) and **divergence** (outward movement).

EXAMINATION

A. **Head position and fixation.** The examination begins with observing the patient while looking at a target. An abnormal head position is characteristic of certain incomitant ocular deviations. Patients with a sixth NP often adopt a head turn toward the side of the lesion, causing the eyes to look out of the field of the paretic muscle. A head tilt away from the side of the weak muscle is characteristic of a fourth NP. Such patients often find that their misalignment is better on up gaze (out of the field of the paretic muscle) and so they adopt, in addition, a chin-down posture. Patients with restrictive orbitopathy (e.g., thyroid eye disease) frequently have limitation of up gaze and so will often adopt a head-back (chin-up) position. It is normal to have an occasional eye movement off the fixation target, but the presence of frequent saccadic intrusions indicates loss of normal inhibition of brainstem pause cells and is characteristic of progressive supranuclear palsy and cerebellar dysfunction. Simple inattentiveness to the target causing larger excursions may indicate frontal lobe disease or more global cerebral dysfunction.

B. **Range of movement.** The patient is instructed to follow a target through the full range of normal eye movements. The range of motion can be quantified using degrees of excursion from primary position, normal being 45 degrees to either side or down and 40 degrees on upgaze. Mild limitation of upgaze is common in elderly patients. Some scleral show on abduction can be normal if it is symmetric between the two eyes and there is no esodeviation. Patients with a true abduction limitation always have a corresponding esodeviation. Limitation can also be graded with a series of hatchmarks from 1 to 4, with 1 indicating mild underaction and 4 signifying no movement past mid-position in that direction, or an estimation of the percentage of normal movement in a particular direction.

C. **Testing saccades.** Limitation of eye movement due to a cranial NP or a supranuclear disorder is associated with saccadic slowing. *In contrast, marked limitation with normal saccadic velocity is characteristic of orbital restrictive disease and of myasthenia.* In myasthenia, large amplitude saccades may exhibit intrasaccadic fatigue, causing slowing at the end of the excursion. Small amplitude saccades will be quite rapid, sometimes appearing as small "quiver" movements in patients with myasthenia. *Slowing of medial rectus saccades is the most* *sensitive sign of internuclear ophthalmoplegia* (INO) and is extremely helpful for distinguishing this condition from other causes of an adduction deficit.

D. **Subjective diplopia testing.** Assessment of alignment based on simple observation of the eyes is extremely insensitive, particularly for vertical misalignments. Some information concerning alignment can be obtained from subjective diplopia testing, which includes red glass and Maddox rod techniques, but objective methods are usually more informative. Whatever techniques are used, it is important to note that *the displacement of the image is always opposite to the displacement of the eye.* For example, when the eye is deviated downward, the image is up. Subjective methods can be useful for identifying which image is coming from which eye in order to determine the direction and pattern of misalignment. For example, viewing a small white light with a red glass held over the right eye, a patient with a right sixth NP will report seeing the red light to the right of the white light and will report that the separation of the two images is greater when looking to the right and less when looking to the left. A Maddox rod transforms a point source of white light into a red line and is useful for demonstrating both phorias and tropias, whereas the red glass technique is less useful for phorias, as the patient may still be able to fuse the two lights. A Maddox rod is an inexpensive and simple device, but a valuable addition to the neurologist's set of tools.

E. **Objective diplopia testing.** Cover tests are the most accurate and preferred method for diagnosing strabismus. In the **cover–uncover test**, one eye is covered and then uncovered, alternating between monocular and binocular vision, while the patient fixates on a target first in primary position and then in different positions of gaze. If a tropia is present, when the fixating eye is covered, the other eye will move to reacquire the target. The direction of this movement of redress will always be opposite to the direction of the deviation. For example, if the eye is exotropic, it will move in to take up fixation. In the alternate (or cross-cover) test, the occluder is quickly transferred from one eye to the other and back, thus preventing binocular viewing. As in the cover–uncover test, any movement of redress is noted. The cover–uncover test reveals tropias, whereas the alternate cover test reveals both tropias and phorias. Although the results of such testing can be quantified with prisms, the examiner may still obtain meaningful information without quantification of the ocular misalignment. In cases of vertical strabismus, ocular alignment can be measured in the upright and supine positions. A decrease in vertical strabismus by at least 50% in the supine position is suggestive of skew deviation as the cause.

F. **Head tilt test.** Diagnosis of vertical diplopia is notoriously difficult if based on ductional deficits alone. **Bielschowsky's three-step test** was designed to determine the paretic muscle responsible for vertical misalignment and is an enormously valuable technique (Fig. 12.1). The ocular alignment results used for the three-step test can be obtained from alternate cover testing, red glass, Maddox rod, patient description, or any other technique that provides the necessary information.

Step 1. Note the vertical deviation in primary position. Take, for example, a patient with a right fourth NP (Fig. 12.1). This individual will have a right hypertropia (RHT) in primary position. This pattern could be due to underaction of the superior oblique or inferior rectus muscle in the right eye (not pulling the right eye down sufficiently) or to underaction of the inferior oblique or superior rectus muscle in the left eye (not pulling the left eye up).

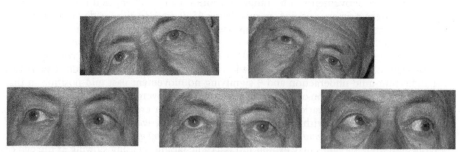

FIGURE 12.1 The three-step test in a patient with a right fourth nerve palsy. Note the right hypertropia is greater on left gaze and with right head tilt.

Step 2. Record the magnitude of the deviation on gaze to either side. In a right fourth NP, the deviation is greater on left gaze, indicating that it must be due to a muscle that has its greatest action in that direction of gaze, either the right superior oblique or the left superior rectus.

Step 3. Compare the deviation with head tilt to either side. In a right fourth NP, the deviation is worse with right head tilt. A right head tilt demands an intorsion movement of the right eye, normally accomplished by the superior oblique and superior rectus muscles. The vertical actions of these two muscles normally cancel each other out but, in the face of a weak superior oblique, contraction of the unopposed superior rectus elevates the eye and worsens the misalignment.

G. **Other examination features.** It is important to look for orbital signs, which are sometimes subtle. These include proptosis, chemosis, conjunctival injection, and globe retraction with attempted eye movement, the latter best observed from the side. Careful inspection for pupil asymmetry or abnormal pupillary function is important, particularly in cases of a suspected mild or partial third NP. It is also helpful to look specifically for evidence of aberrant third nerve regeneration, which may accompany a slow-growing lesion causing a compressive third NP. Lid abnormalities may be helpful, including both retraction (usually indicative of thyroid eye disease) and ptosis (common in myasthenia, third NP, and oculosympathetic palsy). Von Graefe's sign (retarded descent of the upper lid on downward movement of the eye) and lid lag (static higher than normal elevation of the upper lid in downgaze) may be seen with thyroid eye disease. Cogan's lid twitch (twitch of the upper lid on return to primary gaze after prolonged downgaze) may be seen in myasthenia gravis. When eye movements appear limited with voluntary gaze, it is sometimes helpful to also test reflex movements, either with head turning (the vestibulo-ocular or "doll's head" maneuver), Bell's phenomenon (upward eye deviation with forced eyelid closure), or calorics.

LOCALIZATION AND ETIOLOGIES

Binocular diplopia can be caused by disorders of the extraocular muscles, neuromuscular junction, cranial nerves, brainstem, and orbit. In most cases, the pattern of ocular motor dysfunction and the presence of associated abnormalities allow accurate localization.

A. **Brainstem.** Disorders within the brainstem can cause abnormal eye movements by causing nuclear or fascicular cranial nerve palsies, INO, and skew deviation. Most lesions that involve **supranuclear** structures do not produce diplopia because reflex input keeps the eyes aligned. The main exceptions to this concept are disorders that affect vergence: divergence insufficiency causes esotropia at distance, and convergence paresis produces exotropia at near. Common causes of brainstem dysfunction are stroke, demyelinating disease, hemorrhage, inflammation, tumor, trauma, congenital anomalies, and certain metabolic derangements (e.g., Wernicke's encephalopathy).

1. **Nuclear lesions** cause distinctive patterns of oculomotor dysfunction
    a. Unilateral lesions of the oculomotor nucleus cause ipsilateral paresis of the extraocular muscles (EOMs) innervated by the third nerve, plus bilateral ptosis and loss of upgaze. The ipsilateral superior rectus subnucleus projects to the contralateral superior rectus causing loss of upgaze in both eyes. Because the levators are innervated by a single midline central caudal nucleus, a unilateral nuclear palsy causes bilateral ptosis.
    b. The trochlear nucleus innervates the contralateral superior oblique muscle. Head trauma, midbrain tumors, and hydrocephalus may damage both fourth nerves because they decussate in the anterior medullary velum.
    c. A lesion of the abducens nucleus produces an ipsilateral horizontal gaze palsy rather than a sixth NP because, in addition to motor neurons for abduction, the nucleus contains interneurons that supply the contralateral medial rectus subnucleus.
2. **Fascicular** lesions usually affect adjacent brainstem structures and can be localized accordingly. These syndromes are characterized by an ipsilateral ocular motor NP and a contralateral hemi-sensory or hemi-motor deficit and/or ipsilateral cerebellar dysfunction.
3. Damage to the **medial longitudinal fasciculus** produces a disconnection between the ipsilateral abducens nucleus and the contralateral medial rectus subnucleus, resulting in an INO. In addition to a variable degree of ipsilateral adduction deficit, there is slowing of medial rectus saccades and overshoot of contralateral abducting saccades

with abduction nystagmus. Despite limitation of adduction, the eyes are usually aligned in primary position. In young patients, the most common etiology is demyelination and INO is commonly bilateral; in older individuals, the cause is most often stroke and lesions are more often unilateral.

4. Loss of **otolith** input causes vertical strabismus termed **skew deviation**. As otolith input changes with head position, the ocular misalignment of a skew deviation may improve with the patient in the supine position. Unlike misalignment due to a cranial NP, the muscle imbalance in skew is typically comitant, that is, the same in all directions of gaze.

B. Cranial nerves. Common causes of cranial neuropathy are ischemia, compression, meningitis (inflammatory or neoplastic), trauma, and congenital. The most common cause of an isolated ocular motor palsy in older adults is microvascular disease, termed a **vasculopathic palsy**. Most patients have one or more vascular risk factors (diabetes mellitus, hypertension, and hypercholesterolemia). Onset is acute, usually with ipsilateral pain, which resolves spontaneously within 7 to 10 days. Resolution of the motility disturbance takes place within 6 months.

1. **Third (oculomotor) NP**, when complete, causes loss of adduction, supraduction, and infraduction, profound ptosis, and a large, poorly reactive pupil. Unopposed action of the superior oblique and lateral rectus muscles causes a characteristic exotropic and hypotropic eye position. Partial forms are common, however, and recognizing the pattern of ocular misalignment is important (Fig. 12.2). One specific form of partial third NP affects only the **superior division**, resulting in ptosis plus isolated loss of upgaze. Because the pupillomotor fibers travel superficially in the third nerve, the pupil is usually affected early in a compressive third NP, particularly that is due to a posterior communicating artery (pCOM) aneurysm. In contrast, vasculopathic third NP typically spares the pupil (Video 12.1). Thus, the presence of pupil sparing is often taken to "rule out" a pCOM aneurysm as the cause of a third NP. When a third NP is partial, however, pupil sparing is less reassuring because this pattern is occasionally seen with pCOM aneurysms. An otherwise complete but pupil-sparing third NP is never due to a pCOM aneurysm. Pupil sparing is also common in third NPs arising from lesions in the cavernous sinus.

2. **Fourth (trochlear) nerve palsies** result in a limitation of infraduction when the eye is adducted. Patients report vertical and torsional diplopia. The most common cause is trauma, which frequently produces bilateral fourth NPs. Congenital fourth NPs are also common and may present at any age because of decompensation of fusion. A contralateral head tilt on old photographs may be a clue to a history of a congenital fourth NP. It is difficult to test fourth-nerve function in the presence of a third NP because the globe does not move to the position of advantage for the superior oblique muscle; instead the presence of intorsion on attempted downgaze is used to indicate preservation of fourth-nerve function (Video 12.1).

3. **Sixth-nerve (abducens) palsy** causes esotropia and loss of abduction with slowing of lateral rectus saccades (Fig. 12.3). In young adults, multiple sclerosis and tumors are

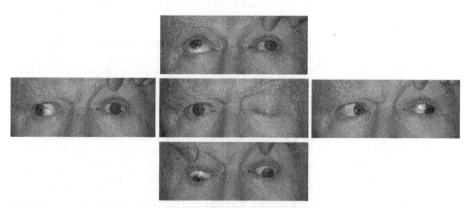

FIGURE 12.2 A 65-year-old man with a diabetic (vasculopathic) left third nerve palsy. There is loss of all third-nerve function with the exception of the pupil.

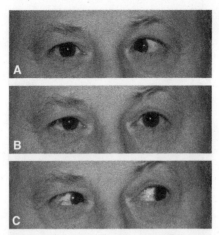

FIGURE 12.3 A 35-year-old man with acute onset of a right sixth nerve palsy secondary to multiple sclerosis. There is a moderate esotropia in primary position (B) that increases on right gaze (A).

important considerations; in older adults, vasculopathic cranial NP is most common. Chronic (greater than 6 months duration) sixth NP is often due to a compressive lesion at the skull base, such as a meningioma. Sixth NP can also be a "false localizing sign" of elevated ICP, caused by downward traction on the nerve.

4. **Combined cranial NP** involving the third, fourth, and sixth nerves localizes to the cavernous sinus or superior orbital fissure. The oculosympathetics and first division of the trigeminal nerve are commonly involved. Etiologies include tumor (primary and metastatic), vascular conditions (cavernous sinus thrombosis, fistula, and aneurysm), pituitary apoplexy, and infection/inflammation.

C. Extraocular muscles.

1. **Neuromuscular junction disease** is most commonly due to **myasthenia**, which causes painless, pupil-sparing, variable ptosis and diplopia. Other etiologies include paraneoplastic disease, botulism, and tick paralysis. Myasthenia is characterized by variability and prominent fatigability, often evident in the history and examination. Symptoms are typically absent upon awakening. Ptosis increases with prolonged upgaze and recovers after rest. Myasthenia may affect just a solitary muscle, several EOMs, or all muscles diffusely. Because of this enormous variability, the disease may mimic a number of different ocular motor conditions, such as cranial nerve palsies, gaze palsy, and INO. Weakness of eyelid closure as well as eyelid opening is a very helpful finding when present because the levators and the orbicularis oculi muscles are innervated by different cranial nerves (third and seventh, respectively).

2. **Chronic progressive external ophthalmoplegia** (CPEO) represents a group of hereditary disorders that causes limitation of eye movements with marked slowing of saccades and ptosis. Most are due to mitochondrial mutations, including Kearns-Sayre, which is sporadic and includes cardiac conduction abnormalities, atypical retinitis pigmentosa, and spongiform CNS changes. CPEO typically evolves over many years and is symmetric. It can be distinguished from myasthenia by its very slowly progressive and chronic course and by atrophy of extraocular muscles on orbital imaging.

3. **Orbital myositis** is occasionally due to a systemic granulomatous or vasculitic disorder but most commonly occurs as a form of idiopathic orbital inflammatory disease (orbital pseudotumor). Acute onset of diplopia is accompanied by pain with eye movement and the diagnosis can be confirmed on neuroimaging.

4. **Graves' ophthalmopathy** causes restriction of eye movements due to inflammatory infiltrates, proliferation of fibroblasts, and edema. The inferior rectus is most commonly affected, producing loss of supraduction. The typical order of extraocular muscle involvement can be remembered by the mnemonic "IM SLO" for inferior rectus, medial rectus, superior rectus, lateral rectus, and obliques. Esotropia is more common

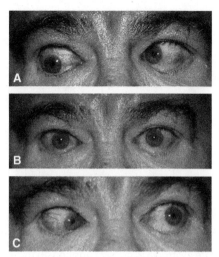

FIGURE 12.4 Esotropia and bilateral abduction deficit in a patient with thyroid eye disease. The presence of bilateral lid retraction and conjunctival injection are helpful signs indicating orbital restrictive disease rather than bilateral sixth nerve palsies.

than exotropia because frequent involvement of the medial rectus causes an abduction deficit, which can mimic a sixth NP (Fig. 12.4).

5. **Giant cell arteritis** (GCA) is an important cause of diplopia in older individuals. Ischemia of extraocular muscles can produce a variety of patterns, sometimes mimicking a cranial NP. GCA can also cause diplopia as a result of ischemic injury to the third, fourth, or sixth cranial nerves.

6. **Sagging eye syndrome** (SES) is a non-neurologic cause of diplopia due to involutional changes in EOMs and orbital connective tissues. It can cause a small-angle distance esotropia (divergence insufficiency) accompanied by cyclovertical strabismus and often ptosis in elderly patients. SES is associated with excyclotropia in the hypotropic eye, whereas a fourth NP exhibits excyclotropia in the hypertropic eye.

D. Orbit.

1. **Masses** in the orbit may displace the globe, mechanically interfere with EOMs, or cause a cranial NP. Specific etiologies include primary or uncommonly metastatic tumors, vascular lesions, and inflammation including lesions of the adjacent paranasal sinuses. Pain, proptosis, chemosis, and conjunctival injection are common.

2. Lesions at the **orbital apex** cause a distinctive combination of ipsilateral optic neuropathy and ocular motor disturbance. Because structures are crowded at the back of the orbit, a relatively small lesion can produce severe dysfunction. Small lesions in this area may not be appreciated on neuroimaging, but the clinical findings should point to the correct localization.

3. **Orbital trauma** often causes fracture of delicate orbital bones. A blowout fracture of the orbital floor can cause entrapment of the inferior rectus muscle, producing a loss of supraduction. Fracture of the medial wall can entrap the medial rectus, which causes an abduction deficit that mimics a sixth NP.

EVALUATION

A. **Clinical diagnosis.** As is so often the case in neurology, the initial step in diagnosis is localization. It is often helpful to start by asking whether the pattern of ocular misalignment fits the pattern of a cranial NP. In the case of a third NP, it is important to be able to recognize ocular alignment patterns that indicate a partial third NP. However, isolated weakness of a single third-nerve muscle is exceedingly rare. Cases with this appearance more likely represent myasthenia, INO, or orbital restriction.

In cases in which the diplopia pattern is not consistent with a single cranial NP, pattern recognition is very helpful. For example, loss of supraduction when the eye is abducted is typical of inferior rectus restriction, such as from Grave's disease or an orbital floor fracture. Limitation of eye movement accompanied by ipsilateral optic neuropathy constitutes the orbital apex syndrome. Any combination of third, fourth, and sixth nerve palsies points to a lesion in the cavernous sinus or superior orbital fissure; there is no other location where these nerves come together. Bilateral sixth NP indicates a lesion (tumor) of the clivus, meningitis (inflammatory or neoplastic), or increased ICP. Certain brainstem disorders create distinctive ocular motor deficit patterns. The one-and-a-half syndrome, for example, causes complete loss of horizontal eye movements in the ipsilateral eye and loss of adduction in the fellow eye, leaving only abduction away from the lesion (unilateral gaze palsy + INO). The combination of a third or sixth NP and contralateral long tract deficit is an example of a "crossed brainstem syndrome" and is highly localizing. In any patient with painless, pupil-sparing diplopia, the possibility of myasthenia should be considered.

B. **Ancillary testing.**

1. **Blood tests.** In all elderly patients with diplopia, giant cell arteritis should be considered. Testing includes complete blood count (CBC), erythrocyte sedimentation rate (ESR), and C-reactive protein (CRP). Testing for acetylcholine receptor antibodies is appropriate if myasthenia is suspected, but antibodies are only positive in 50% to 80% of patients with ocular myasthenia. On the other hand, false-positive antibody testing is so rare that for practical purposes a positive result provides the diagnosis. Similarly, thyroid function tests may be normal in patients with thyroid orbitopathy (termed *euthyroid Graves' disease*). Thyroid-stimulating immunoglobulins (TSIs) correlate with the activity and severity of Graves' ophthalmopathy and can be tested by bioassay.

2. **Radiographic testing** should be directed to the area of interest determined from the clinical findings. Magnetic resonance imaging (MRI) generally provides more information than computed tomography (CT), especially at bone–soft tissue interfaces (skull base) and within the brainstem. However, if an orbital process is suspected, it is important to include dedicated fat-suppressed orbit views with gadolinium. The MRI "orbits" protocol at most institutions consists of coronal and axial thin sections with fat suppression. Alternatively, CT is an effective modality for imaging most orbital structures with the exception of the optic nerve. If optic neuritis is suspected, MRI is the study of choice.

3. The edrophonium chloride (**Tensilon**) test is often useful in patients with suspected myasthenia gravis. The ideal endpoint is an objective finding such as ptosis or a ductional deficit that resolves or substantially improves following injection. A small phoria or a subjective judgment by the patient is unreliable and should be avoided. False-negative results are not uncommon, but false positives are rare.

4. **Single-fiber electromyography (EMG)** is a highly sensitive test for ocular myasthenia gravis, but lacks specificity.

5. **Ice test.** Improvement of ptosis by at least 2 mm after placement of ice on the eyelids for 2 to 5 minutes constitutes a positive ice test for myasthenia. Similar improvement is sometimes seen in diplopia due to myasthenia. Alternatively, myasthenic ptosis often shows dramatic improvement following an interval of sleep or simple rest (eyes closed) for about 20 minutes.

URGENCY OF EVALUATION

In certain conditions, the clinical outcome depends on timely and appropriate treatment. Prompt recognition of these syndromes is thus crucial.

A. **Aneurysmal third NP.** Third NP due to a pCOM aneurysm usually presents with acute onset of ipsilateral pain and pupil involvement. Most pCOM aneurysms can be identified on a good-quality MR angiography (MRA) or CT angiography (CTA); however, even with high-quality imaging an aneurysm may still be missed. If there is high suspicion of an aneurysm on the basis of the clinical features, catheter angiography should be obtained despite a negative MRA or CTA. Features that strongly suggest an aneurysm include patients without vascular risk factors and those with a history suggestive of subarachnoid hemorrhage.

B. **Pituitary apoplexy.** Hemorrhage or infarction of a pituitary tumor usually causes acute onset of severe headache with signs and symptoms related to meningeal irritation. Visual loss, usually with a bitemporal pattern, and diplopia are common. Diplopia is most often due to third-nerve involvement, which may be unilateral or bilateral. In most cases of pituitary apoplexy, a pituitary tumor was not suspected prior to hemorrhage. The diagnosis is usually apparent on MRI, but can be more difficult to visualize with CT, which is often the imaging modality of choice for headache in an emergency department setting. Prompt diagnosis is crucial because of the potential for acute adrenal insufficiency and to improve the visual prognosis in patients with chiasmal compression. Emergency management should include systemic corticosteroids in stress dosages (e.g., hydrocortisone 100 mg IV every 6 to 8 hours) with careful monitoring of electrolyte balance. Surgical decompression is usually indicated, although occasional patients do well with conservative management.

C. **Giant cell arteritis.** In any elderly patient with diplopia, the possibility of GCA should be entertained. In addition to inquiring about typical symptoms, ESR, CRP, and CBC should be obtained. High-dose steroid treatment should be started upon suspicion of the diagnosis and temporal artery biopsy may be obtained thereafter.

TREATMENT

The treatment of diplopia is generally directed toward the underlying condition. Symptomatic treatment of double vision may include simple patching of one eye, which may be an acceptable solution in situations in which the underlying cause of double vision is expected to resolve imminently. In young children, the patch should be alternated to prevent the development of ambylopia; in adults, this is not a concern, and patients are usually most comfortable with the nondominant eye covered. An alternative to patching is to place translucent tape over one eyeglass lens, allowing some blurred vision, but not enough for double vision. A paste-on (Fresnel) prism can be helpful for diplopia that is expected to be temporary or change over time. A ground-in prism is generally preferred for long-term treatment. Patients may complain of excessive blurring, chromatic aberration, and weight of the prism for thick prisms required to correct large-angle ocular deviations. In situations in which the deviation is too large and/or incomitant to treat with prisms, eye muscle surgery may be undertaken after ocular alignment has been stable for a sufficient time period.

Key Points

- Monocular diplopia typically localizes to the ocular media and is very rarely neurologic in origin. Binocular diplopia that resolves with covering either eye is a hallmark of ocular misalignment.
- A complete third NP is characterized by an exotropia and hypotropia with ptosis, with or without pupillary dilation. A pCOM aneurysm can cause a complete pupil-involving or partial third NP. An otherwise complete but pupil-sparing third NP is never from a pCOM aneurysm.
- A fourth NP is characterized by ipsilateral hypertropia worsened with contraversive gaze and ipsilateral head tilt.
- A sixth NP is characterized by esotropia that is worse in the direction of gaze of the palsy.
- INO causes an ipsilateral adduction deficit and contralateral abducting nystagmus. Slowing of adducting saccades is the most sensitive clinical sign for INO.
- Ocular myasthenia gravis is seronegative in 50% to 80% of cases and should be considered with any pupil-sparing ocular misalignment.
- Cranial nerve palsies and supranuclear disorders cause slowing of saccades, while myasthenia and orbital restrictive processes do not.
- The primary treatments for double vision are occlusion of one eye, prisms, and eye muscle surgery.

Recommended Readings

Acierno MD. Vertical diplopia. *Semin Neurol.* 2000;20(1):21–30.

Biousse V, Newman NJ, Oyesiku NM. Precipitating factors in pituitary apoplexy. *J Neurol Neurosurg Psychiatry.* 2001;71:542–545.

Borchert MS. Principles and techniques of the examination of ocular motility and alignment. In: Miller NR, Newman NJ, eds. *Walsh and Hoyt's Clinical Neuro-Ophthalmology.* Vol 1. 6th ed. Baltimore, MD: Lippincott Williams & Wilkins; 2004.

Dinkin M. Diagnostic approach to diplopia. *Continuum (Minneap Minn).* 2014;20(4):942–965.

Jivraj I, Patel V. Treatment of ocular motor palsies. *Curr Treat Options Neurol.* 2015;17(3):338.

Lee AG, Hayman LA, Brazis PW. The evaluation of isolated third nerve palsy revisited: an update on the evolving role of magnetic resonance, computed tomography and catheter angiography. *Surv Ophthalmol.* 2002;47:137–157.

Leigh RJ, Zee DS. *The Neurology of Eye Movements.* 5th ed. Oxford, England: Oxford University Press; 2015.

Richards BW, Jones FR, Jr, Younge BR. Causes and prognosis in 4,278 cases of paralysis of the oculomotor, trochlear and abducens cranial nerves. *Am J Ophthalmol.* 1992;113:489.

Tamhankar MA, Biousse V, Ying TS, et al. Isolated third, fourth, and sixth cranial nerve palsies from presumed microvascular versus other causes: a prospective study. *Ophthalmology.* 2013;120(11):2264–2269.

Vaphiades MS, Bhatti MT, Lesser RL. Ocular myasthenia gravis. *Curr Opin Ophthalmol.* 2012;23(6):537–542.

Wong AM, Colpa L, Chandrakumar M. Ability of an upright-supine test to differentiate skew deviation from other vertical strabismus causes. *Arch Ophthalmol.* 2011;129(12):1570–1575.

Wray SH. *Eye Movement Disorders in Clinical Practice.* Oxford, England: Oxford University Press; 2015.

Yee RD, Whitcup SM, Williams IM, et al. Saccadic eye movements in myasthenia gravis. *Ophthalmology.* 1987;94:219–225.

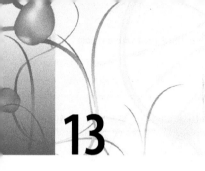

13

Approach to the Patient with Facial Numbness

Arash Salardini and Betsy B. Love

Isolated facial numbness describes impairment of sensation of the face as a result of dysfunction of the trigeminal system or central trigeminal pathways.

STEPS IN THE DIAGNOSIS AND MANAGEMENT OF FACIAL NUMBNESS

Step 1—**History and examination:** It is the basis of all the other steps in our approach.

Step 2—**Localizations:** It is the art of locating anatomically the lesion responsible for the presenting signs and symptoms.

Step 3—**Differential diagnosis:** It is a list of potential pathologies consistent with the semiology of presentation.

Step 4—**Testing based on differential diagnoses:** Appropriate tests are performed depending on the results of the history and examination.

Step 5—**Management and referral:** The wide range of etiologies necessitates multidisciplinary approach to management of facial numbness.

STEP 1: HISTORY AND EXAMINATION

Constituent parts of a thorough history and examination:

A. History. It is important to obtain as much detailed information as possible about the patient's facial numbness. The points that should be addressed include the following:
1. **Sites** of numbness, including whether the numbness is unilateral or bilateral.
2. **Duration** of numbness.
3. **Quality** of numbness.
4. **Associated features** (pain, altered taste, and nasal, dental, and cerebrovascular symptoms).
5. History of **trauma** (accidental, dental, or surgical).
6. History of **malignant disease.**
7. **Medications** used currently and in the past.

B. Physical examination.
1. General physical examination. A thorough, complete examination is necessary to evaluate for a potential cause of the facial numbness. Particular attention must be paid to evaluating for an underlying malignant lesion (including nasopharyngeal tumor), a dental problem, or an underlying rheumatologic condition. Although many different areas need to be assessed, the following areas are especially important.
   a. Head and neck. Inspection of the nose, mouth, and teeth and palpation for adenopathy is important.
   b. Vascular disorders. Bilateral blood pressure should be checked to evaluate for vascular disease. Auscultation for carotid or vertebral bruits should be performed. If there is suspicion of an intracranial aneurysm, listen for cranial bruits.
   c. Breast.
   d. Pulmonary.
   e. Lymphatic.
   f. Rheumatologic.
   g. Skin.

2. **Neurologic examination.** A thorough neurologic examination is necessary. It is particularly important to evaluate all of the functions of the trigeminal nerve and to evaluate for evidence of dysfunction of other cranial nerves.

a. **Clinical evaluation of the trigeminal nerve.**

(1) **Sensory evaluation.** Touch, pain, and temperature are tested in the distribution of the three divisions. Each division is tested individually and compared with the opposite side. The sensation in the nasal and oral mucosa, the anterior two-thirds of the tongue, and the anterior portion of the ear (tragus and anterior helix) should be assessed (Video 13.1).

(2) **Motor evaluation.** The motor functions of the trigeminal nerve are assessed by means of testing the muscles of mastication. By having a patient clench the jaw, the strength of the masseters and temporalis can be tested bilaterally. Weakness is evidenced by absent or reduced contraction of the muscles on the side of the lesion. The lateral pterygoids are tested by having the patient move the jaw from side to side against the resistance of the examiner's hand. The jaw deviates toward the paralyzed side on opening the mouth because of contraction of the intact contralateral lateral pterygoid muscle. It cannot be deviated to the opposite, nonparalyzed side. Finally, the patient should be asked to protrude the jaw. Any evidence of atrophy or fasciculation is noted.

(3) **Reflex evaluation.**

(a) **Corneal reflex.** This reflex is assessed by means of touching a wisp of a sterile cotton-tipped applicator to the edge of the cornea (not the sclera) bilaterally. The afferent portion of the reflex is carried by V_1 (upper cornea) and V_2 (lower cornea), and the efferent portion is carried by cranial nerve VII, both ipsilaterally and contralaterally. Lesions of the trigeminal nerve may cause a diminished or absent response both ipsilaterally and contralaterally.

(b) **Orbicularis oculi reflex (blink reflex).** This reflex is assessed by means of tapping the glabella or supraorbital ridge. This elicits an early ipsilateral blink followed by bilateral blinking.

(c) **Sternutatory reflex.** This reflex is assessed by means of checking light touch sensation of the lateral nasal mucosa with a cotton-tipped applicator. The appropriate response is immediate withdrawal from the irritating stimulus. This reflex may be diminished or absent in lesions of the maxillary division (V_2).

(d) **Masseter reflex or jaw jerk.** This reflex is assessed by means of tapping the slightly opened lower jaw. Lesions of the trigeminal nerve may result in a hypoactive ipsilateral jerk, whereas bilateral supranuclear lesions may result in a hyperactive response.

b. **The rest of the neurologic examination.**

(1) **Speech.** Dysarthria may be present with profound facial, tongue, or oral sensory deficits.

(2) **Cranial nerves.** Careful attention should be paid to associated abnormalities of cranial nerves, especially II, III, IV, VI, VII, and VIII.

(3) Motor and muscle stretch reflexes.

(4) **Sensory loss.** It is important to evaluate for evidence of other regions of sensory loss, especially generalized sensory neuropathy.

(5) **Coordination.** Coordination can be impaired by a process such as a tumor in the cerebellopontine angle.

(6) Gait and station.

Five domains are required for correct diagnosis. These domains are often formulated as "assessment" after the history and examination are completed.

- **Time course.**
  - Is the facial numbness acute, subacute, or chronic?
  - Is it progressive, transient, or stable? Note transient numbness is often due to migraine, epilepsy, or functional complaints.
  - Was the onset abrupt, subacute, or chronic?
- **Quality.**
  - **Paresthesia**—a spontaneous abnormal sensation.
  - **Dysesthesia**—an unpleasant abnormal sensation produced by normal stimuli.

- **Hypoesthesia**—this is classic numbness when the threshold for sensory detection is increased.
- **Pain**—Trigeminal nerve dysfunction associated with pain is discussed in Chapter 14.
- Location.
  - **Bilateral vs. unilateral:** Unilateral numbness is more common. Bilateral numbness can be associated with brainstem involvement, leptomeningeal disease, or systemic diseases, or it can be idiopathic.
  - Partial or complete.
  - **Distribution:** Trigeminal branches or branches of cervical plexus.
  - Does it include the mucous membranes?
- **Associated symptoms.** Brainstem, higher cortical function, headache, and other sensory, for example.
- **Red flags.** These are associated with potentially serious disorders.
  - Brainstem signs:
    - **Horner's syndrome:** This can be seen both in carotid dissection and brainstem pathology.
    - **Cerebellar signs:** These signs, including slurring of speech, can be seen in pontine lesions.
    - **Multiple cranial nerve involvements:** Most commonly VII, VIII.
    - **Hemiplegia:** Points to motor tracts of the brainstem being involved.
  - **Myelopathic signs.** High spine lesions can cause numbness in the C_2 distribution.
  - **Confusion.** May suggest a cortical process.
  - **Numbness not confined to the face.** May suggest lesions of the neuraxis.
  - **Change in vision or diplopia.** May suggest retro-orbital or cavernous etiology.

STEP 2: LOCALIZATION

Facial numbness may be caused by a variety of causes including cortical, subcortical, brainstem, trigeminal nerve, cervical plexus (angle of the jaw numbness) (Table 13.1), and higher cord lesions. Several generalizations may be used to localize the lesion.

1. Lesions of the divisions of cranial nerve V have distinct areas of sensory loss (Fig. 13.1).
2. Lesions proximal to the Gasserian ganglion (GG) cause cutaneous numbness of the entire face and the anterior scalp (Fig. 13.2).
3. Lesions of the brainstem can produce an onionskin distribution of sensory loss (Fig. 13.3).
4. Lesions of cranial nerve V typically spare the angle of the jaw, which is supplied by C2 and C3 (Fig. 13.1).
5. Lesions of the trigeminothalamic pathway above the brainstem are often accompanied by involvement of the trunk because of the involvement of adjacent sensory pathways.
6. Cortical lesions leading to facial numbness may be accompanied by motor symptoms because of the involvement of the adjacent motor cortex.

TABLE 13.1 Types of Numbness Associated with Lesions in Different Areas of the Trigeminal Sensory System

Location of Lesion	Area of Facial Sensory Loss
Ophthalmic (V_1) division	Forehead, scalp, nose (except inferolateral), upper eyelid, upper half of cornea
Maxillary (V_2) division	Lateral nose, upper lip, cheek, lower half of cornea, upper gums, palate, mucosa of lower nasal cavity
Mandibular (V_3) division	Lower lip, lower jaw, chin, tympanic membrane, auditory meatus, upper ear, floor of mouth, lower gums and teeth, anterior two-thirds of tongue
Proximal to GG	Entire face and all structures listed above
Brainstem	Onionskin sensory loss

Abbreviation: GG, Gasserian ganglion.

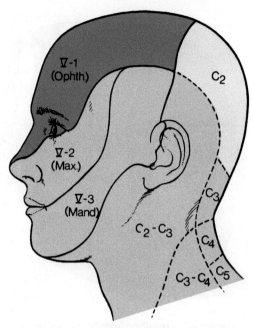

FIGURE 13.1 Regions of the face supplied by the three sensory divisions of the trigeminal nerve (V_1, V_2, and V_3). (Modified from Sears ES, Franklin GM. Diseases of the cranial nerves. In: Rosenberg RN, ed. *Neurology*. New York, NY: Grune & Stratton; 1980, with permission.)

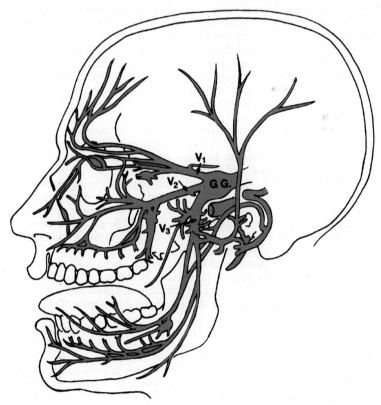

FIGURE 13.2 Relations between the divisions of the trigeminal nerve and the GG.

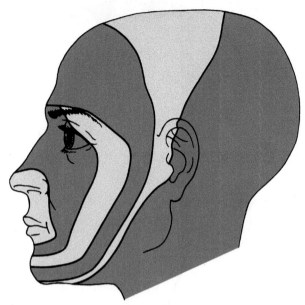

FIGURE 13.3 Onionskin sensory loss resulting from brainstem lesions.

These rules of thumb are based on the neuroanatomy of the trigeminal pain system:

A. Neuroanatomy of the trigeminal sensory system
1. The trigeminal nerve (cranial nerve V) is a mixed sensory and motor nerve.
   a. The sensory portion of the nerve is the largest portion, transmitting sensation from areas of the face, oral cavity, and nasal passages.
   b. There are three divisions of the **sensory portion** of the trigeminal nerve (Fig. 13.1).
      (1) **Ophthalmic (V_1).** The ophthalmic division provides cutaneous supply to the forehead and anterior scalp to approximately the vertex, parts of the nose and the upper eyelid, and the upper half of the cornea. Branches of this division to the facial structures are the nasociliary, infratrochlear, supratrochlear, lacrimal, and supraorbital nerves.
      (2) **Maxillary (V_2).** The maxillary division provides cutaneous supply to portions of the nose, upper lip, cheek, lower half of the cornea, upper gums and teeth, palate, and nasal mucosa. Branches of this division are the zygomaticofacial, zygomaticotemporal, and infraorbital nerves.
      (3) **Mandibular (V_3).** The mandibular division provides cutaneous supply to the lower lip; chin; portions of the jaw, ear, and mouth; lower gums and teeth; and the anterior two-thirds of the tongue. Branches of this division are the auriculotemporal, buccal, and mental nerves. The combined nerve trunk of the mandibular division and the motor portion gives rise to the inferior alveolar nerves and the lingual nerves.
         (a) The **motor portion** of the trigeminal nerve is a smaller division that travels with V_3. It provides motor function to the muscles of mastication and the tensor tympani. This portion is not discussed further. However, it is important to examine the patient for dysfunction of the motor portion of the nerve.
   c. The three sensory divisions (V_1, V_2, and V_3) enter the cranial cavity through the superior orbital fissure, foramen rotundum, and foramen ovale, respectively, to unite in the Gasserian or semilunar ganglion, which lies at the apex of the petrous bones. The first-order neurons for trigeminal nerves are in these ganglia. The exception to this are the proprioceptive fibers, the first-order neurons of which are in the mesencephalic nucleus of trigeminal.

d. Second-order neurons are in the spinal, principal, and mesencephalic nuclei of trigeminal. They synapse on the ventroposteromedial nucleus of thalamus, which projects to the primary and secondary somatosensory cortices.

STEP 3: LOCALIZATION: CAUSES OF FACIAL NUMBNESS

In general, the causes of facial numbness are wide ranging and may include the following (Table 13.2):

A. Tumor
B. Infection
C. Trauma
D. Connective tissue disease
E. Drug or toxin
F. Nontumor mass lesion
G. Vascular disorder
H. Demyelinating disorder
I. Other systemic or rare disease
J. Idiopathic disorder

Since there are so many causes of facial numbness, anatomical localization plays an important role in narrowing down the differentials. The different causes are discussed according to the known or presumed site of involvement of the trigeminal pathway.

1. **Lesions peripheral to the GG** (V_1, V_2, and V_3). The mnemonic VITAMIN D may be used to remember the various causes.
   a. **Vascular disorders.** In rare instances, carotid artery dissection can produce facial numbness.

TABLE 13.2 Causes of Facial Numbness^a

Lesions peripheral to the GG
Trauma (accidental, dental, and surgical)
Infection (leprosy and VZV)
Systemic diseases (sickle cell anemia, diabetes, and diffuse connective tissue disease)
Tumor
Inflammatory
Drugs or toxins (stilbamidine, cocaine, and others)
Idiopathic TSN

Lesions of the GG root
Infection (syphilis, tuberculosis, and VZV)
Tumor
Nontumorous mass lesions (aneurysm and hydrocephalus)
Sarcoidosis
Arachnoiditis
Amyloid
Drug (trichloroethylene)

Lesions of the central trigeminal pathways
Stroke
Tumor
Syringobulbia
Demyelinating disease
Vascular anomaly

^{a}Presumed site of pathologic change.
Abbreviations: GG, Gasserian ganglion, VZV, varicella zoster virus.
Modified from Hagen NA, Stevens JC, Michet CJ. Trigeminal sensory neuropathy associated with connective tissue disease. *Neurology.* 1990;40:891–896.

b. Infection.
  (1) Leprosy. Worldwide, lepromatous leprosy is the most common cause of facial numbness. There can be facial hypalgesia and resultant accidental mutilation of the face.
  (2) Herpes zoster. Although the varicella zoster virus (VZV) resides in the GG, evidence of active infection usually involves a division of the trigeminal nerve. The most commonly affected division is the ophthalmic division.
  (3) Paranasal sinusitis can affect some branches of the trigeminal nerve.
c. Trauma. Injury to the peripheral branches of the trigeminal nerve can occur with head or facial trauma, dental trauma or surgery, or any surgical procedure on the face (e.g., otorhinolaryngologic or dermatologic surgery).
  (1) Head or facial injury. The most frequently affected nerves are the superficial branches, including the supraorbital (branch of V_1), supratrochlear (branch of V_1), and infraorbital (branch of V_2) nerves. The sensory loss is temporally related to the injury. Nerve regeneration can be accompanied by facial pain. The supraorbital branch can be damaged by blunt injury or as a result of a fracture of the upper margin of the orbit. The infraorbital nerve can be injured with closed head injuries or maxillary fractures. The entire ophthalmic division (V_1) can be damaged in fractures through the foramen ovale. Transverse basilar skull fractures can injure the GG, resulting in anesthesia of the entire face and weakness of the masticatory muscles.
  (2) Dental trauma. Facial numbness can occur after tooth extraction. The inferior alveolar or lingual nerve can be damaged, and the result is transient anesthesia. Direct nerve injury also can occur as a result of needle trauma during dental anesthesia. In patients with severe mandibular bone resorption, denture use can cause pressure on the mental nerve, resulting in chin numbness.
  (3) Facial surgery. Any surgical procedure involving the face can lead to trigeminal nerve injury. Facial numbness has been described as a postoperative complication of microvascular decompression for trigeminal neuralgia due to trauma to the trigeminal root.
d. Autoimmune. The presence of facial numbness with a connective tissue disorder is rare. It has been associated with systemic sclerosis, Sjögren's syndrome, mixed connective tissue disease, systemic lupus erythematosus, rheumatoid arthritis, and dermatomyositis.
e. Metabolic and systemic disease.
  (1) Sickle cell anemia. Numbness of the chin and lower lip resulting from mental neuropathy with sickle cell crisis has been described.
  (2) Diabetes. Facial numbness has been reported with diabetes and can accompany other forms of sensory neuropathy.
f. Idiopathic trigeminal sensory neuropathy (TSN). This diagnosis is one of exclusion after serious causes have been ruled out (see section Classic Clinical Syndromes).
g. Neoplastic. Regional spread of a tumor along the trigeminal nerve can occur. Disease (most commonly of the lung and breast) metastasizing to the lower jaw can affect the inferior alveolar or mental nerve and cause numbness of the chin and lower lip. Cheek or malar numbness has been described with local spread of tumors along V_2 or with leptomeningeal involvement with tumors. Meckel cave tumors (Fig. 13.4) may affect one or more divisions of the trigeminal nerve. Numbness of the cheek or malar region (numb cheek syndrome) may herald the recurrence of squamous cell carcinoma of the skin. Nasopharyngeal tumors (squamous cell carcinoma is most common) arise most frequently in the roof of the pharynx. They can encroach on the trigeminal nerve, producing facial numbness. Associated features can include excessive lacrimation, facial pain, proptosis, hearing loss, and Horner's syndrome.
h. Drugs and toxins.
  (1) Stilbamidine is an agent that has been used to treat leishmaniasis and multiple myeloma. Unilateral or bilateral facial numbness and anesthesia have been reported after treatment.

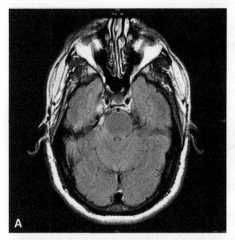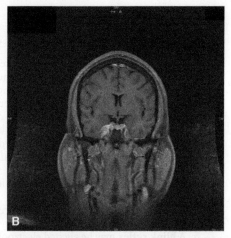

FIGURE 13.4 A and B: Brain MRI with contrast showing enhancing extra-axial mass involving the right Meckel's cave and right cavernous sinus extending into the tentorium. (Courtesy of Drs. Ulises Nobo and José Biller.)

    (2) **Cocaine** abuse by the nasal route is a cause of facial numbness in the territory of the maxillary division (V_2). Usually, there is associated traumatic and ischemic necrosis of the nasal mucosa.

    (3) **Other drugs.** Many drugs can cause facial paresthesia. Circumoral paresthesia has been reported with labetalol, and mandibular neuropathy has been reported with allopurinol.

2. Lesions of the GG or root (mnemonic SAD TINA)
   a. Sarcoidosis.
   b. **Amyloidosis.** In rare instances, the GG or root can be the solitary site of amyloid deposits.
   c. **Drug.** Trichloroethylene is an industrial solvent that has been associated with facial numbness.
   d. **Tumor.** Various tumors can affect the GG or root. Tumors that arise in the ganglion (ganglioneuroma or gangliocytoma) tend to have early, associated pain. Tumors that arise primarily in the root (neurinoma or neurofibroma) tend to have predominant sensory loss without pain. Tumors that can compress or invade the ganglion or root include acoustic neuroma, meningioma, schwannoma, cholesteatoma, pituitary adenoma, chordoma, nasopharyngeal carcinoma, and metastatic lesions.
   e. **Infection** of the GG can occur with syphilis, tuberculosis, and herpes zoster.
   f. Nontumorous mass lesions (aneurysm and hydrocephalus).
   g. Arachnoiditis.

3. **Lesions of the central trigeminal pathways:** Any process affecting the neuraxis can disrupt the trigeminothalamocortical pathway.
   a. **Stroke.** Infarction in the lateral tegmentum of the medulla (Wallenberg's syndrome) can produce ipsilateral facial numbness along with other cranial nerve deficits and long tract signs. In rare instances, lateral pontine hemorrhage causes isolated facial numbness, perhaps as a result of involvement of the main sensory nucleus of the trigeminal nerve.
   b. **Tumor.** Tumors of the pons or medulla can affect the sensory nucleus of cranial nerve V, but there are usually other signs, including long tract and cranial nerve findings.
   c. **Syringobulbia.** This central cavitation of the medulla or pons can be associated with facial numbness.
   d. **Demyelinating disease.** Facial numbness is the initial symptom in 2% to 3% of patients with multiple sclerosis.
   e. **Vascular anomalies.** Isolated facial numbness very rarely results from a posterior fossa aneurysm or other vascular malformation.

STEP 4: TESTING

Testing is used to confirm or rule out differential diagnoses.

1. **Biochemical tests** include complete blood cell count with differential, complete chemistry profile including liver function tests and glucose level, and erythrocyte sedimentation rate. In certain situations, a Venereal Disease Research Laboratory (VDRL) test, antinuclear antibody determination, rheumatoid factor, extractable nuclear antigen antibodies, or an angiotensin-converting enzyme level may be necessary. Skin scraping or biopsy is necessary when leprosy is a consideration.
2. **A purified protein derivative test** should be done if there is suspicion of tuberculosis.
3. A **chest radiograph** should be obtained to evaluate for a malignancy, pulmonary disease, or tuberculosis.
4. **Skull and sinus radiography.** A radiograph of the mandible is indicated if there is a numb chin.
5. **Lumbar puncture** is essential if there is suspicion of infection or a malignant tumor of the leptomeninges.
6. A **blink reflex** may be elicited electrophysiologically by means of electrical stimulation of the supraorbital nerve. It can be helpful in detecting subtle central or peripheral lesions of the trigeminal nerve.
7. **Brain imaging.** Magnetic resonance imaging (MRI) without and with contrast is the imaging test of choice in most instances. The correct imaging protocol to evaluate the area of the suspected lesion should be discussed with the neuroradiologist prior to the test. Computed tomography (CT) with and without contrast enhancement may be indicated if MRI is not available or if there are contraindications to MRI.

STEP 5: TREATMENT AND REFERRAL

Because the range of possible underlying diseases that can cause facial numbness is so wide, it is often necessary to use a teamwork approach to the management of this problem. A **neurologist,** who should be most familiar with localization of lesions of the trigeminal nerve, should be consulted initially. It is often necessary to consult an **otolaryngologist** to evaluate for the presence of a nasopharyngeal tumor, acoustic neuroma, or sinusitis. A **dentist** or an **oral surgeon** may be needed to assist in ruling out a dental cause of facial numbness. In selected instances, a **rheumatologist** may be needed if there is evidence of associated connective tissue disease.

CLASSIC CLINICAL SYNDROMES

A. **TSN.** The literature is rather unclear in its definition of *TSN*. It has been used to describe different populations of patients with facial numbness. Blau et al. in 1969 described a population of patients with TSN who had self-limited facial paresthesia that in one-half of the cases resolved in several months. There were no associated neurologic deficits. At neurologic examination, the corneal response was intact, and the only finding was a subjective decrease in light touch and pinprick over the involved trigeminal distribution. Only 10% of these patients had identifiable causes of TSN, and 10% went on to have trigeminal neuralgia. In contrast to this population, with a seemingly benign course, Horowitz in 1974 found that 88% of a population with facial numbness had an identifiable, usually serious condition. This population almost always had other neurologic deficits (cranial nerve or ataxia). It may be concluded that these two studies involved quite different populations.

TSN is best defined as a general term for facial numbness of which there are many different causes, as previously discussed. Any area of the face can be involved. **Idiopathic TSN** is used to describe purely sensory impairment of unknown causation in a territory of the trigeminal nerve (usually V_2 or V_3) on one or both sides of the face. It can be associated with pain, paresthesia, or dysfunction of taste. Because the data currently available do not allow one to differentiate consistently between facial numbness that is benign and facial numbness that is attributable to a serious condition, idiopathic TSN remains a diagnosis of exclusion after an appropriate, thorough evaluation. Available data do indicate that the presence of associated neurologic signs and deficits usually points to a more ominous process.

B. Numb chin and numb cheek syndromes.

1. **Numb chin syndrome** is an uncommon form of facial neuropathy. However, the occurrence of this syndrome is notable because in the absence of a history of dental trauma, numb chin syndrome is rarely caused by benign lesions and is often a symptom of more ominous processes such as involvement of the mental or inferior alveolar nerves (branches of V_3) by systemic cancer.

   a. Any tumor metastasizing to the jaw can produce this syndrome, but malignant tumors of the breast, lung, and lymphoreticular system are found most commonly. Numb chin syndrome also can be caused by metastasis to the proximal mandibular root at the base of the skull or by leptomeningeal involvement with malignant tumors such as lymphoma.

   b. Most patients already have a known diagnosis of cancer. However, mental neuropathy can be the initial symptom of malignant disease or it can herald tumor recurrence or progression.

   c. The **clinical presentation** involves ipsilateral numbness or anesthesia of the skin and mucosa of the lower lip and chin that extends to the midline. There is usually no associated pain, but there can be lip swelling and ulceration from biting of the numb lip.

   d. The **evaluation** of patients with numb chin syndrome should include radiographs of the mandible with particular attention to the mental foramen, radiographs of the basal skull, MRI of the brain with contrast enhancement, and if there is concern of leptomeningeal infiltration, cerebrospinal fluid analysis.

   e. Although a numb chin is a seemingly benign problem, it should be thoroughly evaluated because of its clinical importance as a possible sign of malignant disease.

2. **Numb cheek syndrome.** Lesions of the maxillary division of the trigeminal nerve in the infraorbital foramen may cause the numb cheek syndrome. Unilateral numbness over the malar region and the upper lip in an infraorbital nerve distribution is typical of this syndrome. These findings can have implications similar to those of numb chin syndrome. Malignancies such as squamous or basal cell carcinoma of the facial skin can spread along the trigeminal nerve. Such tumors also can spread from regional nerves to the skull base and into the intracranial space. Numbness of the anterior gums and teeth suggests a more peripheral lesion, whereas both anterior and posterior gum and teeth involvement suggests leptomeningeal disease.

Key Points

- Diverse etiologies may be responsible for isolated facial numbness (more broad numbness that includes the face is treated elsewhere in the book). For this reason there is a need for a systematic approach to the diagnosis of causes.
- History and examination should concentrate on determining the time course of the symptoms, quality, associated symptoms, and red flags.
- Localization is the basis of narrowing down the large list of differentials.
- The treatment of facial numbness is achieved by addressing the underlying causes and will require expertise outside of neurology.
- Classic trigeminal syndromes include idiopathic trigeminal neuropathy, numb cheek, and numb chin syndromes.

Recommended Readings

Bar-Ziv J, Slasky BS. CT imaging of mental nerve neuropathy: the numb chin syndrome. *AJR Am J Roentgenol.* 1997;168:371–376.

Blau JN, Harris M, Kennett S. Trigeminal sensory neuropathy. *N Engl J Med.* 1969;281:873–876.

Brazis PW, Masdeu JC, Biller J. Chapter 9: Cranial nerve V (the trigeminal nerve). In: Brazis PW, Masdeu JC, Biller J, eds. *Localization in Clinical Neurology.* 6th ed. Philadelphia, PA: Lippincott Williams & Wilkins; 2011:305–319.

Bruyn RPM, Boogerd W. The numb chin. *Clin Neurol Neurosurg.* 1991;93:187.

Burt RK, Sharfman WH, Karp BI, et al. Mental neuropathy (numb chin syndrome): a harbinger of tumor progression or relapse. *Cancer.* 1992;70:877–881.

Campbell WW. The numb cheek syndrome: a sign of infraorbital neuropathy. *Neurology.* 1986;36:421–423.

Gonella MC, Fischbein NJ, So YT. Disorders of the trigeminal system. *Semin Neurol.* 2009;29:36–44.

Greenberg HS, Deck MD, Vikram B, et al. Metastasis to the base of the skull: clinical findings in 43 patients. *Neurology.* 1981;31:530–537.

Hagen NA, Stevens JC, Michet CJ. Trigeminal sensory neuropathy associated with connective tissue disease. *Neurology.* 1990;40:891–896.

Horowitz SH. Isolated facial numbness: clinical significance and relation to trigeminal neuropathy. *Ann Intern Med.* 1974;80:49.

Janjua RM, Wong KM, Parekh A, et al. Management of the great mimicker, Meckel cave tumors. *Neurosurgery.* 2010;67(suppl 2, Operative Neurosurgery):416–421.

Kuntzer T, Bogousslavsky J, Rilliet B, et al. Herald facial numbness. *Eur Neurol.* 1992;32:297–301.

Lecky BR, Hughes RA, Murray NM, et al. Trigeminal sensory neuropathy: a study of 22 cases. *Brain.* 1987;110:1463–1485.

Robinson CM, Addy L, Wylie M, et al. A study of the clinical characteristics of benign trigeminal sensory neuropathy. *J Oral Maxillofac Surg.* 2003;61:325–332.

Sears ES, Franklin GM. Diseases of the cranial nerves. In: Rosenberg RN, ed. *Neurology.* New York, NY: Grune & Stratton; 1980.

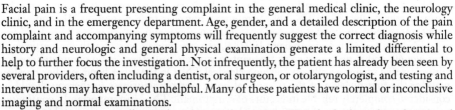

14 Approach to the Patient with Facial Pain

Murray S. Flaster

Facial pain is a frequent presenting complaint in the general medical clinic, the neurology clinic, and in the emergency department. Age, gender, and a detailed description of the pain complaint and accompanying symptoms will frequently suggest the correct diagnosis while history and neurologic and general physical examination generate a limited differential to help to further focus the investigation. Not infrequently, the patient has already been seen by several providers, often including a dentist, oral surgeon, or otolaryngologist, and testing and interventions may have proved unhelpful. Many of these patients have normal or inconclusive imaging and normal examinations.

In this chapter, we will consider trigeminal neuralgia (TN), both idiopathic (classic) and secondary, the much rarer glossopharyngeal neuralgia (GN), migraine, and the trigeminal autonomic cephalgias (TACs), as well as herpetic and postherpetic neuralgia. Temporomandibular joint (TMJ) dysfunction and atypical facial pain (which has been recently renamed persistent idiopathic facial pain [PIFP]) will be briefly considered. Other causes of facial pain, including cranial sinusitis, dental caries, and acute glaucoma, and other causes of orbital and periorbital pain, temporal arteritis, and arterial dissections will be briefly discussed.

The practitioner should bear in mind that patients with facial pain may be in acute distress, and those patients with recurrent chronic pain are frequently distraught, depressed, needy, and clinically quite complex.

TRIGEMINAL NEURALGIA

TN is probably the most common of facial pain disorders effecting adults and, broadly speaking, is among the more severe pain disorders known. Patients complain of very brief, electric-like or lancinating pain involving one or more branches of the trigeminal nerve. Typically the second and third divisions of the trigeminal nerve are involved, contiguously or individually. Rarely, the first division may also be involved, but almost never in isolation. The painful jolt lasts for seconds but can recur multiple times, often in bursts. The pain is almost always unilateral, and its overwhelming severity completely and visibly absorbs the patient when it strikes. Most commonly, there is no pain or paresthesias in between lancinating events and the painful episodes can dissipate as unexpectedly as they appear. The syndrome is often episodic, with painful epochs that stretch for weeks or months, and with spontaneous remissions lasting even years. Over time, typically measured in months or years, there appears to be a tendency toward increasing refractoriness to therapies. Very often, the patient will describe a trigger or aggravating feature, which includes talking, chewing, brushing of teeth, application of makeup, shaving, casual contact with the affected area, or even a stimulus as subtle as an air current. Chewing and swallowing present so much difficulty that the patient loses weight and may even suffer dehydration. The sudden, invasive and miserable nature of TN is captured by the French phrase *tic douloureux*. In some patients, usually years after symptom onset, pain may become longer lasting with duller, more constant pain supervening together with paresthesias in the affected territory. Patients reporting these more complex pain phenomena may also have less predictable responses to invasive treatment, leading many authors to additionally classify these patients as "atypical TN" or "TN type 2."

TN is etiologically divided into classic (or idiopathic) and symptomatic. Symptomatic TN may be due to compressive tumor (meningioma, acoustic neuroma, epidermoid), aneurysm, infiltrative neoplasm or an inflammatory process, typically multiple sclerosis (MS), and rarely sarcoidosis or rheumatologic disorders. Other cited etiologies include vascular malformations, brainstem ischemia, facial trauma, and arteritis. Bilaterality strongly implies a secondary cause although most symptomatic TN cases are unilateral. Younger age favors a secondary cause but classic TN has been described in younger patients. Preferential involvement of the ophthalmic division of the trigeminal nerve suggests a secondary cause may be present. The etiology of classic TN remains uncertain, but most authorities believe that demyelinative damage at the root entry zone due to vascular compression is causal. Pathologic studies support this view. Neuroimaging studies, specifically brain magnetic resonance imaging (MRI), may show a secondary cause in up to 15% of cases. Guidelines suggest that classic TN can be diagnosed on clinical grounds alone. However, this author and others believe at least one neuroimaging study should be encouraged regardless of how typical a patient's presentation may appear. High field strength, and high-resolution MR including diffusion-tensor MR may be able to identify both the offending vessel and intrinsic change within the nerve, and so eventually become a reliable means of confirming classic TN. For the moment, however, high-resolution MR studies lend important support to the vascular compression hypothesis and can aid in surgical planning.

TN has a prevalence of 3 to 6 per 100,000, becomes more frequent with age, particularly after age 60, and is nearly twice as frequent in women. Still, there is no completely secure clinical profile unequivocally establishing classical TN. On the other hand, neither involvement of the first division of the trigeminal nerve nor refractoriness to therapy should be considered completely reliable indicators of symptomatic TN. Most importantly, continuous pain or paresthesias or an abnormal neurologic examination prompts a thorough search for a symptomatic cause.

The general recommendation for initial therapy beyond analgesics is an oral antiepileptic drug (AED), with carbamazepine most commonly considered first-line therapy and where initial favorable response rates in classic TN approach 90%. Treatment with carbamazepine becomes less effective over time, partly because of increased hepatic elimination (auto-induction) but likely involving other, less understood mechanisms. Oxcarbamazepine is a safer agent, does not trigger auto-induction, and may have equal efficacy but has less evidence-based support. Other agents including lamotrigine, gabapentin, or baclofen can be effective in monotherapy or as add-on therapies. Familiarity with these agents, their side effects, and drug–drug interactions on the part of the treating physician are recommended. Internationally accepted detailed guidelines for medical therapy are available.

There is general agreement that surgical intervention should be considered for patients refractory to medical therapy although evidenced-based data are sparse and broad agreement on how soon to seek surgical alternatives is lacking. A very effective approach with high rates of immediate pain relief and very effective long-lasting benefit involves craniotomy with microscopic vascular decompression (MVD) at the trigeminal root. Most authorities now agree that the offending vessel is usually an artery, and most commonly the superior cerebellar but anterior inferior cerebellar and the basilar artery have also been implicated. High-resolution MRI has been employed to detect these offending vessels and predict successful MVD but reliability of presurgical imaging still remains incomplete. Perioperative and postoperative complications occur, but are infrequent in the hands of experienced neurosurgeons. Less invasive partially destructive procedures include radiofrequency thermal rhizotomy, done very commonly, and percutaneous balloon microcompression and less frequently, chemical rhizotomy. Stereotactic radiosurgery should be considered when patient infirmity or patient preference weighs against open surgery. The percutaneous procedures offer degrees of initial pain relief similar to that of MVD but also modestly less reliable sustained benefit. Complications potentially include deafferentation syndromes (anesthesia dolorosa or corneal hypoesthesia with keratitis), hearing loss, or cerebrospinal fluid leak. In the case of the least invasive nonmedicinal approach, stereotactic radiosurgery, the patient must be made aware that pain relief will not become effective for a mean interval of about 1 month. Many experienced neurosurgeons are of the opinion that too many patients have suffered for too long a time before being referred for definitive interventional therapy. There is a concern that inordinate delay reduces procedural effectiveness. The role of invasive therapy in patients with MS remains controversial.

We stress that interventional procedures are effective in patients with classic TN but in patients with other causes of facial pain or frankly equivocal cases of TN, invasive procedures are wisely avoided or approached with appropriate circumspection.

GLOSSOPHARYNGEAL NEURALGIA

GN is similar to TN in that it presents with unilateral lancinating pain, in this case involving the posterior-lateral aspect of the throat (tonsil), the posterior aspect of the tongue, the ear, or larynx. Involvement of the ear implies participation of the auricular branch of the vagus nerve, a purely somatosensory nerve leading some authors to employ the term "vagoglossopharyngeal." As is the case for TN, GN remains a clinical diagnosis. Swallowing is a typical trigger as are speech, cough, or yawn. The lancinating pain appears in some patients to trigger a coughing fit. A rare variant accompanied by syncope has been described, which through presumed influence on vagus nerve outflow can cause recurrent brady-arrhythmia and even asystole. Like TN, GN may remit or relapse spontaneously but it is a far rarer disorder, with an estimated frequency of between one-tenth and one-hundredth that of TN. It may be either idiopathic or symptomatic. Symptomatic causes include tumors of the skull base, infection, an expansile vertebral artery due to large atheroma, vascular malformation, MS, or bony malformations of the skull base, especially an elongated styloid process. Otolaryngologic evaluation as well as neuroimaging evaluation is recommended. Elimination of triggered pain by the application of topical anesthetic may help support the diagnosis. Pharmacotherapy is considered the first-line intervention and preferred agents used are identical to those employed in TN. Data are sparse, however, because of the rarity of the disorder. Microvascular compression at the root entry zone is considered the underlying cause of idiopathic GN by many authorities and so a surgical approach, particularly MVD is often recommended if medical therapy is ineffective. High-resolution MRI lends some support to the theory of microvascular compression. In many cases, severity of GN may be milder relative to TN, and in some instances, patient assurance has proved a sufficient remedy.

HERPES ZOSTER NEURALGIAS

The acute or chronic neuralgia resulting from the segmental (dermatomal) recrudescence of herpes zoster (HZ) virus in the dorsal root ganglia is quite distinct clinically from TN and is generally readily recognized acutely by a characteristic, topographically distinct, unilateral rash. Because involvement of the trigeminal ganglion in reactivated latent herpes virus infection is common, HZ is a frequent cause of facial pain, especially in the elderly.

HZ has an overall incidence of between 1.5 and 3 per 1,000 annually, but this incidence rises to up to 6.5 per 1,000 by age 60 and up to 11 per 1,000 by age 70. Between 20% and 40% of all individuals will experience HZ in their lifetime. HZ affecting the first division of the trigeminal nerve (HZ ophthalmicus) is the second most common form of HZ, second only to involvement of the thoracic dermatomes and comprises 10% to 20% of all HZ cases. The second and third divisions of the trigeminal nerve are rarely if ever affected in isolation. HZ begins with a prodrome that includes fatigue and malaise, headache and photophobia, rarely fever but very frequently includes a vague sensory prodrome in the involved dermatome that consists of tingling paresthesias, sometimes burning paresthesias, sometimes lancinating paresthesias, and sometimes allodynia. The HZ-induced paresthesias are sensed as surface, dermatomal phenomena but a perceived deeper discomfort described as muscle or bone ache or even visceral pain referred to as myotomal phenomena in the older literature also occurs and can be severe. After a period of about 1 to 5 days, the typical rash (shingles), first maculopapular and then frankly vesicular appears, restricted to a primary dermatome and parts of the immediately contiguous dermatomes. As the rash advances, the pain may worsen, and pruritus develops. The pain is mixed and unrelenting; a lancinating component may be prominent but never singular. A patient's scratching will alter the appearance of the rash, with excoriations obscuring vesicles and it is therefore important to remain watchful for secondary bacterial infection. Bilateral or multifocal involvement is seen only in the immune compromised. Rarely, patients perceive a prodrome including sensory symptoms without evidence of rash. This phenomenon together with the sequelae of HZ in the absence of observed rash have been termed "zoster sine herpete." The rash generally subsides over a period of 30 days; pain generally declines with it, but in 10% to 20% of patients the pain persists beyond 30 days. This persistent pain syndrome termed postherpetic neuralgia (PHN) is the most common complication of HZ.

It is important to remember that HZ ophthalmicus often brings with it ocular involvement that can include exposure keratitis and uveitis but may rarely include retinal vasculitis, ischemic optic neuropathy, or necrotizing retinopathy. For these reasons, one should involve an ophthalmologist early in the course of illness, and treat the patient aggressively. The initiation of oral antiviral therapy within 72 hours of the appearance of rash reduces both the duration and severity of an outbreak while delayed treatment may still be beneficial. Intravenous antiviral therapy for the immune incompetent or for severe cases must be considered. Topical antiviral and either systemic or topical corticosteroid may be employed in selected cases.

Although generally self-limited, PHN may last many months or even years. PHN becomes more common in the elderly, and probably more debilitating and more difficult to treat in the older old. Manifestations include burning, lancinating or aching pain, hyperalgesia, and allodynia. Allodynia is prominent and together with other neuropathic pain may severely disturb daily social function. The persistence of pain reflects central nervous system (CNS) changes ("central pain") and possibly persistent low-grade viral activity. Treatment is patient specific. Both gabapentin and pregabalin are US Food and Drug Administration (FDA) approved for the treatment of PHN. A combination of opioid analgesics and AEDs can be used. Tricyclic antidepressants may also be effective. The application of topical sodium channel–directed analgesics such as lidocaine as an ointment or in patch form can be effective and topical capsaicin may be effective. The use of intrathecal corticosteroid is controversial.

The practitioner should be aware of rare but potentially devastating sequelae of HZ including cranial polyneuritis, CNS vasculitis, cerebral infarction, cerebral hemorrhage, postinfectious myelitis, progressive myelopathy, and necrotizing retinopathy. Childhood vaccination against HZ became available in 1995 and may alter the epidemiology of this disorder over time, but in the interim a much higher dose attenuated live virus vaccine approved by the FDA is available to people over age 60. As demonstrated by the initial trial and subsequently confirmed, the vaccine reduces the incidence of HZ by one-half. PHN is reduced by two-thirds.

PRIMARY HEADACHE DISORDERS

Primary headaches, migraine, and its relatives can present with facial pain as a primary or principle feature. Chronic migraineurs, especially those without aura, will not infrequently attribute their problem incorrectly to recurrent sinus infection with infraorbital or retro-orbital pain. In the absence of signs and symptoms of infection and in the absence of unequivocal imaging support, a wary practitioner should consider the diagnosis of chronic migraine or chronic daily headache, even with tension-type characteristics. A careful history of the patient's pain complaint including quality, location, timing, duration, frequency, triggers, associated symptoms, and pattern of drug use or overuse should guide the clinician toward a correct diagnosis and best treatment. Headache of more than 1 hour's duration, pain that is often but not always unilateral, the presence of photophobia, phonophobia, and a reluctance to move, anorexia if not frank nausea with vomiting, the presence of recurrent aura such as bright scotoma or transient hemianopsia or hemifacial or hemibody numbness, or the presence of typical triggers such as bright lights, strong odors, noisy environments, or alcohol should influence the practitioner toward a consideration of migraine as a possible diagnosis. The localization of pain in migraine patients is variable, and although infrequent, it is not unusual for patients to report pain mostly involving the face or even entirely limited to the lower face. Prominent facial pain, especially if infraorbital, can lead to the erroneous diagnosis of recurrent sinusitis (see section **Other Causes of Facial Pain**).

Cluster headache (CH), the less common paroxysmal hemicranial headache and the very rare related headache variant, short-lasting unilateral neuralgiform headache attacks with conjunctival injection and tearing (SUNCT) or its equally rare variant short-lasting unilateral neuralgiform with autonomic features (SUNA) can pose initial diagnostic uncertainty. These pain syndromes are grouped collectively as the TACs.

The pain of CH is always severe, usually peri- and retro-orbital, unilateral, and relatively short lasting in comparison to migraine. The pain is described as stabbing or knife-like, boring or drilling, burning or squeezing, and in some patients may spread to the occiput and posterior cervical regions. Pain is always unilateral but it may shift sides between attacks in about 20% of patients. Attack duration is typically from 15 minutes to 3 hours but most attacks last less than 1 hour. During the attack, the patient appears restless and agitated, a feature that effectively differentiates this form of headache from migraine where ordinary movements are characteristically avoided. More than 80% of patients will show restlessness or manic features. The attacks are cyclical, tend to occur at characteristic times of the day (circadian) and occur on a once up to several times daily basis for weeks or months and then spontaneously resolve. It is the cyclical grouping from which the term "cluster" originates. The most severe headaches are said to wake the patient from sleep early in the night, corresponding to the first rapid eye movement (REM) sleep cycle. The attacks are accompanied by a combination of lacrimation, conjunctival injection, nasal congestion, or rhinorrhea. Sometimes Horner syndrome can be observed. These autonomic manifestations are generally unilateral. Affected individuals are more commonly men, often tobacco smokers and not infrequently alcohol abusers. Alcohol can be an instantaneous trigger during cluster periods. Recent data suggest lifetime prevalence could be as high as 1 in 1,000. Cluster pain is severe, suicidal ideation during attacks is not unusual, and aggressive treatment is mandatory. Multiple abortive therapies can be effective. Rapidly absorbed triptans works; both sumatriptan and zolmitriptan are believed to be effective. High-flow inhaled nasal oxygen can also be an effective abortive therapy. Many different treatments are used by specialty clinics. Transitional and prophylactic therapies are often indicated. Treatment usually requires polypharmacy and ongoing therapy is probably best delivered by a practitioner familiar with the problem. Specialty clinic estimates suggest that 10% of chronic CH patients are resistant to or intolerant of all pharmacotherapy. Interventional therapy such as occipital nerve stimulation or hypothalamic deep brain stimulation may work but efficacy is uncertain and consideration of these therapies should be limited to markedly refractory patients at very experienced centers. Although CH is distinctly clinically recognizable, MRI of the brain with special reference to the skull base is advisable on initial presentation.

Paroxysmal hemicrania consists of multiple severe short-lasting bouts of pain, lasting only minutes, with a pain distribution which is unilateral, often orbital or supraorbital, retro-orbital or temporal. In SUNCT, the pain is even briefer, lasting seconds. The character of the pain in SUNCT and to a lesser degree in paroxysmal hemichrania make it difficult to distinguish these clinically from the pain of TN but both syndromes are accompanied by cranial autonomic features that should distinguish them from TN. Paroxysmal hemicrania responds nearly always to indomethacin as does another headache syndrome with even briefer lasting painful jolts, primary stabbing headache. The extraordinarily rare SUNCT syndrome may respond to lamotrigine or one of the other newer AEDs. In rare patients, headache classifiable as SUNCT may represent a crossover form of TN and could respond to surgical therapy. Distinguishing between SUNCT and TN can in instances be difficult. Both syndromes have cutaneous triggers. Both syndromes are intensely painful with pain equally sharp and brief. SUNCT, however, nearly almost always involves the first division of the trigeminal nerve while TN rarely involves the first division of the trigeminal nerve primarily. SUNCT is rarely observed to cause nocturnal awakenings. Finally, the vast majority of patients with TN would respond favorably to carbamazepine or oxcarbazepine; patients with SUNCT generally have no or very limited response to these agents but a much more favorable response to lamotrigine.

It must be remembered that primary headache including migraine and its variants remains a diagnosis of exclusion. Appropriate neuroimaging must be considered at initial presentation or if the clinical characteristics of the syndrome shift significantly at a later time.

PERSISTENT IDIOPATHIC FACIAL PAIN OR ATYPICAL FACIAL PAIN

Atypical facial pain arose historically as a diagnostic grouping in contradistinction to TN (or "typical" facial pain) and has recently been renamed PIPF by the International Headache Society who have generated a defining set of characteristics. These are chronicity and persistence, dull constant aching (or burning) pain with nonperiodic exacerbations, diffusely localized pain usually unilateral but not conforming to a nerve distribution, and a normal neurologic examination and pain without an attributable cause after adequate clinical and imaging investigation. PIFP patients are less commonly young and less commonly male, are frequently depressed, and frequently have other accompanying somatic complaints. These patients too often come to neurologic attention after one or more interventions, often dental or sinus procedures that have failed to alleviate and may have even aggravated their complaint. A multidisciplinary approach to these patients is advocated and antidepressants are frequently helpful. Amitriptyline is an established therapy but selective norepinephrine and serotonin reuptake inhibitors such as duloxetine may be helpful. Unfortunately, therapy is rarely dramatically successful in patients with PIFP. For patients where duration of the complaint is many years in duration, it is important to obtain a history of the earliest presenting features. Some of these patients may have a chronically evolved form of TN. When the facial pain is relatively new in onset, a rare patient may have an underlying pulmonary malignancy. These patients will be heavy smokers and generally have a prominent periauricular component to their pain syndrome, which may reflect early involvement of the vagus nerve. Nasopharyngeal carcinoma is also a "look-like" that should be considered. Interventional therapies for PIFP are limited to case series and are not particularly encouraging.

LOWER FACIAL AND ORAL PAIN

Both the general practitioner and the neurologist should be familiar with pain disorders involving the lower face. The most common of these are the temporomandibular disorders (TMJ syndromes). Although temporomandibular dysfunction presents principally with pain at the TMJ and its associated musculature, associated symptoms including ear pain, frontal facial pain, more generalized headache, cervical pain, and dizziness make TMJ disorders an important differential consideration in patients presenting with facial pain. Historically, the TMJ dysfunctions have been both overdiagnosed and overtreated. TMJ syndromes present principally with pain involving the TMJ and its associated musculature, is aggravated by jaw function, and is associated with asymmetric movements of the jaw, painfully limited jaw opening and joint sounds. TMJ dysfunction can be usefully divided into primary intra-articular disorders or myofascial disorders. TMJ dysfunction presents most frequently in young adults, with a gender disparity favoring women in ratios of 3 to 1 or more. These disorders are generally self-limiting, and rarely present or persist beyond the age of 40. It is estimated that only 5% of symptomatic patients require any therapy at all, and it is believed that contrary to some historical practices, very few patients require invasive diagnostics or invasive therapies. The vast majority of patients with TMJ syndromes will respond to anti-inflammatory medications and conservative measures such as jaw appliances. The majority of patients refractory to these simple measures have a chronic myofascial pain syndrome and should be considered for multidisciplinary therapy, which may include benzodiazepines and norepinephrine reuptake inhibitors. Narcotic analgesics should be avoided. Physical findings in TMJ dysfunction include tenderness of the TMJ and associated musculature and painful, limited, or asymmetric jaw opening. Evaluation by an appropriate dental or oral surgical practitioner is recommended.

Atypical odontalgia is a rare disorder that mimics common tooth pain. The syndrome is characterized by its chronic nature, by definition more than 4 months duration and is frequently seen following dental extraction (phantom tooth pain), other oral procedures, or oral trauma. On occasion, the syndrome appears to occur spontaneously. The pain is characterized by dull persistence but transient sharp pain is sometimes reported. This pain entity is said not to disturb sleep and may not be present at awakening or briefly thereafter. Hyperpathia and allodynia may be present while spread of the pain to contiguous structures is not uncommon. Once local pathology has been adequately excluded, typical treatments targeting neuropathic pain may prove helpful.

First bite syndrome is a rare complication in the days following parapharyngeal tumor surgery seemingly associated with damage to the sympathetic parotid innervation. The patient experiences severe, lancinating pain along the lower jaw when starting to chew or by just coming into contact with food or drink. The disorder is usually self-limiting. Injection of the parotid gland with botulinum toxin A may be very helpful.

OTHER CAUSES OF FACIAL PAIN

The signs and symptoms of acute infections of the oral cavity, the paranasal sinuses, or the eye are generally obvious. The practitioner must remain alert to the patient who has been treated surreptitiously and unsuccessfully for a poorly documented acute infection where an alternative diagnosis, inflammatory or neurologic, should be considered. Patients and also practitioners frequently mistake migraine without aura and sometimes other primary headaches producing periorbital or maxillary pain for recurrent sinusitis even in the absence of a purulent discharge or fever. In one study of patients with self-diagnosed sinus headaches in the absence of fever or purulent discharge, 70% met formal criteria for migraine. Still, both acute and chronic sinusitis involving the deep sinuses can be clinically inapparent and may present with only vague head or facial pressure and malaise. Modern imaging, either coronal computed tomography (CT) or when needed MRI, is highly sensitive to pathology in or neighboring the ethmoid or sphenoid sinuses. Persistent infection of the sphenoid sinus in particular can lead to catastrophic involvement of the neighboring cavernous sinuses, orbital apex, associated cranial nerves, or the pituitary. The possibility of chronic facial pain heralding the presence of invasive infection in diabetics or the immune compromised must not be overlooked.

Giant cell arteritis should be considered in patients above age 50 who present subacutely with temporal or facial pain coupled with marked fatigue and malaise. These patients may complain of scalp tenderness, jaw claudication on prolonged chewing, and most ominously, visual disturbance. Palpable tenderness of the superficial temporal artery or another branch of the extracranial carotid artery should be present on examination and an elevated erythrocyte sedimentation rate (ESR) will be present in nearly 90% of cases and case series suggest that combined measurement of ESR and C-reactive protein (CRP) increases diagnostic sensitivity to at least 96%. A timely temporal artery biopsy is essential to making the correct diagnosis. Patients suspected of temporal arteritis should be placed on high-dose oral corticosteroids pending biopsy confirmation; biopsy should ideally not be delayed for more than several days once steroid treatment has begun.

Cranial neuropathies can present with pain prior to the development of neurologic deficits. Retrobulbar optic neuritis very frequently presents with pain on eye movement before monocular visual loss becomes apparent. Ischemic neuropathies involving the third or the sixth cranial nerves are typically painful although nonarteritic ischemic optic neuropathy is not. Sjogren's syndrome may present with an isolated trigeminal neuropathy. Neurosarcoidosis not infrequently presents with multiple cranial nerve involvements, which can result in both facial pain and more generalized cephalgia with trigeminal, facial, or vestibular-acoustic nerve involvement common.

Cervical arterial dissection can present with retro-orbital or more diffuse facial or occipital pain. Cervical pain need not be present and Horner syndrome can be either absent or overlooked. Pain frequently precedes cerebral ischemic manifestations, so this entity is important to consider in young adults, especially if there is a recent history of minor head or neck trauma or cervical manipulation (Video 14.1).

Acute glaucoma is associated with orbital and adjacent facial pain but the diagnosis is usually obvious because of corneal clouding and other eye changes. Subacute glaucoma can be more subtle on physical examination and can lead to a late or missed diagnosis.

Facial pain or headache should not be readily attributed to refractive errors or eye strain.

Chronic facial pain accompanied by hyperpathia or allodynia can be a manifestation of a central pain syndrome. The most common of these involves the contralateral thalamus and is usually postischemic. Generally, complete hemisensory loss will be present but on occasion, the loss can be restricted to the trigeminal distribution alone. This form of central pain may readily respond to tricyclic antidepressants such as amitriptyline or to antiepileptic medications such as lamotrigine or gabapentin.

Anesthesia dolorosa is a central pain syndrome that may follow any of the procedures performed to control TN. It is thought to be a consequence of excessive deafferentation and is characterized by the simultaneous presence of a constant, very unpleasant dysesthesia and marked cutaneous facial sensory loss. The syndrome may not surface for weeks or months after an ablative procedure. Neurosurgeons have observed that lessening the degree of deafferentation can lessen the likelihood of anesthesia dolorosa following an ablative trigeminal procedure. This syndrome can be difficult to treat either medically or surgically. Experimental approaches utilizing either invasive or noninvasive brain stimulation technologies could prove quite effective in the near future. A very few patients with significant trigeminal deafferentation may develop self-inflicted and difficult-to-treat ulceration, typically involving the ala nasi and designated "trigeminal trophic syndrome."

Burning mouth syndrome is a chronic and persistent syndrome of bilateral dysesthesias likened to the sensations following exposure to a too hot liquid involving the oral mucosa. Xerostomia and dysguesia may be present. Anxiety, irritability, and other mood changes are frequently present. It is most commonly encountered in perimenopausal or postmenopausal women and is sometimes confused with other facial pain syndromes.

PEARLS FOR FACIAL PAIN

- Only TN responds unequivocally to carbamazepine or oxcarbazepine. TACs should not.
- Pain in the ophthalmic division alone should raise considerable doubts regarding the diagnosis of TN.
- TN sometimes evinces tearing or conjunctival injection but this is not common; when these manifestations are prominent, consider SUNCT as a possibility.
- Paroxysmal hemicranial headache and chronic hemicranial headache very characteristically respond to indomethacin.
- Patients with CH appear restless and agitated. This is in very sharp contrast to migraineurs who very characteristically show a great reluctance to move.
- Migraineurs not infrequently awaken with morning headache or possibly facial pain; if a patient awakens with pain regularly from sleep or experiences pain at another time on a circadian basis, strongly consider CH.
- Patients with SUNCT or SUNA will not respond to medications with the possible exception of lamotrigine.
- Alcohol can be an instantaneous trigger in patients with CH during cluster periods. Alcohol is a more subtle, slower trigger in migraine.
- Migraine is extremely common, CH is not uncommon, TN is not uncommon, paroxysmal and chronic hemicranial headaches are uncommon, and SUNCT and SUNA are very uncommon.
- Frequently recurrent facial pain without fever or purulent discharge is more likely to be migraine, less likely to be sinusitis.

CONCLUDING OBSERVATIONS

It should always be remembered that patients with a chronic complaint, even if that complaint has been thoroughly investigated can develop new symptoms and become refractory to previously effective therapy. Changes in complaint or condition in an otherwise familiar patient could reflect a serious underlying pathology and may merit repeat neuroimaging. Patients with chronic facial pain may harbor an undisclosed malignancy or inflammatory process or a chronic infectious process. The presence of neurologic deficits on examination, be it a cranial nerve palsy, a sensory deficit in the trigeminal distribution, Horner syndrome, or the presence of subjective complaints of dysesthesias, diplopia, hearing loss, or disequilibrium should alert the practitioner to these possibilities. Similarly, the presence of cervical lymphadenopathy, chronic nasal obstruction, proptosis, lid edema, serous otitis, or an objective bruit is a potentially grave sign.

Patients with deficits should be appropriately imaged and referred. If patients with TN do not immediately respond to medication, they should be seen by a neurologist or neurosurgeon. If patients with TN fail medical therapy, consideration of early invasive treatment is generally appropriate. Because of its rarity, the diagnosis of GN should be confirmed by a neurologist or neurosurgeon. Patients with unusual headache syndromes should have their diagnosis confirmed by a neurologist and, if management difficulties are encountered, managed by a neurologist with headache expertise. Patients with HZ ophthalmicus should be seen by an ophthalmologist even if the globe appears uninvolved. Patients with refractory PHN can be expected to do poorly following ablative therapy.

Patients with chronic facial pain would truly benefit from a medical home provided by either their primary care physician or an appropriate specialist, perhaps a neurologist, who can propose new avenues of investigation or therapy and help limit inappropriate interventions.

Key Points

- TN is probably the most common facial pain disorder, is recognized clinically by unilateral bouts of lancinating pain primarily in the second and third divisions of the trigeminal nerve.
- TN is too frequently missed by practitioners but is generally quite treatable.
- GN is relatively rare but pain quality is similar to that in TN but involves the throat, posterior tongue, or ear.
- PHN involving the eye and upper face commonly follows HZ ophthalmicus, which is the second most common site of HZ neuropathy, comprising 10% to 20% of all cases.
- The primary headache disorders presenting as facial pain include CH and the other TACs; however, migraine without aura may present with prominent facial involvement and is not infrequently mistaken for recurrent sinusitis.
- PIFP is a diagnosis of exclusion and should be considered in cases where other causes such as TN, primary headache, or TMJ are poor clinical fits.
- Common causes of facial pain—purulent sinusitis, acute glaucoma, dental infections, sialadenitis—should not be overlooked nor should they be clinically opaque.

Recommended Readings

DeRossi SC, Greenberg MS, Liu F, et al. Temporomandibular disorders evaluation and management. *Med Clin North Am.* 2014;98:1353–1384.

Evans RW, Agostoni E. Persistent idiopathic facial pain. *Headache.* 2006;46(8):1298–1300.

Gronseth G, Cruccu G, Alksne J, et al. Practice parameter: the diagnostic evaluation and treatment of TN (an evidence-based review): report of the Quality Standards Subcommittee of the American Academy of Neurology and the European Federation of Neurological Societies. *Neurology.* 2008;71(15):1183–1190.

Leone M, Bussone G. Pathophysiology of trigeminal autonomic cephalgias. *Lancet Neurol.* 2009;8(8):755–764.

Maarbjerg S, Wolfram F, Gozalov A, et al. Significance of neurovascular contact in classical trigeminal neuralgia. *Brain.* 2015;138(pt 2):311–319.

Obermann M. Update on the challenges of treating trigeminal neuralgia. *Orphan Drugs: Res Rev.* 2015;5:11–17.

Tatli M, Satici O, Kanpolat Y, et al. Various surgical modalities for trigeminal neuralgia: literature study of respective long-term outcomes. *Acta Neurochir (Wien).* 2008;150(5):243–255.

Tseng HF, Smith N, Harpaz R, et al. Herpes zoster vaccine in older adults and the risk of subsequent herpes zoster disease. *JAMA.* 2011;305(2):160–166.

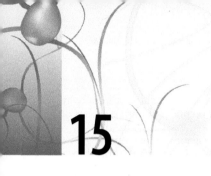

15 Approach to the Patient with Facial Weakness

Sam J. Marzo and John P. Leonetti

The facial nerve has the longest course of any cranial nerve through the skull and is at risk of injury due to inflammatory, infectious, neoplastic, traumatic, and congenital disorders. The most common cause of peripheral facial nerve paralysis is Bell's palsy, with an incidence of 20 per 100,000 people. Bell's palsy has a very favorable prognosis in the majority of patients if treated in a timely fashion with oral steroids. However, other causes of facial nerve injury may require different modalities of treatment, and a delay in proper diagnosis and treatment may result in an adverse facial nerve outcome.

Furthermore, the facial nerve is an important contributor to communication and emotional expression owing to the complex interaction of facial muscle groups innervated by the facial nerve. Facial weakness or paralysis can therefore lead to both physical and psychological distress. These deficits may be both cosmetic and functional. A logical assessment algorithm is required in order to implement timely and effective diagnostic studies and treatment protocols.

ANATOMY

A. **Central pathway.** The somatomotor cortex in the precentral gyrus provides facial nerve projection fibers, and the cell bodies in this area are primarily pyramidal nerve cells. Fascicles of the **corticobulbar** tract project through the internal capsule, through the basal part of the pons within the pyramidal tracts. Most of the nerve fibers decussate to reach the facial nucleus on the opposite side. Some fibers innervate the ipsilateral facial nucleus accounting for emotional control of facial expression.

   The **facial motor nucleus** (7,000 neurons) is within the reticular formation beneath the fourth ventricle. The superior (ventral) facial nucleus receives bilateral cortical input, whereas the inferior (dorsal) portion of the facial nucleus receives only contralateral cortical input for lower facial musculature innervation, hence the **"forehead sparing"** clinical finding in patients with a unilateral cortical (upper motor) versus a peripheral (lower motor) lesion.

   In addition to the motor fibers of the facial nerve responsible for facial expression, there are sensory fibers for taste to the anterior two-thirds of the tongue (**chorda tympanii**), external auditory canal cutaneous sensation, along with parasympathetic fibers to the lacrimal, submandibular, and sublingual glands.

   The facial nerve enters the internal auditory canal with the cochleovestibular nerve (CN VIII) and the nervus intermedius after leaving the pons and traversing the cerebellopontine angle. The segment of the facial nerve within the internal auditory canal is referred to as the meatal segment.

B. **Intratemporal.** The facial nerve is located in the anterosuperior portion of the internal auditory canal. Upon entering its own fallopian canal, the dural covering is replaced with epineurium. The three intratemporal segments of the facial nerve are the labyrinthine, tympanic, and mastoid segments. The labyrinthine segment is the narrowest, and the nerve is particularly at risk here owing to inflammation and trauma. Middle ear disease such as acute and chronic otitis media as well as cholesteatoma can affect the tympanic and mastoid segments of the nerve. The facial nerve exits the skull at the stylomastoid foramen.

C. **Extratemporal.** The facial nerve exits the stylomastoid foramen and divides into the upper (temporofacial) and lower (cervicofacial) segments. A variety of anastomotic branching occurs between the commonly identified temporal, zygomatic, buccal, mandibular, and cervical branches of the facial nerve. Primary and secondary parotid neoplasms as well as facial trauma can injure the nerve in this location.

CLINICAL ASSESSMENT

A. **History.** A detailed history is the most important aspect in the assessment of a patient with facial paralysis and particularly important is the rate of onset of the facial weakness. Acute onset of facial weakness, if nontraumatic, is usually viral or vascular in origin. Subacute onset of facial weakness is usually idiopathic (**Bell's palsy**), whereas delayed, gradual, and progressive facial weakness may be caused by intracranial, intratemporal, or extracranial neoplasms.

Other important factors in the history of facial weakness include whether the deficit is unilateral or bilateral, any past history of similar facial weakness, a history of ipsilateral hearing loss, associated ear or facial pain, trismus, or temporal trauma.

A general medical history can also assist in the evaluation of facial weakness. Predisposing factors include patient's age, arterial hypertension, diabetes mellitus, cigarette smoking, and a prior history of facial weakness. Lyme disease, Sjogren's syndrome, and a history of facial skin cancer may also be associated with facial paralysis.

B. **Physical examination.** Upper motor neuron (UMN) facial weakness caused by a contralateral lesion above the level of the upper medulla oblongata affects only the lower facial muscles. The forehead movement and eye closure are normal. The corneal reflex and emotional facial movements are intact.

Lower motor neuron (LMN) lesions from the facial nucleus to the parotid gland may cause weakness of all branches of the facial nerve. Complete paralysis is apparent with voluntary and emotional (involuntary) attempts to animate the face, and the corneal reflex is impaired (see Table 15.1).

A thorough neurologic examination may identify other focal findings such as other cranial nerve deficits, hemiparesis, hemisensory loss, sensorineural hearing loss (SNHL), or gaze palsy. Facial skin inspection may demonstrate a malignant lesion causing perineural invasion and facial weakness, whereas bimanual parotid palpation, especially in the patient with trismus, can identify a parotid gland malignancy as a cause for facial paralysis. Microscopic otoscopy will help disclose an infectious (acute otitis media) or neoplastic source of facial weakness within the middle ear or mastoid bone.

C. **Diagnostic studies.**
   1. **Computed tomography (CT)** of the temporal bone is useful in cases in which the temporal bone is the suspected site of pathology. The CT will show the intratemporal portion of the nerve. Important areas to focus on are erosive lesions of the middle ear and/or mastoid, which usually suggest chronic otitis media or cholesteatoma. The CT will also show blunt or penetrating trauma as well as facial nerve neoplasms (facial schwannoma, hemangioma) and temporal bone neoplasms such as paragangliomas.
   2. **Magnetic resonance imaging (MRI)** with contrast is useful in patients with suspected brainstem, cerebellopontine angle, or parotid gland lesions. MRI is best at assessing the intracranial and meatal segments of the nerve as well as the extratemporal segment.
   3. **Lumbar puncture** is sometimes used in suspected neoplastic or inflammatory/infectious causes of facial nerve injury such as meningeal carcinomatosis or Lyme disease.
   4. **Electrodiagnostic studies** such as electroneuronography (ENoG) and electromyography (EMG) may have a role in selected cases of facial nerve injury. For example, the ENoG may have prognostic value in patients with complete facial paralysis due to Bell's palsy. Those patients with >90% degeneration within 2 weeks after onset may benefit from a middle fossa facial nerve decompression. In those patients with complete facial nerve injuries longer than 3 weeks, the EMG can assess signs of facial nerve recovery (polyphasic action potentials) or denervation (fibrillation potentials).

TABLE 15.1 House–Brackmann Classification of Facial Function

Grade	Characteristics
I, normal	Normal facial function
II, mild dysfunction	Gross
	Slight weakness noticeable on close inspection
	May have slight synkinesis
	At rest, normal symmetry and tone
	Motion
	Forehead—moderate to good
	Eye—complete closure
	Mouth—slight asymmetry
III, moderate dysfunction	Gross
	Obvious, not disfiguring
	Noticeable synkinesis, contracture, spasm
	At rest, normal symmetry and tone
	Motion
	Forehead—slight to moderate movement
	Eye—complete closure with effort
	Mouth—slightly weak with maximal effort
IV, moderately severe dysfunction	Gross
	Obvious weakness and/or disfiguring asymmetry
	At rest, normal symmetry and tone
	Motion
	Forehead—none
	Eye—incomplete closure
	Mouth—asymmetric with maximum effort
V, severe dysfunction	Gross
	Barely perceptible motion
	At rest, asymmetry
	Motion
	Forehead—none
	Eye—incomplete closure
	Mouth—slight movement
VI, total paralysis	No movement

5. **Audiometric testing** will help determine the type and degree of hearing loss. An asymmetric, ipsilateral SNHL would suggest a cerebellopontine angle or internal auditory canal lesion in patients with LMN facial weakness. A conductive or mixed hearing loss, however, would suggest a middle ear infectious or neoplastic cause for the facial nerve deficit.

DIFFERENTIAL DIAGNOSIS

The most common cause of peripheral facial paralysis is **Bell's palsy.** This is a diagnosis of exclusion. The paralysis can be partial or complete, is unilateral, and usually occurs suddenly over 24 to 48 hours. It is currently believed to be secondary to a herpetic inflammation of the nerve. Approximately 70% of patients recover completely without treatment. Oral steroids and antiviral therapy, when given within the first 10 to 14 days after onset, may have a role in improving the ultimate patient outcome. However, recent data show that antivirals do not provide an added benefit on facial recovery.

    Ramsay Hunt syndrome (herpes zoster oticus) is characterized by aural vesicles, pain, and peripheral facial nerve palsy. The vesicles can also involve the ipsilateral anterior two-thirds of the tongue and soft palate. It differs from Bell's palsy in that vesicles are present, pain may be severe and persistent, there is a higher incidence of vestibular and auditory symptoms, and the prognosis is generally worse. The agent is believed to be **varicella-zoster virus.** Oral steroids and antiviral therapy are the currently accepted treatment.

Melkersson–Rosenthal syndrome is characterized by recurring facial paralysis, and swelling of the face and lips, usually the upper lip. The paralysis may be unilateral or may alternate sides, and may be complete or incomplete. It can occur in males or females, usually in the second decade of life. Associated physical features also include fissuring of the tongue.

Traumatic causes for facial paralysis can be penetrating or blunt. In the patient with a penetrating injury and complete facial paralysis, the nerve should be presumed to be cut unless the facial movement on that side was clearly documented. In these cases the facial nerve should be explored and repaired as soon as the patient is medically stable.

Penetrating injury to the extratemporal, intraparotid facial nerve can be microsurgically repaired if the wound is clean, if performed as soon as feasibly possible, and if the injury involves the main trunk or a primary division of the facial nerve. Individual branch lacerations do not require surgical repair. Penetrating injury to the facial nerve within the temporal bone also requires surgical repair and, if necessary, interposition grafting with the greater auricular nerve. In the patient with a penetrating injury and complete facial paralysis, the nerve should be presumed to be cut unless the facial movement on that side was clearly documented. In these cases the facial nerve should be explored and repaired as soon as the patient is medically stable.

Iatrogenic facial nerve injury can also occur during middle ear and mastoid surgery. The tympanic segment of the facial nerve is particularly at risk during middle ear surgery such as cholesteatoma removal, in which case the bony covering of the facial nerve may be completely absent (Video 15.1). The mastoid segment of the facial nerve may be injured while removing disease in the facial recess and mastoid cavity. In these cases the nerve will usually require repair with a facial nerve graft from the great auricular nerve in the neck.

Blunt trauma to the temporal bone may cause facial paralysis as a result of neural contusion, hematoma, edema, bony impingement, laceration, or avulsion. Delayed-onset facial weakness is usually due to compression with neural edema. These patients generally recover excellent facial function without surgical or medical intervention. Acute-onset facial weakness following blunt temporal bone trauma, however, suggests more serious neural injury requiring transmastoid facial nerve decompression and repair (see Fig. 15.1).

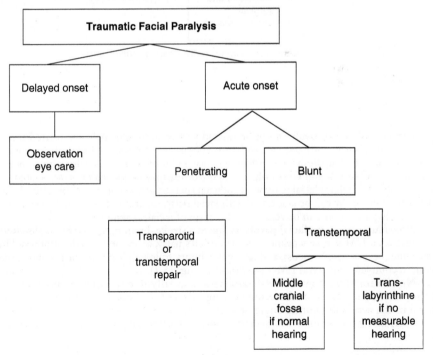

FIGURE 15.1 Clinical assessment algorithm for patients with traumatic facial paralysis.

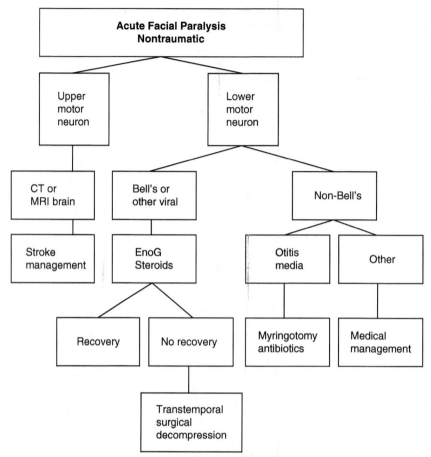

FIGURE 15.2 Clinical assessment algorithm for patients with acute, nontraumatic facial paralysis. Abbreviations: CT, computed tomography; ENoG, electroneuronography; MRI, magnetic resonance imaging.

Congenital facial paralysis can be related to intrauterine or delivery-related trauma, facial nucleus aplasia, and facial musculature aplasia, or be associated with more complex general syndromes. **Cardiofacial syndrome** consists of unilateral facial palsy with congenital heart defects. **Poland's** and **Goldenhaar's syndromes** may occasionally be associated with facial weakness. Bilateral facial palsy with abducens nerve palsy occurs in **Möbius syndrome.** **Myotonic dystrophy** can be associated with facial palsy. An array of medical disorders, such as arterial hypertension, can be related to the onset of facial weakness.

Nontraumatic acute facial paralysis due to a stroke, brain tumor, or brain abscess can manifest as an UMN-type weakness, whereas Bell's palsy, acute otitis media, Ramsay Hunt syndrome (herpes zoster oticus), and iatrogenic injury following otologic or parotid surgery result in complete, unilateral LMN paralysis (see Fig. 15.2).

Nontraumatic, delayed facial paralysis is usually due to a neoplasm (Fig. 15.3). If the patient complains of associated hearing loss and tinnitus, the lesion is likely to be found in the cerebellopontine angle or the internal auditory canal. Slow-growing facial neuromas and glomus tumors may cause a mixed hearing loss if the tumor is isolated to

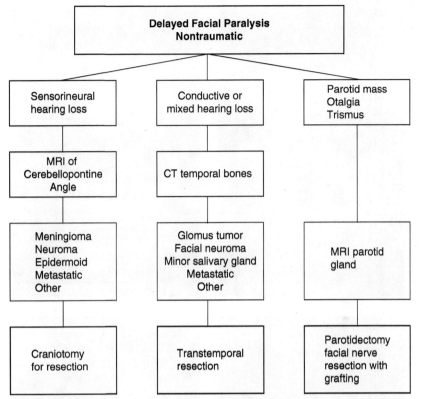

FIGURE 15.3 Clinical assessment algorithm for patients with delayed, nontraumatic facial paralysis. Abbreviations: CT, computed tomography; MRI, magnetic resonance imaging.

the middle ear and/or mastoid bone. Malignant parotid gland tumors also cause gradual onset or segmental facial paralysis in addition to otalgia, facial pain, trismus, and bloody otorrhea (Fig. 15.4). Benign parotid gland tumors, other than intraparotid facial neuromas, rarely cause facial paralysis.

A more inclusive list of causes for facial paralysis is included in Table 15.2.

Care of the eye: A very important aspect of care of the patients with facial nerve injury is the assessment of the patients' ability to protect their ipsilateral eye. Those who can close their eyelid completely usually do very well. Those with incomplete eyelid closure will not be able to adequately lubricate and protect their cornea. These patients may benefit from lubricant eye drops during the day and ointments such as lacrilube at bedtime. The patients can also tape their eyelid closed with paper or silk tape. Care should be taken to not put anything such as a tissue or patch on the cornea. Those patients with corneal irritation or eye pain should be seen by an ophthalmologist.

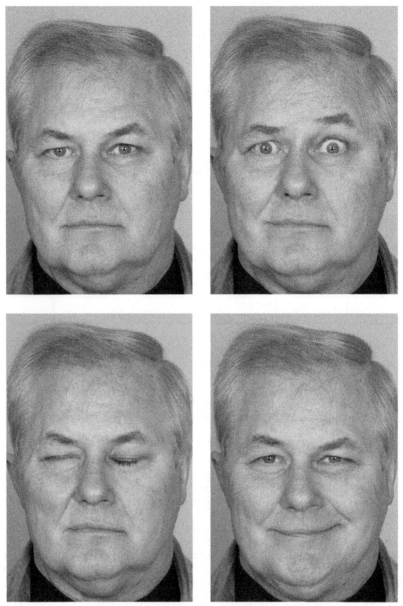

FIGURE 15.4 Long-term facial function following parotidectomy, facial nerve resection, and interposition neural grafting for acinic cell carcinoma of the parotid gland.

TABLE 15.2 Causes of Facial Paralysis

Birth	Molding
	Forceps delivery
	Myotonic dystrophy
	Möbius syndrome (facial diplegia associated with other cranial nerve deficits)
Trauma	Basal skull fractures
	Facial injuries
	Penetrating injury to middle ear
	Altitude paralysis (barotrauma)
	Lightning
Neurologic	Opercular syndrome (cortical lesion in facial motor area)
	Millard–Gubler's syndrome (abducens palsy with contralateral hemiplegia caused by lesion in vertical pons involving the homolateral CN VII nucleus and the descending corticospinal tract)
Infection	External otitis
	Otitis media
	Mastoiditis
	Chickenpox
	Herpes zoster cephalicus (Ramsay Hunt syndrome)
	Encephalitis
	Poliomyelitis
	Mumps
	Infectious mononucleosis
	Leprosy
	Influenza
	Coxsackievirus
	Malaria
	Syphilis
	Scleroma
	Tuberculosis
	Botulism
	Acute hemorrhagic conjunctivitis (enterovirus 70)
	Gnathostomiasis
	Mucormycosis
	Lyme disease
	Cat scratch fever
	AIDS
Metabolic	Diabetes mellitus
	Hyperthyroidism
	Pregnancy
	Hypertension
	Acute intermittent porphyria
	Vitamin A deficiency
Neoplastic	Benign lesions of the parotid gland
	Cholesteatoma
	Seventh nerve tumor
	Glomus jugulare tumor
	Leukemia
	Meningioma
	Hemangioblastoma
	Sarcoma
	Carcinoma (invading or metastatic)
	Anomalous sigmoid sinus
	Carotid artery aneurysm
	Hemangioma of tympanum

(continued)

TABLE 15.2 Causes of Facial Paralysis (*continued*)

	Hydradenoma (external canal)
	Facial nerve tumor (cylindroma)
	Schwannoma
	Teratoma
	Hand–Shüller–Christian disease
	Fibrous dysplasia
	Neurofibromatosis type 2
Toxic	Thalidomide (Miehlke syndrome, cranial nerves VI and VII with congenital malformed external ears and deafness)
	Ethylene glycol
	Alcoholism
	Arsenic intoxication
	Tetanus
	Diphtheria
	Carbon monoxide
Iatrogenic	Mandibular block anesthesia
	Antitetanus serum
	Vaccine treatment for rabies
	Postimmunization
	Parotid surgery
	Mastoid surgery
	Post tonsillectomy and adenoidectomy
	Iontophoresis (local anesthesia)
	Embolization
	Dental
Idiopathic	Familial Bell's palsy
	Melkersson–Rosenthal syndrome
	Hereditary hypertrophic neuropathies
	Autoimmune syndrome
	Amyloidosis
	Temporal arteritis
	Thrombotic thrombocytopenic purpura
	Polyarteritis nodosa
	Guillain–Barré syndrome
	Multiple sclerosis
	Myasthenia gravis
	Sarcoidosis
	Osteopetrosis

Adapted from May M, Klein SR. Differential diagnosis of facial nerve palsy. *Otolaryngol Clin North Am*. 1991;24(3):613–145.

Key Points

- Bell's palsy is the most common cause of peripheral facial nerve paralysis and has a very favorable prognosis.
- The clinical history is the most important factor in the patient assessment.
- The physical examination of the patient with facial paralysis should include otoscopy and parotid gland palpation.
- Imaging may be necessary in some patients in which the history is atypical.
- Timely diagnosis and treatment are important for maximizing facial nerve function.
- Adequate eye care for those who cannot completely close their eyelids can prevent corneal injury.

Recommended Readings

Adour KK. Diagnosis and management of facial paralysis. *N Engl J Med*. 1982;307:348–351.

Bateman DE. Facial palsy. *Br J Hosp Med*. 1992;47:430–431.

Carpenter B, Sutin J. *Pons in Human Neural Anatomy*. Baltimore, MD: Lippincott Williams & Wilkins; 1983:385–389.

Courbille J. The nucleus of the facial nerve: the relation between cellular groups and peripheral branches of the nerve. *Brain*. 1966;1:338–354.

Engström M, Berg T, Stjernquist-Desatnik A, et al. Prednisolone and valaciclovir in Bell's palsy: a randomized, double-blind, placebo-controlled, multicentre trial. *Lancet Neurol*. 2008;7(11):993–1000.

Esslen E. Electromyography and electroneurography. In: Fisch U, ed. *Facial Nerve Surgery*. Birmingham, United Kingdom: Aesculapius Publishing; 1977:93–100.

Finestone AJ, Byers K. Acute facial paralysis: is it a stroke or something else? *Geriatrics*. 1994;49:50–52.

Fisch U, Esslen E. Total intratemporal exposure of the facial nerve: pathologic findings in Bell's palsy. *Arch Otolaryngol*. 1972;85:335–341.

Gupta MK, Kumar P. Reversible congenital facial nerve palsy: an uncommon cause of asymmetric crying facies in the newborn. *Internet J Pediatr Neonatol*. 2007;7(1):1–4. ISSN 1528-8374.

House JW, Brackman DE. Facial nerve grading system. *Otolaryngol Head Neck Surg*. 1985;93:146–147.

Morgan M, Nathwani D. Facial palsy and infections: the unfolding story. *Clin Infect Dis*. 1992;14:263–271.

Nager GT, Proctor B. Anatomical variation and anomalies involving the facial canal. *Ann Otol Rhinol Laryngol*. 1982;(suppl 93):45–61.

Olsen KD. Facial nerve paralysis: all that palsies is not Bell's. *Postgrad Med*. 1984;76:95–105.

Pietersen E. Natural history of Bell's palsy. *Acta Otolaryngol*. 1992;492(suppl):122–124.

Quant EC, Jeste SS, Muni RH, et al. The benefits of steroids plus antivirals for treatment of Bell's palsy: a meta-analysis. *BMJ*. 2009;339:b3354.

Smith JD, Crumley RL, Harker A. Facial paralysis in the newborn. *Arch Otolaryngol Head Neck Surg*. 1981;89:1021–1024.

Sunderland S. *Nerve and Nerve Injuries*. 2nd ed. Edinburgh, United Kingdom: Churchill Livingstone; 1978:31–60.

Terao S, Miura N, Takeda A, et al. Course and distribution of facial corticobulbar tract fibers in the lower brain stem. *J Neurol Neurosurg Psychiatry*. 2000;69:262–265.

Toelle SP, Boltshauser E. Long-term outcome in children with congenital unilateral facial nerve palsy. *Neuropediatrics*. 2001;32:130–135.

Wackym PA. Molecular temporal bone pathology: II: Ramsay Hunt syndrome (herpes zoster oticus). *Laryngoscope*. 1979;107:1165–1175.

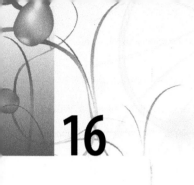

16 Approach to the Patient with Dizziness and Vertigo

Timothy C. Hain and Marcello Cherchi

Dizziness and vertigo are common symptoms. About 2.5% of all primary care visits are for dizziness and about 1% are for vertigo. Dizziness and vertigo have diverse etiologies, spanning multiple organ systems. Thus, a broadly based approach to the dizzy patient is necessary, at times requiring serious and life-threatening medical problems such as cardiac arrhythmia to be distinguished from the more common inner ear diseases and dizziness from unlocalizable sources.

ETIOLOGY

Dizziness and vertigo can be categorized by etiology into four types: otologic, central, medical, and unlocalized (Table 16.1).

TABLE 16.1 Etiologies of Vertigo

Otologic vertigo
BPPV
Vestibular neuritis and labyrinthitis
Ménière's disease
Bilateral vestibular paresis or loss
SSCD and PLF
Tumors compressing the eighth cranial nerve

Central vertigo
Migraine
Stroke and TIA in VB arterial distribution
Seizures
MS
Chiari malformation

Medical vertigo
Postural hypotension
Arrhythmia
Cardiac
Hypoglycemia and diabetes mellitus
Medication effects
Viral syndrome

Unlocalized vertigo syndromes
Anxiety and panic
Posttraumatic vertigo
Hyperventilation
Malingering
Unknown

Abbreviations: BPPV, benign paroxysmal positional vertigo; MS, multiple sclerosis; PLF, Perilymph fistula; SSCD, superior semicircular canal dehiscence; TIA, transient ischemic attack; VB, vertebrobasilar.

A. **Otologic vertigo** is caused by dysfunction of the inner ear. Table 16.1 lists entities that account for about 95% of all cases of otologic vertigo. The distribution of diagnoses varies greatly according to the referral base (e.g., neurology, otolaryngology, general medicine, emergency room), but in all settings otologic vertigo comprises a substantial component.

1. **Benign paroxysmal positional vertigo (BPPV)** has an incidence of about 0.6% per year, making it the most common otologic cause of vertigo (nearly 50%) and accounting for roughly 20% of all cases of vertigo, thus also making it the single most common cause of vertigo over the life span. BPPV presents with brief vertigo provoked by changes in the orientation of the head with respect to gravity. BPPV is caused by loose debris within the labyrinth.

2. **Vestibular neuritis** presents with vertigo, nausea, ataxia, and nystagmus. Limited evidence implicates a viral infection of the vestibular nerve as the etiology. Labyrinthitis presents with the same vestibular symptom complex, combined with aural symptoms of tinnitus and/or hearing loss. Vestibular neuritis and labyrinthitis together account for about 15% of all otologic vertigo cases.

3. **Ménière's disease** presents with intermittent vertigo accompanied by hearing complaints (see the so-called "hydrops" symptom complex in **Section A.3 under Differential Diagnosis**). It accounts for about 15% of otologic vertigo cases.

4. **Bilateral vestibular paresis** presents with oscillopsia and ataxia, usually caused by loss of vestibular hair cells. The typical history is of treatment for several weeks with an intravenous or intraperitoneal ototoxic antibiotic (of which gentamicin is the most commonly used). Bilateral vestibular loss is uncommon.

5. **The superior semicircular canal dehiscence (SSCD) syndrome** exemplifies several conditions in which there is an abnormal opening between the inner ear and a surrounding structure. They generally present with vertigo induced by sound (called Tullio's phenomenon) or as ataxia provoked by activity or straining. The diagnosis of SSCD has been rapidly increasing in recent years because of a combination of improved knowledge about the condition combined with greater use of a new diagnostic modality—vestibular evoked myogenic potentials (VEMPs), and thin-section computed tomography (CT) protocols providing detailed imaging coplanar with the superior semicircular canal. In SSCD, bone over the superior semicircular canal is absent. Similar symptoms are seen in perilymphatic fistula and cholesteatoma.

6. **Tumors compressing the eighth cranial nerve, such as acoustic neuroma,** present with asymmetric hearing loss combined with mild ataxia. Eighth-nerve tumors are very uncommon in the vertiginous population (but are more common in the unilaterally hearing impaired).

B. **Central vertigo** is caused by dysfunction of central structures that process sensory input from the inner ear. Central vertigo accounts for 2% to 50% of vertigo diagnoses, depending on the setting in which patients are seen. In a majority of cases, central vertigo is caused by migraine. Table 16.1 lists entities accounting for about 90% of central vertigo diagnoses, the remainder being made up of individual unusual conditions (e.g., spinocerebellar degeneration).

1. **Migraine-associated vertigo** (also called "vertiginous migraine," "vestibular migraine," and similar labels) ordinarily presents with vertigo and headache, but it can also present as isolated vertigo. Migraine causes about 75% of central vertigo cases, and is the most common cause of vertigo in the pediatric population. It is particularly common in women in their 30s and 50s.

2. **Stroke and transient ischemic attack (TIA) involving the brainstem or cerebellum** is an occasional source of central dizziness. Vertigo can occasionally be the only symptom preceding a posterior fossa stroke; there are not yet reliable means of distinguishing a TIA affecting the vestibular nucleus or cerebellum from another process affecting the vestibular nerve or end organ, although recent research on the head impulse test (HIT) suggests that this may be a promising approach to this diagnostic dilemma.

3. **Seizures** present with vertigo combined with motor symptoms or confusion. About 5% of central vertigo is caused by seizures. Dizziness is a common symptom in persons with known epilepsy.

4. **Multiple sclerosis (MS)** combines vertigo with other central signs such as cerebellar dysfunction. MS is an uncommon source of vertigo. About 2% of central vertigo cases are caused by MS. In persons with known MS, it is important not to attribute vertigo to MS without considering common peripheral causes that might be coincident, such as BPPV.

5. **The Chiari malformation** is a hindbrain malformation wherein the cerebellar tonsils herniate 5 mm or more below the foramen magnum. These patients complain of vertigo, ataxia, and occipital headaches, and often have downbeat nystagmus. Like SSCD, symptoms may be precipitated by straining. Magnetic resonance imaging (MRI) of the posterior fossa establishes the diagnosis. About 1% of cases of central vertigo are caused by the Chiari malformation.

6. **Cervical vertigo** is a controversial syndrome. Diagnosis is most often made after a whiplash injury where findings usually include vertigo, tinnitus, and neck pain. Examination usually demonstrates a nonspecific symptom complex including neck movement limited by pain and nausea or vertigo on neck positioning. Generally, there is no strong nystagmus even using video-recording methods. There are no definitive clinical or laboratory tests for cervical vertigo. MRI of the cervical spine in these patients often shows cervical disks abutting but not compressing the cervical cord. Rare cases have been reported in whom vertigo can be traced to compression of a vertebral artery after neck rotation (bow hunter syndrome). Due to the lack of clarity in the diagnosis of cervical vertigo, its prevalence is unknown.

C. **Medical vertigo** may be caused by altered blood pressure, low blood sugar, and/or metabolic derangements associated with medication or systemic infection. It is largely encountered in the emergency room, where it accounts for about 33% of all cases of dizziness. It is unusual in subspecialty settings (2% to 5%). Table 16.1 lists nearly all causes of dizziness reported in studies of vertigo as it presents to emergency rooms.

1. **Postural hypotension** often presents as giddiness, lightheadedness, or syncope. These symptoms occur only while the patient is upright.

2. **Cardiac arrhythmia** presents with syncope or drop-attacks. Like those of postural hypotension, symptoms are characteristically present only when patients are upright.

3. **Hypoglycemia** and metabolic derangements associated with diabetes present with giddiness or lightheadedness. Hypoglycemia is often accompanied by autonomic symptoms such as palpitations, sweating, tremors, or pallor. Together they account for about 5% of the cases of dizziness in general medical settings.

4. **Medication effects** usually present with giddiness or lightheadedness, but also can present with true vertigo. These diagnoses account for about 16% of the dizzy patients seen in the emergency setting, but are rare outside the emergency room. Medications commonly implicated include antihypertensive agents, especially α_1-adrenergic blockers such as terazosin, calcium-channel blockers such as nifedipine, and sedatives. Benzodiazepines, such as alprazolam, can cause dizziness as part of the withdrawal syndrome. Alcohol intoxication can present as a transient positional nystagmus, cerebellar signs, and direction-changing positional nystagmus.

5. **Viral syndromes** not involving the ear are the reported cause of dizziness in approximately 4% to 40% of all cases seen in the emergency room setting. Such syndromes include gastroenteritis and influenza-like illnesses.

D. **Unlocalized vertigo** patients include those whose symptoms are attributed to psychiatric disorders, those whose symptoms are attributed to events without further definition (such as head trauma), and those with vertigo and dizziness of unknown origin. Common variants of unlocalized vertigo include psychogenic vertigo, hyperventilation syndrome, posttraumatic vertigo, and nonspecific dizziness. Between 15% and 50% of all patients with dizziness or vertigo fall into this category, depending both on referral base and diagnostic diligence.

1. Unknown (nonspecific dizziness). Diagnostic procedures are insensitive, and in dizziness evaluations it is usual to have as many as 50% of patients without any detectable abnormalities on careful clinical examination and thorough testing. Some authors wrongly define psychogenic vertigo as the complaints of patients falling into this category. About 75% of the unlocalized vertigo category consists of patients in whom there are no abnormalities on examination and testing.

2. Psychogenic. Patients with anxiety disorders, panic disorder, and posttraumatic stress disorder may complain of dizziness, ataxia, and autonomic symptoms. This is a common presentation. It is often impossible to determine whether or not anxiety is the sole cause or a reaction. In somatization disorder, symptoms may be present without anxiety.

3. **Posttraumatic vertigo** patients complain of vertigo following head injuries but frequently present no findings on examination or vestibular testing. BPPV is excluded by several

negative Dix–Hallpike maneuvers using an adequately sensitive technique (e.g., video goggles). Posttraumatic vertigo is common. Diagnosis is sometimes complicated by medicolegal proceedings in which secondary gain must be taken into consideration.

4. **Hyperventilation syndrome.** These patients have vertigo after hyperventilation, without other findings or nystagmus. Hyperventilation-induced symptoms without substantial nystagmus are common in normal persons. Hyperventilation-induced symptoms are commonly seen in well-documented structural abnormalities such as acoustic neuroma.

5. **Multisensory disequilibrium of the elderly.** Most elderly people have age-related multisensory impairment. Like the diagnosis of psychogenic vertigo, this diagnosis is often used in situations where examination is otherwise normal.

6. **Malingering.** Because vertigo can be intermittent and disabling, and frequently follows head injury, it may be claimed in an attempt to obtain compensation. Malingering is common only among patients who are being compensated for illness.

CLINICAL MANIFESTATIONS

A. **Primary symptoms.** The primary symptoms listed in Table 16.2 are mainly the result of a disturbed sensorium.

1. Vertigo denotes a sensation of rotation—either of the person or of the world. It can be horizontal, vertical, or rotatory. It can be described as visual "blurring" or "jumping." Horizontal vertigo is the most common type, usually resulting from dysfunction of the inner ear. Vertical vertigo is rarer. When transient, it is usually caused by BPPV. When constant, it is usually of central origin and accompanied by downbeat or upbeat nystagmus. Rotatory vertigo is the least frequent. When transient, rotatory vertigo is usually caused by BPPV. When chronic, it is always central and usually accompanied by rotatory nystagmus.

2. Impulsion denotes a sensation of translation, usually described as brief sensations of being pushed or tilted. Variants include rocking, floating, and perceived changes in the directions of up and down. Impulsion indicates dysfunction of the otolithic apparatus of the inner ear or central processing of otolithic signals. It is often a symptom of Ménière's disease.

3. Oscillopsia is an illusory movement of the world evoked by head movement. Patients with bilateral vestibular loss are unable to see when their heads are in motion because of oscillopsia. Patients with unilateral vestibular loss often complain that "the world

---

TABLE 16.2 Symptoms in Patients with Dizziness and Vertigo

Primary symptoms
Vertigo
Impulsion and rocking
Oscillopsia
Ataxia
Hearing symptoms

Secondary symptoms
Nausea, emesis, diarrhea
Pallor, bradycardia
Fatigue
Headache
Visual sensitivity

Nonspecific symptoms
Giddiness
Lightheadedness

doesn't keep up" or "my eyes lag behind my head" when they rapidly rotate their heads laterally to the side of the bad ear.

4. Ataxia, unsteadiness of gait, is nearly universal in patients with otologic or central vertigo and is variably observed in patients with medical and unlocalized vertigo.

5. Hearing symptoms. Vertigo is often accompanied by tinnitus, hearing reduction or distortion, and aural fullness.

B. **Secondary symptoms** include nausea, autonomic symptoms, fatigue, headache, and visual sensitivity. Visual sensitivity is also known as the "grocery store syndrome." Patients complain of dizziness related to the types of patterned visual stimulation that occur when they traverse grocery store aisles, drive past picket fences or through bridges, or view large-screen movies. The grocery store syndrome is a nonspecific common late symptom in patients with vertigo and is generally thought to be caused by a reweighting of sensory input related to balance (ear, eye, and body) resulting in greater dependence on vision.

C. **Giddiness, wooziness, heavy-headedness, and lightheadedness.** These terms are imprecise although in common usage. They are rarely used by patients with documented inner ear dysfunction but are frequently used by patients with vertigo related to medical problems.

EVALUATION

A. History. The history must either be all-encompassing or follow a heuristic technique whereby questions are selected as the interview progresses. Here we outline the all-encompassing approach.

1. Definition. Does the patient complain of vertigo (spinning), a secondary symptom (such as nausea), a nonspecific symptom (giddiness or lightheadedness), or something entirely different (e.g., confusion)?

2. Timing. Are symptoms constant or episodic? If episodic, how long do they last?

3. **Triggering** or exacerbating factors are listed in Table 16.3. All patients should be queried regarding these factors, either by going through them one by one, or by using an interview heuristic whereby one attempts to rule in or rule out a symptom complex (see section Differential Diagnosis).

4. Otologic history. Ask about hearing loss, tinnitus, and fullness. Positives are indications for an audiogram. The patient's description of tinnitus is sometimes helpful in diagnosis. For instance, "roaring" tinnitus often occurs in Ménière's disease. "Buzzing" tinnitus sometimes occurs in vestibulocochlear paroxysmia. Pulsatile tinnitus suggests a vascular cause.

5. Medication history. Numerous medications can induce dizziness, including ototoxic drugs, antiepileptic drugs, antihypertensives, and sedatives. All current medications, as well as previous exposure to ototoxic agents, should be considered as sources of dizziness.

TABLE 16.3 **Triggering or Exacerbating Factors**

Positional changes of head or body
Standing up
Rapid head movements
Walking in a dark room
Loud noises
Coughing, nose blowing, sneezing, or straining
Underwater diving, elevators, airplane travel
Exercise
Shopping malls, narrow or wide-open spaces, grocery stores
Foods (salt and monosodium glutamate)
Fasting
Alcohol
Menstrual periods
Boat or car travel
Anxiety or stress

6. **Family history.** Has anyone in the immediate family had similar symptoms? Is there a family history of migraines, seizures, Ménière's disease, or early-onset hearing loss? A family history of multiple relatives with conductive hearing loss suggests otosclerosis. The finding of hearing loss on the same side in multiple relatives suggests enlarged vestibular or cochlear aqueduct syndrome.

7. **Review of systems** should explore psychiatric problems (anxiety, depression, and panic), vascular risk factors, cancer, autoimmune disease, neurologic problems (migraine, stroke, TIA, seizures, and MS), otologic surgery, and general medical history (especially thyroid dysfunction, diabetes, Lyme disease, or syphilis).

8. **Previous studies** relevant to dizziness (see **Section C under Evaluation**) should be reviewed.

B. **Physical examination.** The physical examination of the vertiginous patient is outlined in Table 16.4. It is ordered in such a way that procedures may be added on the basis of previous results. Because a full examination may be lengthy, it is most practical to expand or contract the examination dynamically. As an exception to the following procedure, if there is a history of positional vertigo, it is reasonable to go immediately to the Dix–Hallpike test (see **Section B.5.b under Evaluation**).

1. **General examination.** Measure the blood pressure and pulse with the patient standing. Arrhythmia is noted, if present. If the standing blood pressure is low, check blood pressure with the patient lying flat. The heart and the carotid and subclavian arteries are auscultated. Besides, the mastoid is auscultated as well if there is pulsatile tinnitus.

2. **Balance** is assessed via observation of gait (see Chapter 8), and the eyes-closed tandem Romberg test. The tandem Romberg test is extremely useful. Low-normal performance consists of the ability to stand heel-to-toe, with eyes closed, for 6 seconds. Young adults should be able to perform this test for 30 seconds, but performance declines with age. It is helpful to develop a judgment of how much ataxia is appropriate for a given degree of ear injury. Patients with bilateral vestibular loss are moderately ataxic—they make heavy use of vision and are unsteady when their eyes are closed (with a narrow base). No patient with bilateral loss can stand in the eyes-closed tandem Romberg test for 6 seconds. Patients with an additional superimposed position sense deficit are unsteady with eyes open (with a narrow base). Patients with chronic unilateral vestibular loss show very little ataxia, and they are usually normal on the eyes-closed tandem Romberg test. The need to gauge ataxia does not come up in patients with recent unilateral vestibular imbalance because these patients have prominent nystagmus. Patients with cerebellar disorders, such as alcoholic cerebellar degeneration, have greater ataxia than is appropriate for their degree of nystagmus or vestibular paresis. Patients who are malingering also typically emphasize imbalance, which is the disabling aspect of their symptoms. In head injury or where there is other reason to suspect a central nervous system (CNS) origin of imbalance, also test basal ganglia function (pulsion/retropulsion tests).

3. **Otologic examination.** A brief screening test is adequate for hearing. The examiner's thumb and first fingers are rubbed together at arm's length from one of the patient's ears. Persons with normal hearing can perceive this sound at an arm's length. If the sound is not perceived, the source is brought in closer and closer until it is heard, and the distance is recorded. This simple test identifies high-tone hearing loss—for example, most elderly are able to hear at about 6 inches on either side. The tympanic membranes should be inspected for wax, perforation, otitis, discoloration, and mass lesions. Wax should be removed before more sophisticated diagnostic procedures such as audiograms or videonystagmograms are performed.

4. **Neurologic examination.** An abbreviated neurologic examination is adequate, though should be expanded appropriately if abnormalities are discovered. It is usually convenient to check the vestibulo-ocular reflex (VOR) and nystagmus with the ophthalmoscope at this point (see **Sections B.5.a and B.6.b under Evaluation**).

5. **Nystagmus** indicates an inner ear, brain, or (rarely) an ocular muscle disorder. Evaluation of nystagmus optimally requires use of Frenzel's goggles, which are goggles worn by the patient to obscure their vision and magnify the examiner's view of their eyes. Of the two Frenzel's goggle variants available (optical and infrared video), the infrared video goggles are far superior. Without a method of viewing the eyes without fixation, almost all nystagmus procedures are either useless or very insensitive. If you use Frenzel's

TABLE 16.4 Examination Procedures for Dizziness and Vertigo

Procedures	Triggers for Additions
General examination	
Orthostasis	
Arrhythmia	
Balance assessment	
Observe gait	Parkinsonian gait
Eyes-closed tandem Romberg test	
Pulsion and retropulsion	
Otologic examination	
Hearing	
Tympanic membranes	
Neurologic examination	
Cranial nerves	
Long tract signs	
Cerebellar	Fails Romberg test
Position sense testing	
Nystagmus assessment	**("g" indicates that Frenzel's goggles is required)**
Spontaneous nystagmus (use ophthalmoscope if goggles are not available)	
Vibration test (g)	
Vertebral artery test (g)	Dizziness with neck discomfort
Dix–Hallpike positional test	
Head-shake test (g)	Negative exam so far
Valsalva's test (g)	Pressure sensitivity complex of symptoms
Hyperventilation (g)	Negative exam so far
VOR gain assessment	
Dynamic illegible "E" test	Fails Romberg test
Ophthalmoscope test	Fails "E" test
HIT	The presence of:
	• Spontaneous horizontal (±torsional) nystagmus
	• Horizontal nystagmus induced by head shaking or neck vibration
	• Positive dynamic illegible "E" test

Procedures in italics are always performed; procedures not in italics are performed only for certain symptom complexes.
Abbreviation: HIT, Head impulse test.

goggles, mention this in your report. If you do not, indicate in your report that Frenzel's goggles were not available.

a. **Spontaneous nystagmus.** With Frenzel's goggles placed on the patient, the eyes are observed for spontaneous nystagmus for 10 seconds. The typical nystagmus produced by inner ear dysfunction is a primary position "jerk" nystagmus—the eyes slowly deviate off center and then there is a rapid "jerk," which brings them back to the center position. Most nystagmus of other patterns (e.g., sinusoidal, gaze-evoked, saccadic) are of central origin. If Frenzel's goggles are not available, similar information about spontaneous nystagmus can be obtained from the ophthalmoscopic exam. One simply monitors movement of the back of the eye. As the back of the eye moves oppositely to the front of the eye, for horizontal and vertical movement, one must remember to invert the direction of the nystagmus when making notes. Fixation can be removed by covering the opposite eye. Inner ear nystagmus is increased by removal of fixation. Congenital nystagmus is often reduced by removal of fixation.

b. **Dix–Hallpike positional test (Fig. 16.1).** The patient is positioned on the examination table so that, on lying flat, the head extends over the end of the table. The patient is then moved rapidly to this "head-hanging" position. If no dizziness or nystagmus is appreciated after 20 seconds, the patient is sat back up. The head is then repositioned to 45 degrees right, and the patient is brought down to the head-right supine position. After another 20 seconds, the patient is sat up again, and the procedure is repeated to the left (head-left supine position). One hopes to see a burst of nystagmus provoked by either the head-right or the head-left position. The nystagmus of the most common type of BPPV (posterior canal) beats upward and has a rotatory component, such that the top part of the eye beats toward the undermost ear (Video 16.1). The nystagmus typically has a latency of 2 to 5 seconds, lasts 5 to 60 seconds, and is followed by a downbeat nystagmus when the patient is sat up. There are also variant BPPVs with different vectors. The lateral-canal variant of BPPV is associated with a strong horizontal nystagmus that reverses direction between head left and right (Video 16.2). The anterior canal variant is associated with a downbeating nystagmus elicited by the Dix–Hallpike. **The remainder of the nystagmus tests require video Frenzel's goggles.**

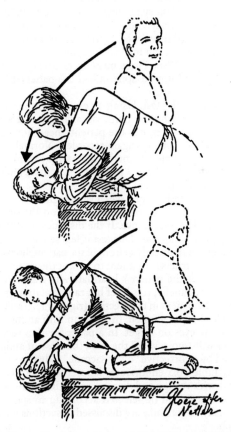

FIGURE 16.1 Dix–Hallpike positional test. To precipitate the characteristic nystagmus of BPPV, the patient is rapidly brought into a head position that makes the posterior canal vertical and also brings it through a large angular displacement. (From Baloh RW, Honrubia V. *Clinical Neurophysiology of the Vestibular System.* 2nd ed. Philadelphia, PA: FA Davis; 1990:124.)

c. Head-shake test. Performed if there is no spontaneous nystagmus or positional nystagmus. Wearing Frenzel's goggles, the patient's head is rotated by the examiner in the horizontal plane, back and forth, for 20 cycles. One aims for a 45 degree excursion of the head to either side and a frequency of 2 cycles per second. A nystagmus lasting 5 seconds or more is an indication of an organic disorder of the ear or CNS and supports further investigation.

d. Neck vibration test. The vibration test is more helpful than the head-shaking test. The eyes are observed in complete darkness while vibration (typically using a massager) is applied to the sternocleidomastoid for 10 seconds, first on one side and then on the other. A strong, direction-fixed nystagmus indicates a compensated peripheral vestibular lesion. The nystagmus beats away from the lesion.

e. Vertebral artery test for cervical vertigo. With the patient upright and wearing the goggles, the head is rotated to the end of rotation on either side and left there for 10 seconds. The eyes remain in the center. A positive test consists of a nystagmus provoked by the position of the head on trunk. Positives are very rare.

f. **Valsalva's test** is performed if there is a pressure sensitivity symptom complex on history (see section Differential Diagnosis). While wearing the goggles, the patient takes a deep breath and strains for 10 seconds, while being observed for nystagmus. A positive test consists of nystagmus at the onset and release of pressure.

g. **The hyperventilation test** is performed if so far the examination has been entirely normal. The patient takes 30 deep, hard breaths. Immediately after hyperventilation, the eyes are inspected for nystagmus with Frenzel's goggles and the patient is asked if the procedure has reproduced the symptoms. A positive test without nystagmus suggests the diagnosis of hyperventilation syndrome. Nystagmus induced by hyperventilation suggests a partially conducting eighth nerve or central vestibular pathways, such as due to a tumor of the eighth cranial nerve, gamma knife radiosurgery for acoustic neuroma, or MS.

6. Assessment of gain of the VOR. These maneuvers are aimed at documenting bilateral vestibular loss. They need not be done unless the patient has failed the eyes-closed tandem Romberg's test.

a. The dynamic illegible "E" test. Using an eye chart at a distance of at least 10 feet, preferably calibrated in LogMar units, visual acuity is recorded with the head still. Then the examiner gently moves the patient's head horizontally at roughly 1 Hz, ±30 degrees, and visual acuity is again recorded. Normal subjects drop from 0 to 2 lines of acuity with head movement. Patients with partial to complete bilateral loss of vestibular function drop from 3 to 7 lines of acuity. Patients with acute complete bilateral loss usually drop 7 lines of acuity.

b. The ophthalmoscope test is done when the illegible "E" test is positive, to obtain objective corroboration. The examiner focuses on the optic disk and then gently moves the head as described above. If the disk moves with the head, this confirms that the VOR gain is abnormal. This test is less sensitive than the illegible "E" test.

c. HIT. The examiner stands directly in front of the patient, holds the patient's head firmly on both sides, and instructs the patient to look at the examiner's nose. The examiner then abruptly rotates the patient's head laterally a small distance (approximately 10 degrees) but very rapidly; this brief but rapid rotation (the "impulse") should be unpredictable to the patient in its direction (right or left) and timing; several impulses toward each side should be tested. In a person with an intact vestibular system, the VOR will keep the eyes on target. In a patient with a recent unilateral vestibular deficit, the eyes will "move with" the head (because of an impaired VOR), and this will be followed by a corrective "overt saccade" to bring the eyes back to the target.

C. Laboratory studies. Table 16.5 enumerates laboratory procedures commonly used for evaluation of patients with vertigo and dizziness, with indications. For efficiency and cost containment, procedures should be selected according to specific symptom complexes and be done sequentially. Algorithms are discussed in sections Differential Diagnosis and Diagnostic Approach.

1. **Audiologic testing** is indicated when there are hearing complaints. If the diagnosis is uncertain audiometry is recommended even for patients who have no hearing abnormalities.

a. Audiogram. The audiogram measures hearing. Abnormalities suggest otologic vertigo.

b. **Otoacoustic emissions (OAEs)** measure sounds generated by the ear itself. This is a quick and simple automated procedure. OAEs are useful in detecting

TABLE 16.5 Laboratory Procedures for Dizziness and Vertigo

Test	Indication
Audiologic tests	
Audiogram	Vertigo, hearing symptoms
OAEs	Hearing symptoms, secondary gain
ECOG	Secondary test for Ménière's disease
Vestibular tests	
VEMP	Vertigo
VNG	Vertigo
Rotatory chair test	Bilateral loss, secondary to confirm VNG
Posturography	Secondary gain
Blood tests	
FTA-ABS	Vertigo with hearing symptoms
Glycosylated hemoglobin	Hydrops symptom complex
ANA	Hydrops symptom complex
TSH	Hydrops symptom complex
Lyme serology	Vertigo in person from endemic area
Radiologic tests	
MRI of head	Central vertigo, abnormal BAER
MRA, VB	TIA
CT scan of temporal bone	Pressure sensitivity or Tullio's sign with asymmetrical VEMP, mastoiditis, congenital abnormality, significant head trauma
Other tests	
EEG	Quick spins, head trauma
Ambulatory event monitoring (Holter monitoring)	Cardiogenic syncope
Tilt table test	Syncope
VHIT	• Suspicion for unilateral or bilateral vestibular loss • VNG and rotatory chair are inconsistent or unavailable

Abbreviations: CT, computed tomography; ECOG, electrocochleography; EEG, electroencephalograph; FTA-ABS, fluorescent treponemal antibody absorption test; MRA, magnetic resonance angiography; MRI, magnetic resonance imaging; OAEs, otoacoustic emissions; TIA, transient ischemic attack; TSH, thyroid-stimulating hormone; VB, vertebrobasilar; VEMP, vestibular evoked myogenic potential; VHIT, video head impulse test; VNG, videonystagmography.

malingering, central hearing deficits, and persons with auditory neuropathy. In these situations, OAEs may be preserved even when subjective hearing is poor. When there is a potential for malingering, audiologists have at their disposal a large assortment of objective hearing tests that can generally detect psychogenic hearing loss. OAEs are usually not helpful in persons older than 60 years old, as OAEs are reduced with age.

c. **Electrocochleography (ECOG)** is an evoked potential in which the recording electrode is positioned on the ear drum. It requires that a patient have no worse than mild to moderate high-frequency hearing loss in the ear being assessed. An abnormal ECOG is suggestive of Ménière's disease. ECOGs are difficult to perform and should not be relied upon for diagnosis by themselves.

2. **Vestibular testing** is not needed for every dizzy patient. The primary study—videonystagmography (VNG) or electronystagmography (ENG) test—is helpful when there is no clear diagnosis after history and examination.

a. **VNG/ENG** is a battery of procedures that can identify vestibular asymmetry (such as that caused by vestibular neuritis) and document spontaneous or positional nystagmus (such as that caused by BPPV). It is a long and difficult test, with little standardization, and an abnormal result that does not fit the clinical picture should be confirmed by rotatory chair testing, ideally in combination with VEMP testing.

b. **VEMP testing** is sensitive to SSCD syndrome, bilateral vestibular loss, and acoustic neuroma. VEMPs are generally normal in vestibular neuritis and Ménière's disease.

c. **Rotatory chair** testing measures vestibular function of both inner ears together. It is highly sensitive and specific for bilateral loss of vestibular function. In unilateral loss, it is sensitive but nonspecific. Also, it does not identify the side of the lesion.

d. Video head impulse test (VHIT). This new vestibular test can quickly diagnose both bilateral vestibular loss and complete unilateral vestibular loss. It can also quantify vestibular compensation and has utility in following progress of persons undergoing treatment.

e. **Posturography** is an instrumented Romberg test. It is very useful in documenting inconsistency (that may be suggestive of malingering) and may also have utility in following the progress of persons undergoing treatment.

3. **Blood tests** are triggered by specific symptom complexes (see section Differential Diagnosis), and there is no "routine" set obtained for every dizzy patient. In particular, chemistry panels, CBCs, glucose tolerance tests, vitamin B_{12} levels, and allergy tests need not be routinely ordered.

4. Radiologic investigations. Skull films, cervical spine films, CT scans of the head, and CT scans of the sinuses are not recommended routinely in the evaluation of vertigo.

a. **MRI scan of the brain** evaluates the structural integrity of the brainstem, cerebellum, periventricular white matter, and eighth-nerve complexes. Coronal high-resolution MRI can also suggest evaluation is needed for SSCD. MRI is not routinely needed to evaluate vertigo without other accompanying neurologic findings (Chapter 32).

b. **CT scan of the temporal bone** provides higher resolution of ear structures than MRI and also is better for evaluating lesions involving bone (see Chapter 32). Temporal bone CT is required to diagnose SSCD. The "high-resolution direct coronal" variant of this scan is best suited for this diagnosis. The temporal bone CT scan involves considerable radiation and for this reason VEMP testing is recommended as an initial screening test for SSCD.

5. Other tests.

a. **Electroencephalography (EEG)** is used to diagnose seizures. Yield is very low in dizzy patients (Chapter 33).

b. **Ambulatory event monitoring, or Holter monitoring**, is used to detect arrhythmia or sinus arrest. Yield is high in persons with episodic orthostatic symptoms, lacking orthostatic hypotension.

c. **Tilt table testing** is sometimes advocated for the diagnosis of neurocardiogenic syncope. When abnormal, treatment should focus on maintenance of blood pressure.

DIFFERENTIAL DIAGNOSIS

We will now discuss symptom complexes, their differential diagnosis, and algorithms used to narrow the differential. Table 16.6 enumerates five specific symptom complexes. When a patient does not fit into a complex in Table 16.6, one may fall back to grouping patients by duration of symptoms only, as in Table 16.7.

A. Approach based on specific symptom complexes.

1. Positional syndromes. Patients complain of a brief burst of rotatory vertigo when getting into or out of bed, or on rolling over from one side to the other. This symptom strongly suggests the diagnosis of BPPV.

a. BPPV. If a typical nystagmus is observed on Dix–Hallpike positional testing, no other diagnoses need to be considered. Because roughly 95% of all positional nystagmus is caused by BPPV, even in cases in which an atypical positional nystagmus is observed, it is usually most efficient to try one of the currently available treatments before considering other diagnoses. Brain MRI is indicated when an atypical BPPV is refractory to treatment.

b. Central disorders. Strong positional nystagmus may also accompany brainstem and cerebellar disorders (e.g., medulloblastoma and the Chiari malformation). Brain MRI is indicated when positional nystagmus is combined with an abnormal neurologic examination or when an atypical BPPV is refractory to treatment.

TABLE 16.6 Specific Symptom Complexes

Positional vertigo
BPPV
Central vertigo
Vestibular neuritis
Postural hypotension
Headaches and vertigo
Basilar migraine
Posttraumatic vertigo
Chiari malformation
Unlocalized vertigo
Hydrops symptom complex (fluctuating hearing loss, vertigo, tinnitus, and ear fullness)
Ménière's disease
PLF
Posttraumatic hydrops
Syphilis
Pressure sensitivity symptom complex
SSCD
PLF
Ménière's disease
Chiari malformation
Stapes malformation or prosthesis
Medicolegal situations
Malingering and disability evaluations

Abbreviations: BPPV, benign paroxysmal positional vertigo; PLF, Perilymph fistula; SSCD, superior semicircular canal dehiscence.

    c. **Vestibular neuritis.** A weak horizontal positional nystagmus may be found in peripheral vestibulopathies. VNG, VHIT, and audiogram are indicated.

    d. **Postural hypotension** also presents with dizziness on getting out of bed, but never occurs in bed. It is diagnosed by a symptomatic decrease in blood pressure between the supine and standing positions. Drops of 20 mm Hg in systolic blood pressure are significant.

2. **Headaches and vertigo.**

    a. **Migraine.** A large group of patients includes women having headaches in their 30s or 50s as these are high-prevalence times for migraine. Food triggers, motion sickness, and positive family history are frequent associations. There is a weak association between BPPV and migraine, and the diagnosis of migraine-associated vertigo should prompt consideration of BPPV. Symptomatic improvement in response to empirical trials of migraine prophylaxis medication supports the diagnosis.

    b. **Posttraumatic vertigo.** Audiometry, VNG, and CT scan of the head are indicated.

    c. **Chiari malformation.** The headache is occipital, and there is downbeat nystagmus and ataxia. Diagnosis is from sagittal T1-MRI of the brain.

    d. **Unlocalized vertigo.** Audiometry and VNG are indicated for the vertigo component. The headache component (tension, migraine, sinus, and so on) is considered separately.

3. **Hydrops.** Patients complain of spells of vertigo, roaring tinnitus, and transient hearing loss, preceded by aural fullness. Audiometry should be obtained in all patients, as well as RPR (rapid plasma reagent), fluorescent treponemal antibody absorption test (FTA-ABS), sedimentation rate, and thyroid-stimulating hormone (TSH) blood tests.

    a. **Ménière's disease.** Usual duration of vertigo is 2 hours, but it can vary from seconds to weeks. Audiometry is crucial to document the fluctuating low-tone sensorineural hearing loss (Fig. 16.2). The diagnosis of Ménière's disease is highly probable when a typical

TABLE 16.7 Typical Duration of Selected Conditions Causing Dizziness

One to three seconds (quick spins)

Vestibular nerve irritation
BPPV variants
Ménière's disease variants
Epilepsy

Less than 1 minute

BPPV
Cardiac arrhythmia
Ménière's disease variants

Minutes to hours

VB TIA
Ménière's disease
Panic attacks, situational anxiety, hyperventilation
Orthostasis

Hours to days

Ménière's disease
Basilar migraine

Two weeks or more

Vestibular neuritis and labyrinthitis
Central vertigo with structural lesion
Anxiety
Malingering
Bilateral vestibular paresis or loss
Multisensory disequilibrium of the elderly
Drug intoxications

Abbreviations: BPPV, benign paroxysmal positional vertigo; TIA, transient ischemic attack; VB, vertebrobasilar.

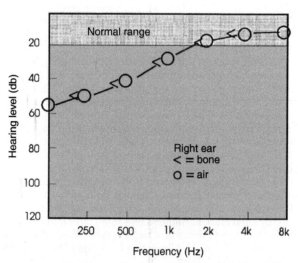

FIGURE 16.2 Low-tone hearing loss. A unilateral low-frequency sensorineural pattern hearing loss is often observed in early Ménière's disease.

history is obtained and when a fluctuating hearing loss (often in the low frequencies) is documented. ECOG testing may be performed in difficult cases, in an attempt to "rule in" the diagnosis. About 10% of all cases of bilateral Ménière's disease are autoimmune. Thyroid disease and/or migraine are very frequent in patients with Ménière's disease. Migraine is a comorbidity in about 50% of patients with Ménière's disease.

b. **Perilymph fistula (PLF).** Occasionally, fistula presents with hydrops rather than the pressure sensitivity symptom complex (see **Section A.4 under Differential Diagnosis**). The only clue may be a history of barotrauma.

c. **Posttraumatic hydrops** is a variant of the Ménière's disease symptom complex that appears after a significant blow to the ear, with presumed bleeding into the inner ear. It is very rare.

d. **Syphilis.** Hearing loss is bilateral. Diagnosis is by rapid plasma reagent followed by FTA-ABS.

4. **Pressure sensitivity.** Patients complain of dizziness or ataxia evoked by nose blowing, high-speed elevators, cleaning of the ear with a cotton swab, straining as at stool, after the landing of an airplane, or after diving. In addition to pressure sensitivity, patients report vertigo induced by loud noises (Tullio's phenomenon) and by exercise. Patients are often extremely motion-intolerant and visually sensitive. Audiometry and the VEMP test are indicated.

a. **SSCD** syndrome is the main source of pressure sensitivity. Vertigo and nystagmus can be provoked by loud noise or pressure. This syndrome is caused by dehiscence of bone overlying the superior semicircular canal. VEMP testing is nearly always abnormal because of both asymmetry and a low threshold on the dehiscent side. Diagnosis is confirmed by a high-resolution CT scan of the temporal bone.

b. **PLF.** Most patients have a history of barotrauma in they were unable to "clear" their ear during scuba diving or airplane travel. Audiometry and ECOG are indicated. A trial of a "ventilation" tube in the suspect ear is often helpful.

c. **Ménière's disease.** Mild pressure sensitivity occurs in about one-third of patients with Ménière's disease. See the hydrops symptom complex description (see **Section A.3 under Differential Diagnosis**) for a differential diagnosis.

d. **Chiari malformation and platybasia.** Vertigo is correlated with straining but not with pressure in the external ear canal. The downbeat nystagmus and abnormal MRI found in the Chiari malformation also separate it from the other entities.

e. **Stapes malformation.** Remarkable pressure sensitivity with torsional movement of the eye occurs in patients in whom stapes prostheses (for otosclerosis) of excessive length have been inserted, or migrated into the inner ear. A high-resolution CT scan of the temporal bone is indicated in this situation.

5. **Medicolegal situations.** The possibility of malingering often comes up in disability evaluations, worker's compensation cases, and legal situations where patients may potentially be compensated for being vertiginous. These patients usually present no objective evidence on physical examination or testing. Often they resist examination, by closing or crossing their eyes at inappropriate times or by refusing to perform key positional maneuvers. Their complaints often cannot be resolved into one of the symptom complexes discussed above. Objective testing (audiometry, OAE, VNG, VEMP, VHIT and/or rotatory chair, and an MRI scan of the head) is nearly always appropriate. In addition, posturography may be helpful. This test can help detect the malingering patient by assessing balance in a series of test conditions of graded difficulty, but presenting those conditions in a random order. The malingerer who is trying to fail the posturography test will frequently perform equally poorly on the easy and difficult subtests, producing a pattern that is neither normal nor typical of vestibular deficits.

B. **Approach based on timing only.** These categories (Table 16.7) are less useful for diagnosis than those based on symptom complexes, but can be used when patients do not fall into any category.

1. **Quick spins are brief spells (1 to 3 seconds) of true vertigo,** unaccompanied by secondary symptoms. EEG should be obtained. A trial of oxcarbazepine may be helpful.

a. **Vestibular nerve irritation** due to the microvascular compression syndrome or a residual from vestibular neuritis. Spells are very brief (often just a fraction of a second) but can be extremely frequent (such as 50 per day). Hyperventilation may induce nystagmus seen with video Frenzel's goggles. Magnetic resonance angiography (MRA) occasionally documents compression of the brainstem by the vertebrobasilar arterial system, but there are many false positives. If the EEG is normal, a good response to oxcarbazepine confirms the diagnosis.

b. **Ménière's disease variants.** Patients complain of "shocks" or "earthquake" sensations. Frequency of spells is daily at most. Hearing is often affected. For diagnosis, see hydrops symptom complex (see **Section A.3 under Differential Diagnosis**).

c. **BPPV variants.** Spells are of no more than daily frequency. Presumably, otoconial debris are caught on a canal wall and suddenly slip down. Diagnosis is by the Dix–Hallpike maneuver. It may take several visits to get a positive result.

d. **Epilepsy.** Spells can be frequent, and there is often a history of head injury. Cognitive impairment is frequent during the dizzy spell.

2. **Less than 1 minute.** These are mainly postural syndromes.

a. **Classic BPPV.** If there is a history of positional vertigo, this diagnosis is easy. However, poor "historians" may omit to mention that they have adopted sleeping strategies (e.g., two pillows) by which bed spins are avoided. BPPV can also be triggered by unusual head positions such as looking up at the "top shelf." Diagnosis is by the Dix–Hallpike maneuver.

b. **Cardiac arrhythmia.** The clue is usually that vertigo spells occur mainly while standing, and that lightheadedness is a more prominent symptom than spinning. Ambulatory event monitoring is the best method of documenting this problem. Holter monitoring may be used in contexts where event monitoring is not available.

c. **Ménière's disease variants.** See **Section B.1.c under Differential Diagnosis**.

3. **Minutes to hours.**

a. **TIA.** Spells of pure vertigo lasting 2 to 30 minutes, of abrupt onset and offset, in a patient with significant vascular risk factors are diagnosed as VB TIA until proven otherwise. Suspicion is reduced if there is a positional trigger. MR angiography (MRA) and CT angiography (CTA) of the VB circulation are the most useful tests.

b. **Ménière's disease.** The typical Ménière's attack lasts 2 hours. If there are hearing symptoms, see the hydrops symptom complex (see **Section A.3 under Differential Diagnosis**). If not, be cautious about proposing this diagnosis. Sometimes the term "vestibular Ménière's disease" is used to denote episodic vertigo having the typical timing of classic Ménière's disease but without any ear symptomatology. It is presently unclear whether this entity exists, and there is no method of confirming this diagnosis.

c. **Panic attacks**, situational anxiety, and hyperventilation may produce symptoms of this duration (minutes to hours). These patients ordinarily are not symptomatic during examination. A detailed history is the most useful diagnostic test. If hyperventilation reproduces symptoms in patients without other findings, the diagnosis is hyperventilation syndrome. If hyperventilation also induces nystagmus, MRI is indicated.

d. **Cardiac arrhythmia and orthostasis.** See Etiology C1, C2 and Evaluation, C5c.

4. **Hours to days.**

a. **Ménière's disease.**

b. **Migraine.** Migraine is so common in the general population that even unusual variants, such as manifestation solely as a vertiginous aura or intractable motion sensitivity with nausea, are relatively common. Diagnosis is suggested by age, female gender, positive family history, attacks provoked by usual migraine triggers, and sensitivity to multiple sensory triggers (e.g., light, sound, motion).

5. **Two weeks or more.**

a. **Vestibular neuritis.** Diagnosis is made by combining a long duration of symptoms, typically more than a week, with spontaneous nystagmus or an abnormal VNG or VHIT test. The VNG should document nystagmus or a significant vestibular paresis (a conservative criterion is a paresis of 40% or more). The VHIT test should be positive for a unilateral weakness. The VEMP test should be normal. After 2 months of vertigo, central vertigo becomes more likely and an MRI is indicated. For labyrinthitis, the diagnosis is made by combining the vestibular neuritis pattern with hearing symptoms. Audiometry, erythrocyte sedimentation rate, and fasting glucose are indicated in addition to the vestibular neuritis battery.

b. **Central vertigo with a fixed structural CNS lesion.** This diagnosis should be considered when there are neurologic symptoms or signs accompanying vertigo. Central vertigo may be permanent. For example, the combination of a peripheral vestibular loss with a cerebellar lesion may occur after acoustic neuroma surgery. Nevertheless, acoustic neuromas are extremely uncommon sources of peripheral or central vertigo owing to their rarity compared with disorders such as BPPV. MRI is the most effective method of diagnosis of central vertigo. There are no examination maneuvers that can always separate peripheral vertigo (such as due to vestibular neuritis) from a central vertigo that lacks any "central signs."

c. **Anxiety.** With this duration of symptoms (2 weeks or more), patients may be complaining of vertigo in your office. If a patient is presently complaining of vertigo, but no spontaneous nystagmus is evident under Frenzel's goggles, if they are not taking vestibular suppressants, one may reasonably conclude that the vertigo is functional in origin. Patients with anxiety typically report that nearly every trigger factor in Table 16.4 exacerbate their symptoms. Interestingly, whereas most patients with inner ear problems report that stress makes their symptoms worse, patients with anxiety frequently claim that everything except stress triggers vertigo. A positive response to a trial of a benzodiazepine supports this diagnosis but does not establish it because many organic vestibular disorders also respond well to these medications.

d. **Malingering.** Malingerers persist in reporting symptoms as long as necessary to accomplish their purpose of obtaining favorable court settlements or disability rulings. Posturography and neuropsychological testing is usually very abnormal. Objective tests of vestibular function such as VHIT, VEMP, and VNG are nearly always normal. Tests that are more vulnerable to lack of cooperation such as rotatory chair tests are variable.

e. **Bilateral vestibular paresis or loss.** These patients fail the dynamic illegible "E" test and the eyes-closed tandem Romberg's test. Their ataxia is worse in the dark. On audiometry, hearing is usually normal. Rotatory chair testing or VHIT testing is the best way to confirm this diagnostic impression.

f. **Multisensory disequilibrium** of the elderly is essentially an unlocalized ataxia in an elderly patient. If the diagnosis is accurate, this is usually a permanent condition.

g. **Drug intoxications.** Diagnosis depends on a positive response to withdrawal of medications.

DIAGNOSTIC APPROACH

A. Perform history and examination as outlined in sections Clinical Manifestations and Evaluation.

B. Approximately 20% to 40% of patients are diagnosed immediately on examination.
1. BPPV patients on Dix–Hallpike maneuver (15% to 20% of vertigo population).
2. Orthostatic hypotension and fixed cardiac arrhythmia such as atrial fibrillation (2% to 5%).
3. Bilateral vestibular paresis or loss on dynamic illegible "E" test (5%).
4. SSCD with positive Valsalva's test (0% to 2%).
5. Acute vestibular neuritis via spontaneous nystagmus and positive HIT test (2% to 5%).

C. For the remaining patients, proceed as follows:
1. If patient fits into a symptom complex category, follow procedures presented in Section A under Differential Diagnosis.
2. If patient does not fit into a symptom complex, follow procedures outlined in Section B under Differential Diagnosis.
   a. If symptoms are intermittent, follow procedures in **Sections B.1 to B.3 under Differential Diagnosis.**
   b. Otherwise, if symptoms are constant, proceed as follows:
      (1) If duration has been <2 weeks, treat symptomatically or simply reassure and have patient return if symptoms persist beyond 2 weeks.
      (2) If duration has been >2 weeks, follow the procedures outlined in **Section B under Differential Diagnosis.**

REFERRALS

A. Otology.
  1. Cerumen disimpaction and ear microscope examination. Ear wax can be safely removed with the examining microscope, a standard piece of otologic equipment.
  2. Progressive or acute hearing loss has potential medicolegal ramifications, and otologic consultation is often helpful.
  3. A perforated tympanic membrane or mass in the canal or behind the tympanic membrane may require otologic referral for closure of the perforation or surgical management of the tumor.
  4. Mastoiditis or chronic otitis media. These patients are commonly managed with a mixture of surgery, cleaning, antibiotics, and antiseptics that requires otologic supervision.
  5. Surgical management of acoustic neuroma, Ménière's disease, fistula, SSCD, and cholesteatoma. Surgical treatment for Ménière's disease has greatly improved in recent years because of greater use of low-dose gentamicin protocols.
B. Internal medicine.
  1. Cardiac or blood pressure problems, especially arrhythmia.
  2. Management of diabetes or thyroid dysfunction.
C. Psychiatry.
  1. Patients with disabling anxiety or panic disorders.
D. Neuropsychology.
  2. Patients who may be malingering.
E. Vestibular rehabilitation (physical therapy).
  1. Treatment for BPPV, bilateral loss, and refractory vestibular neuritis.
  2. Video Frenzel's goggle exam (if examiner does not have this critical piece of equipment).

Key Points

- Dizziness can be broadly categorized as otologic (common causes: BPPV and vestibular neuritis), central (common causes: migraine-associated vertigo), medical (common causes include postural hypotension, adverse effects of medication), and unlocalized (including posttraumatic and psychogenic).
- The most common causes of dizziness in adults include BPPV, migraine-associated vertigo, and vestibular neuritis. The most common cause of dizziness in children is migraine-associated vertigo.
- Aside from the history, general, otologic, and neurologic examinations, the differential diagnosis often relies crucially on clinical examination of eye movements, sometimes supplemented by otologic testing (such as an audiogram) and vestibular testing (such as VEMPs, VNG, and rotatory chair testing).
- Bedside examination maneuvers with high yield include observation for spontaneous unidirectional nystagmus (suggesting vestibular neuritis) and the Dix–Hallpike maneuver (to diagnose posterior canal BPPV).
- Imaging may be helpful in cases where screening otologic and vestibular workups are unrevealing, where specific neuroanatomical abnormalities are suspected (such as Chiari malformation), where medicolegal factors are involved, or when malingering is suspected. Suspicion of acoustic neuroma or congenital inner ear abnormalities warrants MRI of the brain and internal auditory canals without and with contrast. In cases where SSCD is suspected, or where there has been significant head trauma, a temporal bone CT without contrast is appropriate.

Recommended Readings

Baloh RW. *Dizziness, Hearing Loss, and Tinnitus*. New York, NY: Oxford University Press; 1998.

Baloh RW, Halmagyi GM, eds. *Disorders of the Vestibular System*. New York, NY: Oxford University Press; 1996.

Brandt T. Cervical vertigo—reality or fiction? *Audiol Neurootol*. 1996;1(4):187–196.

Drachman D, Hart CW. An approach to the dizzy patient. *Neurology*. 1972;22:323–334.

Fisher CM. Vertigo in cerebrovascular disease. *Arch Otolaryngol*. 1967;85:85–90.

Herr RD, Zun L, Mathews JJ. A directed approach to the dizzy patient. *Ann Emerg Med*. 1989;18:664–672.

Minor LB. Superior canal dehiscence syndrome. *Am J Otol*. 2000;21:9–19.

Nedzelski JM, Barber HO, McIlmoyl L. Diagnoses in a dizziness unit. *J Otolaryngol*. 1986;15:101–104.

Sloane PD. Dizziness in primary care: results from the National Ambulatory Medical Care Survey. *J Fam Pract*. 1989;29:33–38.

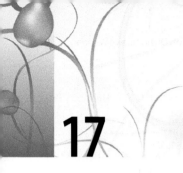

17 Approach to the Patient with Hearing Loss

Richard T. Miyamoto and Marcia J. Hay-McCutcheon

Hearing loss affects almost 17 in 1,000 children under the age of 18 and approximately 314 in 1,000 adults over the age of 65. It has been estimated that 28 million Americans have a hearing impairment. Hearing loss produces substantial communication problems and can be the presenting symptom of serious underlying medical disorders. A detailed medical and audiologic evaluation is required to establish a specific etiology and management plan.

ETIOLOGY

There are various and often complex causes of hearing loss. In many cases, particularly among children, the cause of the hearing loss may remain unknown or idiopathic even after an extensive medical and audiologic workup.

A. Despite the diversity of patients and their presenting symptoms, the causes of hearing loss can be classified as **hereditary** or **acquired.** Occasionally, there is not a clear distinction between the two types. For example, there is a genetic predisposition for certain populations to be more susceptible to noise-induced hearing loss.

B. The **onset** of hearing loss is a useful indicator when describing the cause. Hearing loss is considered **congenital** when it was caused before birth, **perinatal** when the hearing loss occurs during birth or shortly thereafter, and **postnatal** when the onset of the hearing loss occurs more than a month after birth.

C. **Nonorganic** hearing loss may occur in children and adults, and its prevalence varies depending on the clinical situation.

ANATOMY AND PHYSIOLOGY OF THE AUDITORY SYSTEM

The auditory system is divided into four anatomical regions: (1) the external ear, (2) the middle ear, (3) the inner ear, and (4) the central auditory pathway.

A. **External ear.** The external ear consists of the pinna and the external auditory canal. It collects and directs sound to the tympanic membrane. Because of its physical dimensions, the external ear provides an important resonance boost between 2,000 and 5,000 Hz, a frequency range that contributes to the perception of speech.

B. **Middle ear.** The middle ear consists of the tympanic membrane, three ossicles (malleus, incus, and stapes), two middle ear muscles (tensor tympani and stapedius), and the ligaments that suspend the ossicles in the middle ear cavity. The middle ear structures transmit acoustic energy from the external environment to the inner ear and serve as a mechanical transformer recovering energy that would otherwise be lost as sound is transmitted from a gaseous medium (air) to a liquid medium (endolymph). The middle ear structures compensate for this impedance mismatch between the air and liquid mediums. Specifically, the difference in the areal ratio between the relatively large tympanic membrane and the small oval window recovers a substantial portion of the energy lost. Additionally, energy is recovered through the lever action of the handle of the malleus; that is, the handle is slightly longer than the long process of the incus.

C. **Inner ear.** The inner ear is divided into the **vestibular portion** consisting of three semicircular canals as well as the utricle and saccule, and the **auditory portion** consisting of the cochlea. The semicircular canals provide information regarding angular acceleration, and the utricle and saccule provide information regarding gravitational or linear acceleration. The vestibular system, coupled with the visual and proprioceptive systems, functions as the body's balance mechanism. The cochlea is the end organ of hearing and is a shell-shaped cavity placed within the bony labyrinth. This fluid-filled structure is divided into three sections via the basilar membrane and Riessner's membrane. These sections are the **scala vestibuli,** the **scala media** (housing the hair cells), and the **scala tympani.** With the displacement of the stapes, a wave of motion (i.e., **traveling wave**) moves up the basilar membrane, resulting in displacement of the one row of inner hair cells and three rows of outer hair cells. Sitting on the top of the hair cells are tiny cells referred to as **stereocilia,** which make direct contact with the **tectorial membrane,** a structure directly above the hair cells. The shearing action of the stereocilia on the tectorial membrane results in the stimulation of the hair cells. This motion causes the opening and closing of channels, which allows ions to flow into and out of the hair cells, thereby beginning the neural transduction process. The stiffness and mass characteristics of the basilar membrane vary along its length, and, therefore, the traveling wave envelope will reach a peak at different locations. This location corresponds to a specific frequency region equivalent to the frequency of the auditory stimulus. Thus, the inner ear acts as a **low-pass filter,** with high-frequency sounds encoded at the basal region of the cochlea and low-frequency sounds encoded at the apical region of the cochlea. This **tonotopic arrangement** is maintained throughout the central auditory system.

D. Central auditory system. The central auditory system consists of the auditory portion of the eighth cranial nerve, the cochlear nucleus, the trapezoid body, the superior olivary complex, the lateral lemniscus, the inferior colliculus, the medial geniculate body of the thalamus, and finally the auditory cortex. The level of neural complexity increases exponentially with each higher-order neuron or central auditory nucleus.

MEDICAL EVALUATION

Evaluation of the auditory system is accomplished by obtaining a detailed history, performing a physical examination, and conducting audiologic tests. In selected cases, radiologic imaging may be indicated.

A. History. The otologic history includes inquiry into symptoms of ear disease, including hearing loss, ear pain (otalgia), discharge from the ear (otorrhea), tinnitus or other head noises, and vertigo or dizziness (Video 17.1). If any of these symptoms are present, a detailed characterization is performed. The clinical significance of hearing loss is related to the time and acuity of onset, severity, and the tendency to fluctuate or progress. The deleterious effects of hearing loss are particularly great when the onset occurs before the development of spoken language (i.e., prelingual hearing loss).

B. Physical examination.
1. The **otologic examination** begins with inspection of the pinna and palpation of periauricular structures, including the periauricular and parotid lymph nodes.
2. **Otoscopic examination** of the external ear canal and tympanic membranes is performed to identify abnormalities of these structures. Pneumatic otoscopy is helpful in assessing the mobility of the tympanic membrane and is particularly useful in identifying a subtle middle ear effusion.
3. A complete **head and neck examination** is performed, including a cranial nerve and cerebellar testing.
4. **Tuning fork tests** are an important part of the otologic functional examination for hearing acuity. They are particularly useful in differentiation between conductive and sensorineural hearing loss. The most useful tuning forks are those with vibrating frequencies of 512 and 1,024 cycles per second. The two most commonly used tuning fork tests are **Weber's test** and **Rinne's test.**
   a. **Weber's test** is performed by placing the stem of the tuning fork on the midline plane of the skull. The patient is asked to identify the location of the auditory percept within the head. The signal lateralizes to the ear with conductive hearing loss provided normal hearing is present in the opposite ear. This occurs because the ambient room noise present in the usual testing situation tends to mask the normal ear, but the poorer ear with a conductive loss does not hear such noise and better hears bone-conducted sound. If a sensorineural loss is present in one ear and the opposite ear is normal, the fork is heard louder in the better ear.

b. **Rinne's test** is performed by alternately placing a ringing tuning fork opposite one external auditory meatus and firmly on the adjacent mastoid bone. The loudness of the tuning fork in these two locations is compared. The normal ear hears a tuning fork about twice as long with air conduction as with bone conduction. Conductive hearing loss reverses this ratio, and sound is heard longer with bone conduction than with air conduction. Patients with sensorineural hearing loss hear better by means of air conduction than by means of bone conduction, although hearing is reduced with both air and bone conduction.

AUDIOLOGIC EVALUATION

The audiologic evaluation characterizes the type, severity, and configuration of a hearing loss. Loss of hearing can be either partial or total. It can affect the low, middle, or high frequencies in any combination.

A. Range of hearing. Although the human ear is sensitive to frequencies between 20 and 20,000 Hz, the frequency range from 300 to 3,000 Hz is most important for understanding speech.

1. During an audiologic evaluation, pure-tone thresholds are routinely obtained for frequencies at octave intervals between 250 and 8,000 Hz.

2. The range of sound pressure to which the human ear responds is immense. Infinitesimal movement of the hair cells produces a just audible sound, yet a million-fold increase is still tolerable.

3. The large range of numbers needed to describe audible sound pressure is best represented by a logarithmic ratio comparing a sound to a standard reference sound. This is called the decibel. The decibel is defined in relation to the physical reference of sound, or sound pressure level, to the average threshold of normal hearing for young adults, or hearing level (HL), or to a patient's own threshold for the sound stimulus, or sensation level.

4. Speech sounds vary in their acoustic characteristics. Vowels tend to have most of their energy in the low to middle frequencies and are produced at relatively higher intensities than consonants. Thus, vowels carry the power of speech. Consonants tend to contain higher-frequency information and have low power. Much of the actual understanding of speech depends on the correct perception of consonants. Consequently, speech may not be audible for patients with hearing loss across the entire frequency range. Patients with hearing loss in the higher frequencies may hear speech but not understand it.

B. Audiogram. To graphically represent the degree of hearing, pure-tone thresholds are displayed on an audiogram (Fig. 17.1). On this graph, **frequency** (pitch) is represented on the horizontal axis and **intensity** (loudness) is presented on the vertical axis. The 0 dB HL line represents the average threshold level for a group of normal-hearing young adults with no history of otologic disease or noise exposure. Conversational speech at a distance of 1 m has an intensity level of approximately 50 to 60 dB HL. Speech becomes uncomfortable to listen to at approximately 80 to 90 dB HL.

C. Pure-tone threshold audiometry. The audiometric threshold is defined as the softest intensity level of a pure-tone signal that can be detected by the patient 50% of the time. Thresholds are generally obtained for air-conduction stimuli presented through earphones or in a sound field, and for bone-conduction stimuli presented with a vibrator placed on the mastoid or forehead.

For adults and older children, pure-tone testing simply requires a behavioral response to pure-tone stimulation. For infants older than 5 months, **visual reinforcement audiometry** can be used to obtain thresholds. In this operant discrimination task (i.e., yes–no paradigm), infants are trained to turn to their right or left when they hear a signal, where they see an illuminated animated toy. Alternatively, **play audiometry** is used to assess the hearing of preschool children. In this technique, play activities are used as operant reinforcers for a child's response to auditory signals.

The **degree of hearing loss** is classified in terms of audiometric thresholds and are slight (16 to 25 dB HL), mild (26 to 40 dB HL), moderate (41 to 55 dB HL), moderately severe (56 to 70 dB HL), severe (71 to 90 dB HL), and profound (>90 dB HL).

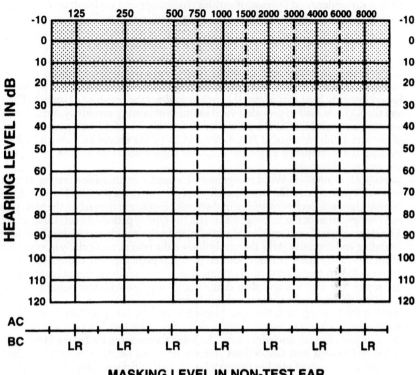

FIGURE 17.1 A sample audiogram. The y-axis represents the intensity level in dB HL and the x-axis represents the pure-tone frequency of the stimulus. The threshold is the softest level that the patient hears the pure-tone signal 50% of the time.

D. **Speech audiometry.** Speech signals can be used to assess hearing sensitivity and the processing capabilities of the auditory system. For some patients, speech can be audible but not easily understood because of various physiologic and environmental factors. The following tests are designed to assess both the audibility and intelligibility of speech.

1. **Speech threshold tests.** A speech recognition threshold (SRT) and a speech awareness threshold (SAT) are used to examine sensitivity to speech. These tests can be obtained for each ear individually or for both ears via sound field testing. The SRT is obtained at the lowest intensity level at which the patient can *repeat* spondee words (i.e., two-syllable words with equal stress on each syllable) 50% of the time. The SAT is the lowest intensity level that allows the patient to *detect* the presence of speech. The SRT and the SAT are used to provide a valid estimate of hearing sensitivity and to verify the accuracy and reliability of the pure-tone thresholds. The SRT and pure-tone average of the thresholds obtained at 500, 1,000, and 2,000 Hz should be within ±7 dB of one another. If a discrepancy exists, the examiner should doubt the validity or accuracy of the patient's thresholds.

2. **Speech discrimination.** Word recognition or speech discrimination testing determines how well a patient can understand speech when the stimuli are presented at suprathreshold intensity levels. Speech recognition or discrimination scores depend on the type, severity, and configuration of the hearing loss and on the type of pathologic condition of the ear. The scores depend on a number of stimulus and response characteristics. The patient's attending and cognitive skills also can influence the results, particularly in examinations of children and elderly persons. Although several pathologic conditions can markedly decrease speech recognition or discrimination scores, a rollover phenomenon in which the scores first increase and then dramatically decrease with increasing presentation levels is a characteristic of retrocochlear lesions.

E. **Screening for hearing loss.** Because hearing is critical for speech and oral language development in children, early identification of hearing loss is a primary concern for health care professionals and educators. The **Joint Committee on Infant Hearing 2007 Position Statement and Guidelines** endorse universal hearing screening of newborn infants before 1 month of age. For infants who fail their initial screening, it is recommended that a comprehensive audiologic evaluation be completed by 3 months of age. For infants with a hearing loss, appropriate health care and educational provisions should be made by 6 months of age. It is also recommended that regular audiologic and communication screenings be conducted within the first 3 years of life for all children.

PHYSIOLOGIC MEASURES OF HEARING

Whenever possible, behavioral measures of hearing should be used to assess the status of the auditory system. However, because of many variables that can affect the validity and reliability of these measures, particularly when testing the hearing of infants and young children, physiologic techniques can be used to assess the integrity of the auditory system.

A. **Immittance audiometry** is an objective means for determining the integrity of the middle and external ear cavities and can provide information about middle ear pressure, the mobility of the tympanic membrane, eustachian tube functioning, the mobility of the ossicles, and acoustic reflex thresholds (ARTs).

1. **Tympanometry** is used to assess disorders of the middle ear that affect the tympanic membrane, middle car space, and ossicular chain. It provides information about the mobility of the tympanic membrane in response to changes in air pressure presented to the external auditory canal. **Tympanograms** typically present the amount of compliance as a function of air pressure and are classified as **Type A** (normal middle ear function—see Fig. 17.2), **Type B** (flat—no change in compliance with change in external ear canal pressure), or **Type C** (negative middle ear pressure that may indicate the presence of fluid in the middle ear). This testing, however, can lack specificity for infants younger than 6 months because of the high compliance of their external ear canal walls.

2. **ART.** When an ear with normal hearing is exposed to an intense auditory signal, the stapedius muscle contracts. This contraction can be measured as changes in ear canal pressure. It can be elicited in normal-hearing individuals using pure-tone signals that vary between

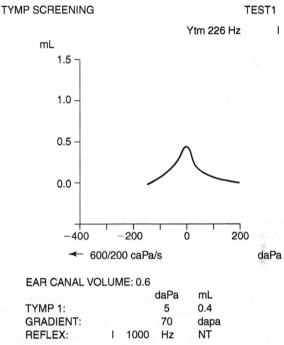

DATE/ TIME : 10/01/2007 10:01 am
CSI TYMPSTAR MIDDLE EAR AYALYZER
PROBE S/N: 20073075

TYMP SCREENING   TEST1

Ytm 226 Hz   I

EAR CANAL VOLUME: 0.6

		daPa	mL
TYMP 1:		5	0.4
GRADIENT:		70	dapa
REFLEX:	I 1000 Hz		NT

FIGURE 17.2 A sample normal (Type A) tympanogram. The compliance of the middle ear system is measured as a function of the presented pressure to the external ear.

70 and 100 dB HL. The lowest intensity level that produces this response is referred to as the ART. This acoustic reflex occurs bilaterally regardless of which ear is stimulated, if the system is functioning normally. The presence or absence of the reflex and the intensity levels at which the reflex is obtained provide information useful in identifying lesions within the auditory system up to the level of the superior olivary complex.

B. **Auditory brainstem response (ABR).** This electrophysiologic response is generated by activation of the neurons within the eighth cranial nerve and lower auditory brainstem. Rapid, short-duration acoustic signals, such as a click stimulus, can elicit this response. Because these responses are relatively small in relation to the noise (both internal and external), signal averaging techniques are used to record the electrical response of the auditory system.

1. An example of an ABR is presented in Figure 17.3. The response is judged by the presence of positive waves (I, II, III, IV, and V) occurring within a specific latency range (i.e., the time after stimulus onset that a response occurs). The latency, amplitude, and morphologic features of the responses depend on the patient's age, the stimulus characteristics, and the recording parameters. Persons with normal peripheral ear and lower auditory brainstem system integrity have a response to clicks at intensities as low as 5 dB normal HL (nHL). When using click stimuli, the response is sensitive to the hearing status between 2,000 and 4,000 Hz. Different methods of evoked potential testing can be used to estimate hearing sensitivity outside this frequency range, but the results typically are less robust than the responses to click stimuli.

2. The test parameters and interpretation criteria for ABR depend on the nature of the questions asked by the clinicians. Because the amplitude measures are highly variable and more susceptible to artifacts, clinicians typically use latency measures to assess

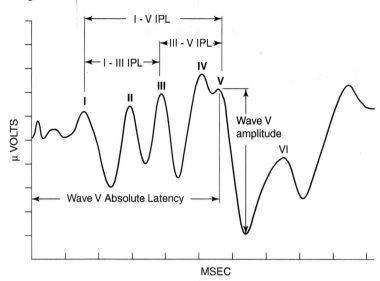

FIGURE 17.3 A sample ABR. Each wave in the response is identified using roman numerals (I, II, III, IV, and V). ABR, auditory brainstem response.

integrity of the system. When screening for hearing loss, the clinician examines the waveform for the presence of distinctive peaks, particularly wave V. As the intensity of the stimulus changes so too should the latency. The obtained latencies are compared with the normative values available for the type of patient. In the differential diagnosis of retrocochlear lesions, a prolonged wave I–V interpeak latency difference becomes the most sensitive indicator of this condition. Also, other prolonged interpeak latencies and interaural latency differences can be enough information for a diagnosis.

3. Although the click-evoked ABR can appear as early as the 25th week of gestation and is typically present at the 27th week of gestation, there are developmental changes in the response until approximately 2 years of age. The decrease in the absolute latency of the response is the most salient change during this maturational period. Therefore, interpretation of the ABR to identify hearing loss depends on age-appropriate norms. If wave V of the ABR is present in a test ear at 35 dB nHL, it is likely that the infant has normal-hearing sensitivity between 2,000 and 4,000 Hz.

C. **Auditory steady-state responses (ASSR)** are brain potentials that are evoked by steady-state stimuli as opposed to short-duration acoustic signals used to generate the ABR. The electroencephalogram (EEG) activity recorded from scalp recording electrodes contains amplitude modulations (AM) and/or frequency modulations (FM) that follow the variations in the recording stimuli. The recorded responses are suspected to arise from the auditory nerve, the cochlear nucleus, the inferior colliculus, and the primary auditory cortex because neurons at these sites are responsive to AM and FM signals.

1. The presence or absence of the ASSR is determined using statistical analyses.

2. As with the ABR, the ASSR can be used to estimate audiometric thresholds. Data have suggested that the ASSR thresholds are correlated with the ABR thresholds. Additionally, there is evidence suggesting that the ASSR can be recorded from individuals without measurable ABR. Consequently, this response has gained popularity as a tool for evaluating children who are being considered for cochlear implantation.

D. **Otoacoustic emissions** are sounds that are generated in the cochlea and propagate back through the middle ear and ear canal where they can be measured with a microphone. Hearing losses due to cochlear or middle ear lesions can be readily identified with otoacoustic emissions; however, these measurements do not define the severity of the hearing loss. There are two classes of otoacoustic emissions—spontaneous otoacoustic emissions and evoked otoacoustic emissions. Evoked otoacoustic emissions can be further divided according to the type of stimulus used during measurement—**stimulus frequency**

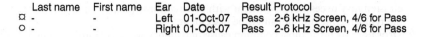

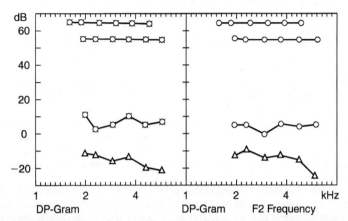

FIGURE 17.4 A sample DPOAE-gram. The left panel displays the results for the left ear (*xs*), and the right panel displays the results for the right ear *(circles)*. The triangles in both panels represent the level of the noise in the ear, and the uppermost lines in each panel indicate the level of signal presentation. DPOAE, distortion product otoacoustic emission.

emissions, transient evoked otoacoustic emissions (TEOAEs), and **distortion product otoacoustic emissions (DPOAEs).** Measurement of DPOAEs and TEOAEs is preferred for clinical purposes.

1. Figure 17.4 illustrates the DPOAE results from a normal-hearing adult. DPOAEs are generated from the presentation of two pure-tone frequencies to the ear, which results in a third "distortion product" response. The nonlinearity nature of the cochlea is responsible for the distortion product. In the figure, the intensity of the response is displayed as a function of the response frequency. The left panel shows the results for the left ear and the right panel shows the responses for the right ear. The triangles in both panels represent the level of the noise and the upper most lines in each panel indicate the level of signal presentation.

HEARING LOSS

It is broadly classified into two types—conductive and sensorineural—and each type has a wide variety of pathologic causes.

A. **Conductive hearing loss** occurs when sound cannot efficiently reach the cochlea. The blockage may be due to abnormalities of the ear canal, the tympanic membrane, or the middle ear ossicles, including the footplate of the stapes.

1. Hearing loss due to **obstruction of the external auditory canal** can result from impacted cerumen, foreign bodies in the canal, and swelling of the canal during infection. Cerumen impaction is the most common cause of conductive hearing loss. It is normally secreted by glands in the outer one-third of the cartilaginous portion of the ear canal. Its function is to clean and lubricate the ear canal and also to provide protection from bacteria, fungi, and insects. Other obstructions include atresia (a complete closure of the ear canal), stenosis (a narrowing of the ear canal), collapsed ear canals, and bony growths within the ear canal.

2. Conductive hearing loss may result from damage to the tympanic membrane or middle ear as a result of trauma or infection. Perforation of the tympanic membrane and ossicular discontinuity are surgically correctable.

3. **Otitis media with effusion** is the most common cause of conductive hearing loss among children. This condition can be associated with adenoid hypertrophy. The middle ear

effusion may necessitate treatment with myringotomy (i.e., creating a small incision in the tympanic membrane) and tube placement.

4. **Otosclerosis** is the most common cause of conductive hearing loss among individuals in the mid-childhood to late middle-adult years. Otosclerotic bone (i.e., growth of spongy bone) progressively fixes the stapes in the oval window. This condition can be successfully managed with a stapedectomy.

B. **Sensorineural hearing loss** results from lesions central to the footplate of the stapes that involve the cochlea or cochlear division of the eighth cranial nerve. When the site of lesion is within the cochlea, the hearing loss is considered sensory. When the site of lesion is within the auditory neural pathway, the hearing loss is neural or retrocochlear. In sensorineural hearing losses, both air- and bone-conduction thresholds are outside the normal range of hearing sensitivity.

1. Hereditary. Sensorineural hearing loss may be hereditary; at least 100 genetic syndromes that involve hearing loss have been identified. It has been estimated that 50% of childhood sensorineural hearing loss is due to genetic factors. Genetic forms of hearing loss may be congenital or delayed in onset, unilateral or bilateral, and progressive or sudden in nature.

2. Infection. A number of viruses, including cytomegalovirus, rubella, and herpes simplex, have been implicated as etiologic agents in congenital and acquired hearing loss. Congenital syphilis and bacterial meningitis are contemporary causes of deafness despite the greatly improved treatment options available.

3. Neoplasm. In patients with unilateral progressive sensorineural hearing loss, acoustic neuroma must be suspected. Bilateral acoustic neuroma is the hallmark of neurofibromatosis type 2 and must be suspected when a patient has a positive family history (autosomal-dominant inheritance).

4. **Other common causes** of sensorineural hearing loss are noise exposure, metabolic and systemic changes in the auditory system, ototoxic medications, aging (presbycusis), and head trauma.

C. **Mixed hearing loss** exists when both conductive and sensorineural hearing losses occur in the same ear. The lesions are additive, resulting in marked air–bone gaps with the bone-conduction thresholds falling outside the normal range of hearing sensitivity.

D. Auditory neuropathy/dyssynchrony. Some patients have normal peripheral auditory systems up to and including the outer hair cells but have hearing difficulties. This condition can result from the absence of the auditory nerve, or more commonly, from dyssynchronous electrical responses that are sent to the brain from the auditory nerve. These patients present with a range of hearing sensitivities but typically have great difficulty understanding speech in degraded listening conditions. These patients typically have normal immittance results and normal otoacoustic emissions, yet they have anomalies in evoked potentials, particularly in the ABR, and in the behavioral response under earphones or in the sound field. The causes of auditory neuropathy/dyssynchrony vary among patients; however, the pathologic process most likely affects the inner hair cell or the auditory processing abilities of the auditory nerve and lower brainstem. Because of the possible dead regions in the cochlea or neural involvement, these patients do not respond typically to some of the traditional treatment protocols.

E. Central auditory processing disorder. Patients with this type of disorder have difficulty perceiving and appropriately using acoustic information because the central auditory system is incapable of adequately processing the signals transduced by the cochlea. Patients with central auditory processing disorders can be taught compensation strategies to improve their ability to comprehend speech. Many adults with sensorineural hearing losses also may have a concomitant central auditory processing disorder, which confounds the evaluation and management of the sensorineural hearing loss.

MANAGEMENT AND REFERRAL LISTS

When any hearing loss is suspected or identified, the patient should be referred for otologic examination and audiologic evaluation to determine the appropriate means of treatment. For conductive hearing loss, medical management is the primary course of treatment. Although many patients with sensorineural hearing loss require medical treatment and follow-up care, the primary course of management of this type of hearing loss is amplification, whether through hearing aids, cochlear implants, or assistive listening devices.

A. **Amplification.** Hearing aids differ in design, size, amount of amplification, ease of handling, volume control, and availability of special features. But they do have similar components, which include a microphone to pick up sound, amplifier circuitry to make the sound louder, a receiver to deliver the amplified sound into the ear, and batteries to power the electronic parts.

1. **Hearing aid styles.** The majority of hearing aids fall into one of four categories. The completely-in-the-canal hearing aid is the smallest and requires some form of automatic signal processing because it is difficult to manipulate controls, which are located deep inside the ear canal. The in-the-canal and in-the-ear aids sit outside the ear canal and allow manual manipulation of various controls on the hearing aid. The behind-the-ear hearing aid rests behind the ear and requires an earmold to direct the flow of sound into the ear. This style is often chosen for young children for safety and growth reasons. Also, the open-fit hearing aid (a behind-the-ear style) is a popular hearing aid for adults. This hearing aid is fit to the ear with a narrow tube as opposed to an earmold, which prevents the occlusion effect (i.e., the booming sensation of one's own voice).

2. **Hearing aid circuitry.** Hearing aids are also differentiated according to technology or circuitry. **Conventional analog** hearing aids are designed with a particular frequency response based on the audiogram. The hearing aid has a series of potentiometers that the dispenser can adjust to approximate the values of amplification needed by the user. **Analog programmable** hearing aids contain a microchip that allows the aid to have settings programmed for different listening environments, such as quiet conversation in the home, noisy situations as in a restaurant, or large areas such as a theater. **Digital programmable** hearing aids have all of the advantages of analog programmable hearing aids, but the dispenser also uses digital signal processing to change the characteristics of the signal to maximize its frequency and intensity characteristics to meet the user's needs at any given moment in time.

3. **Implantable hearing aids.** Implantable aids are typically provided for specific reasons as described below. However, new implantable middle ear hearing aids are being provided to conventional hearing aid recipients to help improve high-frequency hearing, to minimize acoustic feedback, and to improve sound quality. These devices are further described below.

   a. **Bone-anchored hearing aids.** A device is implanted on the mastoid and once in place will use bone vibrations to stimulate the cochlea. These aids are provided for individuals with chronic conductive issues such as draining ears, a large mastoid bowl, otosclerosis, tympanosclerosis, or atresia.

   b. **Middle ear implantable hearing aids.** These devices use an externally placed microphone coupled with an internal transducer that vibrates one of the ossicles. The mechanical energy is converted to electrical energy along the auditory pathway. These devices can be used for individuals with mild to severe sensorineural hearing losses.

   c. **Cochlear implants** are amplification devices used to fit children and adults who have severe and profound hearing losses. Although the external processor is similar to that of a digital hearing aid, the internal components of the cochlear implant directly stimulate the neural cells of the eighth cranial nerve. Sounds sent to the external microphone are processed via the speech processor and then sent directly to the internal electrode array that is placed within the scala tympani of the cochlea. The electrical pulses are directed toward the spiral ganglion cells and the auditory nerve. The peripheral ear, therefore, is completely bypassed with this form of stimulation. Previously, unilateral cochlear implants were commonly provided, but more recently, patients are being provided with bilateral implants. Additionally, some individuals with unilateral implants find the use of a hearing aid in the opposite ear to be beneficial for communication purposes.

4. **Assistive listening devices** are specialized listening systems that may or may not interface with hearing aids and cochlear implants. These devices are designed to augment communication function by improving the signal-to-noise ratio during degraded listening activities. The type of assistive listening device is usually designated by the type of transmission properties the device uses such as FM systems, infrared systems, loop (wire inductance) systems, and hard-wired systems. These devices are particularly

effective for listening in large-group situations such as in classrooms, churches, or public meetings. They are also effective in bridging the gap between many audio devices, such as televisions and radios, with the user's hearing aids or cochlear implants.

B. **Referral.** The following organizations can assist the interested reader in locating patient education materials and appropriate otologic and audiologic service providers in their areas:

American Academy of Otolaryngology—Head and Neck Surgery
1650 Diagonal Road
Alexandria, VA 22314-2859
Phone: (703) 836-4444
Fax: (703) 683-3100
www.entnet.org

American Speech–Language–Hearing Association
10801 Rockville Pike
Rockville, MD 20852
Phone: (800) 638-8255
Fax: (240) 333-4705
www.asha.org

American Academy of Audiology
11730 Plaza America Drive, Suite 300
Reston, VA 20190
Phone: (800) AAA-2336, (703) 790-8466
Fax: (703) 790-8631
www.audiology.org

Key Points

- Hearing loss affects almost 17 in 1,000 children under the age of 18 and approximately 314 in 1,000 adults over the age of 65.
- Hearing loss can result from anatomical/mechanical or neurologic issues.
- Both a medical and an audiologic examination are required to assess the extent and cause of hearing loss.
- Types of hearing loss include conductive (i.e., the outer and middle ear are affected), sensorineural (i.e., the inner ear or auditory nerve is affected), and mixed (i.e., the outer and/or middle ear and the inner ear are affected).
- Management of hearing loss can include the use of amplification, either through the use of a traditional hearing aid, or through the use of implantable hearing aids.
- Implantable hearing aids are surgically implanted in the mastoid bone, the middle ear, or the cochlea depending on the cause and severity of hearing loss.

Recommended Readings

Brown CJ, Johnson TA. Electrophysiologic assessment of hearing. In: Flint PW, Haughey BH, Lund VJ, et al, eds. *Cummings Otolaryngology: Head and Neck Surgery.* 6th ed. Philadelphia, PA: Elsevier Sanders; 2015:chap 134.

Dillon H. *Hearing Aids.* New York, NY: Thieme; 2012.

Durrant JD, Lovrinic JH. *Bases of Hearing Science.* 3rd ed. Baltimore, MD: Lippincott Williams & Wilkins; 1995.

Gorga MP, Johnson TA, Kaminski JR, et al. Using a combination of click- and tone burst-evoked auditory brainstem response measurements to estimate pure-tone thresholds. *Ear Hear.* 2006;27:60–74.

Joint Committee on Infant Hearing. Year 2007 position statement: principles and guidelines for early hearing detection. *Pediatrics.* 2007;120:898–921.

Katz J. *Handbook of Clinical Audiology.* 7th ed. Philadelphia, PA: Lippincott Williams & Wilkins; 2014.

Merchant SN, Nadol JB, eds. *Schuknecht's Pathology of the Ear.* 3rd ed. Shelton, CT: People's Medical Publishing House-USA; 2010.

Miyamoto RT, Miyamoto RC, Kirk KI. Cochlear implants in children. In: Bluestone CD, Stool SE, Kenna MA, et al, eds. *Pediatric Otolaryngology*. 5th ed. Shelton, CT: People's Medical Publishing House—USA; 2014:547–560.

Musiek FE, Rintelmann WF. *Contemporary Perspectives in Hearing Assessment*. Boston, MA: Allyn & Bacon; 1999.

Norton SJ, Gorga MP, Widen JE, et al. Identification of neonatal hearing impairment: evaluation of transient evoked otoacoustic emission, distortion product otoacoustic emission, and auditory brainstem response test performance. *Ear Hear*. 2000;21:508–528.

Pickles JO. *An Introduction to the Physiology of Hearing*. 4th ed. Leiden, The Netherlands: Brill Academic Publishers; 2013.

Ruenes R. *Otologic Radiology with Clinical Correlations*. New York, NY: Macmillan; 1986.

Speaks CE. *Introduction to Sound: Acoustics for the Hearing and Speech Sciences*. 3rd ed. San Diego, CA: Singular Publishing Group; 1999.

Working Group on Cochlear Implants. Cochlear implants. ASHA technical report; 2004.

Yost WA. *Fundamentals of Hearing: An Introduction*. 5th ed. Leiden, The Netherlands: Brill Academic Publishers; 2013.

Yu JKY, Wong LLN, Tsang WSS, et al. A tutorial on implantable hearing amplification options for adults with unilateral microtia and atresia [published online ahead of print on June 2, 2014]. *BioMed Res Int*. doi:10.1155/2014/703256.

Zeng F-G. Trends in cochlear implants. *Trends Amplif*. 2004;8:1–34.

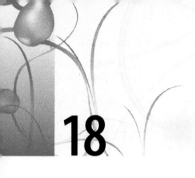

18 Approach to the Patient with Dysphagia

Alejandro A. Rabinstein

Dysphagia is the medical term most commonly used to characterize swallowing difficulties. It has been defined as a subjective or objective abnormal delay in the transit of a liquid or solid bolus during swallowing. It is a symptom or a sign of an underlying disorder, which can be structural (anatomical) or functional (physiologic). Dysphagia can have many causes and the cause is oftentimes neurologic. In fact, many acute and chronic neurologic diseases can affect the swallowing process at various levels. Dysphagia related to neurologic disease is frequently associated with increased risk of aspiration pneumonia because the airway protective mechanisms are concomitantly affected.

ANATOMY AND PHYSIOLOGY OF NORMAL SWALLOWING

Swallowing is an exquisitely complex and precisely regulated function that requires the integration of oral, lingual, pharyngeal, laryngeal, and esophageal muscles controlled by several cranial nerves (V, VII, IX, X, XII) and coordinated by the swallowing center in the medulla oblongata. Although swallowing is smoothly continuous, its physiology has been traditionally described in four sequential phases.

A. Swallowing phases.
   1. Oral preparatory phase. Mastication (effected by masseter, temporalis, and oral medial and lateral pterygoid muscles) breaks down the food into a cohesive bolus while the lips and lateral and anterior sulci are sealed (by contraction of the orbicularis oris and buccinators muscles) and the soft palate is depressed toward the base of the tongue (by contraction of the palatoglossus muscle). The intrinsic muscles of the tongue and genioglossus create a central groove in the tongue to contain the newly formed bolus.
   2. Oral transport phase. Bolus is propelled toward the oropharynx while the soft palate elevates (by contraction of the levator veli palatini and musculus uvulae) to seal off the nasal cavity. Wavelike pressure generated by the tongue muscles moves the bolus centrally and posteriorly as the posterior dorsum of the tongue is depressed (by action of the hyoglossus muscle).
   3. Pharyngeal phase. This is a brief (1 second or less) but critical stage triggered by the passage of the bolus through the anterior faucial pillars. Various characteristics of the bolus can accelerate or delay the pharyngeal triggering (e.g., thicker fluids can delay it while sour foods can accelerate it). During this phase, in close sequence, respiration is held, the pharynx is elevated (by multiple pharyngeal muscles), the tongue base is retracted toward the posterior pharyngeal wall, and pharyngeal constrictor muscles contract in a craniocaudal direction (pharyngeal peristalsis that progresses at a rate of 9 to 25 cm/sec and generates an average pressure of 22 mm Hg) to pass the bolus through the upper esophageal sphincter. At the same time, the larynx is elevated (by the thyrohyoid muscle), which protects the airway against penetration and aspiration and contributes to the swallowing process by augmenting the negative pressure below the bolus and pulling open the lower part of the pharynx and the upper esophageal sphincter.
   4. Esophageal phase. The upper esophageal sphincter opens as the cricopharyngeal muscle relaxes to let the bolus pass and then contracts to prevent regurgitation. The bolus is then propelled downward from its tail by the esophageal peristalsis (3 to 4 cm/sec on average) while the lower esophageal sphincter relaxes to let the bolus enter the stomach. This phase generally lasts 8 to 13 seconds in healthy adults, but the duration changes depending on the characteristics of the bolus (volume and viscosity/texture) and the patient's age.

B. Central neurologic regulation.

1. *Cerebral modulation.* In particular the oral phases of swallowing can be voluntarily controlled through the activity of cortical (primary and supplemental motor and sensory cortices) and subcortical structures. Cortical representation of swallowing is bilateral and asymmetric and the hemispheric dominance is not related to handedness. Volitional prolongation of breath holding can reduce the risk of penetration when drinking large amounts of thin fluid. Rehabilitation techniques rely on voluntary control to improve the safety of swallowing in patients with dysphagia.

2. Medullary. A central pattern generator (known as the **swallowing center**) in the medulla oblongata regulates the oropharyngeal and esophageal phases of swallowing. The dorsal group of neurons receives sensory signals from the pharyngeal trigger (via cranial nerves IX and X and the nucleus of the tractus solitarius) and relays the information to the ventral neurons that produce a motor response via the hypoglossal motor nucleus (activates the muscles of the tongue through the XII cranial nerve), the nucleus ambiguous (activating the IX and X motor fibers that innervate the pharynx, larynx, and striated muscles of the upper esophagus), and the dorsal motor nucleus of the vagus nerve (which innervates the smooth muscle of the lower esophagus). General sensory information from the oral mucosa and the tongue (cranial nerves V and IX) and taste sensation from the tongue (cranial nerves VII and IX) can influence the central regulation of the pharyngeal phase of swallowing.

C. Airway protection.

Multiple mechanisms contribute to ensure that the airway is protected from bolus penetration during swallowing.

1. Breath holding. Respiration ceases during the pharyngeal phase of swallowing.

2. Physical closure of the airway. Through true and false vocal cord adduction and epiglottic deflection.

3. Protective reflexes. Laryngeal adductor response triggered by tactile stimulation of the laryngeal mucosa and the laryngeal cough reflex triggered by tactile or chemical stimulation. Laryngeal sensation is transmitted by the superior laryngeal branch of the recurrent laryngeal nerve bilaterally. Of note, the belief that the gag reflex provides an important contribution to airway safety is a misconception; the risk of aspiration does not correlate well with the presence, reduction, or absence of the gag reflex.

D. Effects of normal aging.

1. Oral transit time slows 0.5 to 1.0 seconds with increasing age, probably because older adults often hold the bolus on the anterior floor of the mouth and must pick it up with their tongue to begin the swallow.

2. Transition from the oral to pharyngeal phase may be slightly delayed after age 60 to 70, probably because of slower neural processing.

3. After age 80, range of motion of pharyngeal structures is reduced and consequently there is less flexibility in the swallow.

4. Over age 60 to 70, esophageal peristalsis becomes less efficient.

5. Healthy elderly individuals do not aspirate more often than young people. Elderly patients (over age 80) who become acutely or chronically ill and develop generalized weakness will demonstrate a weak swallow because of their reduced muscular reserve. This can cause aspiration.

CLINICAL PRESENTATION

1. Patients with dysphagia can present with various different symptoms (Table 18.1).

2. In neurologic cases, odinophagia (i.e., pain with swallowing) is uncommon with the exception of glossopharyngeal neuralgia.

3. Sensation of having a lump in the throat (globus) is typically not associated with true dysphagia or with any neurologic disease.

4. Dysphagia from a neurologic cause is typically oropharyngeal. Esophageal dysphagia is generally caused by non-neurologic disorders.

5. The timing and progression of the dysphagia can help narrow the differential diagnosis: sudden onset with stroke, fluctuating course and worse in the evenings with myasthenia gravis (MG), slowly progressive with neurodegenerative disorders.

TABLE 18.1 Symptoms and Signs of Dysphagia in Patients with Neurologic Disease

Struggling to swallow
Taking longer to eat
Voluntary avoidance of certain food consistencies
Coughing during or after swallowing
Repeated swallowing to clear the food from the throat
Wet, gurgly voice during or after swallowing
Nasal regurgitation during swallowing
Breathing difficulties during or after swallowing
Drooling
Excessive oral or tracheal secretions
Unintended weight loss
Repeated respiratory infections

6. Dysphagia is rarely present in isolation when due to an underlying neurologic disease. Thus, changes in vision, speech, strength, coordination, and sensation should be explored. Speech changes are particularly useful to discriminate among neurologic causes of dysphagia: a spastic dysarthria can indicate motor neuron disease, hypophonia can signal parkinsonism, a nasal speech can be seen with bulbar weakness from neuromuscular disease, nasal regurgitation of fluids points to a problem with the innervation of the soft palate, and stridor may denote a problem involving the recurrent laryngeal nerve or the brainstem (such as in multiple system atrophy).

7. A complete neurologic examination should follow the careful history taking. The most relevant information that should be acquired from the neurologic examination in patients with dysphagia is shown in Table 18.2. The physical examination should also include evaluation of the lungs to exclude signs of aspiration. Specific evaluation for the presence of dysphagia per se is discussed below.

8. Recurrent episodes of pneumonia should always raise the suspicion of aspiration and call for detailed evaluation for possible dysphagia. Remember that dysphagia can be silent in patients with neurologic disease affecting the sensory innervation to the larynx.

COMPLICATIONS

1. *Aspiration pneumonia.* The risk of aspiration pneumonia is greatest in patients with acute neurologic disease, particularly stroke, because these patients have not yet developed any compensatory mechanisms.
2. Malnutrition.
3. Dehydration.

TABLE 18.2 Main Aspects of Neurologic Examination in Patients with Dysphagia

Evaluate	To Exclude
Level of alertness	Drowsiness
Cortical functions	Dementia, neglect, impulsivity, abulia
Bulbar functions	Facial weakness, abnormal extraocular movements, diplopia and ocular fatigability, dysarthria, dysphonia, features of pseudobulbar palsy, tongue wasting and tongue fasciculations, tongue weakness
Muscle tone	Rigidity or spasticity
Muscle strength in the limbs	Weakness from motor neuron disease, polyradiculoneuropathy, myopathy, neuromuscular transmission disorder
Gait	Parkinsonism, ataxia, spasticity

4. Increased dependency.
5. Increased health care costs (gastric feeding, nursing care, hospitalizations for recurrent pneumonia).

COMMON NEUROLOGIC CAUSES OF DYSPHAGIA

A. Acute neurologic disease.
   1. *Stroke.*
      a. Brainstem strokes (pontomedullary infarctions in particular) cause the most severe and persistent forms of dysphagia.
      b. Hemispheric strokes can cause dysphagia by interrupting the cortical or subcortical input to the medullary swallowing center. Dysphagia is more common with large strokes affecting the middle cerebral artery territory, but can also occur with smaller infarctions in cortical and subcortical locations.
      c. Specific hemispheric lesion locations associated with dysphagia include pre- and post-central gyri, operculum, supramarginal gyrus, and respective subcortical white matter tracts. Post-central lesions appear to be associated with more severe dysphagia.
      d. Dysphagia can be a manifestation of advanced subcortical ischemia (particularly with multiple small subcortical infarction).
      e. It is frequently associated with aphasia, dysarthria, and speech apraxia.
      f. Poststroke dysphagia is more common in older patients and especially in the elderly.
      g. Swallowing problems after stroke can include poor coordination of motor function during the oral phases, impaired initiation of the pharyngeal phase, reduced pharyngeal peristalsis with increased pharyngeal transit times, and aspiration.
   2. *Traumatic injury.*
      a. Head trauma can cause dysphagia by disturbing the neurologic control of the oral and pharyngeal phases of swallowing.
      b. Injuries to the head and neck can compound the problem.
      c. Cervical spinal cord injury, especially if treated with an extensive spinal fusion, can also cause dysphagia.
   3. *Acute neuromuscular disorders.*
      a. Severe dysphagia can be seen in patients with Guillain–Barré syndrome. It is more common in patients with generalized weakness, neuromuscular respiratory failure, and dysautonomia. However, it can sometimes be noted in patients with more restricted forms of the disease, such as the Miller Fisher's syndrome.
      b. Acute dysphagia can be a manifestation of botulism and severe forms of inflammatory myositis.
      c. Rarely, dysphagia can be a complication of botulinum toxin injections for treatment of cervical dystonia or spasmodic dysphonia.
B. Chronic neurologic disease.
   1. *Parkinson's disease (PD) and other extrapyramidal disorders.*
      a. Dysphagia is commonly considered a feature of advanced PD, but mild swallowing impairment can be detected in early stages.
      b. Swallowing problems include defective mastication, impaired coordination of the tongue movements (patients with advanced PD often have an involuntary rocking, rolling tongue motion that interferes with the preparation of the bolus), and delayed transfer of the bolus to the pharynx. In turn, the pharyngeal phase is also delayed and the stasis of the bolus in the pharynx increases the risk of aspiration. Furthermore, patients with PD can aspirate silently (i.e., without cough).
      c. Dysphagia and increased risk of aspiration can also be seen with other extrapyramidal disorders, most notably with progressive supranuclear palsy in which swallowing problems can be severe from an early stage of the disease.
   2. *Degenerative dementia.*
      a. Although dysphagia is not often appreciated as a common manifestation of degenerative dementias, epidemiologic studies have reported a fairly high incidence of this complication.
      b. In patients with Alzheimer's disease, studies have reported complaints of dysphagia in 7% and objective evidence of dysphagia in 13% to 29%. Even higher rates of

dysphagia have been reported in patients with frontotemporal dementia (19% to 26% subjective and up to 57% objective).

c. The rates of detection of dysphagia increase proportionally to the severity of the dementia and the age of the patient.

d. Poor insight can increase the risk of aspiration in patients with dementia and dysphagia, thus demanding close supervision.

3. *Multiple sclerosis (MS).*

a. Dysphagia can be an early or more commonly a late manifestation of MS. In late stages, it can be seen in up to two-thirds of patients.

b. Severity of the dysphagia depends on the localization and extension of the demyelinating lesions. It is more severe with brainstem demyelination.

c. Swallowing abnormalities can be multiple, including impaired lingual control and tongue base retraction, delayed pharyngeal trigger, diminished pharyngeal peristalsis, reduced laryngeal closure, and upper esophageal sphincted dysfunction. Sensory impairment in the pharyngeal and laryngeal mucosa can allow silent aspiration. Protective reflexes (laryngeal adduction and cough) may also be affected.

d. Aspiration pneumonia is one of the leading causes of death in advanced MS.

4. *Motor neuron disease.*

a. Dysphagia is a major complication of amyotrophic lateral sclerosis and eventually occurs in all cases.

b. In early stages, the tongue is disproportionally affected and consequently the oral phases of swallowing are predominantly impaired.

c. As bulbar involvement progresses, the dysphagia becomes more severe as the dysfunction extends to other aspects of the swallowing mechanism. The pharyngeal triggering reflex gets delayed and weakened. Meanwhile, laryngeal muscles can become hypertonic and thus lose coordination with pharyngeal movements.

d. Aspiration risk becomes very high over the course of the disease and this should be anticipated.

5. *Chronic neuromuscular disorders.*

a. MG can cause dysphagia because of fatigability of the bulbar muscles. Thus, myasthenic patients should always be interrogated about symptoms of dysphagia (including whether they get tired of chewing toward the end of meals), particularly if the voice is nasal or hoarse.

b. Dysphagia is a very common manifestation of MG exacerbation and, in turn, aspiration pneumonia can precipitate a myasthenic crisis.

c. Rarely, dysphagia can be a presenting symptom of MG.

d. In myasthenic patients, dysphagia can be related to fatigability and weakness of the masticatory muscles, tongue, pharyngeal constrictor muscles, and the muscles responsible for laryngeal elevation.

e. Inflammatory body myositis can cause dysphagia early or later in the course of the disease.

f. Slowly progressive dysphagia is a frequent symptom in patients with oculopharyngeal muscular dystrophy and myotonic dystrophy.

DIAGNOSTIC EVALUATION

After a detailed history and physical examination, patients at risk for dysphagia should have specific testing of their swallowing.

A. Bedside swallowing examination.

1. A bedside screening evaluation of swallowing is necessary in *any* neurologic patient who can be at risk of aspiration and it should be performed as soon as the condition of the patient allows it and before any oral intake.

2. In fact, documentation of performance of a bedside swallowing evaluation before any oral intake is mandatory for patients with acute stroke.

3. The water swallowing test (simply asking the patient to take a few sips of water and watching for signs of choking, coughing, or inability to drink) is quite sensitive for the detection of dysphagia when compared to instrumental gold standards (video fluoroscopic or fiberoptic endoscopic swallowing evaluations). Therefore, although its specificity may be suboptimal, it is a good and practical measure to screen for dysphagia at the bedside.

4. Yet, in some studies the water swallowing test failed to identify high risk of aspiration later proven by video fluoroscopic studies in up to a third of patients. Other bedside tests that incorporate different liquid viscosities and volumes have been proposed (such as the Toronto Bedside Swallowing Screening Test and the Volume Viscosity Swallowing Test); they may have greater diagnostic accuracy than the water swallowing test, but they are less simple to administer (in certain hospitals, these more detailed bedside evaluations, also incorporating foods of different consistency, can be proficiently performed by especially trained therapists). Checklists for dysphagia screening have also been proposed and may be a useful addition.

5. Patients with depressed level of consciousness should not be fed by mouth until they are consistently awake, even if they passed a bedside swallow at one point in time.

6. It is essential to remember that the bedside tests rely on the evaluation of symptoms. Yet, symptoms will be absent in patients with neurogenic dysphagia who have impaired sensory innervation to the pharynx and larynx. Thus, silent aspiration cannot be excluded by a bedside swallowing test.

7. Patients who failed the bedside swallow should be kept NPO (i.e., nothing by mouth) and referred for a video fluoroscopic swallow study.

8. It is prudent to refer also for video fluoroscopic evaluation those patients who passed a water swallowing test at the bedside but have a particularly high risk for aspiration (e.g., brainstem strokes, hospitalized patients with advanced neurogenerative disorders).

B. Video fluoroscopic swallow study.

1. The video fluoroscopic swallow study is the instrument of choice for the evaluation of dysphagia in most practices.

2. It consists of a real-time dynamic X-ray procedure performed during swallows of carefully defined radiopaque fluids and foods (Video 18.1).

3. It allows a detailed analysis of the passage of the bolus, thus providing information to evaluate all the phases of the oropharyngeal swallowing. It also offers indirect visualization of the swallowing structures and a means to assess the outcomes of interventions that can be tried to ameliorate or compensate for the impaired functions.

4. It is typically performed by a therapist and a radiologist and the total radiation exposure averages 3 to 5 minutes. During the study, different volumes of boluses of various viscosities and consistencies are tested following a protocol designed to minimize the risk of aspiration and which is modified according to the individual characteristics of the case. In general terms, a complete study has the steps listed in Table 18.3.

5. The report should contain a description of the oral and pharyngeal anatomy and swallow physiology, the mechanisms responsible for the dysphagia, identification of the types and amounts of foods safely swallowed, whether partial or full nonoral feeding is necessary, and the effectiveness and need for compensatory strategies or swallow therapy.

6. When interpreting the report of a video fluoroscopic swallow evaluation, it is important to understand the differences between **penetration** and **aspiration**. **Penetration** is when the bolus enters the glottis and reaches as far as the vestibule. If the penetration takes a very short course or is very brief before being corrected, it is named "flash penetration." Penetrated boluses should trigger unpleasant sensations from the vestibular walls prompting

---

TABLE 18.3 Video Fluoroscopic Swallow Evaluation

- Patient seated upright and examined in the lateral plane to define speed, efficiency, and safety of the swallow
- Liquids given in 1-, 3-, 5-, or 10-mL drinking amounts (two swallows each) to observe "dose response" of the pharynx and to define optimal tolerated volume for each patient
- If and when the patient aspirates or has a highly inefficient swallow, various treatment strategies are tested to observe their effects radiographically, including postural changes, increased sensory awareness, and increased bolus viscosity (nectar or honey-thickened liquids)
- Pudding (1–2 mL) and a small bite of cookie are given (two swallows each) as tolerated by the patient
- The patient is turned and examined in the anteroposterior plane to define symmetry of the swallow

coughing, choking sensation, or at least tickling. Absence of these responses indicates abnormal sensation. Penetration indicates risk of aspiration. **Aspiration** is when the bolus actually passes the true vocal cords and can move down the tracheobronchial tree potentially reaching the lungs (most commonly bilateral basal segments, right middle lobe and lingual when the aspiration occurs while the patient is erect, and upper lobes and superior segments of the lower lobes when the aspiration occurs while the patient is recumbent or semirecumbent).

C. Additional investigations.

1. The **fiberoptic endoscopic evaluation of swallowing** is performed using a flexible endoscope inserted through the nasopharynx and provides panoramic visualization of the pharynx and larynx. First the examiners should assess the general appearance of the pharynx and larynx and the movement of the vocal cords during phonation and coughing. Puffs of air are blown into the aryepiglottic folds at gradually increasing thresholds until the laryngeal adductor response is triggered. The cough reflex is by direct stimulation of the mucosa or chemical stimulation using brief inhalation of citric acid. Then swallows of different volumes, viscosities, and consistencies are tested.

2. Advantages are greater anatomical definition and direct testing of laryngeal reflexes. It is also advantageous that it can be performed at the bedside. However, it does not permit visualization of the oropharyngeal events during deglutition.

3. Other studies, such as esophageal manometry, barium swallow, and esophageal endoscopy, are necessary when esophageal pathology is suspected, but these investigations are rarely necessary in cases of dysphagia related to neurologic disease.

TREATMENT

The main goal of dysphagia treatment is to minimize the risk of aspiration, maximize safe oral nutrition and hydration, and regain better quality of life, which is undoubtedly compromised in patients with dysphagia. Behavioral treatments represent the mainstay of dysphagia therapy and can be divided into compensatory and rehabilitative treatments. Surgical options (especially placement of a gastrostomy) are indicated in select circumstances and innovative treatment alternatives are being investigated. A summary list of treatment options is provided in Table 18.4.

A. Compensatory treatments.

1. These treatments are the simplest and most commonly used and consist of interventions aimed at modifying the bolus composition, its internal transit, or the conditions of food ingestion.

2. Postural adjustments. Changes in the posture to compensate for the misdirection of bolus transit. The 45-degree angle chin tuck (to slow bolus transit in patients with delayed pharyngeal trigger) is the most frequently employed. A head tilt toward the strong side may be useful in patients with hemiparesis involving the facial muscles.

3. Diet modification. Avoiding the fluid viscosities and food consistencies aspirated during video fluoroscopic swallowing evaluation. Thickened fluids (thin fluids are more frequently aspirated) and softer diets are commonly recommended, yet specific dietary modifications should be individualized based on the results of the diagnostic investigation. Patients restricted to thickened fluids must be carefully monitored for the possibility of dehydration. As the dysphagia improves, reevaluations are necessary to reincorporate more options to the diet.

4. Modification of eating habits. Education to eat slowly, moisten the oropharynx with some fluid before eating food, take small sips and bites, maintain an upright posture while drinking and eating, eliminate distractions while eating, drink fluids during the meal to wash solid residues in the oropharynx, avoid mixing fluids and solids on the same swallow, avoid talking with fluids or food in the mouth, place the food on the strong side of the mouth (if unilateral weakness).

5. Feeding strategies. Using modified cups, wide or one-way valve straws, and long spoons are some examples of useful interventions in select cases.

B. Rehabilitative treatments.

1. Strengthening exercises. Lingual resistance exercises and other focused interventions to strengthen weak deglutory muscles must be guided by trained therapists.

TABLE 18.4 Options for the Treatment of Dysphagia

Compensatory treatments
Postural adjustments
Diet modification
Change of eating habits
Feeding strategies
Rehabilitative treatments
Strengthening exercises
Range-of-motion exercises
Sensory enhancement
Surgical treatments
Correction of structural abnormalities
Treatment of vocal cord paralysis
Cricopharyngeal myotomy or UES dilatation[a]
Gastrostomy (most often percutaneous)
Therapies under evaluation
Transcranial magnetic stimulation
Implantable neuroprosthesis

[a]Only indicated in cases of isolated cricopharyngeal muscle dysfunction, in which this muscle and the UES fail to relax upon swallowing (can be seen as part of the lateral medullary syndrome).
Abbreviation: UES, upper esophageal sphincter.

2. **Range-of-motion exercises.** Examples include a sequence of tongue movements (including elevation, lateralization, gargling, and retraction) several times per day, or the falsetto exercise (raising the vocal pitch to elevate the larynx).
3. **Sensory enhancement.** Most useful in patients with delayed initiation of the pharyngeal phase. Interventions can consist of applying a cold or sour stimuli at specific sites of the oropharyngeal mucosa or swallowing a cold or sour bolus.

C. **Surgical treatments.**
   1. The main surgical intervention in patients with severe and persistent dysphagia is the placement of gastrostomy for nonoral feeding. Percutaneous gastrostomy can be safely performed at the bedside in many cases.
   2. Gastrostomies are reversible and therefore it is always better to proceed with a gastrostomy in patients with dysphagia who have good prognosis for recovery but cannot eat by mouth for the time being or cannot meet caloric requirements because of swallowing difficulties or dietary restrictions. In these cases of acute and potentially reversible dysphagia, it is important to make patients and families understand that a temporary gastrostomy is a small price to pay to avoid the risk of aspiration pneumonia.
   3. Instead, in patients with chronic progressive dysphagia from a neurologic disorder the decision to proceed with gastrostomy needs to be weighed carefully. In such cases the gastrostomy will be permanent and patients or their families should have a clear understanding of the goal and implications of the intervention.
   4. Other surgical interventions are only applicable to very selected cases, such as those with laryngeal incompetence or isolated cricopharyngeal muscle dysfunction.
   5. Surgery may be very useful to treat associated non-neurologic structural conditions that may be contributing to the dysphagia (such as Zenker's diverticula).

D. **Treatments under investigation.**
   1. There is interest in the application of noninvasive brain stimulation to enhance the rehabilitation of patients with dysphagia after stroke. Available information suggests that repetitive transcranial magnetic stimulation (ipsilateral or contralateral to the stroke) may be beneficial.
   2. Implantable neuroprosthesis consisting of intramuscular stimulation of multiple hyolaryngeal muscles that can be controlled by the patient is also being investigated.

Prognosis

The prognosis of neurogenic dysphagia depends on the cause of the problem.

1. In stroke patients, severe deficits, bihemispheric strokes, and brainstem strokes are associated with persistent dysphagia.
2. Less severe strokes are compatible with favorable recovery and can be helped by compensatory and rehabilitative therapies.
3. In neuromuscular diseases, the dysphagia is temporary in patients with acute conditions and in those with myasthenic exacerbation. Dysphagia is irreversible and progressive in patients with muscular dystrophy.
4. In patients with progressive neurologic disorders (parkinsonian syndromes, motor neuron disease, degenerative dementias, progressive MS), the dysphagia worsens over time, generally following the pace of the primary disease.

Key Points

- Dysphagia is a common manifestation of various acute and chronic neurologic disorders putting these patients at risk for aspiration pneumonia.
- Knowledge of the normal anatomy and physiology of swallowing is necessary to understand the causes of dysphagia.
- Stroke, neuromuscular disorders, and chronic progressive neurodegenerative diseases are the main neurologic causes of dysphagia.
- A bedside water swallowing test must be performed to screen for dysphagia before oral intake not only after any stroke but also when evaluating hospitalized patients with neurologic conditions known to be associated with an increased risk of dysphagia and aspiration pneumonia.
- A video fluoroscopic study is necessary to identify silent aspiration (i.e., silent aspiration cannot be detected by a bedside swallow test).
- Compensatory and rehabilitative treatments guided by specialized therapists can improve swallowing safety in many patients with neurologic causes of dysphagia.

Recommended Readings

Altman KW, Richards A, Goldberg L, et al. Dysphagia in stroke, neurodegenerative disease, and advanced dementia. *Otolaryngol Clin North Am*. 2013;46:1137–1149.

Carnaby-Mann G, Lenius K. The bedside examination in dysphagia. *Phys Med Rehabil Clin N Am*. 2008;19:747–768.

Edmiaston J, Connor LT, Steger-May K, et al. A simple bedside stroke dysphagia screen, validated against videofluoroscopy, detects dysphagia and aspiration with high sensitivity. *J Stroke Cerebrovasc Dis*. 2014;23:712–716.

Kertscher B, Speyer R, Palmieri M, et al. Bedside screening to detect oropharyngeal dysphagia in patients with neurological disorders: an updated systematic review. *Dysphagia*. 2014;29:204–212.

Kumar S. Swallowing and dysphagia in neurological disorders. *Rev Neurol Dis*. 2010;7:19–27.

Kumar S, Doughty C, Doros G, et al. Recovery of swallowing after dysphagic stroke: an analysis of prognostic factors. *J Stroke Cerebrovasc Dis*. 2014;23:56–62.

Logemann JA. *Evaluation and Treatment of Swallowing Disorders*. 2nd ed. Austin, TX: Pro-Ed; 1998.

Malandraki G, Robbins J. Dysphagia. *Handb Clin Neurol*. 2013;110:255–271.

Martin-Harris B, Jones B. The videofluorographic swallowing study. *Phys Med Rehabil Clin N Am*. 2008;19:769–785.

Roden DF, Altman KW. Causes of dysphagia among different age groups: a systematic review of the literature. *Otolaryngol Clin North Am*. 2013;46:965–987.

Shaw SM, Martino R. The normal swallow: muscular and neurophysiological control. *Otolaryngol Clin North Am*. 2013;46:937–956.

Suntrup S, Kemmling A, Warnecke T, et al. The impact of lesion location on dysphagia incidence, pattern and complications in acute stroke: Part 1: dysphagia incidence, severity and aspiration. *Eur J Neurol*. 2015;22:832–838.

Yang SN, Pyun SB, Kim HJ, et al. Effectiveness of noninvasive brain stimulation in dysphagia subsequent to stroke: a systemic review and meta-analysis. *Dysphagia*. 2015;30:383–391.

19 Approach to the Patient with Dysarthria

Sarah S. Kramer, Michael J. Schneck, and José Biller

Normal speech production involves integration and coordination of five primary physiologic subsystems: respiration, phonation, articulation, resonance, and prosody. Impairment of any of these elements may lead to dysarthria ("slurring" of speech). Dysarthria may occur secondary to lesions along any part of the neuroaxis that produce motor dysfunction, affecting any of the five speech subsystems. Lesions can be unilateral, or bilateral, and localize throughout the neuroaxis in the cerebral cortex, subcortical structures, brainstem, cerebellum, basal ganglia, cranial nerves, upper cervical nerves, or even the neuromuscular junction or muscles.

DEFINITION

Dysarthria is a speech disorder of neurologic etiology that results from weakness, paralysis, or incoordination of the speech musculature. Words are slurred, but language content is normal. Dysarthria should be recognized as distinct from mutism, dysphonia, aphasia, and speech apraxia.

CLINICAL PICTURE

A normal speech pattern is achieved through smooth coordination of respiration, phonation, articulation, resonance, and prosody. Adequate breath support and forced exhalation give way to changes in vocal fold length, position, and vibratory pattern. As exhalation occurs, changes in the size and shape of the oral cavity, in conjunction with the articulators, produce phonemes for speech production. At the same time, changes in prosody attach meanings to phonemes with alterations in pitch, intonation, stress, and rate. Together, these speech mechanisms allow us to effectively participate in daily conversation. The semiology of dysarthria may include slurred speech, slow or rapid speech, whispering speech, abnormal intonation, and changes in vocal quality. Associated clinical findings include limited or abnormal movements of the tongue, jaw or lips, drooling, and difficulty chewing or swallowing.

TYPES OF DYSARTHRIA

Differentiating among dysarthria types is not simple as there is much overlap in the semiology of the various types, though certain speech characteristics are often associated with specific types of dysarthria. The flaccid, spastic, mixed, ataxic, hypokinetic, and hyperkinetic dysarthria are best characterized and described below (see also Table 19.1).

A. **Flaccid dysarthria** may occur when there is damage to the lower motor neurons (LMNs) or cranial nerves that innervate the muscles of the head and neck. Slowed or imprecise articulations of consonants, breathy vocal quality, hypernasality, and/or nasal emissions are features of flaccid dysarthria. The symptoms may vary, depending on which of the cranial nerves are involved. Muscle weakness, hypotonia, and/or atrophy may be observed. One common cause of flaccid dysarthria is idiopathic peripheral seventh cranial nerve palsy (Bell's). Often these patients complain of changes in speech, drooling, and oral dysphagia. The face may appear asymmetrical during range of motion tasks even if normal at rest. Other diagnoses may include stroke, cerebral palsy, tumor, myasthenia gravis (MG), amyotrophic lateral sclerosis (ALS), or Guillain–Barré syndrome.

B. **Spastic dysarthria,** as seen in pseudobulbar palsy, results from damage to the upper motor neuron (UMN) tracts of the pyramidal and extrapyramidal tracts. Features of spastic dysarthria may include imprecise articulation of consonants, harsh and/or strained

TABLE 19.1 Mayo Clinic Classification of Dysarthria

Dysarthria Type	Neurologic Condition	Location of Lesion	Most Distinctive Speech Deviation
Flaccid	Bulbar palsy	LMN	Marked hypernasality, often with nasal air emission; continuous breathiness; audible inspiration
Spastic	Pseudobulbar palsy	UMN	Very imprecise articulation; slow rate; low pitch; harsh, strained or strangled voice
Ataxic	Cerebellar ataxia	Cerebellum	Excess stress and monostress; phoneme and interval prolongation; dysrhythmia of speech and syllable repetition; slow rate; some excess loudness variation
Hypokinetic	Parkinsonism	Extrapyramidal system	Monopitch, monoloudness, reduced overall loudness; variable rate; short rushes of speech; some inappropriate silences
Hyperkinetic Quick	Chorea	Extrapyramidal system	Highly variable pattern of imprecise articulation; episodes of hypernasality; sudden variations in loudness
	Myoclonus		Rhythmic hypernasality; rhythmic phonatory interruption
	Tourette's syndrome		Sudden tic-like grunts, barks, coprolalia
Slow	Athetosis	Extrapyramidal system	No distinct deviation
	Dyskinesias	Extrapyramidal system	No distinct deviation
	Dystonia	Extrapyramidal system	Prolongations of phonemes, intervals, unsteady rate, loudness
Tremors	Organic voice tremor	Extrapyramidal system	Rhythmic alterations in pitch, loudness, voice stoppages
Mixed	ALS	Multiple motor systems	Grossly defective articulation; extremely slow, laborious rate; marked hypernasality; severe harshness, strained or strangled voice; nearly complete disruption of prosody
	Wilson's disease		Reduced stress; monopitch; monoloudness; similar to hypokinetic dysarthria except no short rushes of speech
	MS		Impaired control of loudness; harshness

Abbreviations: ALS, amyotrophic lateral sclerosis; LMN, lower motor neuron; MS, multiple sclerosis; UMN, upper motor neuron.
Adapted from Johns DF, ed. *Clinical Management of Neurogenic Communicative Disorders.* 2nd ed. Boston, MA: Little, Brown and Company; 1985.
Adapted from Johns DF, ed. *Clinical Management of Neurogenic Communicative Disorders.* 2nd ed. Boston, MA: Little Brown; 1985.

or strangled vocal quality, and hypernasality (Video 19.1). Other findings include muscle weakness with greater than normal tone. Dysphagia may also occur. In addition to spastic dysarthria, the patient with pseudobulbar palsy may often exhibit emotional lability and may exhibit spontaneous outbursts of laughter or crying known as "pseudobulbar affect." Spastic dysarthria may also result from ischemic insults. Isolated or "pure" dysarthria results mainly from small subcortical infarcts involving the internal capsule or corona radiata. Isolated dysarthria, with facial paresis, is considered a variant of the dysarthria-clumsy hand lacunar syndrome. Occasionally, an isolated small subcortical infarct will interrupt the corticolingual fibers from the motor cortex, causing dysarthria without hemiparesis. Other common causes of spastic dysarthria include tumor, traumatic brain injury, spastic cerebral palsy, multiple sclerosis (MS), and ALS.

C. **Mixed dysarthria** is caused by simultaneous damage to two or more primary motor components of the nervous system, involving both UMNs and LMNs. This form of dysarthria

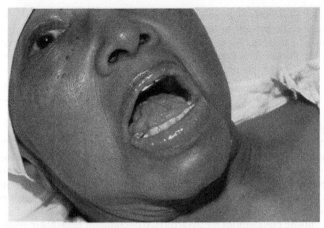

FIGURE 19.1 Diffuse tongue atrophy and fasciculations in a patient with bulbar motor neuron disease.

is common in patients with MS, ALS, or severe traumatic brain injury. The patients may speak very slowly and with great effort. Articulation is markedly impaired with imprecise articulation and hypernasality. Vocal pitch is low with harsh and/or strained, or strangled vocal quality. Prosody is disrupted with intonation errors and inappropriately shortened phrases/sentences. Bulbar involvement in ALS often presents in this fashion with dysarthria, hypophonia, drooling of saliva, and progressive swallowing difficulties (Fig. 19.1).

D. Ataxic dysarthria is usually associated with cerebellar disorders with articulation and prosody most impaired. Patients present with decreased motor coordination for accurate articulation with slow and deliberate articulation, imprecise consonant production, distorted vowel production, and prolonged phonemes. Equal and excessive stress is placed on all syllables. Ataxic dysarthria is caused by damage to the cerebellum, or cerebellar connections to other parts of the brain. Isolated cerebellar dysarthria has also been reported with small infarcts in the left paravermian zone of the ventral cerebellum (lobulus simplex and semilunaris superior).

E. Hypokinetic dysarthria, most typically seen in parkinsonism, is associated with hypophonia or reduced vocal loudness. Furthermore, there is monotonous speech with a slow and flat rhythm. Initiation of speech is difficult, resulting in inappropriate silences intermixed with short rushes of speech. The rate is variable with wide fluctuations in pitch.

F. Hyperkinetic dysarthria also results from secondary to damage to the basal ganglia and is typified by Huntington's disease. Damage to this system causes involuntary movements such as tremors, dyskinesia, athetosis, and dystonia. Vocal quality may be described as harsh, strained, or strangled and is often associated with spasmodic dysphonia.

DIFFERENTIAL DIAGNOSIS

The major clinical distinctions are between dysarthria, dysphonia, apraxia, and aphasia. Both dysarthria and apraxia are motor speech disorders, and it may be sometimes difficult to differentiate among them. Apraxia of speech is a motor programming or planning disorder involving speech production tasks. Automatic and involuntary tasks are usually spared. Errors in articulation are inconsistent and are associated primarily with vowel and consonant distortions. Initiation is difficult with obvious effortful groping in attempts by the patient to achieve accurate movement of the articulators. Patients are often aware of the errors and make specific attempts at correcting the errors. However, the patients are often unsuccessful in achieving initial articulatory configurations or transitioning from one sound to the next.

Aphasia is a loss or impairment of language production and/or comprehension, often accompanied by a loss of ability to read and/or write, whereas dysarthria is a problem in speech articulation. It is not uncommon for aphasia and dysarthria to coexist. A person with aphasia may be able to communicate with adequate breath support, voicing, and articulation, but may be unable to comprehend other persons or name, repeat, or express themselves adequately.

Patients may also have isolated anomia (word-finding difficulty) with inability to state certain words or name specific persons or objects.

Dysphonia is a term that describes voice disorders. It is a characteristic of certain types of dysarthria. Dysphonia, however, may stand alone when describing other voice disorders. Spasmodic dysphonia is a specific type of neurologic voice disorder that involves involuntary tightening or constriction of the vocal cords, causing interruptions of speech and affecting the voice quality, which can be strained or strangled.

DIAGNOSTIC EVALUATION

A detailed history and thorough neurologic examination are essential to determine the possible etiology of the different types of dysarthria. The presenting symptoms, duration, pattern of speech disturbance, and progression of symptoms may help elucidate the mechanism and etiology of dysarthria. In particular, acute onset of symptoms would suggest a possible stroke as the basis of the dysarthria, but one should avoid diagnostic closure and always consider alternative diagnostic explanations for dysarthria. Concomitant neurologic symptoms, medical comorbidities, and knowledge of contributory medications or exposures may all help determine the etiology of the dysarthria. A complete examination is necessary to determine the nature of dysarthria; for example, patients with extrapyramidal disorders have slow, quiet, and monotonous speech, which is gradually progressive and is typically associated with rigidity, bradykinesia, falls associated with postural instability, and characteristic tremors. Scanning speech with dysprosody is often suggestive of a cerebellar disorder, especially when incoordination and gait unsteadiness are present. Patients with an LMN lesion may have pronounced tongue atrophy and fasciculations, with gradual and progressive muscle weakness, whereas an UMN disease is characterized by spastic and explosive speech. Palatal palsy and decreased gag reflex with tongue weakness may indicate bulbar involvement, whereas a brisk jaw jerk, hyperactive gag reflex, and emotional lability are suggestive of pseudobulbar palsy. Mechanical factors contributing to dysarthria include pharyngeal, vocal cord, tracheal, and other airway lesions. Trauma and space-occupying masses in these areas must also be considered.

Neuroimaging studies of the head or neck may be helpful in diagnosing central and peripheral causes (see Chapter 35) with magnetic resonance imaging with contrast enhancement as the preferred modality. Electromyography (EMG) and nerve conduction studies may be an important tool in the diagnosis of motor neuron disease, peripheral nerve injury or focal dystonia, polyneuropathy, myopathy, or neuromuscular junction disorders such as MG or the Lambert–Eaton myasthenic syndrome (LEMS) (see Chapter 36). Repetitive nerve stimulation or single-fiber EMG to help diagnose neuromuscular junction syndromes should be considered in appropriate cases, and EMG of facial, pharyngeal, or tongue muscles may sometimes be useful in elucidating the mechanism of dysarthria. Lumbar puncture and cerebrospinal fluid analysis are discussed in Chapter 33. Pulmonary function testing may be helpful to assess respiratory function and coordination associated with sound production. Specialized serum studies may also be indicated to identify the underlying etiology of dysarthria (for example, serum antibody panels may help diagnose MG or LEMS).

EVALUATION OF SPEECH FUNCTION

In the evaluation of speech disorders, a speech–language pathologist (SLP) is often consulted to differentiate various types of dysarthria and help determine treatment strategies. Several core components are included in the evaluation. The SLP, after reviewing the neurologic and medical evaluation, conducts an interview with the patient and/or caregiver. This interview helps to further define the time of onset, pattern of symptoms, previous assessments completed or treatment received, and the course of symptom improvement of the dysarthria over time.

An examination of the physical structures of the speech mechanism, as well as assessment of articulation, respiration, phonation, resonance, and prosody is performed. This includes a thorough oral mechanism examination to assess strength, rate of movement, range of motion, and coordination of the speech mechanism including the jaw, lips, tongue, and velopharyngeal function. Deviations from the norm give way to articulation errors. Articulation can further be assessed in diadochokinetic rate and by listening to a brief speech sample. Abnormalities are noted with the production of imprecise consonants, producing voiced for voiceless syllables, repeated or prolonged phonemes, or vowel distortions. Speech intelligibility can be rated as well. With decrease in laryngeal control, a patient may be unable to produce voiceless syllables. Abnormalities in respiration are often observed in sustained phonation tasks. A patient may be unable to sustain a vowel, such as "ah," with normal loudness. Verbal output may also be limited to single words or short phrases due to a lack of expiratory effort. Vocal quality may be breathy, and a patient may be unable to maintain voicing throughout the length of a phrase or sentence. Voicing may start strong, but gradually fade with increased phrase or sentence length.

Appropriate phonation is dependent on adequate respiration. Adequate breath support is required to achieve functional vocal fold vibration for phonation. Abnormalities in voicing may be attributed to unilateral or bilateral vocal fold (cord) paralysis, a vocal cord mass, or vocal cord edema. Vocal fold adduction may be compromised resulting in a breathy vocal quality (hypofunction). Excessive adduction of the vocal folds gives way to possible strained or strangled output in addition to increased pitch (hyperfunction). If there is a suspicion of an abnormal approximation of the vocal folds, an ear-nose-and-throat (ENT) specialist consultation should be considered. Assessment of phonation includes sustained phonation tasks. Having the patient sustain a vowel ("ah" or "ee") for as long as they can allows the SLP to discriminate between variations in pitch, breath support, loudness, and voice quality. Of note, measuring maximum length of phonation provides limited direction in differentiating among dysarthria's because sustained phonation is not characteristic of functional conversational speech.

Hypernasality and hyponasality are characterized by abnormalities in resonance. Hypernasality may be evidenced by an excess escape of air into the nasal cavity resulting from reduced velopharyngeal closure or soft palate weakness. It is also important to watch the soft palate at rest, and during sustained phonation, for functional movement or possible fatigue. Hyponasality results from inadequate velopharyngeal opening, which may be caused from a complete or partial blockage of nasal airway. If a blockage is suspected, further ENT evaluation may be required. Prosody can be analyzed by assessing the coordination of respiration, phonation, and articulation. Errors in prosody may present as abnormally slowed or rapid rate of speech, decreased stress or emphasis patterns, intonation errors, or inappropriately shortened phrases/sentences that can be mixed with intervals of silence. Prosody can be assessed within the speech sample or by having the patient imitate various phrases. One sample of stress or intonation variations is "Is THAT your car?", "Is that YOUR car?", and "Is that your CAR?" Clearly, varying the stress/intonation within this short sentence may result in significant changes in the meaning of a sentence.

Impairments to any of the above-listed speech mechanisms resulting in dysarthria often coexist with dysphagia. Current standards require that dysphagia screening be documented on all stroke patients; dysphagia screening should be done on all patients with dysarthria, however. Dysphagia is frequently present with dysarthria in patients with extrapyramidal, motor neuron, or neuromuscular disorders. If dysphagia is noted with a brief swallow screening, a formal swallow evaluation is indicated, and should include a thorough history for possible dysphagia and assessment of oral mechanisms for strength, movement, and coordination of the muscles for swallowing. If then deemed safe, the patient is given various consistencies of liquids and/or solids, and tolerance to the various samples is observed and evaluated. The SLP, through observation and hands-on assessment, notes oral, pharyngeal, and sometimes esophageal difficulties. Depending upon the clinical results of the bedside exam, the SLP may recommend oral feeding with the least-restrictive liquids and/or solids, a video fluoroscopic swallow evaluation, or both. When indicated, a fiberoptic endoscopic evaluation of swallowing may also be helpful for the assessment of swallowing function as well as actual movement of the vocal cords and tracheopharygneal muscles involved in the mechanics of swallowing and speech production.

MANAGEMENT

The underlying etiology of the dysarthria type and overall prognosis for improvement must be taken into careful consideration when devising a treatment plan for the dysarthria. Treatment of the underlying condition (i.e., drugs for neuromuscular or extrapyramidal disorders) will often result in improvement in dysarthria. Treatment also includes patient and family education, and training, about compensatory strategies. Treatment of respiratory/phonatory deficits may include improving breath support to increase vocal volume. Slowing the rate of speech may be necessary to improve articulation and intelligibility. Nonspeech oral-motor training may be recommended for strengthening muscles and increasing mouth, tongue, and lip range of motion and movement. Changes in loudness and prosody, through intonation and stress patterning tasks, may be targets of intervention as well. In severe cases, augmentative and alternative communication devices, such as computerized voice production systems, may be needed.

Key Points

- Normal speech occurs with smooth coordination of respiration, phonation, articulation, resonance, and prosody.
- Components of dysarthria may include slurred speech, slow or rapid speech, whispering speech, abnormal intonation, and changes in vocal quality.
- Six major types of dysarthria have been described: flaccid, spastic, mixed, ataxic, hypokinetic, and hyperkinetic.
- Identification of the underlying cause of dysarthria is imperative; treating the cause will often result in improvement of dysarthria.
- Consider dysphagia screening for all patients with dysarthria, regardless of etiology.
- Speech–language therapy is an integral part of dysarthria treatment.

Recommended Readings

Amarenco P, Cherrie-Muller C, Roullet E, et al. Paravermal infarct and isolated cerebellar dysarthria. *Ann Neurol.* 1991;30(2):211–213.

Biller J, Gruener G, Brazis P. *DeMyer's The Neurologic Examination: A Programmed Text.* 7th ed. New York, NY: McGraw-Hill Medical; 2017.

Brazis PW, Masdeu JC, Biller J. Cranial Nerve XII (The Hypoglossal Nerve) In: *Localization in Clinical Neurology.* 7th ed. Philadelphia, PA: Wolters Kluwer; 2017. Chapter 14; 409-416.

Clebisoy M, Tokucoglu F, Basoglu M. Isolated dysarthria—facial paresis syndrome: a rare clinical entity which is usually overlooked. *Neurol India.* 2005;53(2):183–185.

Darley FL, Aronson AE, Brown JR. *Motor Speech Disorders.* Philadelphia, PA: WB Saunders; 1975.

Duffy JR. *Motor Speech Disorders: Substrates, Differential Diagnosis, and Management.* St. Louis, MO: Mosby; 1995.

Dworkin JP. *Motor Speech Disorders: A Treatment Guide.* St. Louis, MO: Mosby; 1991.

Fisher CM. A lacunar stroke. The dysarthria-clumsy hand syndrome. *Neurology.* 1967;17:614–617.

Gucci MR, Grant LM, Rajamanickam ES, et al. Early identification and treatment of communication and swallowing deficits in Parkinson disease (review). *Semin Speech Lang.* 2013;34(3):185–202.

Hustad KC, Beukelman DR, Yorkston KM. Functional outcome assessment in dysarthria. *Semin Speech Lang.* 1998;19:291–302.

Hustad KC, Jones T, Dailey S. Implementing speech supplementation strategies: effects on intelligibility and speech rate of individuals with chronic severe dysarthria. *J Speech Lang Hear Res.* 2003;46:462–474.

Jani MP, Gore GB. Occurrence of communication and swallowing problems in neurological disorders: analysis of forty patients. *Neurorehabilitation.* 2014;35(4):719–727.

Kaye M. *Guide to Dysarthria Management: A Client–Clinician Approach.* Eau Claire, WI: Thinking Publications; 2005.

Kent RD, Duffy JR, Slama A, et al. Clinicoanatomic studies in dysarthria: review, critique, and directions for research. *J Speech Lang Hear Res.* 2001;44:535–551.

Knuijt T, Kalf JG, deSwart BJ, et al. Dysarthria and dysphagia are highly prevalent among various types of neuromuscular diseases. *Disabil Rehabil.* 36(15):1285–1289.

Kruger E, Teasell R, Salter K, et al. The rehabilitation of patients recovering from brainstem strokes; case studies and clinical considerations. *Top Stroke Rehabil.* 2007;14(5):56–64.

Kuncl RN, ed. *Motor Neuron Disease.* London, UK: WB Saunders; 2002.

Love RJ, Webb WG. *Neurology for the Speech–Language Pathologist.* 2nd ed. Boston, MA: Butterworth–Heinemann; 1992.

Merson RM, Rolnick MI. Speech-language pathology and dysphagia in multiple sclerosis (review). *Phys Med Rehabil Clin N Am.* 1998;9(3):631–641.

Murdoch B. *Dysarthria: A Physiological Approach to Assessment and Treatment*. Frederick, CO: Aspen Publishers; 1998.

Ohtomo R, Iwata A, Tsuji S. Unilateral opercular infarction presenting with Foix-Chavany-Marie Syndrome. *J Stroke Cerebrovasc Dis*. 2014;23(1):179–181.

Okuda B, Kawabata K, Tachibana H, et al. Cerebral blood flow in pure dysarthria. Role of frontal cortical hypoperfusion. *Stroke*. 1999;30:109–113.

Okuda B, Tachibana H. Isolated dysarthria. *J Neurol Neurosurg Psychiatry*. 2000;68:119–120.

Pinto S, Ozsancak C, Tripoliti E, et al. Treatments for dysarthria in Parkinson's disease. *Lancet Neurol*. 2004;3:547–556.

Robert D, Bianco-Blache A, Spezza C, et al. Assessment of dysarthria and dysphagia in ALS patients. *Rev Neurol (Paris)*. 2006;162:445–453.

Robin DA, Yorkston KM, Beukelman DR. *Disorders of Motor Speech*. Baltimore, MD: Paul H. Brookes Publishing; 1996.

Russell JA, Ciucci MR, Connor NP, et al. Targeted exercise therapy for voice and swallow in persons with Parkinson's disease (Review). *Brain Res*. 2010;1341:3–11.

Sellars C, Hughes T, Langhorne P. Speech and language therapy for dysarthria due to non-progressive brain damage. *Cochrane Database Syst Rev*. 2005;3:CD002088.

Urban PP, Rolke R, Wicht S, et al. Left hemisphere dominance for articulation: a prospective study on acute ischaemic dysarthria at different localizations. *Brain*. 2006;129:767–777.

Urban PP, Wicht S, Vukurevic G, et al. Dysarthria in acute ischemic stroke. Lesion topography, clinicoradiologic correlation, and etiology. *Neurology*. 2001;56:1021–1027.

Vogel D, Cannito MP. *Treating Disordered Speech Motor Control*. 2nd ed. Austin, TX: Pro-Ed; 2001.

Yorkston KM, Beukelman DR, Strand EA, et al. *Management of Motor Speech—Disorders in Children and Adults*. 2nd ed. Austin, TX: Pro-Ed; 1999.

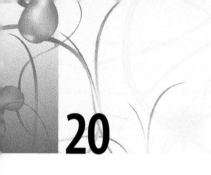

20

Approach to the Patient with Acute Headache

Mark W. Green and Sarah L. Rahal

Headache is the most common neurologic complaint seen in the primary care and emergency department (ED) setting, with a lifetime prevalence of 90% of the general population and representing 5 million ED visits annually. Although primary headache disorders, like migraine and tension-type headache, comprise the vast majority, patients may also present with headaches as a manifestation of underlying disease processes called "secondary headache" disorders. A patient's fear of a secondary headache in the form of brain tumor or cerebral aneurysm is often what drives them to seek medical care. The challenge to the practitioner becomes discerning between these two headache types. Most primary and secondary headaches can be clinically diagnosed without expensive and laborious testing distinguishing those with worrisome pathology, who require more urgent evaluation and possibly treatment. Primary headaches may cause pain and disability, but despite this, it is important to remember that they are almost never dangerous in and of themselves.

Headache is a clinical diagnosis, and most of the clues a practitioner will need lie in the patient's history supplemented by examination findings. In some cases a patient may warrant a thorough workup evaluating for secondary pathology. Moreover, a patient may have both a history of a primary headache disorder as well as a new neurologic disease process. In fact, given how common migraine is, with a lifetime prevalence of 18%, this would not be a rare occurrence. In a patient with a well-documented history of migraines, for instance, new underlying brain pathology may be present only as a change in pattern of the migraine headaches (Video 20.1).

TAKING A HEADACHE HISTORY

Pertinent History

1. Establish an anchor in time: when did the headaches first appear and have they changed since that time? Is there a history of head injury?
2. Burden of headache: number of headache days/month as well as functionally incapacitating headache days. Mild headaches might otherwise not be reported, but may signal a more chronic state. Note that asking how many headaches are experienced can be deceptive as attacks can last seconds to days.
3. If an acute headache, what was the activity at the time the headache occurred?
   Triggers of attacks include sleep (too little or too much), exercise, Valsalva, cough, sex, menstruation, ovulation, stress and relaxation following stress, foods, and dehydration. These triggers in particular can trigger migraine, although headaches triggered by Valsalva should prompt an evaluation for an intracranial lesion. Cluster attacks are often triggered by sleep and alcohol.
4. Individual attacks: first symptom, rate of progression, location of pain (in the beginning of the attack and as it progresses). Some attacks reach full intensity in an instant, and others over hours to days.
5. Are there prodromal symptoms hours to days before the attack? These are typical of migraines.
6. Symptoms associated with headache: photophobia or phonophobia, nausea, vomiting (when do they occur with the attacks; early nausea can alter the route of administration of an acute drug to an injection or nasal spray).
7. Are there focal symptoms accompanying the headache? Migraine auras can involve vision, sensory, or motor symptoms and need to be distinguished from stroke or transient ischemic attack.

8. Were the attacks positional in their onset? Low-pressure headaches generally cause orthostatic headaches at the beginning, but over time this feature may be lost. In low-pressure headache, patients are best as they awaken and the pain worsens as they arise and throughout the day with increased activity.
9. What is the severity of an attack, how is it limiting function? It is most useful to describe the behavior and limitations in functioning that are experienced with an attack. Simply using the 1 to 10 scale often does not yield reliable information.
10. What is the person's behavior during an attack (bed rest, quiet, pacing, lights off)? Migraines, being worse with activity and associated with light and sound sensitivity, cause the sufferer to often seek bed rest in a quiet and dark room. Cluster headache sufferers typically rock and pace, unable to be still.
11. What is the duration of an attack with and without treatment? Migraines typically last 4 hours to 3 days. Cluster headaches typically last 1 to 2 hours.
12. Is there a postdrome? This is a period of time, ranging from hours to days following an attack manifested by fatigue, poor mood, and difficulty in concentration.
13. What is currently being used to prevent attacks and to treat individual attacks? What dose, how many, for how long? How are they used? Are the acute agents used early in the attack, which increases efficacy and reduces the rate of recurrence? Are they being overused, which can lead to an increase in headaches over time? Are preventive agents being used in an adequate dose and for an adequate period of time in order to determine their efficacy? Early on in the use of preventive agents, the side effects are higher and the efficacy lower, which can lead to discontinuation.
14. What treatments have been used in the past? What were the doses of the medications used and how long were they used? Preventive agents often take many weeks to become effective and at an adequate dose so that brief trials do not prove that the agent is ineffective.
15. What laboratory and imaging studies have been performed in the past? Be certain to personally review these results.
16. Is there a family history of headaches? How were their headaches described and what diagnosis was given? Be aware that the assigned diagnosis may be inaccurate.

The Primary Headaches

Primary headache disorders most commonly have onset in childhood and early adult years. Onset in the very young or very old may be worrisome. Migraine prevalence increases steadily until age 40, after which it declines, with peak prevalence from 25 to 55 years of age. Headaches are common in young children. For instance, epidemiologic studies show that by age 7, 37% to 51.5% of children report headache. In the 3-to-5-year-olds, headaches are more prevalent in boys; however, as puberty approaches the incidence and prevalence of headache increases in girls. Age, additionally, may play a role in the manifestation of a primary headache disorder. In particular, children may exhibit "migraine equivalents" such as cyclic vomiting syndrome or benign paroxysmal vertigo, which may presage the development of migraine later in life.

Migraine

Although tension-type headache is the most common variety of headache, a patient presenting to a primary care physician with episodic headache most likely has migraine. Migraine is the phenotypic expression of a large variety of conditions, often with a genetic predisposition. Many adults with migraine also have a history of carsickness, vertiginous spells, and abdominal pain in childhood.

Most attacks, if carefully investigated, begin with a prodrome, which can precede the pain by a day or more. Common prodromes include cold hands and feet, yawning, food cravings, and frequent urination. Recognizing a prodrome may lead to successful preemptive treatment.

Migraine without aura is the most common form comprising about 80% of migraines whereas migraine with aura comprised about 20%.

Migraine without Aura (ICHD-3 Criteria)
A. At least five attacks fulfilling criteria B–D
B. Headache attacks lasting 4 to 72 hours (untreated or unsuccessfully treated)

C. Headache has at least two of the following four characteristics:
1. unilateral location
2. pulsating quality
3. moderate or severe pain intensity
4. aggravation by or causing avoidance of routine physical activity (e.g., walking or climbing stairs)
D. During headache at least one of the following:
1. nausea and/or vomiting
2. photophobia and phonophobia
E. Not better accounted for by another *ICHD-3* diagnosis.

Migraine with Aura (ICHD-3 Criteria)

A. At least two attacks fulfilling criteria B and C
B. One or more of the following fully reversible aura symptoms:
1. visual
2. sensory
3. speech and/or language
4. motor
5. brainstem
6. retinal
C. At least two of the following four characteristics:
1. At least one aura symptom spreads gradually over 5 minutes, and/or two or more symptoms occur in succession.
2. Each individual aura symptom lasts 5 to 60 minutes.
3. At least one aura symptom is unilateral.
4. The aura is accompanied, or followed within 60 minutes, by headache.
D. Not better accounted for by another *ICHD-3* diagnosis and transient ischemic attack has been excluded.

In practice, the diagnosis of migraine is made more liberally as migraineurs have attacks, which vary in location, quality, and duration but are considered to be part of the "spectrum of migraine."

How a migraine presents affects its treatment. Preventive medications are recommended when 6 or more days/month are associated with headache. A realistic expectation is to reduce the attacks by 50% and to render attacks more amenable to treatment. It remains to be determined if aggressive preventive treatment reduces the likelihood of progression.

Individual attacks need to be managed even with successful preventive treatments, as preventive agents are rarely completely successful. Most attacks can be managed with oral medications, but if attacks reach full intensity rapidly or when attacks are associated with early nausea, parenteral medications may be necessary. Auras, should they occur, generally precede the headache, but may begin during the headache period and more than one aura can occur in succession. The headache may develop gradually over several minutes to hours, but at times can reach full intensity rapidly. Attacks tend to last 4 to 72 hours, although there is a great deal of variation. Sleep may terminate attacks, particularly in children. Following the resolution of headache, there can be a postdromal period of several days during which there can be mild but persistent pain and fatigue.

Tension-type Headaches

Although tension-type headaches are the most common headache, by definition they are not disabling, and individuals self-treat and therefore rarely seek medical attention. However, headaches of similar description can occur in an individual as part of the "spectrum of migraine" and are considered to be a variation of migraine. When an individual presents with tension-type headache, it is important to query whether they also suffer other types of headaches, which may uncover the underlying migraine history. Additionally, headaches that are triggered by "tension" are not necessarily tension-type headaches. The usual symptoms are a dull, nonpulsatile headache, often described as constricting. Pericranial tenderness may be present. There is no significant nausea and no vomiting; photophobia or phonophobia, if any, is minimal; and, unlike migraine, these are not worsened with activity.

Treatment of tension-type headaches usually involves the periodic use of simple analgesics. The use of opioids is inappropriate, and the use of butalbital-containing analgesics should be sparing, if at all. Chronic tension-type headache is generally treated with amitriptyline. Small studies suggest that mirtazapine or venlafaxine may be of value. There are no significant studies supporting the use of selective serotonin reuptake inhibitors or muscle relaxants, although anecdotally, tizanidine may be helpful. Onabotulinumtoxin has not shown to be helpful. Electromyography biofeedback, cognitive behavioral therapy, and relaxation therapy may be effective.

Cluster Headaches and Other Trigeminal Autonomic Cephalalgias

A. Cluster headache.

One of the primary headache syndromes, characterized by periods of a few weeks to a few months when one or more headaches are experienced daily, lasting 30 to 120 minutes. A great deal of variation exists. The headaches reach full intensity over minutes, but are not apoplectic in onset. The pain is always unilateral; commonly retro-orbital or temporal, but maxillary pain can exist. The quality is boring and aching often with superimposed sharp pains. Nausea, if present, is generally not prominent. The pain is associated with ipsilateral lacrimation and rhinorrhea. It is often confused with migraine although the quality, associated symptoms, and temporal profile differ. Unlike migraineurs who prefer to be still, cluster attacks are associated with relentless hyperactivity.

1. Treatment. The treatment is only during the active cluster period and there is no evidence that continuing the treatment beyond this prevents the next cluster period.

During this time, both preventive and acute medications are used. Preventive agents include verapamil, which often requires high doses, and may be combined with topiramate or divalproex. Given the severity of cluster attacks and the fact that there may be a considerable latency before preventive agents become effective, a bridge using prednisone is often advised.

Preventive agents are rarely fully effective and acute treatments need to be offered. Sumatriptan subcutaneous injections are likely to be the most effective. Unlike in migraine, 2 or 3 mg subcutaneously may suffice, and since the maximum daily dose is 12 mg, there is an opportunity to treat several attacks with these lower doses. Triptan tablets and nasal sprays are unlikely to be adequate. High-flow oxygen may also be effective; using 10 to 12 L daily with a non-rebreathing mask. This needs to be initiated early in an attack and should be continued for several minutes after the attack appears to be terminated.

Hemicrania Continua

This is a continuous, although variable in intensity, unilateral headache. Exacerbations recur throughout the day associated with ipsilateral lacrimation and rhinorrhea. A dramatic response to indomethacin is seen, which is both a treatment and a diagnostic test.

Episodic and Chronic Paroxysmal Hemicrania

These attacks are very similar to attacks of cluster headaches, except they are brief, usually a few minutes, and recurrent with multiple attacks daily. There is a less common episodic form, with remissions. When pain is severe it is accompanied by ipsilateral lacrimation and rhinorrhea. Unlike cluster, more females suffer from this condition. A dramatic and persistent response to indomethacin is characteristic although some respond to topiramate, which should be attempted given the toxicity of indomethacin.

Secondary Headaches

Headaches Due to Increased Intracranial Pressure

Headaches due to increased intracranial pressure (ICP) include mass lesions in the brain, such as tumors and abscesses.

A. Brain tumors.

Although these have often been characterized as early morning headaches that awaken one from sleep and improve as the day advances, this is not the usual profile. In most cases of secondary headache, the headache is more prominent in those with a preexisting history of a primary headache, such as migraine. The headache experienced is then likely amplification of the preexisting headache type, often associated with more nausea, more frequent, and of longer duration. Therefore, a significant change in a preexisting headache type rather than simply a new headache should prompt a reevaluation. Only 1% of patients with brain tumors have headache as the sole manifestation. Headaches with brain tumors are commonly worse with Valsalva maneuver or exertion, which can also occur as a migraine manifestation. They may awaken the person from sleep, but this is common with cluster headache and migraine as well. Brain abscess may present as a brain tumor and fever is seen with only half of the cases.

B. **Subdural hematoma,** being a mass lesion, has the same features as the headache associated with brain tumors. As they are extra-axial, the lack of focality on examination and a change in sensorium is common. A history of head trauma is not invariable, particularly in the elderly or those with alcoholism.

C. **Idiopathic intracranial hypertension** is a condition of elevated CSF pressure. The most common profile is that of young, obese females with menstrual irregularities. However, thin females and males may also develop the condition. Since there is diffuse pressure elevations, no focality on examination is expected and the headache has the features of a "brain tumor headache." Diplopia, mostly commonly secondary to sixth-nerve palsy, is common, as is pulsatile tinnitus. As the increased pressure is transmitted to root sleeves, radicular pain can accompany the headache. Papilledema is generally, but not invariably, present.

1. Diagnosis. Magnetic resonance imaging (MRI) shows small- or normal-sized ventricles with no masses. Careful evaluation of the globes may demonstrate flattening of the posterior portion of the globe, protruding optic nerve heads, and vertical tortuosity of the optic nerves. Magnetic resonance venography (MRV) excludes a venous sinus thrombosis, although transverse sinuses may be compressed, probably secondary to the swelling, and may be falsely blamed as the cause. There is also a great deal of anatomic variability in venous sinuses. A lumbar puncture (LP) to follow is expected to show normal or low cerebrospinal fluid (CSF) protein and elevated pressure, but is otherwise normal.

2. Etiology. Many cases are idiopathic. Many endocrinopathies, intoxications of vitamin A, tetracycline, and obesity are common triggers of the syndrome.

3. Treatment. The course of the headache and the increased ICP may not run in parallel. Visual field testing needs to be closely monitored even if the headaches improve. Carbonic anhydrase inhibitors or loop diuretics are most commonly employed. Topiramate is a carbonic anhydrase inhibitor commonly effective in the treatment of headache, and also induces weight loss. Serial LPs are not recommended. If the vision is threatened, ventricular shunting or optic nerve fenestration is recommended, which may also improve head pain. In morbidly obese patients, bariatric surgery can be helpful.

Exertional Headaches

The headaches of mass lesions can be triggered by exertion, but other etiologies share this feature. Benign cough headaches are most common in middle-aged males, and headaches have an abrupt onset with cough or sneezing or stooping triggering this pain. The disorder is generally self-limiting and indomethacin can be of value. Other exertional headaches exist, including a pain of abrupt onset with orgasm, and also can be prevented with indomethacin. All of these cases should be evaluated to exclude structural causes. Some cases of benign exertional headaches respond to propranolol or nadolol.

Headaches of Abrupt Onset

Thunderclap headache refers to headache, which reaches it full intensity over seconds. The most worrisome is the headache of subarachnoid hemorrhage. Although "the worst headache of my life" in the emergency room is likely to be a severe migraine, this history should always prompt an evaluation to exclude a subarachnoid hemorrhage with, at the minimum, a noncontrast computed tomography (CT) scan. It is not rare for a subarachnoid hemorrhage to have a more gradual onset. The mortality with each subarachnoid hemorrhage approaches 50% so it is essential to make a rapid diagnosis. Low-volume bleeds, often referred to as "sentinel headaches," commonly precede a catastrophic subarachnoid hemorrhage, and intervention at this point is often life saving. A short-lived headache or a good response to a medication does not exclude a low-volume hemorrhage.

Recurring thunderclap headaches are less likely to be due to recurring subarachnoid hemorrhages, but reversible cerebral vasoconstriction syndrome (RCVS) commonly presents in the way. RCVS is a heterogeneous group of conditions leading to a multifocal narrowing of intracerebral arteries. Magnetic resonance angiography (MRA), computed tomography angiography (CTA), or catheter angiography is used to make this diagnosis, which can be elusive. Each headache tends to resolve over minutes to hours and RCVS tends to be self-limited over a few weeks.

Headache with Stroke

More than a quarter of strokes cause headaches early in the attack, and the number might even be higher with large strokes and those strokes within the posterior circulation. Nausea and vomiting are common in this setting, which may be difficult to distinguish from migraine. Migraineurs, particularly those with aura, are at higher risk of stroke, although migrainous strokes more likely occur interictally than at the time of a migraine.

Venous sinus thrombosis generally has headache of abrupt onset with a subsequent increase in ICP.

Cervical artery dissections arise from an intimal tear with the subsequent development of an intramural hemorrhage. Headache is the presenting feature in about 75% of cases. In a carotid dissection, the pain occurs along the ipsilateral face and neck and head. Almost half have an ipsilateral Horner's syndrome. With a vertebral artery dissection the pain is in the neck and occiput and pulsatile and continuous in quality. Stroke can occur up to 2 weeks later. A history of neck trauma is common, but not invariable.

Headaches Associated with Infection

Headaches can occur with infections of the central nervous system in those with systemic infections, or as a postinfectious headache. Postinfectious headache is suspected when the headache persists 3 months after presumed resolution of an acute intracranial infection. Although unproven, it is suspected that these headaches are due to an inflammatory, immune-mediated source.

Sinusitis is a common diagnosis for headaches, but acute sinusitis is more likely to be the etiology if there is purulent drainage and objective imaging evidence. Chronic sinusitis is an uncommon cause of headache. A study by Schreiber found that in those with self- or physician-diagnosed "sinus headache" migraine was overwhelmingly the cause of their symptoms. The trigeminoautonomic reflex, seen in migraine and other types of head pain, triggers lacrimation and rhinorrhea, often accounting for the confusion.

Orthostatic Headaches

A. Low CSF pressure.
Headache that is worse upon standing is most commonly due to a low CSF pressure, either following an LP, or from a leak in another location. Acute CSF oligemia occasionally presents as a thunderclap headache. This occurs after 30% of LPs, and may be best prevented with the use of atraumatic needles, but prolonged bed rest after an LP is of little value. The treatment involves direct repair of the site of the leak although epidural blood patches or prolonged epidural saline infusions may prove to be effective. Overshunting in one with a ventricular shunt can cause a similar headache and those with a shunt treated with topiramate can become overshunted. Pachymeningeal enhancement on MRI and downward displacement of the cerebellar tonsils strongly suggests a low CSF pressure.

The site of a CSF leak leading to a spontaneous intracranial hypotension is often indeterminate. This can include leaks from meningeal diverticula, erosion of dura from an adjacent lesion, excessive coughing, head trauma, or dural root sleeve tears.

In cases where there is suspected CSF rhinorrhea leading to headache, assaying this fluid for glucose and β_2 transferrin can document that it is indeed CSF and a CT of the paranasal sinuses should be performed.

B. Postural orthostatic tachycardia syndrome (POTS) can also lead to orthostatic headaches, particularly in young thin females. Typically, nonpositional headaches also occur. Coexisting fatigue, exercise intolerance, and attacks that are similar to panic attacks occur. The diagnosis is best made with a tilt table examination and may be treated with hydration, exercise, and increased salt intake, with β blockers, fludrocortisone, or midodrine added.

Giant Cell Arteritis

This condition is rare under the age of 60 and generally causes a diffuse scalp pain, which can be confused with tension-type headache or the scalp allodynia seen in an advanced migraine attack or chronic migraine. This condition can affect any artery before it pierces the dura, so that myocardial infarctions, bowel infarctions, and other ischemic complications can occur aside from blindness. Jaw claudication is commonly seen and queried by asking whether the jaw hurts with *sustained* chewing, in contrast with *acute* jaw pain that can occur with temporo-mandibular joint dysfunction with chewing or jawing.

Elevated erythrocyte sedimentation rate (ESR) and C-reactive protein (CRP) are generally found and a superficial temporal artery biopsy is done to confirm the diagnosis. The treatment is with high dose and prolonged course of corticosteroids. After a prolonged treatment course the condition generally resolves, but recurrences are common and with recurrences the ESR and CRP can be normal.

Hypertension and Headache

Modest hypertension does not cause headache and may actually be protective for head pain. Approximately 20% of patients with hypertensive crises have headaches, and therefore, head pain may accompany severe levels of hypertension.

The Examination of a Headache Patient

1. Vital signs: Are there significant abnormalities in blood pressure, or fever? Fever strongly suggests an infection.
2. Is there evidence of head injury? (Battle's sign, Raccoon's eyes, hemotympanum, CSF rhinorrhea, or otorrhea) Is dentition poor, which might be a local site of infection, which can lead to the development of a cerebral abscess or cerebritis?
3. Is there a disturbance of consciousness? This nearly always suggests a secondary headache.
4. Provocative tests for facet joint pathology, occipital groove, and supraorbital nerve tenderness, is there limitation of neck movement, is there carotid artery tenderness? Anteroposterior neck stiffness suggests a meningeal process.

   Cervical facets may be locally tender or may cause pain radiation locally or into the shoulders or upper back, and rarely radiate in the front or down an arm or into the fingers.
5. Is there purulent drainage from the sinuses? Nasal congestion or clear nasal discharge is commonly seen with migraine and cluster and does not suggest sinusitis.
6. Neurologic examination is clearly important. Elevated ICP can generally be recognized on the funduscopic evaluation with papilledema and lack of spontaneous venous pulsations. Hemiparesis, hemisensory loss, and aphasia strongly suggest a secondary headache even though this can be seen with migraine with aura.

Laboratory tests to be considered:

1. Complete blood count, complete blood chemistries, thyroid panel, ESR, CRP, drug screen.
2. CT scans of sinuses and nasal septum. Chronic sinusitis, rather than acute, is often irrelevant to headache production but can worsen a preexisting primary headache syndrome. Sphenoid sinusitis is an unusual cause of chronic headache and may not be excluded with MRI of the brain and better evaluated on a CT of the paranasal sinuses.
3. CT scan of the brain is the preferred test to exclude acute brain hemorrhage.
4. MRI brain, in general, is the imaging test of choice in headache. In the posterior fossa there may be relevant pathology, and this region may be poorly imaged with CT scanning. Chronic subdural hematomas are better evaluated with MRI compared to CT.
5. MRA or CTA can be used to screen for vascular disease. It is also often used as a screen for cerebral aneurysms. However, small aneurysms can be missed and in cases of known aneurysmal bleed, conventional catheter angiography is still required.
6. MRV is often used to exclude a venous sinus thrombosis as a cause of headache. Negative studies are useful, but these studies frequently demonstrate asymmetries or possible occlusions, which may or may not be relevant.
7. In cases where meningitis needs to be excluded, an LP is mandatory and in critically ill patients should not be delayed for imaging studies.

8. In cases of orthostatic headache, where a CSF leak needs to be excluded, CT myelography is a preferred test although a negative test does not exclude this diagnosis. Although the resolution of the study is high, low-volume leaks are often undetected. In such cases, radionuclide cisternography may prove helpful, scanning for evidence of indium outside of the dura. Nasal pledgets, which are placed during the test, are then scanned for radioactivity, which if found would suggest a CSF leak though the cribriform plate that can occur from a head injury.

Key Points

- Headache is the most common neurologic complaint seen in the primary care and ED setting. While primary headache disorders comprise the vast majority, the challenge to the practitioner lies in discerning which headaches are instead manifestations of more worrisome underlying pathology, deemed secondary headache disorders.
- Key to diagnosis lies in the headache history—establishing an anchor in time and pattern over time, burden of headache, headache features (location, quality, duration, and so on), and associated symptoms in the prodrome, ictal, and postdromal period, as well as treatments trialed and diagnostic studies completed.
- Migraine is the most common episodic headache disorder leading a patient to seek medical attention, and comes in several varieties: either with or without aura, the latter representing 80% of cases.
- Migraine requires at least five attacks of headache lasting 4 to 72 hours, which may include unilateral location, pulsating quality, moderate to severe pain intensity, aggravation by routine physical activity, and must be accompanied by nausea, vomiting, or photophobia and phonophobia.
- Individual attacks are managed with acute medications, and preventive medications are recommended when the patient suffers 6 or more days/month of headache or when acute drugs are ineffective or contraindicated.
- Cluster headache is characterized by episodes of weeks to months of daily, severe unilateral headache of boring quality, lasting 30 to 120 minutes, usually located retro-orbitally or temporally, and is associated with ipsilateral lacrimation and rhinorrhea. Both preventive and acute medication treatments are employed.
- Episodic and chronic paroxysmal hemicrania as well as hemicrania continua are types of side-locked headaches characterized by brief, minutes-long, recurrent attacks of unilateral pain with accompanying lacrimation and rhinorrhea. Hemicrania continua requires an unremitting, underlying headache with episodes of exacerbation. These headaches demonstrate dramatic response to indomethacin.
- Secondary headaches can be associated with increased ICP, as in the case of brain tumor, subdural hemorrhage, idiopathic intracranial hypertension, or brain abscess.
- Headaches of thunderclap onset herald the greatest concern for subarachnoid hemorrhage, though this can also present with a headache of more gradual onset. Noncontrast head CT would be emergent.
- Recurring thunderclap headaches may raise suspicion for RCVS, and should be worked up with MRA, CTA, or catheter angiography.
- Other causes of headache can include stroke (in >25%), sinus venous thrombosis, cervical artery dissection (associated with ipsilateral face and neck pain ± Horner's syndrome with carotid dissection, and ipsilateral neck and occiput pain in vertebral dissection), or infection.
- Orthostatic headaches may be caused by low CSF pressure from trauma or leak, or by POTS, most common in young, thin females and diagnosed with tilt table testing.
- Self- or physician-diagnosed "sinus headaches" are most often migraine.
- Giant cell arteritis most often affects those >60 years old and may lead to ischemic sequelae including blindness. Clues to diagnosis include jaw pain on sustained chewing (claudication) and elevated ESR, and CRP. Temporal artery biopsy should be performed and corticosteroids are the mainstay of treatment.
- On physical examination it is important to assess for evidence of head injury, infection, elevated ICP, or focality on neurologic assessment. Further workup to be considered includes blood work, neuroimaging, vascular studies, and LP.

Recommended Readings

Amendo MT, Brown BA, Kossow LB, et al. Headache as the sole presentation of acute myocardial infarction in two elderly patients. *Am J Geriatr Cardiol.* 2001;10(2):100–101.

Bendtsen L, Evers S, Linde M, et al. EFNS guideline on the treatment of tension-type headache—report of an EFNS task force [abstract]. *Eur J Neurol.* 2010;17:1318–1325. http://www.ncbi.nlm.nih.gov/pubmed/20482606

Bini A, Evangelista A, Castellini P, et al. Cardiac cephalgia. *J Headache Pain.* 2009;10(1):3–9.

Borchers AAT, Gershwin ME. Giant cell arteritis: A review of classification, pathophysiology, geoepidemiology and treatment. *Autoimmun Rev.* 2012;11:A544–A554.

Cumurciuc R, Crassard I, Sarov M, et al. Headache as the only neurological sign of cerebral venous thrombosis: a series of 17 cases. *J Neurol Neurosurg Psychiatry.* 2005;76(8):1084–1087.

Ducros A, Bousser MG. Thunderclap headache. *BMJ.* 2012;345:e8557.

Fischer C, Goldstein J, Edlow J. Cerebral venous sinus thrombosis in the emergency department: retrospective analysis of 17 cases and review of the literature. *J Emerg Med.* 2010;38:140–147.

Graff-Radford S, Schievink WI. High-pressure headaches, low-pressure syndromes, and CSF leaks: diagnosis and management. *Headache.* 2014;54(2):394–401.

Khurana R, Eisenberg L. Orthostatic and non-orthostatic headache in postural tachycardia syndrome. *Cephalalgia.* 2011;31(4):409–415.

Linn FHH, Rinkel GJE, Algra A, et al. Headache characteristics in subarachnoid hemorrhage and benign thunderclap headache. *J Neurol Neurosurg Psychiatry.* 1998;65(5):791–793.

Madsen SA, Fomsgaard JS, Jensen R. Epidural blood patch for refractory low CSF pressure headache: a pilot study. *J Headache Pain.* 2011;12(4):453–457.

Marshall AH, Jones NS, Robertson JJ. An algorithm for the management of CSF rhinorrhea illustrated by 36 cases. *Rhinology.* 1999;37(4):182–185.

Martinez-Lado L, Calviño-Diaz C, Piñeiro A, et al. Relapses and recurrences in giant cell arteritis: a population-based study of patients with biopsy-proven disease from northwestern Spain. *Medicine (Baltimore).* 2011;90(3):186–193.

Mirsattari SM, Powew C, Nath A. Primary headaches in HIV-infected patients. *Headache.* 1999;39(1):3–10.

Mokbel KM, Abd Elfattah AM, Kamal E-S. Nasal mucosal contact points with facial pain and/or headache: lidocaine can predict the result of localized endoscopic resection. *Eur Arch Otorhinolaryngol.* 2010;267(10):1569–1572.

Prakash S, Patel N, Golwala P, et al. Post-infectious headache: a reactive headache? *J Headache Pain.* 2011;12(4):467–473.

Schievink WI, Karemaker JM, Hageman LM, et al. Circumstances surrounding aneurysmal subarachnoid hemorrhage. *Surg Neurol.* 1989;32(4):266–272.

Schreiber C, Hutchinson S, Webster CJ, et al. Prevalence of migraine in patients with a history of self-reported or physician-diagnosed "sinus" headache. *Arch Intern Med.* 2004;164(16):1769–1772.

Silbert PL, Mokri B, Schievink WI. Headache and neck pain in spontaneous internal carotid and vertebral artery dissections. *Neurology.* 1995;45(8):1517–1522.

Tentschert S, Wimmer R, Greisenegger S, et al. Headache at stroke onset in 2196 patients with ischemic stroke or transient ischemic attack. *Stroke.* 2005;36(2):e1–e3.

Terazzi E, Mittino D, Ruda R, et al. Cerebral venous thrombosis: a retrospective multicentre study of 48 patients. *Neurol Sci.* 2005;25(6):311–315.

Wakerly BR, Tan MD, Ting EY. Idiopathic intracranial hypertension. *Cephalalgia.* 2015;35(3):248–261.

Weyand CM, Goronzy JJ. Giant-cell arteritis and polymyalgia rheumatica. *Ann Intern Med.* 2003;139(6):505–515.

Yuh EL, Dillon WP. Intracranial hypotension and intracranial hypertension. *Neuroimaging Clin N Am.* 2010;20:597–617.

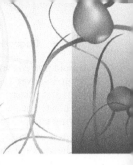

21 Approach to the Patient with Chronic and Recurrent Headache

Robert G. Kaniecki

Headache may represent a sign of biologic dysfunction of the nervous system or a symptom of a secondary process. *The International Classification of Headache Disorders (ICHD-3* beta) organizes headache in primary (defined by symptomatic criteria) and secondary (defined by cause) categories (Table 21.1). Symptomatic overlap between these broad categories is extensive and emphasized by the placement of the following criterion in all primary headache types: "Not better accounted for by another *ICHD-3* diagnosis." Practical headache evaluation may be simplified into three basic steps:

1. Identify those with potential secondary headache disorders warranting diagnostic evaluation. Although this may only represent fewer than 5% of those presenting with chronic headaches, early identification will help limit potential morbidity and mortality.
2. Recognize patients experiencing migraine, since data suggest more than 90% of those presenting to clinicians with recurrent headaches will indeed display migraine.
3. In those without secondary headache or migraine, consider one of the other primary headache disorders such as tension-type headache or one of the trigeminal autonomic cephalalgias (TACs).

CLINICAL ASSESSMENT

HISTORY

A thorough history is the most important element in the evaluation of a patient with chronic or recurrent headache. Temporal profiling assessing frequency and duration of headaches

TABLE 21.1 ICHD-3 Beta Classification of Headache Disorders

Primary headaches
Migraine
Tension-type headache
TACs
Other primary headache disorders

Secondary headaches
Headache attributed to trauma or injury to the head and/or neck
Headache attributed to cranial or cervical vascular disorder
Headache attributed to nonvascular intracranial disorder
Headache attributed to a substance or its withdrawal
Headache attributed to infection
Headache attributed to disorder of homoeostasis
Headache or facial pain attributed to disorder of the cranium, neck, eyes, ears, nose, sinuses, teeth, mouth, or other facial or cervical structure
Headache attributed to psychiatric disorder
Painful cranial neuropathies and other facial pains

should precede and help guide symptomatic assessment. Headaches lasting hours to days and recurring over years should prompt questions probing for migraine, while episodes lasting 1 hour and occurring nocturnally for only the prior 6 weeks should generate questions looking for cluster headaches. The essential elements in headache evaluation would include the following components and questions.

A. **Age of onset.** "How old were you when you had your first memorable headache?" A headache history dating back for years is certainly more comforting, and likely to reflect primary headache, than those histories dating back only a few weeks or months. Most primary headaches develop between the ages of 5 and 50, and onset outside this range should signal the possibility of a secondary headache disorder. In addition, the age–incidence curve for brain tumors displays a bimodal distribution, peaking at ages 5 and 60.

B. **Temporal profile.** *"How long have your headaches been like this—this frequency, this intensity—we are discussing today?"* An accurate assessment of headache frequency is crucial in headache management. Many primary headaches display stable patterns for months or years, while significant secondary headaches are defined by progression or instability of pattern—typically over a period of 6 months or less. Cluster headache patients experience cycles of daily headache for periods of several weeks to months, then often becoming dormant for months or years. Any fundamental change in headache pattern over a period of days to months should signal the possibility of a secondary headache disorder.

1. *"How many days per month do you have headache of any kind, any degree?"* This question is often overlooked but is exceedingly important. The number of total headache days in an average month is important both diagnostically and therapeutically. Those with primary headache disorders such as migraine and tension-type headaches will be designated as "chronic" when there are 15 or more days of headache in an average month. In addition, preventive treatments should be prescribed for migraine or tension-type headache when the patient is averaging at least 8 days of headache per month.

2. *"How many of those headaches become severe? How long do these episodes last, without treatment or if treatment does not work?"* Migraine headaches sometimes become severe, and when untreated in adults last 4 to 72 hours. Tension-type headache episodes are rarely if ever severe and last hours to days. Cluster headache attacks are almost always severe, with typical duration between 15 minutes and 3 hours. Other TACs are characterized by even shorter episodes—chronic paroxysmal hemicranias (CPHs) 2 to 30 minutes, short-lasting unilateral neuralgiform headache attacks with conjunctival injection and tearing (SUNCT) 1 to 600 seconds. Trigeminal neuralgia pains also typically last several seconds at most.

3. *"How many days each month do you take a medication to treat a headache?"* Screening for possible medication overuse, previously known as "rebound" headache, is helpful. Those patients using acute headache medications more than 10 or 15 days per month (based on the medication) may find themselves refractory to preventive measures until the overused agent is discontinued.

C. **Pain characteristics.**

1. *"Where does it hurt?"* Location of head discomfort in both primary and secondary headache disorders is incredibly variable and often unhelpful diagnostically. Migraine is unilateral in 60% of patients, often switching sides, but it may be bilateral or global in 40%. Tension-type headache is most commonly but not universally bilateral, with either frontotemporal or occipital predominance. Cluster headache and other TACs are typically unilateral and involve V_1 distribution pain, trigeminal neuralgia unilateral and V_2, V_3 distribution pain, but both may occasionally occur bilaterally. Structural disease of the orbits and sinuses is typically worse frontally, while that of the cervical spine is worse occipitally. Intracranial vascular or mass lesions and disorders of intracranial pressure may present with pain anywhere in the cranium, with occasional radiation to the face or neck.

2. *"Describe the quality of the pain? What does it feel like? Are the severe headaches steady or throbbing?"* Questions to pain quality do not help distinguish secondary headache syndromes but may help in the diagnosis of primary headaches. Although steady in up to 30%, the pain of migraine is usually throbbing. Tension-type headache is generally described as pressure, aching, or tightness. Cluster headache is classically piercing or boring in nature, but may burn or throb in some. Stabbing pain is characteristic of primary stabbing headache and trigeminal neuralgia.

3. *"On a scale of 1-10, how severe is the pain on bad days? On that same scale, how intense are the minor headaches?"* The usefulness of a linear pain scale is limited, given the variability of pain perceptions and prior pain experiences across patient populations. These values are perhaps most useful in the longitudinal management of individual patients where improvements in headache intensity following treatment may be quantified.

4. *"Is the pain worse with routine physical activity, such as bending over or going up a flight of stairs?"* Disorders of intracranial pressure may worsen with changes in posture or activity. When severe migraine is typically worsened by physical activity, cluster headache is unaffected, and tension-type headache either unaffected or improved. An interesting follow-up question here is, *"What do you do when you get a bad headache?"* Migraine patients tend to resort to bed rest in a quiet and dark environment, tension-type with mild or no alterations in activity, while cluster patients are restless and often pace or participate in some distracting behavior.

D. **Associated features.**

1. *"Do you have any symptoms preceding the pain that suggest a headache is likely to occur?"* Migraine may be preceded by a prodrome characterized by vague constitutional or mood symptoms lasting hours, or aura involving discrete neurologic symptoms lasting minutes. Most patients with other primary headaches and those with secondary headaches have few if any premonitory signs.

2. *"Are you sensitive to light or noise during headaches?"* Significant sensory sensitivities are typical of migraine, common in cluster, and rare in tension-type headache. Photophobia may also be seen in patients with glaucoma or disorders affecting the meninges.

3. *"Are you nauseated or do you vomit with some headaches?"* Similar to the element of sensory sensitivities, nausea and vomiting are typical of migraine, common in cluster, and rare in tension-type headache. Over 70% of patients with migraine will experience nausea, and 30% vomiting. These symptoms are also common in those patients with secondary headache disorders involving increased intracranial pressure.

4. *"Do you experience changes in your vision or speech, or do you have any weakness or numbness during headache attacks?"* Neurologic symptoms lasting 5 to 60 minutes preceding a severe headache may constitute aura. Such complaints typically involve visual, hemisensory, or language functions of the brain (Video 21.1). Brainstem symptoms such as vertigo, diplopia, or ataxia may reflect brainstem aura, and focal weakness hemiplegic migraine, but both of these subtypes of migraine are uncommon. Any patient presenting with headache and neurologic symptoms that are not typical of migraine aura should undergo neuroimaging.

5. *"Do you have tearing, eye redness or drooping, or nasal congestion or drainage associated with headache attacks?"* Cranial autonomic features are seen in up to 50% of patients with migraine. These are often bilateral and frequently lead to a misdiagnosis of sinus headache. The presence of unilateral autonomic features is a hallmark of cluster headache and the other TACs. The absence of such features assists in the distinction between these headaches and trigeminal neuralgia.

E. **Triggers or risk factors.**

1. *"Are there any triggers that seem to cause some of your headaches?"* *"Is there any association with stress, hormone or weather changes, exposures to bright or flashing lights, loud noises, or strong odors?"* Migraine headache patients may describe a variety of internal or external stimuli affecting the likelihood of a subsequent headache attack. Stress, female hormone or weather changes, or exposure to excessive light, noise, or odors may all trigger migraines. Changes in sleep or meal patterns and certain foods or dietary elements such as artificial sweeteners or monosodium glutamate may also be provocative. Stress, neck or eye strain, or sleep deprivation may impact tension-type headache. When in the midst of a cycle, cluster headache patients may report alcohol as a trigger, while between cycles alcohol is not problematic. Some primary headaches are defined by the trigger: primary cough headache, primary exercise headache, and primary headache associated with sexual activity. Certain secondary headaches are also defined by exposure (carbon monoxide) or withdrawal (caffeine) from certain substances.

F. **Family history.**

1. *"Is there any family history of migraine or other headaches?"* Aside from those extended family histories of brain tumor or aneurysm, patients with secondary headache disorders typically

do not possess a family history of relevance. Tension-type and cluster headaches seem to possess only minor genetic influences. A family history of headache is most important in migraine: approximately 50% of patients report a first-degree relative with migraine, and some reports indicate up to 90% will have some family history of headache.

EXAMINATION

1. Pulse and blood pressure should be checked. Uncontrolled hypertension may be associated with secondary headache, although the connection is possibly overstated. Bradycardia or tachycardia may indicate thyroid disease, which may cause headaches. Blood pressure and pulse values may also impact choices of medications used in the prevention or acute management of headache. -blockers may reduce, and tricyclic antidepressants increase, heart rate and blood pressure.

2. The cervical spine musculature should be palpated for spasm or trigger points, and the cervical range of motion assessed. Abnormal cervical spine exam findings could suggest a secondary cervicogenic headache disorder. Tenderness at the occiput could suggest occipital neuralgia.

3. Assessment of the ears, sinuses, mastoids, and cervical glandular tissues may reveal evidence of malignant, infectious, or granulomatous conditions. Thyromegaly may indicate thyroid dysfunction.

4. Temporal artery palpation for pulsation and tenderness should be performed in older adults to screen for giant cell arteritis (GCA). Temporomandibular joint dysfunction as a cause for headache may be suggested by crepitus, diminished range of motion, or tenderness on joint assessment.

5. A thorough examination of the eyes is critical in the evaluation of patients with headache. Ptosis or miosis may be seen with primary headaches such as cluster but also may reflect secondary pathologies such as carotid dissection or stroke. Glaucoma may present with conjunctival injection and pupillary abnormalities. Papilledema on fundoscopic examination arising from increased intracranial pressure may be seen with intracranial mass lesions, venous or sinus thrombosis, obstructive hydrocephalus, or idiopathic intracranial hypertension (IIH). Visual acuity may be affected by glaucoma, optic nerve tumors, or optic neuritis. Visual field defects are typically associated with certain structural lesions along the visual pathways, with bitemporal hemianopsia seen with pituitary tumors and homonymous hemianopsia seen with occipital stroke or mass.

6. Cranial nerve examination helps further identify those patients experiencing headaches from structural lesions. Ophthalmoplegia may occur with intracranial lesions or with structural pathologies in the orbit or cavernous sinus. Chronic sphenoid sinusitis extending to the cavernous sinus or orbital tumor or pseudotumor are some examples. Unilateral or bilateral sixth-nerve palsies may act as a "falsely localizing sign" since either may occur with increased intracranial pressure. Facial palsies and hearing impairment may be associated with lesions in the posterior fossa such as acoustic neuroma, or with intracranial extension of chronic mastoiditis.

7. Focal deficits on sensory or motor testing would typically indicate structural lesions of the central nervous system. Occasionally cervical root compression could result in ipsilateral radicular numbness, focal weakness, or hyporeflexia. Hyperreflexia, Babinski's signs, or ataxia also would be indicative of lesions in the brain or cervical spinal cord.

DIAGNOSTIC STUDIES

1. The majority of patients presenting with chronic or recurrent headache will not require diagnostic evaluation. Most will display a history compatible with a primary headache and a normal neurologic examination. Guidelines recommend against neuroimaging in the setting of a stable pattern of migraine headache. Less than 1% of such patients will have neuroimaging abnormalities, the majority being benign. There are no evidence-based guidelines available for imaging in chronic nonmigrainous headaches. The presence of one of the red flags for secondary headache should prompt neuroimaging as well as other specific diagnostic studies (Table 21.2).

TABLE 21.2 Red Flags for Secondary Headache Disorders

First or worst headache
Abrupt-onset or thunderclap attack
Progression or fundamental change in headache pattern
Abnormal physical examination findings
Neurologic symptoms lasting greater than 1 hr
New headache in persons younger than 5 yr or older than 50 yr
New headache in patients with cancer, immunosuppression, or pregnancy
Headache associated with alteration in or loss of consciousness
Headache triggered by exertion, sexual activity, or Valsalva maneuvers

2. In certain settings blood work may be required to exclude secondary headache disorders. Measurement of the erythrocyte sedimentation rate (ESR) and C-reactive protein is necessary in the evaluation of potential GCA, and subsequent temporal artery biopsy may be indicated to confirm the diagnosis. Serum toxicology, carboxyhemoglobin, and thyroid function tests may also help identify specific secondary headaches.

3. Neuroimaging is the most important diagnostic tool in the assessment of patients with headache. Head computed tomography (CT) is the preferred imaging modality in the setting of acute headache. Skull fracture, acute intracranial hemorrhage, and paranasal sinus disease may be identified. Guidelines now recommend MRI of the brain in the evaluation of patients with chronic or recurrent headache. Although more expensive than head CT, MRI is considered more sensitive in identifying intracranial pathology. Given the absence of radiation exposure MRI is also considered less invasive. Contrast administration may be indicated in settings of malignant, infectious, or inflammatory disease. In addition, most patients with headache from intracranial hypotension will display diffuse non-nodular diffuse meningeal enhancement. CT or MR angiographic or venographic studies may be useful in the settings of suspected vascular occlusion or malformation.

4. Cerebrospinal fluid (CSF) examination is mandatory in the setting of CT-negative subarachnoid hemorrhage. Certain patients with chronic headache disorders may also benefit from lumbar puncture. Measurement of the opening pressure may confirm the presence of either intracranial hypertension or hypotension. Those with subacute meningoencephalitis may show abnormalities in CSF cell count, protein, or glucose. Cultures, gram stains, antibody panels, and polymerase chain reaction analysis may isolate specific organisms. CSF cytology is indicated with suspected leukemic, lymphomatous, or carcinomatous meningitis.

5. There is no role for electroencephalography in the workup of patients with headache unless there is impairment of consciousness or seizure-like activity associated with attacks.

SECONDARY CHRONIC OR RECURRENT HEADACHE DISORDERS

Posttraumatic Headache

Trauma to the head or neck may result in headaches, which may be acute or recur chronically. *ICHD* classification arbitrarily defines acute posttraumatic headache as recurring up to 3 months following an injury, while the term persistent posttraumatic headache is applied to those with headaches extending beyond that time.

1. Traumatic brain injury (TBI) may occur when the nervous system is exposed to either blunt or penetrating trauma. Most patients with obvious structural lesions, such as epidural or parenchymal hemorrhages, will present with acute headaches. Some patients, particularly the elderly or those on anticoagulants, may develop subdural hematomas that present with more subacute or chronic patterns of headache. This may even occur in the setting of relatively insignificant trauma.

2. Headache is a common result of mild TBI, or concussion. This symptom is the most common reported by those with a postconcussion syndrome. Cognitive impairment,

fatigue, sleep disturbances, dizziness, and visual blurring are other typical complaints. Posttraumatic headaches typically resolve within a matter of days to weeks, but some experience headaches lingering for months to years. There is no direct correlation between the degree of trauma and either the duration or severity of the subsequent headache condition. Management of the assorted symptoms of the postconcussion syndrome is largely rehabilitative and symptomatic. It may be helpful to phenotype the headache complaints as either more tension-type or migraine in quality, directing pharmacotherapy accordingly.

3. Cervicogenic headache arises from irritation of upper cervical nerve roots caused by bone, disc, or soft tissue pathology. This is usually but not invariably accompanied by neck pain. Although sometimes atraumatic in origin, cervical sprain or "whiplash" injury is the most common cause of cervicogenic headache. Pain is frequently side-locked, worsened by neck motion, and associated with cervical abnormalities on examination or imaging. Nonsteroidal anti-inflammatory drugs (NSAIDs) and muscle relaxants are often helpful acutely. Physical therapy or manipulation, preventive medications such as amitriptyline or gabapentin, and procedures such as occipital nerve or cervical facet blocks may be helpful in chronic cases.

4. Dysfunction of the temporomandibular joint may occur following facial trauma, possibly arising from airbag deployment during a motor vehicle accident. The pain may be unilateral or bilateral and is typically temporal and aggravated by chewing. The appearance is similar to tension-type headache and the pain often responds to local ice, NSAIDs, and a soft diet. Referral to a dentist or maxillofacial specialist may be required in chronic cases.

5. Occipital neuralgia may present as episodes of severe, shooting pain in the distribution of the greater, lesser, or third occipital nerves. A lingering dull discomfort may persist between paroxysms of severe pain lasting seconds to minutes. The neuralgia may arise from trauma to one of the upper cervical roots or to the nerves themselves in the posterior scalp and may be unilateral or bilateral. Local tenderness or a Tinel's sign may be present. Analgesics are typically unhelpful, while many patients respond to daily amitriptyline or gabapentin. Occipital nerve blocks or cervical facet blocks may be beneficial as well.

HEADACHES SECONDARY TO CEREBROVASCULAR DISEASE

Most patients with headaches of cerebrovascular origin will present acutely. Subarachnoid or intracerebral hemorrhage, ischemic or hemorrhagic stroke, or dissection of the cervical-cephalic vessels will present with acute headache that is frequently abrupt and "thunderclap" in description. Following the acute presentation some may develop ongoing headaches that may resemble migraine or tension-type headache extending for months or years. These are often refractory to medical management but fade with time.

1. Thrombosis of the cerebral veins or sinuses may result in acute or more chronic headaches. Headache is the most common symptom, seen in 80% to 90%, and is the most common presenting symptom. Other symptoms are highly variable, but the majority of cases are associated with papilledema or focal neurologic findings. Suspicion should be raised in the presence of prothrombotic conditions such as malignancy, pregnancy, or the use of oral contraceptives. Management steps include symptomatic care and heparin followed by oral anticoagulation for 3 to 6 months.

2. Unruptured cerebral aneurysms are present in 0.4% to 3.6% of the population. Headache has been reported in up to 20% of these individuals, but usually the aneurysm is an incidental finding. The typical presentation of headache from cerebral aneurysm is an isolated thunderclap attack, but up to 40% will experience a precursor "sentinel leak" headache a few days or weeks prior to aneurismal rupture.

3. Vascular malformations of the brain or dura may be linked with recurrent headaches. Arteriovenous malformations (AVM) may present with headaches in approximately 15% of cases. Atypical presentations of migraine, cluster, and CPHs have been reported. Many may be incidental, with the strongest case for pathophysiologic link made for those with headache locked ipsilateral and neurologic symptoms contralateral to the

AVM. Cavernous angiomas also may be associated with headache in up to 40% of cases, with chronic patterns suggestive of migraine and abrupt headache with acute hemorrhage.

4. Reversible cerebral vasoconstriction syndrome (RCVS) is characterized by recurrent thunderclap headache associated with multifocal segmental cerebral vasoconstriction. Patients may also present with focal neurologic findings, encephalopathy, and seizures. Brain MRI may be normal or show findings consistent with posterior reversible encephalopathy syndrome. CSF is typically normal. RCVS can occur spontaneously or in association with preeclampsia or eclampsia, medications (sympathomimetic agents), blood product transfusions, or pheochromocytoma. Calcium-channel blocker administration (nimodipine or verapamil) is recommended. Intravenous magnesium is added in cases of preeclampsia or eclampsia. The role of corticosteroids is unclear.

5. Primary angiitis of the central nervous system is often confused with RCVS. Headaches, however, are more insidious and progressive. Brain MRI shows subcortical white matter and cortical infarctions in the majority. Over 95% of patients show CSF abnormalities including elevations in cell counts, protein, and opening pressure. Combined immunosuppressive therapy with methylprednisolone and cyclophosphamide is recommended.

6. Headache is the most common presenting symptom of GCA. This condition involves inflammation of the large arteries with a preference for head and neck vessels. Incidence peaks between 70 and 80 years of age, and GCA is more common in Whites and women. Headache is classically temporal but location is highly variable. Other common complaints include myalgias, fatigue, malaise, fevers, anorexia, and weight loss. Jaw claudication is present in only 25% of cases. Cranial nerve palsies and stroke may sometimes occur. ESR is elevated in 95% of biopsy-proven GCA cases, with a mean value of 85 mm/hour. Diagnosis may require bilateral temporal artery biopsies of at least 2 cm in length. Treatment with 1 mg/kg prednisone should be instituted at the first sign of suspicion for GCA, since vision loss is permanent once identified. Prednisone may be necessary for 6 to 24 months, with most patients tapered to 10 mg daily over the first few months. Both clinical and laboratory values are helpful in assessing improvement or relapse.

7. Certain genetic vasculopathies may present with recurrent headache, often exhibiting migrainous features. Cerebral autosomal-dominant arteriopathy with subcortical infarcts and leukoencephalopathy presents with migraine with aura in one-third of cases. It affects small arteries and also results in mood disorder, stroke, and dementia. Mitochondrial encephalopathy, lactic acidosis, and stroke-like episodes may frequently present with migrainous headaches and stroke-like events, in addition to seizures, recurrent vomiting, and sensorineural deafness. Treatment of both is generally symptomatic.

HEADACHE FROM NONVASCULAR INTRACRANIAL DISORDERS

1. Headache associated with brain tumor is highly variable. Approximately 20% of patients will present and 60% eventually develop headache linked to the malignancy. It is more common with infratentorial tumors. Symptoms may arise from the mass lesion, from obstructive hydrocephalus, or from meningeal irritation from carcinomatous meningitis. The classic presentation of headache worse in the morning with associated vomiting is present in approximately 10% of cases. Most will exhibit headaches phenotypically similar to tension-type headache, or occasionally similar to migraine.

2. IIH involves CSF pressure elevation in the absence of an intracranial space-occupying lesion. Approximately 90% of subjects are female, 90% of childbearing age, and 90% with elevations in body mass index. Headache, often tension-type in nature, and visual complaints are most common at presentation. Blurring or episodic darkening of vision, diplopia, pulsatile tinnitus, and neck pain are frequently noted. Papilledema is present nearly universally, and sixth-nerve palsy on occasion. Elevated CSF opening pressure (>250 mm H_2O in adults) in the absence of intracranial lesions confirms the diagnosis. Up to 90% will display blind spot enlargement or peripheral field loss on visual perimetry. Treatment is aimed at preservation

of vision and minimization of headaches. Acetazolamide is the drug of choice, although many now prescribe topiramate for the added benefit of weight loss. Weight reduction through diet and exercise or through bariatric surgery has also been shown to be beneficial. Optic nerve fenestration or shunt procedures may be required in refractory cases.

3. Headache from intracranial hypotension is most frequently seen in the setting of recent lumbar puncture, but may occur spontaneously (SIH) as well. The triad of orthostatic headache, diffuse pachymeningeal enhancement on brain MRI, and low CSF pressure (<6 cm water) is characteristic. The headache may be generalized or focal and develops within 15 minutes after leaving a supine position. Cervical discomfort, stiffness, nausea, vertigo, and hearing changes such as muffling or tinnitus are other common complaints. Diplopia may be seen in the presence of sixth-nerve palsy but most patients present with normal neurologic examinations. Predisposing conditions for SIH include trauma, Marfan or Ehler–Danlos syndromes, and neurofibromatosis. Roles for disc disease or dural diverticula are unclear. In addition to non-nodular diffuse pachymeningeal "thickening" with contrast enhancement, brain MRI may reveal subdural fluid collections, pituitary enlargement, or tonsillar herniation. Identification of the site of CSF leak in cases of SIH can be challenging. CT myelography of the entire spine is the recommended study. Initial management involves bed rest and fluid resuscitation. When required, epidural blood patch is associated with resolution of symptoms in 90% to 95% of cases. Lumbar patches may be helpful both in the settings of postdural puncture headache and SIH, but some with the latter may require cervical or thoracic patches or surgical procedures. The rate of recurrence is approximately 10%.

4. Involvement of the nervous system from noninfectious inflammatory disease may also produce headache. Neurosarcoidosis may present with meningeal involvement or with focal inflammatory lesions in the brain parenchyma or periventricular white matter. Aseptic meningitis may recur in patients with certain autoimmune disorders or with exposure to certain drugs such as NSAIDs, penicillins, or immunoglobulin. Resolution with treatment of the cause is typical. The syndrome of transient headache and neurological deficits with cerebrospinal fluid lymphocytosis is characterized by migraine-like headaches with unilateral sensorimotor or speech deficits of duration greater than 4 hours. CSF analysis reveals >15 lymphocytes. The condition resolves spontaneously within 3 months.

5. Chiari I malformations may be associated with chronic or recurrent headaches. Population prevalence is nearly 1%. Women are more likely to be affected than men, and there may be a slight hereditary component. Chiari I is identified by cerebellar tonsillar descent of >5 mm (below the line connecting the internal occipital protuberance to the basion), or descent of >3 mm with crowding of the subarachnoid space at the craniocervical junction. By definition headache has at least one of the following three characteristics: triggered by cough or other Valsalva-like maneuver; occipital or suboccipital location; duration <5 minutes. Dizziness, ataxia, changes in hearing, and diplopia or transient visual phenomena are not unusual. Neurologic examinations are typically normal but may show brainstem or cerebellar findings. Cervical spine abnormalities may be seen when the Chiari is complicated by a cervical cord syrinx. Significant symptomatic overlap may be seen with migraine. Surgery should be reserved for those patients exhibiting abnormalities on physical exam, or for those with refractory headaches exhibiting features characteristic of a Chiari. The role of Cine MRI CSF flow study is unclear.

HEADACHES ATTRIBUTED TO SUBSTANCES

1. Recurrent headache may be associated with the use of multiple substances or their withdrawal. Although the list of agents potentially causing headache is lengthy, classic perpetrators include nitrates, phosphodiesterase inhibitors, alcohol, and endogenous hormones. Caffeine withdrawal is one of the most common causes of substance-related headaches.

2. Headaches associated with overtreatment with acute medication is now termed "medication overuse" headache (MOH). It is defined as headache occurring on 15 or more days per month developing as a consequence of regular overuse of acute or symptomatic headache medication (on 10 or more, or 15 or more days per month, depending on the medication) for more than 3 months. MOH requires both the presence of an offending agent and susceptible individual. The presence of a primary headache disorder seems crucial, and those with migraine and tension-type headache seem most susceptible. MOH is present in up to 80% of individuals with chronic migraine. Simple analgesics are linked with the 15-day threshold, while the use of triptans, ergots, opioids, or combination analgesics at least 10 days per month is considered excessive. Several studies have associated opioids (critical exposure 8 days per month) and barbiturates (critical exposure 5 days per month) with higher rates of transformation to chronic migraine when compared to NSAIDs or triptans.

TRIGEMINAL NEURALGIA

The most commonly diagnosed recurrent facial pain is trigeminal neuralgia. *ICHD* criteria define those cases arising from structural lesions or trauma as "painful" trigeminal neuralgia, while those without these etiologies are considered "classical." It is characterized by paroxysms of brief electrical shooting pain limited to the distribution of the trigeminal nerve. Approximately 95% of cases involve pain isolated to the second and third branches of the nerve, and 95% are strictly unilateral. By definition the pain lasts only a fraction of a second to 2 minutes and may be triggered by innocuous stimulation of the face. Pains can occur in series, which may be followed by refractory periods of quiescence. Some experience cycles of recurrent pain lasting weeks to months, interrupted by periods of remission, while other patients follow a chronic progressive course. Onset occurs after age 40 in 90%. Those diagnosed at a young age should be evaluated for structural lesions such as multiple sclerosis. Vascular compression of the trigeminal root entry zone in the pons is responsible for most cases of "classical" trigeminal neuralgia. Carbamazepine is the drug of choice. In certain cases oxcarbazepine, baclofen, gabapentin, clonazepam, or lamotrigine may be helpful. Medical therapy fails in approximately 30% of cases. In those who are good surgical candidates, microvascular decompression is the procedure with highest rate of success.

PRIMARY HEADACHE DISORDERS

Migraine Headache

1. The vast majority of patients seen for recurrent or chronic headaches will suffer from migraine. The combination of high population prevalence (13% of US adults) and significant morbidity of the condition leads to the figure that over 90% of patients presenting with recurrent headache in a primary care setting meet criteria for migraine. Incidence peaks in late childhood and early adolescence, and prevalence in the fifth decade of life. It is three times more common in adult women than men. Migraine is characterized by recurrent episodes of severe headache lasting hours to days with associated nausea or sensitivities to light or noise. Although vomiting and aura are held by many as cardinal features of migraine, these symptoms are actually seen in only 25% to 30% of patients. Formal diagnostic criteria are listed in Table 21.3.

2. Because of tremendous phenotypic variations seen in the population, migraine is frequently misdiagnosed. Although absent from diagnostic criteria, neck pain is seen in 75% and nasal congestion or tearing in 50%. The former may lead to a label of "tension" headache, the latter to "sinus" headache. Most patients with migraine will experience both minor and severe attacks, further clouding the picture diagnostically for patients and clinicians.

3. Aura is seen in up to 30% of those with migraine. Aura may come before, during, or completely separate from headache. Any combination of visual, sensory, or language dysfunction without retinal, brainstem, or motor complaints is termed typical aura. Those with aura isolated to one eye are termed "retinal aura." These patients should be screened for retinal issues such as ischemic optic neuropathy or detachment.

TABLE 21.3 ICHD-3 Beta Diagnostic Criteria for Migraine

Migraine without Aura

At least five attacks fulfilling criteria

Headache attacks lasting 4–72 hr (untreated)

Headache has at least two of the four following characteristics:

Unilateral location

Pulsating quality

Moderate or severe pain intensity

Aggravation by or causing avoidance of routine physical activity

During headache at least one of the following:

Nausea and/or vomiting

Photophobia and phonophobia

Not better accounted for by another *ICHD-3* diagnosis

Migraine with Aura

At least two attacks

One or more of the following fully reversible aura symptoms

Visual

Sensory

Speech and/or language

Motor

Brainstem

Retinal

At least two of the following four characteristics:

At least one symptom spreads gradually over >5 min or two or more symptoms occur in succession

Each individual aura symptom lasts 5–60 min

At least one aura symptom is unilateral

The aura is accompanied, or followed within 60 min, by headache

Other *ICHD-3* diagnoses and TIA have been excluded

Migraine with brainstem aura, previously called basilar-type migraine, must possess at least two of the following: vertigo, diplopia, ataxia, tinnitus, hyperacusis, dysarthria, and decreased level of consciousness. Those with any degree of motor weakness are termed hemiplegic migraine, which has both familial and sporadic subtypes. Triptans are contraindicated in those with brainstem or hemiplegic aura.

4. Migraine is subclassified as "episodic" when occurring fewer than 15 days per month. It is termed "chronic" when occurring at least 15 days per month for 3 months and exhibiting migraine features or response to migraine medication on at least 8 days per month. Transformation of episodic into chronic migraine has been shown to occur at a rate of 3% per year in the general population. Risk factors for development of chronic migraine include older age, female sex, major life changes or stressors, obesity, low socioeconomic status, head trauma, excessive caffeine or nicotine exposure, and the presence of pain, sleep, or mental health disorders. Acute treatment may play a role as well. Medication overuse, any exposure to opioid- or butalbital-containing products, and those experiencing inadequate results from acute therapies all have higher risk for chronic migraine.

5. It is often helpful to screen migraineurs for possible comorbidities. Mood disorders such as depression and bipolar disease, generalized anxiety and panic disorders, insomnia, irritable bowel syndrome, and fibromyalgia are all commonly seen. Migraine with aura, particularly in women, also raises the risk of ischemic and hemorrhagic stroke.

Tension-type Headache

1. Tension-type headache is the most common and least distinct of the primary headache disorders. Annual prevalence in US adults approximates 40%, while lifetime prevalence

TABLE 21.4 ICHD-3 Beta Criteria for Episodic Tension-type Headache

Episodes lasting from 30 min to 7 d
At least two of the following four characteristics
   Bilateral location
   Pressing or tightening (nonpulsating) quality
   Mild or moderate intensity
   Not aggravated by routine physical activity
Both of the following
   No nausea or vomiting
   No more than one of photophobia and phonophobia
Not better accounted for by another *ICHD-3* diagnosis

approaches 90%. It is characterized by episodes of nondisabling headache that lack the severity, gastrointestinal issues, and sensory complaints seen with migraine. *ICHD-3* beta diagnostic criteria are outlined in Table 21.4.

2. Tension-type headache is subclassified on the basis of frequency, which appears to be therapeutically helpful, and on the presence or absence of pericranial muscle tenderness, which is not particularly relevant. Episodic tension-type headache is "infrequent" when <1 day per month and "frequent" when 1 to 14 days per month. Chronic tension-type headache occurs on average at least 15 days per month. Those with chronic tension-type headache sometimes develop a picture somewhat similar to migraine and the diagnostic criteria permit one of the following: photophobia, phonophobia, mild nausea.

3. Given significant symptomatic overlap with secondary headaches and migraine, patients with chronic tension-type headaches should have those conditions excluded before the diagnosis is made.

4. Another headache phenotypically similar to chronic tension-type headache is a separate primary headache syndrome known as new daily persistent headache (NDPH). This condition is defined by a daily headache syndrome lasting for at least 3 months with a distinct and clearly remembered onset. NDPH pain begins abruptly, without provocation, and becomes continuous and unremitting within 24 hours. This condition is often seen in younger patients, frequently lasts for years, and has no known effective therapeutic option.

TRIGEMINAL AUTONOMIC CEPHALALGIAS

1. The TACs are a group of headache disorders characterized by episodes of severe pain in the distribution of the first division of the trigeminal nerve accompanied by ipsilateral autonomic features. They are subclassified based on the duration and frequency of attacks.

2. **Cluster headache** is the most prevalent TAC in the population. It is most commonly seen in men. Headache clusters generally last several weeks or months, separated by periods of remission. Circadian rhythmicity of attacks and circannual rhythmicity of cycles is frequently noted. Attacks of pain recur 1 to 8 times per day with duration 15 to 180 minutes. Pain is typically periorbital or temporal, intense, searing, with ipsilateral autonomic features such as ptosis, lacrimation, conjunctival injection, and nasal congestion and rhinorrhea (Table 21.5). Patients are often agitated and restless during acute cluster. Attacks may be triggered by alcohol and often occur nocturnally. Workup should include brain MRI to exclude secondary pathology. The most effective acute treatments are 100% oxygen delivered by face mask and subcutaneous sumatriptan. Steroids can be used to prevent cluster headache transiently, while verapamil is considered the drug of choice for prevention of cycles of greater than 2 weeks in duration.

3. **CPH** is a rare TAC marked by relatively short attacks of very severe lateralized pain with cranial autonomic features and definable response to indomethacin. Attacks usually occur 8 to 20 times daily and last 2 to 30 minutes.

TABLE 21.5 ICHD-3 Beta Criteria for Cluster Headache

At least five attacks
Severe or very severe unilateral orbital, supraorbital, and/or temporal pain
  lasting 15–180 min when untreated
Either or both of the following
  At least one of the following symptoms or signs ipsilateral to the
    headache
    Conjunctival injection and/or lacrimation
    Nasal congestion and/or rhinorrhea
    Eyelid edema
    Forehead and/or facial sweating
    Forehead and/or facial flushing
    Sensation of fullness in the ear
    Miosis and/or ptosis
  A sense of restlessness or agitation
Attack frequency between 1 every other day and 8 per day for more than
half the time when the disorder is active

Though the majority of attacks are spontaneous, 10% of attacks may be precipitated mechanically by bending or rotating the head or via external pressure against the transverse processes of C4–C5 or the greater occipital nerve.

4. **Short-lasting unilateral neuralgiform headache attacks with conjunctival injection and tearing or cranial autonomic symptoms (SUNCT/SUNA)** is an extremely rare condition marked by very short-lasting attacks (1 to 600 seconds) of lateralized severe head pain with prominent cranial autonomic features lingering beyond the period of pain. Attacks may involve isolated brief stabs of pain or series of stabs, and minor discomfort with or without interval. Patients may describe dozens or hundreds of attacks per day. Episodes may be triggered by trigeminal or extratrigeminal stimulation without refractory periods. SUNCT and SUNA are typically refractory to medical management, although case reports suggest possible response to lamotrigine.

5. **Hemicrania continua (HC)** is characterized by a continuous, side-locked, unilateral headache of variable intensity. Exacerbations of sharp pains lasting seconds to hours are common, some with occasional migrainous features. A foreign body sensation affecting the ipsilateral eye is relatively common. Like CPH the diagnosis of HC requires response to indomethacin.

Key Points

- The vast majority of patients presenting with chronic or recurrent headache will meet criteria for migraine.
- Tension-type headache is the most prevalent but least distinct of the primary headache conditions.
- Brain MRI is the imaging modality of choice in the workup of chronic or recurrent headache, but is unnecessary in the setting of typical migraine.
- TACs are subclassified on the basis of the duration and frequency of attacks.
- Migraine aura is classified as "typical" when involving only visual, hemisensory, or language impairment. The presence of any motor weakness leads to the diagnosis of "hemiplegic" aura, and the presence of brainstem symptoms such as vertigo, diplopia, and ataxia to the diagnosis of "brainstem" aura.

Recommended Readings

Bashir A, Lipton R, Ashina S, et al. Migraine and structural changes in the brain: a systematic review and meta-analysis. *Neurology.* 2013;81:1260–1268.

Bellegaard V, Thede-Schmidt-Hansen P, Svensson P, et al. Are headache and temporomandibular disorders related? A blinded study. *Cephalalgia.* 2008;28:832–841.

Cheung V, Amoozegar F, Dilli E. Medication overuse headache. *Curr Neurol Neurosci Rep.* 2015;15(1):509. doi:10.1007/s11910-014-0509.

Ducros A, Blousse V. Headache arising from idiopathic changes in CSF pressure. *Lancet Neurol.* 2015;14(6):655–668. doi:10.1016/S1474-4422(15)00015-0.

Evans R. Diagnostic testing for migraine and other primary headaches. *Neurol Clin.* 2009;27:393–415.

Frishberg B. The utility of neuroimaging in the evaluation of headache in patients with normal neurological examinations. *Neurology.* 1994;44:1191–1197.

Frishberg B, Rosenberg J, Matchar D, et al. Evidence-based guidelines in the primary care setting: neuroimaging in patients with nonacute headache. In: Proceedings from the American Academy of Neurology; April, 2014; Minneapolis, MN. http://tools.aan.com/professionals/practice/pdfs/gl0088.pdf

Fumal A, Schoenen J. Tension-type headache: current research and clinical management. *Lancet Neurol.* 2008;7:70–83.

Gronseth G, Greenberg M. The utility of electroencephalogram in the evaluation of patients presenting with headache: a review of the literature. *Neurology.* 1995;45:1263–1267.

Headache Classification Committee of the International Headache Society. The International Classification of Headache Disorders, 3rd edition (beta version). *Cephalalgia.* 2013;33(9):629–808.

Holle D, Obermann M. Rare primary headaches. *Curr Opin Neurol.* 2014;27:332–336.

Kaniecki R. Headache assessment and management. *JAMA.* 2003;289:1430–1433.

Kaniecki R. Migraine and tension-type headache: an assessment of challenges in diagnosis. *Neurology.* 2002;58(suppl 6):S15–S20.

Lipton R, Diamond S, Reed M, et al. Migraine diagnosis and treatment: results from the American Migraine Study II. *Headache.* 2001;41:638–645.

Lipton R, Fanning K, Serrano D, et al. Ineffective acute treatment of episodic migraine is associated with new-onset chronic migraine. *Neurology.* 2015;84:688–695.

Loder E, Weizenbaum E, Frishberg B, et al; American Headache Society Choosing Wisely Task Force. Choosing wisely in headache medicine: the American Headache Society's list of five things physicians and patients should question. *Headache.* 2013;53:1651–1659.

Maarbjerg S, Gozalov A, Olesen J, et al. Trigeminal neuralgia—a prospective systematic study of clinical characteristics in 158 patients. *Headache.* 2014;54:1574–1582.

May A. Diagnosis and clinical features of trigemino-autonomic headaches. *Headache.* 2013;53:1470–1478.

Nelson S, Taylor L. Headaches in brain tumor patients: primary or secondary? *Headache.* 2014;54:776–785.

Pareja J, Alvarez M. The usual treatment of trigeminal autonomic cephalalgias. *Headache.* 2013;53:1401–1414.

Schwedt T. Chronic migraine. *BMJ.* 2014;348:g1416. doi:10.1136/bmj.g1416.

Smith J, Swanson J. Giant cell arteritis. *Headache.* 2014;54:1217–1289.

Stam J. Thrombosis of the cerebral veins and sinuses. *N Engl J Med.* 2005;352:1791–1798.

Stovner L, Hagen K, Jensen R, et al. The global burden of headache: a documentation of headache prevalence and disability worldwide. *Cephalalgia.* 2007;27:193–210.

Tepper S, Dahlof C, Dowson A. Prevalence and diagnosis of migraine in patients consulting their physician with a complaint of headache: data from the Landmark Study. *Headache.* 2004;44:856–864.

VanderPluym J. Indomethacin-responsive headaches. *Curr Neurol Neurosci Rep.* 2015;15(2):516. doi:10.1007/s11910-014-0516-y.

Wakerly B, Tan M, Ting E. Idiopathic intracranial hypertension. *Cephalalgia.* 2015;35:248–261.

Yu S, Han X. Update of chronic tension-type headache. *Curr Pain Headache Rep.* 2015;19(1):469. doi:10.1007/s11916-014-0469-5.

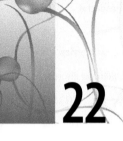

22 Approach to the Patient with Neck Pain and/or Arm Pain

Scott A. Shapiro

TRAUMATIC NECK PAIN WITHOUT ARM PAIN

A. Introduction. Trauma to the neck secondary to a motor vehicle accident, work-related injury, or athletic injury is a common cause of musculoskeletal neck pain. In the vast majority of patients, posttraumatic neck pain is a self-limited problem that is not serious.

B. Etiology. Straining of anterior/posterior cervical muscles and tendons is the mechanism of pain for most posttraumatic neck pain syndromes. The most common cause in clinical practice is vehicular accidents with hyperextension/flexion to the neck (whiplash). Altercations, athletic injuries (especially football), and lifting/tugging work injuries also occur.

C. Evaluation.

1. History and physical examination. The primary complaints are posttraumatic neck pain and neck stiffness. The paracervical muscles are tender with limitation of motion, spinous process point tenderness may be present, and there may be some associated interscapular pain and headache. Complaints of patchy arm numbness are occasionally reported but the neurologic exam is normal for the vast majority of patients.

2. Radiographs.

   a. **Plain X-rays** rule out most fractures and ligamentous instability. In the under-40 age group, the most common finding is loss of the lordotic curve from muscle spasm. In the over-40 age group, X-rays often show degenerative changes such as narrowed disk spaces and osteophyte (bone spur) formation. The accident is not the cause of these X-ray changes but certainly these changes can predispose the patient to more pain than a normal spine.

   b. Computed tomography (CT) scan/magnetic resonance imaging (MRI) scan. Any clinical or radiographic evidence for acute fracture, subluxation (instability), or spinal cord injury requires a thorough evaluation including, a cervical CT scan, consultation with a spine specialist, and, more often than not, a cervical MRI scan.

D. Referral

1. First 2 to 3 weeks (medicate and wait).

   a. Soft collar. Posttraumatic neck pain will usually subside on its own over a week or two. A narrow soft cervical collar can be helpful in taking the weight of the head off the neck and transferring it to the shoulders. The collar should not be so tall that it forces that patient into hyperextension, which is uncomfortable.

   b. Medication. Over-the-counter nonsteroidal anti-inflammatory medication (ibuprofen) with/without acetaminophen is the ideal analgesic. Other analgesics such as propoxyphene, codeine, or codeine analogs are acceptable but no schedule-3 narcotics such as oxycodone, demerol, or morphine should be used. Muscle relaxants such as Robaxin (methocarbamol) 500 mg per os q 6–8 h, Flexeril (cyclobenzaprine) 10 mg PO three times a day, or Parafon Forte (chlorzoxazone) 500 mg PO q 6–8 h can help. Avoid benzodiazepines because of abuse potential. In the patient whose stomach is sensitive to nonsteroidal medication, an evening dose of an H_2 receptor blocker such as cimetidine 300 to 600 mg PO can help prevent gastritis.

   c. Time-off from work. Desk-bound workers with mild to moderate neck pain can work and most ambitious people are able to function. Heavy laborers may benefit from light duty or 1 to 2 weeks off work. Beware of patients who exhibit symptom magnification and functional overlay due for purposes of secondary gain (worker's compensation and litigation). They have the tendency to abuse time-off work. In these scenarios, early referral to a physical medicine and rehabilitation (PM&R) specialist who can scientifically assess for malingering may be helpful.

2. **Weeks 3 to 6 if pain still present.**
   a. **Physical therapy.** If the neck pain does not subside after 2 weeks, physical therapy—heat, ultrasound, massage, and transcutaneous electrical nerve stimulation (TENS)—is reasonable.
   b. **Pain clinic.** Trigger-point injections of anesthetic/steroid can be helpful but are probably best scheduled after evaluation by a spine specialist.
3. **After 6 to 8 weeks.** When neck pain persists after 6 to 8 weeks, despite rest and therapy, and the pain remains severe enough to interfere with work or recreation, the next diagnostic test should be a cervical MRI scan to evaluate the cervical disks. Usually the study is normal or shows mild cervical disk dehydration with disk bulging. Neck pain from cervical disk dehydration can best be treated by cervical traction. Minor cervical disk bulging presenting with chronic pain with a normal neurologic exam is rarely a sufficient indication for surgery. At this point, it is best to get the opinion of a neurosurgeon.

NONTRAUMATIC NECK PAIN OF ARTHRITIC ORIGIN

A. **Introduction.** Neck pain from degenerative arthritis of the neck is of epidemic proportion (60% to 80%) in the elderly population.
B. **Etiology.** Degenerative arthritis of the cervical spine occasionally manifests itself as early as the third decade of life but is much more common with increasing age. Disk dehydration and disk space narrowing with osteophyte formation is a process that occurs naturally with age. Facet arthritis also occurs. Small nerve fibers innervating the disk and facet can be involved leading to neck pain. Dural impingement by osteophytes can also produce neck pain—especially with extension or lateral gaze.
C. **Evaluation.**
   1. **History and physical examination.** Nontraumatic neck pain in the over-40 age group is most often secondary to cervical degenerative arthritis. The pain is gradual in onset and initially intermittent and then becomes more constant. There can be associated occipital headache and interscapular pain. Motion, especially extension or lateral gaze, can aggravate the pain.
   2. **Radiographs.** X-rays show narrowing of disk spaces with bone spur formation. At least 70% of the population over the age of 65 have significant changes of degenerative arthritis. Regardless of how bad the X-rays look, if the patient is neurologically normal, MRI or surgery is not absolutely indicated.
D. **Referral.**
   1. **Medication.** Same as for traumatic neck pain.
   2. **Physical therapy.** Heat, ultrasound, massage, and TENS unit therapy can help.
   3. **Pain clinic.** Trigger-point injections can help.
   4. **Alternative therapies.** Though chiropractors can help many people, we cannot advocate manipulation of the neck when obvious bone spurs exist. Neurologic catastrophes and lawsuits have occurred. Patients can seek chiropractic care at their own risk. Recently magnets have become popular in relieving arthritic complaints with some scientific credence. Finally, oral glucosamine has been shown somewhat effective against arthritis, though its effect on cervical spondylosis remains to be determined.
   5. **Spine specialists.** In the majority of patients with neck pain and no arm pain, surgery is not indicated. The removal of large osteophytes ventral to the spinal cord can improve severe neck pain and occipital headache and actually improve range of motion. Only an experienced spinal surgeon should make this decision on the basis of a CT scan/MRI scan and repetitive physical examinations over a period of time.

NECK PAIN WITH ARM PAIN (RADICULOPATHY) FROM SOFT CERVICAL DISK BULGES/HERNIATIONS

A. Etiology. In the under-50 age group, the most common cause will be a single-level soft cervical disk. The concept of a soft cervical disk means either an eccentric disk bulge or a free fragment herniation compressing a root. A disk consists of an inner water-laden mucoid nuclear material and an outer fibrous annulus. The annulus can fissure, allowing the nucleus either to bulge or to herniate out. There is no osteophyte involved in the compression. The posterior longitudinal ligament extends beneath the entire spinal cord, protecting the cord from disk herniation, and so a disk herniation primarily projects laterally into the foramen, compressing the nerve only. In rare cases, sufficient force, such as in trauma, can lead to a large disk herniation, causing an acute myelopathy.

B. Anatomy. A disk is named by the bordering vertebral bodies. Thus, the disk between vertebral bodies C5 and C6 is named the C5–C6 disk. The nerve root whose number corresponds to that of a given vertebral body exits above that body's pedicle. Thus, a C5–C6 disk compresses the C6 nerve root.

C. Evaluation.

1. History. In the classic story, there is intermittent neck pain, and then severe neck pain and arm pain develop. Rarely is this condition traumatic in origin. The pain radiates down the shoulder and into the arm. There are some dermatomal patterns of radiation that can help discern the level of herniation. Patients may complain of various combinations of suboccipital headache, interscapular pain, numbness, tingling, and weakness. The pain often awakens the patient from sleep.

2. Physical examination.
   a. Neck examination. There is posterior tenderness, especially tenderness at the spinous process near the level of involvement and paracervical tenderness. Painful limitation of motion with extension and lateral gaze to the side of arm pain is classic.
   b. Arm examination.
      (1) C5 radiculopathy (C4–C5 disk herniation). presents with pain and numbness radiating to the shoulder along with a weak deltoid muscle (shoulder abduction). Simultaneous testing of both deltoid muscles by compression on the outstretched upper arms detects minor weakness (Table 22.1). There is no true reflex to test.
      (2) C6 radiculopathy (C5–C6 disk herniation). C5–C6 disk herniation is the second most common cervical disc herniation. Pain and numbness radiate across the top of the neck and along the biceps to the lateral aspect of the forearm and dorsal thumb and index finger. Numbness is usually more distal. A weak biceps, a reduced biceps reflex, and weak wrist extension are observed (Video 22.1).
      (3) C7 radiculopathy (C6–C7 disk herniation). This is the most common disk herniation. Pain radiates across the top of the neck, across the triceps, and down the posterolateral forearm to the middle finger. Numbness again is more distal. A weak triceps and reduced triceps reflex are observed.
      (4) C8 radiculopathy (C7–T1 disk herniation). This is very uncommon. Pain and numbness radiate across the neck and down the arm to the small finger and ring finger. Wrist flexion and the intrinsic muscles of the hand are weak.

3. Radiographic evaluation.
   a. **Plain X-rays** provide very little help. They may show slight narrowing of the disk space involved and loss of lordosis.

TABLE 22.1 Motor Strength Classification (0 to 5 scale)

0 = No movement
1 = Flicker of movement
2 = Able to move but not against gravity
3 = Able to move against gravity but offers no resistance
4 = Offers resistance but able to overcome or easy fatigue
5 = Normal

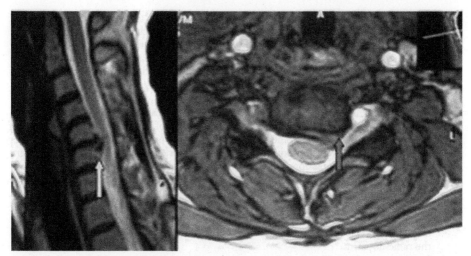

FIGURE 22.1 Sagittal and axial MRI image demonstrating a large eccentric C5–C6 cervical disc herniation causing a left C6 radiculopathy.

  b. **MRI scan** without contrast is the study of choice for demonstrating a soft cervical disk herniation (Fig. 22.1).
  4. Electromyogram and nerve conduction studies (EMG/NCS). An EMG for a single-level disk herniation with a radiculopathy is not absolutely necessary. An EMG can help when other disorders, such as amyotrophic lateral sclerosis, carpal tunnel syndrome, and brachial plexopathy, need to be ruled out.
D. Referral.
  1. Physical therapy. After diagnosis by MRI, a patient with a motor strength rating of 4/5 or more (Table 22.1) can be referred for cervical traction, heat, ultrasound, massage, and a soft collar. Initially, cervical traction should be done by a physical therapist. Inform the therapist that if traction is tolerated; the patient is to be instructed in home cervical traction at 10 lb for ½ hour every night. Approximately 60% to 80% of soft disk herniations improve to the point of resolution of the radiculopathy with traction alone within 4 to 6 weeks. Not every patient can tolerate traction.
  2. Medications. A trial of 4 mg self-weaning methylprednisolone (Medrol) dose pack can be used early in the treatment prior to nonsteroidals with some success. Other medicines were previously discussed in the section on traumatic neck pain.
  3. Time-off from work. Desk-type workers with mild to moderate neck/arm pain can work, and most ambitious people are able to function. Heavy laborers may benefit from light duty or 1 to 4 weeks off work. Beware of patients who exhibit symptom magnification and functional overlay for purposes of secondary gain (worker's compensation and litigation). They have the tendency to abuse time off work. In these scenarios, early referral to a PM&R specialist may be helpful.
  4. Spine specialist. In any patient with three-fifth strength or worse, immediate referral to a spine surgeon is indicated. The longer a root is compressed with severe weakness, the less likely strength will return to normal. If the strength remains four-fifth or better but pain persists after 3 to 6 weeks of traction, then referral to a spine surgeon is also indicated. A well-trained spine surgeon should achieve improvement of arm pain and weakness in 90% to 95% of soft cervical disk herniations.

NECK PAIN WITH ARM PAIN FROM BONE SPURS (HARD DISC, CERVICAL SPONDYLOSIS)

A. Introduction. The combination of neck pain and arm pain in cervical spondylosis is also of epidemic proportions in the elderly population.

B. **Etiology.** Disk dehydration and narrowing lead to bone spur formation at the margins of the vertebral body. The spurs can project into the foramen or canal, compressing the nerve root or the spinal cord, or both. In addition, facet arthritis with resultant hypertrophy and ligamentous hypertrophy also narrow the spinal canal and neural foramina. With progressive age, more than one disc space is usually involved. The center of the process usually extends from C4 to C7.

C. **Evaluation.**

1. **History.** This condition occurs primarily in patients older than soft cervical disk herniation patients, although the two groups overlap. About 90% of patients have gradual onset of neck pain with progression to neck and arm pain. The pain radiates down the shoulder and into the arm. There are some dermatomal patterns of radiation that can help discern the level of root compression. Various complaints of suboccipital headache, interscapular pain, numbness, tingling, and weakness may also be present. The pain often wakes the patient up from sleep. About 10% of patients have asymptomatic degenerative arthritis, and then symptoms of neck pain/arm pain are often precipitated by hyperextension/flexion injuries from trauma (motor vehicle accidents). A large percentage have multiple disk spaces involved, making it more difficult to determine which level or levels caused the radiculopathy.

2. **Physical examination.**

   a. **Neck examination.** There is posterior tenderness, especially tenderness at the spinous process near the level of involvement and paracervical tenderness. Painful limitation of motion with extension and lateral gaze to the side of arm pain is classic.

   b. Arm examination (see Table 22.1) same as discussed in soft cervical disc section.

   c. **Leg examination (Table 22.2).** Gait is usually normal even in the face of significant radiographic evidence of spinal cord compression. Occasionally, myelopathy is present. Early on, the gait is normal in the face of increased muscle stretch reflexes and a Babinski sign. With more severe and prolonged compression, one can observe spastic gait with bowel and bladder problems. In the most severe cases, the patient requires a cane or a walker. Rarely is it allowed to progress to wheelchair dependency.

3. **Radiographs.**

   a. **Plain X-rays** show disk space narrowing with osteophyte (bone spur) formation. Oblique films can exhibit neuroforaminal narrowing.

   b. **MRI scan (Fig. 22.2).** MRI is excellent for demonstrating nerve-root compression and spinal cord compression from bone spurs. It does not provide as much detail about bone anatomy as the CT scan.

   c. **CT scan.** CT shows better bone detail than does MRI but is not as good at showing the neural structures. The two studies together are ideal for this group of patients, but this is obviously not cost-effective, so MRI is the first choice.

4. **EMG and NCS studies.** The EMG can be helpful in discerning which roots are most involved in patients with multilevel spondylosis.

D. **Referral.**

1. **Medication.** As discussed in previous medication sections.

2. **Soft cervical collar.**

3. **Physical therapy.** Heat, ultrasound, massage, traction, and TENS can reduce the symptoms. Approximately 20% of the radiculopathies (arm pain/strength) can be successfully improved with medicine and therapy alone for many years. The majority

TABLE 22.2 **Nurick Classification**

Grade
Signs of spinal cord disease but normal gait
Slight gait abnormality not preventing full-time employment
Gait abnormality severe enough to prevent employment or housework. Still able to ambulate independently
Requires a walker or someone else's help to ambulate
Wheelchair bound

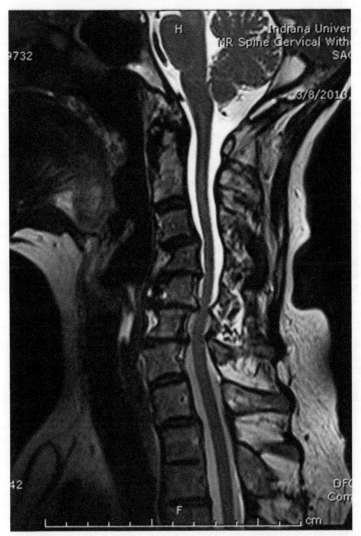

FIGURE 22.2 Sagittal MRI of cervical spondylosis demonstrating multiple level involvement.

of patients have some pain with persistent mild weakness (if any weakness is present). Rarely does myelopathy develop in this group of patients.

4. **Spine specialist.** Surgery for cervical spondylotic radiculopathy is almost always elective. Results of surgery are much better for single-level disease than for multilevel disease—especially for neck pain. Arm strength of 3/5 or worse and any evidence for myelopathy are indications for immediate referral to a spine surgeon. The anterior approach is superior to the posterior approach if bone spurs project under the entire spinal cord. Surgery helps the radiculopathy in 90% to 95% of both single-level and multilevel disease patients, but neck pain improves in only 70% to 75% of multilevel disease patients. Complete relief of radicular pain occurs in approximately 60% to 80%. There is no age cutoff for surgery as long as patient is in reasonable medical condition. The elderly tolerate surgery very well with minimal morbidity. If a myelopathy is present with gait abnormality and an aggressive decompression is performed, an improvement of one grade on the Nurick scale (see Table 22.2) can be expected in 70% to 80% of patients. Duration of symptoms is very important for patients with gait problems. Thus, early referral is indicated.

NECK PAIN WITH/WITHOUT ARM PAIN DUE TO METASTATIC CANCER OF THE CERVICAL SPINE

A. Introduction. As patients live longer with various malignancies, the number of patients who present with spine metastases also increases. The tumors that most commonly involve the spine are lung cancer, breast cancer, prostate cancer, lymphomas, and multiple myelomas. As many as 20% of these tumors will develop symptomatic spinal involvement. In approximately 10% of patients, metastatic spinal involvement will be the mode of presentation with no known primary tumor.

B. Evaluation

1. History and physical examination. Both primary and metastatic tumors of the spine initially present with pain that is often worse at night. The pain continues to worsen over a very short period, and then neurologic symptoms such as radiculopathy and myelopathy develop fairly quickly. It is best to make the diagnosis when neurologic symptoms are minimal.

2. Radiographs.

   a. **Plain X-rays** can show destruction of the vertebral bodies and pedicles (Fig. 22.3). Pathologic compression fractures and lytic pedicles are very common. The sensitivity of plain X-rays is approximately 60%.

   b. **Bone scans** are very sensitive—approaching 100%—in showing spine metastases, including asymptomatic areas with no destruction.

   c. **MRI scans** are ideal for delineating canal involvement, cord compression, and surgical feasibility.

C. Referral.

1. Radiation therapy. Diffuse disease involving large amounts of the spine is treated primarily with steroids and radiation therapy. Radiation is usually reserved for the symptomatic areas only. Dexamethasone 2 to 20 mg PO q6h can be quite helpful in improving pain and neurologic symptoms.

2. Surgery. Early referral to a spine surgeon is warranted following diagnosis regardless of the neurologic examination. If surgery is indicated, it is often best to perform it prior to radiation therapy, because this reduces the wound complication rate. In the face of a cervical myelopathy resulting from diffuse canal involvement and cord compression, a laminectomy can be performed. Patients with lung cancer do very poorly, and it is hard to justify surgery scientifically for metastatic lung cancer unless there is no primary disease and the spine disease is the only systemic metastasis. Other tumors do better, but a good rule is 30% to 50% of all tumors are improved by laminectomy with a 10% mortality rate. Isolated vertebral body disease can be resected from an anterior approach—especially in well-controlled breast cancer, prostate cancer, lymphoma, and renal cell cancer with excellent long-term results that are superior to radiation alone.

MISCELLANEOUS NECK PAIN WITH/WITHOUT ARM PAIN

A. Rheumatoid arthritis.

1. Etiology. Rheumatoid arthritis can affect the C1–C2 articulation leading to erosion of the odontoid process and transverse atlantal ligament, which leads to C1–C2 instability, and cord compression from the developing panus.

2. Evaluation

   a. History and physical examination. Severe neck pain is usually followed by arm pain and a progressive myelopathy.

   b. Radiographs. Plain X-rays and MRI scans are best for showing erosion of the odontoid process with subsequent instability and spinal cord compression (Fig. 22.4).

3. Referral and therapy. Place a soft collar and refer immediately to a spine surgeon. Posterior C1–C2 fusion with transarticular screws is ideal for the problem; occasionally an anterior transoral odontoidectomy is required. These treatments are not without risk and must be individualized.

B. Discitis/osteomyelitis.

1. Introduction. Bacterial discitis/osteomyelitis is extremely uncommon in the cervical spine and fever may not be present.

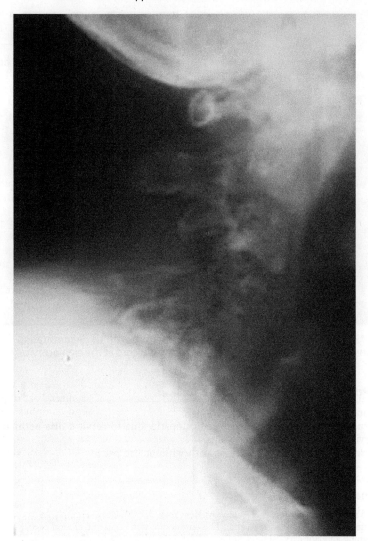

FIGURE 22.3 Lateral radiograph demonstrating lytic destruction of cervical vertebral bodies by tumor.

2. **Evaluation.**
   a. **History and physical examination.** There may be a prior history of skin infection, urinary tract infection, or pulmonary infection. Iatrogenic diskitis/osteomyelitis complicating cervical spine surgery is known to occur. Perhaps the most common cause in urban settings is a history of intravenous (IV) drug abuse. Progressive neck pain with a rapidly progressive myelopathy is the usual presentation.
   b. **Radiographs.** Plain X-rays show disk space collapse with erosion of the bordering vertebral bodies. MRI shows epidural spinal cord compression from kyphosis or epidural abscess.
3. **Referral.** The patient should be immediately referred to either a spine specialist or an infectious disease specialist. An immediate radiology-directed needle biopsy/culture or open biopsy culture, and administration of IV bactericidal antibiotics for at least 6 weeks, are indicated.

   Surgical debridement and decompression are performed for severe kyphosis and neurologic problems.

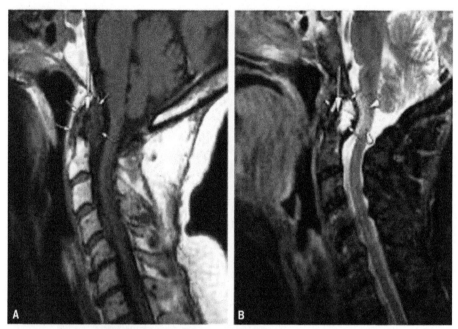

FIGURE 22.4 A and B: Sagittal MRI scans in rheumatoid arthritis demonstrating destruction of the dens with compression of the medulla and spinal cord at the craniocervical junction.

Key Points

- Nonoperative management of neck pain.
- Neurologic findings of cervical radiculopathy due to cervical disc herniation or cervical spondylosis and treatments.
- Miscellaneous causes of neck pain with/without arm pain.

Recommended Readings

Adams R, Victor M, eds. *Principles of Neurology*. New York, NY: McGraw-Hill; 2009.

Burneikiene S, Nelson EL, Mason A, et al. The duration of symptoms and clinical outcomes in patients undergoing anterior cervical discectomy and fusion for degenerative disc disease and radiculopathy. *Spine J*. 2015;15(3):427–432.

DePalma AF, Rothman RH, Levitt RL, et al. The natural history of severe cervical disc degeneration. *Acta Orthop Scand*. 1972;43:392–396.

Melhem E. MR Imaging of the cervical spine and spinal cord. *Magn Reson Imaging Clin N Am*. 2000;8:435–650.

Modic M, Masaryk T, Ross J, eds. *Magnetic Resonance Imaging of the Spine*. Chicago, IL: Yearbook Medical Publishers; 1989.

Patchell R, Tibbs P, Regine W, et al. Direct decompressive surgical resection in the treatment of spinal cord compression caused by metastatic cancer: a randomized trial. *Lancet*. 2005;366:643–648.

Pellicci P, Ranawat C, Tsairis P, et al. A prospective study of the progression of rheumatoid arthritis of the cervical spine. *J Bone Joint Surg*. 1981;63(3):342–350.

Rothman R, Simeone F, eds. *The Spine*. Vols 1 & 2. Philadelphia, PA: WB Saunders; 1992.

Shapiro S. Banked fibula and the locking cervical plate following anterior cervical discectomy. *J Neurosurgery*. 1996;84:161–165.

Shapiro S. Spinal Instrumentation with a low complication rate. *Surg Neurol*. 1997;48:566–574.

Shapiro S, Connolly P, Donnaldson J, et al. Cadaveric fibula, locking plate, and allogenic bone matrix for anterior cervical fusions after cervical discectomy for radiculopathy or myelopathy. *J Neurosurg*. 2001;95:43–50.

Winn HR. *Youmans Neurosurgery*. Vol 1–4. Philadelphia, PA: Elsevier BV; 2011

Wong D, Fornasier V, MacNab I. Spinal metastases: The obvious, the occult and the imposters. *Spine*. 1990;15:1–4.

Approach to the Patient with Low Back Pain, Lumbosacral Radiculopathy, and Lumbar Stenosis

23

Eric M. Horn and Paul B. Nelson

A. **Acute low back pain.** Back pain is extremely common. Most adults can remember at least one episode of back pain sometime in their lives. Approximately 50% of working adults have back pain at least 1 day per year. Back pain has become one of the most expensive health care problems and has become a leading cause of disability among persons younger than 45 years. The estimated annual cost of medical care of patients with low back pain is more than 8 billion dollars.

B. **Lumbar disc disease with sciatica.** Patients with back and leg pain (sciatica) most likely have nerve-root compression secondary to rupture of a lumbar disc. Although it occurs occasionally in the pediatric and geriatric age groups, a ruptured disc generally occurs in the third to fifth decades of life. Approximately 90% of cases of rupture of lumbar discs occur between L4–L5 and L5–S1; 5% occur at L3–L4. The incidence of disc rupture is the same among men and women.

C. **Lumbar spinal stenosis** is any type of narrowing of the spinal canal, lateral recess, or intervertebral foramina secondary to congenital causes, disc degeneration, bony hypertrophy, ligamentous hypertrophy, or spondylolisthesis. Because it is caused primarily by degenerative change, the disease seldom occurs before the fifth decade of life. The mean age of patients undergoing operative procedures for lumbar stenosis is the sixth decade, although it sometimes occurs in the seventh and eighth decades. Lumbar stenosis is most commonly observed at L4–L5 and L3–L4.

ETIOLOGY

A. **Acute low back pain.** Most low back pain is due to mechanical abnormalities (muscle strain, ligamentous injury, annular tears, and so on) and facet joint inflammation. With the disorder being so common and so often mechanical in nature, back pain must be considered a normal part of aging. Degenerative changes in the spine begin in the second decade of life and are extremely common by the fifth decade.

A small percentage of patients have structural abnormalities that account for low back pain. Spondylolisthesis, which is a forward slipping of one vertebral body over another, is caused by defects in the pars interarticularis (spondylolysis) in the younger age group and by degenerative changes in the older age group. Lumbar scoliosis, which is a lateral deformity of the spine, is usually caused by degenerative disease. Primary or metastatic bone tumors or infections of the disc or epidural space are much less common causes of back pain.

B. **Lumbar disc disease with sciatica.** A lumbar disc acts as an articulation between the vertebrae and as a cushion. It is composed of a cartilaginous end plate and an outer annulus that surrounds the nucleus. Degenerative changes begin in the disc by the late 20s and are common by the fourth decade. Alterations in the lumbar disc from age alone and major or minor trauma can cause an intervertebral disc to rupture. The disc most commonly ruptures in a posterolateral direction. Disc extrusions and some protrusions can cause nerve-root or, less frequently, cauda equina compression.

C. **Lumbar spinal stenosis.** Except in patients born with short pedicles, spinal stenosis is secondary to degenerative changes and many years of repetitive trauma. With age, the disc loses its water content and stops functioning as a cushion. There is increased stress on the bony vertebrae, the ligaments, and the facets. There is increased mobility of the vertebral bodies, ballooning of the disc, and hypertrophy of the ligaments. All these changes can cause narrowing of the lumbar canal. Absolute spinal stenosis is defined as a midsagittal diameter of 10 mm or less. A normal lumbar canal is 15 to 25 mm in diameter.

CLINICAL MANIFESTATIONS AND EVALUATION

A. History.
1. **Acute low back pain.** The history interview must determine whether the back pain is mechanical or associated with a more serious problem. It must also determine whether there are any "red flags" that suggest more serious causes of the back disorder (Table 23.1). Symptoms and histories that should alert the physician that there may be a disorder more serious than regular mechanical low back pain include night pain, fever, severe back spasms, leg pain, leg weakness, leg numbness, bladder or bowel dysfunction, major trauma, minor trauma in a patient with osteoporosis, weight loss, lethargy, back pain in a child, history of previous bacterial infection, history of carcinoma, history of intravenous drug use, and a worker's compensation or legal claim.
2. **Lumbar disc disease with sciatica.** A patient with sciatica usually has a history of back pain for several days before the development of leg pain. In L4–L5 and L5–S1 disc disease, the back pain actually may be somewhat relieved as the patient goes on to have burning discomfort in the buttocks and unilateral pain in the posterolateral aspects of both the upper and lower leg. There may also be numbness or tingling in a portion of the foot or toes. The less common L3–L4 disc disease can cause pain in the groin and anterior aspects of the thigh and upper leg. The history occasionally is one of severe sciatic pain from the onset. Bilateral leg pain and bladder or bowel dysfunction suggests cauda equina compression from a large midline disc extrusion.
3. **Lumbar spinal stenosis.** In spinal stenosis, the history is more important than the examination. The patient typically reports back and leg discomfort, numbness, or heaviness with standing or walking. Symptoms improve with rest or forward bending. The leg symptoms are usually asymmetric. Occasional patients have true sciatica (Video 23.1)

B. Physical examination.
1. **Acute low back pain.** Examination of a patient with acute low back pain should begin with inspection and palpation of the low back. Paravertebral muscle spasms may be present. In most cases of mechanical back pain, straight-leg-raise testing causes back pain only. Straight-leg-raise testing that causes back and leg pain suggest root or cauda equina compression. The neurologic examination should include walking on the heels and toes, squatting, and individual testing of the foot and toe dorsiflexors and plantarflexors, the quadriceps, and the iliopsoas muscles. The general examination should include palpation of the abdomen, to rule out an abdominal aortic aneurysm, and a rectal examination.

TABLE 23.1 "Red Flags" That Suggest Serious Causes of Low Back Pain

Symptoms, History	Possible Diagnosis
Night pain	Tumor
Fever, history of recent bacterial infection or intravenous drug use, severe back spasms	Diskitis and epidural abscess
Leg pain	Nerve-root compression
Bilateral lower extremity weakness or numbness, bladder or bowel dysfunction	Cauda equina or conus compression
Major trauma	Fracture, dislocation
Minor trauma in a patient with osteoporosis	Compression fracture
History of carcinoma	Metastatic disease
Systemic symptoms such as fever, weight loss	Multiple myeloma
Back pain in a child	Tumor, tethered cord
Worker's compensation or legal claim	Secondary gain

2. **Lumbar disc disease with sciatica.** The patient walks in a slow, deliberate manner with slight forward tilt of the trunk. Paravertebral muscle tightness can cause decreased range of motion of the back, and asymmetric muscle tightness can cause associated scoliosis. The patient prefers to stand or lie rather than sit. The best position is usually lying on the unaffected side with the affected leg slightly bent at the knee and hip. The pain is frequently worsened by Valsalva's maneuver.

   a. **Straight-leg-raise testing** is important in the diagnosis of lumbar disc disease. The patient is in a supine position with the knee extended and the ankle plantar flexed. The examiner raises the leg slowly. Normally, the leg can be raised to 90 degrees without discomfort or with slight tightness in the hamstring. When the nerve root is compressed by a ruptured disc, the straight leg raise is limited and causes back and leg pain. It worsens with dorsiflexion of the foot. In most cases, the result of the straight-leg-raise test is positive only on the side of the disc rupture. If lifting the leg without symptoms causes pain in the leg with symptoms, one must consider disc rupture in the axilla of the nerve root.

   b. **Motor testing** is directed at the nerve roots most commonly affected. Compression of the L5 nerve root can cause foot and great toe dorsiflexion weakness (tibialis anterior and extensor hallucis longus). When the compression is severe, the patient may have foot drop. Compression of the S1 nerve root can cause plantar flexion weakness. This is difficult to detect at the bedside and is best tested by having the patient do toe raises one leg at a time. Weakness at L4 can cause quadriceps weakness. The patient may have the sensation that the leg is giving way. Disease of the L3–L4 disc decreases the knee reflex, and disease of the L5–S1 disc decreases the ankle reflex.

   c. **Sensory loss** resulting from a disc rupture seldom occurs in a dermatomal pattern. Rupture of the L5–S1 disc can cause relative hypalgesia in the bottom of the foot, lateral aspect of the foot, and little toe. Rupture of the L4–L5 disc can cause relative hypalgesia in the dorsum of the foot and great toe. Rupture of the L3–L4 disc can cause sensory loss in the anterior thigh and shin.

3. **Lumbar spinal stenosis.** Findings at neurologic examination of the lower extremities may be relatively unremarkable at rest. One occasionally may find evidence of mild nerve-root dysfunction such as L5 numbness and weakness.

DIFFERENTIAL DIAGNOSIS

A. **Acute low back pain.**
   1. Lumbosacral sprain
   2. Facet joint inflammation
   3. Degenerative arthritis
   4. Fracture (compression if osteoporotic and minimal trauma history)
   5. Metastatic disease
   6. Primary bone tumor
   7. Diskitis
   8. Epidural abscess
   9. Ankylosing spondylitis
   10. Paget's disease
   11. Tethered spinal cord
   12. Spondylolisthesis
   13. Conversion reaction
B. **Lumbar disc disease with sciatica.**
   1. Ruptured extruded disc
   2. Lateral recess and foraminal stenosis
   3. Synovial cyst
   4. Spondylolisthesis
C. **Lumbar spinal stenosis.**
   1. **Congenital stenosis**
   2. **Stenosis secondary to degenerative damage**
   3. **Synovial cyst**

4. **Peripheral vascular disease.** Arterial vascular insufficiency can cause leg discomfort during walking but is relieved by simply stopping rather than bending forward or sitting.

5. **Degenerative hip disease** can cause limitation of standing and walking. The pain usually comes on with any type of weight-bearing. Examination reveals a decreased range of motion of the hip, and hip rotation may exacerbate the discomfort. The pain associated with degenerative hip disease is most likely to be located in the proximal hip, thigh, and knee.

DIAGNOSTIC APPROACH

A. **Acute low back pain.** In the absence of red flags that suggest a more serious disorder, most testing should be delayed for 4 weeks. If the patient does not respond to conservative treatment in 4 weeks, however, the following studies may be considered.

1. Lumbosacral radiographs of the spine.
2. Magnetic resonance imaging (MRI).
3. Computed tomography (CT) scan if MRI is not available or contraindicated, or if the patient is claustrophobic. CT should include L3–L4, L4–L5, and L5–S1.
4. Lumbosacral myelography and postmyelography CT seldom are needed unless it is impossible to perform MRI (pacemaker).
5. Laboratory tests include complete blood cell count (CBC) with differential and erythrocyte sedimentation rate (ESR).
6. A bone scan can be done, especially if there is a history of carcinoma.
7. Occasionally a discogram may be done in a patient with refracting back pain, a degenerative disc, and no response to extensive conservative therapy.

B. **Lumbar disc disease with sciatica.** Few tests are needed in the first 4 weeks if the signs and symptoms are mild to moderate. Severe sciatica and sciatica associated with marked neurologic deficits and weakness of bladder and bowel movements should be evaluated earlier. The presence of a disc rupture on an imaging study does not necessarily imply nerve-root dysfunction. Approximately 75% of adult patients with symptoms have disc bulges or protrusions. Most severe sciatica is associated with disc extrusion.

1. Plain lumbosacral radiographs of the spine should be performed.
2. MRI is the procedure of choice for evaluating a lumbar disc rupture. L5–S1 disc extrusion causing severe right S1 nerve-root compression is shown in Figure 23.1.
3. CT may be used if the patient is unable to tolerate MRI.
4. Myelography and postmyelography CT can be used occasionally if MRI and CT do not provide enough information for a diagnosis.
5. Diagnostic nerve blocks, if there is doubt about which nerve(s) are involved.
6. Electromyography and nerve conduction velocity studies may be helpful if the signs and symptoms do not correlate well with the MRI or CT findings and if one suspects a peripheral nerve problem.

C. **Lumbar spinal stenosis.** Unless the symptoms are severe, testing may not be done in the early stages of spinal stenosis. A patient who seeks medical therapy for spinal stenosis usually has a walking tolerance of <1 to 2 blocks and a standing tolerance of 20 minutes or less.

1. **Plain radiographs of the lumbosacral spine** are indicated to assess the degree of degenerative change and bone density. Flexion–extension lateral views are needed to detect degenerative spondylolisthesis (Fig. 23.2). Degenerative spondylolisthesis is frequently associated with spinal stenosis.
2. An **MRI** is the best study for evaluating the number of levels involved and the severity of the spinal stenosis. Figure 23.3 is an MRI that shows severe stenosis at L4–L5.
3. **CT** can be used if MRI is not available, but CT does not show the complete lumbar spine and has poorer resolution.
4. A **bone scan** should be obtained if there is a history of malignant disease.
5. **Radiographs of the hip** are needed if there is decreased range of motion of the hip or pain with rotation of the hip.
6. **Laboratory tests.** CBC and differential and ESR should be obtained and possibly serum and urine protein electrophoresis performed if there are systemic symptoms. A prostatic specific antigen assay should be performed for male patients older than 50 years.
7. **Arterial Doppler ultrasonography** should be performed if the patient has diminished or absent peripheral pulses.

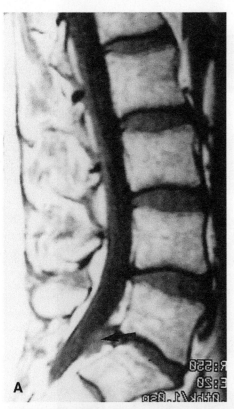

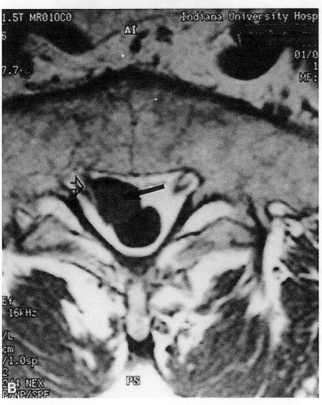

FIGURE 23.1 **A:** T1-weighted sagittal MRI shows a lumbar disc extrusion at L5–S1 that has gone down the lumbosacral canal (*arrow*). **B:** T2-weighted axial MRI shows a large, extruded L5–S1 disc fragment (*solid arrow*) compressing the right S1 nerve root (*open arrow*).

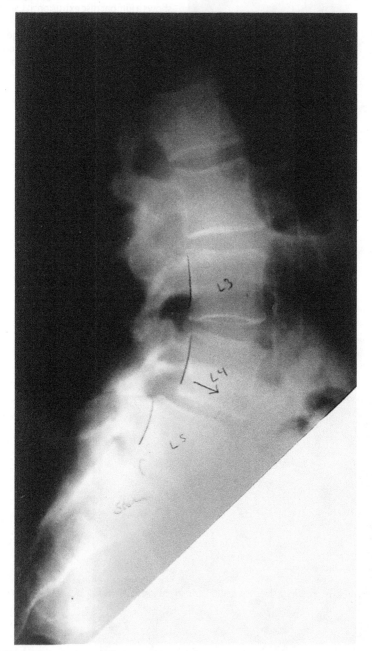

FIGURE 23.2 Lateral plain radiograph of the lumbosacral spine shows spondylolisthesis of L4 on L5.

TREATMENT

A. **Acute low back pain.** Approximately 90% of patients with acute low back pain recover within 1 month. Treatment is as follows:
   1. Restriction of patient activities as tolerated.
   2. Acetaminophen.
   3. Nonsteroidal anti-inflammatory drugs (NSAIDs).

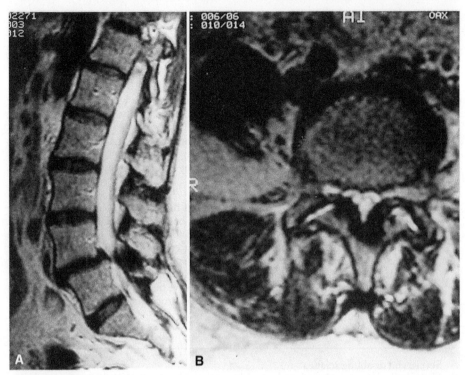

FIGURE 23.3 A: T2-weighted sagittal MRI shows segmental stenosis at L4–L5. **B:** Axial T2-weighted MRI shows severe stenosis at L4–L5. There is marked facet and ligamentous hypertrophy.

4. Opioids, but for no longer than 2 weeks.
5. Short course of steroids (3 to 5 days).
6. Muscle relaxants.
7. Heat.
8. Epidural and/or facet steroid/lidocaine injections.
9. Limit lifting to 20 lb (9 kg) for moderate to severe back pain. Activity restrictions at work should seldom be extended beyond 3 months.
10. Surgery may be considered if the back pain is associated with a more serious problem (Table 23.1). Rarely surgery is done for refractory back pain that is associated with a degenerative disc, a positive discogram of the level of the degenerative disc, and no response to conservative therapy.

B. **Lumbar disc disease with sciatica.** The initial management of sciatica is similar to that of acute low back pain. At least one half of patients with sciatica improve within 1 month.

1. Two to four days of rest with gradual return to normal activities.
2. Acetaminophen.
3. NSAIDs.
4. Short course of opioids (no more than 2 weeks).
5. Short course of steroids (3 to 5 days).
6. Muscle relaxants.
7. Heat.
8. Epidural steroid injections are of limited value in patients with extruded discs.
9. Limit lifting to 20 lb (9 kg). Try to keep work-related activity restrictions to no more than 3 months.
10. Surgery for lumbar disc disease should be considered for patients with severe pain that do not respond to conservative therapy, patients with significant weakness such as a foot drop, and a patient with bladder or bowel dysfunction. Surgery should be considered in a more urgent basis if there is significant cauda equina compression.

Conservative therapy can be tried for a longer period of time when you are dealing with primarily nerve-root compression.

There has been an increased interest using minimally invasive techniques when surgical intervention is required. Some surgeons have made use of a tubular retractor system when performing microdiscectomies.

C. **Lumbar spinal stenosis.**

1. Conservative therapy requires that patients be taught to live within the limits of their walking and standing tolerances. They need to realize that they should get off their feet, if possible, when symptoms occur.
2. **Patient with severe** limitation of walking may benefit from the use of license plates for persons with disabilities.
3. **Patients with degenerative** spondylolisthesis may benefit from lumbosacral support.
4. **Core strengthening** experiences.
5. **Epidural steroid** injections have limited use.
6. **Surgical treatment** should be considered only if the patient's condition is medically stable and the patient can no longer live with his or her degree of spinal claudication. Patients with true sciatica that does not respond to conservative therapy also can be considered for surgery. Surgical procedures that can be considered include lumbar laminectomy, lateral recess decompression, and spinal fusion. Seldom is surgery for spinal stenosis necessary in the first 3 months of symptoms. In most cases, the patient has symptoms for 12 to 18 months. Minimally invasive techniques are now also available for both lumbar decompression and lumbar fusion procedures.

SURGICAL REFERRAL

A. Severe and disabling sciatica.
B. Neurologic deficits such as foot drop or bladder and bowel disturbance.
C. Poor response to at least 4 weeks of conservative therapy.
D. Other red flags (Table 23.1).

Key Points

- Low back pain is extremely common and in 90% of cases will respond to conservative therapy within a month.
- Patients with back and leg pain (sciatica) most likely have nerve-root compression secondary to a ruptured lumbar disc.
- Patients older than 50 with back and leg discomfort and/or numbness and/or heaviness with standing and walking may have lumbar stenosis.
- Diagnostic workup may include plain L–S x-rays with flexion and extension lateral views and L–S MRI if the patient remains symptomatic after an appropriate trial of conservative therapy.
- Microlumbar discectomy for ruptured discs, lumbar laminectomy for spinal stenosis, and lumbar laminectomy and spinal fusion for patients with both spinal stenosis and spondylolisthesis may be needed in patients who do not respond to conservative therapy and/or have associated severe neurologic deficits.

Recommended Readings

Bigos SJ, Bowyer R, Braen GR, et al. *Clinical Practice Guidelines, Acute Low Back Problems in Adults: Assessment and Treatment.* Washington, DC: U.S. Department of Health and Human Services; 1994. AHCPR publication no. 95-0643.

Foley KT, Smith MM. Microendoscopic discectomy. *Tech Neurosurg.* 1997;3:301–307.

Friedly JL, Comstock BA. A randomized trial of epidural glucocorticoid injections for spinal stenosis. *N Engl J Med.* 2014;371(1):11–21.

Jensen MC, Brant-Zawadzki MN, Obuchowski N, et al. Magnetic resonance imaging of the lumbar spine in people without back pain. *N Engl J Med*. 1994;331:69–73.

Malmivaara A. The treatment of low back pain-bed rest, exercise, or ordinary activity? *N Engl J Med*. 1995;332:351–355.

McCafferty R, Khoo L, Perez-Cruet M. Percutaneous pedicle screw fixation of the lumbar spine using the PathFinder system. *Surg Tech (Lumbar Spine)*. 2006;34:591–614.

Mimran R, Perez-Curet M, Fessler R, et al. Endoscopic lumbar laminectomy for stenosis. *Surg Tech (Lumbar Spine)*. 2006;31:569–582.

Mixter WJ, Barr JS. Rupture of the intervertebral disc with involvement of the spinal canal. *N Engl J Med*. 1934;211:210–215.

Palmer S, Turner R, Palmer R. Bilateral decompression of lumbar spinal stenosis involving a unilateral approach with microscope and tubular retractor system. *J Neurosurg (Spine 2)*. 2002;97:213–217.

Parker SL, Godil SS. Two-year comprehensive medical management of degenerative lumbar spine disease (lumbar spondylolisthesis, stenosis, or disc herniation): a value analysis of cost, pain, disability, and quality of life: clinical article. *J Neurosurg Spine*. 2014;21(2):143–149.

Perez-Cruet M. Percutaneous pedicle screw placement for spinal instrumentation. *Surg Tech (Lumbar Spine)*. 2006;32:583–590.

Resnick DK, Watters WC 3rd, Sharan A, et al. Guideline update for the performance of fusion procedures for degenerative disease of the lumbar spine. Part 9: lumbar fusion for stenosis with spondylolisthesis, *J Neurosurg Spine*. 2014;21(1):54–61.

Rihn JA, Hilibrand AS, Zhao W, et al. Effectiveness of surgery for lumbar stenosis and degenerative spondylolisthesis in the octogenarian population: analysis of the Spine Patient outcomes Research Trial (SPORT) data. *J Bone Joint Surg Am*. 2015;97(3):177–185.

Rockman RH, Simeone FA. *The Spine*. Philadelphia, PA: WB Saunders; 1992.

Weinstein JN, Tosteson TD, Lurie JD, et al. Surgical versus nonsurgical therapy for lumbar spinal stenosis. *N Engl J Med*. 2008;358:794–810.

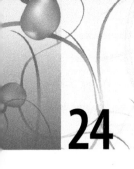

24

Approach to the Patient with Upper Extremity Pain and Paresthesias and Entrapment Neuropathies

Mark A. Ross

Upper extremity (UE) pain and **paresthesias** are common clinical complaints, which often accompany reversible peripheral nervous system (PNS) or musculoskeletal (MSK) disorders. Common PNS disorders causing these symptoms include cervical radiculopathy, brachial plexopathy, and peripheral nerve entrapment syndromes (mononeuropathies). Muscle weakness and atrophy may complicate these PNS disorders but typically do not occur with MSK disorders. The location of symptoms and signs of these PNS disorders usually reflects PNS anatomy and thus helps to suggest the diagnosis. Electrodiagnostic studies (EDS) are regularly used to clarify a specific diagnosis. Ultrasound of peripheral nerves can also help to identify focal nerve abnormalities. The cause of UE complaints can be determined by integrating clinical history, physical findings, and diagnostic study results.

DIFFERENTIAL DIAGNOSIS AND ETIOLOGY OF UE PAIN

For differential diagnosis and etiology of UE pain, see Table 24.1.

EVALUATION

A. History.
  1. Symptoms. The patient's description of symptoms should be obtained. Clarification of reported symptoms is helpful as patients may misuse terms, for example, saying weakness to describe numbness. The examiner should inquire about symptoms in the unaffected UE and legs, as well as performing a general review of systems to address the possibility of a generalized process or a systemic disorder.
    a. Sensory symptoms.
      (1) Pain. Pain descriptions are never pathognomonic of specific disorders. Tingling or radiating pain suggests a peripheral nerve, plexus, or root disorder, whereas dull, aching, nonradiating pain is typical of MSK disorders. Exceptions to this rule occur frequently. Acute onset of excruciating pain in the shoulder or arm is common with idiopathic brachial plexopathy. Pain radiating from the neck to the arm or hand suggests radiculopathy. The pain location may suggest the root involved—for example, lateral arm (C5), lateral forearm or thumb (C6), middle finger (C7), or medial hand and forearm (C8). Pain localized to the shoulder may result from MSK disorders, such as bicipital tendinitis, rotator cuff injury, and adhesive capsulitis, or from PNS disorders, such as C5 radiculopathy, brachial plexopathy, or entrapment of the suprascapular or dorsal scapular nerves (DSNs). Pain radiating distant from the site of pathology may belie the location—for example, carpal tunnel syndrome (CTS) occasionally manifests as forearm or shoulder pain. Forearm pain may occur with C6 radiculopathy, plexopathy, or nerve entrapment in the forearm. Pain involving specific digits may help localization. Pain involving the thumb, index finger, or middle finger suggests a median mononeuropathy, a C6 or C7 radiculopathy, or middle brachial plexus disorder. Pain involving the ring and little fingers suggests an ulnar mononeuropathy, a lower plexus disorder, or C8–T1 radiculopathy. Digital pain may also result from local MSK disorders—for example, arthritis. Bizarre descriptions of pain are typical of psychological or functional disorders.

TABLE 24.1 Differential Diagnosis and Etiology of Upper Extremity Pain

Disorder	Common Etiologies
PNS disorders	
Radiculopathy	Root compression (disk, bone), trauma
Brachial plexopathy	Idiopathic, trauma, tumor, radiation, compressive (TOS)
Mononeuropathy	
Suprascapular n.	Trauma, IBP
Dorsal scapular n.	Trauma, IBP
Long thoracic n.	Trauma, IBP
Musculocutaneous n.	Trauma, IBP
Median n.	
Anterior interosseous n.	Compression, trauma
Pronator teres syndrome	Compression, trauma
CTS	Compression
Ulnar n.	
Cubital tunnel syndrome	Compression, trauma
Guyon's canal	Compression, trauma
Radial n.	
Spiral groove	Compression, trauma
Posterior interosseous	Compression, trauma
Superficial radial	Compression, trauma
MSK disorders	
Rotator cuff injury	Overuse, trauma
Biceps tendinitis	Overuse, trauma
Adhesive capsulitis	Immobility, shoulder weakness
Lateral epicondylitis	Overuse, trauma

Abbreviations: CTS, carpal tunnel syndrome; IBP, idiopathic brachial plexopathy; MSK, musculoskeletal; PNS, peripheral nervous system; n., nerve; TOS, thoracic outlet syndrome.

(2) Paresthesias and sensory loss. Paresthesias are spontaneous sensations originating from nerve fibers, which patients describe as "tingling" or "pins and needles." Sensory loss indicates absence of normal sensation, which patients may describe as "numbness" or "like Novocain." Paresthesias and sensory loss may occur together or independently, and either suggests PNS disease is more likely than an MSK disorder. The distribution of paresthesias or sensory loss can help to localize a nerve disorder. However, patients may report a distribution of sensory symptoms that varies from the precise anatomic distribution of an affected nerve or nerve root. Patients with CTS may complain of sensory symptoms in any of the first three hand digits and often report the entire hand is numb. Thus, failure of sensory symptoms to localize precisely to a specific nerve or nerve-root distribution should not exclude these disorders. The differential diagnosis of paresthesias and sensory loss should include central nervous system (CNS) disease, especially when pain is absent. Intermittent paresthesias also occur in normal individuals, usually related to a specific activity or limb position resulting in nerve compression, stretch, or irritation. Thus, paresthesias in isolation do not always indicate a pathologic state.

  b. Motor symptoms. Patients complaining of weakness should be asked to describe specific activities that cause difficulty. Impaired fine motor skills—for example, buttoning buttons—indicate distal muscle weakness and suggest involvement of C8 or T1 roots, lower plexus, or nerves supplying hand muscles (median or ulnar nerves). Difficulty with arm and shoulder movements indicates proximal muscle weakness, suggesting involvement of the C5 or C6 roots, upper plexus, or nerves supplying proximal muscles (e.g., long thoracic, suprascapular, axillary nerves). Patients with pain or sensory loss may misconstrue impaired motor performance as weakness. This possibility may be clarified during the exam, or asking the patient to state which factor chiefly limits physical performance. CNS disorders can also produce weakness of either the proximal or distal musculature.

2. **Onset and precipitating factors.** The history should seek to identify specific activities the patient participated with during or just preceding the onset of symptoms and whether or not physical activity exacerbates the symptoms.

   a. **Physical activities.** Some physical activities may predispose to specific PNS disorders. Heavy lifting may precipitate cervical disk herniation and resultant radiculopathy. Head turning often exacerbates pain or paresthesias associated with radiculopathy. Arm abduction or shoulder rotation exacerbates the pain of MSK shoulder disorders and also the pain associated with brachial plexopathy. Repetitive flexion and extension movements of the elbow or sustained elbow flexion may predispose to ulnar mononeuropathy at the elbow (cubital tunnel syndrome). Repetitive flexion and extension movements at the wrist or fingers may predispose to median mononeuropathy within the carpal tunnel. Repetitive pronation and supination may lead to hypertrophy of the pronator teres muscle and median nerve entrapment in the forearm (pronator teres syndrome). The radial nerve may be compressed in the axillary region by improper use of a crutch, or in the arm when pressure is applied by a tourniquet, a hard surface, or the body's weight. Radial nerve compression in the arm is especially likely to occur when consciousness is reduced by anesthesia, sedatives, or alcohol intoxication. Handcuffs or other tight-fitting objects at the wrist—for example, watchbands or bracelets—may injure the median, ulnar, or superficial radial sensory nerves. The history should include review of occupation, hobbies, and recent changes in physical activity. Sporting activities, playing musical instruments, gardening, and knitting are examples of physical activities that could predispose to compressive nerve injuries.

   b. **Trauma** often causes UE pain and sensorimotor complaints. Even remote trauma may contribute to UE pain or sensorimotor symptoms. Examples include entrapment of a nerve by the callus of a healing fracture and development of a central cavity in the spinal cord (syringomyelia).

      (1) **Motor vehicle accident (MVA).** The severe trauma of a MVA may cause multiple neurologic complications including vertebral fracture with direct spinal cord injury, nerve-root avulsion, radiculopathy, brachial plexus injury, peripheral nerve injury, or late development of syringomyelia. Arm traction or stretching the arm and neck in opposite directions may cause cervical root avulsions or a stretch injury to the brachial plexus. An MVA may cause more than one PNS disorder—for example, cervical nerve-root avulsions and concomitant peripheral nerve injury. After an MVA, attention to multiple life-threatening injuries, or casting for multiple limb fractures, may preclude detection of PNS disorders until late in the course of recovery.

      (2) **Fractures and dislocations** may cause specific nerve injuries. Shoulder dislocation or fracture of the humerus may injure the axillary nerve. Fracture of the clavicle may injure components of the brachial plexus. Fracture of the humerus predisposes to radial nerve injury in the spiral groove, whereas fracture or dislocation of the radius may injure the posterior interosseous nerve (PIN) branch of the radial nerve. Fracture of the elbow predisposes to ulnar mononeuropathy, which may not manifest until years after the trauma, hence the name "tardy ulnar palsy." A wrist fracture may cause either median or ulnar mononeuropathy.

      (3) **Laceration.** When UE pain or sensorimotor symptoms begin after a skin laceration or puncture wound, direct injury to a nerve needs to be considered. Exploration is needed to determine if the nerve requires repair.

   c. **Physiologic compression sites.** The median and ulnar nerves are vulnerable to injury at specific sites where normal ligamentous and bony structures predispose to physical compression. The common compression sites are the wrist for the median nerve (carpal tunnel) and the elbow for the ulnar nerve (cubital tunnel). At these locations, the nerves are particularly susceptible to compression injury, hence the term "physiologic compression sites." A patient with UE sensorimotor symptoms, without any clear predisposing factors, is likely to have an abnormality of one of these nerves.

d. **Systemic illnesses.** Systemic illness may predispose to development of PNS disorders that manifest as UE sensorimotor symptoms. A complete listing of systemic illnesses with PNS complications exceeds the scope of this chapter, but several common examples are given.

   (1) **Endocrine disorders.** Patients with diabetic polyneuropathy are more vulnerable to development of mononeuropathies at physiologic compression sites. Patients with hypothyroidism are prone to developing CTS.

   (2) **Rheumatologic disorders.** Several rheumatologic disorders predispose to UE nerve or nerve-root injury. Rheumatoid arthritis causes joint and degenerative bone disease, which may lead to cervical radiculopathy, CTS, and PIN injury. Systemic vasculitis may involve individual peripheral nerves in either the upper or lower extremities. Abrupt onset of a mononeuropathy is occasionally the presenting manifestation of systemic vasculitis. Primary amyloidosis and some hereditary forms are associated with CTS.

   (3) **Renal failure and dialysis.** Patients receiving chronic hemodialysis are particularly likely to develop CTS, owing to deposition of amyloid material (β_2 microglobulin) within the carpal tunnel. Placement of arteriovenous fistulas for hemodialysis may cause median or ulnar neuropathies and, less often, a severe distal ischemic injury to all UE nerves, called ischemic monomelic neuropathy. Diabetic patients seem particularly prone to this severe nerve injury.

   (4) **Malignancy.** A patient with a history of cancer—particularly of the breast or lung—who develops UE sensorimotor complaints needs to be evaluated for metastases to the brachial plexus. Patients with radiation therapy to the brachial plexus region can develop radiation-induced brachial plexopathy, which may begin many years after radiation therapy.

3. **Other history.** The medical history should also inquire about symptoms of depression and a review of the social situation for factors that might influence the patient's symptoms. Specific questions should be asked regarding employment, accidents, work injuries, and possible litigation. Evidence of CNS disease should be sought, which might include seizures, disturbed consciousness, personality change, or problems with cognition, language, or vision.

B. **Physical examination.**

1. **Motor examination.**

   a. **Muscle inspection.** Muscles are inspected for atrophy and spontaneous muscle contractions. Muscle atrophy is present when reduction of the normal muscle bulk is revealed by visual inspection or direct measurement of limb circumference. Atrophy of specific muscles helps localize the disorder. Atrophy of the thenar eminence alone suggests a disorder of the median nerve or the deep terminal branch of the ulnar nerve. Atrophy of the thenar and hypothenar areas and the interossei muscles should raise considerations of combined median and ulnar mononeuropathies, lower trunk brachial plexopathy, C8–T1 radiculopathy, or C8–T1 spinal cord disease. Winging or elevation of one scapula suggests a long thoracic nerve mononeuropathy. Muscle inspection also involves a careful search for fasciculations, which are fine muscle twitches visible through the skin. Fasciculations may occur infrequently as an isolated finding in asymptomatic individuals. However, when present in conjunction with muscle weakness and atrophy, fasciculations are a sign of a lower motor neuron process. The exam should include inspection for fasciculations in all four limbs, as well as in the back and abdomen. Fasciculations occur most commonly with anterior horn cell diseases—for example, amyotrophic lateral sclerosis—but can also occur with diseases affecting the motor root, plexus, or peripheral nerve.

   b. **Muscle strength ratings.** Muscle strength is assessed with manual muscle testing using the Medical Research Council strength rating scale (Table 22.1). Muscle strength should be tested in proximal and distal muscles in all four limbs. This allows quantification of weakness and may reveal weakness the patient was not aware of. Muscles that should be tested bilaterally in the UE include muscles for arm abduction (deltoid and supraspinatus), arm external rotation (infraspinatus), elbow flexion (biceps), elbow extension (triceps), wrist flexion (flexor carpi radialis and flexor carpi ulnaris), wrist extension (extensor carpi radialis), finger flexion (flexor digitorum superficialis and flexor digitorum profundis), finger extension (extensor digitorum communis), finger spreading (interossei), thumb abduction (abductor pollicis brevis), and grip strength.

Patients with MSK disorders and patients with depression, psychological disturbances, or malingering may exhibit a type of weakness known as "breakaway" weakness, in which incomplete effort gives the appearance of weakness. Features suggesting breakaway weakness include pain complaints during muscle strength testing, reasonable initial strength that decreases, variability in motor performance on serial exams, improved strength with encouragement, and absence of other objective signs of motor impairment. Patients with breakaway weakness due to a psychological disturbance or malingering often make facial expressions or body contortions to convey that great effort is being made.

c. **Muscle tone** is assessed by noting how easily the patient's limbs can be passively moved while the patient is asked to relax the limb tested. The tone is rated according to the Ashworth scale, in which normal tone is assigned a value of 1, and values 2 to 5 represent increasing degrees of abnormal stiffness. Muscle tone should be normal with all of the common PNS disorders causing UE pain and sensorimotor symptoms. Increased muscle tone raises the question of a CNS disorder. When increased muscle tone occurs with UE weakness and atrophy, the possibility of upper motor neuron disease needs to be considered. Considerations should include a compressive lesion of the cervical spine such as spinal stenosis, metabolic disorders such as B_{12} deficiency or copper deficiency, or amyotrophic lateral sclerosis.

2. **Reflexes** are tested bilaterally in all four limbs, including the brachioradialis (C5–C6), biceps (C5–C6), triceps (C7–C8), quadriceps (L2–L4), and soleus (S1) tendons. Reflexes are rated as normal, decreased, or increased. A significant reflex asymmetry suggests an abnormality of the nervous system. Radiculopathy involving a cervical root typically depresses the corresponding UE reflex on the affected side. Brachial plexopathy causes decreased reflexes corresponding to the part of the plexus involved. Patients with C8–T1 radiculopathy or lower trunk brachial plexopathy may exhibit normal UE reflexes. Mononeuropathies of the UE do not usually influence the UE reflexes, unless the nerve involved supplies the muscle tested in the reflex arc—for example, musculocutaneous nerve mononeuropathy may cause a reduced biceps reflex. Reflexes are preserved in MSK disorders and increased in CNS disorders.

3. Sensory examination. The sensory examination involves testing of light touch, pain (pinprick), vibration, and joint position sensations in the upper and lower extremities. Particular attention is paid to cutaneous areas where there are sensory complaints.

4. Maneuvers. Several maneuvers may aid in the evaluation of UE sensorimotor complaints. Tinel's sign, originally described for assessment of regenerating nerve fibers, is now commonly employed to elicit paresthesias radiating in a nerve's cutaneous distribution. It is elicited by gentle tapping over a nerve. It may be observed in association with regenerating nerve fibers, neuroma, focal demyelination, and even in normal individuals. Tinel's sign is easier to elicit from a diseased nerve than from a normal nerve, and thus it may help to localize an abnormal nerve. It is commonly used to assess for CTS by tapping over the median nerve on the volar surface of the wrist. With Phalen's maneuver, the wrist is flexed for up to 1 minute to elicit paresthesias in the median nerve distribution. A positive Phalen's maneuver provides supportive evidence for CTS. Adson's maneuver refers to assessing the radial pulse when the arm is abducted and extended. Loss of the radial pulse with this maneuver is alleged to indicate compression of the subclavian artery by a cervical rib or a hypertrophied scalenus muscle. However, it is not a useful test because it is subjective and may cause normal individuals to lose their radial pulse.

C. Diagnostic studies.

1. **EDS** consist of nerve conduction studies (NCS) and electromyography (EMG). These tests permit an objective and quantitative assessment of individual peripheral nerves and muscles. They can substantiate a clinically suspected diagnosis or reveal unsuspected abnormalities. With rare exceptions, all patients with symptoms of UE pain and sensorimotor symptoms should have EDS as part of the initial diagnostic evaluation. When performed in the first few days after onset of nerve injury, EDS do not reveal as

many abnormalities as when performed 7 to 10 days later. However, performing EDS early after injury allows the opportunity to document preexisting abnormalities. This may be important for complicated diagnostic cases or when medicolegal issues occur. Detailed discussion of EDS is found in Chapter 36.

2. Radiologic studies.

   a. Plain films. After head or neck trauma, cervical spine films are necessary to evaluate for fractures. When cervical radiculopathy is suspected, cervical spine films may reveal narrowing of specific neural foramina. Cervical spine films may also be useful in detecting a cervical rib, which should be investigated when clinical and EDS evidence suggests a neurogenic thoracic outlet syndrome (TOS). The patient with brachial plexopathy should have a chest film to evaluate for malignancy. If clinical evidence suggests Pancoast's syndrome, apical chest film views should be included to search for an apical tumor. Plain films may also be useful in evaluation of MSK disorders, by revealing evidence of degenerative arthritis or tendon calcifications.

   b. Magnetic resonance imaging (MRI). Cervical spine MRI studies are usually performed to evaluate cervical radiculopathy. Myelography combined with computerized tomography may be used when MRI is not an option. MRI of the brachial plexus is often used to search for evidence of tumor as the cause of brachial plexopathy. MRI can also demonstrate enlargement or increased signal within the brachial plexus.

   c. Ultrasound can be used to evaluate focal peripheral nerve abnormalities. It has been particularly helpful for evaluating the median nerve at the wrist in patients with suspected CTS. The typical ultrasound finding in patients with CTS is enlargement of the median nerve cross-sectional area (CSA) at the wrist. Ultrasound can also demonstrate focal enlargement of other nerves, for example, ulnar nerve enlargement in the elbow region. Video 24.1 demonstrates ultrasound of the median nerve at the wrist in a normal individual. The CSA is measured by tracing the outline of the median nerve with the ultrasound machine. The upper limit of normal CSA for the median nerve at the wrist is 10 mm² (or 0.1 cm²).

3. Laboratory studies for investigation of systemic illnesses are obtained for patients with UE sensorimotor complaints, depending on individual case circumstances. Tests that may be useful include complete blood count (CBC) with differential, chemistry panel, blood sugar, erythrocyte sedimentation rate, antinuclear antibody, urinalysis, serum immunofixation electrophoresis, thyroid function, and, occasionally, spinal fluid tests.

D. Unexplained Symptoms. When thorough evaluation of UE pain or sensorimotor symptoms does not reveal a specific PNS or MSK disorder, alternative explanations must be considered. Possibilities include positional nerve compression, CNS disease, depression, psychological factors, or malingering. The symptoms and signs of CNS and PNS diseases may overlap, particularly for slowly progressive conditions—for example, brain tumor or multiple sclerosis. Clues suggesting CNS disease include painless weakness or sensory disturbance, upper motor neuron signs, altered consciousness or personality, or problems with cognition, language, or vision. Depression may present with unexplained UE pain or sensorimotor symptoms. Some patients may not have frank depression but unhappiness or conflict in the psychosocial realm, which manifests as neurologic symptoms. Often patients with this cause of symptoms are unable to identify a relationship between their psychological state and neurologic symptoms. Others have onset of symptoms after accidents or injuries, and either the process of litigation or the power of suggestion from inquisitive physicians distorts the usual concept of wellness and perpetuates the symptoms. Patients with unexplained symptoms should have neurologic consultation, and may need to be followed and observed over time.

DIAGNOSTIC APPROACH

The history provides initial hypotheses about the cause of the symptoms, and these hypotheses are tested during the physical examination. Knowledge of PNS anatomy is essential for interpreting UE sensorimotor symptoms and signs. In almost all cases, EDS are performed to help localize or exclude a suspected PNS disorder. When a PNS disorder is present, EDS help determine the severity and type of pathologic process. Additional diagnostic assessments may include radiologic studies or laboratory tests, depending on individual patient circumstances.

SELECTED DISORDERS AND CRITERIA FOR DIAGNOSIS

A. PNS disorders.
   1. Mononeuropathy.
      a. Median nerve.
         (1) CTS
            (a) Anatomy and etiology. CTS is a very common disorder caused by compression of the median nerve at the wrist within the unyielding space known as the carpal tunnel. Many disorders compromise this space, resulting in median nerve compression. The most common cause is flexor tenosynovitis, which may be associated with excessive physical use of the hands. Patients with primary carpal stenosis—that is, a narrow carpal tunnel—may be especially prone to CTS. Other local factors causing CTS include vascular lesions, abnormal tendons, ganglion cysts, tumoral calcinosis, pseudoarthrosis, and infection. Systemic disorders associated with CTS include endocrine disorders such as hyperparathyroidism, acromegaly, and hypothyroidism, and rheumatologic disorders such as rheumatoid arthritis, systemic lupus erythematosus, polymyalgia rheumatica, temporal arteritis, scleroderma, and gout. Other conditions predisposing to CTS include diabetic and other polyneuropathies, chronic hemodialysis, shunts for hemodialysis, and pregnancy.
            (b) **Clinical features of CTS** include numbness or tingling involving one or more of the first four digits (thumb through ring finger), although occasionally the entire hand is involved. There may be pain in the fingers or wrist, and occasionally in the forearm or shoulder. Patients are often awakened at night by these symptoms, and physical activity with the hands may exacerbate symptoms. Advanced cases can develop weakness and atrophy of the thenar muscle. Physical examination reveals decreased sensation in the volar aspect of the first four digits. Because the median nerve innervation frequently supplies only the lateral half of the ring finger, sparing of sensation on the medial half of the ring finger is a helpful sign. CTS typically spares sensation over the thenar eminence. Advanced cases show weakness and atrophy of the abductor pollicis brevis. Tinel's and Phalen's signs may be present.
            (c) **Diagnosis** of CTS is established by clinical history, physical findings, and EDS. The EDS findings vary with the severity of the disorder. In mild cases, the amplitude of the median compound muscle action potential (CMAP) and sensory nerve action potential (SNAP) are normal, and the wrist latency values are prolonged. The median NCS reveals focal slowing across the wrist. Slowing of NCS in proximal median nerve segments should not exclude the diagnosis of CTS. In some cases, there may be conduction block at the wrist level. In more advanced cases, the median CMAP and SNAP amplitude values are reduced, and fibrillation potentials may occur in the abductor pollicis brevis muscle. The ulnar nerve studies in the same hand are normal. Ultrasound can also be used to diagnose CTS. The typical ultrasound finding in patients with CTS is enlargement of the median nerve CSA at the wrist. Most studies indicate median nerve CSA at the wrist greater than 10 mm^2 is abnormal. Comparison of the wrist and forearm median nerve CSA is considered the most sensitive ultrasound measurement for CTS with a wrist-to-forearm ratio greater than 1.4 being abnormal. Additional ultrasound abnormalities in CTS include increased hypoechoic signal in the median nerve, disproportionate flattening of the median nerve, bowing of the flexor retinaculum, and reduced excursion of the median nerve with digit movement. Some patients with typical symptoms of CTS have normal EDS. Within this group of "EMG negative CTS patients," some will have enlarged CSA by ultrasound. In patients with positive EDS studies, the degree of enlargement of median nerve CSA by ultrasound correlates with

the severity of the EDS abnormalities. Some patients may have multiple entrapment neuropathies, such as bilateral median neuropathies at the wrist and bilateral ulnar neuropathies at the elbows. In this circumstance, it is necessary to evaluate lower extremity nerves for the possibility of an underlying polyneuropathy.

(2) Pronator teres syndrome

(a) Anatomy and etiology. The pronator teres syndrome refers to compression of the median nerve in the forearm where it passes between the heads of the pronator teres muscle. This uncommon disorder is usually related to an occupation involving repetitive pronation of the forearm, which leads to hypertrophy of the pronator teres muscle. Other causes include a fibrous band from pronator teres to flexor digitorum superficialis, or local trauma.

(b) Clinical features. The predominant symptom is pain in the volar forearm. Median innervated muscles, including the pronator teres, remain strong. Median sensory function is typically normal. Examination may show tenderness in the region of the pronator teres muscle, and there may be a Tinel's sign over the pronator muscle.

(c) **Diagnosis** is established primarily by clinical features. EDS are often normal, but occasionally slow median NCS may be observed in the forearm segment.

(3) Anterior interosseous syndrome

(a) Anatomy and etiology. This relatively uncommon median nerve disorder involves compression of the anterior interosseous branch of the median nerve in the forearm, usually by a fibrous band from the pronator teres or the flexor digitorum superficialis muscles. Other forearm anomalies or forearm trauma may also cause the disorder. The anterior interosseous nerve (AIN) is a purely motor nerve that supplies the flexor pollicis longus (FPL), flexor digitorum (FD) I and II, and pronator quadratus muscles.

(b) **Clinical features** include forearm or elbow pain combined with weakness of flexion of the distal phalanx of the thumb (FPL) and the index and middle fingers (FD). Patients note inability to pinch the thumb and index finger together. Pronation strength is preserved as the pronator teres muscle is unaffected.

(c) **Diagnosis** is established by the abovementioned clinical features and EDS. The median NCS are normal. The EMG shows fibrillation potentials confined to one or more of the above muscles supplied by the AIN. When AIN causes weakness confined to the FPL, EMG is extremely helpful for differentiating a partial AIN syndrome from rupture of the FPL tendon.

b. Ulnar nerve.

(1) Cubital tunnel syndrome

(a) Anatomy and etiology. The ulnar nerve may become compressed in the elbow region either in the condylar groove or the cubital tunnel. The cubital tunnel is formed on the sides by the two heads of the flexor carpi ulnaris muscle with a floor (medial ligament of the elbow), and roof (aponeurosis of the flexor carpi ulnaris muscle) completing the boundaries. The ulnar nerve runs through this space, and then underneath the flexor carpi ulnaris muscle. Remote elbow trauma, with or without fracture, predisposes to later development of entrapment neuropathy in the elbow region (tardy ulnar palsy). However, many patients develop ulnar neuropathy without antecedent trauma. Repetitive movement at the elbow or prolonged flexion of the elbow may be predisposing factors.

(b) **Clinical features** include sensory complaints in the ulnar division of the hand (the fifth digit and the medial half of the fourth) and the ulnar-innervated portion of the hand and wrist. Sensory complaints may include decreased sensation, paresthesias, and pain. Pain may involve the medial forearm and elbow. Weakness involves the interossei, abductor digiti minimi, adductor pollicis, and flexor pollicis brevis. When weakness is chronic, atrophy may occur, and a claw hand deformity may develop. Most often, the flexor carpi ulnaris muscle remains strong. A diagnosis of ulnar neuropathy requires normal strength in C8–T1 muscles innervated by the median and radial nerves.

(c) **Diagnosis** is established by the characteristic history and physical findings, and EDS. Ulnar neuropathy at the elbow may show reduction of the ulnar CMAP and SNAP. There may be evidence of conduction block in motor fibers that can be localized to the elbow region. Ulnar NCS may be focally slow across the elbow. The EMG may show fibrillation potentials and/or abnormal motor unit potentials (MUPs) in ulnar-innervated hand muscles. Usually the flexor carpi ulnaris does not show fibrillation potentials, although it may if its motor branch is also compressed.

(2) Compression at the wrist (Guyon's canal)

(a) Anatomy and etiology. Guyon's canal is a fibro-osseous tunnel connecting the pisiform and hamate wrist bones through which the ulnar nerve travels. As the ulnar nerve emerges from Guyon's canal, it divides into motor and sensory branches. The deep terminal branch is purely motor and supplies all of the ulnar-innervated hand muscles. The superficial terminal branch supplies sensation to the medial distal half of the palm and the palmar surfaces of the fourth and fifth digits. Sensation to the medial proximal half of the palm is supplied by the palmar cutaneous branch of the ulnar nerve, which arises in the mid-forearm and does not pass through Guyon's canal. Sensation to the medial dorsal half of the hand is supplied by the dorsal cutaneous branch of the ulnar nerve, which arises above the wrist and does not pass through Guyon's canal. Factors predisposing to ulnar neuropathy at the wrist include chronic compression, which may occur in cyclists and local trauma—for example, wrist fracture.

(b) **Clinical features** vary depending on the precise level of abnormality. Compression of the entire ulnar nerve within Guyon's canal or of the two branches as they leave the canal causes weakness of all ulnar-innervated hand muscles and sensory loss in the superficial terminal branch distribution. Sensation of the dorsal medial hand and the proximal half of the medial palm is spared because sensation is supplied by other branches. Compression of the deep terminal motor branch may occur in isolation either before or after it supplies the hypothenar muscles, producing ulnar-innervated hand muscle weakness with no sensory loss. Finally, compression of only the superficial terminal branch causes sensory loss in its palmar distribution with normal hand strength.

(c) **Diagnosis** is established by clinical examination and EDS. The EDS findings vary depending on which of the abovementioned ulnar nerve branches is involved. If the superficial terminal sensory branch is involved, NCS will show a reduced or absent ulnar SNAP recorded from the fifth digit, but the SNAP from the dorsal ulnar cutaneous nerve remains normal. If the abnormality involves the deep terminal branch, ulnar CMAP amplitude may be reduced and there may be fibrillation potentials or abnormal MUPs in ulnar-innervated hand muscles.

c. Radial nerve.

(1) Axilla or spiral groove compression

(a) Anatomy and etiology. The radial nerve may be compressed against the humerus by external pressure in the axilla or the spiral groove. Compression in the axilla can be caused by improper use of crutches. Compression in the spiral groove is likely to occur when an individual falls asleep with the arm hanging over a chair, or with a partner's head against the arm. Radial nerve compression is especially likely if use of alcohol or sedatives prevents the patient from normal turning during sleep. The term "Saturday night palsy" has been used for such a radial nerve palsy. A similar outcome may follow use of an arm tourniquet during surgery. The radial nerve may also be injured in the spiral groove by blunt trauma, fractures of the humerus, and rarely by vigorous arm exercise.

(b) **Clinical features** are weakness of radial-innervated muscles and sensory loss on the dorsal aspects of the hand, thumb, and index and middle fingers. Radial-innervated muscles include triceps, brachioradialis, supinator, and the wrist and finger extensors. The triceps is affected by radial nerve compression in the axilla but spared with spiral groove compression. Weakness of wrist extensors causes wrist drop. Inability to stabilize the wrist prevents normal hand interossei muscle function giving the false impression that ulnar-innervated hand muscles are weak.

(c) **Diagnosis** of radial mononeuropathy is confirmed by clinical features and EDS. Nerve conduction studies show a reduced-amplitude radial CMAP and reduced or absent SNAP. The presence or absence of fibrillation potentials in triceps helps to localize the compression site (axilla or spiral groove).

(2) PIN

(a) Anatomy and etiology. The PIN is the purely motor termination of the radial nerve in the forearm. The PIN supplies the supinator muscle and the wrist and finger extensors. Entrapment of the PIN is relatively uncommon. When this occurs, it is usually at the level of the supinator muscle. Predisposing factors include vigorous use of the arm, fracture of the head of the radius, and other local traumas. Hypertrophied synovia of the elbow joint in patients with rheumatoid arthritis may compress the PIN.

(b) **Clinical features** are weakness of the wrist and finger extensors. Some patients have pain in the elbow or dorsal forearm. There are no sensory abnormalities apart from pain, because the PIN is purely motor.

(c) **Diagnosis** is established by the abovementioned clinical features and EDS. NCS show a reduced-amplitude radial CMAP and normal radial SNAP. The EMG exam shows fibrillation potentials and abnormal MUPs in the aforementioned radial-innervated muscles.

(3) **The superficial sensory branch**

(a) Anatomy and etiology. The superficial sensory branch of the radial nerve arises in the vicinity of the elbow and supplies sensation to the dorsolateral hand and the dorsal aspects of the first three digits. It may be injured at the wrist level by local trauma or compression from tight objects around the wrist, such as watchbands or handcuffs.

(b) **Clinical features** are purely sensory, with paresthesias and sensory loss in the radial sensory distribution.

(c) **Diagnosis** is made by the history, physical findings, and NCS evidence of a reduced or absent superficial radial SNAP.

d. Axillary nerve.

(1) Anatomy and etiology. The posterior cord of the brachial plexus divides into the radial and axillary nerves. The axillary nerve travels below the shoulder joint and supplies the teres minor muscle, which externally rotates the arm. The axillary nerve then courses behind and lateral to the humerus before dividing into anterior and posterior branches, which supply corresponding portions of the deltoid muscle. The posterior branch gives a cutaneous nerve that supplies the skin over the lateral deltoid. The axillary nerve may be injured by shoulder dislocation or fractures of the humerus. It may be the only nerve affected by idiopathic brachial plexopathy (see **Section A.2.a under Selected Disorders and Criteria for Diagnosis**).

(2) Clinical features. The main clinical manifestation is impaired shoulder abduction resulting from deltoid weakness. The supraspinatus initiates arm abduction, so patients may retain limited arm abduction. Weakness of the teres minor muscle may be difficult to demonstrate on physical examination because of normal infraspinatus muscle function. Sensory loss may be demonstrated over the lateral portion of the deltoid muscle.

(3) **Diagnosis** is confirmed by weakness limited to the deltoid muscle and EMG abnormalities restricted to the deltoid and teres minor muscles. An axillary NCS study with surface recording from the deltoid muscle may show delay or reduced amplitude of the axillary nerve CMAP.

e. Musculocutaneous nerve.

(1) Anatomy and etiology. The musculocutaneous nerve arises from the lateral cord of the brachial plexus and supplies the coracobrachialis, biceps, and brachialis

muscles. It continues in the forearm as the purely sensory lateral antebrachial cutaneous nerve. Mononeuropathy of the musculocutaneous nerve is uncommon, but it may occur with shoulder dislocation, direct trauma or compression, or sudden extension of the forearm.

(2) **Clinical features** include impaired arm flexion resulting from weakness of the biceps and the other musculocutaneous-innervated muscles. The biceps reflex may be normal or reduced, depending on the severity of the biceps weakness. Sensory loss is present over the lateral forearm.

(3) Diagnosis. The clinical features of musculocutaneous neuropathy closely parallel those of C5 radiculopathy. Diagnosis is established by the abovementioned clinical features and EDS results that differentiate C5 radiculopathy from musculocutaneous nerve mononeuropathy. The lateral antebrachial SNAP is reduced or absent in musculocutaneous neuropathy but normal in C5 radiculopathy. EMG shows involvement of only muscles supplied by the musculocutaneous nerve.

f. **Long thoracic nerve.**

   (1) Anatomy and etiology. The long thoracic nerve is a purely motor nerve arising from the ventral rami of the C5, C6, and C7 spinal nerves. It courses along with other brachial plexus components underneath the clavicle, and then travels down the chest wall anterolaterally to supply the serratus anterior muscle. This large muscle fixes the scapula to the chest wall, providing general stability for the shoulder during arm movements. Injury of the long thoracic nerve may occur with trauma or with vigorous physical activities involving shoulder girdle movements. Long thoracic neuropathy may be caused by idiopathic brachial plexopathy.

   (2) **Clinical features** of long thoracic mononeuropathy include pain and weakness in the shoulder. Patients have difficulty abducting the arm or raising it above the head. Winging of the scapula is demonstrated by having the patient extend the arms forward and push against a wall. The scapula elevates from the chest wall because the weak serratus muscle cannot hold it.

   (3) **Diagnosis** is established by the abovementioned clinical features and EMG showing fibrillation potentials involving only the serratus anterior muscle. Long thoracic nerve NCS are technically difficult and other NCS are normal.

g. **Suprascapular nerve.**

   (1) Anatomy and etiology. The suprascapular nerve is a purely motor nerve arising from the upper trunk of the brachial plexus and passing through the suprascapular notch on the upper border of the scapula to supply the supraspinatus and infraspinatus muscles. The suprascapular nerve is most often injured by trauma in which there is excessive forward flexion of the shoulder. It may be involved in idiopathic brachial plexopathy.

   (2) **Clinical features** are pain in the posterior shoulder and weakness of the spinati muscles. The supraspinatus initiates arm abduction, whereas the infraspinatus externally rotates the arm.

   (3) **Diagnosis** is established by clinical history, physical findings, and EDS. Routine NCS are normal, but motor NCS with recording from the supraspinatus muscle may show reduced amplitude or prolonged latency relative to the unaffected side. The EMG exam shows abnormalities confined to the spinati muscles on the affected side.

h. **Dorsal scapular nerve.**

   (1) Anatomy and etiology. The DSN is a purely motor nerve arising from the upper trunk of the brachial plexus and passing through the scalenus medius muscle to supply the rhomboid and levator scapulae muscles. Injury to the DSN is uncommon.

   (2) **Clinical features** include pain in the scapular region and weakness of the rhomboid and levator scapulae muscles.

   (3) **Diagnosis** is established by clinical features and EMG showing fibrillation potentials restricted to the muscles supplied by the DSN. There is no satisfactory NCS for the DSN.

2. Brachial plexopathy.
   a. Idiopathic brachial plexopathy.
      (1) Anatomy and etiology. Idiopathic brachial plexopathy, also known as Parsonage–Turner syndrome or neuralgic amyotrophy, is an uncommon condition believed to represent an immune-mediated neuropathy affecting various portions of the brachial plexus. An antecedent event such as an upper respiratory infection or immunization is present in about half of the cases.
      (2) Clinical features. The main clinical features are abrupt onset of severe pain in the shoulder and proximal arm followed at a variable interval (hours to weeks) by shoulder and arm muscle weakness. The pain is exacerbated by movement of the arm, shoulder, or neck, which may give the false impression of an MSK disorder. Any combination of muscles innervated by nerves arising from the brachial plexus may be involved, but there is a predilection for proximal muscles. Muscles supplied by the axillary, suprascapular, long thoracic, radial, musculocutaneous, and AINs are commonly involved. The nerve involvement may be extensive or restricted to a single nerve. Asymmetric contralateral involvement occurs in one-third of patients. Sensory loss or paresthesias may be present, but these features are relatively minor.
      (3) **Diagnosis** is established by the characteristic clinical history, physical findings, and EDS. Patients with this disorder typically present early for evaluation and treatment of the severe pain. If EDS are performed early, abnormalities of MUP recruitment may be observed, but the studies may be otherwise normal. If EDS are repeated 7 to 10 days after weakness begins, the NCS show evidence of axonal injury, with the distribution varying according to the specific nerves involved. EMG shows fibrillation potentials in clinically weak muscles, and often in muscles that were not judged weak by physical examination. For this reason, EMG is essential for determining the extent of injury.
   b. Neurogenic TOS.
      (1) Anatomy and etiology. The "true" neurogenic TOS is a very rare disorder in which the lower trunk of the brachial plexus is compressed by an elongated transverse process of C7, a rudimentary cervical rib, or a fibrous band running from either of these to the first rib.
      (2) **Clinical features** are weakness and wasting of the intrinsic hand muscles, most markedly affecting the abductor pollicis brevis muscle; pain involving the medial forearm or hand; and sensory loss involving the fourth and fifth fingers and the medial hand and distal forearm.
      (3) **Diagnosis** is established by clinical features and characteristic EDS results. Radiographic evidence of an elongated C7 transverse process or a rudimentary cervical rib is helpful but not mandatory for diagnosis, because the structural problem may be a fibrous band that cannot be detected on imaging studies. The nerve conduction findings include severely reduced or absent median CMAP, normal median SNAP, reduced or absent ulnar SNAP, and mildly reduced or normal ulnar CMAP. The EMG exam shows fibrillation potentials in lower trunk–innervated muscles, particularly those supplied by the median and ulnar nerves. In contrast to the rare and well-defined true neurogenic TOS is a condition commonly misdiagnosed as TOS, which has various UE sensorimotor symptoms but no consistent clinical history. Patients said to have this form of TOS have no objective neurologic abnormalities and no abnormalities on EDS. This form of TOS has been aptly referred to as "disputed" neurogenic TOS and its existence as an entity remains controversial. Patients erroneously diagnosed with this type of TOS are often subjected to first-rib resection, and, unfortunately, severe brachial plexopathy may be a complication.
   c. Brachial plexopathy in patients with malignancy.
      (1) Anatomy and etiology. Metastasis to the brachial plexus needs to be considered whenever a patient with a history of malignancy (especially breast or lung cancer) develops UE pain or sensorimotor symptoms. Brachial plexopathy is usually not the presenting feature of malignancy, except in Pancoast's syndrome, in which

an apical lung carcinoma invades the lower trunk of the brachial plexus. For patients who have undergone prior chest wall radiotherapy, brachial plexopathy from radiation injury may occur as a later complication.

(2) Clinical features of brachial plexopathy resulting from tumor invasion are pain, weakness, and sensory changes that more commonly affect the lower plexus. Unlike idiopathic brachial plexopathy, malignant brachial plexopathy has a gradual onset of symptoms, and lymphedema of the arm is common. In Pancoast's syndrome, patients usually first have pain in the medial arm, and may develop sensorimotor abnormalities in the lower trunk distribution. Horner's syndrome (ipsilateral ptosis, miosis, and facial anhidrosis) often results from a tumor invading the inferior cervical sympathetic ganglion. Malignant plexopathy is more likely than radiation plexopathy to be painful and involve the lower trunk.

(3) Diagnosis. A patient with a history of malignancy and new onset UE sensorimotor symptoms or pain should have EDS to exclude common conditions such as mononeuropathy or radiculopathy, which might cause symptoms identical to those of brachial plexopathy. The EDS can determine if there is evidence of brachial plexopathy and clarify the locations of abnormalities within the plexus. This information can help in planning and interpreting MRI studies of the plexus, which should be performed to look for evidence of tumor. Patients with lower trunk plexopathy should have apical chest film views to look for an apical lung tumor. Myokymic discharges detected by EDS in patients with prior chest wall radiotherapy support a diagnosis of radiation plexopathy but do not conclusively exclude tumor metastases.

3. **Cervical radiculopathy.** The clinical and electrodiagnostic features of cervical radiculopathy are mentioned above, and thoroughly reviewed in Chapter 22.

B. **MSK disorders** share in common the predominant symptom of pain and an absence of other neurologic manifestations. In general, EDS are normal when MSK disorders are the cause of UE pain symptoms. However, it is common for an underlying neurologic disorder affecting the PNS to result in a secondary MSK disorder, in which case EDS may be abnormal as a result of the underlying neurologic disorder.

1. **Rotator cuff injury.** The rotator cuff comprises the tendons of the supraspinatus, infraspinatus, teres minor, and subscapularis muscles, which fix the humeral head in the glenoid fossa during shoulder abduction and provide internal and external arm rotation. Rotator cuff inflammation (tendinitis) and tear are common causes of shoulder pain. Tendinitis results from repetitive minor trauma to the cuff, and tear may occur as a chronic stage of this degenerative process, or acutely from abrupt trauma. With tendinitis or tear, there is shoulder pain on arm abduction or on internal or external arm rotation. With tear, there may be weakness of rotator cuff functions, but EMG studies are negative. Plain films may reveal tendon or subacromial bursa calcifications. Ultrasound or an arthrogram of the shoulder may confirm a rotator cuff tear.

2. **Bicipital tendinitis.** Inflammation of the biceps tendon causes pain and tenderness in the anterior shoulder region. The pain may be reproduced by supination of the forearm against resistance or by flexion and extension of the shoulder. There are no neurologic abnormalities, and the diagnosis is established clinically.

3. **Adhesive capsulitis (frozen shoulder).** Loss of motion at the shoulder joint may result in adhesion of the joint capsule to the humerus. Shoulder pain from any cause can lead to immobility and subsequent adhesive capsulitis. Alternatively, weakness of shoulder girdle muscles from either PNS or CNS disorders may cause this problem. Whatever the cause, the joint becomes stiff, and attempted motion causes severe shoulder pain. Muscle atrophy may result from PNS disease, or secondarily from disuse. The diagnosis is usually made by the clinical features.

4. **Lateral epicondylitis (tennis elbow).** Overuse of the extensor carpi radialis muscles (wrist extensors), or direct trauma to their tendinous insertion on the lateral epicondyle, may lead to inflammation, degeneration, or tear of the tendons. This produces pain localized over the lateral epicondyle, which may be exacerbated by use of the forearm-wrist extensor muscles.

REFERRAL

Patients should be referred to a reliable EMG laboratory for EDS, as these studies facilitate accurate diagnosis. Establishing the diagnosis guides subsequent diagnostic testing and treatment decisions. In addition, EDS can estimate the severity of the abnormality, which can help to estimate prognosis. Neurologic consultation for UE pain or sensorimotor symptoms is appropriate at any stage of the evaluation process if there are questions concerning diagnosis or management.

Key Points

- UE pain may occur with PNS disorders and MSK disorders. The presence of additional sensory symptoms such as paresthesias suggests a neurologic etiology.
- Knowledge of PNS anatomy is critical for identifying patterns that suggest specific nerve disorders. However, occasionally patient's complaints do not respect known anatomical distributions; for example, it is not unusual for patients with CTS to complain of numbness involving the entire hand.
- UE pain and paresthesias may be associated with systemic disorders and these must be considered with the evaluation of the primary complaint. Common examples include diabetes, thyroid disorders, rheumatoid arthritis, and renal disease.
- Evaluation for UE pain and paresthesias may occasionally not reveal a specific diagnosis. In this setting, a broad differential should include positional paresthesias, central nervous system disease, psychiatric disease, and psychological factors.
- EDS are an essential diagnostic test used to diagnose UE neurologic disorders. EDS are typically normal in MSK disorders and abnormal in neurologic disorders.
- Ultrasound may be helpful for evaluating UE peripheral nerve disorders. It is particularly helpful for demonstrating enlargement of the median nerve at the wrist in patients with CTS.

Recommended Readings

Cailliet R, ed. *Neck and Arm Pain: Pain Series*. 2nd ed. Philadelphia, PA: F. A Davis; 1981.

D'Arcy CA, McGee S. The rational clinical examination. Does this patient have carpal tunnel syndrome? *JAMA*. 2000;283(23):3110–3117.

Dawson DM. Entrapment neuropathies of the upper extremities. *N Engl J Med*. 1993;329:2013–2018.

Hobson-Webb LD, Massey JM, Juel VC, et al. The ultrasonographic wrist-to-forearm median nerve area ratio in carpal tunnel syndrome. *Clin Neurophysiol*. 2008;119:1353–1357.

Klauser AS, Halpern EJ, De Zordo T, et al. Carpal tunnel syndrome assessment with US: value of additional cross-sectional area measurements of the median nerve in patients versus healthy volunteers. *Radiology*. 2009;250(1):171–177.

Nakano KK. The entrapment neuropathies. *Muscle Nerve*. 1978;1:264–279.

Pecina MM, Krmpotic-Nemanic J, Markiewitz AD, eds. *Tunnel Syndromes*. 3rd ed. Boca Raton, FL: CRC Press; 2001.

Stewart JD. *Focal Peripheral Neuropathies*. 4th ed. West Vancouver, BC: JBJ Publishing; 2009.

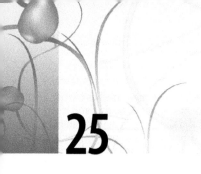

25

Approach to the Patient with Lower Extremity Pain, Paresthesias, and Entrapment Neuropathies

Gregory Gruener

Lower extremity pain and paresthesia are common symptoms of peripheral nervous system (PNS) disorders. Diagnosing a mononeuropathy requires that the motor, reflex, and sensory changes be confined to a single nerve and can, if necessary, be supported by electrodiagnostic studies (EDX).

Diagnosis and management of PNS disorders was once the sole domain of specialists. However, "reemergence" of generalists in health care has resulted in at least two major trends. The first, as expected, is that persons with such disorders are no longer under the sole care of a specialist. The second, somewhat "unintentional" effect, is that the role of specialists has become more demanding. Specialists need to develop a greater proficiency in differentiating neuropathy from radiculopathy, plexopathy, and other non-neurologic syndromes of pain, disturbed sensation, or weakness. This increasing competency occurs in the setting of fewer and more carefully selected laboratory investigations.

Fortunately, recognition of a neuropathy has always necessitated careful attention to the history and examination, skills that are expected of specialists, but "within reach" of a generalist. After localization, a ranking of potential etiologies is formulated, and further diagnostic evaluation is planned.

This chapter provides an outline of common as well as some infrequent forms of lower extremity neuropathy. Symptoms and findings are emphasized, and the most frequent etiologic considerations are mentioned. The importance of bedside examination is assumed throughout, but the application of general diagnostic tests is also reviewed.

EVALUATION

A. **History.** Various aspects of the history help in narrowing the etiologies of a mononeuropathy. The nature of onset (abrupt or insidious), preceding events (injury, surgery, or illness), associated symptoms (fever, weight loss, or joint swelling), and aggravating or alleviating features (joint position or specific activities) are all important. Because the observed deficit can be similar regardless of etiology, historical information is instrumental in limiting the differential diagnosis.

B. **Physical examination.** Although motor and sensory symptoms and signs correspond to the distribution of a single peripheral nerve or branch, the degree of deficit and constellation of findings can vary. Motor signs may be clinically absent, or varying degrees of weakness, atrophy, or fasciculations may be found. Likewise, sensory symptoms can be positive (e.g., tingling, pricking, and burning), negative (hypoesthesia), or, while corresponding to a sensory distribution of a nerve, may be most pronounced in its distal distribution. Therefore, the sensory examination should begin with the **patient's description** of the area of involvement. The **course of the nerve** should be evaluated and local areas of discomfort or the presence of a Tinel's sign (pain or paresthesia in the cutaneous distribution of a nerve elicited by light percussion over that nerve) sought. The relationship of sites of discomfort to adjacent anatomic structures helps in identifying sites of nerve entrapment or compression. It is also prudent to remember that anatomical variations exist in spinal nerve contributions to individual nerves as well as their course.

C. **Diagnostic studies.** Further evaluation may be necessary in confirming the presence and severity of a mononeuropathy and excluding more proximal sites of involvement (plexus or root) that can clinically mimic a mononeuropathy.

1. **EDX.** An electromyogram (EMG) and nerve stimulation studies (NSS) are quite useful in the evaluation of a mononeuropathy. They can aid in localization, detect bilateral but asymmetric nerve involvement (or detect an underlying polyneuropathy), define severity, and provide prognostic information.
2. **Laboratory testing** is directed at identification of a systemic or generalized disease that may be a predisposing factor and with newer imaging techniques, at times, targeted fascicular nerve biopsy. Owing to the practical nature of this section, an exhaustive listing of the medical, systemic diseases, or structural disorders that can cause a mononeuropathy is not provided. The Recommended Readings provide extensive tabulations of frequent as well as unusual etiologies.
3. **Imaging studies.** Radiographic imaging was previously undertaken to identify intrathoracic, abdominal, retroperitoneal, or pelvic masses that may lead to nerve root, plexus, or nerve injury, but now it is also applied to imaging the PNS directly. This role for imaging considerably advanced with MRI, now the method of choice for delineating a focal site of involvement, characterizing and at times assisting in the diagnosis of a nerve lesion. However, its effectiveness not only depends on the necessary MRI hardware and software, but clinical expertise through an interdisciplinary and collaborative effort among physicians and clinical departments. Routine X-ray studies play a less significant role. Recently, high-resolution ultrasound has been used in diagnosis and possibly establishing prognosis of entrapment neuropathies.

SPECIFIC FORMS OF MONONEUROPATHY

A. **Femoral and saphenous neuropathy.** Formed within the psoas muscle by fusion of the dorsal (posterior) divisions (branches) of the ventral (anterior) rami of the L2–L4 spinal nerves, the femoral nerve exits from the lateral border of the psoas and descends between it and the iliacus muscles (which it may also innervate), but under the fascia of the iliacus. Emerging under the inguinal ligament, lateral to the femoral artery, the nerve divides into motor branches, which supply the quadriceps muscles, and sensory branches to the anterior portion of the thigh (Fig. 25.1). One major division, the saphenous nerve, descends medially within Hunter's (adductor) canal, accompanying the femoral artery. At the medial superior aspect of the knee, it emerges from the canal and, accompanying the saphenous vein, descends medially down the leg, ending at the medial aspect of the foot. The saphenous nerve supplies the sensory innervation to the medial aspect of the leg and foot.

1. **Femoral neuropathy** is usually caused by trauma from surgery (intrapelvic, inguinal, hip operations, or lateral retroperitoneal transpsoas surgery for lumbar spine fusion), stretch or traction injuries (prolonged lithotomy position in childbirth), or direct compression (hematoma within the iliacus compartment). Although diabetes mellitus is described as a frequent etiologic factor, such cases are misnomers and represent a restricted plexopathy or more diffuse lesions, but predominantly affecting femoral nerve function. **Saphenous neuropathy** is most often attributable to injury following surgery (peripheral vascular, saphenous vein removal, or knee operations).
2. **Clinical manifestations.**
   a. **History.** The patient reports leg weakness (as if the leg will "fold under") on attempting to stand or walk. Pain in the anterior part of the thigh accompanied by the abrupt onset of leg weakness is a frequent presentation of an iliacus (retroperitoneal) hematoma. A similar pattern of pain, but usually subacute in onset, can be observed in cases of "femoral neuropathy" occurring in diabetes mellitus. With the exception of pain, sensory involvement tends to be infrequent and a minimal symptom of femoral neuropathy. Because of its association with surgery, sensory loss in saphenous neuropathy may initially go unnoticed or be of little concern to the patient. However, pain may be prominent, and in such cases, it usually appears sometime after the assumed injury to the nerve.
   b. **Physical examination.**
      (1) **Neurologic.** Examination reveals weakness of the quadriceps muscles, absent or diminished patellar reflex, and sensory loss over the anterior thigh and, with saphenous nerve involvement, the medial aspect of the leg and foot.

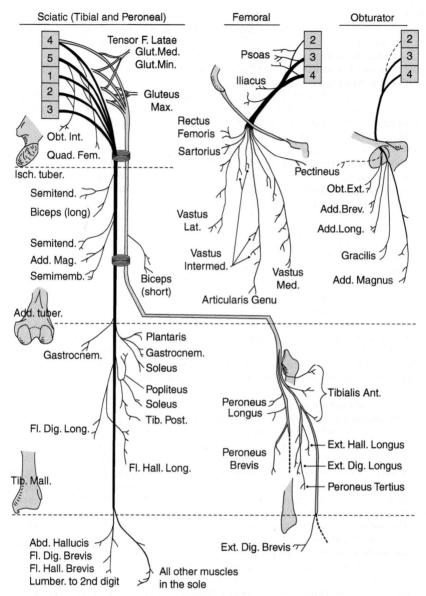

Sciatic (Tibial and Peroneal)

| 4 |
| 5 |
| 1 |
| 2 |
| 3 |

Tensor F. Latae
Glut. Med.
Glut. Min.

Gluteus
Max.

Obt. Int.
Quad. Fem.

Isch. tuber.

Semitend.

Biceps (long)

Semitend.
Add. Mag.
Semimemb.

Add. tuber.

Gastrocnem.

Fl. Dig. Long.

Tib. Mall.

Abd. Hallucis
Fl. Dig. Brevis
Fl. Hall. Brevis
Lumber. to 2nd digit

Plantaris
Gastrocnem.
Soleus

Popliteus
Soleus
Tib. Post.

Biceps
(short)

Fl. Hall. Long.

All other muscles
in the sole

Femoral

| 2 |
| 3 |
| 4 |

Psoas

Iliacus

Rectus
Femoris

Sartorius

Vastus
Lat.

Vastus
Intermed.

Vastus
Med.

Articularis Genu

Peroneus
Longus

Peroneus
Brevis

Ext. Dig. Brevis

Obturator

| 2 |
| 3 |
| 4 |

Pectineus

Obt. Ext.
Add. Brev.

Add. Long.

Gracilis

Add. Magnus

Tibialis Ant.

Ext. Hall. Longus
Ext. Dig. Longus
Peroneus Tertius

FIGURE 25.1 Motor distribution of the nerves of the lower limb. (Modified from Basmajian JV. *Grant's Method of Anatomy*. 9th ed. Baltimore, MD: Williams and Wilkins; 1975.)

(2) **General.** Examination or palpation within the inguinal region and, in cases of saphenous nerve involvement, the medial aspect of the knee may identify focal areas of pain and perhaps the site of involvement. The proximity of a surgical scar or point of injury can provide additional etiologic clues. In cases in which retroperitoneal hemorrhage is suspected, peripheral pulses may be normal, but there is characteristic posturing of the leg (held flexed at the hip), and attempts to extend or perform a reverse straight-leg test exacerbate the pain.

3. **Differential diagnosis.** Discovery of hip adduction weakness suggests a more proximal process, plexus, or root as the site of involvement, although a superimposed obturator neuropathy cannot be excluded.

4. **Evaluation.**
   a. **EDX.** NSS are not as helpful as EMG in the evaluation of a suspected femoral neuropathy. EMG includes study of other L2–L4 innervated muscles and paraspinal muscles because they should not be involved in isolated femoral neuropathy.
   b. **Imaging.** CT or MRI of the retroperitoneum helps to identify cases resulting from retroperitoneal hemorrhage or suspected mass lesion.

B. **Obturator neuropathy.** Arising within the psoas muscle from ventral (anterior) divisions of the ventral rami of L2–L4 spinal nerves, the obturator nerve exits from the psoas muscle at its lateral margin, descends into the pelvis, and exits through the obturator foramen. It innervates the gracilis, adductor magnus, longus, and brevis muscles and supplies sensation to the upper medial aspect of the thigh.
   1. **Etiology.** Isolated neuropathy of the obturator nerve is unusual. In cases resulting from pelvic or hip fracture, involvement of other nerves to the lower extremity or lumbosacral plexus also occurs. Benign and malignant pelvic masses can result in obturator neuropathy, as can surgical procedures performed on those masses or within the pelvis.
   2. **Clinical manifestations.**
      a. **History.** Leg weakness and difficulty walking are the most common first symptoms and usually overshadow sensory loss, if present.
      b. **Physical examination.**
         (1) **Neurologic.** Motor evaluation shows weakness of hip adduction, and sensory loss may be found along the upper medial thigh. The patellar reflex should be intact.
         (2) **General.** Careful pelvic and rectal examinations can identify an intrapelvic tumor and are necessary when obturator paralysis occurs without trauma.
   3. **Differential diagnosis.** The presence of hip flexor or knee extensor weakness or an impaired patellar reflex suggests a lumbosacral plexopathy or L3–L4 radiculopathy. In addition, sensory loss, which extends below the knee, is inconsistent with the expected sensory deficit. (Cases of obturator neuropathy with minimal gait disturbance have been attributed to more prominent sciatic nerve, tibial portion, and innervation of the adductor magnus muscle.)
   4. **Evaluation.**
      a. **EDX.** NSS are not as helpful as EMG where involvement of other L2–L4 muscles or paraspinal muscles identifies a more proximal lesion.
      b. **Imaging.** When obvious trauma is not a consideration, radiologic imaging of the pelvic cavity is helpful when a mass or infiltrative lesion is suspected.

C. **Lateral femoral cutaneous neuropathy.** Dorsal divisions of the ventral rami of the L2–L3 spinal nerves contribute to the lateral femoral cutaneous nerve, which emerges from the lateral border of the psoas major muscle. It then crosses laterally, within the fascia of the iliacus muscle, and crosses over the sartorius muscle before passing under the lateral border of the inguinal ligament. Piercing the fascia lata, it divides into anterior and posterior branches that provide sensory innervation to the anterolateral aspects of the thigh. Anatomic variation is frequent in regard to origin (it can arise as a branch of the femoral or genitofemoral nerve), course of its branches, and extent of its sensory innervation.
   1. **Etiology.** In most cases, entrapment or compression at or near the inguinal ligament is the assumed etiologic factor. However, entrapment or compression at other sites (i.e., retroperitoneal mass), surgical procedures (especially those involving retroperitoneal structures, pelvis, or inguinal sites), and trauma to the thigh can also injure the nerve.
   2. **Clinical manifestations.**
      a. **History.** Pain (burning or a "crawling" sensation) with variable loss of sensation on the anterolateral aspects of the thigh and exacerbated by walking or arising from a chair **(meralgia paresthetica).** Frequently, the patient rubs their thigh for relief.
      b. **Physical examination.**
         (1) **Neurologic.** The area of sensory change is usually small and over the lateral aspect of the thigh.
         (2) **General.** Careful palpation along the inguinal ligament and anterior pelvic brim will infrequently detect an area of tenderness or precipitate symptoms.
   3. **Differential diagnosis.** The primary differential diagnosis is a femoral neuropathy. Lumbar plexopathy and L2 radiculopathy are considerations, but limited sensory impairment, lack of motor involvement, and intact reflexes help in their exclusion.

4. Evaluation. Although clinical features usually provide enough support for a diagnosis, when uncertainty or a preexisting illness complicates the issue (retroperitoneal mass), further testing may be needed.

Unlike the situation with other entrapment syndromes, responsiveness to treatment may help to "confirm" the diagnosis of lateral femoral cutaneous neuropathy. Subcutaneous injection of an anesthetic agent or steroid at the assumed exit point of the lateral femoral cutaneous nerve (medial to the anterior superior iliac spine and under the inguinal ligament) or at a site of local tenderness may relieve symptoms and support but does not confirm the diagnosis.

a. EDX. Difficulty in eliciting a response from healthy or control subjects during NSS has limited the use of such testing. However, EMG studies play a more important role by clarifying unusual or unclear symptoms, because detection of clinically silent motor involvement implies involvement of more than the lateral femoral cutaneous nerve.

b. Imaging. Radiographic imaging is not indicated. However, unexplained or concomitant gastrointestinal or urogenital symptoms should raise suspicion of a retroperitoneal or pelvic mass and then further evaluation is appropriate.

D. Sciatic neuropathy. The sciatic nerve arises from the ventral divisions of the ventral rami of the L4–L5 spinal nerves, which, by way of the lumbosacral trunk, fuse with those from S1 to S3. Passing along the inner wall of the pelvis, it exits through the sciatic notch and passes under the piriformis muscle, where it lies between the ischial tuberosity and greater trochanter. Remaining in this deep location, the sciatic nerve descends into the extremity and proximal to the knee, divides into the peroneal and tibial nerves. The sciatic nerve itself is clearly divisible into two trunks—the medial, which receives contributions from the L4 to S3 rami and gives rise to the tibial nerve, and the lateral, the contributions of which are from L4 to S2 and from which the common peroneal nerve is derived. The sciatic nerve itself has no sensory branches. The lateral trunk provides innervation to the short head of the biceps femoris muscle and, by way of the medial trunk, the semitendinosus, semimembranosus, and long head of the biceps femoris muscles. With the obturator nerve, the adductor magnus muscle is also innervated.

1. Etiology. Most cases of sciatic neuropathy, whether involved at the gluteal level or the thigh, are secondary to trauma. (The sciatic nerve is possibly second to the peroneal nerve as the most common neuropathy of the lower extremity.) This includes injury to adjoining or neighboring structures in fractures of the pelvis, hip, or femur as well as from direct injury. Injection injuries are no longer as frequent, but compression injuries are increasing and often occur in the setting of prolonged immobility such as in various operative procedures (e.g., cardiac bypass graft surgery). Miscellaneous causes include entrapment by fibrous constricting bands, local hematoma, or tumor.

Mention must be made of the **piriformis syndrome.** At this time, few cases rigorously support the assumed pathogenesis of this syndrome, compression of the sciatic nerve by the overlying piriformis muscle, and treatment remain unclear, but it remains a frequent clinical diagnosis. Point tenderness of the sciatic nerve at the level of the piriformis muscle can be found among patients with plexopathy or lumbosacral radiculopathy and does not necessarily confirm pathologic compression of the sciatic nerve by the piriformis muscle.

2. Clinical manifestations.

a. History. Complete lesions are associated with paralysis of the hamstring muscles and all muscles below the knee. Sensory loss occurs in the tibial and peroneal distributions. Partial lesions, especially those of the lateral trunk, make up most cases of sciatic neuropathy and often manifest as foot drop.

b. Physical examination.

(1) Neurologic. Although variable paralysis of muscles innervated by both the medial and lateral trunk can be present, involvement of muscles innervated by the lateral trunk is the most frequent presentation. Sensory loss is variable, but restricted to the distribution of the sensory branches of the peroneal and tibial nerves. The muscle stretch reflexes of the hamstring and Achilles' tendons can be depressed.

(2) General. Palpation along the course of the nerve may help identify masses or locate points of pain and tenderness, but cannot entirely exclude more proximal nerve lesions.

3. **Differential diagnosis.** Care must be taken to ensure that a radiculopathy (especially L5–S1) is not masquerading as a sciatic neuropathy. The straight-leg-raise test, frequently positive in radiculopathy, can also be present in cases of lumbosacral plexopathy and sciatic neuropathy. A careful rectal and pelvic examination is indicated when sciatic neuropathy is suspected because involvement of the sacral plexus by a pelvic mass may not otherwise be identified. Finally, an isolated common peroneal or tibial neuropathy must be considered.

4. **Evaluation.**
   a. **EDX.** Both NSS and EMG are useful in differentiating sciatic mononeuropathy from L5 to S2 radiculopathies or plexopathy and require careful study of the paraspinal and gluteal muscles. Yet at times there can still be diagnostic confusion. When the lateral division of the sciatic nerve is "selectively" involved, EMG and NSS may show a pattern that suggests peroneal nerve involvement, whereas tibial nerve studies may appear to be normal.
   b. **Imaging.** In cases in which radiculopathy and plexopathy cannot be excluded, further radiologic studies can provide useful information. In addition, in cases in which only sciatic nerve involvement is found, MRI with gadolinium infusion may effectively depict the course of the nerve and help in identifying focal abnormalities.

E. **Peroneal neuropathy.** Arising from dorsal divisions of the L4–S2 ventral rami of spinal nerves, the common peroneal nerve descends into the leg as the lateral division of the sciatic nerve. At the level of the popliteal fossa, it branches from the sciatic nerve and moves toward the lower lateral portion of the popliteal fossa. Two cutaneous sensory branches arise at this point, one to the sural nerve and the other, the lateral (sural) cutaneous nerve of the calf, providing sensation to the upper lateral calf. Exiting laterally from the popliteal space, the peroneal nerve is in close juxtaposition to the fibula, winds below its head, and passes through a tendinous arch formed by the peroneus longus muscle. At its exit from the arch, the nerve divides into the superficial and deep peroneal nerves. The superficial peroneal nerve descends adjacent to the peroneus longus and brevis muscles, which it innervates, and in the distal third of the leg, it pierces the fascia. The terminal branches (medial and lateral) of the superficial peroneal nerve provide sensation to the lateral dorsal surface of the foot. The deep peroneal nerve enters the extensor compartment of the leg and with the tibial artery descends on the interosseous membrane, innervating the tibialis anterior, extensor hallucis longus, and extensor digitorum longus muscles. The terminal portion of this nerve then passes under the extensor retinaculum at the ankle, where a lateral branch innervates the extensor digitorum brevis muscle and a medial branch provides sensory innervation to the first and second toes.

   1. **Etiology.** Most cases of peroneal neuropathy are caused by external compression (anesthesia and casts), trauma (blunt injury, arthroscopic knee surgery, and fractures), and less frequently by other etiologies (e.g., tumor, constriction by adjacent structures, involvement in systemic disease, and traction injuries from severe ankle strain).
   2. **Clinical manifestations.**
      a. **History.** Most patients present with foot drop, and sensory disorders are usually minimal or of no concern. Less prominent degrees of weakness or only affecting intrinsic foot muscles may not elicit alarm in the patient. On review of the history, careful attention needs to be paid to possible episodes of trauma, compression, or unusual sustained postures that may have preceded the problem (e.g., squatting and kneeling).
      b. **Physical examination.**
         (1) **Neurologic.** The characteristic presentation is foot drop, and with complete involvement of the common peroneal nerve, paralysis of ankle dorsiflexion, ankle eversion, and toe extension (dorsiflexion). Sensory loss occurs over the anterolateral lower leg and the dorsum of the foot and toes. (See Video 25.1.)
         (2) **General.** Palpation in the popliteal fossa and along the fibular head may elicit signs of tenderness or discovery of a mass and define the site of involvement and possible etiology. Examination of the dorsum of the ankle and distal lateral leg, where the terminal branch of the deep peroneal nerve emerges, may reveal similar signs and suggest a distal injury. The most common sites at which focal pathologic processes can affect the nerve or its branches include the fibular head and its proximal neck, the outer compartment of the leg, and the superior and inferior extensor retinaculum at the ankle, beneath which branches of the

peroneal nerve pass. However, the peroneal nerve serves as a reminder that, in cases of focal compression, there can be variable fascicular involvement. Motor impairment of only the deep or superficial component, sensory dysfunction only, or various combinations may be the result of nerve compression at the fibular head.

3. **Differential diagnosis.** The primary differential diagnoses are other causes of foot drop: involvement of the L5 root, the lumbosacral trunk, and the lateral division of the sciatic nerve.

4. **Evaluation.** The extent of evaluation depends on the history. In cases in which an identifiable episode of compression is present, supportive care, after elimination of continuing compression, is often all that is needed. When disruption (laceration) of the nerve is suggested, the onset of the problem is insidious, or physical findings are inconclusive (incomplete common peroneal neuropathy), further evaluation is indicated.

   a. **EDX.** NSS assist in identification of the site of involvement, extent of axonal injury, and prognosis by comparison to the asymptomatic leg, but could also identify bilateral, although asymmetric, nerve involvement suggesting an underlying generalized nerve disorder (polyneuropathy). EMG helps to further define the extent of axonal injury or evidence of a different etiology of the patient's symptoms, if abnormalities are found in other L4–L5 innervated muscles or paraspinal muscles.

   b. **Imaging.** Although X-ray studies can be useful when joint trauma or a mass is detectable at examination, CT and MRI are more useful in defining lesions of the nerve and delineating the relationship of adjacent structures.

F. **Tibial neuropathy.** Ventral divisions of the ventral rami from the L5 to S2 spinal nerves contribute to the tibial nerve, which descends into the extremity as part of the medial trunk of the sciatic nerve. At the distal portion of the extremity, the sciatic nerve bifurcates into both the tibial and peroneal nerves. Entering the calf, the tibial nerve descends to the depth of the gastrocnemius, which it innervates, and provides innervation to the soleus, tibialis posterior, flexor digitorum, and hallucis longus muscles. At the level of the ankle, it divides into its terminal branches (plantar nerves), which innervate all intrinsic foot flexor muscles as well as providing sensation to the sole.

1. **Etiology.** Tibial neuropathy is infrequent partly because of the deep anatomic location of the nerve but, severe ankle injuries can cause proximal or distal tibial nerve injuries through traction on the nerve. Major knee trauma is surprisingly an infrequent cause of severe tibial nerve injury.

2. **Clinical manifestations.**
   a. **History.** Sensory loss is evident along the lateral side of the foot and extends proximally if the contribution of the tibial nerve to the sural nerve is also involved. Weakness may not be noticed unless ankle plantar flexion is involved.

   b. **Physical examination.**
      (1) **Neurologic.** Sensory loss is present along the sole of the foot. Weakness may be limited to intrinsic toe flexor muscles, or, with more proximal nerve involvement, weakness of ankle dorsiflexion and inversion.
      (2) **General.** Careful palpation over the course of the nerve, especially within the popliteal space, should be performed. The finding of a mass or precipitation of paresthesia or pain on palpation helps in localization and may suggest the cause as a tumor involving the tibial nerve (or any nerve) that may increase the sensitivity of the nerve to such maneuvers.

3. **Differential diagnosis.** Because of its infrequent occurrence, any suspicion of tibial neuropathy should prompt a search for a more proximal lesion. Radiculopathy, plexopathy, or sciatic neuropathy can manifest clinically as an "isolated" tibial neuropathy. Careful examination of more proximal muscles, reflexes, as well as the sensory examination can help identify or suggest those conditions as more appropriate diagnoses.

4. **Evaluation.**
   a. **EDX.** Plays a crucial role in identifying as well as excluding a tibial neuropathy by identifying involvement of other nerves on NSS or EMG evidence of muscle involvement other than those innervated by the tibial nerve. At times, plantar nerve involvement rather than a more proximal tibial lesion is the cause of the observed sensory or motor deficits.

    b. Imaging. Identification of a mass or point of tenderness in cases of unclear causation may necessitate MRI to identify the anatomic structure of the nerve and its relations to adjacent structures.

G. Medial and lateral plantar neuropathy. At the level of the ankle, the terminal portion of the tibial nerve is medial to the Achilles tendon. As it descends, it passes under the flexor retinaculum (lacinate ligament), which comprises the ligamentous roof of the tarsal tunnel. Within the distal part of this tunnel and at the upper edge of the abductor hallucis muscle the tibial nerve divides into the medial and lateral plantar nerves, which descend toward the foot, and a calcaneal or sensory branch, which provides sensation over the heel (a palpable "soft spot" along the medial border of the heel and distal edge of the abductor hallucis muscle overlies the origin of these divisions). Both plantar nerves then cross under the abductor hallucis muscle (which the medial plantar nerve innervates) and go on to innervate all the muscles of the foot as well as providing sensation to the sole and the toes (the medial nerve supplies the medial and the lateral supplies the lateral portion) through their distal divisions, which give rise to the digital nerves. Muscles innervated by the medial plantar nerve include the flexor hallucis brevis and digitorum brevis. The lateral plantar nerve innervates the interossei, the flexor and abductor digiti minimi, and the adductor hallucis.

1. **Etiology.** The proximity of the plantar nerves to osseous and fibrous structures predisposes them to injury or compression. At the level of the tarsal tunnel, external compression and ankle injury are the most frequent etiologic factors. A multitude of other less frequent structural abnormalities (synovial or joint changes and mass lesions) can also lead to nerve injury. Within the foot itself, the medial and lateral plantar nerves are susceptible to the effects of trauma or fracture of the foot bones.

2. **Clinical manifestations.**
   a. **History.** The first recognition of disorder occurs when sensory impairment develops, because foot pain or discomfort is more frequently assumed to have an "orthopedic" origin. Sensory loss can be present in the sole or heel and at times can be precipitated by specific foot positions. Weakness of foot muscles usually produces no significant symptoms.
   b. **Physical examination.**
      (1) **Neurologic.** Sensory loss in the distribution of the plantar nerves or their distal divisions (digital nerves) should be sought. If foot involvement is asymmetric, changes in foot muscle bulk can be appreciated, as can weakness, although usually only toe flexion can be reliably evaluated clinically.
      (2) **General.** Careful examination of the course of the nerve along the ankle into the foot accompanied by attempts to elicit discomfort or a Tinel's sign by means of light percussion over its course may confirm the presence and location of plantar nerve involvement. Joint changes, deformity, or swelling can also help to suggest a site of nerve involvement.

3. **Differential diagnosis.** One needs to consider a more proximal nerve (tibial) or root (S1) lesions that can cause foot pain or paresthesia. Motor and reflex changes should aid in this distinction. Polyneuropathy can be considered when bilaterality, depressed reflexes, and sensory involvement outside of the plantar sensory nerve distribution are found.

4. **Evaluation.**
   a. **EDX.** Are helpful in demonstrating findings consistent with nerve entrapment (tarsal tunnel) of the medial or lateral plantar as well as calcaneal nerves. Because of the technical difficulty of such recordings, further study of asymptomatic or contralateral nerves clarifies the findings. An EMG is needed to exclude more proximal disorders (tibial neuropathy, sciatic neuropathy, or radiculopathy).
   b. **Imaging.** Studies of possible sites of involvement (ankle) are not usually indicated. However, in cases of marked discomfort or disability, such studies may identify underlying orthopedic abnormalities and guide treatment.

H. Iliohypogastric, ilioinguinal, and genitofemoral neuropathy. The iliohypogastric, ilioinguinal, and genitofemoral nerves are described as a group because of the similarity of their origins, sensory innervation, and causes of dysfunction. These nerves arise predominantly from or have major contributions from the L1 ventral rami of the spinal nerves (the genitofemoral nerve also has an L2 contribution), but the ilioinguinal may have additional contributions from T12, L2, and L3 while the iliohypogastric from T12 ventral rami. These nerves first pass through and then close to the psoas muscle in their intra-abdominal course. The iliohypogastric nerve emerges above the iliac crest and supplies sensation to an area of skin over the lateral upper buttock and another area over the pubis or symphysis. The ilioinguinal nerve enters the inguinal canal at its lateral border and supplies the area above the inguinal ligament and the base of the genitalia. Both the iliohypogastric and ilioinguinal nerves also supply the muscles of the lower abdominal area. Clinically evident weakness of the lower abdominal musculature can occur, but perhaps more common with loss of function of both of those nerves. After it emerges from the psoas muscle, the genitofemoral nerve is retroperitoneal and descends to the inguinal ligament while resting on the surface of the psoas muscle. It supplies sensation to a small area over the proximal genitalia and anterior proximal thigh.

1. Etiology. Because of the location and course of these nerves, neuropathy usually results from surgical procedures (inguinal herniorrhaphy, laparoscopic surgery, or lumbar sympathetic blocks). The development of neuralgia is not infrequent after injuries to these nerves.
2. Clinical manifestations.
    a. History. Patients have varying sensory problems, including numbness, paresthesia, or pain within the ipsilateral inguinal and perineal areas. If the cause is related to surgery, these difficulties may be evident immediately after the operation or may not become evident for several weeks.
    b. Physical examination.
        (1) Neurologic. Iliohypogastric neuropathies are infrequent, but result in sensory loss over the lateral upper buttock and suprapubic area. Ilioinguinal impairment results in sensory loss over the inguinal area and the base of the genitalia but typically resolves or results in minimal disability. In other cases, pain may appear both here and in the inferior abdomen and upper thigh and be worsened or precipitated by changes in leg position. Genitofemoral neuropathy usually accompanies inguinal nerve involvement because of the anatomic proximity of the genitofemoral and inguinal nerves. Symptoms and precipitating factors are similar as well, but sensory problems can extend into the medial and proximal areas of the genitalia.
        (2) General. In ilioinguinal and genitofemoral neuropathy, areas of tenderness that often conform to the site of injury may be found in the inguinal region.
3. Differential diagnosis. In these cases, nerve involvement predominantly causes sensory impairment, and the differential diagnosis is directed at detecting other causes of sensory impairment outside the typical boundaries of these nerves, including abnormalities in the medial thigh (obturator nerve), anterior thigh (femoral nerve), and lateral thigh (lateral femoral cutaneous nerve), as well as dermatomal involvement caused by T12 or L1 radiculopathy. Because of these overlapping sensory innervations, the presence of motor deficits or reflex changes provides the strongest clue to the presence of one of these other disorders. Back pain, which can suggest a radiculopathy, or the absence of a previous operative procedure, which is the usual cause of these neuropathies, suggests another etiologic factor.
4. Evaluation.
    a. EDX. Plays little role in the identification of these neuropathies. However, they become indispensable in helping to identify more proximal lesions (plexus or root) or other forms of neuropathy (femoral) that may clinically resemble iliohypogastric, ilioinguinal, or genitofemoral neuropathy in regard to sensory deficits.
    b. Imaging. Is performed if there is suspicion of radiculopathy or if a retroperitoneal, intra-abdominal, or pelvic lesion is under consideration.

MISCELLANEOUS NEUROPATHIES

This grouping and brief review are based on their infrequent occurrence or isolated involvement.
1. Superior gluteal neuropathy. Arising from and receiving its contributions from the dorsal divisions of the L4 to S1 ventral rami components of the sacral plexus, the nerve passes through the sciatic notch above the piriformis muscle and innervates the gluteus medius and minimus muscles. Its isolated involvement is unusual and is most often the result of injury by a misplaced injection.

2. **Inferior gluteal neuropathy.** Arises from the L5 to S2 dorsal divisions of the ventral rami components of the sacral plexus and exits through the sciatic notch. Its proximity to the sciatic, pudendal, and posterior cutaneous nerves of the extremity results in their concomitant involvement from local injuries.

3. **Posterior cutaneous nerve of the thigh.** Arising from the dorsal divisions of S1 and S2 and the ventral divisions of S2 and S3 of the ventral rami components of the sacral plexus, it descends through the sciatic notch close to the sciatic nerve and supplies sensation to the posterior portion of the buttock and thigh. At times it is susceptible to local compression, but its isolated involvement is unusual.

4. **Pudendal neuropathy.** Derived from the ventral divisions of the S2 to S4 ventral rami components of the sacral plexus, it passes through the sciatic notch and descends toward the perineum. Supplying muscles of the perineum, including the anal sphincter and erectile tissue, it also provides sensory innervation to the perineum. Its deep location protects it, but prolonged compression or stretch injuries related to prolonged labor can cause dysfunction and manifested as fecal and urinary incontinence as well as persistent pain.

REFERRALS

I. Indications for and purposes of neurologic consultation.
1. Site of involvement unclear from examination or history, and discrepancy between severity of the underlying disease and the neuropathy.
2. Progressive deterioration despite appropriate treatment.
3. Problem precipitated by trauma or injury.
4. Prior to more expensive or invasive evaluation (MRI or nerve biopsy) or more aggressive intervention (surgery).
5. Confirmation of diagnosis, etiology, or treatment plan.

J. EMG and NSS evaluation.
1. Basic tenets of such testing
   a. Extension of the clinical examination and not a replacement
   b. Intended to clarify the clinical question to be answered (e.g., carpal tunnel syndrome or C6 radiculopathy)
   c. Sensitivity and specificity vary according to the etiologic factor and process in question.
2. Role in the evaluation of neuropathy
   a. Confirmation of diagnosis or characterization, localization, and quantification of a disease process
   b. Defining prognosis
   c. Detection of subclinical disease
   d. Planning treatment or determining need for further evaluation or consultation

Key Points

- To limit confusion, when localizing a peripheral nerve lesion it is best to keep in mind that there are anatomical variations in spinal nerve contributions to individual nerves and variability in the terminal distribution and course of their sensory divisions.
- Sensory deficits with peripheral nerve lesions are often not complete, may only involve the distal sensory nerve distribution and are often best defined/outlined by the patient.
- Sciatic nerve lesions are often partial, involve the lateral trunk of the nerve and can present as foot drop, suggesting a peroneal neuropathy.
- At times an obturator neuropathy may result in little gait impairment and believed to represent the occurrence of significant innervation of the adductor magnus by the tibial division of the sciatic nerve.
- There is significant variability within the terminal divisions of the lateral femoral cutaneous nerve that at times can hamper localization or therapeutic interventions.
- The overlapping sensory innervation territories of the ilioinguinal, iliohypogastric, and genitofemoral with other lower extremity nerves can impact clinical localization, but the presence of weakness or reflex changes should clinically raise that suspicion.

Recommended Readings

Bradshaw AD, Advincula AP. Postoperative neuropathy in gynecologic surgery. *Obstet Gynecol Clin North Am.* 2010;37:451–459.

Cassidy L, Walters A, Bubb K, et al. Piriformis syndrome: implications of anatomical variations, diagnostic techniques, and treatment options. *Surg Radiol Anat.* 2012;34:479–486.

Distad BJ, Weiss MD. Clinical and electrodiagnostic features of sciatic mononeuropathies. *Phys Med Rehabil Clin N Am.* 2013;24:107–120.

Donovan A, Rosenberg ZS, Cavalcanti CF. MR imaging of entrapment neuropathies of the lower extremity: part 2: the knee, leg, ankle and foot. *Radiographics.* 2010;30:1001–1019.

Fridman V, David WS. Electrodiagnostic evaluation of lower extremity mononeuropathies. *Neurol Clin.* 2021;30:505–528.

Gould JS. Tarsal tunnel syndrome. *Foot Ankle Clin.* 2011;16:275–286.

Hart MG, Santarius T, Trivedi RA. Muscle and nerve biopsy for the neurosurgical trainee. *Br J Neurosurg.* 2013;27:727–734.

Khoder W, Hale D. Pudendal neuralgia. *Obstet Gynecol Clin North Am.* 2014;41:443–452.

Klassen Z, Marshall E, Tubbs RS, et al. Anatomy of the ilioinguinal and iliohypogastric nerves with observations of their spinal nerve contributions. *Clin Anat.* 2011;24:454–461.

Laughlin RS, Dyck PJB. Electrodiagnostic testing in lumbosacral plexopathies. *Phys Med Rehabil Clin N Am.* 2013;24:93–105.

Marcinial C. Fibular (peroneal) neuropathy: electrodiagnostic features and clinical correlates. *Phys Med Rehabil Clin N Am.* 2013;24:121–137.

Matejčík V. Anatomical variations of lumbosacral plexus. *Surg Radiol Anat.* 2010;32:409–414.

Mirilas P, Skandalakis JE. Surgical anatomy of the retroperitoneal spaces: part IV: retroperitoneal nerves. *Am Surg.* 2010;76:253–262.

Moore AE, Stringer MD. Iatrogenic femoral nerve injury: a systematic review. *Surg Radiol Anat.* 2011;33:649–658.

O'Brien M. *Aids to the Examination of the Peripheral Nervous System.* 5th ed. New York: WB Saunders; 2010.

Patijn J, Mekhail N, Hayek S, et al. Meralgia paresthetica. *Pain Pract.* 2011;11:302–308.

Petchprapa CN, Rosenberg ZS, Sconfienza LM, et al. MR imaging of entrapment neuropathies of the lower extremity: part 1: the pelvis and hip. *Radiographics.* 2010;30:983–1000.

Shin JH, Howard FM. Abdominal wall nerve injury during laparoscopic gynecologic surgery: incidence, risk factors, and treatment outcomes. *J Minim Invasive Gynecol.* 2012;19:448–453.

Zappe B, Glauser PM, Majewski M, et al. Long-term prognosis of nerve palsy after total hip arthroplasty: results of two-year-follow-ups and long-term results after a mean time of 8 years. *Arch Orthop Trauma Surg.* 2014;134:1477–1482.

26 Approach to the Patient with Failed Back Syndrome

Tarik F. Ibrahim, Russ P. Nockels, and Michael W. Groff

Although commonly used as a diagnostic term, failed back syndrome (FBS) is a misnomer. The term "syndrome" should not be applied to patients with a "failed back" because it gives the perception that patients with FBS have a group of symptoms that commonly occur together. Taken as such, the danger exists that a clinician may disregard important signs and symptoms that will lead to the proper treatment of a patient. Fortunately, a set of diagnostic principles can be used to clarify these issues and, from a practical standpoint, be used methodically to achieve a more appropriate diagnosis.

FAILED BACK SYNDROME

The FBS is a clinical condition experienced by patients who undergo a surgical procedure, typically in the lumbosacral region, with unsatisfactory results. Back pain is the second most common reason, behind asthma, for patients to seek medical help. It has been estimated that 300,000 laminectomies were performed last year. With the advent of modern instrumentation systems, an increasing number of lumbar fusions are being performed each year. Unfortunately, not every operation is successful, and the success rate ranges from 50% to nearly 100% depending on the indication. Consequently, the prevalence of FBS is quite high.

Categories of FBS include the following:

A. **Failure to improve due to misdiagnosis.** By definition, FBS implies previous surgery. Therefore, the first priority in the evaluation of these patients is to understand the indication for the original operation. It is often helpful to ask the patient to compare current symptoms with those experienced prior to surgery in terms of location, frequency, and intensity. A patient who fails to improve at all following surgery is more likely to have been misdiagnosed than a patient who improves for a period of time. If the original indication for surgery is suspect, it is extremely unlikely that further surgical intervention will be helpful.

B. **Failure to improve due to improper treatment.** Patients who do not improve or worsen immediately after surgery may have suffered a technical error during surgery. These errors include inadequate decompression, wrong-level surgery, or nerve-root injury. Frank instability of the operated level may also worsen if an unstable spinal motion segment such as a mobile spondylolisthesis is not stabilized or fused at the time of decompression.

C. **Recurrent pathology.** A patient who experiences identical recurrent symptoms after a postoperative period of significant improvement will likely harbor recurrent pathology. Disc herniations, for example, carry a lifelong risk of recurrence because the majority of the anatomical intervertebral disc remains after a discectomy and the annular tear that permits the herniation never completely heals. An infection may also be present, frequently becoming apparent within the first 4 weeks of surgery. Infections may cause recurrent symptoms as well as the new onset of significant back pain. These infections can be occult, and imaging studies should be performed to determine if endplate erosion or a fluid collection is present.

D. **Progression of pathologic changes at unoperated sites.** Surgical procedures of the lumbar spine are commonly performed for degenerative diseases. Spondylosis, or bony overgrowth of the facet joints and intervertebral endplates, in association with soft tissue ligamentous hypertrophy can cause significant stenosis. Spondylolisthesis, or malalignment of the spine, can progress after decompression alone, causing recurrent nerve-root entrapment. Additionally, progression of degenerative changes at a level adjacent to a lumbar fusion may occur, resulting in stenosis and/or spondylolisthesis.

SIGNS AND SYMPTOMS THAT WILL AID IN THE ASSESSMENT OF FAILED BACK SYNDROME

A. **Radiculopathy** is a pain that shoots like a jolt of electricity and follows a particular dermatomal distribution. This is most often caused by a herniated disk, but not exclusively so. Many times there is associated sensory loss in the same dermatome. The associated myotome can manifest weakness in some cases. Abnormal reflexes can also help to localize the level of involvement in the spinal canal.

   1. Imaging is helpful in this context to confirm the level implicated by the history and physical examination findings. However, it has been well shown that healthy persons without back pain can harbor disks that would be concerning from a purely radiographic perspective. Therefore, imaging findings without a clinical correlate can typically be ignored.

   2. The most common cause of the pathogenesis of radiculopathy is herniation of a disk followed closely by degenerative foraminal stenosis. Other entities, such as synovial cyst, are distinctly less common.

   3. Whatever the cause, surgery for radiculopathy is focused on decompressing the affected nerve root. The prognosis is quite good; early good results are achieved in >95% of cases.

   4. When this type of surgery is unsuccessful, strong consideration should be given to the possibility that the diagnosis was incorrect, the wrong level was operated on, or the patient has secondary issues that are preventing improvement.

   5. Radiculopathy can be confused with hip disease in some cases. A positive **Patrick's test** should be followed with an evaluation to rule out hip arthrosis.

B. **Claudication** is a cramping pain or sense of fatigue in the legs caused by exertion. Most patients report the onset of symptoms after walking a particular distance. The pain typically abates after several minutes of rest, such that the person can continue.

   1. It is important not to confuse **neurogenic** and **vascular** claudication. Patients with neurogenic claudication exhibit a "shopping cart sign," which is the ability to walk further when leaning forward. This flexed position slightly diminishes the ligamentous compression of the cauda equina, allowing the patient to walk further. For the same reason, a patient with neurogenic claudication will do much better on exercising bicycle than they would on walking. Patients with vascular claudication show no such improvement.

   2. **Neurogenic claudication** is most commonly managed with lumbar laminectomy over the stenotic levels. The goal of surgery is to decompress the thecal sac by removing hypertrophied ligamentum flavum, the medial facet, and occasionally disc material. Foraminotomies are required to decompress the exiting nerve roots, and this may result in iatrogenic instability causing some patients to require fusion as well.

   3. Imaging with either MRI or **CT myelography** shows a markedly compressed thecal sac with a characteristic trefoil configuration and amputation of the exiting nerve-root sleeves.

C. **Instability** is another common indication for lumbar surgery. From both a theoretical and a practical standpoint, instability is distinct from stenosis and radiculopathy. Management of radiculopathy and stenosis is decompression; management of instability is fusion. The success of fusion operations is distinctly less than that of decompression. For this reason, many patients with FBS have experienced failed fusion.

   1. **Instability** is defined as the ability of the bony components of the spine to withstand physiologic loads without mechanical pain or compromise of nerve-root function.

   2. Although instability is often thought of in a binomial way as either present or absent, in clinical practice there is a spectrum of instability ranging from **gross instability,** most often the result of trauma, to **microinstability,** which is found in the context of degenerative disease.

   3. The underlying hypothesis in offering fusion to patients with degenerative spondylosis is that instability represents a painful dysfunctional motion segment. The pain is characteristically exacerbated by prolonged sitting or standing and is often relieved by recumbency. Because the pain does not radiate, it is not possible to localize the responsible spinal level by means of history or physical examination.

   4. The pathogenesis of mechanical back pain is controversial and is likely multifactorial. There is evidence implicating the disk space as well as the facet joints. Many patients who improve after lumbar fusion fail to demonstrate overt instability on preoperative

dynamic studies. Therefore, the specific pain generator is unknown, and the lumbar segment inclusive of the disc and facet joints is thought to be dysfunctional.

5. If **flexion–extension radiographs (dynamic radiographs)** show movement of >4 mm, the diagnosis is more certain. However, a large number of patients with movement in excess of 4 mm also do not have mechanical pain. Plain radiographs can provide indirect evidence of instability in the form of traction spurs that result from the tension placed on the bone from **Sharpy's fibers** of the annulus or loss of disk height indicative of disk degeneration. MRI often shows **Modic's changes** at the interspace thought to represent inflammatory reaction in the adjacent vertebral bodies secondary to disk disruption. Many of these findings are present in patients who are pain free, and therefore their utility is suspect.

6. In an attempt to better determine whether instability is present in a particular patient and whether it is responsible for the back pain being reported, several strategies have emerged. The trial use of a temporary **external orthosis** or percutaneous **pedicle screws** before surgical fusion has fallen out of favor.

   a. Use of diagnostic facet blocks targeting a spinal level thought to be unstable can be helpful. Epidural steroids, although clinically beneficial, are of no diagnostic significance because they are not specific to an anatomic level.

   b. **Provocative diskography** has been championed because it shows the disk disruption anatomically and functionally. Great care must be taken to inject both normal and diseased levels in a patient-blinded fashion in order to determine whether the targeted level(s) have pain concordant with the patient's primary complaints of back pain.

7. Technical aspects of lumbar fusion have improved outcomes such as the use of supplemental interbody devices, less rigid implants, and bone morphogenic protein (BMP). However, it is still not possible to predict who will benefit from lumbar fusion and who will not with a high degree of certainty. This explains, in part, the relative lack of success with fusion operations compared with decompression operations for radiculopathy or stenosis. Most series have favorable outcome in 50% to 70% of cases when lumbar fusion is performed for degenerative disease.

8. If the indication for fusion was not present at the time of the first operation, revision surgery will be futile. Moreover, even when the original procedure is well conceived, revision surgery is effective only if a problem amenable to surgical correction is identified preoperatively. Examples consistent with a successful operation include pseudoarthrosis and degeneration at the level adjacent to the fusion. The plan should be well defined preoperatively.

SOMATIC PROBLEMS NOT RELATED TO THE SPINE

Many somatic problems not related to the spine can manifest as back pain. These must be excluded in a thorough review of systems.

A. **Abdominal causes** include aortic aneurysm, cholelithiasis, and pancreatitis. Pyelonephritis most often manifests as flank pain but can also lead to referred back pain.

B. In female patients, **endometriosis** can manifest as low back pain.

C. **Sacroiliac joint (SIJ) pain** is increasingly common because of abnormal shifting of the pelvis in patients with lumbar degenerative disease. Injections of the SIJ can be both diagnostic and therapeutic.

D. **Osteoarthritis of the hip** can be easily confused with back pain radiating into the buttock. Patrick's test is useful to differentiate the two. Severe radiation of the pain to the groin is diagnostic of hip pathology.

E. **Major depression** has been shown to exacerbate the severity of back pain. It is also a poor prognostic sign for outcome after surgical intervention. Ongoing worker's compensation litigation has also been shown to be an independent predictor of poor outcome.

NONSURGICAL MODALITIES

After the rationale for the primary operation or previous operations is understood, emphasis should be given to nonsurgical modalities. In any cohort of patients with FBS, only a small number should ever come to revision surgery.

A. It should be well understood that **lumbar spondylosis** is a degenerative disease. As such, surgery can ameliorate the most severe manifestations of the problem, but it can never address the underlying cause. For this reason, treatments such as weight loss, smoking cessation, and physical therapy offer the patient a better outcome, if successful, and can often make surgery unnecessary. Moreover, even when surgery is entertained, it should only be in the context of a complete treatment plan that embraces these other aspects of care. At the same time, the efficacy of surgery decreases with each subsequent operation, unless significant additional pathology has been uncovered.

B. Degenerative changes in the spine are often associated with deformities. These deformities can be focal such as spondylolisthesis, or more global, such as scoliosis. Recently, sagittal deformities have been demonstrated to have a significant impact on outcome. If these sagittal imbalances are fixed, that is, not amenable to postural changes by the patient, surgical correction of the deformity may be required. In the past, lumbar fusion surgeries focused less on sagittal issues and may have resulted in **flat back syndrome,** whereby the lumbar spine was fused in a hypolordotic position. Patients with FBS due to fixed sagittal imbalance require long cassette standing scoliosis studies to accurately assess the condition.

C. In most cases of FBS, the patient comes to medical attention with the chief symptom of pain. Pain is a subjective symptom. Considerable progress has been made in the development of **outcome instruments** (Oswestry, SF36) that attempt to quantify pain and functional level in an objective way. This has given spine specialists a means of comparing of the clinical effectiveness of various interventions.

D. The pain that patients report and the disability they experience have a great deal to do with their expectations. Pain is ordinarily an important protective phenomenon. When pain becomes chronic, as in FBS, the noxious percept that reaches consciousness serves no productive purpose. The assumption of many patients that the pain they are experiencing is evidence of ongoing damage is incorrect. When patients understand this, their perception of pain can become less noxious, and their functional abilities can improve. Therefore, patient education can play a therapeutic role.

E. As a clearer understanding emerges of the nature of pain in FBS, more effective, interdisciplinary treatments are being developed. It is increasingly recognized that depression not only exacerbates the symptoms of FBS but is also a consistent consequence of FBS. If relatively severe, depression should be addressed before surgical intervention is planned.

PAIN MANAGEMENT

The nonsurgical therapies discussed in section Nonsurgical Modalities address the causes of FBS in just as direct a manner as surgery does. In some cases, indirect measures can be considered purely with the intent of ameliorating a patient's pain. Although these modalities are not directed at the underlying cause, they do enhance functional ability and improve quality of life.

A. There is increasing experience with **narcotics** in the management of chronic pain of a nonmalignant causation, such as FBS. This is an expansion of experience with **cancer pain.** Subsequently, some authors have expanded the indications to include patients with **chronic pain of benign causation.** Because the life expectancy of patients with FBS is much longer than that of patients with cancer, the duration of treatment is considerably longer. These patients must be followed for the development of toleration and habituation. Topical forms of opiates such as Fentanyl have been increasingly used for chronic pain because their pharmacokinetic profile lacks the peak and trough levels of oral opiates. Serum chemistries with liver function tests should be checked on a regular schedule. Moreover, it has been estimated that as many as 45% of patients with FBS are being medicated excessively, and this treatment remains controversial.

B. **Intrathecal pumps** for the administration of opioids have been used to minimize the side effects of systemic opiate therapy, such as sedation, lethargy, and decreased libido. Because the drug is delivered directly to the opiate receptors within the dorsal horn of the spinal cord, effective analgesia can be obtained at much lower doses. This leads to a much lower incidence of side effects. However, the use of intrathecal pumps has increasingly been reserved for patients with pain due to cancer, as oral and topical analgesics have become more effective.

C. The **gate-control theory** of pain proposed by Melzack and Wall was the inspiration for **spinal cord stimulation.** Modern implantable and rechargeable systems are much more effective and easier to insert than earlier versions. Most studies demonstrate favorable early and late success for these implants in treating FBS, although the cost effectiveness of these procedures is currently under debate. The complication rate is low, with neurologic injury occurring in <1% of patients.

SURGICAL MANAGEMENT

When conservative therapy is unsuccessful, operative intervention should be considered (Video 26.1).

A. In cases of **immediate failure,** the patients never improve after surgery. This universally implies an **error in diagnosis** or a **technical deficiency** with the surgery. After the protocol outlined in sections Nonsurgical Modalities and Pain Management has been implemented, these patients require MRI with and without contrast material. The prognosis for these patients is very good when an error is identified. If no deficiency is found, the outcome is considerably more discouraging. Surgery has no role in those cases.

B. The next group of failures manifests **days to weeks** after surgery. It is quite common, however, for patients who have initial improvement postoperatively in the hospital to experience a setback as they become more active on arriving home. This is a normal although not universal finding and is best managed expectantly. Patients who experience initial improvement and then experience clear deterioration need a more deliberate evaluation. These cases can represent **recurrent disk herniation, iatrogenic instability,** or **sagittal imbalance.** The physical examination and pain signature favor one diagnosis over the other. Recurrent nerve-root compression is best evaluated with MRI with and without contrast material. Instability should be evaluated with CT to assess the bony removal, and dynamic plain radiographs. Standing long cassette studies in both the coronal and sagittal plane are required to rule out deformity. In this time frame, some patients have progressive **causalgia-type** or **neuropathic pain.** This may result from a prolonged preoperative duration of nerve compression or injury during surgery. This condition is very refractory, although recent success has been reported with gabapentin, pregabalin, and a variety of antidepressants.

C. Another group of failures manifests **weeks to months** after surgery. The description of clear radiculopathy suggests recurrent herniation. **Arachnoiditis** manifests most often at this time. Patients often describe back and leg pain, which can be similar to the presenting problem. Classic cases manifest as symptoms of claudication or lower extremity causalgia. CT myelography is the study of choice and typically shows clumping of nerve roots and restricted flow of intrathecal contrast material. Surgery directed at the arachnoiditis is unsuccessful. There has been some success with spinal cord stimulators in these cases. Thankfully, the incidence has decreased dramatically with the advent of water-soluble contrast agents and the relatively infrequent use of myelography in the MRI era.

D. The last group of failures manifests after a pain-free interval of **months to years.**

1. Many of these cases have developed either iatrogenic lumbar instability because decompression was too wide or lumbar instability caused by the intrinsic disease. The incidence of **post-laminectomy spondylolisthesis** is somewhere between 2% and 10%. Even simple discectomy has been associated with a 3% incidence of postoperative instability that necessitates subsequent fusion. It has been widely circulated that the medial half of the facet joint can be removed bilaterally without inducing instability. However, this admonishment is not consistent with the fact that the medial half of the joint comprises the descending facet almost exclusively and that removal of the medial half can leave the facet completely incompetent. There is consensus that complete laminectomy and bilateral facetectomy consistently produce instability. In cases in which this extent of resection is needed to accomplish decompression, fusion should be incorporated into the surgical plan.

2. **Pseudoarthrosis** after lumbar fusion manifests in a time frame similar to that of postlaminectomy spondylolisthesis. In part, the timing of presentation may represent the fact that most spine surgeons are not prepared to give up on a fusion for 9 to 12 months after surgery. There are also no commonly accepted criteria for diagnosis of pseudoarthrosis. Dynamic radiographs often appear normal, and bone scans are equivocal. The incidence of symptomatic pseudoarthrosis after a posterolateral lumbosacral fusion is between 5% and 15%. The cause can be either technical deficiency of the surgery or biologic deficiency of the patient. There is good evidence that smoking negatively

affects the rate of fusion. The rate of pseudoarthrosis increases with the number of levels of arthrodesis. The use of BMP, external bone stimulators, and allograft bone graft extenders has decreased the rate of pseudoarthrosis. Hardware implanted in the patient may also become symptomatic during this time frame. The modulus of elasticity of metal rods is 10 to 20 times stiffer than bone, so that even following a successful fusion, these implants may loosen at the bone–implant interface or break. Recent experience suggests that alternate biomaterials, such as PEEK, may be a more suitable implant because of its near-identical stiffness to bone, and resistance to breakage.

RADIOGRAPHIC EVALUATION OF FAILED BACK SYNDROME RADIOGRAPHY PLAYS AN IMPORTANT ROLE IN THE EVALUATION OF FBS

A. In the evaluation of recurrent disk herniation, **contrast-enhanced CT** or **MRI** is vital (Figs. 26.1 and 26.2). Postoperative scar becomes homogeneously enhanced. A herniated disk may have some peripheral enhancement, but because it is avascular, the disk does not become centrally enhanced. Although scar and disk can both cause compressive symptoms, surgery to remove scar tissue is rarely successful.

B. Radiographic evaluation of a fusion is more difficult. In short, there is no universally accepted way to assess successful fusion after arthrodesis.

1. **Dynamic** or **flexion and extension radiographs** are specific for instability if motion is detected. However, these studies are very insensitive. Fibrous nonunion or the instrumentation itself can prevent the flexion–extension radiographs from appearing abnormal.

2. **Plain radiographs** can show a robust fusion mass, but it is often impossible to know whether the bony mass is in continuity. Lucency or halos around pedicle screws suggest instability. CT with sagittal and coronal reconstruction can be helpful. Special techniques must be used to minimize artifact of the instrumentation.

3. **Bone spectroscopy** has been advocated, but this modality is unreliable for at least several years after surgery.

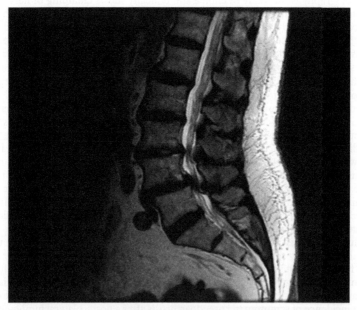

FIGURE 26.1 Preoperative lumbar MRI showing stenosis at L3–L5 with an L4–L5 spondylolisthesis.

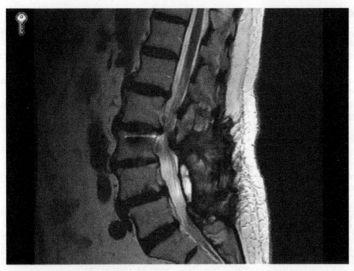

FIGURE 26.2 Repeat lumbar MRI obtained 3 years following L3–L5 laminectomies and fusion, and recurrent symptoms. Note junctional stenosis at the L2–L3 level.

4. **Three-dimensional CT** has been advocated by some authors in the evaluation of FBS. It has the advantage of clearly imaging the bony resection and can clearly delineate the extent of bony fusion.

REFERRALS

A. Referral to a neurologist or spine surgeon is indicated for any patient with a new or progressive neurologic deficit. In the context of FBS and chronic pain, it is important not to miss this dramatic change in the patient's course.

B. Imaging should be performed only in response to a significant change in the symptoms. When dramatic changes are found at imaging studies, patients with FBS should be reevaluated.

C. Often the job of weaning narcotics is left to an internist or general neurosurgeon. This can be appropriate; however, when reduction goals are not being met and the program becomes stalled, these patients should be referred to specialized centers. Long-term use of narcotic analgesics can be acceptable treatment in some cases, but it should be chosen explicitly, not as an ad hoc default.

D. FBS is a difficult management problem, and all these patients should be seen by a spine surgeon or pain center. In general, patients with FBS should be cared for by a multidisciplinary team. It is important to maintain vigilance in case new important symptoms arise, which may alter the treatment regimen.

Key Points

- FBS typically occurs following lumbosacral surgery.
- Etiology includes initial misdiagnosis, recurrent pathology, new spondylosis or spondylolisthesis at the site of previous surgery or adjacent levels, or pseudoarthrosis.
- Symptoms include radiculopathy, neurogenic claudication, and back pain.
- Evaluation with a combination of CT with or without myelography, MRI and flexion–extension X-rays is required.

Recommended Readings

Burton AK, Waddell G, Tillotson KM, et al. Information and advice to patients with back pain can have a positive effect. *Spine*. 1999;24:2484–2491.

Canos A, Cort L, Fernandez Y, et al. Preventive analgesia with pregabalin in neuropathic pain from "failed back surgery syndrome": assessment of sleep quality and disability. *Pain Med*. 2015;1–9.

Chou R. Nonsurgical interventional therapies for low back pain: a review of the evidence for an American Pain Society clinical practice guideline. *Spine*. 2009;34:1078–1093.

Frey M, Manchikanti L, Benyamin R, et al. Spinal cord stimulation for patients with failed back surgery syndrome: a systematic review. *Pain Physician*. 2009;12:379–397.

Hussain A, Erdek M. Interventional pain management for failed back surgery syndrome. *Pain Pract*. 2014;14(1):64–78.

Jee-Soo J, Sang-Ho L, Jun-Hong M, et al. Surgical treatment of failed back surgery syndrome due to sagittal imbalance. *Spine*. 2007;32:3081–3087.

Line J. Spinal cord stimulation versus conventional medical management for failed back surgery syndrome: long-term results from the PROCESS study. *Neurosurgery*. 2008;62:1426–1427.

Melzack R, Wall PD. *The Challenge of Pain*. New York, NY: Basic Books; 1983.

Van Buyten J, Linderoth B. "The failed back surgery syndrome": definition and therapeutic algorithms—an update. *Eur J Pain Suppl*. 2010;4:273–286.

Weinstein J, Lurie JD, Tosteson TD, et al. Surgical versus nonoperative treatment for lumbar disc herniation. *Spine*. 2008;33:2789–2800.

Weinstein J, Lurie JD, Tosteson TD, et al. Surgical compared with nonoperative treatment for lumbar degenerative spondylolisthesis. *J Bone Joint Surg*. 2009;91:1295–1304.

27 Approach to the Patient with Acute Sensory Loss

Eoin P. Flanagan and Neeraj Kumar

Evaluation of **acute sensory loss** involves clinical assessment of the nature of the sensory loss (section Clinical Manifestations), localization of the pathologic process (section Localization of the Pathologic Processes), association of other neurologic signs (section Association of Other Neurologic Signs), evaluation of possible etiologies (section Etiology of Acute Sensory Loss), and diagnostic testing (section Diagnostic Approaches to Acute Sensory Loss).

CLINICAL MANIFESTATIONS

The location, extent, and quality of the sensory deficit can help to localize the lesion and narrow the differential diagnosis. During the history taking, it is important to clarify the meaning of sensory symptoms; some patients who report an extremity going "numb" or "dead" are actually trying to describe weakness. The sensory examination is a crude procedure and inconsistent responses are commonly encountered. A reliable technique can minimize errors. The sensory examination may be normal in persons reporting acute sensory disturbances. Conversely, it is rare for examination to reveal sensory loss that a patient is not aware of, except in the situation of sensory neglect. Sensory testing should be performed in a systematic fashion but varying the interval between stimulus application can minimize patient anticipation, which can result in automatic responses and errors in the examination.

A. **Examination of sensory modalities in acute sensory loss.**

Touch sensation is tested with a wisp of cotton or the light touch of a finger. The patient is asked to say yes when they feel the touch. The stimulus should be compared with that applied to the contralateral corresponding area with expected normal sensation.

1. **Pain sensation** is tested by indicating the intensity of the pinprick sensation (sharp or dull) initially by demonstration in an area of known sensory preservation (e.g., upper sternum) and then throughout the body by comparison of each region assessed with a corresponding area with normal pain sensation. If responses to pinprick testing are inconsistent, assessing temperature sensation (hot or cold) is an excellent alternative. It must be determined if an area of decreased sensation suggests **nerve-root** or **peripheral nerve** involvement. Dermatomal charts showing typical peripheral nerve or nerve-root distributions vary somewhat from one book or study to another, but a general awareness of these sensory distributions is essential for accurate localization of sensory deficits. Loss of pinprick sensation is best determined by proceeding from the area of decreased or absent sensation to the area of normal sensation. A sensory level is both a symptom and a sign. Patients with myelitis often complain of ascending sensory loss up to a level across the trunk frequently with associated genital numbness and such symptoms should be considered reliable even if not fully reproducible on examination.

2. **Position sense** in fingers or toes is examined by holding the digit perpendicular to the direction of movement. The patient is asked to identify the directions of passive flexion and extension. It is important to isolate a single joint, to avoid detection of movement in more proximal joints. Small-amplitude fast movements are best and even the slightest movement should be detectable in those with normal position sensation. Loss of proprioception results in sensory ataxia, which can be compensated for by using visual input. Patients often complain of worsened balance in the dark or when they close their eyes in the shower as removal of visual input worsens joint position sensation markedly. Pseudoathetosis indicates joint position dysfunction and occurs when abnormal writhing movements of the fingers are evident with the arms outstretched and eyes closed.

Romberg's sign is positive when a patient is able to stand steady with the feet together (which patients with cerebellar ataxia typically cannot do) but falls or sways markedly when the eyes are closed (because of loss of visual input) indicating problems in joint position (or vestibular function) rather than cerebellar function.

3. **Vibration sense** is a composite sensation requiring preserved touch and deep pressure sensation. It is important to begin testing by demonstrating the presence and absence of vibration in a region known to be preserved (e.g., the sternum). A 128-Hz tuning fork should be used and placed over a bony prominence distally in each extremity and if absent more proximal bony prominences are assessed; mild vibratory loss in the toes is common in the elderly.

4. Cortical sensation. Perception of sizes and shapes of objects (stereognosis), ability to recognize numbers or letters drawn on the patient's skin (graphesthesia), and two-point discrimination can be impaired with lesions in the sensory cortices. Double simultaneous sensation is a quick and reliable test of sensory neglect, most useful in acute stroke, in which the double simultaneous bilateral stimuli (usually touch) are perceived only on the normal side but testing individually on both sides reveals normal sensation.

B. Positive sensory symptoms.
1. **Paresthesia** means spontaneous abnormal sensation frequently described as burning, tingling, prickling, "pins and needles," or cutting. Chronic paresthesias do not always indicate a primary neurologic disorder and is a common complaint of fibromyalgia patients and in those with anxiety (perioral and in the fingertips during hyperventilation).
2. **Dysesthesia/allodynia** is discomfort or pain triggered by normally painless stimuli.
3. **Hyperesthesia** indicates abnormally increased sensitivity to light touch, pinprick (also known as hyperpathia), or thermal sensation.

C. Negative sensory symptoms.
1. **Numbness** indicates decreased or absent sensation.
2. **Anesthesia** is complete loss of sensation.
3. **Hypesthesia** is decreased sensation.
4. **Pallesthesia** indicates loss of vibratory sensation.

D. Functional sensory loss. It is often difficult to establish with certainty that sensory impairment is functional, meaning inorganic or nonphysiologic. Functional sensory loss frequently occurs in a nonanatomic distribution, but similar findings may occur with demyelinating disease. Losses of touch, pinprick, and vibration sensation exactly at the midline over the chest or abdomen, or in the entire limb with sharp delineation of the sensory loss or poor reproducibility of the demarcation of the sensory deficits with repeated exams, all suggest functional sensory loss. Hearing loss on the side of hemisensory loss or differences in the sensation of vibration on both sides of the forehead are additional clues of functional sensory loss.

LOCALIZATION OF THE PATHOLOGIC PROCESSES

A. Sensory receptors.
1. **Exteroceptors** (free nerve endings) are localized in the skin and subserve superficial sensation to touch (Merkel's discs, Meissner's corpuscles) and pain and temperature (free nerve endings). The cutaneous sensory fibers run in sensory or mixed sensory and motor nerves. Sensory neurons have their cell bodies in the dorsal ganglia with their central projections to the posterior roots.
2. **Proprioceptors** (muscle spindles, Golgi tendon organs, Pacinian corpuscles) are localized in deeper somatic structures, including tendons, muscles, and joints and travel through the dorsal columns of the spinal cord and terminate in the gracile and cuneate nuclei of the medulla. The secondary afferent fibers from these nuclei cross the midline in the medulla and ascend in the brainstem as the medial lemniscus to the ventral posterolateral thalamic nucleus.

B. Nerve roots. Individual nerve roots mediate sensation in segments oriented longitudinally in the extremities and horizontally over the trunk. Dermatomal charts depict typical nerve-root distributions.

C. Peripheral nerves. Knowledge of peripheral nerve and nerve branch sensory distributions and distinguishing these from dermatomal patterns of sensory loss is helpful with localization (Video 27.1).

D. **Brachial and lumbosacral plexus.** Acute sensorimotor deficits indicating multiple nerve or nerve-root distributions in an arm or leg suggest plexopathy.

E. **Spinal cord.** Most fibers conducting pain and temperature sensation decussate over several segments by way of the ventral white commissure and ascend in the lateral spinothalamic tract to terminate eventually in the ventral posterior lateral nucleus of the thalamus. Fibers conducting light touch, vibration, joint position, and two-point discrimination ascend in the ipsilateral posterior column of the spinal cord and decussate in the medial lemniscus of the medulla.

F. **Cranial nerve and brainstem.** Cutaneous sensation from the face and mucous membranes is carried to the brainstem by the trigeminal nerve; cell bodies for pain, temperature, light touch, and pressure are located in the gasserian ganglion. After entering the pons, part of the sensory fibers descend as a bundle to form the spinal tract of the trigeminal nerve, which reaches the upper cervical segment of the spinal cord (therefore patients with upper cervical cord lesions may exhibit ipsilateral facial numbness). The spinal tract of the trigeminal nerve, located laterally in the brainstem/upper cervical cord, gives off pain and temperature fibers to the more medially located nucleus of the spinal tract of the trigeminal nerve. Touch, vibration, and pressure sensation terminate in the chief sensory nucleus within the pons. Proprioception fibers from the muscles of mastication bypass the gasserian ganglion and ascend terminating in the mesencephalic nucleus in the midbrain (the only sensory ganglion located within the central nervous system [CNS]), which is the afferent component of the jaw jerk. Fibers from the spinal nucleus and many fibers from the chief sensory nucleus cross the midline (some also ascend ipsilaterally to the thalamus) and ascend in the contralateral trigeminothalamic tract terminating in the ventral posterior medial nucleus of the thalamus.

G. **Cortex.** The cortical projections of the posterior ventral thalamic complex ascend to reach the postcentral cortex in a somatotopic arrangement with the face in the lowest area and the leg in the parasagittal region. In addition to the postcentral cortex, the cortical thalamic projections include the superior parietal lobule (Video 27.2). The fine sensory discrimination and fine location of pain, temperature, touch, and pressure (so-called primary modalities) require normal functioning of the sensory cortex. The cerebral cortex of the postcentral gyrus also subserves cortical sensory processes, including perception of sizes and shapes of objects (stereognosis), ability to recognize numbers or letters drawn on the patient's skin (graphesthesia), and two-point discrimination, all of which can be impaired with cortical lesions in this region. Sensory neglect often accompanies a lesion of the nondominant sensory cortex. Pain fibers also project to limbic regions, hypothalamus, and brainstem reticular formation by complex pathways and are involved in the autonomic, endocrine, arousal, and emotional response to pain.

ASSOCIATION OF OTHER NEUROLOGIC SIGNS

Pure sensory loss is unusual. Accompanying signs referable to brainstem, motor loss, associated cortical signs, and reflex abnormalities can help localize a lesion and narrow the diagnostic considerations and evaluation.

A. **Acute sensory disturbance in the face** usually indicates a lesion in a branch or branches of the trigeminal nerve, the trigeminal nucleus in the brainstem, or in the lemniscal pathways of the brainstem. Involvement of the ophthalmic branch of the trigeminal nerve can also cause a decreased corneal reflex.

1. **Acute onset of facial paresthesia** manifesting as numbness, tingling, or ill-defined discomfort, if lasting only several seconds or minutes in a person who is exposed to stressful circumstances, is often idiopathic and self-limited. Paresthesia in the perioral area can be caused by and reproduced by hyperventilation. Trigeminal neuralgia (also known as tic douloureux) is a severe form of recurrent lancinating facial pain lasting seconds and frequently triggered by a breeze hitting the face or brushing ones teeth; similar recurrent lancinating pain in the back of the throat occurs with glossopharyngeal neuralgia. Sjögren's syndrome is a well-recognized cause of trigeminal neuropathy. Sensory disturbance in the area of the mandibular division of the trigeminal nerve can reflect inflammatory or traumatic events involving the mandible or fracture of the base of the skull in the area of the foramen ovale. Sensory disturbance in the area of the chin

can be caused by **numb chin syndrome** because of neoplastic invasion of the inferior alveolar or mental nerve from mandibular metastases of lymphoma, breast or prostate cancer, or melanoma.

2. Involvement of other cranial nerves may occur with **idiopathic peripheral facial nerve (Bell's) palsy;** trigeminal nerve involvement on that side may result in ipsilateral numbness of the face.

3. Alteration in sensation in the ophthalmic and/or maxillary division of the trigeminal nerve and accompanying abrupt onset of fever, proptosis, chemosis, diplopia, and papilledema suggest **cavernous sinus thrombosis,** which can be caused by suppurative processes involving the upper half of the face, orbits, or nasal sinuses. Septic cavernous sinus thrombosis is life-threatening, necessitating immediate hospitalization. Sensory deficit in the ophthalmic division can also accompany meningitis.

4. A relatively sudden onset of numbness over the first two divisions of the trigeminal nerve can result from a low-grade inflammatory process involving the cavernous sinus **(Tolosa–Hunt syndrome),** which also causes eye movement abnormalities from involvement of one or more of the third, fourth, and sixth cranial nerves. Orbital pseudotumor is another inflammatory process that can involve similar regions. IgG4-related disease can manifest with either of these syndromes and should be considered as a potential etiology.

B. **Facial sensory disturbance in association with hemibody sensory disturbance, either ipsilateral or contralateral.**

1. Abrupt onset of pain and temperature loss over the entire half of the face and contralateral half of the trunk and extremities indicates involvement of the lateral medulla. The acute sensory loss is often associated with dysphagia, dysarthria, vertigo, vomiting, ipsilateral cerebellar signs, and ipsilateral Horner's syndrome. The most frequent cause of the lateral medullary (Wallenberg) syndrome is ipsilateral posterior inferior cerebellar artery infarction.

2. Acute onset of bilateral or unilateral facial numbness rapidly extending into the contralateral half of the face and associated with or followed by progressive weakness of facial muscles can be the earliest manifestation of acute inflammatory-demyelinating polyneuropathy or **Guillain–Barré syndrome (GBS).** Cases that begin in the face may have a triad of sensory ataxia, areflexia, and ophthalmoplegia called the **Miller-Fisher variant of GBS.** Typical GBS starts with numbness, paresthesia, and weakness in the distal portion of the legs and ascends to eventually involve the face. The Miller-Fisher variant of GBS tends to involve the respiratory centers of the brainstem more quickly than typical GBS, making surveillance of respiratory status particularly important in this variant. The diagnosis of GBS should be especially considered in persons with histories of respiratory or gastrointestinal viral infection, immunization, or surgical procedures preceding the onset of neurologic symptoms.

3. Recurrent hemifacial sensory disturbances, particularly among older patients with a clinical history of arterial hypertension, cardiovascular disease, diabetes, and cigarette smoking, may represent a carotid artery territory transient ischemic attack (TIA). The TIA episodes are of variable duration, usually lasting less than 30 minutes.

4. Loss of pain and temperature sensation in the face with preserved light touch sensation suggests **syringobulbia,** with an expanding syrinx involving the spinal nucleus of the trigeminal nerve.

5. The rostral part of the nucleus of the spinal tract of the trigeminal nerve represents the midline facial areas, whereas the sensation fibers from the lateral facial areas terminate in the more caudal part of the nucleus at the level of the medulla and spinal cord. In acute intraparenchymal processes involving the brainstem, facial sensory loss can occur in an "onionskin" distribution with decreased sensation in the central facial areas, indicating a pontine or pontomedullary lesion. Acute presentation of **"onionskin-like" sensation deficits** in the face can accompany acute brainstem encephalitis.

C. **Acute sensory loss over the scalp and neck,** that is, the "top of the head." Some patients, after exposure to cold or for no obvious reason, may experience the sudden onset of lateralized discomfort or pain associated with decreased sensation in the occipital area, in the distribution of the greater or lesser occipital nerves, which both arise from the C2 cervical nerve root; the C1 cervical nerve root is entirely motor. Acute sensory impairment in the area over the angle of the mandible, the lower part of the external ear, and the upper neck below the ear suggests neuropathy involving the great auricular nerve.

D. **Acute sensory loss over half of the face, trunk, and corresponding extremities.** Acute primary modality sensory loss over the entire half of the body is often a manifestation of a stroke or a traumatic CNS lesion.

1. Hemisensory loss can indicate damage rostral to the upper brainstem up to the postcentral gyrus and parietal area of the cerebral hemisphere contralateral to the side of the sensory deficit.

2. Acute onset of numbness, tingling, prickling, or a crawling sensation starting in the lips, fingers, or toes and spreading in seconds over half of the body and typically lasting less than 1 minute may represent a partial seizure. Etiologies include tumors or vascular malformations involving the contralateral hemisphere.

3. Transient hemisensory impairment can be caused by TIAs. The diagnosis of TIA is more probable if the hemisensory impairment is accompanied by motor deficits.

4. A patient with an acute vascular event in the nondominant, right parietal lobe may be unable to give a reliable history because of decreased ability to appreciate motor or sensory deficits in the contralateral extremities **(anosognosia).**

5. Hemisensory impairment manifesting as a tingling sensation, numbness, or ill-defined pain can accompany an acute vascular lesion involving the contralateral thalamus. Thalamic paresthesia and pain (Dejerine–Roussy syndrome) are disabling and difficult to manage. Vascular lesions of the thalamus are typically lacunar infarcts of small thalamoperforate vessels coming off the basilar artery and proximal posterior cerebral arteries.

E. Clinical aspects of acute sensory loss in the area of the trunk. Acute unilateral or bilateral sensory loss with a horizontal sensory level over the chest or abdomen localizes a lesion to the spinal cord and necessitates urgent evaluation to minimize residual neurologic impairment secondary to a possible spinal cord lesion.

1. **Complete transection of the spinal cord** results in bilateral weakness of legs or arms and loss of all forms of sensation immediately below the level of the lesion. Absence of vibration sense at the spinous process below the lesion can be helpful in localizing the spinal cord damage. A zone of increased pinprick or light touch sensation at the upper border of the anesthetic zone may be established. Urinary and fecal incontinence or urinary retention is typically present.

2. Muscle weakness in a leg, with ipsilateral loss of vibration and proprioception immediately below the lesion and contralateral loss of pain and temperature sensation one to two segments below, suggests a hemispinal cord lesion on the side of the weakness, also known as a **Brown–Séquard syndrome.**

3. Acute loss of pain and temperature sensation can accompany **occlusion of the anterior spinal artery** although rapid-onset paraplegia/quadriplegia usually predominates. Light touch, position, and vibration senses remain intact. Anterior spinal artery syndrome can occur during aortic surgery or in advanced atherosclerotic disease of the aorta. It also can develop in the course of meningovascular syphilis, as a manifestation of collagen-vascular disease, from a fibrocartilaginous embolism (which may be preceded by trauma and have an accompanying collapsed disc space) or from watershed infarction in the setting of vertebral artery occlusion and thus anterior spinal artery hypoperfusion. The midthoracic spinal cord is a "watershed" area at increased risk for infarction. However, the most common region affected by spinal cord infarction is the lower thoracic cord.

4. Acute ascending numbness is a characteristic manifestation of **acute transverse myelitis.** Functional alteration in sphincters with urinary and fecal incontinence can be present. Symmetric, severe muscle weakness in the lower extremities can develop over hours to days, particularly when caused by neuromyelitis optica spectrum disorders; magnetic resonance imaging (MRI) in such cases characteristically reveals a longitudinally extensive lesion ≥3 vertebral segments and serum testing positive for aquaporin-4-IgG is often diagnostic. Viral diseases or vaccinations may precede the onset of neurologic symptoms in acute idiopathic transverse myelitis by 1 to 3 weeks. Demyelinating lesions in the cervical cord often result in Lhermitte's phenomenon (shooting tingling sensation down the spine or into finger tips with neck flexion) or a **sensory useless hand syndrome** with proprioceptive deficits in the hand resulting from a focal lesion in the ipsilateral dorsal column.

5. Posterior column dysfunction with sparing of temperature and pinprick occurs with vitamin B_{12} deficiency and may be accompanied by spastic weakness when corticospinal tracts are involved (**subacute combined degeneration**). Acute sensory loss can occur with nitrous oxide use precipitating vitamin B_{12} deficiency. Methylmalonic acid should be assessed in those with low normal vitamin B_{12} levels as it is more sensitive for detecting cellular deficiency. Copper deficiency causes a similar syndrome and zinc-containing denture creams or malabsorption syndromes (e.g., celiac disease) should be considered as potential underlying causes. Human immunodeficiency virus, human T-lymphotrophic virus type 1, and syphilis are infectious etiologies that have a predilection for the dorsal columns.

6. Pain and temperature first-order neurons typically ascend ipsilaterally for one or two segments within the spinal cord in the tract of Lissauer before synapsing on their second-order neurons. These second-order neurons then cross to the opposite side through the commissural fibers just anterior to the central canal. Lesions of the spinothalamic tracts thus cause contralateral loss of pain and temperature sensation one or two vertebral segments below the lesion and may have ipsilateral loss of pain and temperature at the level of the lesion.

7. Dissociated sensory loss with loss of pain and temperature sensation but preservation of light touch, proprioception, and vibration occurs when the crossing pain and temperature fibers in the anterior commissure adjacent to the central canal are damaged in syringomyelia or from trauma (hematomyelia). The dissociated sensory deficit can extend over several segments and often occurs in a hallmark "cape like" distribution when cervical cord involvement occurs.

8. The spinothalamic fibers are arranged in a laminar fashion with sacral fibers most lateral and hence a central cord lesion may result in loss of pain and temperature sensation below a lesion with "**sacral sparing.**"

9. **Acute "saddle" sensory loss** localizes a lesion to the tip of the spinal cord at the conus medullaris. Sphincteric disturbance of bowel and bladder function is often associated.

10. Individual **nerve roots** are typically affected by trauma from spondylotic vertebral bone spurs or disc herniation. Increased intraspinal pressure during coughing, sneezing, or Valsalva can worsen the associated radicular pain. Acute **cauda equina syndrome** with bilateral lumbosacral radiculopathies resulting in rapidly progressive weakness, sensory loss (saddle anesthesia), and urinary retention is a neurologic emergency requiring emergent lumbosacral spine MRI and neurosurgical consultation.

11. A sensory neuronopathy (or sensory ganglionopathy) with disease affecting the dorsal root ganglia presents with numbness, sensory ataxia (positive Romberg sign), areflexia, and pseudoathetosis, and is classically associated with Sjögren's syndrome and paraneoplastic disease (most often anti-nuclear-neuronal-autoantibody-type-1 or anti-Hu antibodies in association with an underlying small-cell lung cancer). Cisplatin toxicity may also present in this manner.

12. The **brachial plexus** can be affected by local trauma during surgery in this region or in accidents involving the shoulder or birth injuries. Prolonged positioning during surgery is another well-recognized cause of brachial plexopathy from compression or stretching and usually resolves over days to weeks. Acute onset of severe pain (often requiring opiates for relief) accompanied by numbness and tingling and usually followed in several hours or days by muscle weakness and patchy hypoesthesia in the area of the shoulder girdle and proximal arm muscles is typical of brachial plexus neuritis (also known as neuralgic amyotrophy or Parsonage–Turner syndrome). It can follow infection, vaccination, or recent surgery. Hereditary autosomal-dominant recurrent brachial plexitis is described with *SEPT9* gene mutations. Neoplastic involvement of the brachial plexus is often very painful and infiltration may be evident on MRI of the plexus.

13. The **lumbosacral plexus** can be affected by operations in the area, including those that cause retroperitoneal hematoma. Diabetic lumbosacral radiculoplexus neuropathy (diabetic amyotrophy) is a well-recognized cause of pain, lower extremity numbness, and weakness in type 2 diabetics; the diabetes is usually well controlled and severe weight loss is commonly associated.

14. Mononeuritis multiplex causes sensory and motor deficits in multiple peripheral nerves, and underlying systemic diseases such as diabetes, vasculitic disorders, and paraneoplastic disorders are among the diagnostic possibilities.

15. Small-fiber neuropathies typically cause positive sensory symptoms in the feet and they are associated with normal nerve conduction studies and electromyography (EMG) (which are much better at detecting large-fiber neuropathies). Autonomic testing is helpful in such cases. An accompanying autonomic neuropathy is common and may result in orthostatic hypotension, decreased sweating, visual difficulty during transition from dark to light (pupil dysfunction), early satiety and bowel and bladder dysfunction. Common causes of small-fiber neuropathy include type 1 diabetes (including diabetic treatment–induced neuropathy [previously termed insulin neuritis]), amyloidosis, autoimmune disorders associated with antibodies directed against the 3 subunit of the ganglionic acetylcholine receptor, Sjögren's syndrome, and Fabry's disease (in young males with associated angiokeratomas of the skin and caused by -galactosidase deficiency).

16. **Peripheral nerves** are susceptible to trauma or compression in certain classic areas. Hereditary neuropathy with liability to pressure palsy (from peripheral myelin protein 22 gene deletion) can also result in a general susceptibility to recurrent compressive neuropathies.

   a. **Axillary nerve.** Dislocation of the shoulder joint, injury to the humerus, or prolonged pressure, stretching, or traction involving the arm during anesthesia or sleep can result in lesions of the axillary nerve.

   b. **Median nerve.** The median nerve can be damaged by injuries involving the arm, forearm, wrist, and hand, including stab and bullet wounds. Procedures involving needle insertion, particularly in the cubital fossa, can also result in median nerve damage. In rare instances, prolonged compression during anesthesia or sleep can cause acute median nerve involvement that manifests as sensory and motor deficits. Numbness and tingling in the distribution of the median nerve that wakes a person from sleep and is relieved by shaking the hand and arm are classic signs of carpal tunnel syndrome, which typically results from repetitive motion injury around the wrist. Persons with diabetes, hypothyroidism, arthritis, or acromegaly, or those who are pregnant are particularly predisposed.

   c. **Ulnar nerve.** This is most frequently injured in the cubital tunnel at the elbow (e.g., during olecranon fractures or from recurrent or prolonged compression) or in Guyon's canal at the wrist (e.g., acutely during blunt injury or more chronically from a ganglion cyst).

   d. **Radial nerve.** The radial nerve is probably the most commonly injured peripheral nerve. Sensory loss over the first web space with an accompanying wrist drop is characteristic. Injuries including dislocation and fracture of the shoulder, extended pressure on the nerve such as when a person falls asleep with their arm over a chair compressing the radial nerve at the spiral groove ("Saturday night palsy"), and fractures of the neck of the radius are the most frequent causes of radial nerve damage.

   e. **Femoral nerve.** Acute femoral nerve injury with sensory loss in the anterior thigh and quadriceps weakness may follow fractures of the pelvis and femur, dislocation of the hip, pressure or traction during hysterectomy, forceps delivery, femoral artery catheterization for coronary angiographic procedures, or pressure in hematoma in the area of the iliopsoas muscle or groin. Paresthesia and sensory loss in the area of the saphenous nerve can occur as a result of injury in the area above the medial aspect of the knee in medial arthrotomy or as an iatrogenic complication during venous graft harvesting for coronary artery bypass graft surgery.

   f. **Obturator nerve.** The nerve can be damaged during surgical procedures involving the hip or pelvis, or secondary to iliopsoas hematoma, and sensory loss is in the medial thigh and accompanied by weakness of hip adduction.

   g. **Lateral femoral cutaneous nerve.** The lateral femoral cutaneous nerve can be damaged by compression from the inguinal ligament, tightly fitting garments in obese individuals, or during pregnancy, causing tingling, numbness, and pain and is termed **meralgia paresthetica**.

   h. **Sciatic nerve.** Acute sciatic nerve damage results in variable sensory and motor dysfunction depending on the site of injury and can occur in association with fractures or dislocations of the hip, hip joint surgery, and other pathologic conditions of the pelvis including gunshot wounds or injections in the vicinity of the sciatic nerve.

i. **Peroneal nerve.** Peroneal nerve lesions are most often caused by compression (e.g., habitual leg crossing, leg casting, or positioning during surgery) and may be precipitated by recent weight loss. Fibular fracture is another cause and iatrogenic injury may occur during knee surgery. Sensory loss is on the dorsum of the foot and lateral calf region sparing the fifth toe is typical. It can be distinguished from an L5 radiculopathy by its sparing of inversion strength. Fascicular involvement of the peroneal division of the sciatic nerve (which seems to be more susceptible to injury than the tibial division) can occur, mimicking a common peroneal neuropathy. EMG abnormalities found in the short head of the biceps femoris suggests involvement of the peroneal division of the sciatic nerve.

j. **Tibial nerve.** The tibial nerve is injured mostly in the popliteal fossa or at the level of the ankle or foot. Tarsal tunnel syndrome, most common in athletes, results from compression of the tibial nerve as it passes through the tarsal tunnel behind the medial malleolus. Numbness and pain in the first three toes, dorsum of foot, and heel are typical.

ETIOLOGY OF ACUTE SENSORY LOSS

A. **Infectious–parainfectious neurologic diseases** are preceded by or associated with acute febrile diseases involving the upper respiratory or gastrointestinal system or the lower urinary tract. Parainfectious involvement of the CNS or peripheral nervous system (PNS) typically follows the onset of clinical symptoms of the infectious process by 1 to 3 weeks.

B. **Inflammatory-demyelinating disease** can be parainfectious or postinfectious but can also be idiopathic or autoimmune.

C. **Ischemic–hemorrhagic neurologic disorders** manifesting as acute CNS or PNS involvement usually occur among older persons with vascular risk factors.

D. **Traumatic–compressive lesions** of the CNS and PNS can manifest as acute sensory loss. Complications of surgical procedures, venipuncture, or intravascular injection and prolonged positioning during surgery can cause acute sensory loss, usually secondary to peripheral nerve damage.

DIAGNOSTIC APPROACHES TO ACUTE SENSORY LOSS

Diagnostic approaches to acute sensory loss are focused by the localization of the lesion (sections Clinical Manifestations, Localization of the Pathologic Processes, and Association of Other Neurological Signs) and by suspected etiologic factor (section Etiology of Acute Sensory Loss).

A. **PNS evaluation.** If a lesion localizes to a particular peripheral nerve, the extremity and nerve can be evaluated radiographically and electrophysiologically.

1. Radiographs of the involved limb can help identify fractures or bony deformities that can cause focal compression of damage to the nerve. MRI of the brachial or lumbosacral plexus can be useful in identifying the nature of damage.

2. **EMG with nerve conduction velocity (NCV) studies** can be helpful in documenting and localizing damage to a peripheral nerve, a plexus, or a nerve root and in providing prognostic information (see Chapters 24 and 25). In a traumatized nerve or root, abnormalities may not appear immediately on nerve conduction studies. It also takes approximately 3 weeks for denervation change to occur in muscles innervated by damaged nerves, so an initially unremarkable or borderline EMG must be repeated if there is continued suspicion of damage. Sensory axon potentials are spared in radiculopathies as the cell body in the dorsal root ganglion is typically proximal to the lesion. In the acute period, a demyelinated nerve can show slowing of nerve conduction, conduction block across demyelinated nerve segments, and slowing of F waves that reflect proximal nerve-root damage. The greater the denervation and axonal dropout found at subacute EMG/NCV studies, the worse the prognosis. EMG/NCV is normal in small-fiber neuropathy and autonomic testing should be performed if this diagnosis is being considered.

3. MRI neurography and ultrasound of the nerve are additional imaging modalities that may be useful in the evaluation of acute sensory loss.

B. **Spinal cord evaluation.** Localization of a lesion to the spinal cord necessitates neuroimaging of the cord. Traumatic lesions necessitate immediate imaging of an immediately stabilized spine by means of traditional radiographs and subsequent imaging of the spinal cord parenchyma by means of MRI or computed tomography (CT) myelography.

  1. **MRI** is the preferred technique for imaging the spinal cord parenchyma, and use of gadolinium can be helpful in identifying acute inflammatory lesions.

  2. **CT myelography** is typically used in patients with contraindications to MRI (e.g., pacemaker) and is especially good at depicting bone, disc, and ligamentous structures that may impinge on the spinal cord.

  3. **Somatosensory-evoked responses** can help determine whether there is slowed conduction of somatosensory stimuli from arms or legs in the somatosensory pathways from peripheral nerve to cortex and can crudely localize the lesion.

  4. **Formal spinal angiography** is the gold standard to identify dural-arterio venous fistula in those with a suspicious presentation and MRI (e.g., MRI showing a longitudinally extensive swollen thoracic cord lesion with flow voids dorsal to the cord).

C. **Brain evaluation.** Acute sensory loss that localizes to the brain, including cerebral cortex, thalamus, or brainstem, can be evaluated by several techniques.

  5. **Computed tomography** of the head can be helpful, particularly acutely such as in a suspected acute stroke; CT is particularly effective at evaluating for acute hemorrhage.

  6. **MRI** can most precisely localize a lesion and can include MR angiography and MR venography to examine blood vessels. Diffusion-weighted imaging has very high specificity for acute stroke (see Chapter 35). For suspected inflammatory-demyelinating or postinfectious processes, MRI is the procedure of choice. Gadolinium contrast material should be administered to assess whether there is acute enhancement, which suggests active inflammation and breakdown of the blood–brain barrier. The presence of typical demyelinating white matter lesions on MRI brain during a clinically isolated syndrome of demyelination (e.g., transverse myelitis) indicates increased risk of development of multiple sclerosis.

  7. **Cerebral angiography** may be necessary to diagnose vascular abnormalities such as ruptured aneurysm, atherosclerotic narrowing, and vasculitis.

  8. **Electroencephalography** (EEG) can aid in the diagnosis of seizures (see Chapter 36). However, in patients with simple partial sensory seizures the discharges may not be detectable with scalp EEG.

D. **Blood work** can be used to diagnose infectious, inflammatory, or metabolic conditions that can cause acute sensory loss, including complete blood cell count, blood cultures when indicated, erythrocyte sedimentation rate, vitamin B_{12}, and methylmalonic acid, copper, antinuclear antibodies, SSA and SSB antibodies, antineutrophil cytoplasm autoantibodies, rheumatoid factor, angiotensin-converting enzyme, rapid plasma reagin, Lyme disease serology, HIV, HTLV-1, lactate dehydrogenase, peripheral smear, glucose level, and hemoglobin A_{1c}, serum protein electrophoresis and immunofixation, and paraneoplastic autoantibody evaluation. Serum testing for aquaporin-4-IgG is useful in the diagnosis of neuromyelitis optica spectrum disorders.

E. **Nerve biopsy** may be considered in PNS disorders suspected to be from neoplasia, inflammation (e.g., sarcoid), vasculitis, or amyloidosis (fat pad biopsy is also a useful test of amyloidosis).

F. **Examination of cerebrospinal fluid (CSF)** for cell count, protein, glucose, and inflammatory markers helps in the evaluation of acute sensory loss (see Chapter 36). An elevated white blood cell count is seen with infectious and inflammatory etiologies and the differential of the white cells can help suggest the underlying cause (neutrophilic predominance favors bacterial infection; lymphocytic favors viral infections or inflammatory etiologies). A markedly elevated protein with normal cell count known as **albuminocytologic dissociation** is typical of GBS, but is also seen with spinal block such as may occur in severe cervical stenosis. Hypoglycorrhachia (low CSF glucose) can indicate infectious (bacterial, fungal, or mycobacterial) etiologies but is also seen with neurosarcoidosis and lymphoma. CSF cytology and flow cytometry should be performed in cases suspicious for lymphoma. A positive IgG index or elevated oligoclonal bands are seen in greater than 85% of multiple sclerosis patients, but may also occur in other inflammatory/autoimmune disorders. For suspected infectious causes, cultures and smears for bacteria, acid-fast bacilli, and fungus are important. Serologic and polymerase chain reaction tests also can be done for many viruses, including herpes simplex types 1 and 2, Epstein–Barr virus, cytomegalovirus (a common cause of polyradiculopathy in immunosuppressed patients [e.g., HIV]), and varicella zoster virus. A CSF venereal disease research laboratory test can be undertaken if syphilis is suspected.

REFERRALS

Cases of acute sensory loss should be referred to a neurologist if:

A. Sudden onset or resolution suggests TIAs or seizures.
B. Radiculopathy is suspected and focal neurologic deficits are present (weakness and reflex loss).
C. Fever is present, and there is a suspicion of epidural abscess, encephalitis, or cortical sinus thrombosis.
D. Deficits progress rapidly, ascend, or evolve to include motor signs and symptoms, suggesting GBS.
E. Acute deficit localizes to the spinal cord. Emergency MRI is important in this situation and if a compressive lesion is found, an urgent neurosurgical referral is appropriate.

Key Points

- The sensory examination is crude and responses may be inconsistent, but a reliable neurologic examination technique helps minimize this inherent variability.
- Knowledge of sensory dermatomes of nerve roots and peripheral nerve sensory distributions and the pathways they take from the PNS to the cortex is essential for neurologists to be able to accurately localize lesions.
- The distribution and types of sensory modalities impaired vary depending on lesion location: cortical lesions cause agraphesthesia, astereognosis, difficulty with two-point discrimination, and sensory neglect (in nondominant lobe); thalamic lesions cause hemisensory deficits; lateral medullary lesions cause ipsilateral face and contralateral body pain and temperature loss; spinal cord lesions typically result in a complete sensory level or a Brown–Séquard syndrome; dorsal column loss and sensory ganglionopathy cause numbness and a sensory ataxia; nerve-root and peripheral nerve sensory loss varies by dermatomal innervation.
- Sensory loss is usually accompanied by other neurologic symptoms and signs whose presence helps with determining the location of the nervous system involved.
- The differential diagnosis of sensory loss can be narrowed by knowledge of its localization and allow investigations be tailored toward a limited number of diagnoses.

Recommended Readings

Benarroch EE, Daube JR, Flemming KD, et al. *Mayo Clinic Medical Neurosciences Organized by Neurologic Systems and Levels.* 5th ed. Florence, KY: Informa Heathcare; 2008.

Biller J, Gruener G, Brazis PW. *DeMyer's The Neurologic Examination: A Programmed Text.* 7th ed. New York, NY: McGraw-Hill; 2017.

Brazis PW, Masdeu JC, Biller J. *Localization in Clinical Neurology.* 7th ed. Philadelphia, PA: Wolters Kluwer; 2017.

Daroff RB, Fenichel GM, Jankovic J, et al. *Bradley's Neurology in Clinical Practice.* 6th ed. Philadelphia, PA: Elsevier Saunders; 2012.

Fisher CM. Pure sensory stroke and allied conditions. *Stroke.* 1982;13:434–447.

Kimura J. *Electrodiagnosis in Diseases of Nerve and Muscle.* Philadelphia, PA: FA Davis; 1984.

Patten J. *Neurological Differential Diagnosis.* New York, NY: Springer-Verlag; 1980.

Polman CH, Reingold SC, Banwell B, et al. Diagnostic criteria for multiple sclerosis: 2010 revisions to the McDonald criteria. *Ann Neurol.* 2011;69:292–302.

Ropper AH, Samuels MA, Klein JP. *Adams and Victors Principles of Neurology.* 10th ed. New York, NY: McGraw-Hill Education; 2014.

Wiebers DO, Dale AJ, Kokmen E, et al. *Mayo Clinic Examinations in Neurology.* 7th ed. Philadelphia, PA; Mosby, Elsevier's Health Sciences; 1998.

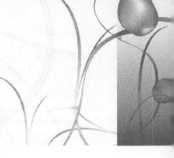

28 Approach to the Hyperkinetic Patient

Javier Pagonabarraga and Christopher G. Goetz

Hyperkinetic movement disorders are abnormal involuntary movements characterized by excessive movement. Two complementary and intersection classification systems are utilized:

A. Phenomenology.
1. Tremor
2. Dystonia
3. Chorea
4. Myoclonus
5. Tics (Table 28.1)

B. Etiology.
1. Hereditary
2. Nonhereditary primary hyperkinetic movement disorders
3. Degenerative
4. Secondary: ischemic or posthypoxic, demyelinating, tumoral, posttraumatic, inflammatory, infectious, immunologic, endocrinologic, or metabolic
5. Drug-induced

TREMOR

A. Definition. Tremor is a rhythmic, involuntary back-and-forth oscillation of part of the body. It is described clinically by the location where it develops (hands, feet, back, neck, face, and voice), and the situations, postures, or movements that trigger or enhance it (action, at rest, and maintenance of a posture), and electrophysiologically by the frequency, amplitude, and pattern of muscle activation, as assessed by accelerometry and surface electromyography.

B. Phenomenologic classification.
1. Rest tremor. Tremor that occurs in a body part that is not voluntarily activated and is completely supported against gravity. Rest tremor amplitude always diminishes during target-directed movements, which helps to separate rest tremor from postural tremors

---

TABLE 28.1 Hyperkinetic Movement Disorders

Term	Clinical Manifestations
Tremor	Rhythmic oscillation of agonist and antagonist muscles
Dystonia	Sustained or intermittent muscle contractions causing patterned, abnormal, and repetitive movements or postures, which are usually initiated or worsened by voluntary action
Chorea	Irregular, rapid, and continuous flow of random muscle contractions from one part of the body to another
Ballismus	Violent flinging movements of the limbs, usually affecting only one side of the body (hemiballismus)
Myoclonus	Sudden, lightning-like, and jerky involuntary movements caused by muscular contractions or inhibitions
Tics	Repeated and stereotyped movements or sounds that are preceded by an urge or sensation in the affected muscle group, and a sense of temporary relief once the movement is made

that continue when the limb is supported. It increases with mental stress (counting backward), or when movements of another body part are performed (especially walking). It is mostly found in Parkinson's disease (PD), but also in other parkinsonian syndromes, including drug-induced parkinsonism. Its presence indicates dysfunction of the nigrostriatal dopamine pathway or its efferent projections to basal ganglia-thalamo-cortical circuits.

  2. **Action tremor.** Any tremor that is produced by voluntary contraction of muscle, and it includes postural, simple kinetic, intention tremor, and task-specific kinetic tremor.

    a. **Postural tremor.** Tremor that is present while voluntarily maintaining a position against gravity. It is usually documented by having the patient outstretch the arms.

    b. **Simple kinetic tremor.** Tremor that occurs during voluntary action that is not target-directed.

    c. **Intention tremor.** Action tremor whose amplitude increases substantially during the pursuit of a target or goal. Its presence suggests a disturbance of the cerebellum or its afferent/efferent pathways.

    d. **Task-specific kinetic tremor.** Tremor that occurs during specific activities such as the primary writing tremor and occupational tremors. These tremors are often associated with dystonia.

C. **Etiologic classification.**

  1. Physiologic and enhanced physiologic

  2. Hereditary (familial, fragile X-associated tremor/ataxia syndrome [FXTAS], Wilson's disease, spinocerebellar ataxias [SCAs], hereditary hemochromatosis, and acute intermittent porphyria)

  3. Nonhereditary primary tremor: essential and orthostatic

  4. Degenerative: PD and other parkinsonisms

  5. Ischemic and posthypoxic

  6. Demyelinating disease

  7. Inflammatory, infectious, or immunologic: AIDS and brain abscesses

  8. Neuropathic

  9. Endocrinologic/metabolic: thyroid and hypoglycemia

  10. Posttraumatic

  11. Drug-induced or toxic: valproate acid, amlodipine, selective serotonin reuptake inhibitors (SSRIs), prednisone, cyclosporine A, and tacrolimus **(also see section Tardive Syndromes)**

D. **Pathophysiology.** Tremor is not associated with any uniform brain lesion or clear histopathologic changes in the brain. However, two regions within the central motor pathways, the inferior olive and the relay nuclei of the thalamus, demonstrate oscillatory behavior, and their pharmacologic manipulation in the harmaline mouse model may produce or improve tremor. These regions are functionally interconnected with the cerebellum. Thus, the inferior olive, relay nuclei of the thalamus, and the cerebellum are the principal candidates for the origin of any pathologic central tremor.

E. **Selected clinical syndromes.**

  1. **Physiologic tremor** is a low-amplitude and high-frequency (8 to 12 Hz) postural tremor that is most prominent in outstretched hands. It can be present in normal subjects but can be enhanced under certain circumstances, including fever, drugs, excited mental states, alcohol withdrawal, and caffeine use.

    a. **Differential diagnosis.**

      (1) Metabolic or endocrine derangements

      (2) Essential tremor

      (3) Cortical myoclonus

      (4) Drug-induced or withdrawal

      (5) Anxiety

    b. **Evaluation.**

      (1) Blood tests to rule out metabolic problems: hyperthyroidism, hypercorticism, hyperparathyroidism, hypocalcemia, hepatic encephalopathy, hypoglycemia, and pheochromocytoma

      (2) Review of medications (most common cause): thyroid drugs, corticosteroids, lithium, theophylline, $_2$-adrenergic receptor agonist, SSRIs, and sodium valproate

      (3) Assessment for anxiety

2. **Essential tremor** is the most frequent neurologic disease causing tremor in the general population. It is an action tremor, mainly postural and kinetic. It is bilateral, largely symmetric, but it can be also asymmetric or even unilateral. The frequency is usually 4 to 12 Hz but may decrease with age. Conversely, amplitude increases during the follow-up. Its major clinical feature is postural tremor of the hands, but it can also be present in other body parts (distal legs, voice, and head). About 5% of patients may present with tremor almost exclusively in the head and voice. Improvement of tremor amplitude with alcohol is a characteristic feature of the disease but is not present for most patients.

Although most patients have strong family histories, and different gene loci (*ETM1* on *3q13*, *ETM2* on *2p24.1*, a locus on *6p23*, *Lingo-1* overexpression, and missense mutations in *TENM4*) have been identified in patients and families with the disorder, the cause of essential tremor is unclear. In recent years, systematic postmortem studies have shown essential tremor to be associated with clearly identifiable structural changes, including Purkinje's cell loss, development of torpedoes in the cerebellum and, in some patients, deposition of Lewy bodies in the brainstem.

a. Differential diagnosis.
   (1) Physiologic tremor **(see above)**
   (2) Metabolic or endocrine derangements
   (3) Wilson's disease (when age of onset of essential tremor is under 40 years)
   (4) Rhythmic myoclonus and cortical tremor
b. Evaluation.
   (1) Review medication and blood tests to rule out metabolic problems **(see Section E.1 under Tremor)**.
   (2) Assess history of caffeine use, smoking, or alcohol withdrawal.
   (3) Evaluate serum ceruloplasmin to rule out Wilson's disease (under 40 years).

3. **PD** is the most frequent cause of rest tremor. It is typically defined by bradykinesia, rigidity, and impairment of postural reflexes. The neural correlates of rest tremor in PD are unknown, and the participation of other neurotransmitter systems apart from the dopaminergic dysfunction is likely. **Parkinsonian tremor** occurs at 3 to 7 Hz. It may be unilateral in the early stages of the disease, but it soon spreads to the contralateral side. Characteristically, it remains asymmetric through the course of the disease. Mental stress or movements of another body part (contralateral hand and gait) typically trigger the rest tremor or increase tremor amplitude. Parkinsonian tremor can be also present while maintaining a posture. Postural tremor in PD has been designated as a reemergent tremor, with a latency for the tremor to appear about 9 seconds, which is significantly longer than the latency observed in patients with essential tremor (1 to 2 seconds).

a. Differential diagnosis.
   (1) Other parkinsonian syndromes: multisystem atrophy (MSA), progressive supranuclear palsy (PSP), corticobasal degeneration (CBD), dementia with Lewy bodies (DLB), Alzheimer's disease (AD) with extrapyramidal features, and frontotemporal dementia with parkinsonism
   (2) SCA (SCA2, SCA3, SCA8, and SCA12)
   (3) Vascular parkinsonism
   (4) Drug-induced parkinsonism
   (5) Structural lesions involving the substantia nigra pars compacta
b. Evaluation.
   (1) Review of drugs: dopamine receptor–blocking drugs (haloperidol, risperidone, olanzapine, and metoclopramide), calcium-channel blockers, and trimetazidine
   (2) Computed tomography (CT) scan or brain magnetic resonance imaging (MRI) to rule structural lesions involving the substantia nigra, basal ganglia, or diffuse cerebral white matter disease
   (3) Transcranial ultrasonography can show distinctive patterns in PD versus MSA, PSP, or CBD.
   (4) Dopamine transporter SPECT, a marker of the integrity of the presynaptic nigrostriatal pathway, is increasingly used to separate PD from vascular parkinsonism, essential tremor, or psychogenic parkinsonism

4. **Cerebellar tremor** is clinically defined by pure or dominant intention tremor. It may be uni- or bilateral. Postural tremor may be present, but no rest tremor. Typically, tremor frequency is below 5 Hz. Cerebellar tremor is often associated with dysmetria (finger-to-nose and heel-to-shin testing maneuvers) and hypotonia. This kind of tremor can be considered a symptomatic tremor produced by any disease that affects the functionality of the cerebellum or its afferent/efferent pathways.

   a. Differential diagnosis.

      (1) Alcohol or drug abuse

      (2) Drug-induced

      (3) Multiple sclerosis

      (4) SCA, autosomal-recessive hereditary ataxias, and FXTAS

      (5) Space-occupying mass, or an ischemic, toxic, or infectious disorder in the brainstem, the cerebellum, or the frontal lobes (due to diaschisis)

   b. Evaluation.

      (1) Brain MRI to rule out structural lesions in the posterior fossa or the frontal lobes

      (2) Review of drugs: phenytoin, carbamazepine, and phenobarbital

5. **Holmes' tremor** is clinically defined by rest and intention tremor, with postural tremor present in many patients. It is mostly unilateral. Postural tremor tends to be more severe than tremor at rest, and intention tremor more severe than the postural tremor. Tremor frequency is usually <4.5 Hz. This is also a symptomatic tremor that occurs after a brainstem, midbrain, or thalamic lesion, when two systems, the dopaminergic nigrostriatal system and the cerebellothalamic system, are lesioned. A variable delay (4 weeks to 2 years) between the lesion and the appearance of the tremor is typical.

   a. **Differential diagnosis and evaluation** (see **Section E.4 under Tremor**).

   b. Treatment. Holmes' tremor and thalamic tremor do not usually respond to pharmacologic treatments. Although the effects of thalamic deep brain stimulation in the ventral intermediate nucleus are incomplete, functional surgery in complex tremor syndromes appears as the only available therapeutic option and provides significant and lasting functional improvement.

6. FXTAS. Over the past decade, it has been shown that premutation carriers (especially males) of the *FMR1* mutation (55 to 200 CGG repeats) are at risk of developing the FXTAS. Core clinical features of FXTAS are progressive cerebellar gait ataxia, mild parkinsonism, autonomic dysfunction, peripheral neuropathy, and intention tremor. Postural and rest tremor may be also present. FXTAS is often misdiagnosed as essential tremor and PD. As the diagnosis of FXTAS has substantial implications regarding genetic counseling, it is important to consider FXTAS as a cause of tremor when ataxic symptoms are also present (Videos 28.1 and 28.2).

   a. Differential diagnosis.

      (1) Essential tremor

      (2) PD

      (3) Atypical parkinsonian disorders (MSA, PSP, and CBD)

      (4) SCAs and other hereditary ataxic syndromes

      (5) DLB

   b. Evaluation.

      (1) The presence of combined essential-like tremor, along with gait ataxia or parkinsonism in an adult (usually male) with a grandchild with intellectual disability, should prompt genetic testing for FXTAS.

DYSTONIA

A. Definition. Dystonia is a syndrome characterized by sustained or intermittent muscle contractions causing abnormal, often repetitive, movements, postures, or both. Dystonic contractions are mainly characterized by the following:

   1. Consistent directionality. The movements are patterned and repeatedly involve the same muscle groups.

   2. Aggravation by voluntary movement (action exacerbation). Dystonia may be also triggered by particular actions such as writing or playing a musical instrument (task-specific dystonia).

3. Presence of a "sensory trick," the use of a tactile or proprioceptive stimulus, generally in some particular spot in the same area where the dystonic movements are present, which can improve the muscle contractions.

B. **Phenomenologic classification.**

1. **Focal.** The abnormal movements affect single body region such as cervical dystonia, blepharospasm, spasmodic dysphonia, oromandibular dystonia, or brachial dystonia.

2. **Segmental.** The abnormal movements affect two or more contiguous body parts, as in Meige's syndrome (blepharospasm plus oromandibular dystonia), craniocervical dystonia, or bibrachial dystonia.

3. **Multifocal.** Two or more noncontiguous body areas are involved.

4. **Hemidystonia.** The abnormal movements affect one side of the body.

5. **Generalized.** Abnormal movements are present in the legs (or in one leg and the trunk) plus at least one other area of the body.

C. **Classification by age of onset.**

1. **Early-onset.** ≤26 years.

2. **Late-onset.** >26 years.

D. **Etiologic classification.**

1. **Primary, or idiopathic, dystonia.**
   a. Primary torsion dystonia (PTD). DYT1 (Oppenheim's dystonia), DYT2, DYT4, DYT6, DYT7, and DYT13

2. **Secondary dystonia.**
   a. **Dystonia-plus syndromes.** Dystonic syndromes with other neurologic features in addition to dystonia, in which clinical and laboratory findings suggest neurochemical disorders, with no evidence of neurodegeneration.
      (1) Dopa-responsive dystonias (DRDs)
          (a) Segawa's disease (DYT5) = GTP cyclohydrolase 1 deficiency
          (b) Tyrosine hydroxylase deficiency, other biopterin deficiencies, and dopamine-agonist-responsive dystonia due to deficiency of aromatic l-amino acid decarboxylase
      (2) Myoclonus-dystonia (DYT11)
      (3) Rapid-onset dystonia-parkinsonism (DYT12)
   b. **Associated with heredodegenerative.** Neurodegenerative diseases in which dystonia is sometimes a prominent feature
      (1) Huntington's disease (HD), pantothenate kinase-associated neurodegeneration (PKAN—formerly known as Hallervorden–Spatz disease), neuroacanthocytosis, SCA, dentatorubropallidoluysian atrophy, and mitochondrial diseases associated with parkinsonian disorders (PD, CBD, PSP, and MSA)
   c. **Acquired dystonia.** When dystonic movements are symptomatic of an exogenous or environmental cause
      (1) **Main causes.** Cerebrovascular diseases, central nervous system (CNS) tumor, central trauma, infectious or postinfectious encephalopathies, toxins (CO and manganese), metabolic diseases (Wilson's disease and GM1 gangliosidosis), paraneoplastic syndromes, perinatal anoxia, kernicterus, and peripheral trauma

E. **Pathophysiology.** Dystonia is attributed to basal ganglia abnormalities and to a dysfunction of the cortico-striatothalamo-cortical circuits. Idiopathic dystonia is not associated with any particular structural brain lesion. However, neurophysiologic and neuroimaging techniques have shown a correlation between the cocontraction and overflow of electromyogram (EMG) activity of inappropriate muscles, with reduced pallidal inhibition of the thalamus due to lower firing rates, large sensory receptive fields, and irregular discharges in bursts or groups of bursts in neurons of the medial globus pallidus. Supporting the theory of basal ganglia dysfunction, secondary dystonia is mostly observed in patients with lesions of the putamen and connections with the thalamus and cortex.

F. **Selected clinical syndromes.**

1. **PTD.** It refers to those syndromes in which dystonia is the only phenotypic manifestation (except for tremor). In cases of PTD, there is no history of brain injury, no laboratory findings exclusive of genetic tests to suggest a cause for dystonia, no consistent associated brain pathology, and no improvement with a trial of low-dose levodopa. Some of these cases can be attributed to a genetic cause. **Early-onset PTD (Oppenheim's dystonia)**

is inherited as an autosomal-dominant trait with reduced penetrance (30% to 40%). The genetic mutation for the most frequent and severe form of early-onset PTD, named DYT1, was mapped to chromosome 9q34, which encodes the protein TORSIN, whose function remains unknown. The disorder develops before 26 years of age in nearly all cases. It normally begins in one arm or a leg, and spreads to other limbs and trunk, leading to the most severe generalized form of the disease in most cases. Selective or pronounced craniocervical or orofacial involvement is unusual. Conversely, late-onset PTD (>26 years—DYT4, DYT6) normally involves the upper part of the body (cranial–cervical region) and usually remains focal or segmental. In spite of this archetypical pattern, dystonia may remain localized as writer's cramp in some patients with early-onset PTD.

a. **Differential diagnosis.**
   - **(1)** Perinatal hypoxia
   - **(2)** Head trauma
   - **(3)** DRD
   - **(4)** Wilson's disease
   - **(5)** PKAN and neuroferritinopathy
   - **(6)** **Other metabolic disorders.** Glutaric acidemia type 1, GM1 and GM2 gangliosidosis, metachromatic leukodystrophy, sialidosis, Krabbe's disease, Niemann–Pick type C (NPC), vanishing white matter disease, and biotinidase deficiency
   - **(7)** HD (Westphal's variant)
   - **(8)** Ataxia telangiectasia
   - **(9)** Leigh's syndrome

b. **Evaluation.**
   - **(1)** Brain MRI
     - **(a)** Primary dystonia usually has normal MRI.
     - **(b)** "Eye of the tiger" sign (globus pallidus central hyperintensity with surrounding hypointensity on T2-weighted images) is due to iron deposition in the globus pallidus and very suggestive of PKAN.
     - **(c)** Wilson's disease has also distinctive neuroimaging findings, with T2-weighted globus pallidal hypointensity, T2-weighted "face of giant panda" sign (hyperintensity of the midbrain, hypointensity of the aqueduct, and relative sparing of red nucleus, superior colliculus, and substantia nigra pars reticulata), and T1-weighted striatal hyperintensity (bilateral thalamus and lenticular nucleus).
   - **(2)** Patients with onset before 26 years of age should be always considered for trial of low-dose levodopa, to exclude DRD.
   - **(3)** **Wilson's disease.** To exclude this disorder, slit-lamp eye examination for Kayser–Fleischer rings and determination of serum ceruloplasmin level should be performed in dystonia patients younger than 50 years.
   - **(4)** Screening of metabolic inherited diseases, when atypical features of DYT1 are present (bulbar and orofacial symptoms, cognitive impairment, behavioral disturbances, and polyneuropathy)
   - **(5)** Patients with onset before 26 years of age should be considered for genetic testing for the *DYT1* gene. A detailed family history should be obtained.

2. **Focal dystonia.**
   a. **Blepharospasm** is a disorder that consists of uncontrollable involuntary spasms of the eyelids causing spontaneous closure. It often interferes with vision, resulting in functional blindness. It may be worsened by bright light or stress.
   b. **Oromandibular dystonia** consists of grimacing of the lower part of the face, usually involving the mouth, jaw, and platysma muscle. Depending on the nature of the oromandibular movements, jaw closing, jaw opening, and jaw deviation oromandibular dystonias are differentiated.
   c. **Cervical dystonia** or spasmodic torticollis consists of intermittent uncontrollable spasms of the neck muscles. The neck may involuntarily turn, tilt, or rotate forward, sideways, or backward.
   d. **Spasmodic dysphonia** involves only the vocal cords. There are two types of spasmodic dysphonia. With **adductor-type** spasmodic dysphonia, hyperadduction of the cords produces an intermittent strain and strangle quality to the voice. Often patients also

report tightness in the throat during the spasms. With the rarer **abductor type** of spasmodic dysphonia, there is a whispering quality to the voice.

e. **Task-specific dystonia.** The dystonic movements are brought out by performing a specific task such as writing, typing, or playing a musical instrument. Writer's cramp is the most common and most underdiagnosed form of limb dystonia. Examples of task-specific dystonia include a secretary who has dystonic hand cramps only while typing, and a violinist who has finger spasms only while playing.

(1) Differential **diagnosis of focal dystonia.**

(a) Drug-induced (most common cause of secondary focal dystonia)

(b) Pseudodystonias

(1) **Sandiffer's syndrome.** Torticollis and paroxysmal dystonic postures induced by gastroesophageal reflux

(2) Posterior fossa tumors

(3) Chiari's malformation

(4) Atlantoaxial subluxation

(c) Structural lesions involving the basal ganglia, thalamus, brainstem, or the cervical spinal cord (ischemic, demyelinating, inflammatory, infectious, immunologic lesion, and space-occupying mass)

(2) Evaluation.

(a) Review of medication record for dopamine receptor–blocking drugs (metoclopramide, clebopride, haloperidol, risperidone, and tiapride), flupenthixol, melitracene, antidizziness drugs (tietilperazine, sulpiride, and veralipride).

(b) MRI of the brain including the posterior fossa and the cervical spinal cord. To rule out structural lesions, or images suggestive of metabolic inherited disorders, or of neurodegeneration with brain iron accumulation (PKAN and neuroferritinopathy).

3. Acquired dystonia. These disorders relate usually to lesions in the CNS, mostly in the basal ganglia, although peripheral trauma in the neck or limbs can result in dystonic posturing of that body part. Stroke, CNS tumor or demyelinating disease, perinatal anoxia, and trauma are the most frequent causes of acquired dystonia. Acquired dystonia typically involves one side of the body (hemidystonia) or only one extremity and may be accompanied by impairment of different neural systems: weakness, sensory disturbances, or pyramidal signs. Peripherally induced dystonia may show atypical dystonic features, such as fixed postures and maintenance of dystonia during sleep, and a worse response to botulinum toxin than seen with other acquired forms.

a. **Evaluation.** MRI of the brain including the posterior fossa and the cervical spinal cord to rule out structural lesions

4. Wilson's disease. It is the most common known metabolic defect causing secondary dystonia. It is an inherited deficit in copper metabolism.

a. **Differential diagnosis and evaluation** (see **Section F.1 under Dystonia**).

(1) Neurologic symptoms affecting the basal ganglia, including bradykinesia, dysarthria, dystonia, tremor, ataxia, and abnormal gait, occur in 40% to 60% of patients. Spasmodic dysphonia is a common feature.

(2) Wing-beating tremor is classically described in patients with Wilson's disease (55%). This tremor is absent at rest and develops after the arms are extended. Rest tremor may also be present in 5% of the patients.

(3) Psychiatric symptoms (65%) (psychosis, depression, irritability, agitation, and disinhibition), mild cognitive impairment (70%), and dementia (5%) can be associated with the motor manifestations.

Early treatment can reverse the liver involvement in Wilson's disease and stop the neurologic impairment.

5. DYT6. Mutations in the *THAP1* gene have been identified as a cause of autosomal-dominant primary dystonia. Families described over the past years have shown the clinical picture of DYT6 patients to be heterogeneous, but some features can help to distinguish them from DYT1 mutation carriers. The combination of cervical, upper limb, or generalized progressive dystonia with spasmodic laryngeal dystonia or oromandibular involvement may guide the clinician to the diagnosis.

6. **Dopa-responsive dystonia—DYT5.** This childhood-onset disease usually begins with leg dystonia that gradually progresses to other parts of the body. Typical features are a diurnal fluctuation of the symptoms, so that they worsen as the day progresses or after intense exercise, and they improve after sleep. Patients may also show extensor plantar responses with hyperreflexia in the lower limbs, tremor, and parkinsonism. The most characteristic feature of DRD is a dramatic and sustained response to low-dose levodopa, without the typical complications of motor fluctuations and dyskinesias.

7. **Myoclonus-dystonia (DYT11).** This disorder is characterized by involuntary jerks and dystonic movements and postures, both of which may be dramatically alleviated with alcohol. It normally begins in the first or second decade of life (5 to 18 years), with myoclonic jerks and dystonic movements most frequently involving the arms, neck, and face. Although spread to axial muscles and the legs is typical, the condition is compatible with an active life of normal span. Obsessive-compulsive disorder, anxiety/panic/phobic disorders, and alcohol dependence are frequently associated with the motor manifestations.

8. **Rapid-onset dystonia-parkinsonism (DYT12).** This very rare condition involves dystonic spasms, bradykinesia, postural instability, severe dysarthria, and dysphagia that develop abruptly over a period ranging from several hours to weeks. Some patients report specific triggers consisting of either physical or psychological stress. There is little response to dopaminergic drugs, and the neurologic sequelae remain stable over time.

9. **Anti-N-methyl-D-aspartate (NMDA) receptor encephalitis.** Encephalitis due to NMDA receptor antibodies has been recently associated with the development of jaw opening and other orofacial dystonias. Distonic movements have been reported in combination with opisthotonic posturing, seizures, psychosis, and other behavioral changes. Anti-NMDA receptor antibodies have been even found to cause isolated hemidystonia. As NMDA receptors are present in the neuronal membrane, discovery and treatment of neoplasias producing anti-NMDA receptor antibodies (ovarian and mediastinic teratoma, breast cancer, and pancreatic cancer), and immunotherapy can improve and even resolve the neurologic condition.

10. **NPC.** Some neurometabolic disorders may be treatable. In these cases, early diagnosis may slow the degenerative process or even halt the process. Patients with the adult form of NPC, which usually start between the third and fifth decades of life, have specific clinical features very useful in the differential diagnosis of secondary dystonias. The combination of bibrachial dystonia with facial dystonia ('facial grimacing'), ataxia, and supranuclear vertical gaze palsy usually precede the development of more severe features of the disease like schizophrenia-like symptoms and dementia. NPC can be diagnosed by genetic testing or the Filipin test (analysis of cholesterol perinuclear vesicles in skin fibroblasts culture).

CHOREA

A. **Definition.** Chorea is characterized by arrhythmic involuntary movements resulting from a continuous flow of random muscle contractions. When choreic movements are more severe, assuming a large amplitude and sometimes violent character, they are called ballism. Although typical choreic movements are predominantly distal, ballistic movements are more proximal. Athetosis is a related writhing and twisting movement that manifests predominantly in distal arms. Regardless of its cause, chorea has very distinctive clinical features. The differential diagnosis of choreic syndromes relies on differences in the presence of other accompanying findings.

B. **Etiologic classification.**
1. Genetic choreas.
   a. HD
   b. Huntington's disease–like 2 (HDL2) and other HD-like symptoms
   c. Neuroacanthocytosis (chorea-acanthocytosis, X-linked McLeod syndrome)
   d. PKAN
   e. Neuroferritinopathy
   f. Ataxia telangiectasia
   g. SCA, types 2, 3, or 17

    h. Dentatorubropallidolyusian atrophy
    i. Benign hereditary chorea
    j. Paroxysmal kinesigenic choreoathetosis
    k. C9orf72 hexanucleotide expansion: recent studies have indicated that this is the most common genetic cause of HD phenocopies

2. Structural basal ganglia lesions.
    a. Vascular chorea in stroke
    b. Hemodynamic ischemia secondary to carotid stenosis
    c. Mass lesions (lymphoma and metastatic brain tumors)
    d. Multiple sclerosis plaques
    e. Extrapontine myelinolysis
    f. Polycythemia vera (generally not related to focal vascular lesions in the basal ganglia)
    g. Moyamoya disease
    h. Postpump chorea (generalized chorea immediately after extracorporeal circulation. Benign prognosis with spontaneous remission in most cases.)

3. Parainfectious and autoimmune disorders.
    a. Sydenham's chorea
    b. Systemic lupus erithematosus (SLE)
    c. Chorea gravidarum (chorea during pregnancy)
    d. Antiphospholipid antibody syndrome
    e. Behçet's disease
    f. Postinfectious or postvaccinal encephalitis
    g. AntiGAD65, antiLGi1 antibodies
    h. Paraneoplastic choreas (anti-CV2/CRMP5, antiCASPR2, or anti-Hu antibodies, associated with small-cell lung cancer, Hodgkin's lymphoma, or thymoma)

4. Infectious chorea. HIV primoinfection, toxoplasmosis, cysticercosis, diphtheria, infective endocarditis, neurosyphilis, viral encephalopathies (mumps, measles, and varicella), herpes simplex, and parvovirus B19

5. Metabolic or toxic encephalopathies.
    a. Hyperglycemic-induced hemichorea–hemiballismus
    b. Acute intermittent porphyria
    c. Hyponatremia/hypernatremia
    d. Hyperthyroidism
    e. Hypoparathyroidism
    f. Hepatic/renal failure
    g. CO, manganese, mercury, and organophophorate intoxication
    h. Hyperhomocysteinemia ± vitamin B_{12} deficiency

6. Drug-induced chorea.
    a. **Antiparkinsonian drugs.** L-Dopa and dopamine agonists
    b. Dopamine receptor–blocking agents (chronic exposure)
    c. **Antiepileptic drugs.** Phenytoin, carbamazepine, valproic acid, and gabapentin
    d. **Psychostimulants and other drugs.** Amphetamines, cocaine, heroin, and methylphenidate
    e. Methadone
    f. **Calcium-channel blockers.** Cinnarizine, flunarizine, and verapamil
    g. Oral contraceptives (likely to induce chorea in patients with previous choreic episodes—such as SLE or Sydenham's chorea)
    h. Steroids
    i. Antihistamine drugs
    j. **Others.** Lithium, baclofen, digoxin, tryciclic antidepressants, cyclosporine, theophylline, ribavirine, and α-interferon

C. Pathophysiology. Chorea results from facilitation of the striato-pallido-thalamic output pathway, leading to thalamo-cortical disinhibition of previously learned and patterned movements. This failure of control comes from dysfunction of neural networks in the basal ganglia that are interconnected with the motor cortical areas. Neurophysiologic and lesional studies and cases of chorea in patients with focal lesions in the basal ganglia have shown that failure of inhibition of movements relates mainly to dysfunction of the caudate nucleus and the subthalamic nucleus.

D. Selected clinical syndromes.

1. HD is an autosomal-dominant progressive neurodegenerative disease characterized by chorea, dystonia, loss of balance, cognitive decline, and behavioral changes. Neurodegeneration primarily affects the head of the caudate nucleus and the frontal cortex. The genetic disorder is caused by a trinucleotide (CAG) repeat expansion in the gene encoding huntingtin on chromosome *4p16.3*. Polyglutamine expansions are the main component of Huntington that lead to neuronal degeneration, a pattern also seen in several SCA. Healthy individuals have fewer than 35 CAG repeats, and repeats of 40 or above cause HD with 100% penetrance. Individuals with 36 to 39 repeats can develop the disease, but penetrance is incomplete (Videos 28.3, 28.4, 28.5, and 28.6).

   The mean age at onset is 40 years. Although chorea is the main feature of the disease, the full spectrum of motor impairment includes eye-movement abnormalities, parkinsonism, dystonia, myoclonus, tics, cerebellar ataxia, spasticity with hyperreflexia, dysarthria, and dysphagia. Features of chorea are very variable, but choreic orofacial movements and mild slow, sinusoidal, and flowing distal movements in the four extremities are very common in the early stages of the disease. With progressing illness, dystonia and parkinsonism may become the main motor features. Behavioral and cognitive impairment affect almost all patients, with depression, anxiety, apathy, irritability, agitation, obsessive-compulsive symptoms, and social disinhibition accounting for the most frequent disorders. Young-onset disease (<20 years, so-called Westphal's variant) is associated with >55 CAG repeats and is characterized by predominant dystonic symptoms, myoclonus, parkinsonism, and seizures.

2. Sydenham's chorea. It is the most common cause of acute chorea in children worldwide. It has a female preponderance, and the typical age of onset is 8 to 9 years. Sydenham's chorea represents the prototype of chorea resulting from immune mechanisms, related to rheumatic fever. Up to 25% of patients with rheumatic fever develop generalized chorea 4 to 8 weeks after an episode of β-hemolytic streptococcal pharyngitis, although it can be manifested as hemichorea in 20% of patients. Molecular similarities between streptococcal and basal ganglia antigens seem to be the main pathogenetic mechanism leading to chorea.

   Chorea is frequently accompanied by hypotonia, tics, motor impersistence, and behavioral abnormalities (attention-deficit hyperactivity disorder [ADHD] and obsessive-compulsive symptoms). Mitral valvulopathy is also present in up to 60% to 80%. Sydenham's chorea has a good prognosis. Spontaneous remission often occurs after 8 to 9 months, although in 50% of patients some chorea may persist after 2 years, and recurrences may appear. A medical history of Sydenham's chorea seems to be a risk factor of development of chorea gravidarum or chorea related to use of oral contraceptives or antiepileptic drugs.

3. Chorea-acanthocytosis (ChAc), also known as neuro-acanthocytosis. This autosomal-recessive disease is characterized by generalized chorea and severe orofacial dystonia with tongue and lip biting that produce orofacial self-mutilations. Neuropathy, subclinical or mild myopathy, and seizures, along with hepatic disease, are common associated features. X-linked inherited McLeod's syndrome has indistinguishable clinical findings, with otherwise less frequent orofacial dystonia, and more frequent seizures and severe hepatic failure.

4. PKAN. This disorder has onset during childhood, with the hallmarks of chorea and generalized dystonia that typically affect bulbar and orofacial muscles, with speech difficulties as a prominent clinical feature. Chorea and dystonia are associated with cognitive impairment and behavioral disorders, parkinsonian, and pyramidal tract features.

5. Hyperglycemic-induced hemichorea–hemiballismus. This condition occurs mostly in women, ranging from 50 to 80 years of age, and chorea develops in association with nonketotic hyperglycemia in type 2 diabetes mellitus. Patients usually have no previous history of diabetes mellitus but develop choreic or ballistic movements on one side of the body, in the setting of elevated serum glucose levels (range of 400 to 1,000 mg/dL). CT scans may reveal a hyperdense lesion involving the right caudate and lentiform nucleus, but sparing the internal capsule, without mass effect. MRI scans reveal hyperintensity and hypointensity in the same structures in T1- and T2-weighted images, respectively.

In most patients, lowering serum glucose levels to the normal range completely reverses the movements within 24 to 48 hours. In some cases, however, chorea persists after correction of the metabolic abnormality.

E. **Differential diagnosis and evaluation.** Although classification of chorea is based on etiology, differential diagnosis and evaluation of choreic patients are based primarily on age of onset.

1. **Adult-onset chorea.**
   a. **Positive family history.**
      (1) **Genetic testing for HD.** Up to 25% of newly diagnosed HD patients have a negative family history because of nonpaternity or ancestral death before disease manifestation.

      SCA2, SCA3, and SCA17, neuroferritinopathy, and *C9orf72* hexanucleotide expansions must be considered when genetic testing for HD is negative.

      (2) **Wilson's disease.** See **Section F.1.b under Dystonia.**
   b. **No family history.**
      (1) MRI scan should be done in all cases to exclude vascular, neoplastic, infectious, or inflammatory pathology in the basal ganglia or adjacent structures.
      (2) Rule out other causes of chorea.
         (a) Pregnancy testing
         (b) Review of medication record and drug abuse (**see classification**)
         (c) Metabolic and autoimmune disorders. Blood testing considering SLE, antiphospholipid antibody syndrome, thyrotoxicosis, or other metabolic disorders (**see classification**)
         (d) Polycythemia must be considered, especially in the elderly. Chorea associated with polycythemia seems to be related to blood hyperviscosity throughout the brain. Chorea may be the presenting symptom of polycythemia or a sign of hematologic deterioration of the disease. Therapy with repeated phlebotomies may be an effective treatment of chorea in this condition.
         (e) Diagnosis of ChAc must be suspected in young-adult patients with suggestive symptoms, even in the absence of family history. Analysis of acanthocytes in fresh blood samples has very low sensitivity, and repeated measurements must be done. Recently, determination of chorein in peripheral blood samples offers a markedly higher sensitivity and specificity for the diagnosis of ChAc. Western blot detection of chorein strongly supports the clinical diagnosis of ChAc when chorein is low or absent in the erythrocyte membrane.

2. **Childhood-onset chorea.**
   a. **Positive family history.**
      (1) **Wilson's disease.** See **Section F.1.b under Dystonia.**
      (2) Genetic testing for HD
      (3) Genetic testing for benign hereditary chorea, usually associated with slowly progressive ataxia, should be investigated.
      (4) When there is a history of progressive cerebellar ataxia and choreoathetosis, with and without ocular motor apraxia, ataxia telangiectasia should be ruled out by measuring fetoprotein in serum, even if telangiectasias are not observed in the conjunctiva, oral mucosa, or the skin.
      (5) **Acanthocytes in blood testing.** As acanthocytes are not specific of neuroacanthocytosis (also present in 10% of HDL2 and PKAN patients), they will not be ordered if neuroacanthocytosis is not clinically suspected.
   b. **No family history.**
      (1) MRI scan
      (2) **Sydenham's chorea.** Antistreptolysin-O may be increased, but due to the long latency between streptococcus infection and the onset of chorea, most laboratory tests indicative of preceding streptococcal infection are not useful. Anti-DNase-B titers may be increased up to 1 year after the infection. Echocardiography may be very useful in supporting the diagnosis, when mitral valvulopathy is detected.
      (3) Rule out other autoimmune disorders like SLE and infectious chorea associated with viral (mumps, measles, and varicella) or postvaccination encephalitis.

MYOCLONUS

A. **Definition.** Myoclonus is a clinical sign defined as sudden, brief, lightening-like, involuntary movements caused by muscular contractions or inhibitions. Muscular contractions produce so-called positive myoclonus, whereas muscular inhibitions produce negative myoclonus or asterixis.

B. **Etiologic classification.** In clinical practice, treatment of myoclonus is mainly based on the treatment of the underlying disorder. However, it can also be classified according to examination findings or neurophysiologic testing.

1. **Physiologic myoclonus.** Sleep jerks, anxiety induced, exercise induced, hiccups (singultus), and benign infantile myoclonus with feeding
2. **Palatal myoclonus.** Idiopathic or symptomatic
3. **Epileptic myoclonus.** Seizures dominate the disease.
    a. Epilepsia partialis continua
    b. Idiopathic stimulus-sensitive myoclonus
    c. Myoclonic absences in petit mal epilepsy
    d. **Childhood myoclonic epilepsy.** Lennox–Gastaut syndrome, Aicardi's syndrome, and juvenile myoclonic epilepsy (awakening myoclonus epilepsy of Janz)
4. **Progressive myoclonus encephalopathies.**
    a. Baltic myoclonus (Unverricht–Lundborg disease)
    b. Neuronal ceroid lipofuscinoses (Kufs disease)
    c. **Sialidosis.** cherry-red spot myoclonus
    d. Lafora body disease
    e. PRICKLE-2-related progressive myoclonus epilepsy with ataxia
5. **Symptomatic or secondary myoclonus.**
    a. **Metabolic.** Hyperthyroidism, hepatic failure, renal failure, dialysis syndrome, ion alterations (Na^+, K^+, Ca^{+2}, and Mg^{+2}), hypoglycemia, nonketotic hyperglycemia, metabolic acidosis, or alkalosis
    b. **Myoclonus in the setting of renal failure.** Uremic encephalopathy, dialysis encephalopathy, drug-induced (acyclovir, ciprofloxacin, dobutamine, cephalosporins, amantadine, gabapentin), May–White syndrome, Galloway–Mowat syndrome, action myoclonus-renal failure syndrome due to *SCARB2* mutations.
    c. **Infectious or postinfectious.** HIV, subacute sclerosing panencephalitis, progressive multifocal leukoencephalopathy, herpes simplex encephalitis, postinfectious encephalitis, malaria, syphilis, Cryptococcus, and Lyme's disease
    d. Hashimoto's encephalopathy
    e. **Malabsorption.** Celiac disease and Whipple's disease
    f. **Other encephalopathies.** Posthypoxia (Lance–Adams syndrome), posttraumatic, and electric shock
    g. **Drug-induced myoclonus.** Tricyclic antidepressants, selective serotonin uptake inhibitors, monoamine oxidase inhibitors, lithium, antipsychotics, narcotics, anticonvulsants, anesthetics, contrast media, calcium-channel blockers, antiarrhythmics, and drug withdrawal
    h. **Basal ganglia degenerations.** Wilson's disease, PKAN, HD, MSA, CBD, PSP, and dentatorubropallidoluysian atrophy
    i. **Dementias.** Creutzfeldt–Jakob disease, AD, DLB, frontotemporal dementia, and Rett's syndrome
    j. Focal **central** or **peripheral** nervous system damage. This category includes propriospinal or segmental spinal myoclonus.
    k. **Spinocerebellar degenerations.** Ramsay–Hunt syndrome, Friedreich's ataxia, and ataxia telangiectasia
    l. **Storage disease.** Lafora's body disease, GM2 gangliosidosis, Tay–Sachs disease, Gaucher's disease, Krabbe's leukodystrophy, ceroid-lipofuscinosis, and sialidosis
    m. **Opsoclonus-myoclonus syndrome.** Idiopathic, paraneoplastic (neural crest tumors)

C. **Pathophysiology.** Cortical myoclonus is produced by an imbalance between inhibitory and excitatory systems in the sensorimotor cortex rapidly conducting to the pyramidal tracts. Cortical myoclonic activity spreads relatively rapidly from an initial focus in one sensorimotor cortex to other ipsilateral sensorimotor cortical areas through corticocortical pathways and to the opposite sensorimotor cortex through the corpus callosum. Propriospinal myoclonus is explained by changes in spinal cord excitability, probably due to dorsal horn interneuron hyperactivity. In brainstem myoclonus, muscle jerks arise from activity in neuronal centers within the lower brainstem, probably involving the same circuitry as the normal startle reflex.

D. Selected clinical syndromes.

   1. **Cortical myoclonus** is multifocal, but predominantly affects body parts with the largest cortical representations such as the hands and face. Patients with cortical myoclonus may have purely focal or multifocal jerks, but they may have additional bilateral or generalized jerks, suggesting the spread of excitatory myoclonic activity between the cerebral hemispheres and across the sensorimotor cortex. As the motor cortex is most involved in voluntary action, the jerks are usually most marked during action. Metabolic encephalopathies cause generalized and spontaneous myoclonus that, like other forms of myoclonus, is triggered or enhanced by sensitive stimuli (light touch or stretch lead to reflex jerks of the stimulated area). **Epilepsia partialis continua** is a myoclonic epilepsy caused by focal cortical lesions, and myoclonic rhythmic jerks usually occur in the hands or face. Rhythmic forms of the myoclonic jerks can be misinterpreted as tremor.

      a. Differential diagnosis.

         (1) Clonic tics

         (2) Myokymia

         (3) Startle syndromes (hyperekplexia)

         (4) **Parkinsonian disorders.** Mainly CBD

         (5) **Dementing conditions.** Creutzfeldt–Jakob disease, DLB, CBD, and AD

      b. Evaluation.

         (1) MRI of the brain including the posterior fossa and the cervical spinal cord, to rule out structural lesions

         (2) Blood tests, to rule out metabolic disturbances. Antithyroid antibodies, to rule out Hashimoto's encephalopathy

         (3) Review of medication records

         (4) EEG, to rule out epileptogenic discharges

         (5) Lumbar puncture (LP), to rule out encephalitis, Creutzfeldt–Jakob disease, or postinfectious encephalopathies (HIV and subacute sclerosing panence-phalitis)

   2. Brainstem myoclonus. Brainstem motor systems are particularly involved in axial and bilateral movements. Jerks in brainstem myoclonus are generalized, especially axial, with long-lasting electromyographic bursts (>100 ms) and may be provoked by many different types of sensory stimuli, although cutaneous taps around the nose and face are particularly effective. The hallmark is auditory reflex jerks, known as hyperekplexia.

      a. Differential diagnosis.

         (1) Brainstem structural lesions

         (2) Startle syndromes

         (3) Creutzfeldt–Jakob disease

      b. Evaluation.

         (1) MRI of the brain including, to rule out structural lesions

         (2) Family history of startle syndrome

         (3) LP

   3. Propriospinal myoclonus. Spinal segmental systems may become hyperexcitable, often by viral irritation or the isolation of anterior horn cells from inhibitory influences by disorders such as syringomyelia, glioma, or spinal ischemia. The result is myoclonus involving one or two contiguous spinal myotomes. Propriospinal myoclonus leads to predominantly axial flexion and extension jerks that, unlike brainstem myoclonus, spare the face and are not provoked by sound. This form of myoclonus is usually caused by damage to the spinal cord through cervical trauma, inflammation, or a tumor.

      a. Evaluation.

         (1) MRI of the cervical, thoracic, and lumbar spine to rule out structural lesions

         (2) Evaluation for multiple sclerosis

         (3) Personal history of cervical trauma

4. **Palatal myoclonus.** This nomenclature is historically respected but phenomenologically inaccurate, and more properly it should be designated as palatal tremor. Palatal movements are fast and rhythmic and can spread to the throat, face, and diaphragm. Patient may hear an "ear click" due to contraction of the tensor veli palatini muscle. Palatal myoclonus/tremor may be idiopathic or symptomatic. Although the presence of the ear click had been classically associated with the idiopathic cases, it can be also present in secondary cases, in patients with structural brainstem lesions. Idiopathic cases have been related to hypertrophy of the inferior olive, and symptomatic cases to lesions (ischemic, neoplastic, and inflammatory) in the triangle of Guillain–Mollaret, which includes the red nucleus, the inferior olive, and the dentate nucleus.

   a. **Evaluation.** MRI of the brain including the posterior fossa to rule out structural lesions involving the triangle of Guillain–Mollaret.

5. **Posthypoxic action (intention) myoclonus, or Lance–Adams syndrome.** This form of cortical myoclonus occurs in survivors of anoxic brain injuries. The jerks are triggered by voluntary movement, and specially, when movements are directed to a particular goal or target. Action-intention myoclonus is the most disabling form of myoclonus associated with provocative factors, with jerks that prevent or disrupt the movement. The myoclonic movements range from simple, localized focal jerks to generalized, disabling jerks.

TICS

A. **Definition.** Tics are brief, intermittent, and repetitive, involuntary or semivoluntary movements and sounds. They are preceded by an urge or sensation in the affected muscle group and a sense of temporary relief once the movement is performed. Although tics may resemble other types of hyperkinetic movements (e.g., myoclonus and dystonia), the urge is considered a key characteristic that suggests that the movement is a tic. The patient's ability to transiently suppress the movements by conscious effort and an increased frequency of tics after efforts to suppress have ceased are additional supportive features of the diagnosis. Onset of tic disorders usually occurs during childhood (before age 18).

B. **Phenomenologic classification.**

1. **Anatomic distribution.**

   a. **Simple motor tics.** Focal movements involving one group of muscles (eye blinking, mouth movements, and shoulder elevation)

   b. **Complex motor tics.** Coordinated or sequential patterns of movement involving various groups of movements. They may resemble usual motor tasks or gestures (jumping and throwing) and include echopraxia (imitating others' gestures) and copropraxia.

   c. Simple phonic tics are elementary, meaningless noises or sounds (sniffing, grunting, clearing the throat, coughing, and belching).

   d. Complex phonic tics are meaningful syllables, words, or phrases ("okay" and "shut up") and include pallilalia, echolalia, and coprolalia.

   e. Sensory tics are uncomfortable sensations (pressure, cold, warmth, or paresthesias) localized to certain body parts that are relieved by the performance of an intentional act in the affected area.

2. **Speed of movement.**

   a. Clonic tics are brief, sudden, and jerk-like.

   b. Dystonic tics involve sustained twisting, or posturing is present.

   c. Tonic tics involve tensing contraction of muscles (abdominal or limb muscles).

3. **Natural history.**

   a. **Transient tic disorder.** Multiple motor and/or phonic tics with duration of at least 4 weeks, but <12 months. These tics occur in 20% of children during the first decade of life.

   b. **Chronic tic disorder.** Single motor and/or phonic tics, but not both, which are present for >1 year.

   c. **Tourette's syndrome.** Both motor and phonic tics are present for >1 year.

C. **Etiologic classification.**

   1. **Primary.**

      a. Tourette's syndrome, transient tic disorder, and chronic tic disorder

   2. **Secondary.**

      a. **Hereditary disorders with tics as one manifestation of another primary neurologic condition.** HD, neuroacanthocytosis, PKAN, Wilson's disease, and tuberous sclerosis complex

      b. **Infections.** Encephalitis, neurosyphilis, and Sydenham's chorea

      c. **Drugs.** Methylphenidate, antiepileptic drugs, dopamine receptor–blocking drugs (see section Tardive Syndrome), psychostimulant drugs (amphetamines, pemoline and cocaine), and levodopa

      d. Head trauma

      e. **Toxins.** Carbon monoxide

      f. **Developmental.** Autistic spectrum disorders (Rett's syndrome and Asperger's syndrome), intellectual disability syndromes, chromosomal disorders (Down's syndrome, Klinefelter's syndrome, fragile X syndrome, and triple X)

      g. **Focal brain lesions.** Stroke and multiple sclerosis

D. **Pathophysiology.** Dopaminergic imbalance in the ventral part of the cortico–striatal–thalamocortical pathways (medial prefrontal cortex connecting to the ventral striatum—ventral part of the globus pallidus, and the dorsomedial thalamus) is involved in the expression of tics. However, some data suggest an associated cortical dysfunction in Tourette's syndrome. In volumetric and functional MRI studies, children with Tourette's syndrome have shown larger dorsolateral prefrontal regions, increased cortical white matter in the right frontal lobe, and activation of the prefrontal cortex related to tic suppression. Likewise, transcranial-magnetic-stimulation studies suggest that tics originate from impaired inhibition in the motor cortex.

E. **Selected clinical syndromes.**

   1. **Tourette's syndrome.** Tourette's syndrome is characterized by multiple motor tics plus one or more phonic tics that wax and wane over time. Diagnosis is made according to the *DSM-IV* clinical criteria.

      a. Multiple motor and one or more phonic tics (not necessarily concurrently)

      b. Onset before age 21 years

      c. Variations in anatomic location, number, frequency, complexity, and severity of the tics occur over time.

      d. Tics occur many times a day, nearly every day or intermittently for more than a year, with symptom-free intervals not exceeding 3 months.

      e. Tics are not related to intoxication with psychoactive substances or CNS disease (e.g., encephalitis).

      f. Tics cause distress to the patient.

        The average age at the onset of tics is 5 years, become more severe at 10 years of age, but half of patients are free of tics by 18 years. Although tics may persist into adulthood, their severity is gradually diminished.

        Tourette's syndrome is commonly associated with behavioral comorbidities such as ADHD (15% to 50%), obsessive-compulsive disorder (35% to 45%), addictive and aggressive behaviors (related to poor impulse control), anxiety, depression, and decreased self-esteem. Obsessive-compulsive symptoms in Tourette's syndrome are characterized by ritualistic behaviors, and need for completion, symmetry, and perfection. In severe cases, self-injurious behaviors may be also present.

      g. **Differential diagnosis.**

        (1) Myoclonus **(see above)**

        (2) HD, neuroacanthocytosis, and PKAN

      h. **Evaluation.**

        (1) MRI of the brain to rule out structural brain lesions or to disclose images suggesting a metabolic disorder, if neurologic examination demonstrates other findings besides tics

        (2) Review of medication record for drug exposure

(3) History of drug exposure (psychostimulant drugs)

(4) Genetic testing for HD if other neurologic symptoms are present (cognitive impairment and ataxia)

(5) Review of family background for other examples of tics, attention deficits, or OCD

TARDIVE SYNDROMES

A. Definition. Tardive syndromes refer to a group of disorders characterized by persistent abnormal involuntary movements caused by chronic exposure to a dopamine receptor–blocking drug within 6 months of the onset of symptoms and persisting for at least 1 month after stopping the offending drug.

Tardive syndromes cover the gamut of hyperkinetic movement disorders, often with multiple types. Choreic and stereotypic bucco-linguo-masticatory dyskinesias are characterized by repetitive and predictable or unpredictable movements involving the oral, buccal, and lingual areas (tongue twisting and protusion, lip smacking or elevation, and chewing). Dystonic facial grimacing, and neck and trunk arching movements are also common and can mix with choreic movements. Myoclonus, tics, and restless purposeful movements (akathisia) have also been related to chronic exposure to dopamine receptor–blocking agents. Tardive tremor has been described but is controversial, and parkinsonism in a patient on neuroleptic medication is usually due to an increased dose of neuroleptic (drug-induced parkinsonism), and therefore not considered a tardive syndrome. Tardive syndromes may occur on steady doses of dopamine receptor–blocking agents or also induced by withdrawal.

B. Drugs reported to cause tardive syndromes.

1. Neuroleptic drugs. Haloperidol, risperidone, olanzapine, chlorpromazine, pimozide, levomepromazine, thioridazine, tiapride, fluphenazine, perphenazine, among others

2. Anxyolitics. Flupenthixol and melitracene

3. Calcium-channel blocker. Cinnarizine and flunarizine

4. Dihydropiridines. Amlodipine, nifedipine, and nimodipine

5. Antiemetic drugs. Metoclopramide, clebopride, and cinitapride

6. Antidizziness drugs. Tietilperazine, sulpiride, amisulpride, and veralipride

7. Trimetazidine

C. Risk factors for tardive dyskinesia.

1. Age older than 65 years

2. Female sex

3. Concomitant extrapyramidal symptoms

4. Basal ganglia lesions on neuroimaging

D. Selected clinical syndromes.

1. Typical orofacial buccolingual dyskinesia

2. Tardive dystonia. This syndrome may be indistinguishable from idiopathic dystonia and can be focal, segmental, or generalized. The movement can improve with sensory tricks. However, contrary to idiopathic dystonia, tardive dystonia often improves with voluntary actions such as walking. When involving the neck, predominates retrocollis, and when the trunk is affected, predominates tonic lateral flexion of the trunk (Pisa syndrome or pleurothotonus), or bench arching (opisthotonus).

3. Tardive akathisia. Akathisia is characterized by a feeling of inner restlessness. Subjectively, the most common complaint is the inability to keep the legs still and feeling fidgety, but patients can also describe a vague inner tension or anxiety. Objectively, patients are seen rocking from foot to foot, walking in place while sitting, and, occasionally, grunting, or trunk rocking. Characteristically, akathisia may improve with low doses of propranolol.

Key Points

- PD is the most frequent cause of rest tremor, but other diagnoses must be considered because of their different associated signs and prognoses: MSA, PSP, DLB, frontotemporal dementia with parkinsonism, SCAs, vascular parkinsonism, and drug-induced parkinsonism.
- FXTAS, characterized by ataxia and intentional tremor, is important to include within the considerations of adult ataxias. According to epidemiologic studies, FXTAS is more frequent than SCAs and has important genetic counseling implications.
- DYT6 patients can be identified clinically by the combination of cervical, upper limb, or generalized progressive dystonia with spasmodic laryngeal dystonia and/or oromandibular involvement.
- The combination of bibrachial dystonia with facial dystonia ('facial grimacing'), ataxia, and supranuclear vertical gaze palsy may guide the clinician to the diagnosis of NPC, a treatable cause of ataxia and dystonia.
- Chorea may dominate the neurologic picture of multiple, treatable disorders, and these conditions must be carefully considered in patients with an absence of a family history of chorea or with negative tests for HD.
- ChAc is characterized by generalized chorea and severe orofacial dystonia with tongue and lip biting and feeding dystonia, and can be easily diagnosed by determination of chorein in peripheral blood samples.
- *C9orf72* hexanucleotide expansions appear as the most frequent cause of HD phenocopies.

Recommended Readings

Albanese A, Bhatia K, Bressman SB, et al. Phenomenology and classification of dystonia: a consensus update. *Mov Disord.* 2013;28:863–873.

Berardelli A, Rothwell JC, Hallett M, et al. The pathophysiology of primary dystonia. *Brain.* 1998;121:1195–1212.

Bhatia K, Marsden MD. The behavioural and motor consequences of focal lesions of the basal ganglia in man. *Brain.* 1994;117:859–876.

Caviness JN, Brown P. Myoclonus: current concepts and recent advances. *Lancet Neurol.* 2004;3:598–607.

Deuschl G, Bain P, Brin M; Ad Hoc Scientific Committee. Consensus statement of the Movement Disorder Society on Tremor. *Mov Disord.* 1998;13(suppl 3):2–23.

Deuschl G, Elble R. Essential tremor—neurodegenerative or nondegenerative disease towards a working definition of ET. *Mov Disord.* 2009;14:2033–2041.

Djarmati A, Schneider SA, Lohmann K, et al. Mutations in THAP1 (DYT6) and generalised dystonia with prominent spasmodic dysphonia: a genetic screening study. *Lancet Neurol.* 2009;8:447–452.

Dobson-Stone C, Velayos-Baeza A, Filippone LA, et al. Chorein detection for the diagnosis of chorea-acanthocytosis. *Ann Neurol.* 2004;56:299–302.

Espay AJ, Chen R. Myoclonus. *Continuum (Minneap Minn).* 2013;19:1264–1286.

Ferioli S, Dalmau J, Kobet CA, et al. Anti-N-methyl-D-aspartate receptor encephalitis: characteristic behavioral and movement disorder. *Arch Neurol.* 2010;67:250–252.

Fernandez HH, Friedman JH. Classification and treatment of tardive syndromes. *Neurologist.* 2003;9:16–27.

Geyer HL, Bressman SB. The diagnosis of dystonia. *Lancet Neurol.* 2006;5:780–790.

Louis ED. Essential tremor: evolving clinicopathological concepts in an era of intensive post-mortem enquiry. *Lancet Neurol.* 2010;9:613–622.

Rubio-Agustí I, Dalmau J, Sevilla T, et al. Isolated hemidystonia associated with NMDA receptor antibodies. *Mov Disord.* 2011;26:351–352.

Singer HS. Tourette's syndrome: from behaviour to biology. *Lancet Neurol.* 2005;4:149–159.

Walker RH, Jung HH, Dobson-Stone C, et al. Neurologic phenotypes associated with acanthocytosis. *Neurology.* 2007;68:92–98.

Wild EJ, Tabrizi SJ. The differential diagnosis of chorea. *Pract Neurol.* 2007;7:360–373.

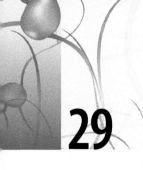

29 Approach to the Ataxic Patient

Adolfo Ramirez-Zamora

Ataxia is a syndrome characterized by lack or impaired coordination with disorganized movements, postures, and impaired balance. The initial evaluation of patients with progressive cerebellar ataxia is challenging. Numerous acquired, hereditary, paraneoplastic, toxic, and neurodegenerative conditions need to be considered in the broad differential diagnosis. An organized and systematic approach is critical to identify treatable conditions requiring early intervention and to arrive to correct diagnosis. When patients present with disequilibrium, the initial step is to determine the anatomical localization leading to imbalance. The neurologic examination provides clues to exclude weakness, spasticity, or musculoskeletal complaints as the cause of patient's symptoms. Particular attention should be given to exclude the presence of sensory ataxia secondary to proprioceptive loss with impaired cortical sensory feedback or vestibular ataxia that is characterized by loss of balance and coordination in the setting of vestibular system dysfunction or its connections. If proprioceptive ataxia is present, patients have reduced vibratory and position sense in distal extremities commonly associated with paresthesias or distal sensory loss impairment. Patients with chronic bilateral loss of vestibular function report a sense of unsteadiness, dizziness, vertigo, postmovement gaze variability, and oscillopsia. Conversely, patients with cerebellar ataxia present with poor balance with falls, imprecise hand coordination, postural or kinetic tremor of the extremities or trunk, dysarthria, dysphagia, vertigo, and diplopia. Once cerebellar ataxia is identified, the initial assessment requires careful evaluation of the patient's neurologic and non-neurologic features with emphasis on particular historical and examination details that can provide powerful information to narrow the differential diagnosis. The initial diagnostic evaluation should always include assessment for potential acquired causes—even if a hereditary ataxia is suspected—because acquired and hereditary causes can coexist.

HISTORY AND EXAMINATION

A. Speed of onset and progression of symptoms.

Recognizing the time of onset and subsequent progression of neurologic symptoms provides the initial framework to investigate potential etiologies responsible for cerebellar ataxia as these conditions greatly differ in etiology.

1. Acute onset.

The presence of acute-onset cerebellar ataxia should always alert the clinician to the presence of a toxic exposure, cerebrovascular event, structural lesions, or acute demyelinating disease affecting the cerebellum or its connections.

a. Alcoholic cerebellar degeneration is one of the most common forms of cerebellar ataxia. The ataxia can evolve rapidly within weeks to months, but most patients have a slow and steady course. Acute exposure to lithium, phenytoin, amiodarone, toluene, 5-fluorouracil, and cytosine arabinoside, as well as heavy metals, including organic lead compounds, mercury, and thallium, can present with acute onset of ataxia. Immediate cessation of toxic exposure is the most important therapeutic intervention.

b. When infarctions are restricted to the cerebellum, patients typically experience nonspecific symptoms (i.e., dizziness, nausea, vomiting, unsteady gait, and headache) and show neurologic signs (i.e., dysarthria, ataxia, and nystagmus) that might be absent, subtle, or difficult to distinguish from benign disorders of the peripheral vestibular system needed neuroimaging. Clues to the diagnosis to cerebellar stroke include older age of onset (>50 years), prior history of stroke or transient ischemic attack, stroke risk factors, recent head or neck injury, dizziness that persists more than 24 hours or in association with sudden hearing loss at onset, normal vestibular–ocular reflex by head impulse test (absence of a corrective saccade), spontaneous nystagmus that is direction-changing or dominantly vertical or torsional, skew deviation (vertical ocular misalignment), and severe difficulty or inability to stand or walk.

c. Several infectious agents can cause acute cerebellopathy/cerebellitis, with the most common ones being Epstein–Barr virus and Varicella-Zoster virus. Cerebellitis is more common in children and patients typically report a prodromal infectious phase followed by acute or subacute onset of cerebellar symptoms. Cerebrospinal fluid (CSF) analysis is required for the diagnosis. Other infections causing prominent ataxia are syphilis, human immunodeficiency virus (HIV), and Whipple's disease.

2. **Subacute onset.**

   The presence of subacute onset and progression of cerebellar symptoms and ataxia indicates a neurologic syndrome leading to marked functional disability over weeks.

   a. **Steroid-responsive encephalopathy associated with autoimmune thyroiditis (SREAT),** often referred to as Hashimoto encephalopathy, is an autoimmune syndrome characterized by subacute onset of confusion with altered level of consciousness, seizures, and myoclonus with elevated serum levels of thyroperoxidase (TPO) and thyroglobulin antibodies. Cerebellar ataxia is observed in more than 75% of patients. The rapid progression of multiple neurologic symptoms should prompt additional assessment. Treatment with high-dose intravenous methylprednisolone followed by oral prednisone taper can provide marked improvement in symptoms.

   b. **Creutzfeldt–Jakob disease (CJD)** is characterized by a rapidly progressive multifocal neurologic dysfunction, myoclonic jerks, and severe cognitive impairment. A subgroup of patients with sporadic CJD present with a virtually isolated cerebellar syndrome, and in some, cognitive decline may be delayed for weeks or even months. Cerebellar features are common in patients with CJD but these largely accompany pervasive and generalized cognitive decline and other neurologic features. The association of acute ataxia, severe cognitive impairment, and movement disorders should prompt consideration of this disorder. Increased CSF concentrations of 14-3-3 and prominent basal ganglia MRI signal changes on diffusion-weighted and fluid-attenuated inversion-recovery images are common in the ataxic variant, whereas typical electroencephalographic signs (periodic sharp-wave complexes) are usually absent.

   c. **Paraneoplastic cerebellar degeneration** represents a clinical syndrome characterized by progressive ataxia and cerebellar findings due to antineuronal antibodies in response to an immunologic trigger to tumor antigens that are similar to intracellular neuronal proteins (molecular mimicry). The most common associated malignancies are ovaries, breast, uterine cancers, Hodgkin's lymphoma, and small-cell carcinoma of the lung. Computed tomography scan of chest and abdomen, whole-body positron-emission tomography scans, and paraneoplastic panels are indicated in patients with a suspect paraneoplastic cerebellar syndrome. Treating the underlying tumor, combined with immunomodulatory treatment, might improve or stabilize symptoms. For most people, the prognosis is poor with up to 80% of patients never walking unaided.

   d. **The Miller Fisher variant of Guillain–Barré syndrome** presents with the triad of ophthalmoplegia, areflexia, and proprioceptive ataxia that develops over 1 to 2 weeks. Serum anti-GQ1b antibodies are commonly elevated. Treatment is with intravenous immunoglobulins (IVIGs) or plasma exchange.

   e. **Cerebellar ataxia associated with antibodies against glutamic acid decarboxylase (GAD65-Abs)** is one of the best characterized cerebellar syndromes. Autoimmune mechanisms probably have a relevant pathogenic role. Up to 38% of patients present with subacute presentation of ataxia lasting for weeks, although most cases have a chronic course progressing during months or years. Muscle rigidity and spasms are identified in many patients along with fluctuating vertigo before developing ataxia. Most patients are middle-age women (~90%) with or without type 1 diabetes mellitus, thyroiditis, or pernicious anemia. Immunosuppressive treatments with IVIG or corticosteroids have been used in most cases with good clinical response.

3. Chronic onset

Most metabolic, idiopathic, or neurodegenerative causes of progressive ataxia follow a slowly progressive, chronic course. Hereditary forms of cerebellar ataxia should be considered in the differential diagnosis. Several etiologies are important to recognize early, as maximal therapeutic benefit is only possible when done early.

a. **Gluten ataxia** is defined as insidious onset sporadic ataxia with positive serologic markers for gluten sensitivity including antigliadin antibodies, endomysial antibodies, and antibodies directed to surface cell transglutaminase 2. Transglutaminase-6 primarily expressed in neural tissue appears to be a sensitive and specific marker of GA found in up to 32% in idiopathic sporadic ataxia, and 73% in patients with GA. However, controversy remains about the specificity and sensitivity of these antibodies, as they have not been reproduced among all research laboratories. Patients often present in adulthood with an insidious onset, progressive, pure cerebellar ataxia syndrome. Less than 10% of patients will have any gastrointestinal symptoms, but a third will have evidence of enteropathy on biopsy. Treatment includes strict adherence to gluten-free diet. The best marker of strict adherence to a gluten-free diet is serologic evidence of elimination of circulating antibodies related to gluten sensitivity, although serum antibodies might be present for 6 to 12 months after initiation of the diet.

b. **Ataxia with vitamin E deficiency (AVED)** is an autosomal-recessive disease caused by mutations in the alpha tocopherol transfer protein on chromosome 8q13. It presents as a slowly progressive spinocerebellar ataxia syndrome (SCA) resembling Friedreich's ataxia (FRDA). Symptoms include ataxia, loss of muscle stretch reflexes, vibratory and sensory disturbances, muscle weakness, dysarthria, and upper motor neuron signs. A high dose of vitamin E (800 mg/d) is the specific treatment.

c. **Cerebrotendinous xanthomatosis (CTX)** is an uncommon, autosomal-recessive lipid storage disorder caused by a mutation of the mitochondrial enzyme 27-sterol hydroxylase on chromosome 2, which is a part of the hepatic bile-acid synthesis pathway. Neurologic symptoms include cerebellar ataxia, spastic paraparesis, extrapyramidal signs, sensorimotor peripheral neuropathy, seizures, psychiatric problems, and dementia, along with congenital/juvenile cataracts, tendon xanthomas, pulmonary insufficiency, and endocrinopathies. The disease is treated with oral chenodeoxycholic acid 250 mg three times per day.

d. **Niemann–Pick disease type C** is a rare neurodegenerative autosomal-recessive lipid storage disorder characterized by unique abnormalities of intracellular transport of endocytosed cholesterol with sequestration of unesterified cholesterol in lysosomes and late endosomes. Clinical presentation is extremely heterogeneous but the adult and juvenile forms of the disease initially present with progressive cerebellar ataxia, vertical supranuclear ophthalmoplegia, and cognitive impairment. Additionally, movement disorders, psychiatric symptoms, splenomegaly, and dysphagia are common. Miglustat, at doses of 200 mg three times daily, can modestly stabilize disease progression and improve quality of life.

e. **Abetalipoproteinemia** is caused by mutations in the gene for the large subunit of microsomal triglyceride transfer protein presenting with a neurologic phenotype similar to FRDA in addition to lipid malabsorption, hypocholesterolemia, acanthocytosis, and retinitis pigmentosa. Treatment involves dietary modification and vitamin replacement. Large doses of vitamin E and A supplementation are required for treatment.

f. **Refsum disease** is a rare autosomal-recessive disorder of fatty acid metabolism, mostly caused by mutations of the peroxisomal enzyme phytanoyl-CoA hydroxylase gene. A diagnostic tetrad of retinitis pigmentosa, cerebellar ataxia, polyneuropathy, and high CSF protein content without pleocytosis has been found in almost all patients with phytanic acid storage disease. Parosyxmal symptoms typically occur, sometimes triggered by infection or pregnancy or rapid weight loss. The goal of treatment is reduction of normal daily intake of phytanic acid to a maximum of 10 mg per day.

g. **Episodic ataxia type 2 (EA2)** is caused by a variety of point mutations in the same calcium-channel gene (CACNA1A) associated with SCA type 6 and familial hemiplegic migraine. EA2 is characterized by insidious onset of episodes of ataxia and nystagmus lasting for hours to days, and ranging in frequency from a few times a year to three to four episodes per week. Episodes are commonly triggered by emotional or physical stress. Symptoms vary from a pure ataxia to combination of symptoms including nausea, vertigo, dysarthria, and truncal ataxia. EA2 patients commonly respond to acetazolamide treatment with doses between 250 and 1,000 mg/d or 4-aminopyridine, 5 mg three times daily.

h. **Superficial CNS siderosis** results from recurrent hemorrhages into the subarachnoid space with hemosiderin deposition in the subpial layers of the cranial nerves, cerebellum, brainstem, and spinal cord leading to neurologic dysfunction. The classic clinical triad is cerebellar ataxia, sensorineural hearing loss (SNHL), and myelopathy. Symptoms usually progress from cranial nerve dysfunction (nearly always SNHL) and ataxia, to signs of brainstem and spinal cord dysfunction. The source of hemorrhage encompasses dural vascular abnormalities, trauma, other vascular lesions, tumors, or neurosurgical procedures. However, the source of bleeding is only found in about 50% of cases. MRI findings include T2-weighted and gradient echo hypointensities in affected regions consistent with hemosiderin deposition.

i. **Multiple system atrophy (MSA)** is a late-onset, sporadic neurodegenerative disorder characterized by autonomic failure, parkinsonism, cerebellar ataxia, and pyramidal tract signs in various combinations pathologically defined by widespread neurodegeneration in striatonigral and olivopontocerebellar structures with distinctive glial cytoplasmic inclusions formed by fibrillized -synuclein. MSA is an important cause of sporadic cerebellar ataxia. The diagnostic challenge arises, in considering cases of a pure or predominantly cerebellar ataxia coming on in adulthood with no family history and negative evaluation for acquired causes. The main differential diagnosis is the syndrome of sporadic adult-onset ataxia of unknown etiology/idiopathic late-onset cerebellar ataxia, which presents with a number of extracerebellar symptoms that overlap with features of MSA, including erectile dysfunction, bladder urgency, dysphagia, restless leg syndrome, and rapid eye movement sleep behavior disorder. Approximately 30% of patients diagnosed with sporadic idiopathic ataxia develop MSA over time. However, the natural histories of the two diseases differ with MSA average survival of 7 to 9 years. In contrast, in half of the patients with sporadic adult-onset ataxia their lifespan reportedly is most likely to be normal. The presence of muscular rigidity, tremor, dysphagia, and bladder dysfunction is significantly more frequent in patients with MSA than in patients with unexplained ataxia. Decreased and absent muscle stretch reflexes are more predominant in patients with unexplained ataxia. Although not pathognomonic, the presence of the "Hot cross bun" sign or posterior putaminal hypointensites can indicate MSA.

j. **Fragile-X-associated tremor/ataxia (FXTAS)** syndrome is a unique hereditary disorder associated with sporadic adult-onset ataxia caused by FMR1 premutations with a repeat length of 55 to 200. FXTAS is characterized by progressive cerebellar ataxia with prominent tremor, often accompanied by cognitive decline, parkinsonism, neuropathy, and autonomic failure. The penetrance of FXTAS is dependent on gender and age with >75% of all FMR1 premutation carriers having symptoms at age 80. MRI scans of patients with FXTAS show highly characteristic hyperintense signal changes lateral to the dentate nucleus that extend into the middle cerebellar peduncles, and are often accompanied by signal changes in the supratentorial white matter and generalized brain atrophy.

FAMILY HISTORY

Hereditary ataxias are a clinically and genetically heterogeneous group of disorders characterized by slowly progressive cerebellar dysfunction and atrophy of the cerebellum. Obtaining a three-generation family history with attention to other relatives with neurologic symptoms is critical for diagnosis. Hereditary ataxias can be inherited in an autosomal-dominant, autosomal-recessive, X-linked manner or through maternal inheritance if part of a mitochondrial genetic syndrome. Patients with AD ataxia typically present in third or fourth decade in contrary to most AR ataxias with onset of symptoms before 25 years of age.

A. Autosomal-dominant ataxias (ADCAs). The age of onset and physical findings in the ADCAs greatly overlap and cannot be differentiated by clinical or neuroimaging studies. Many of the ADCAs in addition to limb and truncal ataxia present with dysarthria, dysphagia, and neuropathy (Video 29.1). Upper motor neuron signs (hyperreflexia and spasticity) are commonly found in patients with SCA1 and SCA3; cognitive impairment has been reported in association with SCA2, SCA12, SCA13, and SCA17; chorea may manifest in patients with SCA17 or dentatorubral-pallidoluysian atrophy (DRPLA). Saccadic velocity is clearly abnormal in SCA3 and SCA2. Extremely slow saccades are very common in SCA2. Except for tics, all types of movement disorders can been observed in many of the SCAs. Dystonia is mainly associated with SCA17, SCA3, and SCA2. Parkinsonian features can be observed in SCA2, SCA3, or SCA17. Myoclonus has been observed in many of the SCA subtypes, but is most frequent in SCA2 and SCA14.

B. Autosomal-recessive ataxias (ARCAs). ARCAs may present with additional extra–central nervous system signs and symptoms. ARVE deficiency, abetalipoproteinaemia, CTX, and Refsum disease should always be considered in the differential as discussed above. Coenzyme Q10 (CoQ10) deficiency presents with seizures, cognitive decline, pyramidal track signs, and myopathy but may also include prominent cerebellar ataxia. Symptoms may respond to CoQ10 supplementation.

1. **Friedreich ataxia (FRDA)** is the most common AR ataxia. FRDA is characterized by slowly progressive ataxia with onset usually before 25 years of age associated with depressed tendon reflexes, dysarthria, Babinski sign, and loss of position and vibration sense. About 25% of affected individuals have a presentation with later onset (age >25 years) with retained muscle stretch reflexes and marked cerebellar atrophy on MRI or unusually slow progression of disease.

2. **Ataxia telangiectasia (AT)** presents with progressive, childhood-onset, cerebellar dysfunction and oculomotor apraxia, frequent infections, choreoathetosis, telangiectasias of the conjunctivae, immunodeficiency, and an increased risk for malignancy, particularly leukemia and lymphoma.

3. **Ataxia with oculomotor apraxia type 1 (AOA1)** is characterized by childhood onset of slowly progressive cerebellar ataxia followed by oculomotor apraxia that progresses to external ophthalmoplegia associated with severe primary motor peripheral neuropathy and cognitive impairment. Hypoalbuminemia is observed on laboratory investigations.

4. **Ataxia with oculomotor apraxia type 2** presents with a similar phenotype as type 1, but age at onset is in the early teens and there is perhaps a lesser degree of certain features. In further contrast to type 1, laboratory studies show normal albumin and high serum α-fetoprotein concentrations.

5. **Autosomal-recessive mutations in polymerase γ-1 (POLG mutations)** are associated with a broad spectrum of CNS and systemic phenotypes, including a mitochondrial recessive ataxic syndrome characterized by cerebellar ataxia, nystagmus, dysarthria ophthalmoplegia, and frequently epilepsy, neuropathy, and dysarthria. Sporadic adult-onset ataxia is most frequently encountered in myoclonic epilepsy associated with ragged-red fibers, mitochondrial myopathy, encephalopathy, lactic acidosis, and stroke-like episodes (MELAS), and neuropathy, ataxia, and retinitis pigmentosa. Progressive external ophtalmoplegia might point toward the diagnosis of a mitochondrial cytopathy.

C. Associated neurologic signs.

Identifying additional neurologic signs in addition to features of cerebellar dysfunction (dysmetric and saccadic eye movements with nystagmus, dysarthria, a coarse kinetic tremor, dysdiadochokinesia, and a wide-based unstable gait) can provide powerful insight into potential causes of ataxia and dictate secondary investigations).

1. Ataxia and myelopathy.
   a. Structural or vascular pontocerebellar abnormalities
   b. Inflammatory CNS diseases
   c. Multiple sclerosis
   d. Superficial CNS siderosis
   e. Paraneoplastic syndromes
   f. Nutritional deficiencies (vitamin B_{12}, vitamin E, copper)
   g. Hereditary conditions including Alexander's disease, spastic paraplegia 7, autosomal-recessive spastic ataxia of Charlevoix–Saguenay (ARSACS), adult-onset FRDA, or SCA3

2. Ataxia and retinitis pigmentosa/vision loss
   a. Refsum disease
   b. Vitamin E deficiency
   c. SCA7.
   d. Mitochondrial disease
3. Ataxia and ocular apraxia
   a. AOA1
   b. AOA2
   c. Whipple's disease
   d. AT
4. Ataxia and chorea
   a. Huntington disease
   b. SCA17
   c. SCA1
   d. SCA2
   e. DRPLA
   f. AT
   g. AT type 2
   h. Neuroacanthocytosis syndromes
   i. Glucose transporter type 1 deficiency
5. Ataxia and tremor
   a. FTAX
   b. Wilson's disease
   c. SCA12
6. Ataxia and early cognitive impairment
   a. CJD
   b. GAD ataxia
   c. POLG mutations
   d. Ataxic variant of SREAT
   e. SCA17
7. Ataxia and parkinsonism
   a. SCA2
   b. SCA3
   c. SCA17
   d. SCA1
   e. MSA
8. Ataxia and polyneuropathy
   a. Late-onset Tay–Sachs disease
   b. CTX (axonal, demyelinating, or mixed)
   c. AT
   d. AOA2
   e. ARSACS (axonal or demyelinating)
   f. Refsum disease (demyelinating)
   g. POLG mutations (demyelinating)
   h. Late-onset Tay–Sachs disease
   i. Several ADSCs including SCA1, SCA2, SCA3, SCA4, SCA8, SCA12, and SCA18.
D. Brain MRI.

Brain MRI is required in the evaluation of all patients presenting with cerebellar ataxia to assess for cerebellar atrophy or structural lesions. MRI is also the method of choice to detect cerebellar malformations, such as Chiari malformation, which can be a cause of sporadic adult-onset ataxia. Global cerebellar atrophy is commonly seen in most causes of chronic inflammatory or degenerative ataxias. Additionally, severe other specific abnormalities can be seen with high-yield diagnostic values as described in previous sections and below (Fig. 29.1).

1. Cerebellar and cerebral white matter disease hyperintensities
   a. Metabolic leukodystrophies
   b. Alexander's disease
   c. POLG mutations

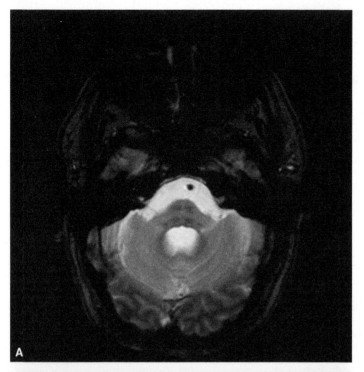

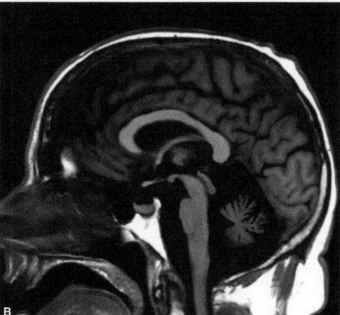

FIGURE 29.1 **A** shows the "hot-cross bun" sign consisting of a cruciform pattern of hyperintensity in the basis pontis visible on T2-weighted sequences in patients with MSA. **B** shows marked atrophy of the pons, middle cerebellar peduncles, and cerebellum in the same patient. **C** shows linear hypointensity on midbrain surface on T2-weighted sequences in a patient with superficial CNS siderosis. **D** illustrates moderate to severe cerebellar atrophy in a patient with ADCA. ADCA, autosomal-dominant ataxias; CNS, central nervous system; MSA, multiple system atrophy.

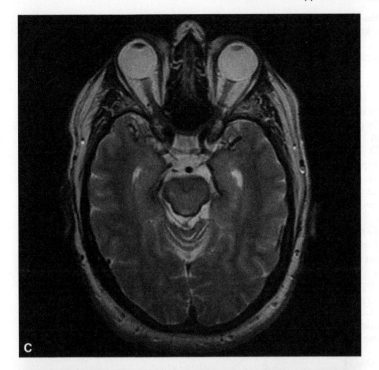

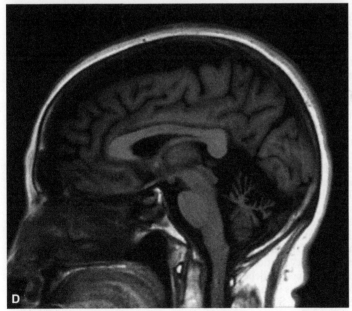

FIGURE 29.1 (*continued*)

    d. Langerhans histiocytosis
    e. Adrenoleukodystrophy
    f. CTX
2. Severe spinal cord atrophy
    a. FRDA
    b. Alexander's disease
3. In patients with suspected AR ataxia, MRI can stratify patients in different categories narrowing the differential and prompting specific testing.
    a. FRDA-like phenotype *without* cerebellar atrophy
        (1) FRDA
        (2) AVED
        (3) Abetalipoproteinemia
        (4) Refsum disease
    b. FRDA-like phenotype *with* cerebellar atrophy
        (1) Late-onset Tay–Sachs disease
        (2) CTX
        (3) POLG mutations
        (4) Spinocerebellar ataxia with axonal neuropathy
    c. Early-onset ataxia *with* cerebellar atrophy
        (1) AT
        (2) AOA type 1
        (3) AOA type 2
        (4) ARSACS
        (5) Infantile-onset spinocerebellar ataxia
        (6) Marinesco–Sjögren's syndrome

PRACTICAL APPROACH

A rational strategy for investigating potential etiologies and to dictate further testing is necessary when evaluating patients with cerebellar ataxia. Assessment should start discerning from other causes of unsteadiness including musculoskeletal conditions, vestibular or proprioceptive ataxia, or cognitive dysfunction. At initial visit, the diagnostic evaluation should be directed to in-depth assessment for acquired conditions with hierarchical selection of laboratory testing with focus on potentially treatable conditions. It is important to recognize that in the elderly, multifactorial disease is rather common. Alcohol consumption, exposure to possible toxic agents, chronic infections (including HIV), and history of current or prior malignancies should be obtained. Initial testing should include serum electrolytes and complete blood count, erythrocyte sedimentation rate, antinuclear antibody, Ds-DNA Abs, vitamin B_{12}, methylmalonic acid, homocysteine, thyroid-stimulating hormone, liver enzymes, parathyroid function, vitamin E levels, and serum copper to exclude common metabolic or inflammatory conditions in conjunction with brain MRI. Secondary investigations including lactate and pyruvate, antigliadin antibodies, transglutaminase 2 and 6 antibodies, TPO Abs, paraneoplastic panel, anti-GAD65 Abs, electromyogram/nerve conduction velocities studies, or CSF analysis should be considered based on clinical phenotype.

    Additionally, evaluation should focus on obtaining a detailed family history to determine if a hereditary ataxia is present and the suspected mode of inheritance particularly if initial investigations for acquired cases are unrevealing. Age of onset, temporal profile, and associated clinical findings are critical for evaluation. When considering testing for hereditary ataxias, genetic tests should be individualized depending on family history and clinical phenotype. If no acquired cause of the ataxia is identified, the probability is about 13% that the affected individual has SCA1, SCA2, SCA3, SCA6, SCA8, SCA17, or FRDA. If an AR cause of ataxia is possible, testing for elevated α-fetoprotein, serum cholestanol, hypoalbuminemia, or phytanic acid levels should be entertained. Finally, investigating for other rare causes of ataxia including muscle biopsy, CoQ10 in skeletal muscle, amino acids and organic acids in serum or CSF to exclude mitochondrial disease, CoQ10 deficiency, or inborn errors of metabolism can be considered. In cases of late-onset cerebellar ataxia that are found to lack a specific acquired or genetic etiology after complete evaluation, the diagnosis of idiopathic late-onset cerebellar ataxia should be entertained. Clinical exome sequencing is an evolving, newer diagnostic tool that can identify pathogenic gene variants in patients with unexplained ataxia but ancillary testing should be individualized based on clinical presentation.

Key Points

- The key features of cerebellar dysfunction include dysmetria and saccadic eye movements with nystagmus, dysarthria, action tremors, impaired coordination of targeted and rapid-alternating movements, and a wide-based unstable gait.
- Diagnostic evaluation of ataxia should always include assessment for acquired and causes as acquired and hereditary causes can coexist.
- Age of onset, symptom's temporal profile, and associated clinical findings are essential elements of ataxia evaluation.
- Brain MRI is required in all patients presenting with cerebellar ataxia to assess for cerebellar atrophy, structural lesions, and high-yield specific abnormalities.
- Initial testing should be individualized based on clinical presentation and aim to exclude common or treatable conditions followed by hereditary and neurodegenerative etiologies.

Recommended Readings

Fogel BL, Perlman S. An approach to the patient with late-onset cerebellar ataxia. *Nat Clin Pract Neurol.* 2006;2:629–635; quiz 621–635.

Fogel BL, Perlman S. Clinical features and molecular genetics of autosomal recessive cerebellar ataxias. *Lancet Neurol.* 2007;6:245–257.

Jayadev S, Bird TD. Hereditary ataxias: overview. *Genet Med.* 2013;15:673–683.

Klockgether T. Sporadic ataxia with adult onset: classification and diagnostic criteria. *Lancet Neurol.* 2010;9:94–104.

Koeppen AH. Friedreich's ataxia: pathology, pathogenesis, and molecular genetics. *J Neurol Sci.* 2011;303:1–12.

Paulson HL. The spinocerebellar ataxias. *J Neuroophthalmol.* 2009;29:227–237.

Ramirez-Zamora A, Zeigler W, Desai N, et al. Treatable causes of cerebellar ataxia. *Mov Disord.* 2015;30:614–623.

van Gaalen J, van de Warrenburg BP. A practical approach to late-onset cerebellar ataxia: putting the disorder with lack of order into order. *Pract Neurol.* 2012;12:14–24.

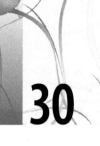

30 Approach to the Hypokinetic Patient

Ergun Y. Uc and Robert L. Rodnitzky

Hypokinesia is defined as a decrease in the amount and amplitude of both volitional and automatic movements and is almost always associated with *bradykinesia* (slowness of movement). The term *akinesia* is sometimes used to imply a severe reduction in the amount or amplitude of movement. *Parkinsonism* refers to a motor syndrome with the following cardinal features: bradykinesia, rigidity, rest tremor, and postural instability. Idiopathic Parkinson's disease (IPD) is the most common cause of *parkinsonism*. Other forms of *parkinsonism* are histologically different and often accompanied by additional neurologic signs and symptoms (Fig. 30.1).

Through careful questioning, clinicians can distinguish a history of neuromuscular weakness from a movement disorder causing parkinsonism such as IPD. It is also essential to determine whether slowness or lack of movement is caused by a psychiatric disorder (catatonia or severe depression), neuromuscular condition producing stiffness (e.g., stiff person syndrome), endocrine disorders such as hypothyroidism with resulting global slowing, or a rheumatologic condition such as ankylosing spondylitis with mechanical restriction of movements.

EVALUATION OF PARKINSONISM: HISTORY

A. **Direct motoric manifestations of parkinsonism.** What a patient perceives as weakness or poor balance may actually be a manifestation of hypokinesia. Conversely, slowness in performing motor functions such as dressing, walking, feeding, or writing may actually relate to incoordination, weakness, or dementia. Difficulty in rising from a chair, hesitancy in initiating gait, and a change in the legibility and size of handwriting, falls, freezing, hypophonia, and hypomimia are common symptoms of hypokinesia.

Bradykinesia (slowness of movement), rest tremor, stiffness (rigidity), and postural imbalance in the absence of other neurologic complaints suggest an IPD (Video 30.1). On the other hand, the association of hypokinesia/bradykinesia with neurologic symptoms outside the motor realm usually suggests a condition other than IPD. Such symptoms include seizures, sensory loss, paresthesias, headache, early dementia, visual loss, apraxia, and early or severe autonomic symptoms such as impotence, orthostatic hypotension, or urinary incontinence. Another useful historical fact in differentiating IPD from other forms of parkinsonism is the sequence in which otherwise typical parkinsonian symptoms appear. Although postural imbalance and severe gait disturbance often appear late in the course of IPD, their appearance as presenting symptoms in a hypokinetic patient suggest a different etiology of parkinsonism.

B. **Response to medications.** Absence of benefit from adequate dosages of dopaminergic drugs, especially levodopa, casts doubt on the diagnosis of IPD and suggests a diagnosis of secondary causes of parkinsonism or one of the Parkinson-plus syndromes. Equally important is determining whether, early in the illness, these medications produced psychiatric side effects such as hallucinations or autonomic symptoms such as severe orthostatic hypotension. The former suggest the possibility of dementia with Lewy bodies (DLB), and the latter indicate possible multiple-system atrophy (MSA). In IPD, psychiatric and autonomic side effects from dopaminergic drugs are not uncommon but usually appear when the illness is at least moderately advanced.

C. **Cognitive symptoms.** Even early in the course of the disease process, patients with IPD may have mild executive and visuospatial dysfunction. Dementia in IPD is largely related to cortical -synuclein deposits in the form of Lewy bodies and Lewy neurites, but cortical amyloid can also contribute to an already impaired patient. Frank dementia is more common

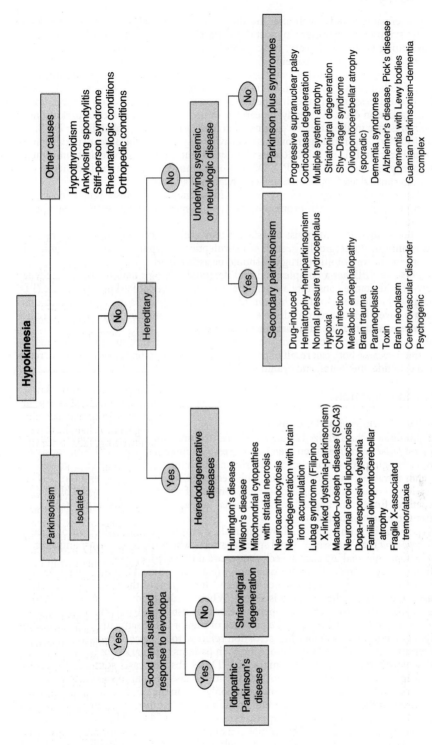

FIGURE 30.1 Algorithm for differential diagnosis of hypokinesia.

among older patients and usually after the illness is moderately advanced. Mild to moderate cognitive symptoms are present in most of the Parkinson-plus syndromes but are seldom the presenting symptom. Severe, early cognitive abnormalities may indicate a primary dementing disorder such as Alzheimer's disease (AD) or vascular dementia.

D. Psychiatric symptoms. Symptoms suggestive of depression or anxiety may precede the onset of IPD. If hallucinosis (typically visual) is present, determine if it began early or late in the course of the illness and whether it appeared in response to the institution or escalation of an anti-Parkinson drug. Very early appearance of hallucinations in cases of parkinsonism or their presence in an untreated parkinsonian patient raises the probability of DLB.

E. Sleep disorders. The rapid eye movement behavior may precede the onset of parkinsonism by several years in IPD or DLB. Restless legs syndrome and/or periodic limb movements of sleep may be associated with IPD. Discomfort because of rigidity and inability to turn in bed can cause sleep fragmentation (see Chapters 9 and 60).

F. Dysautonomia. Constipation, urinary urgency, impotence, and orthostasis may accompany or even precede IPD. When prominent early, and especially if severe, these symptoms may suggest MSA.

G. Medication usage. Patients must be asked if they are currently taking or have recently received antidopaminergic drugs such as neuroleptics, reserpine, or metoclopramide. In addition, any history of illicit drug use should be ascertained.

H. Family history. IPD has a complex and multifactorial etiology. Patients with Mendelian pattern of inheritance constitute a small minority of the overall Parkinson's disease (PD) population. Heritable disorders that can mimic PD include Wilson's disease (autosomal recessive), juvenile Huntington's disease (HD; autosomal dominant), and essential tremor (ET; autosomal dominant with variable penetrance).

I. Toxic exposure. Exposure to toxins such as manganese or carbon monoxide must be ascertained because both can result in parkinsonism. Less common causes include mercury, carbon disulfide, methanol, and cyanide.

PHYSICAL EXAMINATION

A. The clinical findings of parkinsonism.
   1. **Hypomimia** is characterized by diminished facial expression with infrequent eye blinking. *A fixed facial expression*, often seen in progressive supranuclear palsy (PSP), consists of an unchanging expression such as surprise in which the forehead may be furrowed, the eyelids retracted, and the nasolabial folds deepened. *Myerson's sign*, present in IPD and a variety of other basal ganglia disorders, consists of persistent reflex eyelid blinking to repetitive finger taps applied to the glabella, instead of the normal rapid habituation after the fourth or fifth tap.
   2. **Hypophonia** is characterized by diminished amplitude and inflection of speech. *Tachyphemia* is an excessively rapid speech pattern, which is a common accompaniment of hypophonia, making such speech even more unintelligible.
   3. **Rigidity** may be predominant in axial muscles (e.g., neck or trunk), in the limbs, or equally severe in both. Increased resistance to passive movement of the involved body part is easily appreciated when rigidity is severe. When subtle, rigidity can be reinforced by asking the patient to alternately open and close the fist of the hand on the side opposite of the arm or leg being tested. The presence of tremor in the same limb demonstrating rigidity gives rise to a rachet-like sensation referred to as *cogwheel rigidity*.
   4. **Tremor** may appear in one or more forms in patients with parkinsonism.
      a. **Resting tremor** is the hallmark of IPD. Its absence casts some doubt on the diagnosis but certainly does not rule it out. It is also present in some other forms of parkinsonism. The tremor is most commonly seen in the hands and to a slightly lesser extent in the lower extremities and mandible. **Rest tremor** rarely involves the head and never affects the voice. It appears at a frequency of 4 to 5 Hz and is often at least temporarily extinguished by volitional movement. A subtle tremor can be uncovered by asking the patient to perform difficult mental arithmetic, a mildly stressful task.
      b. **Action tremor** may also be present in IPD as well as in other parkinsonian syndromes, especially those associated with cerebellar dysfunction. It can be present as a *postural tremor* while the arms are outstretched in front of the patient or as a *kinetic tremor*

while the patient is performing a task such as the finger-to-nose test. Postural tremor alone, in the absence of parkinsonian signs, suggests a diagnosis of ET.

c. **Positional tremor.** Some tremors are particularly prominent when the involved body part is placed in a specific position. The *wing beating tremor* of Wilson's disease is an example of this phenomenon. This tremor is noted when the arms are abducted at the shoulders while flexed at the elbow.

5. **Bradykinesia** can be documented by simply observing the speed, amplitude, and amount of ordinary movements made by the patient such as gestures or shifting of body position. Repetitive motion tasks such as tapping the index finger against the thumb demonstrate slowness of movement and a progressive loss of amplitude.

6. **Impairment of automatic movements** is noticeable as a decrease in gesticulation and head movement during conversation, a reduction in the automatic repositioning of limbs while sitting in a chair or reclining in bed, and as a decrease in the amplitude of arm swing while walking. In severe hypokinesia, the affected arm(s) may not swing at all, but rather be held in a semiflexed posture across the trunk.

7. **Impairment of repetitive movements** such as handwriting or buttoning a shirt is not only performed slowly, but the amplitude of each successive movement typically becomes progressively smaller. This may account for the progressively smaller letters (micrographia) seen when a hypokinetic patient is asked to write a long sentence.

8. **Impaired initiation of movement** is manifested by difficulty in arising from a chair or hesitancy in taking the first step while attempting to walk. Many patients with IPD have difficulty initiating two motor acts simultaneously such as standing up and shaking hands. Rising from a chair is tested by asking the patient to rise with arms crossed in front of the body to prevent pushing off. The patient may require several attempts to succeed or may be totally unable to arise without using his arms. If the patient is unable to rise without assistance, a judgment must be made as to whether the cause is weakness (which can be tested independently).

9. **Gait and posture** should be evaluated by having the patient walk a distance of at least 20 feet in an area free from obstacles. Parkinsonian patients often display reduced stride length and arm swing, stooped posture, difficulty in initiating gait, and turns with the body moving as a single unit (en bloc). In more advanced cases, progressively more rapid, small steps as the body leans forward (festination) and "freezing" in midgait may be observed.

10. **Freezing** is a sudden involuntary cessation of a motoric act, usually walking, while other functions remain intact. This phenomenon is confined to basal ganglia disorders. It may occur spontaneously or may be provoked by external circumstances such as attempting to turn midgait or pass through a narrow space such as a doorway. Emotional stimuli including anger or fear can provoke freezing as can the prospect of entering a room filled with people. A variety of sensory or motor tricks such as marching to a cadence are effective in overcoming freezing.

11. **Postural reflexes** are evaluated by asking the patient to establish a comfortable base, with feet slightly apart and then, while standing behind the patient, applying a brisk backward sternal perturbation. A normal response is to take up to one corrective step backward to prevent falling. When postural reflexes are impaired, more than one step will be needed before balance is reestablished. When postural reflexes are absent, the patient will continue to reel backward and fall if not checked by the examiner.

B. Non-Parkinsonian neurologic signs. Several neurologic findings are associated with one or more forms of atypical parkinsonism, but most of these signs are uncommon in IPD.

1. **Apraxia** should be tested independently in both upper extremities. The patient should be asked to perform such tasks as saluting, throwing a kiss, or demonstrating how to use an imaginary tooth brush. Inability to perform these tasks in the face of normal strength and coordination, or the use of a body part such as a finger in place of an imagined implement, suggests apraxia. Apraxia and parkinsonism can be seen in cases of corticobasal degeneration (CBD) and AD.

2. **Cortical sensory functions** such as graphesthesia, stereognosis, and tactile localization are sometimes abnormal in CBD.

3. **The alien limb phenomenon** is present when a patient manifests uncontrollable grasping and manipulating of objects or when a hand exhibits interfering involuntary

movement with one of the other limbs (intermanual conflict). This phenomenon may be present in CBD, ischemic strokes, or Creutzfeldt–Jakob disease (CJD).

4. **Ocular motility abnormalities.** Inability to generate normal saccadic eye movements, especially downward, with preservation of the same movements when eliciting the oculocephalic reflex, indicates a *supranuclear gaze palsy*. This finding is most characteristic of PSP but can be found in other forms of atypical parkinsonism as well. It is important to remember that limited upgaze is not an uncommon finding in the normal elderly patient, but impaired downgaze is always abnormal. Excessive *macro square wave jerks* and spontaneous repetitive small horizontal oscillations of the eyes from the midline are also seen in PSP.

5. **Reflex myoclonus,** elicited by tapping the arm, leg, or fingertip with the examiner's own fingertip or with a percussion hammer, may be present in cases of CBD.

6. **Blood pressure** must be measured in the recumbent and standing positions while recording the concurrent heart rate. Orthostatic hypotension is an early and common manifestation of MSA but occurs later in the course of IPD, especially with the use of dopaminergic or anticholinergic drugs.

7. **Mental status evaluation.** Evaluation should include functions such as immediate and short-term recall, orientation, constructional praxis, calculation, and comprehension of three-step commands.

8. **Other neurologic signs.** To determine the full extent of involvement of the central nervous system (CNS), a complete neurologic examination should be performed to establish the presence of hyperactive or hypoactive muscle stretch reflexes, sensory loss, cranial nerve dysfunction, cerebellar signs, pathologic reflexes (especially Babinski's sign), weakness, or muscle atrophy.

LABORATORY STUDIES

A. **Neuroimaging.**
   1. **IPD.** In classical IPD where the diagnosis is strongly suggested by the history and physical examination, neuroimaging is not necessary. IPD is commonly asymmetric, but if symptoms or signs of parkinsonism are remarkably asymmetric resulting in severe involvement on one side and virtually no involvement on the other, a CNS imaging study, preferably magnetic resonance imaging (MRI), is indicated to evaluate for the possibility of unilateral structural basal ganglia pathology such as a neoplasm, arteriovenous malformation, infarction, or the presence of brain hemiatrophy.
   2. **Other forms of parkinsonism.** In patients with insufficient findings to make a diagnosis of IPD (e.g., a patient with hypokinesia only) or with additional neurologic findings not usually seen in IPD, a brain imaging procedure is indicated, preferably an MRI. Not all degenerative forms of parkinsonism are associated with demonstrable MRI abnormalities and those that are may demonstrate the characteristic abnormality infrequently or only in the advanced stages of the illness (see **Section C under Diagnostic Approach**). Therefore, a normal MRI or computed tomography (CT) scan of the brain does not rule out syndromes such as PSP or MSA but does usually rule out normal pressure hydrocephalus (NPH), brain tumor, or stroke.

B. **Laboratory and genetic tests** are not useful in establishing a diagnosis of IPD except in few genetic forms, but can be of benefit in diagnosing several other causes of parkinsonism (see **Section G under Diagnostic Approach**).

DIFFERENTIAL DIAGNOSIS

A. **IPD.** This is the most common cause of parkinsonism with a prevalence 0.2% and increasing with age (4% among those patients older than 80 years). IPD is a degenerative disorder of unknown but probable multifactorial etiology, with genetics likely conferring susceptibility to the effects of the environment and aging in most cases. More than 10 mutations (e.g., *Parkin, PINK1, LRRK2*) with Mendelian pattern of inheritance have been identified, leading to an IPD picture ranging from young onset with some atypical features to typical presentation and course in old age. Yet, patients with single-gene disorders constitute a small minority of the overall PD population. Consideration of single-gene inheritance is most important in young-onset patients. Metabolic dysfunction of mitochondrial complex I has been demonstrated in PD, whether acquired or hereditary. The predominant abnormality is in the substantia nigra pars compacta and nigrostriatal pathway leading to dopamine deficiency in the striatum. The wide spectrum of symptoms and the resistance of some nonmotor symptoms (such as depression, sleep disorders, cognitive impairment, and autonomic dysfunction) to levodopa support the pathologic observations that the degenerative process also involves other brainstem nuclei and subcortical structures.

1. **Clinical.** The cardinal symptoms are resting tremor, bradykinesia, rigidity, and impairment of postural reflexes. The onset is usually asymmetric, and tremor is the most common presenting sign. Postural instability, gait difficulty, and dysautonomia appear with progression of the disease. Depending on the age of the cohort and follow-up period, 30% to 78% of patients have been reported to develop dementia, but it is seldom severe and is never a presenting symptom. The incidence of an IPD increases sharply with age, although it can present at any age. Arbitrarily, patients with onset between ages 21 and 39 are classified as young-onset IPD. They exhibit a more gradual progression of symptoms and are more likely to experience dystonia as an early sign. Levodopa-induced dyskinesias and motor fluctuations that can occur in IPD at any age are more frequently observed in this age group. The differential diagnosis of juvenile parkinsonism (before the age of 21) is broad and includes hereditary and metabolic conditions.

2. **Neuroimaging.** MRI and CT of the brain are usually unremarkable in IPD. A positron-emission tomography (PET) scan shows decreased fluorodopa uptake in the striatum but no striatal abnormality in fluorodeoxyglucose scans. Single photon emission computed tomography (SPECT) shows decreased dopamine transporter density, although it must be kept in mind that some other forms of parkinsonism, such as MSA and PSP, can also result in an abnormal SPECT scan.

3. **Neuropathology.** Lewy bodies (eosinophilic intra cytoplasmic inclusions), mainly in the substantia nigra, are the pathologic hallmark of this disorder. In IPD, these inclusions stain for alpha-synuclein, the protein produced by the mutant gene in the rare autosomal-dominant form of PD.

4. **Other tests.** There is no specific test for the diagnosis of IPD.

B. **Secondary parkinsonism.** Parkinsonism can be induced by a wide spectrum of disease processes affecting the brain, especially the basal ganglia. These include infection, cerebrovascular disorders, toxins, metabolic disorders, trauma, neoplasm, drugs, hypoxemia, and hydrocephalus. Selected causes include the following:

1. **Drug-induced parkinsonism.** Neuroleptics and metoclopramide block striatal D-2 dopamine receptors, whereas reserpine depletes dopamine from presynaptic vesicles. Each of these drugs can result in motoric symptoms indistinguishable from IPD. The "atypical" neuroleptic clozapine mainly blocks extrastriatal (D-4) receptors and does not cause parkinsonism; quetiapine also seems to have a low potential to cause this adverse effect. Other atypical neuroleptics, such as risperidone, olanzapine, and aripiprazole, can cause parkinsonism. An underlying predisposition to PD may be in part responsible for the emergence of this syndrome. The resolution of drug-induced parkinsonism may take several months after discontinuation of the offending medication.

   a. **Neuroimaging.** SPECT scan of the dopamine transporter protein is very useful in distinguishing drug-induced parkinsonism from IPD in that SPECT is normal in the former condition.

2. **Normal pressure hydrocephalus.**

   a. **Clinical.** This is a form of communicating hydrocephalus. Approximately one-third of patients with this disorder have a history of spontaneous or traumatic subarachnoid hemorrhage or meningitis. Although, as measured by lumbar puncture, the cerebrospinal fluid (CSF) pressure is normal, there is excessive force on the walls of the dilated lateral ventricles, especially the frontal horn, leading to the compression of surrounding structures. The clinical triad of NPH consists of gait apraxia (magnetic gait), subcortical dementia (which may later include cortical features), and urinary incontinence, often appearing late in the illness. The hesitant gait may resemble that seen in IPD, but the absence of rest tremor, the appearance of incontinence, and the absence of significant benefit from levodopa allow the two conditions to be distinguished. Early recognition of this syndrome is important because in some cases shunting the ventricles can reverse it (see Chapter 8).

b. **Neuroimaging.** Enlarged lateral ventricles, especially the frontal and lateral horns, which are disproportionate to cortical atrophy, are seen. A proton density MRI demonstrates periventricular hyperintensity suggesting transependymal flow.

c. **Other tests.** Fisher's test consists of removing 30 to 50 cc of CSF and observing for improvement in symptoms over the next 24 hours. It is a useful test and does not require sophisticated laboratory techniques. Intracranial pressure monitoring allows demonstration of periods of high CSF pressure (b-waves) and is used widely as a predictor of response to shunting.

3. **Hemiatrophy–hemiparkinsonism.** These patients present at a relatively early age with markedly asymmetric parkinsonism affecting the side of their body manifesting hemiatrophy. They may have a history of abnormal birth and contralateral hemisphere hemiatrophy, both of which raise the possibility of an early childhood brain insult, which later in life manifests as delayed-onset parkinsonism. The slow progression of this disorder, its occasional association with dystonia, and the striking asymmetry form the basis of its distinction from IPD.

4. **Toxins.**

   a. **Carbon monoxide (CO).** Acute or chronic CO poisoning causes globus pallidus or striatal necrosis. The onset of parkinsonism can be immediate after the incident, but more commonly develops days to weeks after an initial recovery from coma. Response to levodopa is poor or absent.

   b. *Manganese* intoxication can result in a parkinsonian state, and in addition is often associated with unusual behavioral symptoms such as hallucinations and emotional lability or other movement disorders such as dystonia.

   c. *Cyanide* and *methanol* intoxication can also cause bilateral basal ganglia necrosis and parkinsonism.

5. **Cerebrovascular disease.** Either a lacunar state with multiple small infarcts of the basal ganglia or subacute arteriosclerotic encephalopathy affecting basal ganglia connections can lead to parkinsonism. In either condition, dementia is also common. Resting tremor is usually absent in these patients. Gait disorder can be very prominent and occasionally constitutes the only neurologic symptom, giving rise to the term "lower-body parkinsonism." The response to levodopa is limited, but occasional patients do show benefit.

10. **Trauma.** Pugilistic encephalopathy is a progressive neurologic syndrome characterized by parkinsonism, dementia, and ataxia. It is seen in boxers with a history of repeated head trauma. Treatment is usually unsatisfactory.

   Focal acute injury to the midbrain and substantia nigra and subdural hematoma are two other possible causes of posttraumatic parkinsonism.

C. **Parkinson-plus syndromes.** This is a group of parkinsonian syndromes distinguished from IPD by the presence of additional prominent neurologic abnormalities. In these conditions, there may be cerebellar, autonomic, pyramidal, oculomotor, cortical sensory, bulbar, cognitive, and psychiatric dysfunction, as well as apraxia and movement disorders not typically seen in untreated IPD such as myoclonus, dystonia, or chorea. Any of these neurologic or psychiatric abnormalities can appear early in the course of the illness. Early falls with gait disturbance or postural instability, absence of resting tremor, early dementia, and supranuclear gaze palsy are signs that should always prompt consideration of a Parkinson-plus syndrome. The parkinsonian components of these disorders such as akinesia and rigidity are usually not responsive to levodopa, although early transient responsiveness can be observed. The onset of these diseases is generally in the fifth or sixth decade of life with average survival of 5 to 10 years. The cause of death is usually pneumonia, other intercurrent infections, or sepsis. The etiology of this entire group of disorders is largely unknown.

   Despite the apparent clinical differences between IPD and the Parkinson-plus syndromes, differentiation between the two can be difficult. In a clinicopathologic study, 24% of patients who were clinically diagnosed with IPD were found to have a different type of parkinsonism at autopsy. In Parkinson-plus syndromes, the brain MRI can occasionally be helpful. An electroencephalogram (EEG) may show nonspecific abnormalities such as slowing of the background activity. The specific clinical and imaging features of individual Parkinson-plus syndromes are described below. Although each of these conditions has characteristic clinical findings, it is important to remember that there is significant overlap in signs and symptoms among them.

1. PSP.
   a. Clinical. Early onset of gait difficulty, loss of postural reflexes resulting in backward falls, and freezing of gait, coupled with supranuclear gaze palsy (initially downgaze), are suggestive of PSP. Axial rigidity and nuchal dystonia with extensor posture of the neck, generalized bradykinesia, "apraxia" of eyelid opening and closing, blepharospasm, a furrowed forehead leading to a fixed facial expression, and a monotonous, but not hypophonic voice are additional features suggesting the diagnosis. There is variable, but often mild, cognitive decline, especially in executive functions. The presence of prominent bradykinesia in association with the fixed facial expression raises the possible diagnosis of IPD in these patients, but the ocular motility abnormalities, the early gait instability, the frequent absence of tremor, and the absence or loss of levodopa response suggest the correct diagnosis.
   b. Neuroimaging. Midbrain and, later, pontine atrophy are sometimes apparent on MRI.
   c. Neuropathology. PSP is a tauopathy. Globose neurofibrillary tangles composed of tau filaments are present affecting mainly the cholinergic neurons of the basal ganglia and brainstem nuclei with apparent sparing of the cortex.
2. CBD.
   a. Clinical. More recently, this has often been referred to as **cortical basal syndrome**, to emphasize the point that different pathologies, most notable PSP, can result in a nearly identical clinical syndrome, which can only be determined at autopsy. This syndrome can present as a strikingly asymmetric or unilateral akinetic-rigid syndrome associated with limb apraxia, alien limb phenomenon, cortical sensory signs, stimulus sensitive myoclonus, dystonia, and postural or action tremor. Supranuclear gaze palsy, cognitive impairment, and pyramidal tract signs can also be seen.
   b. Neuroimaging. MRI or CT of the brain is abnormal in some patients and reveals asymmetric frontoparietal atrophy.
   c. Neuropathology. CBD is also a tauopathy. Neuronal loss and gliosis are found in the frontoparietal regions and substantia nigra pars compacta. Swollen achromatic neurons and basophilic nigral inclusions, which represent an overlap with Pick's disease, are characteristic. Abundant cytoplasmic inclusions consisting of aggregated hyperphosphorylated tau protein are found.
3. MSA.
   a. Clinical. Sporadic, progressive disease in adults (onset after 30 years of age) characterized by autonomic failure, including urinary incontinence (with erectile dysfunction in men), or an orthostatic decrease in blood pressure by at least 30 mm Hg systolic or 15 mm Hg diastolic within 3 minutes of standing, plus one of the following:
      (1) Parkinsonism (slowness of movements, rigidity, and tendency to fall) with poor response to levodopa (parkinsonian subtype [MSA-P]). MSA-P was referred to as striatonigral degeneration before.
      (2) A cerebellar syndrome (wide-based gait, uncoordinated limb movements, action tremor, and nystagmus) (cerebellar subtype [MSA-C]). MSA-C was referred to as olivopontocerebellar atrophy before.
         From a diagnostic point of view, MSA should always be suspected in the hypokinetic patient with little response to levodopa who also manifests prominent autonomic or cerebellar dysfunction.
   b. Neuroimaging. MRI of the brain shows putaminal hypointensity in MSA-P, probably because of excessive iron deposition in this structure. Cerebellar atrophy can be seen in MSA-C.
   c. Neuropathology. Common to all the MSA syndromes is the presence of characteristic glial cytoplasmic inclusions. Like Lewy bodies seen in IPD, these inclusions stain for the protein alpha-synuclein. Especially in SDS, additional neuronal loss and gliosis are seen in the structures responsible for autonomic functions such as the intermediolateral cell column of the spinal cord and the dorsal motor nucleus of the vagus.

(1) **Dementia syndromes.** AD, Pick's disease, and DLB are degenerative CNS disorders whose predominant manifestation is dementia. Familial frontotemporal dementia and parkinsonism linked to chromosome 17 (FTDP-17) are associated with mutations in the tau gene. Although the degenerative process in these disorders has a predilection for certain cortical regions, subcortical structures may also be involved leading to extrapyramidal manifestations including parkinsonism. The key to identifying a primary dementing disorder as a cause of parkinsonism is the early appearance of dementia, often antedating the onset of parkinsonism (e.g., dementia occurs before or within 1 year after the onset of parkinsonism in DLB).

D. Heredodegenerative diseases.

1. Wilson's disease. An autosomal-recessive condition associated with impairment of copper excretion caused by a genetic defect in a copper-transporting ATPase, resulting in copper accumulation in different organ systems including the CNS, liver (cirrhosis), cornea (Kayser–Fleischer ring), heart, and kidney.

   a. Clinical. The age of presentation ranges from 5 to 50, peaking between 8 and 16. Neurologic symptoms are present at the onset of the disease in about 40% of patients. Extrapyramidal symptoms such as dystonia, rigidity, and bradykinesia are more common in children, whereas tremor and dysarthria are more likely to appear in adults. A variety of psychiatric symptoms can be seen in Wilson's disease. An especially important clue to the diagnosis is the presence of liver dysfunction such as cirrhosis or chronic active hepatitis, especially in a young patient. The combination of bradykinesia and tremor in these patients may suggest PD, but the very young age of onset, and the presence of psychiatric symptoms, liver dysfunction, or dystonia should prompt a search for laboratory signs of Wilson's disease. As the consequences of Wilson's disease are preventable and the neurologic symptoms are reversible with early treatment using copper chelating drugs, this condition should always be kept in the differential diagnosis of atypical parkinsonism, especially that appearing below the age of 50.

   b. Neuroimaging. MRI of the brain shows ventricular dilation as well as cortical and brainstem atrophy. The basal ganglia, especially the putamen, may appear either hypo- or hyperintense on T2-weighted studies, and hypodense on CT examinations. Occasionally, there is the characteristic "face of the giant panda" appearance of the midbrain on MRI studies.

   c. Neuropathology. There is generalized brain atrophy. The putamen, globus pallidus, and caudate nucleus are cavitated and display a brownish pigmentation reflecting copper deposition.

   d. Other tests. Plasma ceruloplasmin is the most useful screening test and is usually below 20 mg/dL (normal: 25 to 45 mg/dL). Plasma copper is decreased and 24-hour urinary copper excretion is increased. Slit lamp examination of the cornea reveals Kayser–Fleischer ring in almost all neurologically symptomatic patients and represents a very specific but not pathognomonic finding. If one or more of these tests are normal and the diagnosis is in doubt, it should be confirmed by liver biopsy that shows increased copper content. Because of abundance of disease-specific mutations and their location at multiple sites across the genome, genetic diagnosis is limited to kindreds of known patients.

2. HD. A relentlessly progressive autosomal-dominant disorder characterized by dementia, psychiatric disturbance, and a variety of movement disorders.

   a. Clinical. The major clinical components of HD are cognitive decline, various psychiatric abnormalities (personality changes, depression, mania, and psychosis), and movement disorder. Although chorea is the most common motoric symptom, bradykinesia usually coexists with chorea and may explain the occasional exacerbation of the motor impairment when control of the chorea is attempted with antidopaminergic medications. An abnormality of saccadic eye movement, particularly slow saccades, is often one of the earliest neurologic signs of this disorder. The typical age of onset is in the fourth or fifth decade, but 10% of the patients develop symptoms before age 20 (juvenile Huntington's). Successive generations may develop symptoms at a progressively earlier age, especially if they have inherited the disease from their father, reflecting the genetic phenomenon of anticipation. The juvenile form presents with a combination of a progressive akinetic-rigid syndrome (Westphal's variant), dementia, ataxia, and seizures. It is these akinetic-rigid patients that are most likely to be confused with IPD, but the autosomal-dominant inheritance pattern, the early age of onset, and the presence of seizures should suggest the correct diagnosis. The duration of illness from onset to death is about 15 years for adult-onset HD and 8 to 10 years for those with onset in childhood.

   b. **Neuroimaging.** Atrophy of the head of the caudate is the principal finding on neuroimaging. It can be appreciated on either MRI or CT scan.

   c. **Neuropathology.** There is loss of medium spiny striatal neurons, as well as gliosis in cortex and striatum (particularly the caudate). This striatal neuronal loss accounts for the drastic decrease in the two neurotransmitters associated with these cells, -aminobutyric acid, and enkephalin.

   d. Other tests. HD can be diagnosed and presymptomatic individuals can be identified with great certainty using DNA testing. The genetic abnormality has been localized to chromosome 4 and consists of an expansion of the usual number of repeats of the trinucleotide sequence CAG. The presence of 40 or more CAG repeats confirms the diagnosis of HD. Reduced penetrance is seen with 36 to 39 CAG repeats. Because of the ethical, legal, and psychological implications of presymptomatic predictive testing, it should only be carried out by a team of clinicians and geneticists fully sensitive to these issues and aware of published guidelines.

3. **Other neurologic conditions,** occasionally associated with parkinsonism, include neuroacanthocytosis, neurodegeneration with brain iron accumulation (NBIA, formerly known as Hallervorden–Spatz syndrome), Machado–Joseph disease (spinocerebellar ataxia type 3), Fragile X-associated tremor/ataxia syndrome (FXTAS), and familial calcification of the basal ganglia.

DIAGNOSTIC APPROACH

A. **Clinical.** Careful history taking and physical examination are essential. A meticulous survey of the past medical and psychiatric history, family history, and occupational or environmental exposure to toxins will reveal most causes of secondary parkinsonism. Disease onset at a young age, a strong family history of the same disorder, lack of resting tremor, absent response to levodopa and early appearance of postural instability, gait disorder, dysautonomia, or dementia should be considered red flags in the history suggesting a diagnosis other than IPD. The general physical examination is important because it may reveal signs of a systemic disease that is contributing to secondary parkinsonism. Neurologic examination establishes whether parkinsonism is isolated or associated with involvement of other neuronal systems in the CNS. The presence of aphasia, apraxia, supranuclear gaze palsy, cortical sensory loss, alien limb phenomenon, pyramidal signs, lower-motor neuron findings, myoclonus, chorea, or dystonia indicates more widespread CNS involvement than is the case in IPD.

B. **General laboratory tests.**

1. **CBC and peripheral blood smear.** Acanthocytes are found on a fresh peripheral blood smear in neuroacanthocytosis. A low hemoglobin level and elevated reticulocyte count consistent with hemolytic anemia may be present in Wilson's disease.

2. Blood chemistry. Abnormal liver function tests may be found in Wilson's disease. Hypocalcemia, hypomagnesemia, and a low parathormone level are present in hypoparathyroidism. Elevated creatine kinase is associated with neuroacanthocytosis, and elevated serum lactate, suggesting lactic acidosis, is found in mitochondrial cytopathies. Low thyroxin and high thyroid-stimulating hormone (TSH) levels point to hypothyroidism.

3. **Serology.** Elevated ESR, C-reactive protein, or rheumatoid factor may be found in inflammatory or rheumatologic conditions. Antibodies against glutamic acid decarboxylase are present in stiff person syndrome.

C. **Radiology.**

1. **Plain X-rays.** Spine X-rays may reveal ankylosing spondylitis or osteoarthritis as the cause of mechanical limitation of movement.

2. **CT or MRI of the brain.** CT may demonstrate a neoplasm, stroke, hydrocephalus, basal ganglia calcification, atrophy, or sequelae of trauma. It has some limitations, in that the

resolution is not always adequate to evaluate density changes or storage materials in the basal ganglia, and brainstem or cerebellar cuts may suffer from bone artifact (see Chapter 35). In these circumstances, an MRI of the brain is more desirable. Several characteristic MRI patterns that are suggestive of specific hypokinetic disorders are listed below:

a. **Many lacunar strokes.** vascular parkinsonism
b. Large ventricles, out of proportion to cerebral atrophy; transependymal flow: NPH
c. **Caudate atrophy.** HD
d. **Decreased T2 signal in striatum.** MSA
e. Homogeneous decreased T2 signal or decreased T2 signal with a central hyperintensity (Tiger's eye) in the globus pallidus: NBIA
f. **Striatal necrosis.** Wilson's disease, Leigh's disease, and CO intoxication
g. **Midbrain atrophy.** PSP
h. **Asymmetric frontoparietal atrophy.** CBGD

3. PET or SPECT. With modern analysis techniques, fluorodeoxyglucose PET, by characterizing the regional cerebral metabolism pattern, can distinguish PD, MSA, and PSP from one another with >90% accuracy. These techniques are not readily available at many hospitals, however. The status of nigral dopaminergic neurons can be determined using fluorodopa PET or $[I^{123}]$FP-CIT (Ioflupane) SPECT. In IPD, either of these two modalities demonstrates a loss of dopaminergic nigral cells. Although both of these techniques identify nigral dopaminergic dysfunction, they do not clearly differentiate between IPD and other causes of parkinsonism such as MSA, PSP, and CBD. The major clinical usefulness of Ioflupane SPECT is that it is very accurate in distinguishing IPD from mimicking conditions that do not involve dopamine-producing cells such as ET, dystonic tremor, or drug-induced parkinsonism. Of additional importance, SPECT imaging equipment is available at many hospitals.

D. Electrophysiology.

1. ECG. Heart block may be present in mitochondrial cytopathy.
2. EEG. Epileptic activity or focal slowing may appear with focal lesions (stroke and tumor). Slow background activity is seen in some primary dementias. Periodic triphasic complexes may be present in CJD (see Chapter 36).
3. EMG/nerve conduction studies. Mild nerve conduction slowing suggestive of axonal polyneuropathy is seen in neuroacanthocytosis. Myopathic findings on EMG (see Chapter 36) may be present in cases of mitochondrial cytopathies.

E. Neuropsychological testing. If there is clinical suspicion of dementia, formal testing should be employed to plot the profile of cognitive decline (see Chapter 4).

F. CSF analysis. Elevated protein and pleocytosis can be detected in CNS infections. The presence of high levels of the 14-3-3 protein in CSF is highly suggestive of CJD (see Chapter 36). A large volume of CSF can be removed (Fisher's test) with observation for improvement in neurologic signs as one means of corroborating the diagnosis of NPH.

G. Special diagnostic tests.

1. Wilson's disease. Low ceruloplasmin, low serum copper, increased 24-hour urinary copper excretion, and Kayser–Fleischer ring on slit lamp examination of the cornea are all suggestive of Wilson's disease. Liver biopsy for copper content is performed only if the diagnosis is in question.
2. NPH. Intracranial pressure monitoring shows episodic appearance of high-pressure waves.

H. Genetic testing. Monogenic PD is found in approximately 3% of IPD patients and mutations in these PD genes are most common in those with an early age of onset or those belonging to certain ethnic groups. Commercial testing is available for *LRRK2*, *PINK1*, *DJ-1*, *SNCA* (alpha-synuclein), *GBA* (glucocerebrosidase), and *Parkin* genes. In patients with onset before age 51, almost 20% have a mutation in one of these genes, most commonly *Parkin*, followed by *LRRK2*. The mutation rate is still higher for those with onset prior to age 30. In individuals developing PD under the age of 20, as many as 77% have a mutation of the *Parkin* gene. Jewish PD patients are more likely to harbor a mutation of the *GBA* gene. Although genetic testing does not affect patient management, it can clarify prognosis and allow genetic counseling. Genetic testing is also increasingly more available for other conditions where parkinsonism can be a clinical component of the overall syndrome such as HD, FXTAS, SCA3, and other SCA subtypes, dystonia subtypes, and various mitochondrial conditions.

I. **Therapeutic trial.** A brisk and unequivocal beneficial response to a trial of levodopa therapy is strongly suggestive of IPD. It must be kept in mind, however, that in some of the Parkinson-plus syndromes there can be a positive response, although seldom remarkable, frequently only present with large doses, and often not persistent over time.

WHEN TO REFER

Patients with new-onset hypokinesia who have the following characteristics are less likely to have IPD and would benefit from referral to a movement disorders specialist:

A. Early onset, for example, before 50 years of age
B. Early gait difficulty and postural instability
C. Prominent dementia
D. A family history of parkinsonism
E. Supranuclear gaze palsy
F. Apraxia, alien limb phenomenon, cortical sensory loss, myoclonus, marked asymmetry of neurologic involvement
G. Bulbar, cerebellar, or pyramidal dysfunction
H. Marked dysautonomia
I. Absent, limited, or unsustained response to levodopa.

Key Points

- IPD is the most common cause of hypokinesia.
- Aside from IPD, the differential diagnosis of hypokinesia includes the Parkinson-plus syndromes, NPH, fragile X tremor ataxia syndrome, some spinocerebellar ataxia syndromes, Wilson's disease, and (especially juvenile) Huntington's disease.
- In addition to hypokinesia, IPD is characterized by rigidity, rest tremor, loss of postural reflexes, and a great number of nonmotor features including, but not limited to, autonomic dysfunction, depression, dementia, and sleep disorders.
- SPECT imaging of the dopamine transporter is very useful in establishing a diagnosis of non–drug-induced parkinsonism, but not in distinguishing IPD from Parkinson-plus syndromes.
- Genetic analysis of patients with hypokinesia is becoming increasingly important and more available in the case of IPD, especially in those patients with a very young age at onset or a strong family history. It is extremely important for the evaluation of spinocerebellar ataxia syndromes, Huntington's disease, dystonia, and fragile X tremor ataxia syndrome.
- An unequivocal and lasting response to levodopa therapy is generally an important feature that distinguishes IPD from most other conditions presenting with hypokinesia.

Recommended Readings

Clarke CE. Parkinson's disease. *BMJ*. 2007;335(7617):441–445.

de Lau LM, Breteler MM. Epidemiology of Parkinson's disease. *Lancet Neurol*. 2006;5(6):525–535.

Fahn S, Oakes D, Shoulson I, et al. Levodopa and the progression of Parkinson's disease. *N Engl J Med*. 2004;351(24):2498–2508.

Fanciulli A, Wenning GK. Multiple-system atrophy. *N Engl J Med*. 2015;372(14):1375–1376.

Klein C, Djarmati A. Parkinson disease: genetic testing in Parkinson disease-who should be assessed? *Nat Rev Neurol*. 2011;7(1):7–9.

Lee SE, Rabinovici GD, Mayo MC, et al. Clinicopathologic correlations in corticobasal degeneration. *Ann Neurol*. 2011;70(2):327–340.

Poewe W, Mahlknecht P. The clinical progression of Parkinson's disease. *Parkinsonism Relat Disord*. 2009;15(4):S28–S32.

Uc EY, Rizzo M, Anderson SW, et al. Visual dysfunction in Parkinson disease without dementia. *Neurology*. 2005;65(12):1907–1913.

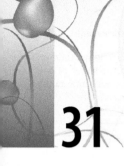

31

Approach to the Patient with Acute Muscle Weakness

Holli A. Horak

Muscular weakness implies lack or diminution of muscle strength, which leads to an inability to perform the usual function of a given muscle or group of muscles. Muscle weakness should be differentiated from fatigue, which is a subjective perception of being "weak." In other words, weakness is the objective evidence of lack of strength, and fatigue is a subjective symptom. After the existence of "true" weakness is established, an etiologic search should be conducted. Muscular weakness has diverse causes. This chapter emphasizes the diagnostic evaluation of the leading neurologic causes of acute weakness involving the peripheral nervous system (PNS).

EVALUATION

A. **History.** Determine the onset, course, and distribution of weakness and any associated neurologic findings (such as sensory symptoms, which implies a peripheral nerve disorder rather than muscle). Ask if there is a history of recent febrile illness, change of medications, or exposure to toxic agents. Ask the patient if he/she has had prior episodes of weakness or if there is a family history of muscle disease.

B. **General physical examination.** Examine the skin for evidence of dermatomyositis (DM)-associated skin changes (Gottron papules, heliotrope rash). Evaluate the patient for thyroid enlargement and ocular proptosis, assessing for hyperthyroidism. Evaluate the respiratory system, including neuromuscular parameters such as cough and ability to count up to 30 during exhalation. More objective measurements are "bedside" forced vital capacity (FVC) and negative inspiratory force (NIF).

C. **Neurologic examination.** The neurologic examination focusing on the muscular system is highlighted.

1. **Distribution of weakness.**
   a. **Proximal symmetric muscle weakness** is usually found among patients with primary muscle diseases such as polymyositis (PM) or DM or occasionally in patients with acute polyradiculoneuropathy, such as the Guillain–Barré syndrome (GBS).
   b. **Proximal asymmetric muscle weakness** occurs among patients with nerve root trauma or acute brachial or lumbosacral plexopathies.
   c. **Distal symmetric muscle weakness** is rarely acute but may be seen with GBS or a subacute onset of chronic inflammatory demyelinating polyneuropathy.
   d. Predominantly **distal asymmetric muscle weakness** occurs in patients with acute mononeuropathy such as foot drop secondary to peroneal nerve palsy. Mononeuritis multiplex (vasculitis of the PNS) manifests as a multifocal asymmetric peripheral weakness. Focal weakness also occurs with anterior horn cell involvement such as acute anterior poliomyelitis.
   e. **Acute diffuse muscle weakness** is found among patients with rhabdomyolysis, GBS, myasthenia gravis (MG), periodic paralysis, or tick paralysis.

2. **Muscular findings.**
   a. **Muscle bulk** is decreased in chronic neuromuscular diseases, such as muscular dystrophy, motor neuron disease (MND), or chronic neuropathy. Muscle bulk is usually normal during the acute stage of PM, MG, or acute demyelinating polyneuropathy (such as GBS).
   b. **Muscle tone** is often normal in patients with muscle (PM) or neuromuscular junction diseases (MG). Tone is decreased (flaccid) in disorders of nerves such as MND and GBS.

    c. **Key muscle examination** can aid in narrowing the differential. For example, neck flexor and extensor muscles are compromised early in both MG and PM.

    d. **Muscle stretch reflexes** are normal in patients with neuromuscular junction disease or primary muscle disease and are diminished or absent in patients with acute polyneuropathies such as GBS.

3. Sensory features.

    Sensory symptoms occur among patients with peripheral nerve dysfunction: polyneuropathy (GBS) or plexopathy. Sensory examination is normal among patients with primary muscle disease, MND, or neuromuscular junction disease.

4. Pain.

    Pain is not the same as sensory loss or sensory disturbance. Pain typically indicates inflammation in acute muscle weakness. Pain is often present in rhabdomyolysis, less so in PM, and rarely present in MG.

DIFFERENTIAL DIAGNOSIS

A useful approach in the evaluation of acute muscle weakness is to localize the site of lesion along the "motor unit." The motor unit is all muscle fibers innervated by a single anterior horn cell. The following discussion is limited to the most frequent conditions causing acute muscle weakness.

A. Acute anterior horn cell disease.

    1. **Acute anterior poliomyelitis** does not occur in the United States but is endemic in other countries. It typically follows a prodrome of systemic symptoms such as fever, nausea, vomiting, constipation, muscle pain, and headaches. Muscle weakness develops a few days after the prodromal stage with asymmetric weakness.

    2. **The West Nile virus (WNV)** is associated with many disorders of the neurologic system. One of the neurologic manifestations of WNV infection is acute anterior horn cell myelitis. Rarely (0.1%), patients infected with WNV will develop acute flaccid paralysis in a focal or segmental distribution. Electromyography/nerve conduction studies (EMG/NCS) reveal evidence for MND. Cerebrospinal fluid (CSF) analysis reveals a pleocytosis, elevated protein, and elevated immunoglobulin M (IgM) West Nile titers. The prognosis is poor.

B. Acute polyradiculoneuropathy.

    1. **GBS** is an acute inflammatory demyelinating polyradiculoneuropathy. It begins with lower-extremity paresthesia followed by ascending symmetric muscle weakness. Rarely, proximal muscles weakness is more prominent.

        Muscle stretch reflexes are universally absent or diminished. Bifacial peripheral weakness is frequent. Labile blood pressure, tachycardia, and other autonomic disturbances may occur as a result of involvement of the autonomic nervous system. Early in the course of the disease, the only EMG abnormality may be the absence of F-waves as a result of proximal root involvement; later, the EMG shows changes consistent with demyelination. CSF examination shows elevation of protein with minimal or no pleocytosis.

    2. HIV infection. Acute inflammatory demyelinating polyneuropathy similar to GBS can occur in patients with HIV infection. CSF pleocytosis is common.

    3. Cauda equina syndrome. This is an acute polyradiculoneuropathy of the conus medullaris and lumbosacral nerve roots. Cauda equina syndrome manifests as lower extremity neuropathic pain, sensory disturbance, bowel and bladder dysfunction, and asymmetric both lower extremities (BLE) weakness. There are many causes, including neoplastic invasion, cytomegalovirus (CMV) infection, and acute compression, such as from an epidural hematoma. Evaluation includes emergent imaging by magnetic resonance imaging (MRI), often followed by lumbar puncture to evaluate the CSF.

C. Acute plexopathy.

    1. **Acute idiopathic brachial plexopathy** is an uncommon disorder characterized by shoulder pain followed by weakness of shoulder girdle muscles, although distal arm muscles can be involved as well. Pain is a very important part of this syndrome. There is sensory disturbance in affected plexus distributions. There are familial (hereditary) and sporadic cases. It is diagnosed clinically, but can be confirmed by EMG.

2. **Acute lumbosacral plexopathy,** sometimes known as diabetic amyotrophy, is an acute inflammatory lesion of the lumbosacral plexus. Patients have weakness, sensory changes, and severe neuropathic pain, which can be asymmetric, because of unequal involvement of the various roots within the plexus. It sometimes occurs in the setting of poorly controlled diabetes. Other settings include carcinomatous infiltration, vasculitis, or idiopathic. Diagnosis is made with clinical examination, EMG, and lumbar puncture.

3. **Other acute forms of plexopathy.** Acute plexus lesions can occur in patients who have sustained closed or open trauma to the plexi, as in traction injuries. Neoplastic involvement, radiation, and orthopedic procedures also can cause plexus damage. Traumatic plexus injuries may follow gunshot wounds or retroperitoneal hematomas.

D. **Acute neuropathy.**

1. **GBS.** See Section **B** under Laboratory Studies.

2. **Lyme disease.** Acute demyelinating polyneuropathy can occur among patients with Lyme disease. Lyme disease can manifest with peripheral facial palsy and an ascending-type paralysis from the lower extremities, similar to GBS. CSF is abnormal, showing elevation of protein; but unlike GBS, there is a moderate degree of lymphocytic pleocytosis. Lyme titers indicating active infection are needed. The US Centers for Disease Control and Prevention recommends a two-step testing procedure.

3. **Mononeuritis multiplex.** An asymmetric form of acute sensorimotor polyneuropathy is common among patients with vasculitis. EMG shows evidence of multiple mononeuropathies. The diagnosis is established by clinical presentation; EMG; nerve biopsy; and appropriate laboratory evaluation for vasculitis, including HIV and hepatitis C.

4. **Acute motor axonal neuropathy (AMAN)** was first recognized in northern China and was referred to as the *Chinese paralytic syndrome*. This condition has many similarities to GBS. Pathologically, it is an axonopathy without demyelination. CSF examination shows few cells but an increased protein level. Patients have flaccid, symmetric paralysis and areflexia. The clinical course is usually rapidly progressive and may cause respiratory failure. EMG shows decreased compound motor action potentials, consistent with a motor axonopathy. Latencies and F-waves are normal. Sensory nerve action potentials are within normal ranges. Rare variants include acute motor and sensory neuropathy, which includes sensory involvement.

5. **Acute intermittent porphyria (AIP).** Weakness usually starts in the proximal upper extremities, but all limbs may become involved. Muscle tone will be reduced, with areflexia, except for ankle jerks, which may be preserved. Bulbar muscle function is usually preserved. Consistent with an acute neuropathy, paresthesia and autonomic dysfunction may be present. Attacks of AIP are usually associated with abdominal pain and cramping. NCS show reduced amplitudes in motor and sensory nerves. Needle examination shows evidence of denervation consistent with axonal neuropathy. During attacks of AIP, there are increases in urinary excretion of both Δ-aminolevulinic acid and porphobilinogen (PBG). The increase in PBG excretion (in milligrams per gram of creatinine) is greater than the increase in aminolevulinic acid excretion.

6. **Acute critical illness neuropathy** often manifests in the intensive care unit (ICU) as failure to wean from the ventilator. The patient has weakness and atrophy with amplitude loss on EMG and NCS. Overlap with acute quadriplegic myopathy may be present (see **Section F.5 under Differential Diagnosis**).

E. **Acute neuromuscular junction disorders.**

1. **Presynaptic disorders.** Only selective disorders are considered. Lambert–Eaton myasthenic syndrome, which has a more insidious presentation, is not discussed (see Chapter 48).

   a. **Botulism** is caused by ingestion of toxins produced by *Clostridium botulinum*. This disease often manifests as weakness of extraocular muscles followed by dysarthria, limb, and respiratory muscle weakness. This diagnosis is suggested by a history of ingestion of contaminated food, acute diffuse weakness, and no sensory symptoms. Repetitive nerve stimulation at high frequency (50 Hz) will show an incremental response. Botulism intoxication may be seen in infants, whose gastrointestinal tract can be colonized by *C. botulinum*.

   b. **Tick paralysis** is a rare disease caused by the female tick Dermacentor andersoni. Neurologic symptoms begin with walking difficulty and imbalance followed by ascending flaccid paralysis with areflexia. Ocular and bulbar muscles may be involved. EMG shows reduced amplitude of muscle action potentials and an incremental response to high-frequency stimulation. Removal of the tick may dramatically improve the weakness.

   c. **Organophosphate poisoning** causes muscle weakness. Extraocular and bulbar muscles are involved. Muscarinic symptoms such as miosis, increased salivation, and generalized fasciculations are present. EMG findings are usually normal. Repetitive nerve stimulation may show incremental responses at high-frequency stimulation.

   d. **Drug-induced MG.** Certain medications adversely affect neuromuscular transmission. Weakness usually involves proximal limb muscles rather than ocular or bulbar muscles. Drug-induced MG may be associated with the use of kanamycin, gentamicin, procainamide, primidone, or hydantoins.

2. Postsynaptic disorders: MG. Adult-onset autoimmune generalized acquired MG begins with fluctuating weakness; proximal muscle weakness is prominent (see <u>Video 31.1</u>). Eventually, dysarthria, dysphagia, and respiratory distress may occur. Ocular myasthenia will present with asymmetric ptosis and diplopia. There is fatigability induced by repetitive exercise. Muscle tone, bulk, reflexes, and sensory examination are normal. Diagnosis is based on clinical examination, single-fiber EMG/repetitive nerve stimulation, and laboratory assessment for acetylcholine receptor antibodies (AchR Abs). AchR-binding antibodies are the most sensitive; blocking and modulating antibodies do not significantly increase the sensitivity. MuSK antibody MG occurs more often in females, with oculobulbar onset.

F. **Primary myopathy.**

1. PM/DM. Acute inflammatory myopathy usually begins with proximal symmetric weakness involving the muscles of the shoulder and hip girdle. Muscle tone, bulk, and muscle stretch reflexes are normal. There are no sensory deficits. PM is usually painless or may have an achy nonspecific muscular pain. Consider DM if typical skin lesions are present (erythematous rash in the periorbital, malar, forehead, or chest region, and a scaly, erythematous rash over the knuckles and extensor surfaces). Serum creatine kinase (CK), lactic acid dehydrogenase (LDH), and aspartate aminotransferase (AST) levels are often elevated. Erythrocyte sedimentation rate (ESR) may be increased. NCS and amplitude are normal. Needle EMG will show a myopathic pattern in affected muscles. Muscle biopsy shows an inflammatory response, which differs depending on the pathologic process present: perimysial inflammation is noted in DM and intrafascicular inflammation is present in PM. The biopsy will also show muscle fiber necrosis and a variable degree of muscle fiber regeneration.

2. **Rhabdomyolysis** occurs after severe injury to muscles: it may be focal or generalized depending upon the injury. Patients will have swelling and pain in the affected muscles, demonstrate weakness, and have markedly elevated CKs. Acutely elevated CKs may put the patient at risk for renal failure and focal injury may cause compartment syndrome. These patients need to be hospitalized for monitoring and careful hydration.

3. Acute infectious myositis. Postviral myositis is associated with myalgia and weakness, which may be severe. HIV infection can manifest as proximal muscle weakness.

4. Acute toxic myopathy. Most drug-induced myopathies are subacute in onset. Amiodarone can cause acute myopathy and paralysis. Hyperthyroidism can cause acute weakness in severe cases.

5. **Acute periodic paralysis** is a group of primary muscle diseases associated with acute transient quadriparesis without respiratory compromise. Patients may have had attacks for years but will present to the emergency room for a particularly severe attack. The episodes of quadriparesis typically resolve spontaneously, although, over the years, patients may develop a chronic myopathy/weakness. These diseases are also known as channelopathies because the etiology is a defect in an ion pore of the muscle membrane. Hyperkalemic periodic paralysis (Hyper PP) is caused by a defect in the gene coding for a muscle sodium channel (SCN4A) and hypokalemic periodic paralysis (Hypo PP) is caused by either a gene defect in a calcium channel of the muscle (CACNA1S) or the sodium SCN4A channel. There is significant overlap between the presentations of both conditions and diagnosis is best confirmed by genetic testing. Patients with Hyper PP may have clinical myotonia. The diagnosis is suspected if the patient has a history of intermittent weakness induced by exertion or a high-carbohydrate diet, a family history, and abnormal serum potassium levels during attacks. EMG/NCS may be normal or may show decreased compound muscle action potentials (CMAPs); the prolonged exercise test can be used to demonstrate a reduction in CMAP amplitude. Muscle biopsy may show a vacuolar myopathy.

6. **Acute critical illness myopathy** occurs in the ICU setting. Patients will have flaccid paralysis and difficulty weaning from the ventilator. Sometimes, this disease is associated with treatment for status asthmaticus using high-dose steroids and neuromuscular blockade agents. The EMG shows either myopathic features or an electrically silent muscle; it is differentiated from ICU neuropathy by normal sensory NCS. Muscle biopsy typically shows loss of myosin filaments at electron microscopic examination. Patients may recover from this process, unlike acute critical illness neuropathy.

LABORATORY STUDIES

A. Blood tests. If myositis is suspected, measurement of serum CK, ESR, LDH, and AST is useful. Anti-Jo antibody test results are positive in approximately 30% of cases of PM. The presence of this antibody is a marker of risk for pulmonary fibrosis. Other autoantibodies associated with inflammatory myopathy are insensitive and not diagnostically useful.

If vasculitis is suspected, measure ESR, serum complement, antinuclear antibodies, antineutrophil cytoplasmic antibodies, and cryoglobulins. Consider evaluating the patient for HIV and chronic hepatitis infection.

If MG is suspected, check AchR Ab (binding) titers and thyroid function tests. If these results are negative, consider testing MuSK antibodies and antibodies to the voltage-gated calcium channel (Table 31.1).

In conditions such as periodic paralysis, serum potassium and thyroid function tests may or may not be helpful. Potassium (K^+) levels can fluctuate greatly during the course of an attack. The genetic defects for some channelopathies are known. Commercial testing is available for the genes encoding for the SCN4A channel (Hyper PP/paramyotonia congenital and Hypo PP, type 2) and the CACNA1S channel (Hypo PP, type 1).

Patients affected with AMAN may have had a recent *Campylobacter jejuni* infection. The anti-GQ1b ganglioside antibody is both sensitive and specific for the Miller Fisher variant of GBS. This variant manifests as ophthalmoparesis, ataxia, and areflexia.

In suspected cases of West Nile viral infection, acute and convalescent titers should be drawn (serum IgG and IgM levels).

B. **Lumbar puncture** is indicated in the evaluation of patients with suspected GBS, in which CSF may show protein elevation with minimal or absent pleocytosis (albuminocytologic dissociation). In patients with an acute poliomyelitis picture (acute MND), the lumbar puncture may show lymphocytic pleocytosis and protein elevation. Check for WNV-IgG antibodies, and, if the patient is immunocompromised, check the CSF for herpes simplex virus, varicella zoster virus, and CMV infections as well.

C. Electrodiagnostic studies. EMG and NCS are extremely useful in the evaluation of disorders of motor neurons, peripheral nerves, neuromuscular junctions, and muscles. The value of electrodiagnostic tests is discussed in Chapter 33.

D. Muscle biopsy. Muscle tissue can be obtained by means of open incision. The site of muscle biopsy should involve a weak but not atrophic muscle. Specimen handling and interpretation of muscle biopsy findings by an experienced pathologist are crucial. Muscle biopsy aids in diagnosis of acute primary muscle pathologies such as PM/DM.

E. **Nerve biopsy** is most often performed on the sural nerve. This procedure should be performed only when the biopsy results will influence management. One of the leading indications for nerve biopsy is the suspicion of vasculitis (mononeuritis multiplex).

F. **MRI** of the affected muscles may indicate inflammation in an infectious/inflammatory myositis. Atrophy of the muscles will be noted in subacute to chronic processes, such as dystrophy or MND.

DIAGNOSTIC APPROACH

Diagnosis begins with establishing the presence of weakness and then determining whether the weakness reflects upper or lower motor neuron involvement. After exclusion of upper motor neuron weakness, further localization within the motor unit is needed. Diagnosis often requires support by laboratory studies. Elevated CK is the easiest way to identify muscle inflammation. An EMG/NCS will further localize the lesion. Muscle biopsy is recommended for evaluation of PM/DM. Nerve biopsy is indicated mainly in cases of suspected vasculitic neuropathy.

TABLE 31.1 Diagnostic Table for Selected Diseases Causing Acute Muscle Weakness

	GBS	MG	PM/DM
Features			
Initial weakness	Typically distal	Ocular and bulbar	Proximal
Fatigability with repeated testing	Not present	Prominent	Not present
Wasting/atrophy	Not in acute phase	Not typically present	Can occur late in disease
Sensory loss	Present	Not present	Not present
Reflexes	Diminished/absent	Normal	Normal
Fasciculations	Not typically noted	Rarely present in severe disease	Not present
CSF protein	Elevated	Normal	Normal
EMG			
Fibrillations	Occur late in disease	Occur with long-standing disease	Present
Fasciculations	Can be present	Occur with long-standing disease	Not present
Motor unit recruitment	Marked decrease	Variable	Increased
CK	Normal	Normal	Increased
AchR Ab	Negative	Elevated	Negative
Muscle biopsy	Not indicated	Not indicated	InflammationAbbreviations: AchR Ab, acetylcholine receptor antibody; CK, creatine kinase; EMG, Electromyography; GBS, Guillain–Barré syndrome; MG, myasthenia gravis; PM/DM, polymyositis/dermatomyositis.

MANAGEMENT

Patients with acute onset of generalized neuromuscular weakness need to be hospitalized, particularly those with acute paralysis or paresis. If respiratory or bulbar muscles are compromised, patients need admission to an ICU. Bedside pulmonary function tests (FVC and NIF) are used to monitor respiratory function. A sustained drop in FVC, or an FVC <1 L, indicates impending respiratory failure, and intubation is indicated. Neuromuscular diseases with a subacute onset may sometimes be managed in the outpatient setting. Many of the therapies for neuromuscular weakness require careful monitoring and follow-up assessment, especially if steroids and immunosuppressive agents are used.

Key Points

- Muscular weakness must be distinguished from fatigue, lethargy, and tiredness, which are not neuromuscular in origin.
- Physical examination should focus on determining the pattern of weakness; localizing the deficit along the motor unit; and assessing for sensory involvement.
- CK testing will assess for muscle inflammation.
- Patients with respiratory or bulbar involvement and those with acute rhabdomyolysis need to be hospitalized and monitored carefully.

Recommended Readings

Amato AA, Greenberg SA. Inflammatory myopathies. *Continuum.* 2013;19(6):1615–1633.

Barohn RJ, Mazen MD, Jackson CE. A pattern recognition approach to patients with a suspected myopathy. *Neurol Clin.* 2014;32:569–593.

Dalakas MC. Therapeutic approaches in patients with inflammatory myopathies. *Semin Neurol.* 2003;23(2):199–206.

Davis LE, DeBiasi R, Goade DE, et al. West Nile virus neuroinvasive disease. *Ann Neurol.* 2006;60:286–300.

Keesey JC. Clinical evaluations and management of myasthenia gravis. *Muscle Nerve.* 2004;29:484–505.

Latronico NN, Bolton CF. Critical illness polyneuropathy and myopathy: a major cause of muscle weakness and paralysis. *Lancet Neurol.* 2011;10:931–941.

Ridley A. The neuropathy of acute intermittent porphyria. *QJM.* 1969;38:307–333.

Wilbourn AJ. Plexopathies. *Neurol Clin.* 2007;25(1):139–171.

32

Approach to the Patient with Neurogenic Orthostatic Hypotension, Sexual and Urinary Dysfunction, and Other Autonomic Disorders

Emilio Oribe

The autonomic nervous system (ANS) maintains the body's internal homeostasis and regulates its protective responses. ANS modulation of body functions is achieved through autonomic reflex pathways and an extensive vasomotor, visceromotor, and sensory innervation. Parasympathetic (PS) and sympathetic (S) efferent autonomic pathways, each with their pre- and postganglionic neurons, synapse with their target effector organs. The ANS enteric nervous system (ENS), with its local neural networks within the gut walls, regulates the gastrointestinal (GI) tract. The baroreflex, an example of an autonomic reflex, exquisitely regulates blood pressure (BP), heart rate (HR), and extracellular fluid volume (Fig. 32.1).

The site of an autonomic reflex pathway lesion determines if ANS dysfunction is focal or generalized. ANS dysfunction may be "central" due to lesions involving neurons of the central nervous system (CNS), brainstem, spinal cord, and preganglionic neurons, or "peripheral" due to efferent pathway lesions involving peripheral ganglia and postganglionic neurons, or to lesions involving afferent reflex pathways (Fig. 32.1). Selected autonomic clinical features are summarized in Table 32.1. Autonomic dysfunction may be present with many disorders (Table 32.2). Common causes include ANS neuropathies (diabetes mellitus [DM] and amyloid small-fiber neuropathies), ganglionopathies, and multiple system atrophy (MSA).

EVALUATION OF THE PATIENT WITH AUTONOMIC NERVOUS SYSTEM SYMPTOMS

The aims are to confirm the presence of autonomic dysfunction, determine the extent of autonomic involvement, localize the site of a lesion in the ANS reflex arc, and to distinguish primary from secondary autonomic disorders. The site of an autonomic lesion, the clinical course, and the presence or absence of accompanying somatic neurologic and/or systemic or localized manifestations of disease help establish a cause of autonomic dysfunction. Typically, acute/subacute ANS manifestations suggest autoimmune (i.e., acute autonomic ganglionic neuropathy, paraneoplastic), or toxic causes; pain and neuropathy, a peripheral autonomic neuropathy; and involvement of the CNS, a central cause (i.e., MSA).

A. History. Important elements of the autonomic history include the following:
1. **Chief autonomic complaints.** Severity of symptoms, their distribution and frequency, progression, the presence of aggravating and alleviating factors, accompanying symptoms, and a measure of the degree of disability
2. **Medical, surgical, and psychiatric history.** To define any underlying/associated illness
3. **Review of ANS systems.** Cardiovascular, urinary, sudomotor, secretomotor, sexual, vasomotor, GI, thermoregulatory, pupillomotor, and sleep functions
4. **Medication and toxin review.** Antihypertensive, psychotropic, antiandrogenic, laxative medications, and alcohol and recreational drugs and toxins. Medications are the most frequent cause of ANS symptoms.
5. **Family history** (inherited autonomic disorders)

B. Physical examination.
   The physical and neurologic examinations determine the nature, site, and extent of the neuroanatomical lesions responsible for ANS dysfunction and define associated disorders. The examination may also demonstrate the extent to which a patient can participate in their own care. The ANS examination includes supine and upright BP and HR (Table 32.2), and comprehensive neurologic and multisystem examinations.

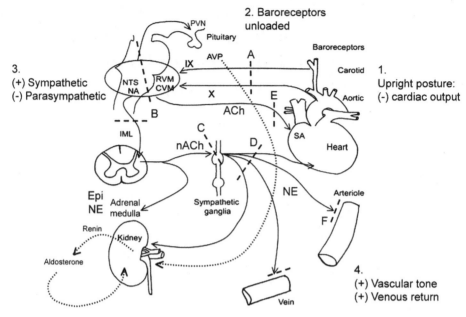

FIGURE 32.1 Baroreflex pathways. Efferents from arterial carotid sinus baroreceptors travel to the CNS with the glossopharyngeal (IX) nerve and those from the arterial aortic arch baroreceptors travel with the vagus (X) nerve. S preganglionic efferents travel in the intermediolateral cell column of the spinal cord (IML) to synapse with postganglionic neurons (nicotinic acetylcholine receptors) of the S ganglia. Postganglionic neurons travel to innervate vascular smooth muscle, the heart, and the adrenal glands. Vagal preganglionic neurons are situated in the ventrolateral medulla and the dorsal vagal nucleus and vagal innervation of the cardiac sinus node travels with the vagus nerve. **The baroreflex. 1, Standing** produces a shift or "pooling" of 600–1000 mL of blood to the lower body (mainly limb and splanchnic capacitance circulation), reducing venous return and cardiac output; **2,** This is sensed by specialized stretch receptors (arterial and cardiopulmonary baroreceptors) that in turn activate (unload) baroreflexes. Inputs from carotid and aortic baroreceptors travel with the glossopharyngeal (IX) and vagus nerves (X) to converge on cardiovascular centers in the brainstem and medulla (mainly nucleus of the tractus solitarius) and their projections; **3,** The physiologic baroreceptor reflex response to the volume shifts produced by upright posture is a compensatory increase in S tone with a decrease in PS outflow; **4,** S nerve terminals release NE that produces increased vasoconstriction of skeletal and mesenteric muscle vessels, HR, and cardiac contractility. Additional increases in venous return occur through a "pumping" effect of contracting limb and abdominal muscles engaged by the effort of standing (not shown); **5,** A longer-term response promoting extracellular fluid volume expansion includes baroreflex-mediated release of renin, angiotensin, and aldosterone, leading to increased renal Na^{++} absorption, and release of vasopressin, with an increase in free-water absorption. **A,** Afferent baroreflex limb dysfunction is present when lesions involve baroreceptors and IX and X cranial nerves (neck surgery, radiotherapy, trauma, neuropathies, and autonomic disorders such as baroreflex failure, Holmes–Adie syndrome, and HSAN III); **B,** Central lesions involve the ventrolateral medulla (MSA), descending S pathways (medullary lesions, spinal cord lesions above T5), and IML (MSA, Lewy body disorders); **C.** S ganglia lesions involve S ganglia (autoimmune ganglionopathies associated with nAChR antibodies or paraneoplastic, Lewy body disorders); **D, E,** Postganglionic S and efferent PS lesions are present with small-fiber neuropathies (diabetes, amyloidosis, Sjögren's syndrome, HSAN III). **F:** Efferent S neuroeffector junction dysfunction occurs with dopamine β-hydroxylase deficiency and α-1 adrenoceptor blocking drugs. AVP, arginine vasopressin; CNS, central nervous system; CVM, caudal ventrolateral medulla; HR, heart rate; IML, intermediolateral cell columns of the spinal cord; NA, nucleus ambiguus; MSA, multiple system atrophy; nAChR, nicotinic acetylcholine receptor antibodies; NE, norepinephrine; NTS, nucleus tractus solitarius; RVM, rostral ventrolateral medulla; S, sympathetic; SA, sinus node.

TABLE 32.1 Selected Clinical Features of ANS Dysfunction

	Common Symptoms	Examination
Cardiovascular autonomic	Orthostatic intolerance: syncope, near-syncope, lightheadedness, confusion and impaired cognition, weakness, slurring, visual disturbances, tremors, neck and shoulder ("coat hanger") aches Exercise intolerance, silent myocardial infarction, intraoperative cardiovascular liability, increased mortality	OH, hypotension, orthostatic tachycardia Tachycardia, loss of HR respiratory sinus arrhythmia. Intraoperative hypothermia, reduced hypoxic-ventilatory drive
Vasomotor	Skin discoloration	Flushing, pallor, distal cyanosis, trophic changes. Changes in skin blood flow absent
Sudomotor and thermoregulatory	Hypohidrosis, hyperhidrosis, heat/cold intolerance	Abnormal temperature regulation, hypothermia, hyperthermia
Secretomotor	Dry mouth, excessive salivation, gustatory sweating, tearing, dry eyes	Dry mouth, dry eyes
Gastrointestinal	Difficulty swallowing, constipation, early satiety, bloating, nausea, vomiting, abdominal pain/cramping, diarrhea, fecal incontinence, weight loss	Abnormal bowel sounds, abdominal distention, reduced anal tone. Gastroparesis, esophageal enteropathy
Bladder	Incontinence, urgency, weak stream, dribbling, hesitancy, retention, recurrent infection	Distended bladder, increased postvoid residual
Sexual	Loss of libido, decreased genital engorgement, ED, ejaculatory dysfunction, dyspareunia	Decreased penile or clitoral and labial engorgement, decreased genital lubrication
Pupillomotor	Glare, blurred vision, poor night vision	Impaired pupillary responses

Abbreviations: ANS, autonomic nervous system; ED, erectile dysfunction; HR, heart rate; OH, orthostatic hypotension

TABLE 32.2 Selected Autonomic Disorders

	Autonomic Disorders
Central autonomic failure	MSA
	Disorders of various causes (cerebrovascular, epileptic, tumoral, demyelinating, traumatic, infectious, degenerative) and autonomic presentations. Lesions may involve frontal lobes, limbic system, hypothalamus, brainstem, cerebellum, spinal cord
Peripheral autonomic failure	Pure autonomic failure (peripheral involvement predominant), Parkinson's disease, Lewy body disorders
	Autonomic neuropathies and ganglionopathies:
	Acute and subacute:
	Isolated ANS involvement: AAG, paraneoplastic autonomic neuropathy
	ANS and somatic involvement: Landry–Guillain–Barré syndrome, botulism, porphyrias, drug induced and toxic
	Chronic peripheral autonomic neuropathies
	S and PS: diabetic, amyloid, autoimmune autonomic neuropathy (paraneoplastic), sensory neuronopathy with autonomic failure, distal small-fiber neuropathies, hereditary neuropathies, cobalamin deficiency, HIV, leprosy, Chagas disease
Catecholamine dysfunction	Baroreflex failure, tumors that secrete catecholamines (pheochromocytoma, neuroblastoma, chemodectoma, familial paraganglioma syndrome), disorders affecting neurotransmitter metabolism (tetrahydrobiopterin deficiency, L-aminoacid decarboxylase deficiency, dopamine β hydroxylase deficiency and Menkes disease, monoamine oxidase deficiency states, dopamine metabolism disorders)
Orthostatic intolerance and hypotension	POTS
	Mitral valve prolapse dysautonomia
	OH of the elderly and after deconditioning and bed rest
	Drug-induced (nitrovasodilators, sympatholytics, neuroleptics, tricyclic antidepressants, insulin [i.e., hypoglycemia-associated autonomic failure]) and toxin-induced (alcohol, vincristine, cis-platinum, heavy metals, solvents, pyrinuron)
	Reflex syncope: vasovagal, situational syncope
Miscellaneous	Hyperhidrosis (generalized, focal) and anhidrosis (CNS, peripheral nerve, dermatologic)
	Horner's syndrome, Holmes–Adie syndrome, Ross' syndrome, crocodile tears
	Hirschsprung's disease

Abbreviations: AAG, autoimmune autonomic ganglionopathy; ANS, autonomic nervous system; CNS, central nervous system; HIV, human immunodeficiency virus; MSA, multiple system atrophy; OH, orthostatic hypotension; PS, parasympathetic; POTS, postural orthostatic tachycardia syndrome; S, sympathetic.

C. **Autonomic testing.** ANS testing is an extension of the physical examination. Conclusions arising from ANS testing are of most value when the selection of tests is guided by the clinical findings. As an abnormal test does not always imply disease, several tests are usually required to confirm autonomic dysfunction. Combing several autonomic test results and BP values into a composite scale (composite autonomic scoring scale) has been used as a reliable measure of autonomic function. Autonomic labs should have standardized testing conditions and normative test data.

    Most ANS tests assess the integrity of an autonomic reflex indirectly by recording stimulus-evoked effector organ responses. Bedside ANS tests (Table 32.3) measure those effector organ responses that are most easily recorded (i.e., changes in HR, BP, pupillary size, sweating patterns, SSR, and so on). Sophisticated tests such beat-to-beat arterial

TABLE 32.3 Blood Pressure and Heart Rate Responses to Posture

Cause	Blood Pressure	Heart Rate	Comments
Neurogenic OH	↓ SBP >20, ↓ DBP >10 after 3 min of standing or 60 degrees head up tilt	=	Efferent S vasomotor and vagal dysfunction due to autonomic failure. Supine hypertension is frequent
Initial OH on standing	↓ SBP >40, ↓ DBP >20 (symptomatic), within 15 s. Absent OH >3 min of standing	↑	Temporary cardiac output and vascular resistance mismatch on standing (only detected with beat-to-beat BP recordings). No ANS failure
Delayed OH	↓ SBP >20, ↓ DBP >10 beyond 3 min of standing or tilt table testing	=, ↑	Efferent S vasomotor dysfunction (mild/early)
Postprandial hypotension	↓ SBP >20 after 3 min of standing 1 hr after meal intake	=, ↑	Efferent S vasomotor dysfunction, with insufficient vasoconstriction to oppose postprandial blood pooling
Neurally mediated ("vasovagal")	↓	↓ (paradoxical, in the setting of ↓ BP)	Reflex withdrawal of efferent S and enhanced efferent PS tone. Typically with autonomic activation (pallor, cold sweats, nausea, vomiting), followed by prompt recovery
POTS	=, ↑	↑ (>30 beats/min)	Exaggerated efferent S response to upright posture
Extracellular volume depletion	↓	↑	Volume depletion. Intact baroreflexes
Drugs	↓	↓, =, ↑ (depending on the drug)	Drugs with vasomotor and/or chronotropic effects. Drugs that produce dehydration
Supine hypertension	↑ (>150 SBP, ↑ >90 DBP)	↓, =, ↑	Impaired baroreflex, inappropriate residual supine S, drugs with hypertensive effect. Risk of end-organ damage
Orthostatic hypertension	↑ (>20 SBP, ↑ >10 DBP)	↓, =, ↑	Excessive pooling, with increased S tone and impaired baroreflex function (proposed). Increased risk of HTN, CNS ischemia and neuropathy in DM
Exercise hypotension	↓	↓, =, ↑	Failure to compensate for exercise-induced skeletal muscle vasodilatation

Neurogenic OH may be "uncovered" under certain conditions, such as volume depletion and with vasodilatation (in hot environments, with exercise, alcohol, and medications). BP values may vary following a circadian pattern (i.e., lower in the early mornings), and may be exacerbated by prolonged bed rest, physical deconditioning, and with aging.
Abbreviations: ANS, autonomic nervous system; BP, blood pressure; CNS, central nervous system; DBP, diastolic blood pressure; DM, diabetes mellitus; DM, diabetes mellitus; HTN, hypertension; OH, orthostatic hypotension; POTS, postural orthostatic tachycardia; PS, parasympathetic; SBP, systolic blood pressure; S, sympathetic. BP in mm Hg.

pressure recordings during different challenges (i.e., changes in posture, Valsalva-like and other maneuvers—Video 32.1) and measurement of sweat output and its latencies (i.e., quantitative sudomotor axon reflex test [QSART]), to assess efferent sudomotor function, require more complex and expensive instruments.

The release of autonomic neurotransmitters (and their metabolic byproducts) in response to different challenges (i.e., by maneuvers, changes in posture, pharmacologic stimuli) may be helpful in some diagnostic situations (Table 32.4).

Cardiac S innervation, as measured by the uptake of radionuclide tracers (i.e., [123]-meta-iodo-benzylguanidine—a guanethidine analog) into cardiac S neurons, helps discriminate central (it is preserved with MSA) from peripheral ANS dysfunction (it is impaired with ANS peripheral neuropathies, pure autonomic failure (PAF), Lewy body dementia (LBD), Parkinson's disease (PD) patients with OH, and in some PD patients without OH).

D. Laboratory and other evaluations.
   1. Screening tests.
      a. Complete blood count
      b. Erythrocyte sedimentation rate
      c. Blood urea nitrogen (BUN)/creatinine (Cr)
      d. Glucose, fasting (hemoglobin A1C, glucose tolerance test if diabetes suspected)
      e. Thyroid-stimulating hormone
      f. Vitamin B_{12}/folate
      g. Immunoelectrophoresis/immunofixation (serum and urine)
      h. Urinalysis (U/A)
      i. Human immunodeficiency virus (HIV)
      j. Testosterone levels (in patients with erectile dysfunction [ED])
   2. Additional testing is usually directed by the clinical presentation.
      a. Autoantibodies.
         (1) Ganglionic nicotinic α3 acetylcholine receptor antibodies (α3-AChR) (see section Autonomic Neuropathies, below), paraneoplastic autoantibodies (anti-Hu [ANNA-1]), and voltage-gated P/Q type and N-type calcium channel and potassium channel [VGKC], in particular with autonomic symptoms of subacute onset. Anti-Hu and anti-CV2/collapsin response mediator protein 5 (CV2/CRMP-5) are frequently present in autonomic neuropathies.
         (2) VGKC and anti-N-methyl-D-aspartate antibodies when limbic encephalitis is present.
         (3) Antinuclear antibodies, rheumatoid factor, anti-Ro/SS-A, and anti-La/SS-B (Sjögren's, and other connective tissue disorders) when autonomic dysfunction is associated with somatic peripheral neuropathy.
      b. Electrophysiologic studies. Nerve conduction studies (NCS) and electromyography (EMG), sphincter and pelvic floor EMG to detect denervation potentials of spinal cord anterior horn cells (MSA), polysomnography (MSA), and urodynamic studies.
      c. Imaging studies include magnetic resonance imaging (MRI) of brain and spine, which determine CNS and spinal cord lesions and pelvic imaging structural lesions.
      d. Histopathologic tests include amyloid staining in fat aspirate, rectal or gingival biopsy, intraepidermal sweat gland nerve fiber density, and sural nerve biopsy.
      e. Other testing includes aminolevulinic acid, porphobilinogen, and porphyrins (24-hour urine collection), erythrocyte porphobilinogen deaminase activity (porphyria), testing for deficient α-galactosidase A enzyme activity in males, and genetic testing (inherited neuropathies).

SELECTED CLINICAL PRESENTATIONS OF AUTONOMIC DYSFUNCTION

Orthostatic Hypotension and Orthostatic Intolerance Syndromes

NEUROGENIC ORTHOSTATIC (POSTURAL) HYPOTENSION

Orthostatic hypotension (OH), defined as a sustained decrease in systolic pressure of at least 20 mm Hg (30 mm Hg in patients with supine hypertension) and of diastolic pressure of at

TABLE 32.4 Selected Bedside Autonomic Tests Assessing Baroreflex Pathways

Test	Methods	Normal	Abnormal	Site of Lesion
Active standing (supine rest for >3 min, or until BP, HR stable followed by unaided standing)	BP and HR supine and standing after 3 min	↑ HR < 30 beats/min; ↓ SBP < 30 mm Hg	= HR[a]; ↓↓ SBP	S vasomotor efferents(α_1 adrenergic)
	HRmax/HRmin during first 30 s of active standing (30:15 ratio)	>1.02	1.00	Cardiovagal efferents(M_2 cholinergic)
Deep breathing(6 breaths/min)	HRmax-HRmin or R-Rmax in expiration/R-Rmin in inspiration (E/I ratio)	>10 beats/min; >1.10	<8 beats/min; <1.05	Cardiovagal efferents (M_2 cholinergic)
Valsalva's maneuver (blow into a mouthpiece with small leak, maintaining 40 mm Hg for 15 s)	R-Rmax after maneuver/R-Rmin	>1.15	<1.10	No rebound bradycardia (phase IV): Cardiovagal efferents; No tachycardia (phase II): S vasomotor efferents
NE release in response to upright posture	Supine and upright plasma NE[b]	↑	=	S efferents (S ganglion, adrenergic fibers)
Mental stress (cortical/CNS afferents, independent of baroreflex afferents)	HR and BP 2 min into the stress of mental arithmetic (i.e., serial 7 subtractions for 2.5 min)	↑ HR > 12	=	S efferents (require intact baroreflex afferents)
BP response to head down tilt	BP after 10 min of head down tilt	=	↑	Barorefex afferents
Baroreflex release of vasopressin	Supine and upright AVP vasopressin[b]	↑	=	Baroreflex afferents (AVP released by posterior pituitary; does not require efferent pathways)

Abbreviations: AVP, arginine vasopressin; BP, blood pressure; CNS, central nervous system; EMG, electromyography; HR, heart rate; HRmax, maximum HR; HRmin, minimum HR; M_3, cholinergic muscarinic M_3 receptors; NE, norepinephrine; PAF, pure autonomic failure; R-R, electrocardiographic R-R intervals; R-Rmax, maximum R-R; R-Rmin, minimum R-R; S, sympathetic; α_1, adrenergic, α_1 adrenergic receptors.

Autonomic tests are used to explore the integrity of whole or of portions of autonomic reflex arcs, in this case the baroreflex. Bedside tests require a sphygmomanometer and ECG or EMG instruments (typical settings: low-frequency filter = 1 to 5 Hz and high-frequency filters = 500 Hz) and plasma NE and vasopressin determinations (available through commercial laboratories). Testing should be performed in a quiet, comfortable environment.

[a]Exaggerated increases in HR suggest hypovolemia, deconditioning. POTS.
[b]Particularly valuable in the setting of marked upright hypotension. May help distinguish PAF from MSA.

Abbreviations: AVP, arginine vasopressin; BP, Blood pressure; CNS, central nervous system; EMG, electromyography; HR, Heart rate; HRmax, maximum HR; HRmin, minimum HR; NE, norepinephrine; PAF, pure autonomic failure; R-R, electrocardiographic R-R intervals; R-Rmax, maximum R-R; R-Rmin, minimum R-R; S, sympathetic; α_1, adrenergic, α_1 adrenergic receptors; M_3, cholinergic muscarinic M_3 receptors.

least 10 mm Hg within 3 minutes of standing or head up tilt to at least 60 degrees on a tilt table, is a frequent and disabling manifestation of autonomic disorders. It may be the initial sign (i.e., "tip of the iceberg"), heralding the onset of autonomic disorders.

A. **Diagnosis.** BP measured with a sphygmomanometer and pulse rate recorded while in supine rest (once BP values are stable) and after standing for 2 to 3 minutes determine if OH is present. HR responses add valuable data and help determine a diagnosis (Table 32.3). OH standing times (the maximum time a patient is able to stand) replace BP in patients with severe OH who do not tolerate standing for enough time to allow BP measurement.

B. **Pathophysiology.** Hemodynamic responses to shifts in volume produced by changes in posture are complex, and depend on intact baroreflexes (Fig. 32.1). Neurogenic orthostatic hypotension (NOH) is due to deficient vasoconstriction, occurring because of failure to appropriately release norepinephrine (NE), the S postganglionic neurotransmitter that innervates blood vessels. This may be due to impaired afferent baroreflex pathways or to impaired efferent S outflow at central or peripheral sites. (Chronic OH due to autonomic failure should not be confused with episodic hypotension caused by the acute reflex withdrawal of S vascular tone occurring with vasovagal syncope—see section Reflex Syncope, Neurally Mediated Hypotension, and Bradycardia.)

C. **Causes.**
1. **Medications** (in particular antihypertensive agents)
2. **Autonomic neuropathies**
3. **Spinal cord lesions,** above T4 or T5 (complete transection and higher levels impair more S efferent nerves).
4. **Brainstem and medulla lesions**
5. **MSA, PD, dementia with Lewy bodies (diffuse Lewy body disease [DLB]),** and PAF should be considered in the differential diagnosis of OH (Fig. 32.1).
6. **Exacerbating factors.** Extracellular volume depletion (dehydration), physical deconditioning, and aging.

D. **Treatment.**

Treatment of OH is directed at improving a patient's symptoms and functional capacity and quality of life, rather than treating BP "numbers." Recording symptoms and BP and HR while supine and after standing for >2 to 3 minutes, before and 1 hour after meals, to determine if postprandial (postcibal) hypotension is present, facilitates management. Neurally mediated (vasovagal) hypotension and bradycardia, postural orthostatic tachycardia, OH in the elderly, orthostatic intolerance associated with prolonged bed rest, and deconditioning and spaceflight also respond to these treatments.

7. **Nonpharmacologic treatment** (Table 32.5, Video 32.1) is indicated for all patients with orthostatic intolerance (i.e., NOH, vasovagal syncope, and postural tachycardia). Countermeasures are used to acutely raise BP when symptoms of cerebral hypoperfusion are present.
8. **Pharmacologic treatment (Table 32.6).** Fludrocortisone acetate is considered the first-line drug in the treatment of OH.

Drugs with vasoconstrictor effects are administered during the patient's active hours (and withheld in evenings) to minimize supine hypertension. Supine hypertension is a manifestation of impairment of the baroreflex, with failure to prevent excessive BP rise in response to increased venous return when supine. It is sometimes severe enough to lead to hypertensive end-organ damage. Recommendations include avoiding supine postures, always sleeping with the head of the bed elevated (reverse Trendelenburg ~30 degrees), and having bedtime meals (to produce postprandial BP drop). Short-acting antihypertensive drugs (nitroglycerine, nifedipine, losartan, clonidine) are helpful.

POSTURAL ORTHOSTATIC TACHYCARDIA SYNDROME

Postural orthostatic tachycardia syndrome (POTS) is characterized by excessive tachycardic response to upright postures (Table 32.3). It may be accompanied by various ANS, psychiatric, and somatic complaints. Some forms are associated with alterations in adrenergic (sudomotor and vascular tone) function (pheochromocytoma should be considered). Many hemodynamic features are similar to those of deconditioning produced by bed rest and exposure to microgravity.

TABLE 32.5 Nonpharmacologic Treatment of Orthostatic Hypotension

Objective	Intervention
Understand mechanisms of OH and recognize factors that trigger/worsen OH	Avoid: abrupt standing, prolonged motionless standing, Valsalva-like maneuvers, hyperventilation, excessive exercise, hot environments, alcohol, large meals (recommend six small meals), high-carbohydrate meals, and drugs with hypotensive effects
Increase venous return and cardiac output	Counter-maneuvers with "muscle pumping" effect: leg and arm crossing, muscle tensing, handgrip, squatting, sitting, lying down and raising limbs Mechanical compression of capacitance vessels of abdomen and lower limbs: muscle toning exercises, abdominal and thigh binders
Expand plasma volume (goal: light urine color, low urine specific gravity)	Adequate water intake (2–2.5 L fluid/d), adequate salt intake (>8 g/d) with additional 4–6 g/d if symptomatic from OH and 24-hr urinary volume <1.5–2.5 L and $[Na^{++}]$ <170 mmol/L Exercise (as tolerated)
Enhance vasoconstriction	Activate osmopressor reflexes (vasoconstriction in response to acute hypo-osmolarity): 500 mL water by mouth over ~5 min. Sustained pressor response 5–60 min Tilt training by standing 30 min leaning with low back against a wall and feet 15 cm away from the wall, once or twice a day (as tolerated)
Plasma and red blood cell volume expansion	Stimulate renin and vasopressin release: head up at night in reverse Trendelenburg position with head of bed elevated by 10–20 degrees, and out of bed while awake Exercise (as tolerated)

Abbreviation: OH, orthostatic hypotension.

REFLEX SYNCOPE, NEURALLY MEDIATED HYPOTENSION, AND BRADYCARDIA

Reflex syncope is a short-duration, self-terminating loss of consciousness that results from a chain of ANS events (i.e., neurally mediated) that lead to hypotension and cerebral hypoperfusion. Onset is rapid and is followed by spontaneous, prompt, and complete recovery. Vasovagal syncope is the most common cause of reflex syncope. Prodromal symptoms of autonomic activation (sweating, pallor, nausea) are typical. Vasovagal syncope is reflexly triggered by emotion (i.e., emotional syncope) and by gravitational volume shifts produced by upright postures. Other causes of reflex syncope are situational (i.e., cough, micturition). All forms of reflex syncope require relatively preserved PS and S pathways as the typical hemodynamic response involves reflex vasodilatation (due to S withdrawal) and slowing of the HR (due to PS activation via the vagus nerve). The diagnosis is clinical and cardiac (and sometimes epileptic) causes should be considered. Treatment includes educating the patient to avoid triggering situations and how to apply some of the counter-maneuvers outlined above for OH. Some medications may be effective in reducing the risk of recurrent reflex syncope.

SEXUAL DYSFUNCTION AND URINARY BLADDER DYSFUNCTION

A wide range of neurologic diseases are associated with sexual and urinary bladder dysfunction.

TABLE 32.6 Selected Pharmacologic Treatment of Neurogenic Orthostatic Hypotension

Objective	Mechanism	Drug	Comments
Expand plasma volume	Mineralocorticoid	Fludrocortisone	>0.1 mg/d + adequate fluid and dietary salt intake and potassium supplementation. Potassium-rich diet and monitor plasma [K+] (decreased in up to 50%). Titrate weekly. May cause fluid overload
	Antidiuretic (V$_2$ receptor agonist)	Desmopressin	Reduces nocturnal polyuria
Expand red blood cell volume	↑ Red blood cell mass, blood viscosity	Erythropoietin alpha	Improves orthostatic tolerance in patients with OH and anemia. 25–50 U/K s.c. t.i.w.
	↑ Adrenoceptor sensitivity	Fludrocortisone	<0.1 mg/daily. At these lower doses combine with high-salt diet and sleeping with the head of the bed elevated (i.e., reverse Trendelenburg)
Enhance vasoconstriction	α-adrenoceptor agonists	Midodrine	Monotherapy (or combined with fludrocortisone): 2.5–10 mg b.i.d or t.i.d. As supine hypertension is common, give <4 hr before bedtime
		Droxidopa (DOPS)	NE precursor, used for DBH deficiency, OH. Begin: 200 mg/daily
		Phenylpropanolamine	10–25 mg q.i.d.
		Atomoxetine	NET blockade, pressor effect in "central" (i.e., MSA) NOS with intact peripheral S efferents. 18 mg given 1 hr before activities and >4 hr before going to sleep
	↑ S ganglionic transmission (by increasing ACh)	Pyridostigmine	Modest increase in BP, with less supine hypertension as compared with other agents. 60 mg t.i.d.
	Vasodilatatory gut peptide antagonist	Octreotide	Reduces PPH and tachycardia in POTS. Does not increase supine hypertension. Has been used in combination with midodrine
	Delaying intestinal glucose absorption	Acarbose	Reduces PPH. 50 mg/daily before largest meal and titrate up

Abbreviations: ACh, acetylcholine; BP, blood pressure; b.i.d. or t.i.d., twice a day or three times a day; DBH, dopamine-α-hydroxylase; MSA, multiple system atrophy; NE, norepinephrine; NET, norepinephrine transporter; PPH, postprandial OH; V, Vasopressin; POTS, Postural orthostatic tachycardia syndrome; q.i.d., four times a day; S, sympathetic; s.c., subcutaneously; t.i.w, three times per week.

SEXUAL DYSFUNCTION

Male and female sexual dysfunction is common. Sexual dysfunction may manifest as disorders of libido, of arousal and orgasm in women, and of erection and ejaculation in men. Sexual dysfunction in men may be an early sign of autonomic dysfunction, first with ED (discussed here) and later by failure of ejaculation.

Pathophysiology

The sexual response cycle of excitement, plateau, orgasm, and resolution is mediated through the integrated and coordinated activity of the somatic and ANSs. Central ANS networks and pathways involved in controlling sexual function include the medial preoptic area, amygdala, periventricular nucleus, periaqueductal gray, and the ventral tegmentum. They project onto S fibers originating from T12–L2 that synapse in the hypogastric plexus to travel to the pelvic plexus, where they meet PS fibers from S2–S4 segments. From here, S and PS travel together in pelvic nerves to innervate the pelvic organs.

Sexual response cycles begin with smooth muscle relaxation with vasodilatation and an increase in pelvic blood flow and genital engorgement. Genital engorgement is a neurovascular event dependent on spinal autonomic centers, enhanced by genital stimulation and by supraspinal sexual centers. Ejaculation depends on two different spinal reflexes. One results in emission of semen into the urethra, and another, in ejaculation.

Erectile Dysfunction

A. **Diagnosis.** ED is the persistent inability to develop and maintain an erection sufficient enough to permit satisfactory sexual performance. ED is a common and sometimes early presentation of autonomic dysfunction. In addition to autonomic causes, ED may result as a side effect of medications, or because of mechanical, endothelial, endocrine, metabolic, vascular, and psychogenic causes, frequently acting in combination. Depression and anxiety are common causes of sexual dysfunction and frequent complicating factors. Particular attention should be paid to the history of symptoms of leg claudication and cardiovascular symptoms as ED is a strong predictor of future cardiovascular disease in younger men. Abdominal examination is necessary as 1% of patients with ED have abdominal aortic aneurysm.

B. **Physiology.** Penile engorgement and erection result from endothelium-mediated engorgement of the corpora cavernosa (and less so, of the corpora spongiosum) with venous blood. Erection is triggered by **somatosensory stimulation** (reflexive erection, disrupted by lesions of the sacral cord and intermediolateral cell columns—as in MSA), **audiovisual stimulation** (psychogenic erection, disrupted by lesions above the sacral cord), and by **nocturnal cortical stimulation** during rapid eye movement (REM) sleep ("morning erection," nocturnal penile tumescence, disrupted by disturbed REM sleep).

For erection to occur, appropriate stimuli trigger the release of neurotransmitters from efferent cholinergic PS and noncholinergic, nonadrenergic fibers originating from the pelvic plexus. Key to erection is the release of nitric oxide (NO) from nitrergic nerves in the corpora cavernosa and from cavernous vascular endothelium. NO results in an increased cyclic guanosine monophosphate (cGMP)-dependent dilatation of trabecular arteries. Dilated trabecular arteries in turn compress the cavernous vein against the tunica albuginea, obstructing venous outflow to produce engorgement of the penis with venous blood. Concurrent contractions of the ischiocavernosus and bulbospongiosus muscles compress corpora cavernosa veins to limit venous outflow and maintain erection. Most ED results from deficient release of NO. Penile detumescence occurs when corpus cavernosa phosphodiesterase-5 (PDE-5) hydrolyzes cGMP, ending arteriolar vasodilatation. Understanding of this pathway has led to treatment of ED by using reversible competitive inhibitors of PDE-5 (see section **D.2** under Erectile Dysfunction, Sexual Dysfunction below).

C. **Laboratory testing.** In men who do not respond to treatment with PDE-5 inhibitors, when specific neurologic causes are considered, or when the cause of ED is not apparent:
  1. Free testosterone, luteinizing and follicle-stimulating hormone and prolactin levels, glucose tolerance, liver function, prostatic specific antigen, BUN, creatinine, and thyroid function tests.
  2. **Consultations.** Psychiatric, urologic, and vascular consultations in the appropriate clinical settings.

D. Treatment of ED.
  1. **Nonpharmacologic treatment.**
    a. **Lifestyle changes.** Exercise (>18 MET/hour/week), weight loss (goal: BMI <30 kg/m^2), and smoking and alcohol cessation are recommended for all patients with sexual dysfunction. Pelvic floor muscle strengthening exercises may be helpful.
    b. b. Treatment of underlying endocrine, metabolic, vascular, and psychogenic causes, and management or withdrawal of any offending medications. Psychosexual counseling is important in many cases.

2. **Pharmacologic treatment.** PDE-5 (see section **B** under Erectile Dysfunction above) inhibitors are the mainstay of the pharmacologic treatment of ED. By blocking the destruction of cGMP, they potentiate penile vessel smooth muscle relaxation and, thus, penile engorgement. PDE-5 inhibitors require sexual stimulation to be effective (they do not increase libido). PDE-5 inhibitors are not effective where ED is due to significant endothelial dysfunction with deficient NO bioavailability. NO-mediated smooth muscle relaxation is androgen-dependent and supplementing testosterone in those who are deficient (i.e., morning testosterone <300 ng/dL) may offer benefit.

Sildenafil (50 to 100 mg) and vardenafil (10 to 20 mg) taken 1 hour prior to intercourse have a duration of effect up of to 4 hours. Tadalafil (10 to 20 mg), taken 1 to 12 hours prior to intercourse, has a duration of effect of up to 36 hours. As it has a long half-life, tadalafil should be avoided in patients in whom cardiac risk from sexual activity is high. As interactions between PDE-5 inhibitors and NO donors (i.e., nitrates) may precipitate serious hypotension, the ongoing use of nitrates is an absolute contraindication to their use. Significant hypotension may result from the use of PDE-5 inhibitors in patients with MSA.

3. **Local treatments.** Used in patients in whom PDE-5 inhibitors are ineffective or contraindicated. Vacuum constriction devices and constriction rings applied to the base of the penis produce unnatural but effective erections. Alprostadil, a prostaglandin E-1 (PGE-1) analog inserted into the urethra, produces penile smooth muscle relaxation and penile erection. Medications (papaverine, alprostadil, phentolamine, and PGE-1) self-injected into the corpus cavernosa to cause an erection are very effective. A normal erection in response to the intracavernosal injection of vasoactive agents (i.e., papaverine) indicates that vascular mechanisms involved in erection are intact, suggesting psychogenic impotence (although approximately 30% of men with normal erections may lack a response). Penile implants are beneficial and well tolerated and are usually reserved for those who PDE-5 inhibitors and other methods are unsatisfactory.

URINARY BLADDER DYSFUNCTION

A wide range of neurologic diseases are associated with urinary bladder dysfunction. Common conditions are stroke, dementia, PD, multiple sclerosis, DM, and other forms of neuropathy with autonomic involvement. Tumoral, infectious, traumatic, and congenital (i.e., spina bifida, tethered cord) causes are less frequent.

Anatomy

The cerebral cortex, basal ganglia, cerebellum, and brainstem pontine detrusor nuclei influence the sacral spinal nuclei involved in urinary bladder control via peripheral nerves. Peripheral nerves innervate the external sphincter, periurethral muscles, and other abdominal and pelvic muscles. **Micturition** relies on a brainstem and spinal cord autonomic reflex that includes periaqueductal gray and the pontine micturition center (PMC), regulated by the hypothalamus and prefrontal cortex and their inputs from other areas (i.e., with the right insula providing interoception and limbic system providing hedonic valance). Micturition is initiated by the hypothalamus and prefrontal cortex (i.e., consciousness about the appropriateness of voiding) by withdrawing their inhibition of the PMC. The PMC activates relaxation of the external sphincter striated muscle followed by relaxation of the bladder detrusor muscle. **Urinary storage** depends on a sacral cord autonomic reflex arc. It is tonically facilitated by the pontine storage center, hypothalamus, cerebellum, basal ganglia, and frontal cortex.

Bladder filling triggers the micturition reflex. Micturition is primarily a PS function with S2–S4 efferents stimulating bladder (detrusor muscle) contraction while inhibiting the internal bladder sphincter. The S nervous system is involved in urine storage and bladder capacity. S T10–L2 efferents inhibit the detrusor while stimulating the internal sphincter. Bladder contraction occurs with stimulation of PS cholinergic muscarinic receptors and relaxation with stimulation of β-adrenoceptors. Contraction of the urethra occurs with stimulation of α-adrenoceptors and relaxation with stimulation of nicotinic acetylcholine receptors.

Clinical Evaluation

A. **History.** Patterns of urinary incontinence and frequency and urgency of urination are determined. Desire to void, ability to initiate and terminate urination, force of urinary stream and urine volume, and sensations associated with urination are other important aspects of the history. Particular attention must also be paid to medication.

B. **Examination.**

The neurologic examination and the postvoid urine residual, complemented by urodynamic studies, determine the site of an autonomic lesion.

1. **Lesion sites.**
   a. Lesions above the PMC produce an uninhibited bladder. There is lack of awareness of bladder filling and of the passage of urine. There is urinary retention with elevated residual bladder urine volumes.
   b. Lesions below PMC and above the S2–S4 produce an upper motor neuron bladder. There is lack of awareness of urinary sensations. Bladder and sphincter contractions occur simultaneously (detrusor-sphincter dyssynergia). Residual bladder urine volumes are low, and detrusor is hypertrophic (may produce vesicourethral reflux). With thoracolumbar spinal cord lesions there is loss of S control of the bladder neck resulting in retrograde ejaculation. Spinal cord lesions above T6 result in disinhibition of S neurons and patients with these lesions are at risk of autonomic dysreflexia (see section **B** under Autonomic Crisis below). With lesions above S2–S4, the voiding reflex is preserved, and there is frequency of micturition, and reduced bladder capacity.
   c. Sacral cord or sacral nerve root lesions produce a lower motor neuron bladder. The bladder is flaccid (the PS nucleus is affected), and bladder residual volumes are elevated. There is stress incontinence, and lack of awareness of urinary sensations (although hypogastric nerves transmit pain from a distended bladder).
   d. d. Peripheral nerve lesions produce a flaccid bladder (the PS nucleus connections with the bladder are affected), and bladder residual volumes are elevated. There is stress incontinence. If the motor nerves are preferentially involved, volitional voiding may be severely compromised even though bladder sensation may be largely preserved.

C. **Evaluation of urinary dysfunction.**

1. Urinalysis and urine culture with appropriate sensitivity studies (many patients have associated urinary tract infection), postvoid urine residual. Renal function is monitored as vesicoureteral reflux may cause renal failure.
2. Ultrasound determines postvoid residual and anatomy.
3. **Urodynamic investigations.** Cystometry provides information about the pressure–volume relation on filling (bladder compliance), bladder capacity, volume at first sensation and at urge to void, voiding pressure, and if uninhibited detrusor contractions are present (Table 32.7). Endoscopy allows direct visualization of the bladder neck during voiding.
4. Spinal and brain imaging, as directed by the clinical features.
5. Sphincter and pelvic floor EMG detects denervation potentials in selected muscles in lesions of the anterior horn cells in the S2–S4 spinal cord, and is helpful in patients in whom there is suspicion of cauda equine syndrome, and when MSA is suspected (it is abnormal).

TABLE 32.7 Urodynamic Findings in Various Types of Neurogenic Bladder Dysfunction

Spastic Bladder	Atonic Bladder	Sphincter Dyssynergia
Decreased capacity	Increased capacity	Fluctuating voiding pressure
Reduced compliance	Increased compliance	Intermittent flow rate
Uninhibited detrusor contractions	Low voiding pressure and flow rate	

D. **Clinical presentations.**
1. **Urinary incontinence** is defined as failure to store urine normally.
   a. **Stress urinary incontinence** occurs when intra-abdominal pressure rises. It occurs because of weakened ligaments supporting the urethra (i.e., damage with childbirth) or because of a weak urinary sphincter due to lesions involving sacral neurons (Onuf's nucleus).
   b. **Urinary urgency incontinence** occurs when there is an overactive bladder resulting from decreased inhibition from the brain ("upper motor neuron bladder"). Incontinence occurs when bladder contraction pressure overcomes bladder neck outlet resistance. Urodynamic studies demonstrate detrusor overactivity (DO), with inappropriate bladder contractions during storage. Symptoms include frequency, nocturia, intermittent bladder contractions with incontinence, and urgency if sensation is preserved. Patients with urinary incontinence with urgency usually have upper motor neuron signs at neurologic examination. There are many causes: dementias, PD, hydrocephalus, bilateral frontal lobe lesion, spinal cord disease, syphilis, and tethered cord. In the elderly, there may be impaired cortical ability to inhibit the voiding reflex with urge incontinence. The non-neurologic cause of urgency is usually cystitis secondary to infection or inflammation with another cause.
2. **Voiding difficulties with urinary retention** result from an underactive detrusor (atonic bladder and bladder weakness), manifesting as a "lower motor neuron bladder." Urodynamic study confirms a large, low-pressure bladder, and absent contractions. It is due to lesions affecting peripheral nerves or S2–S4 neurons innervating the bladder (acute upper neuron lesions can also cause detrusor weakness). There may be lack of awareness of bladder filling and inability to initiate voiding, producing urinary retention with overflow incontinence. Causes include spinal shock, myelitis, conus medullaris and cauda equina lesions, and neuropathy. Other causes are MSA, Friedreich's ataxia, tabes, diabetes, alcoholic neuropathy, plexopathy, and after pelvic radiation.
3. **Urgency incontinence and difficulty voiding** with incomplete bladder emptying. Lesions in both the storage-facilitating areas of the brain (basal ganglia and pontine storage center) and the voiding-facilitating areas (PMC and sacral preganglionic intermediolateral cell column neurons) result in a combination of DO in the filling phase and underactive detrusor in the voiding phase, accompanied by urgency incontinence and difficulty voiding with incomplete emptying (detrusor hyperactivity with impaired contractile function—DHIC). DHIC is typical of MSA.

E. **Treatment.**
1. Bladder training. Timed bladder emptying, intermittent catheterization, and biofeedback techniques are helpful. Pelvic floor muscle strengthening with training exercises lead to decreased detrusor contractions and increased internal sphincter tone, with improvement of urinary frequency.
2. Bladder catheterization.
3. Pharmacotherapy for urinary storage dysfunction (Table 32.8). Injection of botulinum toxin type A has been used when there is no response to antimuscarinic drugs.
   a. Urologic consultation is recommended.

GASTROINTESTINAL DYSFUNCTION

Esophageal, Gastric, and Intestinal Dysfunction

The ENS reflex pathways organized as myenteric (Auerbach's) and submucosal (Meissner's) plexus regulate gut motility, secretion and absorption, and vascular tone. ENS function is modulated by PS and S efferents.

Symptoms

Depending on the GI tract site affected, GI dysfunction manifests as esophageal dysphagia, gastroparesis, constipation, intestinal pseudo-obstruction, colonic inertia, megacolon, and defecatory dysfunction. Symptoms range from dysphagia, early satiety, fullness, bloating, nausea, postprandial vomiting, diarrhea, constipation, and fecal incontinence.

TABLE 32.8 Selected Drugs Used to Manage Neurogenic Bladder Dysfunction

Class of Drug	Drug Name	Dosage
Antimuscarinic anticholinergic agents	Oxybutynin	2.5–20 mg/d
	Darifenacin	7.5–15 mg/d
	Solifenacin	5–10 mg/d
	Tolterodine	2–4 mg/d
	Trospium	20–40 mg/d
β-adrenergic agonists	Mirabegron	25–50 mg/d
S α-antagonists	Doxazosin	1–8 mg/d
	Tamsulosin	0.4–0.8 mg/d
Tricyclic antidepressants	Imipramine	10–50 mg/d

Dosages of each drug must be individualized to achieve optimum effect with minimum adverse effects. Some may be used in combination for better effects.
Abbreviation: S, sympathetic.

Causes

A. Drugs: opioids, tricyclic antidepressants, and dopamine agonists are frequent causes.
B. Mechanical obstruction and gut inflammation.
C. Neurologic: PD, MSA, spinal cord lesions, neuropathies (i.e., diabetic, amyloid), autoimmune ganglionopathies (paraneoplastic and primary), neuromuscular transmission defects, and myopathy are notable causes.
D. Other: Chagas disease is a common cause of autonomic GI dysfunction and should be considered with exposure to *Trypanosoma cruzi*-endemic areas. Rare causes include inherited neuropathies.

Fecal Incontinence

Fecal incontinence is associated with aging, reflecting a decline in muscle strength, mobility, and cognitive functioning. Typically there is loss of the sphincter's endovascular cushion, thickening of external and internal sphincters, loss of resting and squeeze sphincter pressures, and reduced rectal sensation. Pudendal nerve stretch injury and direct trauma to the sphincter may produce pelvic floor dysfunction and fecal incontinence.

Typical symptoms range from insensible loss to sensory urge fecal loss, including complaints limited to perianal irritation.

Upper motor neuron lesions rostral to the sacral cord produce increased anal sphincter tone, loss of voluntary control, inability to relax or contract the sphincter on command, and result in fecal retention. With lesions of the sacral cord, conus medullaris, or cauda equina, there is a weak and areflexic anal sphincter with a patulous anus. Sensory loss may be present. Pelvic nerve lesions produce incontinence with loss of formed stool (diarrheal) with denervated external and internal anal sphincters.

Evaluation of Gastrointestinal Dysfunction

1. Physical examination with inspection of perineum, rectum, and vagina.
2. Direct observation via videoendoscopy.
3. Imaging studies: Dynamic imaging includes video-fluoroscopy, barium swallow studies, radionuclide gastric emptying studies, breath tests using radiolabeled substances (duodenal transit), colonic transit (markers, radionuclide), and defecography (barium, dynamic MRI). Anatomical imaging includes MRI of the spine (spinal cord lesions), pelvic computed tomography and/or MRI (malformations and structural abnormalities), endoanal ultrasonography (anal canal musculature and sphincter defects), and radiographic measurement of the rectoanal angle.
4. Manometry assesses GI sphincter function by measuring pressures.

5. Neurophysiologic studies. EMG of anal sphincter and puborectalis muscle and pudendal nerve terminal motor latency may help determine the type of neurologic disorder causing fecal dysfunction.

Management of Gastrointestinal Dysfunction

Gastroparesis

1. Diet with low-fat, low-fiber (to prevent bezoar), small and frequent meals
2. Prokinetic drugs: metoclopramide (also antiemetic), erythromycin
3. Pyloric sphincter botulinum

Constipation

1. Increase colonic content volume and maintain a near-normal consistency: high fiber content (>15 g/day), psyllium dietary fiber, methylcellulose, docusate sodium stool softener, lubiprostone (produces Cl-rich fluid secretion).
2. Laxatives: magnesium salts, lactulose, polyethylene glycol, bisacodyl (stimulates colonic contraction and increases fluid and NaCl secretion)
3. To prevent bacterial overgrowth due to slowed GI transit: metronidazole, ciprofloxacin, doxycycline (antibiotics are given for 1 week each month)

Fecal Incontinence

1. Techniques to achieve orderly defecation. Straining with Valsalva's maneuvers, pressing on the abdomen (for patients with some preserved rectal sensation and able to feel the urge to defecate), digital stimulation of the rectum (most effective after glycerin suppositories, and in the sitting position). Scheduled enemas
2. Biofeedback training with EMG
3. Neuromodulation: anterior sacral root stimulators
4. Surgery: Replacement sphincter and pelvic floor reconstruction.

HYPO- AND HYPERHIDROSIS

Sweating abnormalities are frequent ANS symptoms. Sweating disorders may be idiopathic or part of small-fiber neuropathies, ANS ganglionopathies (see section Anhidrosis), MSA, and many other disorders. In addition to the potential disruption of thermoregulation, sweating disorders may be a source of disabling social embarrassment (hyperhidrosis).

Sweating is mediated by S cholinergic postganglionic neurons activating M_3 muscarinic receptors of the eccrine sweat gland (vasointestinal peptide is also released to produce vasodilatation enhancing sweat production). Sweating stimuli may be thermoregulatory or emotional. Thermoregulatory sweating produces cutaneous vasodilatation and sweating distributed over the face, trunk, and proximal limbs, whereas emotional sweating produces vasoconstriction and seating is distributed over the palms and soles.

The pattern of the sweating abnormalities helps determine a cause. Distal patterns occur with length-dependent neuropathies, and generalized patterns reflect widespread ANS dysfunction as with MSA, ganglionopathies, and the effect of offending medication. Segmental S innervation helps to localize a spinal cord lesion. S innervation to the face originates from the T1–T2 spinal cord, the upper limbs from T4–T8, the trunk from T4–T12, and the lower limbs from T10–T12. Thermoregulatory sweat testing (where sweat produces changes in the color of substances—typically starch/iodine applied to the skin) provides clear anatomical sweating maps. Silicone imprint (sweat droplets are counted) and other more sophisticated tests provide indication of sweat production. QSART permits discrimination between preganglionic and postganglionic lesions.

Anhidrosis

Typically it is distributed over the upper body, head, and face. It may be accompanied by compensatory hyperhidrosis in proximal unaffected areas. Anhidrosis accompanies multiple ANS disorders, including MSA, PAF, peripheral neuropathies, autoimmune ganglionopathies, and CNS lesions (i.e., contralateral hypohidrosis with stroke) and the effect of various drugs.

Acquired idiopathic anhidrosis selectively affects sweating, likely due to immune-mediated disruption of muscarinic sweat gland receptors.

Treatment relies on avoiding situations or environments that raise body temperature (i.e., adjusting clothing, exercising in cool environments), maintaining optimal hydration, and avoiding medication with anticholinergic effects, caffeine, and alcohol.

Hyperhidrosis

Generalized hyperhidrosis is usually associated with disorders producing S overactivity (i.e., alcohol withdrawal, thyrotoxicosis, pheochromocytoma, hypoglycemia, voltage-gated potassium channel antibodies, baroreflex failure, and HSAN III). It may also result from the effect of malignancies (i.e., lymphomas) and infections (i.e., tuberculosis), altering the thermoregulatory sweating threshold. Focal hyperhidrosis is frequent, and produces excessive sweating with mental stress and physical activity. It involves axillae, palms, and soles, and may be severe enough to cause significant social embarrassment. There are multiple syndromes associated with hyperhidrosis, many beyond the scope of this chapter.

Symptomatic treatment includes avoiding triggering factors (i.e., anxiety), topical preparations with aluminum chloride, tap water iontophoresis (palms, soles, axillae), oral medication (antimuscarinic anticholinergic drugs, clonidine, and topiramate), local injection of botulinum toxin, and in selected situations sympathectomy.

AUTONOMIC DISORDERS

Primary Autonomic Failure

A. Alpha-synucleinopathies. The ANS is typically involved with intracellular α-synuclein inclusions. In central ANS disorders (i.e., MSA), they are distributed in the CNS, and in peripheral ANS disorders they are mainly postganglionic (i.e., in LBD and PD, LBD), or exclusively postganglionic (i.e., PAF).

   1. **PAF** (previously progressive autonomic failure, idiopathic OH, or Bradbury–Eggleston syndrome) is a sporadic degenerative disorder of middle to late life, affecting men more often. The cardinal manifestation is OH, with variable urinary sphincter and ED and constipation. Supine NE is low, and fails to increase with upright postural challenge (despite symptomatic hypotension).

      In PAF postganglionic efferent S and PS autonomic neurons are impaired. The pathology is similar to that of idiopathic PD and DLB, with Lewy bodies in the CNS, S and PS ganglia, and in pre- and postganglionic neurons. Abnormalities in spinal cord and peripheral nerves are more prominent in PAF, perhaps explaining clinical differences between these disorders. Occasionally PAF may progress clinically to PD with OH and DLB with OH, and may develop dementia.

      The differential diagnosis includes other causes of NOH (peripheral neuropathies with ANS disease, PD, and MSA). With PAF there are no parkinsonian, cerebellar, corticospinal, sensory, or lower motor neuron features, and ganglionic AChR are absent (autoimmune autonomic ganglionopathy [AAG] may be clinically similar to PAF). The clinical diagnosis requires the absence of symptoms other than autonomic >5 years, to distinguish PAF from cases of early MSA with isolated OH. Progression is slow, and, despite prominent OH, is less disabling than MSA.

   2. **MSA** is a progressive, adult-onset neurodegenerative synucleinopathy involving both autonomic and somatic nervous systems, causing autonomic cardiovascular, urinary, and anorectal dysfunction, parkinsonism, and ataxia, in any combination. Onset is typically in the sixth decade of life, and men are affected more frequently. Early urinary and anorectal and ED with an abnormal sphincter EMG (due to loss of neurons of the sacral nucleus of Onuf) is typical. In many patients, chronic OH precedes other neurologic involvement, making differentiation of MSA from PAF difficult (Table 32.9). Pathology demonstrates abnormal oligodendroglial filaments of α-synuclein (glial cytoplasmic inclusions) mainly in substantia nigra, striatum, locus ceruleus, pons, inferior olives, cerebellum, and spinal cord, with neuronal degeneration and gliosis at multiple sites within the brain and spinal cord, but no Lewy bodies.

TABLE 32.9 Differential Diagnosis of MSA

	Clinical Features	Differential Diagnosis
MSA-P	Non- or poorly levodopa responsive akinetic-rigid syndrome with pyramidal signs, with autonomic dysfunction	• Idiopathic PD • PAF (when MSA has a purely autonomic presentation) • PD presenting with autonomic failure (most MSA with autonomic failure develop other neurologic features within 5 yr, but the interval can be longer) • Progressive supranuclear palsy, corticobasal degeneration, primary lateral sclerosis, amyotrophic lateral sclerosis (slowing, spasticity, and pyramidal signs may be confused with a levodopa-unresponsive akinetic-rigid syndrome with pyramidal signs similar to MSA. The characteristic eye movement findings of these are absent in MSA) • Cerebrovascular disease
MSA-C	ILOCA syndrome with autonomic dysfunction	• ILOCA syndrome (25% have MSA) • Friedreich's ataxia (atypical, late-onset form) • SCA2, SCA3, and SCA6 (cerebellar features and parkinsonism, with family history in SCA2 and SCA3, sporadic in SCA6) • Primary progressive multiple sclerosis, fragile X tremor ataxia syndrome, sporadic adult-onset ataxia, and sporadic cerebellar-olivary atrophy

Abbreviations: ILOCA, idiopathic late-onset cerebellar ataxia; MSA, multiple system atrophy; MSA-P, multiple system atrophy(parkinsonism); MSA-C, multiple system atrophy(cerebellar); PAF, pure autonomic failure; PD, Parkinson's disease; SCA, spinocerebellar ataxia.

MSA is classified as either **MSA-P (parkinsonism)** or **MSA-C (cerebellar)**, depending on the presence of predominant parkinsonism or cerebellar ataxia. As some clinical features of MSA are shared with other chronic progressive disorders such as PD and PAF, the clinical diagnosis may be difficult.

a. Clinical features. Patients with MSA typically have OH, erectile and urinary dysfunction, hypohidrosis, early instability, rapid progression, abnormal postures, bulbar and respiratory dysfunction, and emotional incontinence and Parkinsonism and cerebellar features.

b. Laboratory evaluation.
   (1) Autonomic testing (Table 32.3)
   (2) EMG may suggest involvement of the anterior horn cells in MSA. Abnormal sphincter muscle EMG (denervation potentials of spinal cord anterior horn cells) can distinguish MSA from PD (Onuf's neurons are spared) in the first 5 years after the onset of symptoms and signs, and from PAF, as well as from cerebellar ataxias, if other causes for sphincter denervation have been ruled out. Normal EMG is unlikely in MSA.
   (3) MRI. Linear hyperintense putaminal border rim, putaminal atrophy, and putaminal hypointensity relative to the globus pallidus signal, and cruciform pontine hyperintensities ("hot cross bun" pattern) are specific to MSA, but sensitivity is low. Cerebellar atrophy may be present in some patients even without clinical cerebellar signs.

c. Management (Tables 32.5 and 32.6). Only symptomatic treatment is available. One-third of patients have temporary response to levodopa; some may respond to amantadine. Side effects, especially accentuation of hypotension, must be kept in mind.

AUTONOMIC NEUROPATHIES

Autonomic neuropathies are peripheral neuropathies where ANS fibers are prominently affected. Impairment of the lightly myelinated or unmyelinated ANS fibers may interfere with the normal functioning of many organ systems, leading to various cardiovascular, urogenital, GI, sudomotor, thermoregulatory, and pupillomotor autonomic symptoms. Injury and dysfunction of ANS innervation may be secondary to diabetes, alcoholism, infections, amyloidosis, connective tissue disorders, and paraneoplastic syndromes, or occur in isolation without evident underlying disease (primary autonomic neuropathies). Depending on the extent and location of an autonomic lesion, ANS neuropathy may be widespread or limited to neurotransmitter type (cholinergic and adrenergic neuropathies), an organ system, or to distal small fibers. Selected examples are discussed here.

Diabetic autonomic neuropathy (DAN), a chronic autonomic neuropathy, is a common complication of diabetes. DAN may involve cardiovascular, GI, urogenital, and thermoregulatory (sweating) functions. As a length-dependent neuropathy, DAN affects the vagus nerve early on with abnormal cardiovascular autonomic function, manifested as reduced HR variation, the earliest indicator of cardiac autonomic neuropathy (CAN). The 5-year mortality rate is five times higher for those with CAN than for individuals without cardiovascular autonomic involvement. Clinical symptoms of DAN generally do not occur until long after the onset of diabetes, and are more common with worse glycemic control. In patients with long-standing diabetes, esophageal transit is delayed in 50% and gastroparesis is present in 40%. Symptoms are variable and more common in patients with worse chronic glycemic control and with psychological disorders. Other common GI symptoms include constipation, diarrhea, and fecal incontinence. Impaired glucose regulation (impaired glucose tolerance [IGT], nondiabetic hyperglycemia, prediabetes) with small-fiber neuropathy is accompanied by mild autonomic neuropathy (sudomotor fibers tend to be affected earlier with IGT).

AAG is a primary acute and subacute autonomic neuropathy characterized by a rapid onset of **isolated diffuse ANS dysfunction** associated with ganglionic nicotinic $\alpha 3$-acetylcholine receptors ($\alpha 3$-AChR) autoantibodies. AAG may follow respiratory and GI infections, vaccines, surgery, treatment with interferon, and may be a paraneoplastic presentation (30% have malignancies, mostly adenocarcinoma). Typical features of the classic form of AAG are acute/subacute widespread and frequently severe involvement of the S, PS, and ENSs (GI dysmotility is prominent). It is a monophasic disorder with high (>0.5 nmol/L) antibody levels (ANS manifestations are more pronounced with higher levels). Other forms are slowly progressive and chronic, ANS involvement is more localized, and $\alpha 3$-AChR antibody levels are low. As slowly progressive and chronic forms of ANS dysfunction (including PAF) may be due to AAG, these patients should be screened for AAG. Postural tachycardia, chronic idiopathic anhidrosis, isolated GI dysmotility, and distal small-fiber neuropathies may have low $\alpha 3$-AChR antibody levels. Symptoms may improve with immunotherapy, although in acute and subacute forms improvement (usually partial) may also be spontaneous. Chronic forms of AAG should be treated early on in an attempt to prevent disease progression.

Paraneoplastic autonomic neuropathy is frequently present with paraneoplastic disorders. Anti-Hu, anti-CV2/CRMP-5, and $\alpha 3$-AChR antibody are frequently associated with autonomic involvement (GI dysmotility is prominent). Various antineuronal (typically anti-Hu, anti-VGCC, and antiganglionic acetylcholine receptor) antibodies associated with underlying disease (usually a paraneoplastic syndrome associated with lung, thymus, gyn, and breast cancer) may be detected. Treatment of the underlying tumor is the main therapeutic approach. Immunomodulatory therapy can be beneficial in some cases

Enteric ganglionitis (EG) is an example of an autonomic disorder affecting the gut exclusively. It is characterized by inflammatory or immune dysfunction of intrinsic GI innervation causing dysmotility and delayed transit. Lymphoid infiltration of the small intestine produces intestinal pseudo-obstruction; infiltration of the myenteric ganglia causes achalasia. EG is usually associated with paraneoplastic neurologic syndromes, but may be also present with CNS disorders and with Chagas disease.

AUTONOMIC CRISIS

A. Autonomic crises. Acute autonomic dysfunction occurs in many conditions and a hypersympathetic state is most often encountered. Examples of such neurologic conditions are as follows.

  1. Cerebral lesions. Ischemic stroke, intracerebral hemorrhage, subarachnoid hemorrhage, intracranial mass lesion, Cushing's response

2. Spinal cord lesions (in particular with an injury at level T6 or above)
3. **Peripheral nerve disease.** Guillain–Barré syndrome (GBS)
4. **Systemic diseases.** Tetanus, episode of acute intermittent porphyria
5. **Drug-related conditions.** Neuroleptic malignant syndrome, sympathomimetic drug overdose, tricyclic antidepressant overdose

B. **Autonomic dysreflexia** is a life-threatening "sympathetic storm" that occurs in cases of spinal cord transection. The spinal cord lesion is usually above the midthoracic level. The episodes are paroxysmal and start several months after the acute spinal cord injury as recovery occurs. They are characterized by sudden onset of severe hypertension, headache, sweating and flushing, piloerection, and sometimes chills due to uninhibited activity of spinal S neurons. A precipitating cause can often be identified, and is usually a noxious stimulus. Urinary bladder distention, constipation, and fecal impaction are common causes. Elimination of the precipitating cause often results in resolution of the episode, and prevention is the best therapy. Hypertension is treated with antihypertensive agents with rapid onset and short-duration effects.

C. **Anesthetic complications.** Patients with autonomic dysfunction may have unpredictable, life-threatening, intraoperative hypotension and cardiovascular collapse. Caution and close operative and postoperative observation and monitoring are necessary, and including with spinal anesthesia may result in hypotension because of volume shifts (it may produce further loss of autonomic control of splanchic bed volumes).

Mechanisms

A. Impaired cardiovascular reflexes with inadequate compensation for anesthetic-induced vasodilatation and volume shifts, unpredictable responses to vasoactive agents due to denervation supersensitivity, and impaired response to atropine (due to cardiac PS denervation, as in DAN)
B. Impaired central respiratory reflexes with hypopnea and apnea
C. GI autonomic dysfunction with gastroparesis and increased risk for aspiration
D. Impaired temperature regulation with hyperthermia (due to impaired sweating) or hypothermia (due to deficient vasoconstriction)
E. Decreased hepatic clearance of drugs due to liver hypoperfusion during hypotension

Prevention

Prevention includes:

1. Optimal hydration and BP management
2. Rapid sequence induction of anesthesia and volatile anesthetics in high-risk patients with autonomic dysfunction
3. Caution and close operative and postoperative observation and monitoring. Particular attention is given when switching ventilation parameters, as this may precipitate acute hypotension because of changes in venous return. Hyperventilation should be avoided as it aggravates hypotension.

Key Points

- The ANS maintains the body's internal homeostasis and regulates its protective responses.
- Symptoms of ANS dysfunction reflect the widespread ANS innervation, and their differential diagnosis is broad.
- The site of an autonomic lesion, the clinical course, and the presence or absence of accompanying somatic neurologic and/or systemic or localized manifestations of disease help establish a cause of autonomic dysfunction.
- NOH is a frequent and disabling manifestation of ANS dysfunction.
- Nonpharmacologic management of symptomatic OH is key to successful treatment.
- ANS dysfunction may be serious and life threatening in certain instances, and these should be sought and managed appropriately.

Recommended Readings

Asahina M, Vichayanrat E, Low D, et al. Autonomic dysfunction in Parkinson's disorders: assessment and pathophysiology. *J Neurol Neurosurg Psychiatry*. 2013;84:674–680.

Benarroch E, ed. *Autonomic Neurology*. London, England: Oxford University Press; 2014.

Freeman R. Autonomic peripheral neuropathy. *Neurol Clin*. 2007;25:277–301.

Garg BP. Disorders of micturition and defecation. In: Swaiman KF, Ashwal S, Ferriero DM, eds. *Pediatric Neurology: Principles and Practice*. 4th ed. St. Louis, MO: Mosby; 2006.

Gibbons CH, Freeman R. Antibody titers predict clinical features of autoimmune autonomic ganglion-opathy. *Auton Neurosci*. 2009;146:8–12.

Kaufmann H, Hague K, Perl D. Accumulation of alpha-synuclein in autonomic nerves in pure autonomic failure. *Neurology*. 2001;56:980–981.

Oribe E. Testing autonomic function. In: Appenzeller O, ed. *The Autonomic Nervous System. Part 1—Normal Functions*. In: Vinken PJ, Bruyn GW, eds. *Handbook of Clinical Neurology*. Amsterdam: Elsevier Science; 1999;74:595–648.

Robertson D. The pathology and diagnosis of orthostatic hypotension. *Clin Auton Res*. 2008;18(suppl 1):2–7.

Robertson D, Biaggioni I, Burnstock G, et al. *Primer on the Autonomic Nervous System*. 3rd ed. London, England: Academic Press; 2012.

Seth JH, Panicker JN, Fowler C. The neurological organization of micturition. In: Aminoff MJ, Boller F, Swaab DF, eds. *Handbook of Clinical Neurology* (117, 3rd Series). Amsterdam: Elsevier Science; 2013:111–117.

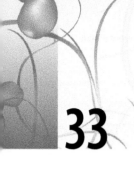

33

Approach to the Patient with Functional Disorders in the Neurology Clinic

Jeannette M. Gelauff and Jon Stone

Functional neurologic disorders (also commonly called psychogenic or "nonorganic") exist at the interface between neurology and psychiatry and are characterized by symptoms such as movement disorders (tremor/dystonia/jerks), limb weakness, sensory disturbance, and attacks of unconsciousness with or without jerking (dissociative [nonepileptic] attacks). The symptoms are genuine but do not relate to a defined disease process. They are defined by the presence of physical signs that demonstrate internal inconsistency or incongruity with recognized neurologic disease. Psychological factors and comorbidity are common but not universal. They account for between 15% and 30% of neurology outpatients depending on how they are defined and may coexist with neurologic disease. Functional disorders such as irritable bowel syndrome or fibromyalgia are similarly common throughout primary and secondary health care.

CLASSIFICATION AND TERMINOLOGY

A. **Terminology.** Over time, many different names have been fashionable:
   1. **Psychosomatic, psychogenic, somatization, and conversion disorder** all imply psychological etiology or the conversion of psychological distress in to physical symptoms. Studies show higher rates of psychological comorbidity, and some useful treatments are psychological but in many patients it is not possible to pinpoint a clear psychological etiology.
   2. The ancient term *hysteria* is still sometimes used but is pejorative.
   3. **Nonorganic (e.g., nonepileptic) and medically unexplained** label the problem by what it is not. This is not helpful for patients and also contrary to our known ability to make a positive and stable diagnosis in this group of patients. In the case of "medically unexplained" many conditions in neurology have an unknown etiology.
   4. **Dissociative** refers to a dissociation of nervous system or psychological functioning.
   5. **Functional symptom/disorder**, also an old term, which emphasizes a disorder of function without assuming etiology. It arguably allows for a broader biopsychosocial model but has been criticized for being too vague.
B. **Classification.** Classification has shifted hand in hand with the shifting terminology.
   1. *DSM-5* criteria (*Diagnostic and Statistical Manual of Mental Disorders*, Fifth Edition) classify these symptoms as **"Conversion Disorder/Functional Neurological Symptom Disorder."** There must be motor or sensory symptoms, positive clinical features related to assessment of the target symptom (e.g., limb weakness, tremor, blackouts), and impairment. In *DSM-IV* a psychological stressor was required but this criterion has now been removed, although may still remain relevant for some patients.
   2. *ICD-10* (*International Classification of Diseases*, Tenth Edition) identifies them as **Dissociative (Conversion) Disorder** in the psychiatry section. In *ICD-11* functional neurologic symptoms will appear in both neurology and psychiatric sections.
   3. **Factitious disorder**—refers to patients who consciously simulate symptoms for medical attention and *is not a functional disorder*. Most experts agree that factitious disorder and/ or malingering is rare among patients with functional disorders presenting to routine health services. Neurologists understandably still worry about this because the symptoms are diagnosed partially because of their similarity to normal voluntary movement.
   4. **Malingering**—refers to patients who consciously simulate symptoms for financial or other material gain and is *not a medical or psychiatric diagnosis*.

ETIOLOGY AND MECHANISM

A. Etiology. Functional neurologic symptoms are considered to be multifactorial. Their etiology is best understood with a biopsychosocial model, in which biologic, psychological, and social factors can be all be involved to a certain extent, varying between individuals (Fig. 33.1). In this model predisposing factors and precipitating factors are responsible for the onset of symptoms and perpetuating factors prevent patients from getting better. The diagnosis of functional neurologic disorders is not based on these etiologic factors, but a formulation on these lines can be helpful in explanation and as targets in treatment.

   1. Predisposing factors. Childhood adversity, psychiatric disorders, and adverse life events are more common than in controls but are not present in many individuals. They should be regarded in a similar way to the relationship between smoking and stroke. Look for them but do not be surprised if they are absent. Others include the presence of neurologic disease in the patient or others, previous functional disorders, migraine, and probably genetic factors.

   2. Precipitating factors. Common triggers for functional movement disorders include physical (head or limb) injury (often minor and in the affected body part), acute experience of derealization or depersonalization, pain, fatigue, extensive bed rest, sleep paralysis, anesthetics, infection, side effects of medication, and panic attacks. Dissociative (nonepileptic) attacks often start with syncope or vertigo as a first episode associated with panic. The experience of a minor pathophysiologic or physiologic event such as these provides the focus for a pattern of learned or conditioned involuntary symptom experience or behavior.

   3. Perpetuating factors. probably include most of the following: Unhelpful illness beliefs (including ongoing uncertainty about the diagnosis, typically worsened by the lack of a clear diagnosis from treating physician), the presence of a welfare system, neuroendocrine and immunologic abnormalities similar to those seen in depression and anxiety, not feeling believed, avoidance of symptom provocation, stigma of mental illness, altered plasticity in motor and sensory pathways in the central nervous system, and deconditioning.

   4. Mechanism. The genesis of symptoms, symptom distribution in the body (e.g., when incompatible with normal physiology), variability of symptoms in time, and the influence of distraction are all in line with the idea that the symptoms are not caused by a lesion of the nervous system. Symptoms utilize voluntary motor pathways but are experienced as involuntary. Experimental (neurophysiologic and imaging) and clinical evidence supports a hypothesis that there is a mismatch of higher-order expectations ("My leg is weak") and lower-order sensory input and motor output. This is based on dysfunctional attentional processes (symptoms temporarily abate when attention is

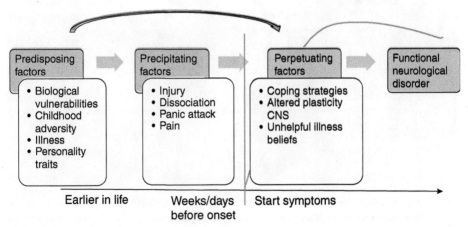

FIGURE 33.1 Factors that are associated with origination of a functional neurologic disorder. Predisposing factors are general factors in life that cause susceptibility. Precipitating factors trigger the onset of symptoms. Perpetuating factors prevent the symptoms from resolving and thereby induce symptoms to become chronic.

diverted), altered self-agency ("It's not me that's making my arm shake"), and beliefs ("It feels like I have had a stroke").

CLINICAL MANIFESTATIONS AND DIAGNOSTIC APPROACH

Although there will often be clues in the history, the diagnosis of a functional neurologic disorder **should be based mainly on positive signs** on examination (Video 33.1). **It should not be a diagnosis of exclusion.** Sharing these signs with the patient is also a useful step in treatment (see section Evaluation below). Some patients are monosymptomatic for one of the problems described below. More commonly patients present with mixtures of more than one symptom. Pain, fatigue, sleep disturbance, and/or impaired concentration are also present in more than 50% of patients. The findings described below have variable sensitivity and specificity. They are sufficient in the hands of a neurologist to lead to a diagnosis with good stability over time but as with any physical finding are more reliable when considered in the context of the rest of the history and examination. Positive evidence of a functional disorder also does not exclude an additional comorbid neurologic diagnosis, which should always be considered. There is female preponderance for most presentations of a functional neurologic disorder, although as patients get older gender ratios become more equal. Although anyone over 5 years may develop these problems the peak age for seizures is mid-20s, and for weakness and movement disorder late-30s.

A. Functional limb weakness/paralysis.
1. Symptoms.
   Functional limb weakness, or paresis, usually presents as unilateral weakness, but monoparesis and paraparesis also occur. Complete paralysis is rarer. About 50% of patients present acutely. Left-sided symptoms are not clearly more common than right. Patients may report dropping things, knees giving way, or that their limb feels alien or "not part of them."
2. Physical examination.
   a. **Hoover's sign** is positive when there is weakness of hip extension, which improves when the patient flexes their contralateral unaffected hip against resistance (Fig. 33.2). It can be performed with the patient sitting or lying. The patient may need to be asked to focus attention on the unaffected limb.
   b. **Hip abductor sign** is similarly positive when there is weakness of hip abduction, which improves when the patient abducts their contralateral hip against resistance.

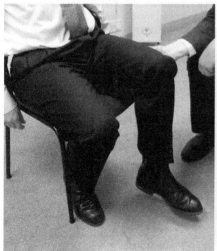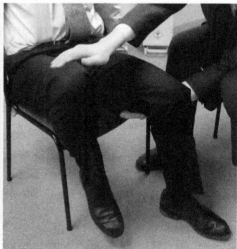

Test hip extension – it's weak   Test contralateral hip flexion against resistance – hip extension has become strong

FIGURE 33.2 Hoover's sign for functional weakness. (Adapted and reproduced by permission from Stone J. Bare essentials: functional symptoms in neurology. *Pract Neurol.* 2009;9:179–189.) (See color plates.)

c. **Dragging gait.** A typical dragging gait of functional leg weakness involves the forefoot remaining in contact with the ground rather than the circumducting gait of an organic hemiparesis. There may be internal or external hip rotation.

d. **Global pattern of weakness** involving flexors and extensors equally

e. **Give-way weakness** describes transiently normal power, which then gives way and is a feature of variable weakness.

f. **Discrepancies of movement.** For example, inability to plantarflex ankles but able to stand on tip toes and walk from the waiting room or inability to grip examiner's hand compared to getting an object out of a bag.

g. **Drift without pronation.** There is some evidence that drift without pronation, the downward drift of an arm without the pronating movement seen in pyramidal lesions, is more common in functional arm weakness than in patients with neurologic disease.

3. **Investigations.**

No specific positive neurophysiologic findings although "reduced recruitment" may be seen on electromyography. Most patients require other investigations such as magnetic resonance imaging (MRI) of brain and/or spine to assess for comorbid neurologic disease.

B. **Functional movement disorders.**

1. **Symptoms.** Functional movement disorders include tremor, myoclonus (jerks), dystonia (abnormal posturing), and parkinsonism.

a. **Tremor.** Functional tremor is characterized by variable frequency and amplitude, often subsides for certain periods, and may occur at rest, action, or posture. Tremor may be synchronous in body parts. This is in contrast to tremor in Parkinson's disease (rest tremor), essential tremor (posture and action), or dystonic tremor (posture).

b. **Myoclonus.** or jerky movements. In functional myoclonus the duration of each jerk is often relatively long. Jerks that occur as a synchronous bilateral movement of both legs or in the abdomen/trunk are very likely to be functional. Jerks that start after the age of 20 and are localized in several body parts (generalized) are also relatively likely to be functional. Some patients report unpleasant prodromal symptoms, which are temporarily relieved by the jerk and/or the ability to suppress or provoke jerks (unlike myoclonus caused by neurologic disease).

c. **Dystonia.** is abnormal posturing of a body part. The most typical feature of functional dystonia is a fixed posture, usually a flexed arm and clenched fist or an inverted plantar flexed ankle (Fig. 33.3). This in contrast to organic dystonia, where the posturing is mobile and reversible. Pain and abnormal body schema are common in functional dystonia versus organic dystonia. Phenomenology overlaps with complex regional pain syndrome.

d. **Facial dystonia.** Functional facial dystonia or spasms are usually unilateral and may cause eye closure or pull the mouth or jaw to one side giving a superficial appearance of facial weakness (Fig. 33.4).

e. **Parkinsonism.** The combination of functional tremor (described above) and general slowness can lead to a Parkinsonian appearance.

2. **Physical examination.**

a. **Tremor.**

(1) **Variable tremor frequency** (variable amplitude or response to stress is not specific)

(2) **Entrainment test.** Ask the patient to copy, with one hand, a rhythmic movement (e.g., tapping of index finger and thumb), which the examiner varies in frequency. Positive evidence of a functional tremor arises when (a) tremor in the contralateral hand stops; (b) the tremor "entrains" to the same rhythm as the examiner or (c) the patient is unable to copy the movement.

(3) **Pause with ballistic movements.** For example, asking the patient to touch the tip of your finger as it is moved around in space.

(4) **Distraction.** Patients may have less or no tremor when they are distracted.

(5) **Cocontraction** of agonist and antagonist muscles may be seen.

(6) **Worsening of tremor with loading or spread of the tremor elsewhere when the limb is immobilized.**

b. **Myoclonus.** The effect of distraction can be observed in some patients (although the intermittent nature is a challenge). Long-duration jerks, especially axial jerks, favor a functional origin. Most patients previously thought to have propriospinal myoclonus probably have a functional movement disorder.

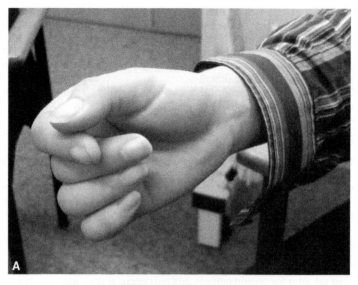

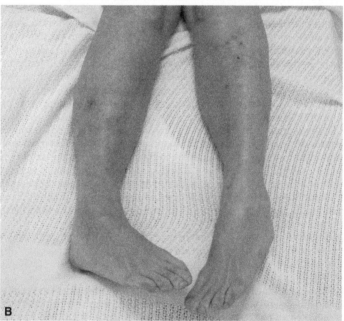

FIGURE 33.3 Functional dystonia typically presents with a clenched fist/flexed fingers **(A)** or inverted and plantar flexed foot **(B)**. (Reproduced with permission from Stone J. Bare essentials: functional symptoms in neurology. *Pract Neurol.* 2009;9;179–189; Stone J, Carson A. Functional neurological disorders. *Continuum.* 2015;21:818–837.) (See color plates.)

c. Dystonia. A fixed acquired dystonia (clenched fist, inverted ankle) is characteristic but is harder to definitively diagnose unless there is resolution.

d. Facial spasms. Characteristic unilateral contraction of platysma often associated with jaw deviation or persistent unilateral contraction of orbicularis oculis (vs. transient contraction seen in hemifacial spasm or bilateral orbicularis contraction seen in blepharospasm). Tongue may deviate to the affected side also.

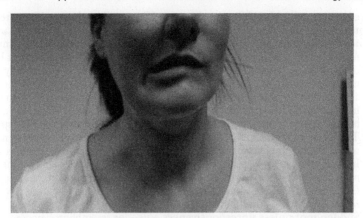

FIGURE 33.4 Functional facial spasm involves unilateral platysmal or orbicularis oculis contraction typically with jaw deviation and may give the appearance of facial weakness. (Reproduced with permission from Stone J. Functional neurological disorders: the neurological assessment as treatment. *Neurophysiol Clin.* 2014;44:363–373.) (See color plates.)

    e. Parkinsonism. In addition to features of functional tremor there may be slowness without diminishing amplitude while tapping and impaired eye movements in all directions.

3. Investigations.

    a. Tremor. Polymyography with tremor registration can be performed to confirm the features above. This is especially useful in long-standing functional tremor where these features may be harder to see at the bedside.

    b. Myoclonus. Polymyography with back-averaging should show evidence of Bereitschaftspotential (readiness potential) before the jerk, in functional myoclonus. This may be technically difficult and depends on jerks being frequent, but not too rapidly successive. Variable pattern of recruitment of the muscles in each jerk and burst duration of over 300 also makes functional myoclonus more likely.

    c. Dystonia. No additional investigations available

    d. Facial spasms. No additional investigations available

    e. Parkinsonism. A normal dopamine transporter–single-photon emission computed tomography scan may be useful although does not exclude a wide range of alternative "organic" extrapyramidal disorders (scans without evidence of dopaminergic dysfunction) and reminds us that the diagnosis of a functional disorder must be made on positive grounds, not because tests are normal.

C. Functional gait disorder.

    1. Symptoms. Gait disorders can be caused by a movement disorder like tremor, myoclonus, or weakness in functional neurologic disorder. However, some patients do not suffer from any of those symptoms, but still have difficulties walking. Common abnormal walking patterns include ataxia-like problems with instability and/or fear of falling; gait with small steps, which may look Parkinsonian, or as if the person is "walking on ice"; ability to stand without ability to walk (abasia without astasia) or vice versa.

    2. Physical examination. If unsteady while standing then the patient may improve when asked to repeat numbers drawn on their back, follow eye movement, or play a game on a smartphone. Tandem gait may appear abnormal, but in fact require good balance control to maintain the adopted posture. Walking may improve with encouragement such as fingertip support from the examiner, or normalize when the patient is asked to walk backwards or adopt a "skating" motion. Caution is warranted in diagnosing gait disorder as functional because it is "bizarre," as many "organic" movement disorders, for example, chorea or dyskinetic gait in Parkinson's disease can be "bizarre."

D. Dissociative/Psychogenic (nonepileptic) attacks/seizures.

    1. Symptoms. Dissociative attacks or seizures (terminology from *ICD-10*) present with episodes with jerking and unresponsiveness or events in which there is motionless

unresponsiveness (either falling to the ground lying still or absence-like states). In this context dissociation describes the patients' experience of losing awareness and having amnesia for an event, regardless of whether they experience dissociative symptoms.

    a. **Aura or warning symptoms** are present in more than 50% of patients, at least some times although patients are often reluctant to describe them. Commonly there is a mixture of symptoms of autonomic arousal (feeling hot, clammy with a tight chest, and altered breathing) combined with dissociative symptoms, the feeling of being detached from yourself (depersonalization) or the world around you (derealization). This may be described as feeling "not there," "feeling far away," "disconnected," or "spaced out." There may be panic and fear, but particularly in patients with many attacks, no fear, but nonetheless an unpleasant, "horrible" or "unbearable" feeling that precedes the attack. In some patients the attack itself comes as a relief of this distressing feeling. In many patients no warning symptoms are discernible or the warning signs have stopped.

    b. **Generalized shaking attacks,** with hyperkinetic limb movements, typically tremor rather than clonic movements

    c. **Sudden motionless unresponsiveness episodes** resembling syncope.

    d. **Blank spells** resembling absence seizures.

2. **Physical examination.** As with all attack disorders, the initial diagnosis should be suggested with a witness history, preferably supplemented with a home video, which makes the diagnosis more reliable. A sudden fall to the floor with motionless unresponsiveness and eyes closed for more than 2 minutes is a dissociative attack unless proven otherwise. Specific features of dissociative seizures include long-duration attacks (more than 3 minutes) (compared with tonic-clonic epileptic events that typically last 60 to 90 seconds); closed eyes +/– resistance to eye opening (vs. eyes open in epilepsy); ability to recall generalized shaking; crying directly after the attack; side-to-side head movements; tremor-like asynchronous movements and hyperventilation (vs. clonic movements and apnea in epilepsy). Features that do NOT distinguish dissociative and epileptic seizures well include falls and injury, urine incontinence, breath-holding spells leading to desaturation, tongue biting, and seizures that arise from sleep.

3. **Investigations.** Video electroencephalography (EEG) during an attack is the gold standard. There should be typical semiology of a dissociative attack recorded during the EEG. In epilepsy there will be typical clinical features of epilepsy accompanied by epileptiform abnormalities on EEG. The semiology is crucial though, for example, surface EEG can be normal in frontal lobe epilepsy or epilepsy with a deep focus.

E. **Functional sensory symptoms.**

  1. **Symptoms.** Hypersensitivity, numbness, tingling, and loss or altered proprioception can occur. Patients with limb weakness may report circumferential numbness at the shoulder or top of the leg. Hemisensory disturbance is also a common pattern. Dense sensory loss to all modalities including pain is sometimes striking.

  2. **Physical examination.** Positive sensory signs of a functional disorder on examination (e.g., midline splitting of vibration sense) are not specific, although may be more so if the sensory disturbance is dense. Typically mild functional weakness is also present.

  3. **Investigations.** Somatosensory evoked potentials may be useful in patients with dense sensory loss.

F. **Speech symptoms.**

  1. **Symptoms.** Functional dysphonia presenting with a whispering speech is the commonest type. Acquired onset of stuttering in adulthood is often functional in nature. Less commonly patients may present with telegrammatic speech omitting conjunctions, prepositions, and definite articles, a foreign accent syndrome or mutism.

  2. **Physical examination.** Variability is the hallmark. Resolution under hypnosis or sedation can also help to positively identify the problem.

  3. **Investigations.** Assessment of variability in speech is best assessed by a speech pathologist who can recognize internal inconsistencies. Foreign accent syndrome can occur from organic brain lesions.

G. **Visual symptoms.**

  1. **Signs and symptoms.** More commonly seen by ophthalmologists than neurologists. Symptoms include impaired vision, blindness, intermittent blurred vision, and altered visual fields including tunnel vision and diplopia.

2. **Physical examination.** Patients with functional blindness may have difficulty signing their name or touching their index fingers in front of their face. Unilateral visual loss or impaired vision can be positively diagnosed as functional using tests such as a fogging test in which lenses of progressive opacity are placed in front of the good eye until vision can be demonstrated to occur in the affected eye. A tubular visual field (the same width at 1 and 2 meters) is evidence of a functional visual field deficit (organic visual fields expand conically). Functional diplopia is associated with convergent spasm, which can sometimes look like a sixth nerve palsy.

3. **Investigations.** Cortical blindness should be considered in someone with limited "blindsight."

H. **Cognitive symptoms.**

1. **Symptoms.** Not strictly part of Functional Neurological Symptom Disorder (*DSM-5*) but common in association with other symptoms. Memory symptoms range from impaired concentration and memory as seen in depression and anxiety to profound retrograde amnesia lasting years. Language problems such as using the wrong word or spoonerisms are often reported by patients. Executive impairments are commonly found on formal testing.

2. **Physical examination.** Patients may perform poorly on tests of attention and executive function with "blanks" in their performance. Marked retrograde amnesia in the presence of normal anterograde memory or disproportionate loss of memory for personal identity is usually functional/psychogenic. Cognitive "effort" tests can be useful at identifying patients who are performing at or below chance. In a legal setting this should increase suspicion of malingering.

3. **Investigations.** Functional cognitive symptoms are common but clinicians should be wary of patients presenting in the prodrome of neurodegenerative conditions.

I. **Dizziness.** Chronic subjective dizziness, also called phobic postural vertigo or persistent perceptual postural dizziness (PPPD), describes a fairly common group of patients who present with disequilibrium and increased focus on bodily movement and sensation without evidence of vestibular or neurologic disease. They have usually experienced vertigo because of migraine, minor head injury, or a transient vestibular pathology, which has become persistent as part of a functional disorder. Additional anxiety and dissociative symptoms are common.

EVALUATION

The neurologic evaluation of patients with a functional neurologic disorder can itself be the beginning of treatment.

A. **History.**

1. **List of all symptoms.** It is both informative and potentially therapeutic to make a list of all current physical symptoms including fatigue, sleep, concentration problems, and dizziness.

2. **Day-to-day functioning.** What does a normal day look like? Patients often focus on what they cannot do, but try to establish what they actually spend time doing. This provides clues about anxiety and mood disorders.

3. **Symptom onset.** Symptoms or events at onset can be helpful in later explanation of mechanism (e.g., minor injury or a panic attack leading to unilateral attentional focus). We would suggest, however, leaving questions about life events or trauma for later assessments unless volunteered by the patient.

4. **Illness beliefs.** What does the patient think is wrong? Any particular conditions they were wondering about? Discuss previous medical experiences and their expectations of treatment. Are they motivated to change? This helps tailor your explanation and onward referral to meet the patients' concerns.

5. **Discussing anxiety, depression, and other psychiatric symptoms.** Although these are common they are not universal and not necessary in order to make a correct diagnosis. This patient group is typically sensitive to the idea that they are faking the symptoms or that the symptoms might be a result of them having a psychiatric disorder. Physical symptoms and day-to-day activity often strongly suggest psychological comorbidity. If asked directly it is often better to ask "Do your symptoms make you anxious?" rather than "Do you have anxiety?".

B. **Physical examination.** The diagnosis of a functional neurologic disorder rests on demonstrating positive physical signs on examination (described above).

C. **Investigations.** It is not a diagnosis of exclusion or a diagnosis made by performing multiple negative tests. Investigations will usually be necessary, but the purpose is to look for comorbid neurologic disease, not to disprove a clinically definite diagnosis of a functional disorder. Studies show that anticipating negative results, and discussing the potential for incidental abnormalities (such as high-signal T2 lesions on MRI brain) or changes that are simply normal for age (degenerative disease of the spine) are helpful for later understanding.

DIFFERENTIAL DIAGNOSIS

In principle all neurologic disorders could be listed as a differential diagnosis of functional neurologic disorders. We, therefore, discuss common issues and diagnostic pitfalls. **Misdiagnosis** occurs in less than 5% of patients in studies, which is the same rate as for other neurologic and psychiatric disorders.

A. **Factitious disorder and malingering are defined at the start of this chapter.** Clues to either are listed below. Some patients exist on a spectrum between a genuine functional disorder and willful exaggeration.

1. **Major discrepancy between reported and observed function** (i.e., seen jogging when they had reported requiring a walking aid). Note that a discrepancy between reported symptoms (e.g., telling a doctor they have 10/10 severity pain but relatively normal day-to-day function) is not evidence of willful exaggeration but a common feature of functional disorders.

2. **Evidence of previous lying to health professionals.**

3. **Obvious financial incentive (e.g., a legal case).** Most patients in legal cases have genuine disorders but this situation should encourage greater scrutiny of the possibility of willful exaggeration.

4. **Failure of cognitive effort testing.** Examples of this are scoring a) well below chance or b) lower than someone with severe dementia. Even here it can be argued that patients may subconsciously aim to fail a test in order to demonstrate their complaints to a health professional.

   Arguments against willful exaggeration as an explanation for the vast majority of patients include similarity of patient experiences across countries and across time; clustering of typical symptoms including pain, anxiety, cognitive symptoms, and fatigue; strong desire for investigations in many patients; response to treatment when delivered with expertise; persistence of symptoms on long-term follow-up in a high proportion of untreated patients.

B. **General diagnostic pitfalls.**

1. **Assuming that a functional disorder is a diagnosis of exclusion.** It is not, it requires positive evidence for a diagnosis and can be diagnosed in a patient with a neurologic disease.

2. **Forgetting to look for comorbid neurologic disease.** Disease is a strong risk factor for functional disorders. Patients in the early stages of neurodegenerative diseases, especially Parkinson's disease, may present with functional symptoms that are disproportionate to their developing pathology.

3. **Assuming that because something is bizarre it is functional.** Many neurologic diseases look bizarre, for example, "sensory tricks" in focal dystonia, bizarre axial posturing in clear consciousness during frontal lobe seizures, or chorea.

4. **Placing too much weight on psychiatric comorbidity, abnormal personality traits, stress.** All of these are common in neurologic disease and may be absent in neurologic disease.

5. **Assuming that a patient who is male, older, or appears to be psychologically "normal" cannot have a functional disorder.** They can!

6. **Assuming that long-standing diagnoses such as epilepsy, multiple sclerosis, or stroke are correct.**

7. **La belle indifference.** This refers to cheerful indifference to neurologic impairment has often been cited as evidence of a functional disorder. Studies show it has no diagnostic value and is common in patients with frontal lobe disorders. When present in a functional

disorder it typically represents a patient "putting on a brave face" to avoid anyone thinking they are distressed or low in mood.

8. **Secondary gain.** This refers to the benefits of being ill, and occurs in patients with functional disorders (when it is often a focus of attention by the clinician) and disease (where it is often overlooked). It has never been convincingly demonstrated to be a specific feature in this patient group.

9. **Attributing symptoms incorrectly to minor radiologic or laboratory test abnormalities** in the presence of clear evidence of a functional disorder. For example, degenerative changes are universal in the population over 40 and high-signal lesions become more common as people age.

C. **Motor symptoms.** Specific pitfalls include the following:

   1. **Tics.** Tourette syndrome normally begins in childhood and can be voluntarily suppressed.
   2. **Orthostatic tremor.** Tremor only when standing often with gait abnormality. Patients feel the tremor, but it does not always present visibly.
   3. **Axial (propriospinal) myoclonus.** Is mostly functional, but can be caused by spinal abnormalities.
   4. **Higher cortical lesions, for example, parietal stroke.** Problems such as inattention or neglect may present with apparent inconsistent symptoms or unusual gait.
   5. **Stiff person syndrome and autoimmune encephalitis.** These are examples of neurological conditions associated with a high rate of psychiatric symptomatology, and variable and sometimes bizarre symptoms, which can obscure the neurologic diagnosis.
   6. **Urinary retention in a patient with weak legs.** This should always be investigated but in many cases appears to relate to a combination of acute pain, opiates, and a functional disorder.

D. **Seizure symptoms.** Specific pitfalls include the following:

   1. **Frontal seizures.** These often look strange with axial twisting movements, including pelvic thrusting, verbalization, and hard-to-characterize hyperkinetic movements. Surface EEG may be normal. They are, however, typically very brief.
   2. **Temporal lobe seizures.** These can last several minutes and may be associated with ictal fear and dissociation that make them appear clinically similar to panic or dissociative attacks.
   3. **Self- or stress-induced epilepsy.**
   4. **Atypical features of dissociative nonepileptic seizures.** These include olfactory hallucinations, physical injury, tongue biting, incontinence, and desaturation (because of breath holding).
   5. **Response to anticonvulsants.** This does not necessarily indicate a diagnosis of epilepsy and "therapeutic trials" should be avoided for this reason.

TREATMENT BY THE NEUROLOGIST AND ONWARD REFERRAL

The prognosis is often poor when left untreated for functional motor and seizure disorders.

A. **The role of the neurologist.** The neurologist, as the doctor who usually makes the diagnosis, has a central role in treatment. This includes explaining the nature of the disorder to the patient, providing follow-up and coordinating onward care.

B. **Why neurologist attempts at treatment fail.** Communication of the diagnosis and treatment of a functional disorder may go wrong in neurologic settings for many reasons including delay in considering the diagnosis failure to name the disorder (either by giving no diagnosis or simply telling the patient the conditions they do not have); failure to explain the rationale for the diagnosis and that it is not a diagnosis of exclusion; jumping too quickly to speculative discussions of etiology, for example psychological factors that are then interpreted by the patient as an accusation of faking the symptoms and failure to offer a rational program of treatment. Failure at this stage normally means that other health professionals will be unlikely to help the patient.

C. **Using the normal model of neurologic treatment.** Communication of the diagnosis works best when physicians stick to the normal model use in any other consultation. Name the disorder, explain the rationale (in the case of functional disorder, the positive clinical signs), and something about the mechanism (a problem with nervous system functioning or "dissociation") but leave discussions about etiology for later (as we do for most neurologic disease) and take responsibility for onward treatment—it is unlikely anyone else will if the neurologist does not.

D. Elements of successful diagnostic communication.

1. Name the diagnosis (tell them "You have a Functional Movement Disorder with Dissociative attacks"). Avoid an initial focus on telling the patient what they do not have. Although at some stage this will be helpful this is not what we do for other disorders (e.g., "You have migraine" comes before "You do not have a brain tumor").

2. Underline that this diagnosis is common.

3. Tell the patient you believe him/her. Patient with a functional neurologic disorder often have the feeling physicians do not believe their symptoms are real. Explicit discussion that the symptoms are genuine can help.

4. Explain the rationale for the diagnosis. Convincing the patient that the diagnosis is correct is not something trivial: patients have often seen many physicians before you and may be skeptical that no scans or blood tests are needed to make this diagnosis. We would strongly suggest sharing the positive clinical signs with the patient. For example, demonstrate Hoover's sign in limb weakness or entrainment in tremor. This needs to be done supportively to demonstrate unequivocally that this is a clinical diagnosis in which normal functioning is still, transiently, possible and therefore the disorder is potentially reversible.

5. Explain the mechanism. "It is a problem in the functioning of the nervous system. Nothing is damaged, but it is not working properly." For seizures: *"You are having episodes in which you are spontaneously going into a trance like state called dissociation."* You can use metaphors like *"It is a software problem, not a hardware problem."*

6. The symptoms are potentially reversible if there is active participation from the patient. Recovery is possible as there is no damage to the nervous system; however, there is no magic quick fix. Patients need to relearn normal functioning. Active involvement of the patient is essential for that. *"These attacks have developed as an involuntary habit. You'll need help to learn how to retrain out of this habit. Treatment can help you retrain the brain to change these habits".*

7. Provide self-help information. For example, www.neurosymptoms.org, http://www. nonepilepticattacks.info

8. Send the patient a copy of your clinic letter. To ensure transparency and to maximize the patient's understanding

E. Second neurologic consultation. A second visit allows an assessment of the patients' understanding of a complex diagnosis that they are unlikely to have previously heard of and their motivation to read self-help material. This in turn influences further management. Patients with good understanding and motivation are more likely to benefit from further treatment. Those with little understanding who cannot repeat back any information or who disagree with the diagnosis probably will not benefit. Patients with a positive experience from the first visit will often disclose additional relevant information at a second visit.

F. Triaging and coordinating further treatment.

1. First-line treatment. Explanation and provision of self-help, simple rehabilitation advice, and follow-up by a neurologist

2. Second-line treatment. Should be offered to patients who have engaged with their diagnosis and are motivated for treatment

   a. Functional movement disorders including limb weakness. Referral to a physiotherapist with expertise in functional motor disorders. Physiotherapy techniques differ from those used in stroke or multiple sclerosis, are well described, and show benefit in randomized clinical trials. A skilled physiotherapist will use treatment to reinforce the rationale for the diagnosis and incorporate graded exercise and cognitive behavioral techniques for symptoms such as fatigue and pain.

   b. Dissociative (nonepileptic) seizures. Referral for education and psychotherapy. The best evidence is for cognitive behavioral therapy.

3. Third-line treatment includes multidisciplinary inpatient treatment, hypnosis, therapeutic sedation (which may be particularly relevant for patients with functional dystonia), and psychodynamic or other types of psychotherapy. There is no evidence for pharmacotherapy although comorbid depression and anxiety or pain can be treated in the usual way.

Key Points

- Diagnose a functional neurologic disorder primarily on positive examination signs such as Hoover's sign or the Tremor Entrainment sign, not by exclusion.
- The diagnosis should not be made just because tests are normal, the presentation is bizarre, or there is psychosocial comorbidity.
- The neurologist has a key role in explaining the diagnosis, preferably by sharing positive evidence of the diagnosis and providing written information.
- Further treatment involves both physical and psychological therapy but this is dependent on a successful neurologic consultation.
- Current models encompass both neurologic factors (e.g., abnormally focused attention, amplification of physiologic stimuli) and psychological factors (e.g., "top down" beliefs and emotional dysregulation).

Recommended Reading

Baizabal-Carvallo JF, Jankovic J. Speech and voice disorders in patients with psychogenic movement disorders. *J Neurol.* 2015;262(11):2420–2424. doi:10.1007/s00415-015-7856-7.

Chen CS, Lee AW, Karagiannis D, et al. Practical clinical approaches to functional visual loss. *J Clin Neurosci.* 2007;14:1–7.

Edwards M, Bhatia K. Functional (psychogenic) movement disorders: merging mind and brain. *Lancet Neurol.* 2012;11:250–260.

Edwards MJ, Adams RA, Brown H, et al. A Bayesian account of 'hysteria'. *Brain.* 2012;135(pt 11):3495–3512.

Edwards MJ, Stone J, Lang AE. From psychogenic movement disorder to functional movement disorder: it is time to change the name. *Mov Disord.* 2014;29(7):849–852.

Goldstein LH, Chalder T, Chigwedere C, et al. Cognitive-behavioral therapy for psychogenic nonepileptic seizures: a pilot RCT. *Neurology.* 2010;74:1986–1994.

Jordbru AA, Smedstad LM, Klungsøyr O, et al. Psychogenic gait disorder: a randomized controlled trial of physical rehabilitation with one-year follow-up. *J Rehabil Med.* 2014;46(2):181–187.

Lafrance WC, Baker GA, Duncan R, et al. Minimum requirements for the diagnosis of psychogenic nonepileptic seizures: a staged approach: a report from the International League Against Epilepsy Nonepileptic Seizures Task Force. *Epilepsia.* 2013;50(11):2005–2018.

Nielsen G, Stone J, Matthews A, et al. Physiotherapy for functional motor disorders: a consensus recommendation. *J Neurol Neurosurg Psychiatry.* 2015;86:1113–1119.

Schrag A, Trimble M, Quinn N, et al. The syndrome of fixed dystonia: an evaluation of 103 patients. *Brain.* 2004;127(pt 10):2360–2372.

Staab, JP. Chronic subjective dizziness. *Continuum (Minneap. Minn).* 2012;18:1118–1141.

Stone J, Reuber M, Carson A. Functional symptoms in neurology: mimics and chameleons. *Pract Neurol.* 2013;13(2):104–113.

Stone J, Carson A. Functional neurologic disorders. *Continuum (Minneap Minn).* 2015;21(3):818–837.

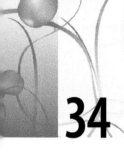

34 Approach to the Patient with Suspected Brain Death

Christopher P. Robinson and Eelco F. M. Wijdicks

Brain death is defined as the complete, irreversible loss of brain function, leading to viscero-somatic and cardiopulmonary failure. The diagnosis and confirmation of such pathology require a unique combination of interpersonal communication skills and clinical knowledge. Physicians must have a deep understanding of the ethical consequences, evidence-based guidelines for diagnosis, and have a firm background in the criticism and interpretation of confirmatory tests. The key factors in making an accurate diagnosis include a detailed neurologic examination, accurate laboratory evaluation, historical context of symptoms, neuroimaging, and specific neurophysiologic assessments. The first attempts at defining diagnostic criteria for brain death can be traced back to 1968 as defined by the Harvard criteria. Since their development, several international collaboratives in both the United Kingdom and the United States have further developed stricter definitions related to both clinical examination and objective confirmation. In 2010 the American Academy of Neurology (AAN) published the now widely accepted and widely used evidence-based guidelines for determining brain death in adults. The use of such guidelines is justified when patients with altered states of consciousness cease to have evidence of all neurologic functions. In these cases, initiation of a thorough brain death assessment is indicated.

ETIOLOGY

A. **Background.** The clinical diagnosis of brain death is uncommon and accounts for less than 1% of annual deaths in the adult and pediatric populations. It occurs in the setting of an acute irreversible brain injury and often progresses rapidly. More common than brain death is the comatose patient who has suffered catastrophic injury, but retains some brainstem function. Brain death accounts for only a few intensive care–related deaths on a monthly basis. Adequate differentiation between brain death and coma is imperative, and requires a knowledgeable physician and careful neurologic examination.

B. **Causes.** Brain death progresses through a common mechanism following severe injury. Both destructive and compressive pathologies can lead to shift and displacement of the brainstem, altering its functionality. Such lesions can be either supratentorial or infratentorial.

1. **Supratentorial compressive lesions** include intracranial hemorrhage, tumor, meningitis, encephalitis, and abscess formation. Lesions can singularly or in combination involve the epidural, subdural, subarachnoid, and intracerebral compartments. Compression results in parenchymal displacement, intracranial pressure (ICP) elevation, and hydrocephalus, leading to herniation.

2. **Supratentorial destructive lesions** include traumatic brain injury, cerebral venous sinus thrombosis, distal basilar artery occlusion, bilateral carotid artery occlusion, and encephalitis. Lesions with the capability to cause herniation typically involve both cortical and bilateral diencephalic structures.

3. **Infratentorial compressive lesions** include cerebellar infarction or hemorrhage, cerebellar abscess, or infratentorial tumors. Lesions can involve the epidural, subdural, and subarachnoid spaces, the brainstem, or the cerebellum itself. Compression tends to lead to displacement and herniation of mesopontine structures with associated obstructive hydrocephalus and elevated ICP.

4. **Infratentorial destructive lesions** include pontine hemorrhage, intramedullary tumors, leptomeningitis, and brainstem infarction. Lesions include various and multiple brainstem

structures. Destruction results in altered and nonreversible physiologic drive including respiration and vasomotor tone. Associated hemorrhage and obstructive hydrocephalus predispose to herniation and brain death.

PATHOPHYSIOLOGY

A. **Mechanism.** The major pathophysiologic mechanism behind terminal cortical destruction is due to herniation of the thalamic–brainstem complex leading to progressive loss of function and malignant increases in ICP. Herniation may occur via downward displacement, medial displacement, or a combination of the two. Displacement of the thalamic–brainstem complex will initially result in damage to the mesopontine structures leading to impaired consciousness and dysfunctional breathing drive. Further displacement will result in medullary destruction, coupled by the termination of all breathing drive and loss of vasomotor tone. Simultaneously, compressive edema and ventricular obstruction result in an equilibration of ICP and mean arterial pressure (MAP), leading to absent cerebral perfusion and irreversible termination of cerebrovascular blood flow. This termination of flow is permanent and leads to diffuse cerebral necrosis. Once these changes occur, cerebral blood flow and brainstem function will cease to function and do not return.

B. **Neuropathology.** Varying neuropathologic changes can be seen following brain death. The most common findings include a herniated, diffusely edematous cerebrum, with autolysis of herniated cerebellar tonsils. Additionally, diffuse neuronal changes are found exclusionary from the primary pathologic lesion leading to brain death. Microscopic evaluations have shown that pathology can vary widely and exclude well-known areas susceptible to ischemia such as the CA-1 and CA-3 regions of the hippocampus and the Purkinje cells of the cerebellum. The spinal cord is typically spared from damage, but in rare occasions upper cervical ischemia may occur with tonsillar herniation. The early detailed pathologic descriptions of brain death, which described diffuse brain necrosis, have not held true. This was likely due to pathologic specimens from patients with chronic no-flow vascular states such as persistent vegetative state, which eventually progressed to brain death. It is now widely accepted that neuronal loss may occur in one-third of the cortex and thalamus, and one-half of the brainstem.

EVALUATION

A. **Guidelines** for the determination of brain death in both the adult and pediatric populations have been strictly defined. Each guideline encourages a strict adherence to the literature and a thorough evaluation of all pertinent clinical aspects. To date, there are a minimum of 25 specific tests and verifications that must be met to clinically diagnose brain death (Table 34.1).

1. **Adult guidelines** for brain death were originally established by the AAN in 1995 and further revised in 2010. The guidelines are both comprehensive and practical, and must include all of the following:
   a. Exclusion of confounders
   b. Established etiology of coma
   c. Ascertain the futility of interventions
   d. All clinical prerequisites are met
   e. Test for the absence of motor responses
   f. Test for absence of brainstem reflexes at all levels
   g. Test for conclusive lack of respiratory drive
   h. Confirmatory apnea test with $Paco_2 \geq 60$ mm Hg *or* $Paco_2$ increase >20 mm Hg from normal baseline value

2. **Pediatric guidelines** for brain death were first published in 1987 and again revised in 2011 by the American Academy of Pediatrics (AAP) and the Child Neurology Society (CNS). The guidelines define the minimum standards that must be met in all clinical situations for brain death to be considered. There are three distinct differences in

TABLE 34.1 25 Assessments to Declare a Patient Brain Dead

Prerequisites (all must be checked)
 1. Coma, irreversible, and cause known
 2. Neuroimaging explains coma
 3. Sedative drug effect absent (*if indicated, order a toxicology screen*)
 4. No residual effect of paralytic drug (*If indicated, use peripheral nerve stimulator*)
 5. Absence of severe acid–base, electrolyte, or endocrine abnormality
 6. Normal or near-normal temperature (*Core temperature ≥36°C*)
 7. SBP >100 mm Hg
 8. No spontaneous respirations
Examination (all must be checked)
 9. Pupils nonreactive to bright light
10. Corneal reflexes absent
11. Eyes immobile, oculocephalic reflexes absent (*tested only if C-spine integrity ensured*)
12. Oculovestibular reflexes absent
13. No facial movement to noxious stimuli at supraorbital nerve or temporomandibular joint or absent snout and rooting reflexes (*neonates*)
14. Gag reflex absent
15. Cough reflex absent to tracheal suctioning
16. No motor response to noxious stimuli in all four limbs (*spinally mediated reflexes are permissible and triple flexion response is most common*)
Apnea Testing (all must be checked)
17. Patient is hemodynamically stable (*SBP ≥100 mm Hg*)
18. Ventilator adjusted to normocapnia (*$Paco_2$ 35–45 mm Hg*)
19. Patient preoxygenated with 100% Fio_2 for 10 min (*Pao_2 ≥200 mm Hg*)
20. Patient maintains oxygenation with a PEEP of 5 cm H_2O
21. Disconnect ventilator
22. Provide oxygen via an insufflation catheter to the level of the carina at 6 L/min or attach T-piece with CPAP valve at 10 cm H_2O
23. Spontaneous respirations absent
24. Arterial blood gas drawn at 8–10 min, patient reconnected to ventilator
25. $Paco_2$ ≥60 mm Hg, or 20 mm Hg rise from normal baseline value
or
Apnea test aborted and ancillary test (EEG or cerebral blood flow study) confirmatory
Documentation
Time of death (*use time of blood gas result or time of ancillary test*)
Brain Death Guideline Recommendations
• Newborn (≥37 wk gestational age) to 30 d: 2 examinations, 2 separate physicians, 24 hr apart
• 30 d to 18 yr: 2 examinations, 2 separate physicians, 12 hr apart
• ≥18 yr: 1 examination (*a second examination is needed in 8 US states: AL, CA, CT, FL, IA, KY, LA, VA*)

Wijdicks EF. *The Comatose Patient.* New York, NY: Oxford University Press; 2014. (Courtesy of Wijdicks.)
Abbreviations: CPAP, continuous positive airway pressure; EEG, electroencephalography; PEEP, positive end-expiratory pressure; SBP, systolic blood pressure.
Abbreviation: SBP, systolic blood pressure.

comparison to the adult guidelines that include apnea test requirements, number of examinations, and an observation period. The guidelines are as follows:
a. Exclusion of confounders
b. Established etiology of coma
c. Ascertain the futility of interventions
d. All clinical prerequisites are met
e. Test for the absence of motor responses
f. Test for absence of brainstem reflexes at all levels
g. Test for conclusive lack of respiratory drive
h. Confirmatory apnea test with $Paco_2$ ≥60 mm Hg *and* $Paco_2$ increase >20 mm Hg from normal baseline value

   i. Two separate neurologic and apnea examinations performed by different qualified examiners

   j. Interexaminer observation periods of:

      (1) 24 hours for term newborns up to 30 days of age

      (2) 12 hours for infants and children up to 18 years of age

B. **Prerequisites.** For each patient, the clinical assessment of brain death should be performed in an orderly and repetitive fashion. A step-by-step approach should be developed by the examiner that creates an unbiased and objectively confident diagnosis. With this approach, prior to examination, the clinician should define a set of prerequisites that rule out all medical and neurologic cofounders that mimic brain death.

   1. **Coma** should be evaluated and assessed early on in the clinical course. Both etiology and irreversibility are key factors in determining the need for a brain death examination. A thorough review of the history, a complete neurologic examination, and adequate assessment of ancillary data are necessary. In approach to the patient, some period of time should be allowed to pass following acute presentation to exclude the possibility of recovery. Some conditions that may mimic brain death and reverse with appropriate management include hypothermia, drug intoxication, basilar artery occlusion, nonconvulsive status epilepticus, Guillain–Barré syndrome, and botulism. The etiology of acute presentations can be established with a variety of objective assessments including examination, neuroradiologic testing, and neurophysiologic testing. The concept of irreversibility is established not only with examination, but by the assurance that all necessary interventions for a given etiology have been performed. Such interventions can include ventriculostomy placement, hematoma evacuation, craniectomy, osmotic diuresis, and intoxication reversal. If these considerations have been met, then consideration of brain death may be necessary.

   2. **Neuroimaging** should be performed and strictly evaluated with every patient suspected of brain death. Typical patterns with cause for concern include mass lesions with hemispheric shift, subdural hematoma with multiple parenchymatous contusions, diffuse subarachnoid hemorrhage, generalized loss of gray–white junction, and diffuse brain edema alone with effacement of the basal cisterns. In specific situations, such as early cardiac arrest, initial computed tomography scans may be normal. In such cases, repeat imaging should be performed to confirm or exclude the presence of advancing pathology. In cases of repeated normal neuroimaging, other confounders including intoxication and metabolic disturbance should be considered.

   3. **Pharmacologic interventions** are a commonly overlooked confounder in the assessment of brain death. A detailed historical and objective examination into the history and administration of sedative, analgesic, and paralytic agents should be performed. It is recommended that all patients undergo a urine and plasma drug screen in addition to an adequate medication reconciliation. Examiners should consider the half-life clearance of all medications administered, and in situations of impaired renal and hepatic function, adjust appropriately. In patients who have undergone therapeutic hypothermia, metabolic clearance rates are slower and should be accounted for during examination. In patients who have received paralytic agents, confirmation of clearance with either facial nerve stimulation or the presence of muscle stretch reflexes is imperative.

   4. **Metabolic** parameters should be adequately assessed in all patients prior to procession of the neurologic examination. Reversible metabolic conditions such as uremia, renal failure, hepatic failure, and hyponatremia should be worked up and treated. The presence of a severe acid–base disturbance may suggest an alternate underlying pathology. Metabolic acidosis is typically seen following drug intoxication. Respiratory acidosis may be seen following sedative and analgesic administration. Consideration of such factors and appropriate reversal should be considered. Finally, absence of all endocrine abnormalities, such as Hashimoto's encephalopathy, should be confirmed to rule out such confounders that may mimic comatose or brain death states.

   5. **Physiologic** parameters such as blood pressure and core temperature should also be considered in the assessment of brain death. In general, the diagnosis of brain death should never be made in an individual whose core temperature is <36°C. With every 1° drop in temperature, there is some decrease in brainstem responses, and at <20°C, all brainstem responses may be lost. In terms of blood pressure, it is recommended to

achieve a baseline systolic blood pressure (SBP) of >100 mm Hg or an MAP >80 mm Hg. This can be achieved with either volume resuscitation or vasoactive medications. If overt arterial hypotension and shock are present, the brain death examination should not continue until all morbidities have been treated.

6. **Respiratory** analysis should be performed to ensure that no spontaneous respirations occur. The absence of physiologic respiratory patterns confirms suspected pontomedullary dysfunction and is necessary when testing apnea. In specific situations, including tidal volume mismatch, triggering of the ventilator may not be indicative of a breathing patient. If some form of ventilatory triggering is present, the examiner should consider further analysis using decreased sensitivity or a pressure support setting to confirm all absence.

C. **Neurologic examination.** Following confirmation that all prerequisites have been met and all confounders have been excluded, procession with the neurologic examination is warranted. The assessment of brain death should include a detailed evaluation of the following: pupillary response, corneal reflexes, oculocephalic reflexes, oculovestibular reflexes, facial movement, gag reflex, cough reflex, and motor responses.

1. **Pupillary responses** are the first examination technique in the assessment of brain death, measuring the integrity of the afferent limb of cranial nerve II and the efferent limb of cranial nerve III. The examiner should use a bright light in both eyes to determine the presence or absence of a pupillary response. The typical pupillary patterns associated with brain death are the midposition (4 mm) fixed pupils and dilated (6 mm) fixed pupils. Pupillary dilation, in some cases, is still present in brain death because of intact ascending cervical sympathetic input. With initial assessment prior pupillary trauma or surgery should be distinguished from history. Many drugs are known to influence pupillary size. However, such agents do not inhibit the total contraction or dilation of the ciliary muscle and with careful examination can be excluded.

2. **Corneal reflexes** assess the integrity of the afferent limb of cranial nerve V and the efferent limb of cranial nerve VII, to elicit a blink response. Such response requires a distinct interplay between cranial nerves and an intact brainstem is vital. The examiner should induce corneal stimulation by squirting water on the cornea or by stimulating with a cotton swab. Stimulation of this pathway should produce a bilateral blink response. Facial trauma and edema may preclude adequate examination. The complete absence of blink response is compatible with brain death.

3. **Oculocephalic reflexes** assess the functionality of cranial nerves III, IV, and VI. This technique, also referred to as the doll's eyes technique, requires the examiner to initiate quick turning of the head from midposition to 90 degrees in either direction. Turning of the head should stimulate horizontal ocular movements. The examiner should also observe the eyes initially at rest with the lids open, assessing presence or absence of spontaneous ocular movements. The presence of forced deviation (vertical, horizontal, or skew) and nystagmus at rest would otherwise imply intact brainstem or cortical function. The absence of all ocular movements at rest and with motion is compatible with brain death.

4. **Oculovestibular reflexes** are used to assess the integrity of cranial nerves III, IV, VI, and VIII. In contrast to the oculocephalic reflex, the oculovestibular reflex requires the use of cold caloric testing with ice water. The examiner should elevate the patient's head 30 degrees from supine position to ensure verticality of the horizontal canal. Next, a small suction catheter should be attached to the end of a 50-cc syringe filled with ice water and instilled into the patient's auditory canal. Following injection, 1 minute should be allowed for observation of response, and 5 minutes should be given between examinations of either canal. Instillation of cold water into the tympanum induces an inhibition of the ipsilateral vestibular complex. In a comatose patient, a forced deviation of the eyes would ensue toward the cold stimulus. Certain pharmacologic agents including anticholinergics, tricyclic antidepressants, ototoxic antibiotics (aminoglycosides), and antiepileptics (phenytoin) may diminish such response, but are rarely relevant confounders. In brain death the oculovestibular response is completely absent.

5. **Facial movements** are a less common examination technique used in the assessment of brain death, but should be considered in all patients. Noxious stimulation should be

performed with either deep nail bed pressure or bilateral condylar temperomandibular pressure. Stimulus in a comatose patient should cause activation of cranial nerve VII and elicit a grimace response. Supraorbital pressure may also be applied, stimulating both cranial nerve V and VII. The complete absence of facial grimacing following noxious stimulation is compatible with brain death.

6. **Gag and cough reflexes** are used to assess the functionality of cranial nerves IX and X. Determination of the gag and cough reflexes in an intubated patient can at times be difficult. The examiner should attempt stimulation by using bronchial suctioning. The catheter should be advanced completely through the endotracheal tube, followed by suctioning pressure for several seconds. In a comatose patient, a cough or gag reflex is typically initiated. Simultaneously, the clinician should also observe for physiologic responses to suctioning including tachycardia and change in respiratory rate. The complete absence of physiologic response and cough reflexes during bronchial suctioning is consistent with brain death.

7. **Motor responses** are used to assess functionality of the cortical and brainstem pathways required for movement. The examiner should apply a noxious stimulus, such as deep nail bed pressure, sternal rubbing, or condylar temperomandibular pressure, to the patient. In brain death, noxious stimulation should produce no motor response at all. The presence of spinally mediated reflexes to noxious stimulus can be seen, but is not indicative of an intact brainstem. The spinal reflexes can include brief movements of the upper limbs, finger flexion, finger tremors, and arm elevation. Differentiation between normal motor responses and spinal reflexes can be difficult and requires much expertise. Typically repetitive stimulation will cause spinal reflexes to diminish and help the examiner define a response. Fasciculations may also be noted on examination, and are likely due to pathologic anterior horn cells. Plantar reflexes are typically absent in brain death, but may be seen with instances of triple flexion. The absence of all motor movements is consistent with brain death (Video 34.1).

D. **Apnea testing** uses the mechanics of oxygen diffusion to assess ventilatory drive and is the most commonly used technique in the assessment of brain death. The apnea test itself, like that of the overall brain death assessment, requires a definable set of prerequisites be met to ensure that performance and interpretation of the test is adequate (Table 34.2). Prior to initiation, the patient must be hemodynamically stable with a SBP >100 mm Hg. The ventilator should then be adjusted to achieve normocapnea ($Paco_2$ 35 to 45 mm Hg) and a consistent positive end-expiratory pressure (PEEP) of 5 cm H_2O should be initiated. The patient is then preoxygenated with 100% Fio_2 to a goal of Pao_2 >200 mm Hg to ensure adequate oxygenation. Once all prerequisites have been met, the ventilator is disconnected and an oxygen insufflation catheter is inserted. After 8 minutes, an arterial blood gas is drawn and the patient is reconnected to the ventilator. The defined criteria for determining brain death with the apnea test includes the absence of all spontaneous respirations, a $Paco_2$ >60 mm Hg, or an increase in the baseline $Paco_2$ >20 mm Hg.

In rare instances, complications may arise during the apnea test. The two most common complications include hypotension and hypoxemia. If the patient's SBP drops below 70 mm Hg, the apnea test should be aborted and the patient should be reconnected to the ventilator. In general, cases of hypoxemia can be avoided by the use of a tracheal insufflation catheter to supply oxygen following disconnection from the ventilator. Cardiac arrhythmias, another concern, are very uncommon and can also be avoided with oxygen supplementation. If the examiner concludes that all criteria for the apnea test have been met, a diagnosis of brain death is confirmed. However, if the patient fails to meet all criteria, further investigation with ancillary testing should be considered.

E. **Confirmatory tests.** The use of confirmatory tests in the assessment of brain death is reserved for instances when the apnea test cannot be performed, the test itself was inconsistent, or the neurologic examination was unreliable. The current available confirmatory tests aim at the evaluation and interpretation of two distinct categories: cerebral blood flow and neuronal function. Confirmatory tests alone should never be used to diagnose brain death, but rather confirm findings from the neurologic examination. To date, only electroencephalography (EEG), transcranial Doppler (TCD), and cerebral scintigraphy have consensus statements regarding testing in brain death. The use of other ancillary studies including conventional

TABLE 34.2 Apnea Testing Prerequisites

SBP > 100 mm Hg
Ventilator adjustment to normocapnea ($PaCO_2$ 35–45 mm Hg)
PEEP setting of 5 mm H_2O

Preoxygenation with 100% FiO_2 for 10 min to PaO_2 >200 mm Hg
Oxygen supplementation with insufflation catheter (6 L/min) or CPAP (10 mm H_2O)
Baseline arterial blood gas prior to disconnection

Abbreviations: CPAP, continuous positive airway pressure; PEEP, positive end-expiratory pressure; SBP, systolic blood pressure.

cerebral angiography, and somatosensory evoked potentials (SSEPs) may be considered, but true evidence is lacking. It should also be noted that confirmatory testing may provide false-negative results with an otherwise convincing neurologic examination. The usual explanation in these cases is that testing was performed too early in the determination of brain death, and details that timing of ancillary testing is a crucial concept.

1. **EEG** is the most used ancillary test in the determination of brain death worldwide. Diffuse isoelectric activity is the EEG pattern consistently observed with brain death. Prior to interpretation of the EEG, consensus criteria must be met and consistent throughout the recording (Table 34.3). The overall sensitivity and specificity of EEG in brain death is 90%; however, limitations do exist. Confounders including electrical interference in the intensive care unit, posterior fossa lesions, and preserved subcortical function with ischemic cortex should all be considered. If all stated criteria are not met and a definitive isoelectric pattern is not observed, the EEG may not be considered valuable when assessing brain death.

2. **TCD** is used in brain death to identify and transmit signals from both middle cerebral arteries (MCAs) and is a validated ancillary test. The sensitivity and specificity are 91% to 99% and 100%, respectively. Performing the exam in the assessment of brain death requires the confirmation of intracranial circulatory arrest on two separate occasions at least 30 minutes apart. The typical pattern seen with cerebrovascular arrest is oscillating flow with early systolic peaks and a high pulsatility index. It should be noted, however, in normal population studies that sonography of the MCAs cannot be obtained in 10% of patients. This limits its use for definitive diagnosis in brain death. The major advantage of TCD is its portability; however, its major disadvantage is interpretive, relying on expertise of the sonographer and the clinician experience. All variables must be taken into account when TCD analysis is considered in the assessment of brain death.

3. **Cerebral scintigraphy** is a dynamic nuclear scan that utilizes radioisotope gamma monitoring to identify cerebral circulation patterns. The tracer isotope is injected into the patient 30 minutes before initiation of the scan. In clinical instances of brain death, the scan will display complete cerebrovascular circulatory arrest at the skull base.

TABLE 34.3 Isoelectric EEG: Brain Death Requirements

Minimum of eight scalp electrodes
Impedances between 100 and 10,000 Ω
Interelectrode distance of at least 10 cm

Sensitivity $\leq 2\ \mu V$
Time constant of 0.3–0.4 s

High-frequency filter >30 Hz

Low-frequency filter <1 Hz

$\geq$30 min recording time
Testing of EEG reactivity to noxious stimuli and bright light

From American Electroencephalographic Society.
Abbreviation: EEG, electroencephalography.

Comparison with the spleen or internal carotid arteries should be performed to assess the viability of intracranial tracer uptake. The specificity in brain death is 96%. In certain instances, small amounts of uptake may be seen in cortical venous or subcortical parenchymal structures, rendering the scan inconclusive. Nuclear scanning can also be difficult to obtain institutionally, and with its reported false-positive and false-negative rates, is not a preferred test in the assessment of brain death.

4. **Conventional digital subtraction cerebral angiography (DSA)** is a dynamic vascular study utilizing contrast injection to visualize the anterior and posterior circulation. In healthy individuals, filling follows normal anatomic and physiologic variables, with internal carotid artery (ICA) and intracranial filling first, followed by external carotid artery filling. In brain death, this normal filling pattern is reversed with extracranial filling occurring first, and arrest of ICA flow at the skull base. This reversal is due to the ICP gradient created at the base following brain death. Of note, DSA has also been shown to correlate quite well with cerebral scintigraphy. To date, no criteria for confirmation of brain death have been established by neuroradiologic societies, implying lack of standardization and perhaps limitation.

5. **Electrophysiological studies** used in brain death include SSEPs and brainstem auditory evoked potentials (BAEPs). Both studies utilize the generation of electric potentials to assess the functionality and connectivity of specific neural circuits. Several studies have evaluated the use of SSEPs and BAEPs in the assessment of brain death and have found very poor predictive values. With SSEPs, cortical responses are shown to be absent bilaterally in up to 20% of comatose patients. With BAEPs, patients with anoxic ischemic encephalopathy are shown to have absent wave forms, while wave forms are present in brain death. Although certain institutions recommend the use of electrophysiologic studies in brain death, they should truly be reserved for unique instances with otherwise inconsistent confirmatory tests.

ETHICAL CONSIDERATIONS

A. **Legal background.** Traditionally, the legal definition for death was defined as the complete cessation of all cardiopulmonary function. Early in the literature there was no mention of brain functionality as a definitive criterion. In 1981, the President's Commission on Bioethics reinterpreted the definition of death as either irreversible cessation of cardiopulmonary function, or irreversible cessation of all brain functions. This Uniform Determination of Death Act was widely adopted by both medical and legal authorities in the United States. All states have also either adopted identical or similar legislation defining brain death as a mortal qualifier. These laws, given their correct use and interpretation, allow a clinician to cease all physiologic support when brain death is confirmed. There are, however, two qualifiers that continue to exist prohibiting termination of resuscitative care. These include preparedness for organ procurement and accommodation of specific family wishes. In three states (California, New Jersey, and New York), law currently protects all family wishes following a diagnosis of brain death, and they must be accommodated regardless of medical opinion.

B. **Religious beliefs.** Religion in the United States and throughout the modern world plays an integral part in the determination of brain death. Each major religion has long-standing traditions of defining death. Traditional language for most includes the cessation of the beating heart. Over time, however, general acceptance of brain death as a definition of death has been established. Both Christianity and Islam have held international summits that have come to the consensus that no brain function qualifies as death. In Judaism or Jewish Law, brain death is somewhat less defined and divided. Jewish Orthodoxy accounts only cardiopulmonary function as a qualifier, but less-conservative Judaism accepts brain death as a true entity. In general, the qualification of brain death is dependent on religious leaders and their acceptance of both the medical examination and objectivity used to determine diagnosis. In Buddhism, the prolongation of suffering is against standard practice, and brain death is widely accepted. The religious stance of organ procurement is a completely separate topic and again dependent on specific organizations. As an examiner, it is imperative that religious preference is known during the assessment of brain death to accommodate all parties involved.

C. **Social background.** Family and social support in the initial, intermediate, and late assessment of brain death is vital. Family-centered care and communication go a long way in understanding the diagnosis and willingness to accept death. Studies have shown that only half of families who have undergone an experience with brain death are able to define its criteria and show understanding of the process. Traditional cultural thinking defines the heart as the ultimate living being and the keeper of the soul. With its failure, then and only then is death imminent. A clinician must be able to approach these conflicting beliefs with care and compassion as well as clarity.

Ethnicity also plays an important role in communication and education in brain death. It is crucial to develop a multidisciplinary team approach for the care of the patient and the family that is sensitive to all beliefs and cultures. This will create a unique understanding and sense of respect with the family that may otherwise be lacking. Use of the clergy is also recommended as a safe go-between in the evaluation of brain death.

COMMON PRACTICAL PROBLEMS

A. **Examiner qualification.** To date, there are no specific studies detailing the accuracy of examination and diagnosis among different specialties. In the majority of tertiary care centers across the United States, the brain death examination is performed by either a neurologist, neurosurgeon, or a critical care physician. Other subspecialties likely participate in other institutions. Legally, all physicians in the United States are allowed to diagnose brain death. There are no adult guidelines recommending qualified examiners; however, the pediatric guidelines allow only for intensivists, neonatologists, trauma surgeons, neurologists, and neurosurgeons. Currently, there exists no standardized competency test to determine qualification. The most common portions of the examination left unchecked are the oculovestibular responses and the apnea test. Moving forward, two separate examinations may need to be considered in the adult population to ensure accurate diagnosis and qualification of examiners. Institutions may also consider implementation of standardized training and evaluation ensuring uniform certification. In general, most physicians do not feel comfortable with or have never performed the brain death examination. Further consideration should be made in the future to allow for only qualified interpretation in the assessment of brain death.

B. **Primary brainstem lesion.** Acute, destructive lesions to the brainstem can mimic brain death. In primary brainstem lesions, the cerebral hemispheres usually remain intact, precluding a diagnosis of brain death. Typical lesions that will cause catastrophic injury include basilar artery occlusion, pontine hemorrhage, compression from cerebellar hemorrhage, and direct brainstem trauma. In most common instances, a detailed neurologic examination will show some preservation of brainstem function. In most typical brainstem lesions, the medulla oblongata will be spared. The patient will have preserved respiratory drive and lack signs of autonomic failure. In instances when examination is concerning for brain death, patients will pass an apnea test. Ancillary studies such as EEG and intracranial vascular studies will show alpha coma pattern and preserved blood flow, respectively. Generally speaking, brain death examinations in patients with catastrophic brainstem injuries should be reserved for highly qualified clinicians.

C. **Spinal reflexes** are a polysynaptic, polysegmental reflex that can occur in brain death. Such reflexes are described as slow, short-duration movements that can be diminished by repetitive stimulation. Typical descriptions of such reflexes include triple flexion, finger jerks, head turning, abduction or adduction of the arms, and even attempts at sitting up. The frequency of movements in brain death varies, but has been reported as high as 39%. Review of spinal reflexes compared to complex motor movements has shown no correlation. Typical decerebrate and decorticate motor responses have no clinical correlation with spinally mediated responses, and are thus differentiated. The presence of spinal reflexes on examination does not preclude the diagnosis of brain death. Both experience and careful assessment will allow an examiner to reach a correct conclusion.

D. **Difficulty with the apnea test.** The final step in the confirmation of brain death is completion of the apnea test. There are several clinical scenarios in which the apnea test may be difficult to ascertain.

1. **Chronic CO_2 retention** is commonly encountered in patients with a history of chronic obstructive pulmonary disease (COPD). It is well documented that chronic hypercapnia (pco_2 50–70 mm Hg) results in a reduction of the chemoreceptor response. In such clinical instances, it is impossible to set target pco_2 values with the apnea test. Although rare, situations may arise where brain death determination is warranted in a patient with COPD. In such cases, the apnea test cannot be reliably performed and further ancillary testing is indicated.

2. **Breathing during the apnea test** is usually seen in comatose patients with a catastrophic neurologic injury. Brain death exclusively implies that all respiration is absent. Careful re-examination may reveal a cough reflex or other brainstem function that excludes brain death as a diagnosis. In a small number of documented patients, small gasps and agonal breathing have been seen. In such instances a repeat of the apnea test 24 hours later resulted in a positive test. Once the apnea test is positive, breathing effort will not return. If breathing during the apnea test has truly been established, family conversation should switch to determine further goals of care.

3. **Termination of the apnea test** is a common concern that continues to exist. Factors associated with the need for early termination include insufficient preoxygenation, hypotension, pretest acidosis, and polytrauma. Review of most clinical scenarios demonstrates that patients are inadequately preoxygenated. Additionally, all test prerequisites are not typically met including SBP >90 mm Hg and PEEP supplementation (5 mm Hg) following disconnection from the ventilator. If hypotension occurs during testing, a trial of intravenous phenylephrine may be considered. In situations where adequate oxygenation is difficult to overcome, apnea testing may not be reliable and other investigations should be considered.

E. **Cardiopulmonary resuscitation and hypothermia.** Therapeutic hypothermia following cardiac arrest has become a standardized practice in most institutions. Brain death occurs in around 5% of patients following arrest. The institution of hypothermia has shown to be beneficial in improving long-term neurologic outcomes and thus utilized today. Most protocols use a combination of benzodiazepines, opioid analgesics, and neuromuscular blocking agents to achieve cooling goals. Such medications are confounders in the examination of brain death and can present a diagnostic challenge. Additionally, hypothermia itself changes the pharmacokinetics of most drugs and delays objective neurologic findings on exam. Some authors recommend delaying a definitive neurologic examination up to 1 week following therapeutic hypothermia compared to the typical 3 days. The clearance of most medications during this time has been shown to be delayed up to five times the norm. Following therapeutic hypothermia it is important that examiners allow for adequate time to pass in order to exclude all major confounders and proceed with assessment of brain death. The use of a checklist prior to examination is highly recommended.

Key Points

- Brain death is defined as the complete, irreversible loss of brain function, leading to viscerosomatic and cardiopulmonary failure.
- A definable set of evidence-based guidelines for the diagnosis of brain death are widely available and should be used consistently during evaluation.
- Clinicians should have a firm background in the criticism and interpretation of confirmatory testing in brain death.
- Physicians must have a deep understanding of the ethical, religious, and legal implications of a brain death diagnosis.
- Effective communication and education are vital in brain death, and a multidisciplinary care team should be used to achieve such goals.

Recommended Readings

Burkle CM, Pope TM. Brain death: legal obligations and the courts. *Semin Neurol.* 2015;2:174–179.

Datar S, Fugate J, Rabinstein A, et al. Completing the apnea test: decline in complications. *Neurocrit Care.* 2014;3:392–396.

Fugate JE, Wijdicks EF, Mandrekar J, et al. Predictors of neurologic outcome in hypothermia after cardiac arrest. *Ann Neurol.* 2010;6:907–914.

Kompanje EJ. Families and brain death. *Semin Neurol.* 2015;2:169–173.

Kramer AH. Ancillary testing in brain death. *Semin Neurol.* 2015;2:125–138.

Mathur M, Ashwal S. Pediatric brain death determination. *Semin Neurol.* 2015;2:116–124.

Wijdicks EF. *Brain Death.* New York, NY: Oxford University Press; 2011.

Wijdicks EF. *The Comatose Patient.* New York, NY: Oxford University Press; 2014.

Wijdicks EF. Brain death guidelines explained. *Semin Neurol.* 2015;2:105–115.

Wijdicks EF, Pfeifer EA. Neuropathology of brain death in the modern transplant era. *Neurology.* 2008;15:1234–1237.

Wijdicks EF, Varelas PN, Gronseth GS, et al; American Academy of Neurology. Evidence-based guideline update: determining brain death in adults: report of the Quality Standards Subcommittee of the American Academy of Neurology. *Neurology.* 2010;23:1911–1918.

35 Neuroimaging of Common Neurologic Conditions

Jordan Rosenblum

Most common neurologic conditions are imaged using computed tomography (CT), magnetic resonance imaging (MRI), or both. In the emergent setting, CT is still the most commonly utilized modality. Patients with trauma or a suggestion of acute intracranial hemorrhage are routinely imaged with CT scans, whereas those with findings suggestive of ischemic stroke may be triaged to either CT or MRI. Frequently, the decision rests on the availability of the modality and the time needed to obtain the study. Advances in neuroimaging allow greater specificity in identifying metabolic and physiologic differences between normal tissue and pathology. Some of the most exciting advances include the use of diffusion-weighted imaging (DWI) with MRI that can demonstrate physiologic change within minutes of ischemic change, MR spectroscopy (MRS) that can identify abnormal metabolites and help in differentiating pathology such as recurrent tumor versus radiation necrosis, and functional MRI (fMRI) that can be used to localize specific functional areas in the brain. The choice of most appropriate imaging modality is presented according to clinical presentation. The information available with medical imaging carries with it specific risks that must be balanced against diagnostic gain. Ionizing radiation from CT may result in significant radiation dose, especially when multisequence scans are performed. Although the actual risk of cancer induction is still an open debate, it is clear that scans should only be ordered that are absolutely necessary and that will affect patient management. Other risks to consider from imaging have been described from contrast use in both CT and MRI. Iodinated contrast can lead to a contrast-induced nephropathy in patients with preexisting renal insufficiency. Gadolinium contrast has been linked to nephrogenic systemic fibrosis (NSF), a rare scleroderma-like systemic disease that can occur in patients with preexisting renal insufficiency. Current recommendations are to either forgo gadolinium contrast in patients in moderate renal insufficiency, or, if medically indicated, reduce the dose and use one of the agents believed to be associated with less risk of NSF. Patients with severe renal failure should in most cases not receive gadolinium contrast.

TRAUMA

CT is the primary imaging modality in trauma because of ready availability, speed, ability to detect bony abnormalities, and superior accuracy in detecting acute intracranial blood. High-resolution, fast CT scanners are frequently installed either within emergency departments or in close proximity. CT is performed routinely in trauma patients, often including those without focal neurologic signs to screen for occult injury. Widely accepted standards for patient selection in this setting are still controversial. MRI in the setting of acute trauma is still a secondary modality. The most important indication is in evaluating for diffuse axonal injury in which diffuse brain injury may be seen in the presence of a normal head CT. MRI may also demonstrate small extra-axial hemorrhages not seen by CT, particularly in the subtemporal and subfrontal regions. MRI is also indicated in the evaluation of changes secondary to chronic changes and demonstrates the extent of injury better than CT (Video 35.1).

A. **Closed head injury.** CT imaging parameters in trauma should include a narrow window (for acute blood), an intermediate window (for subacute blood), and a wide (bone) window. Acute blood may be present in the form of intracerebral (contusion), epidural, or subdural hematomas and subarachnoid hemorrhage (SAH). Fractures are well evaluated on bone windows and from coronal and sagittal reconstruction images. Patients with acute trauma and favorable initial coma scores usually fare well and do not require extensive follow-up imaging. In patients with moderate or severe trauma, or low initial Glasgow Coma Score,

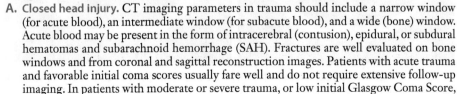

sequential CTs allow evaluation of the course of the initial trauma and the effects of therapy, including extension of initial hemorrhage, rehemorrhage, cerebral edema, herniation, response to external ventricular drainage, and intracranial pressure monitors. Diffuse cerebral edema, more common in younger patients, causes effacement of cerebrospinal fluid (CSF) spaces and may result in herniation (tonsillar, transtentorial, or subfalcine). In patients who come to medical attention several days or weeks after head trauma, with worsening headaches or seizures, MRI may be preferred as subacute hematomas may be isodense on CT, and therefore difficult to see. MRI is superior in evaluating for the presence of blood products in the brain parenchyma (Fig. 35.1A and B).

B. **Penetrating head injury.** CT is the modality of choice in patients with penetrating head injuries. Metallic objects (shrapnel) and glass appear hyperdense on CT, whereas wood objects generally appear hypodense. CT permits an excellent evaluation of the extent of bone damage, and that of the underlying parenchyma, including hematomas, edema, infarction, and herniation.

C. **Cervical spine injury.** Plain X-rays remain the first-line imaging method in patients with cervical spine trauma and should include at least anteroposterior, lateral, and open-mouth (odontoid) views. Cervical spine CT offers submillimeter resolution allowing the detection of subtle fractures not seen on plain films. MRI is used to evaluate for spinal cord injury, which appears bright on T2 pulse sequences and dark on gradient echo sequences because of the magnetic susceptibility effect of acute blood.

D. **Vascular injury.** Blunt injury to the neck may result in traumatic arterial dissections, pseudoaneurysms, or occlusions. In stable patients, magnetic resonance angiography (MRA) and CT angiography (CTA) are excellent imaging methods. Unstable patients may go directly to angiography, particularly if endovascular management is contemplated. Penetrating injuries may result in similar lesions, in addition to significant bleeding from both arterial and venous (jugular vein) injuries. CTA is the imaging method of choice in these patients because current fast scanners allow the evaluation of large anatomical areas with high-resolution and limited-contrast administration. Unstable patients may also require emergency angiography and possibly lifesaving endovascular occlusion of a bleeding vessel.

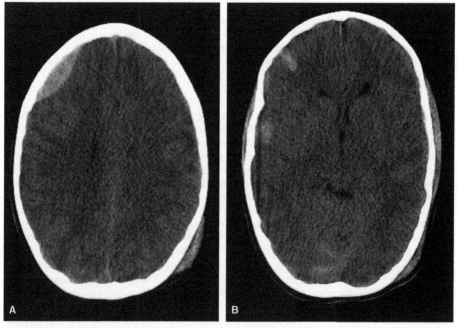

FIGURE 35.1 CT of a 10-year-old boy who fell from a tree. Noncontrast head CT demonstrates a right frontal epidural hematoma **(A)** and parenchymal contusions **(B)**. CT, computed tomography.

HEADACHES

Headache is one of the most common indications for neurologic consultation, with 50% of adults being seen for a severe headache at least once in their life. Fortunately, the vast majority have a benign origin. Pain-sensitive structures in the cranial area include the scalp, the scalp blood vessels, head and neck muscles, dural sinuses, the dura and large cerebral arteries at the skull base, meningeal arteries, and pain-sensitive fibers of the fifth (CN V), ninth (CN IX), and tenth (CN X) cranial nerves. Serious conditions that cause headaches include hemorrhage (subarachnoid, subdural, and intracerebral), infections (meningitis and brain abscess), tumors (primary or metastatic), hydrocephalus, and hypertensive crises. Patients at higher risk for significant pathology include those with (1) severe headache of sudden onset; (2) mental status changes, fever, focal neurologic deficits, or seizures; and (3) onset after the age of 50.

A. **Acute headaches.** Acute headache associated with nausea, vomiting, nuchal rigidity, and transient alteration in mental status is suggestive of SAH and should prompt immediate evaluation. CT is currently the preferred neuroimaging method for SAH, with reported accuracy rates in the 98% to 99% range.

1. **SAH and aneurysms.** Nontraumatic SAH is caused by a ruptured intracranial aneurysm in 80% to 85% of adult patients (Fig. 35.2A and B). About 10% of patients with SAH, usually in the younger age group, have a nonaneurysmal perimesencephalic hemorrhage, a benign and self-limiting venous hemorrhage. Catheter cerebral angiography remains the gold standard to evaluate SAH, followed by endovascular or surgical aneurysm obliteration if an aneurysm is identified. CTA is increasingly used as a reliable replacement for cerebral angiography, including for the surgical planning of ruptured and unruptured aneurysms. Uncommon causes of SAH include cerebral and dural arteriovenous malformations (AVMs), arterial dissections, cerebral tumors, vasculitides, and moyamoya disease.

2. **Intracerebral hemorrhage and other causes of acute headache.** Intracerebral hemorrhage is most commonly caused by arterial hypertension and may be putaminal, thalamic, lobar, cerebellar, or pontine. Cerebral amyloid angiopathy may cause lobar hemorrhage in the nonhypertensive elderly. CT is the primary method of evaluation. In younger, nonhypertensive patients, a cerebral or dural AVM may be the cause of hemorrhage, requiring further workup with MRI and cerebral angiography, which may need to be repeated or delayed if there is a large and compressive hematoma. Contrast-enhanced MRI and possibly MRS may be useful if a tumor is suspected.

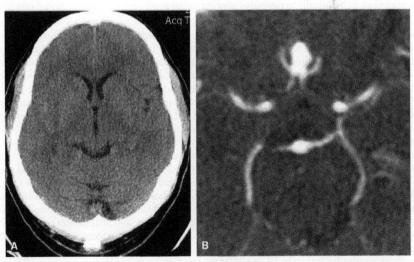

FIGURE 35.2 CT of a 38-year-old woman with acute-onset severe headache. Noncontrast head CT demonstrates subtle subarachnoid blood in right Sylvian fissure **(A)**. CTA demonstrates an anterior communicating artery aneurysm **(B)**. CTA, CT angiography.

Severe unilateral headache with cervicalgia and/or a Horner's syndrome may be caused by an acute carotid or vertebral arterial dissection. MRI/MRA, especially with precontrast fat-saturated axial T1 imaging, is diagnostic, showing the true lumen as a flow void and the mural thrombus as a bright crescent, so that there is generally no need for conventional angiography unless intracranial extension is suspected or endovascular treatment is contemplated. Migraines can cause severe acute headaches, usually periorbital, hemifacial, and frontal. The diagnosis is clinical, and CT may be sufficient to rule out hemorrhage in typical cases. Sinusitis is also diagnosed clinically; coronal CT shows soft tissue material obstructing sinus drainage pathways and filling the sinuses, and air–fluid levels in acute sinusitis. Glaucoma, retrobulbar optic neuritis, hydrocephalus, and infection may also cause acute headaches, evaluated with CT in clinically uncertain cases.

B. **Subacute headaches.** MRI is generally the modality of choice in the evaluation of subacute headache; however, CT may be more readily available and in many cases can provide the necessary information. Subacute headaches, particularly in the elderly, may be caused by a subdural hematoma. CT is usually adequate for both the initial evaluation and the follow-up, showing subdural space crescentic collections. Acute blood is hyperdense, whereas chronic collections are hypodense. CT is also a reasonable choice to diagnose hydrocephalus (the temporal horns and the third ventricle are early reliable indicators of hydrocephalus). In children, modified MRI scans can be performed in less than 5 minutes to identify hydrocephalus, or to assess changes in ventricular size without the risk of ionizing radiation. Cerebral tumors and infections may be evaluated with postcontrast CT (although contrast-enhanced MRI is superior). Spontaneous intracranial hypotension, possibly associated with a chronic CSF leak, is a potential cause for headaches causing recurrent emergency room (ER) visits; postcontrast MRI (particularly in the coronal plane) may be diagnostic, showing thickened and densely enhancing meninges as well as "sagging of the midbrain" and decreased volume in the suprasellar and basilar cisterns.

C. **Chronic headaches.** Unruptured AVMs, temporal arteritis, vasculitides, colloid cysts of the third ventricle, and cervical spondylosis are all potential causes of chronic headaches, in addition to migraine, cluster headaches, and chronic sinusitis. MRI has the highest yield in screening patients with a suspected structural intracranial anomaly.

CEREBRAL ISCHEMIA

Cerebral ischemia may be the result of acute arterial occlusion, hypoxic or anoxic injury, or may result from venous occlusion with increased venous pressure. Arterial occlusion may be an acute event, a chronically progressive process, or an acute process superimposed on chronic.

A. **Acute stroke.** Acute stroke is a true emergency (time is brain). There is a 4.5-hour window after the ischemic stroke onset for the delivery of intravenous tissue plasminogen activator. In appropriate cases, endovascular therapy may be of benefit up to 6 hours after symptom onset. In light of the urgent nature of imaging and because treatment guidelines recommend noninvasive vascular imaging before treatment, it is desirable to include such studies in the initial evaluation as well as ensuring a reliable method of evaluation of the studies obtained. One proposed algorithm for the emergency evaluation of acute stroke is to obtain a plain CT, followed (if no hemorrhage) by a contrast CTA and, possibly, a CT perfusion study to evaluate the perfusion deficit. The Alberta Stroke Program Early CT Score (ASPECTS) is a quantitative scoring system for assessing early ischemic changes in the MCA territory on CT in a reliable and reproducible fashion. Multiphase enhanced CT can also be utilized to grade collateral flow in the anterior and posterior MCA distribution. Vessel occlusion and success in revascularization after thrombolysis can be graded using the Thrombolysis in Cerebral Infarction grades, which are modeled after the Thrombolysis in Myocardial Infarction grading scheme, in which no perfusion is a grade 0, minimal perfusion a grade 1 and grade 2 is divided into 2a with partial filling of less than 2/3 if vascular territory, and 2b indicates complete filling of territory but in delayed fashion. Normal filling is a grade 3. In some centers, MRI, MRA, and MR perfusion are utilized in acute stroke patients. DWI is positive for acute stokes as early as 30 minutes and up to 10 days after the onset and is therefore particularly well suited to differentiate acute and subacute from chronic events. In most institutions, CT is more readily available and is thus still the predominant imaging modality (Fig. 35.3A–C).

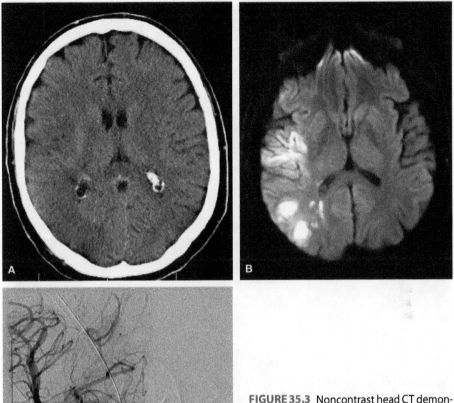

FIGURE 35.3 Noncontrast head CT demonstrates an area of hypodensity in the right temporal region **(A)**. Diffusion-weighted MRI scan **(B)** demonstrates larger area of restricted diffusion, consistent with acute ischemic change. **(C)** Cerebral angiogram demonstrates filling defect at proximal M1 segment with stent retriever device in place across the thrombus. CT, computed tomography; MRI, magnetic resonance imaging.

B. **Dural sinus and cortical vein thrombosis.** The venous intracranial circulation should always be evaluated, particularly if the patient's neurologic deficit is accompanied by headache or does not fit a recognizable vascular distribution. Recent thrombus within a dural sinus may be difficult to identify on plain CT (although possibly seen as a spontaneously hyperdense filling structure) or on plain MRI (hyperacute blood may appear gray on both T1 and T2 sequences). Therefore, postcontrast imaging (CT and MRI) has higher accuracy, showing clots as filling defects within a dural sinus or cortical vein. An MR venography (MRV) provides three-dimensional visualization of the venous system, which may be selectively imaged owing to its lower velocity profile compared with arterial structures. Unilateral cranial nerve symptoms in association with sinusitis, or facial infection can be seen with cavernous sinus thrombosis, which generally presents unilaterally, but can spread to be bilateral via intercavernous connecting veins (Fig. 35.4A–D).

C. **Intermittent and chronic deficits.** Transient ischemic attacks (TIAs) and chronic ischemic deficits are best evaluated with MRI/MRA. DWI MRI is most often normal in TIAs and ischemic lesions 10 days or older. MRI is superior to CT in evaluating stroke mimics including demyelinating disease and tumor. MRA is effective in screening the intracranial

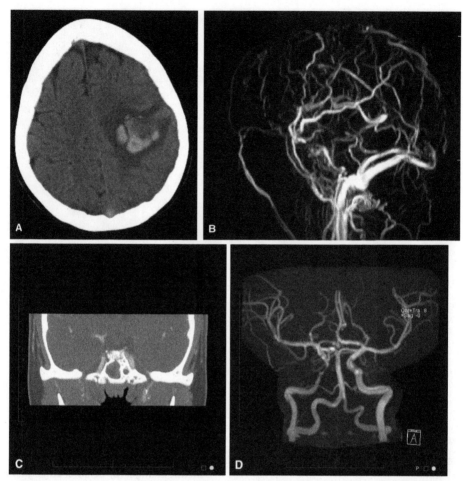

FIGURE 35.4 Severe headache and mental status changes. Noncontrast head CT demonstrates parenchymal hemorrhage in the left hemisphere with high density noted in the superior sagittal sinus **(A)**. MRV demonstrates absent signal in the superior sagittal sinus consistent with sinus thrombosis **(B)**. Different patient, with right eye swelling and painful range of motion, coronal postcontrast CT, demonstrates cavernous sinus thrombosis with lack of enhancement of right cavernous sinus **(C)** and irregular narrowing of the cavernous carotid artery on MR angiogram consistent with arteritis **(D)**. CT, computed tomography; MRV, MR venography.

and cervical arterial vasculature although the resolution of CTA (0.625 mm with current 64-detector scanners) provides excellent definition, nearing that of conventional angiography in certain locations. Severe arterial stenoses are a known pitfall of MRA, which exaggerates the degree of the lesion owing to signal loss. Therefore, conventional angiography remains useful in equivocal cases whenever corrective therapy is contemplated.

ALTERED LEVEL OF CONSCIOUSNESS

Evaluation of a patient with an altered level of consciousness (LOC) is a common indication for neurologic consultation requiring immediate neuroimaging. Causes of altered LOC may include intracranial hemorrhage (including traumatic), stroke, metabolic disorders, toxic substance ingestion (suicide attempts or accidental), and cerebral tumors (primary or metastatic).

The immediate concern in these patients is to rule out a major indication for emergent intervention, including intracranial hemorrhage, acute infarctions, impending tonsillar or transtentorial herniation, or other life-threatening conditions. CT scanning is the preferred modality in these patients because of ready access and accuracy in identifying intracranial hemorrhage (intracerebral, SAH, subdural hematoma (SDH), and epidural). It is also possible to assess the risk for herniation if a lumbar puncture is indicated to rule out SAH or infection. In patients without CT evidence of acute abnormal findings, MRI should be obtained as soon as possible to detect CT occult process including dural sinus thrombosis, acute basilar artery thrombosis, and posterior reversible encephalopathy syndrome, which show characteristic T2 and FLAIR cortical and subcortical lesions.

DEMENTIA

Cognitive decline may be related to a number of clinical conditions including (1) depression, (2) structural lesions (cerebral tumor, subdural hematoma, and hydrocephalus), (3) chronic cerebral ischemia, or (4) primary neurodegenerative conditions, the most common of which is dementia of the Alzheimer's type (Major or Mild Neurocognitive Disorder due to Alzheimer's Disease—*Diagnostic and Statistical Manual of Disorders*, Fifth Edition [*DSM-5*]). A thorough clinical evaluation plays a major role in these patients who are often in the older age group. Neuroimaging detects correctable causes of dementia, found in about 5% of patients with progressive cognitive decline. CT is adequate to identify severe hydrocephalus and chronic subdural hematomas. MRI is superior to CT in the vast majority of patients. Assessment of generalized cerebral and focal hippocampal atrophy in major or mild neurocognitive disorder due to Alzheimer's disease is more easily done with MRI, including computerized volumetric measurements of the hippocampus. Positron emission tomography and single photon emission computed tomography may allow detection of Dementia Alzheimer's type (DAT) earlier by showing decreased hippocampal glucose metabolism. MRS may show increased myo-inositol and decreased N-acetyl-aspartate peaks in the gray matter. Vascular dementia is also well evaluated by MRI, particularly FLAIR imaging, which demonstrates lacunar infarcts and white matter abnormalities. Cerebral autosomal-dominant arteriopathy with subcortical infarcts and leuko-encephalopathy (CADASIL) may have a typical distribution (periventricular, anterior temporal, and subinsular) that may suggest the diagnosis (Fig. 35.5A and B). In cases of major or mild frontotemporal neurocognitive disorder (*DSM-5*) the predominance of frontal lobe atrophy is well evaluated on multiplanar MRI. In suspected normal pressure hydrocephalus, transependymal CSF flow may be present, seen as periventricular bright T2 signal. The pattern and velocity of CSF flow may be evaluated at the foramen magnum using phase-contrast flow techniques.

SEIZURES

A. **New-onset adult seizures.** Although patients presenting with seizures are often scanned initially with CT to rule out hemorrhage or tumor, MRI is the preferred initial imaging method to investigate new-onset adult seizures, owing to its superior contrast resolution and multiplanar capability. Magnetoencephalography (MEG) is a technique that measures magnetic fields caused by neuronal activity, with a spatial resolution of a few millimeters and a temporal resolution of milliseconds. Magnetic source imaging uses MEG in combination with MRI in the same machine and has currently the highest yield detecting epileptogenic foci. New-onset adult seizures may be caused by tumors (primary or metastatic), AVMs, inflammatory conditions, vasculitides, ischemic lesions, and gliosis from prior injury (Fig. 35.6A and B).

B. **Known seizure disorder.** In patients with temporal lobe epilepsy, coronal MRI (FLAIR and T2) has a high overall detection rate (up to 80%) for mesial-temporal sclerosis, showing an atrophic hippocampus with high T2 signal and indirect signs including dilated choroidal fissure and forniceal atrophy. Presurgical evaluation includes the evaluation of hemispheric language dominance, usually obtained by Wada testing (selective internal carotid artery injection of sodium amobarbital). The fMRI has been used to detect language dominance.

C. **Pediatric seizures.** Infants with germinal matrix and traumatic hemorrhages, intracranial neonatal infections, and perinatal ischemia may be evaluated and followed with CT. In stable,

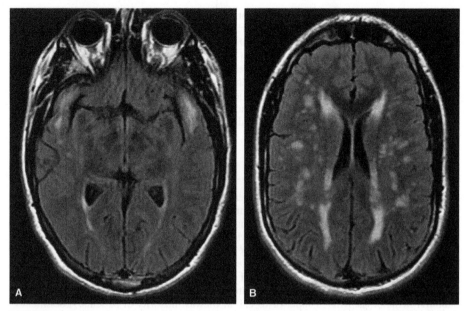

FIGURE 35.5 Forty-one-year-old man with migraines with aura, TIAs, and cognitive decline diagnosed with CADASIL. Axial FLAIR images at the level of the lateral ventricles **(A)** and through the temporal lobes **(B)** demonstrate scattered areas of signal abnormality. The symmetric anterior temporal lobe abnormalities are typical in this disease. CADASIL, cerebral autosomal-dominant arteriopathy with subcortical infarcts and leukoencephalopathy; TIAs, transient ischemic attacks.

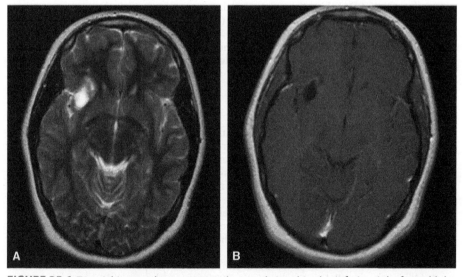

FIGURE 35.6 T2 axial image demonstrates abnormal signal in the inferior right frontal lobe **(A)**. Postcontrast T1 axial image **(B)** demonstrates a minimally enhancing cystic ganglioglioma in this 19-year-old with a history of seizures.

nonfebrile infants, most neonatal seizures are related to congenital disorders (migrational anomalies and structural defects), which are best evaluated with MRI, although traumatic lesions are detectable on CT. In childhood-onset seizures, clinical and electroencephalogram (EEG) evaluations are usually adequate and imaging may not be necessary for certain forms of seizure activity, including febrile, absence (petit mal) seizures, infantile spasms (Lennox–Gastaut syndrome), and benign focal epilepsy, unless the child has abnormal physical findings or delayed development. Certain forms of childhood epilepsy, like juvenile myoclonic epilepsy, are associated with a higher frequency of structural anomalies requiring MRI evaluation.

HEARING LOSS AND TINNITUS

A. **Hearing loss.** Clinical and audiometric data should guide neuroimaging. The deficit may be (1) sensorineural (SNHL), conductive (CHL) or mixed; (2) unilateral or bilateral; and (3) congenital or acquired.

1. **SNHL.** Unilateral or asymmetrical SNHL in adults is best evaluated with MRI. The most common cause is a vestibular schwannoma (acoustic neuroma). Even small lesions of the internal auditory canal and cerebellopontine angle are diagnosed with thin T1, T2, and postcontrast axial and coronal MRI, and the addition of a high-resolution volume acquisition such as FIESTA (Fast Imaging Employing Steady sTate Acquisition, GE Medical Systems). MRI should also evaluate the remainder of the acoustic pathway for possible ischemic or demyelinating lesions, particularly the medullary cochlear nuclear complex (the lesions that mimic those caused by vestibular schwannomas), thalamus, and temporal lobe.

   SNHL in children, unilateral or bilateral, is usually related to congenital inner ear diseases, requiring high-resolution noncontrast CT as the initial evaluation to assess the cochlea, vestibule, semicircular canals, vestibular aqueduct, and endolymphatic duct and sac. Enlarged vestibular aqueduct syndrome is a common cause of SNHL.

2. **CHL.** CHL is caused by disruption of the mechanical components of the auditory apparatus. CHL is therefore best evaluated by noncontrast high-resolution CT. It is most commonly caused by temporal bone inflammatory disease, particularly otomastoiditis and otitis media. Otospongiosis, in which there is replacement of endochondral bone by spongious bone at the oval window (fenestral) or the cochlea (retrofenestral), causes both CHL and SNHL (bilateral in 80%) and tinnitus. Other causes for CHL include middle ear cholesteatomas, tumors (glomus tympanicum), and traumatic ossicular dislocations, all well evaluated with CT.

B. **Tinnitus.** Tinnitus may be very disturbing to patients. It may be pulsatile or nonpulsatile. Objective tinnitus, heard by both the patient and the examiner, commonly leads to findings. Subjective tinnitus, only heard by the patient, has a low diagnostic yield.

1. **Pulsatile tinnitus.** Pulsatile (pulse synchronous) tinnitus is best evaluated by MRI/MRA, whether or not direct otoscopic examination shows a retrotympanic mass. A vascular-appearing tympanic membrane may be associated with arterial (aberrant carotid artery, carotid stenosis or dissection, and petrous carotid artery aneurysms), venous (dehiscent or high-riding jugular bulb), inflammatory (cholesterol granuloma, middle ear mastoiditis) causes, or tumors (glomus tympanicum or jugulo tympanicum and meningioma). Tinnitus with a normal otoscopic examination should raise suspicion for a dural arteriovenous fistula (of the transverse or sigmoid sinus or the tentorium); MRI may show suspicious flow voids, MRA source images may demonstrate trans-osseous arterial structures, and postcontrast MRI and MRV may demonstrate an occluded dural sinus. Confirmation (and therapy) is provided via catheter angiography. Other conditions include venous sinus stenosis, idiopathic intracranial hypertension (pseudotumor cerebri), chronic anemia, and thyrotoxicosis.

2. **Nonpulsatile tinnitus.** It is most commonly caused by Ménière's disease, which also manifests as episodes of vertigo and SNHL. Increased volumes of endolymph causing enlarged endolymphatic spaces have been incriminated. The diagnosis is clinical, but when indicated, neuroimaging should be done with CT. Other causes include otosclerosis and middle ear inflammatory disease, also best studied with CT.

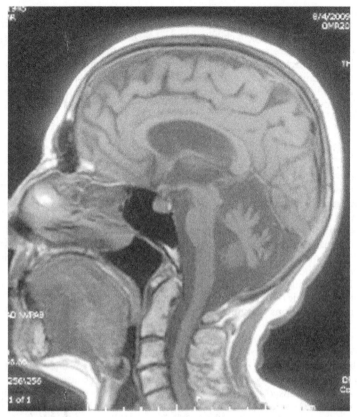

FIGURE 35.7 Sagittal T1 image demonstrates prominent volume loss of the cerebellum, pons, and brainstem, in this patient with multiple system atrophy of the cerebellar type (olivopontocerebellar atrophy).

VERTIGO AND ATAXIA

Vertigo and ataxia may indicate posterior fossa lesions where MRI is the modality of choice because of superior contrast resolution and beam-hardening artifact with CT.

Causes of vertigo that may be diagnosed with imaging include vestibular schwannomas, viral labyrinthitis, or perilymphatic fistulae. Central vertigo may be caused by posterior fossa lesions including demyelinating disease, tumors, strokes, Chiari 1 malformation, and trauma. The preferred neuroimaging method to investigate vertigo is MRI. Even small vestibular schwannomas may be diagnosed with a good quality MRI, appearing as small enhancing masses. Rarely, viral labyrinthitis may be seen as T1 hyperintensity within the vestibular apparatus indicative of hemorrhagic products. Small multiple sclerosis plaques and ischemic lesions appear as bright lesions on T2 and FLAIR imaging.

Ataxia usually reflects cerebellar dysfunction, although it may also be sensory or vestibular in origin. Again, MRI is the preferred imaging modality to study patients with ataxia because of its superior contrast resolution in demyelinating diseases, ischemia, and tumors. Other causes of ataxia include chronic ethanol and phenytoin intoxication, a number of degenerative conditions, paraneoplastic syndromes, all accompanied with cerebellar atrophy, well demonstrated on sagittal and coronal MRI (Fig. 35.7).

DISTURBANCES OF VISION

The optic pathways and the globe are both well evaluated with MRI, which is the preferred neuroimaging study in patients with visual disturbance.

A. Visual loss (including amaurosis fugax). Gradual monocular vision loss is usually related to ocular pathology like cataract. Sudden unilateral vision loss most commonly results from diabetic retinopathy, followed by ocular ischemic syndrome, which may be caused by retinal vein occlusion, retinal artery occlusion, anterior ischemic optic neuropathy, an ischemic syndrome of the anterior ciliary vasculature, and rarely to demyelinating disease of the optic nerve, well evaluated with pre- and postcontrast MRI. Amaurosis fugax designates vision loss caused by reduced blood flow to the eye, heralding a stroke and prompting therapy. The most common cause of amaurosis fugax is carotid artery stenosis, which is well evaluated by MRA. CTA is an excellent alternative to evaluate carotid disease, although heavily calcified plaques remain a limitation.

Visual field deficits related to lesions affecting the optic chiasm, tracts, and radiations should be studied with contrast-enhanced MRI. Lesions affecting the chiasm, like pituitary adenomas, and suprasellar lesions are particularly well suited for coronal and sagittal MRI. Most demyelinating and inflammatory conditions and tumors involving the postchiasmatic optic pathways appear bright on T2 and FLAIR imaging and enhance after contrast administration. Cerebral AVMs of the temporal and occipital lobes appear as dark, tortuous flow voids on T1 and T2 imaging.

B. Impairment of ocular motility. Ocular motility dysfunction most commonly results from diabetic cranial neuropathy and traumatic lesions of the orbit or the superior orbital fissure. Traumatic lesions involving bony structures are best evaluated with thin-cut CT with coronal reconstructions. Nontraumatic pathology may result from a variety of lesions affecting the oculomotor, trochlear, and abducens nerves anywhere between their brainstem nuclei and the orbit including brainstem strokes, demyelinating and inflammatory lesions, tumors, petrous apex lesions, cavernous sinus and orbital apex tumors, aneurysms, and inflammatory lesions. MR is the modality of choice in evaluating all of these possibilities. A sudden third cranial nerve (CN III) palsy suggestive of an internal carotid artery–posterior communicating artery junction aneurysm may be initially evaluated with either MRI/MRA or CT/CTA. The extraocular muscles are also well evaluated with coronal MRI of the orbits.

C. Chemosis and proptosis. Carotid-cavernous fistulae (CCFs) are the most common causes of ophthalmic venous system flow reversal and engorgement. Direct CCFs are caused by arterial wall rupture of the intracavernous carotid segment, most commonly from a traumatic arterial laceration, less commonly from spontaneous rupture of a small aneurysm, Ehlers–Danlos syndrome type IV (vascular type), fibromuscular dysplasia, or a spontaneous arterial dissection. Indirect CCFs are because of spontaneous arteriovenous shunting to the ophthalmic vein from dural arterial branches of the external carotid. The most common associations are pregnancy, dehydration, and sinus infections. Contrast-enhanced CT and MRI show dilated ophthalmic vein and cavernous sinus in direct CCFs. Indirect CCFs may be much more subtle, sometimes only suspected on the basis of small flow voids around a dural sinus. Catheter angiography is diagnostic and provides the route for transvascular therapy.

NECK PAIN AND CERVICAL RADICULOPATHY

Cervical spondylosis is the most common cause of neck pain and cervical radiculopathy, and its incidence increases with age. It is characterized by hypertrophic arthropathy of the facet joints, osteophyte formation at the disk margins, and progressive intervertebral disk degeneration and herniation. All these changes result in central canal and neural foraminal stenoses, with resulting restriction of the spinal cord and the nerve roots. In younger patients, sudden disc herniation may cause acute symptoms. Other causes of cervical pain and radiculopathy

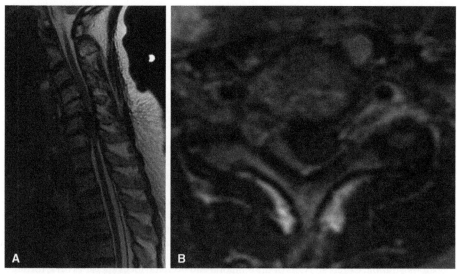

FIGURE 35.8 T2 sagittal image **(A)** and axial image **(B)** demonstrate a large left paracentral disc protrusion at the C5–C6 level with marked deformity of the underlying cord with increased signal in the cord that may represent edema or myelomalacia.

include syringomyelia with or without Chiari malformation, benign tumors of the spinal canal or the neural foramina like schwannomas and meningiomas, demyelinating disease, and posttraumatic myelomalacia. MRI is the preferred method to image these patients because it allows superior evaluation of the cervicomedullary junction, the cord, the spinal canal, and the neural foramina. CT myelography may be useful in patients with cervical spondylosis and contraindications or intolerance to MRI (Fig. 35.8A and B).

BACK PAIN

Low back pain is one of the most common presenting complaints to physicians with up to 85% of the population having experienced symptoms at least once.

A. General causes and evaluation. Most causes of transient low back pain are benign and related to degenerative disease, muscle strain, mild trauma, excess weight, and poor posture. Imaging is recommended for back pain associated with certain findings, including radiculopathy or lower motor neuron deficit, sudden onset, older age, signs of systemic infection, known or suspected malignancy, and trauma. MRI is the preferred study in these cases. The relationship between persistent back pains including radicular pain may be striking. Instability may be defined as loss of support of a segment of the spine, subjecting it to abnormal displacement during physiologic movements. Plain X-rays of the spine, in neutral position, flexion, and extension are the most widely used screening method and allow identification of patients who are likely to benefit from corrective surgery, that is, those with spondylolisthesis and lumbar intervertebral instability. CT may be useful to provide further detail.

B. Lumbar radiculopathy (sciatica). It is pain that originates along the course of the sciatic nerve, which runs from the lumbar spine to the posterior thigh. Lumbar disc herniation, the most common cause of sciatica, is a break in the annulus fibrosus with subsequent displacement of nucleus pulposus, cartilage, or bone beyond the disc space. Other causes of sciatica include degenerative disease (including synovial cysts) and spinal stenosis, tumors (primary and metastatic), infections (osteomyelitis and abscess), and hematomas (epidural, subdural, and psoas). MRI is the study of choice for the initial evaluation of lumbar radiculopathy, as it demonstrates the conus, cauda equina, nerve roots, bony elements, and discs with exquisite contrast in multiple planes. Contrast enhancement is utilized in evaluating infections and tumors. Disc herniations are well evaluated with MRI, although

CT myelography may allow greater detail of bone abnormalities. MRI is inferior to CT in spondylolysis and spondylolisthesis.

MYELOPATHIES

MRI is the preferred imaging method in myelopathies, both acute and chronic, providing multiplanar imaging, superior contrast between normal and abnormal spinal cord, CSF, fat and bony structures. Gating techniques help reduce artifacts from breathing and CSF, and cardiac and vascular pulsations. Patients with acute myelopathy and major contraindications to MRI (pacemakers) may be evaluated with plain CT or CT myelography.

Nontraumatic acute myelopathy may result from spinal cord compression by a retropulsed neoplastic vertebral compression fracture, usually in an elderly patient with an unknown (or known) cancer, best evaluated by noncontrast whole spine MRI. Acute inflammatory myelopathy caused by transverse myelitis or demyelinating conditions are also best evaluated with MRI, with the addition of contrast (Fig. 35.9A–D). Less commonly, acute myelopathy is caused by spontaneous epidural hematoma. In the setting of trauma, possible cord contusions are best evaluated by MRI using T2, short T1 inversion recovery (STIR), and gradient echo sequences.

Causes of chronic myelopathy include spinal cord tumors, degenerative disease and disc herniations, syringomyelia, congenital anomalies, inflammatory and demyelinating disease, and spinal dural arteriovenous fistulae. Initial evaluation of these patients is also best undertaken with pre- and postcontrast MRI. CT myelography should be reserved for the rare patient with a major contraindication to MRI.

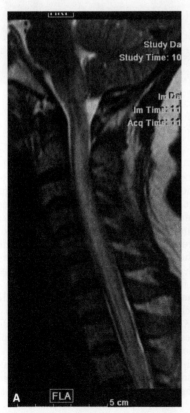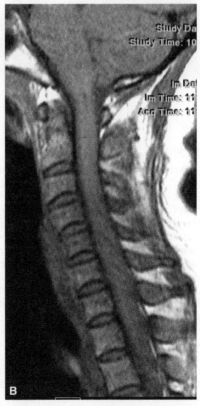

FIGURE 35.9 T2 sagittal **(A)**, T1 sagittal **(B)**, T1 sagittal with contrast **(C)**, and T2 axial **(D)** of the cervical spine demonstrate increased signal on T2 with slight cord enlargement. Postcontrast T1 sagittal images demonstrate enhancement in the areas of signal abnormality in this 42-year-old woman with Devic's disease.

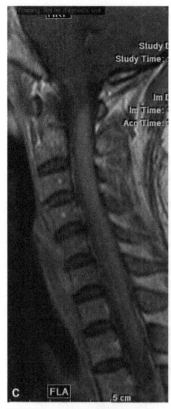

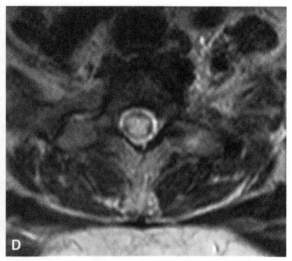

FIGURE 35.9 *(continued)*

Key Points

- The choice of most appropriate imaging modality is a function of suspected pathology, availability of types of imaging, and a balance of potential risk versus diagnostic gain.
- In most cases, acute trauma of either the head or spine is most appropriately imaged with CT with MR as a secondary modality depending on the results of initial CT scan.
- Potential risks to consider with CT include the risk of ionizing radiation and, if contrast is utilized, the potential risk of contrast nephropathy. With MR imaging, risks are predominantly associated with the high magnetic fields. Caution must be used to screen for cardiac or implanted electronic devices, other metallic implants, or history of injury with possible metallic foreign bodies.
- Most suspected intracranial pathology other than trauma is best imaged using MRI, including seizures, headache, suspected ischemic changes, and visual symptoms.
- Advanced imaging techniques including MRS, diffusion tensor imaging, and perfusion imaging (CT and MR) are potential sources of physiologic imaging, which may play a role in imaging a variety of pathologic conditions of the CNS.
- In the spine, CT is the primary modality in most cases of acute trauma, and at times in surgical planning, but for most other indications, MR is far superior in its ability to depict soft tissue abnormalities including signal abnormality within the cord and extra-axial soft tissue abnormalities.

Recommended Readings

Brazis PW, Masdeu JC, Biller J. *Localization in Clinical Neurology*. 7th ed. Philadelphia, PA: Wolters Kluwer; 2017.

Faro SH, Mohamed FB. *Functional MRI: Basic Principles and Clinical Applications*. 2nd ed. New York, NY: Springer; 2012.

Fugate JE, Klunder AM, Kalmes DF. What is meant by "TICI." *AJNR*. 2013;34:1792–1797.

Grossman RI, Yousem DM. *Neuroradiology: The Requisites*. 3rd ed. St Louis, MO: Mosby; 2010.

Osborn AG. *Osborn's Brain: Imaging, Pathology, and Anatomy*. 1st ed. Philadelphia, PA: Lippincott Williams and Wilkins; 2012.

Powers WJ, Derdeyn CP, Biller J, et al. 2015 American Heart Association/American Stroke Association focused update of the 2013 guidelines for the early management of patients with acute ischemic stroke regarding endovascular treatment: a guideline for healthcare professionals from the American Heart Association/American Stroke Association. *Stroke*. 2015;46:3020–3035.

Simpson JR. DSM-5 and neurocognitive disorders. *J Am Acad Psychiatry Law*. 2014;42:159–164.

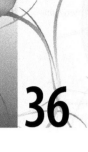

36

Approach to the Selection of Electrodiagnostic, Cerebrospinal Fluid, and Other Ancillary Testing

Maria Baldwin and Matthew A. McCoyd

Neurophysiologic electrodiagnostic studies define alterations in the functions of the nervous system that may not be visualized by imaging procedures. The major areas of study include electroencephalography (EEG), nerve conduction studies (NCS), electromyography (EMG), and evoked potentials (EPs). The clinical usefulness of these examinations is here discussed, followed by brief descriptions of other ancillary neurologic tests such as polysomnography and the multiple sleep latency test (MSLT), and finally the indications, contraindications, and utility of performing lumbar puncture (LP) for cerebrospinal fluid (CSF) analysis.

ELECTROENCEPHALOGRAM

A. **Introduction.** The EEG involves recording of the spontaneous electrical activity of the brain from the scalp and activity elicited by activation procedures, including sleep, hyperventilation, and photic stimulation. This electrical activity is the summation of both excitatory and inhibitory postsynaptic potentials from cortical neurons aligned perpendicular to the surface. Small metal disks containing conductive gel are attached to the scalp and ear lobes according to a system of measurements, termed the 10 to 20 system and are connected by flexible wires to a recording instrument that amplifies the brain activity about a million times. The EEG is sampled on moving paper or on a computer simultaneously from 16 to 21 pairs of electrodes (derivations) in selected combinations (montages).

B. **Normal EEG activity.**
   1. **EEG rhythms.** The EEG is a composite of several different types of activity, each with characteristic factors of frequency, amplitude, morphology, reactivity, topography, and quantity. The frequency bands of activity are as follows:
      a. **Delta activity** (<4 Hz)
      b. **Theta activity** (4 to 7 Hz)
      c. **Alpha activity** (8 to 13 Hz)
      d. **Beta activity** (>13 Hz)
   2. The most characteristic feature of a normal EEG in an adult during relaxed wakefulness is the **alpha rhythm,** which occurs over the posterior regions of the head while the eyes are closed (Fig. 36.1). Judgments of normality for various EEG activities depend on the age and state of alertness of the subject because complex changes in the EEG patterns occur throughout life and patterns evolve when going from wakefulness through different stages of sleep.
   3. **Activation procedures** are used to elicit abnormal activities that may not occur spontaneously.
      a. **Hyperventilation** for 3 minutes is most effective for activating generalized epileptiform and seizure activities such as the spike–wave paroxysms of absence seizures. It may less frequently activate focal abnormalities (e.g., slowing) and focal epileptiform activity. It is contraindicated in a patient with cardiac infarction, recent subarachnoid hemorrhage (SAH), or significant pulmonary disease.
      b. **Photic stimulation** consists of repetitive brief flashes of light generated by an electronic apparatus and delivered at frequencies of 1 to 30 Hz. This procedure evokes responses over the occipitoparietal regions of the EEG and is termed photic driving. It is a normal response seen in much of the population. However, lack of a photic driving response is not considered abnormal. An asymmetry to the response or generation of epileptiform discharges or seizures is considered abnormal. The most frequent

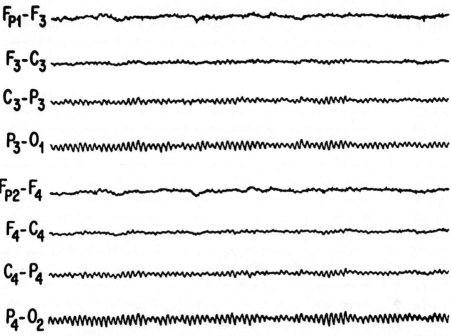

FIGURE 36.1 Normal EEG in an adult man at rest with eyes closed. Four rows—EEG activity from frontal to occipital regions on *left* (**top**). Four rows—EEG activity from frontal to occipital regions on *right* (**bottom**). Note normal alpha activity over posterior head regions. EEG, electroencephalography.

abnormal response is diffuse paroxysms of spike–wave complexes (photoparoxysmal or photoconvulsive response) that often indicate a seizure propensity.

    c. **Sleep recordings** are most useful for recording paroxysmal abnormalities in patients with epilepsy. Sleep may activate focal or generalized epileptiform activity. Sleep deprivation on the night before the study may facilitate sleep, and the deprivation itself may activate epileptiform activity.

C. **Abnormal EEG activity.** Many EEG changes are nonspecific, but some are highly suggestive of specific entities such as epilepsy, herpes simplex encephalitis (HSE), and metabolic encephalopathies. In general, neuronal damage or dysfunction is suggested by the presence of **slow waves** (activity in the theta or delta range) in a focal or diffuse location, whereas the presence of **sharp waves** or **spikes** (epileptiform activity) in a focal or diffuse pattern suggests a seizure tendency. Localized slowing is highly sensitive and significant for local neuronal dysfunction or focal brain damage but is quite nonspecific because it cannot distinguish the pathologic type of lesion. Thus, cerebral infarction, brain tumor, brain abscess, and head trauma may all cause similar focal EEG changes (Fig. 36.2). Diffuse slowing also indicates organic rather than psychiatric disease but again is nonspecific because such slowing may occur with any significant toxic, metabolic, degenerative, or even multifocal disease process. The EEG is also useful in following the courses of patients with altered states of consciousness and may, in certain circumstances, provide prognostic information. Finally, the EEG can be important in the determination of brain death as an ancillary test.

    1. **Epilepsy.**

        a. Some types of interictal EEG patterns are termed *epileptiform* because they have a distinct morphology and occur in a high proportion of EEGs from patients with seizures but rarely in records from asymptomatic patients. Epileptiform discharges are not seizures in themselves. Epileptiform patterns include sporadic spikes, sharp waves, and spike and slow-wave complexes. Epileptiform findings must always be

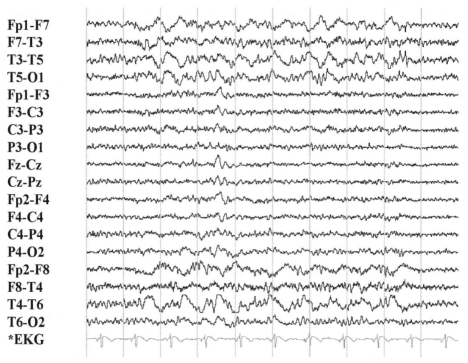

FIGURE 36.2 Left focal frontotemporal slow-wave abnormality in an adult patient with a recent large left frontotemporal infarction. (Image courtesy of Dr. David Chabolla.)

interpreted with caution because, though they may support a diagnosis of epilepsy, they are poorly correlated with frequency and likelihood of recurrence of epileptic seizures. One must always treat the patient and never "treat" the EEG. Not all spike or sharp-wave patterns indicate epilepsy; 14- and 6-Hz positive spikes, sporadic sleep spikes, wicket spikes, 6-Hz spike–wave complexes, and the psychomotor variant pattern are all spike patterns that are of no proven clinical significance. These patterns are termed **benign normal variants** and can be seen in the general population with no association with epilepsy. **Seizures** are electrographically defined as an evolution in frequency, location, or morphology of epileptiform discharges and typically last >10 seconds. An example of an electrographic seizure is demonstrated in Figure 36.3.

b. A substantial portion of patients with unquestioned epilepsy have normal EEGs. However, epileptiform activity has a high correlation with clinical epilepsy. Only about 2% of nonepileptic patients exhibit epileptiform EEG activity, in contrast with 50% to 90% of patients with epilepsy, depending on the circumstances of recording and on whether more than one EEG has been obtained. The most conclusive proof of an epileptic basis for a patient's episodic symptoms is obtained by recording an EEG seizure during the typical clinical event.

c. The EEG helps establish whether the seizure originates from a limited or focal area or network in the brain (**focal seizures**) (Fig. 36.4) or involves the brain as a whole from the onset (**generalized seizures**). This distinction is important because of the different possible causes of these two basic epilepsy types, possibly different medical management and because the clinical manifestations of both types may be similar.

d. In general, location of the epileptiform activity on the EEG may be helpful in classifying the patient's seizure type.

(1) Generalized seizures originate within networks involving both hemispheres and are typically associated with bilaterally synchronous bursts of spikes and spike–wave discharges.

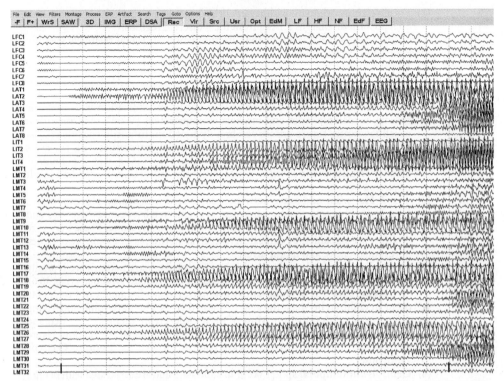

FIGURE 36.3 Focal seizure recorded with intracranial electrodes resting atop cortical surface. Note focal onset of rhythmic discharges, which spread and alter in frequency and morphology. (Image courtesy of Dr. Maria E. Baldwin.)

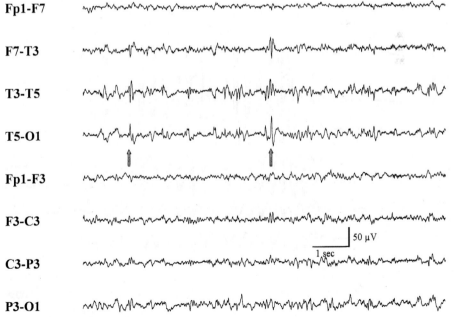

FIGURE 36.4 Focal epileptiform activity (spike) *(arrows)* in left posterior temporal region of an adult with partial seizures.

(2) Focal seizures originate within networks limited to a single hemisphere with epileptiform discharges arising from focal discrete regions.

e. The EEG analysis may permit further discrimination of several relatively **specific electroclinical syndromes.**

(1) **Hypsarrhythmia** refers to a high-voltage, arrhythmic EEG pattern with a chaotic admixture of continuous, multifocal spike–wave and sharp-wave discharges and widespread, high-voltage, arrhythmic slow waves.

This infantile EEG pattern usually occurs in association with infantile spasms, myoclonic jerks, and intellectual impairment (West's syndrome) and usually indicates severe diffuse cerebral dysfunction. **Infantile spasms** consist of tonic flexion or extension of the neck, body, or extremities with the arms flung outward and typically last 3 to 10 seconds. The EEG and clinical findings do not correlate with a specific disease entity but reflect a severe cerebral insult occurring before 1 year of age.

(2) The **3-Hz spike-and-wave activity** is associated with typical absence attacks (Fig. 36.5). This pattern most often occurs in children between the ages of 3 and 15 years and is enhanced by hyperventilation and hypoglycemia. These bursts are typically accompanied by clinical signs such as staring, brief clonic movements, unresponsiveness, and motor arrest.

(3) **Generalized multiple spikes and waves** (polyspike–wave pattern) are typically associated with myoclonic epilepsy or other generalized epilepsy syndromes (Fig. 36.6).

Generalized slow spike-and-wave patterns at a frequency of 1 to 2.5 Hz occur in children between the ages of 1 and 6 years who have some underlying diffuse cerebral dysfunction. Most of these children are mentally retarded and have poorly controlled seizures. The clinical triad of mental retardation, severe seizures, and the slow spike-and-wave pattern is called the **Lennox–Gastaut syndrome.**

(4) **Central–midtemporal spikes** occur in childhood and are associated with benign rolandic epilepsy. These seizures are often nocturnal and consist of focal clonic movements of the face or hand; tingling in the side of the mouth, tongue, cheek, or hand; motor speech arrest; and excessive salivation. The spells are easily controlled with anticonvulsants and disappear by 12 to 14 years of age.

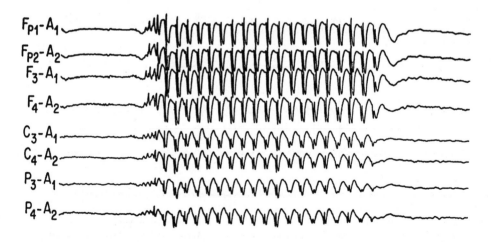

FIGURE 36.5 Burst of generalized 3-per-second spike-and-wave discharges in a child with absence (petit mal) seizures.

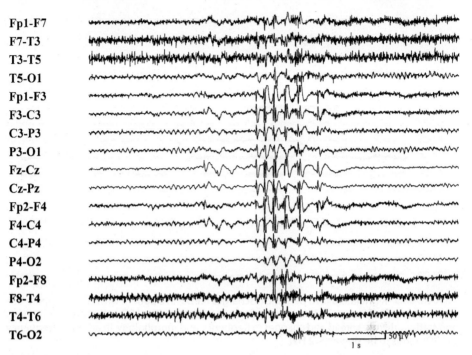

Fp1-F7
F7-T3
T3-T5
T5-O1
Fp1-F3
F3-C3
C3-P3
P3-O1
Fz-Cz
Cz-Pz
Fp2-F4
F4-C4
C4-P4
P4-O2
Fp2-F8
F8-T4
T4-T6
T6-O2

1 s   30 μV

FIGURE 36.6 Burst of generalized multiple spike-and-wave discharges in a patient with generalized tonic–clonic seizures.

(5) **Lateralized periodic discharges (LPDs)** are high-voltage, sharply contoured complexes that occur over one cerebral hemisphere with a particular periodicity. These complexes are not necessarily epileptic and usually correlate with acute destructive cerebral lesions, including infarction, rapidly growing tumors, and HSE (Fig. 36.7). In the past, there was much debate if LPDs constituted seizure activity. A consensus has now been reached in which LPDs is not considered an ictal pattern, especially if the discharges occur at slower frequencies of 2 Hz or less.

(6) **Focal slowing (delta activity)** in the interictal period usually indicates an underlying structural lesion of the brain as the cause of the seizures. However, such focal slowing may be a transient aftermath of a focal seizure and may not indicate a gross structural lesion. Such slowing may correlate with a clinical transient postictal neurologic deficit (Todd's phenomenon).

f. The EEG can make a critical contribution to the diagnosis of a patient who is obtunded when prolonged subclinical seizures with only brief interruptions are recorded, signifying **nonconvulsive status epilepticus.**

g. **Ambulatory EEG** is the recording of an EEG in a freely mobile patient outside of the EEG laboratory, or hospital. The main indication is to determine whether a spell is a seizure or some other phenomenon, especially in patients whose spells occur at unusual times or in association with specific events or activities. The yield depends on the type of patient selected, but the absence of EEG seizure activity during a spell does not fully exclude a seizure disorder, because surface electrodes may not record some mesial temporal, basal frontal, or deep midsagittal seizure discharges.

h. Patients with intractable focal seizures are sometimes candidates for surgical removal of the area of dysfunction causing the seizure. Precise identification of the epileptogenic brain area requires special inpatient monitoring facilities for simultaneous video and EEG recording **(VEEG)**. Prolonged inpatient VEEG monitoring is also often used to document whether a patient's clinical spells are epileptic or nonepileptic. This is especially invaluable for patients with nonepileptic behavioral (psychogenic) spells.

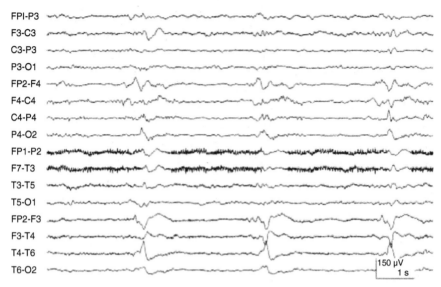

FIGURE 36.7 Right lateralized periodic discharges (LPDs) in a patient with HSE. Compare this figure with that of Figure 33.3 demonstrating a focal seizure. The LPD activity is monotonous and static with little spread and changes in frequency and morphology. In addition, frequency of LPDs tends to be slower (<2 Hz).

2. Altered states of consciousness.
   a. For most causes of acute encephalopathy (e.g., toxic–metabolic disease), the EEG changes are nonspecific, consisting of diffuse slowing. There is, however, a generally good correlation between the degree of EEG slowing and the clinical state.
   b. An abnormal EEG confirms an organic rather than a psychogenic cause for a patient's altered state of consciousness. It is also required to document unrecognized epileptic activity as a cause of depressed consciousness (nonconvulsive status epilepticus).
   c. **Certain** EEG patterns increase the likelihood of specific metabolic disorders.
      (1) Prominent **generalized fast (beta) activity** in the EEG of a comatose or obtunded patient should raise the suspicion of drug intoxication most commonly seen with benzodiazepines.
      (2) Broad **triphasic waves** that are bilaterally symmetric and synchronous and have a frontal predominance may occur during an intermediate stage of hepatic encephalopathy (Fig. 36.8). However, such a pattern may also occur with other metabolic disorders.
      (3) Severe generalized voltage depression may suggest hypothyroidism if anoxia and hypothermia can be excluded.
      (4) Patients with uremia and hyponatremia, and taking various psychotropic medications may exhibit paroxysmal spike–wave discharges and a photoparoxysmal response to photic stimulation in addition to the diffuse slow-wave abnormality. There are also specific drugs that can also induce epileptiform discharges and disorganized slowing of the EEG background such as cefepime.
      (5) Focal epileptiform activity is commonly seen in hyperosmolar coma.
   d. **Cerebral hypoxia** produces diffuse nonspecific slow-wave abnormalities on the EEG that may be reversible. More severe hypoxia may cause EEG abnormalities that may be paroxysmal and associated with clinical myoclonus. An EEG obtained 6 hours or more after a hypoxic insult may demonstrate patterns of prognostic value in determining the likelihood of neurologic recovery. A poor neurologic outcome is suggested by the presence of the following abnormalities.

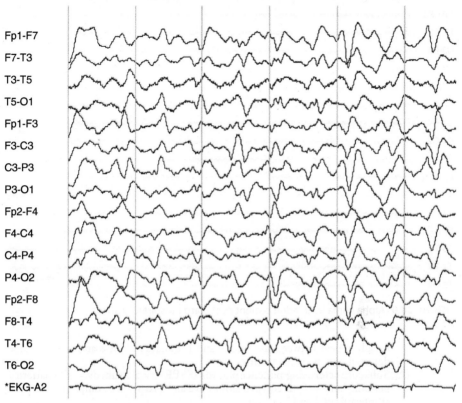

Fp1-F7

F7-T3

T3-T5

T5-O1

Fp1-F3

F3-C3

C3-P3

P3-O1

Fp2-F4

F4-C4

C4-P4

P4-O2

Fp2-F8

F8-T4

T4-T6

T6-O2

*EKG-A2

FIGURE 36.8 Frontal predominant triphasic waves and diffuse slow-wave abnormality in a patient with hepatic encephalopathy. (Image courtesy of Dr. David Chabolla.)

(1) Alpha coma refers to the apparent paradoxical appearance of the monorhythmic alpha frequency activity in the EEG of a comatose patient (Fig. 36.9). However, in contrast to normal alpha activity, that observed in alpha coma is generalized, often most prominent frontally, and completely unreactive to external stimuli.

(2) The **burst–suppression pattern** consists of occasional generalized bursts of medium- to high-voltage, mixed-frequency slow-wave activity, sometimes with intermixed spikes, with intervening periods of severe voltage depression or cerebral inactivity. The bursts may be accompanied by generalized myoclonic jerks involving the face, torso, or extremities.

(3) A generalized **periodic pattern**, which consists of generalized spikes or sharp waves that recur at a relatively fixed periodicity of 1 to 2 per second. The periodic pattern is usually accompanied by myoclonic jerks.

(4) Electrocerebral silence. See section **C.3.a** under Electroencephalogram.

e. Infectious and autoimmune disease processes of the central nervous system (CNS) produce predominantly diffuse and nonspecific slow-wave activity. However, certain EEG patterns assist in the diagnosis of specific infectious etiologies.

(1) The EEG is extremely important in the initial assessment of **HSE**, often showing abnormalities before lesions detected by computed tomography (CT) or magnetic resonance imaging (MRI) are recognized. A majority of patients show temporal or frontotemporal slowing that may be unilateral or, if bilateral, asymmetric. **Periodic sharp complexes** over one or both frontotemporal regions add relative specificity to the EEG findings (Fig. 36.7). These diagnostic features

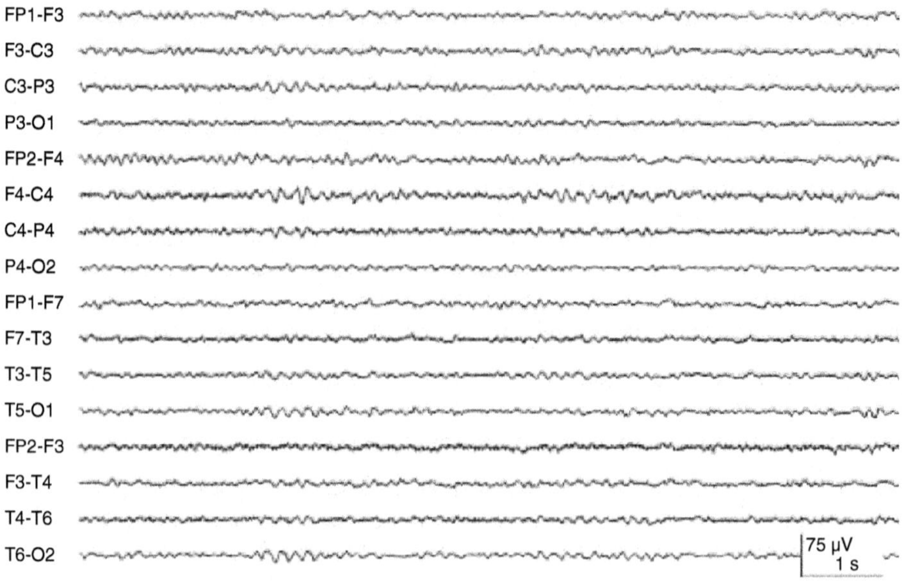

FP1-F3
F3-C3
C3-P3
P3-O1
FP2-F4
F4-C4
C4-P4
P4-O2
FP1-F7
F7-T3
T3-T5
T5-O1
FP2-F3
F3-T4
T4-T6
T6-O2

75 μV
1 s

FIGURE 36.9 Alpha coma in an adult patient post–cardiorespiratory arrest.

usually appear between the second and 15th days of illness and are sometimes detected only on serial tracings.

(2) **Subacute sclerosing panencephalitis (SSPE)** has a distinctive EEG pattern of periodic bursts of stereotyped slow-wave and sharp-wave complexes occurring at intervals of 3 to 15 seconds.

(3) **Transmissible spongiform encephalopathy** is associated with a relatively specific EEG pattern of diffuse high-voltage diphasic and triphasic sharp-wave complexes occurring at a periodicity of approximately 1 per second (Fig. 36.10). This periodic pattern is noted only in the end state of the disease process. Myoclonic jerks are also frequently seen and can correlate with the periodic discharges.

(4) **Paraneoplastic syndrome-**anti-N-methyl-D-aspartate (NMDA) receptor antibody encephalitis is clinically characterized by altered mental status, abnormal facial movements, and an EEG with a specific pattern referred to as "extreme delta brush" consisting of a fast activity overriding a slow wave (Fig 36.11).

3. Brain death.

a. Because the EEG is a measure of cerebral, especially cortical, function, it has been widely used to provide objective evidence of loss of that function. With cortical death, the EEG demonstrates complete loss of brain-generated activity and is termed **electrocerebral silence**. The determination of electrocerebral silence is technically demanding and requires strict adherence to a standard special recording protocol (see Chapter 34).

b. Rarely, temporary and reversible loss of cerebral electrical activity may be observed immediately following cardiorespiratory arrest, overdose of CNS depressants, and severe hypothermia. Therefore, electrocerebral silence in these circumstances does not indicate irreversible cortical dysfunction.

c. Patients in a chronic vegetative state with preserved brainstem function may have an isoelectric EEG, probably reflecting total neocortical death.

d. Thus, the establishment of **brain death** (cerebral plus brainstem death) requires the following criteria.

(1) Irreversible structural brain damage
(2) Apneic coma
(3) Loss of brainstem reflexes and signs of brainstem function
(4) Electrocerebral silence on EEG (best viewed as a confirmatory test).

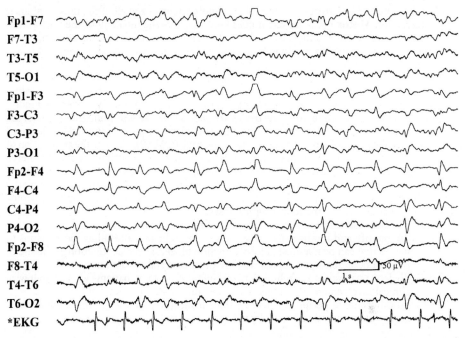

FIGURE 36.10 Generalized periodic (approximately 1 per second) diphasic and triphasic sharp waves seen in patient with biopsy-proven prion disease of spongiform encephalopathy.

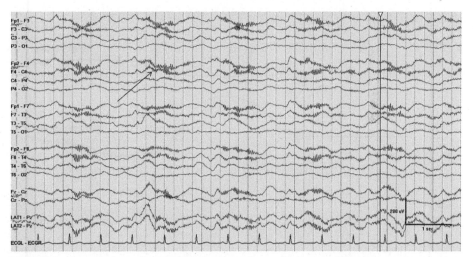

FIGURE 36.11 *Arrow* denoting extreme delta brush in patient with NMDA encephalitis. NMDA, *N*-methyl-ᴅ-aspartate. (Image courtesy of Dr. Maria E. Baldwin.)

NERVE CONDUCTION STUDIES AND THE ELECTROMYOGRAM

A. Introduction.
　　1. **NCS** comprise a simple and reliable method of testing peripheral nerve function. An impulse initiated by electrical stimulation of the nerve travels along motor, sensory, or mixed nerves, and the conduction characteristics of the impulse are assessed by recording potentials either from the muscle innervated by the motor nerve or from the nerve itself.

2. The **motor unit** consists of a single-lower motor neuron and all of the muscle fibers it innervates. **Motor NCS** are techniques used to assess the integrity of the motor unit. Information about the function and the structural status of the motor neuron, nerve, neuromuscular junction, and muscle is acquired. Quantitative information can be obtained regarding the location, distribution, time course, and pathophysiology of lesions affecting the peripheral nervous system (PNS). Prognosis, response to treatment, and the status of repair of the motor unit may also be obtained. For motor conduction studies, recording electrodes are placed on the skin over the motor point of a muscle and over the tendon of the muscle, and stimulating electrodes are placed over the skin along the course of the nerve to be tested. The response of the muscle to electrical stimulation can be measured by recording the compound muscle action potential (CMAP), which is the summation of the electrical potentials of all muscle fibers that respond to the stimulation of the nerve (Fig. 36.12). The time it takes for the electrical impulse to travel to the muscle (latency) can be measured, and by stimulating the nerve at various locations and measuring the distance the stimulus travels, motor nerve conduction velocities are attained. Motor NCS can be used for the following purposes.

a. To obtain objective evidence of disease of motor units

b. To identify and localize sites of compression, ischemia, and other focal lesions of nerves that can be manifested by conduction block, slowed conduction at the site of the lesion, or abnormal conduction proximal or distal to the lesion

c. To detect widespread subclinical involvement of nerves in patients who present with clinical involvement of a single nerve (i.e., mononeuropathies)

d. To differentiate peripheral neuropathies from lower-motor neuronopathies (e.g., amyotrophic lateral sclerosis) from myopathies in patients with weakness

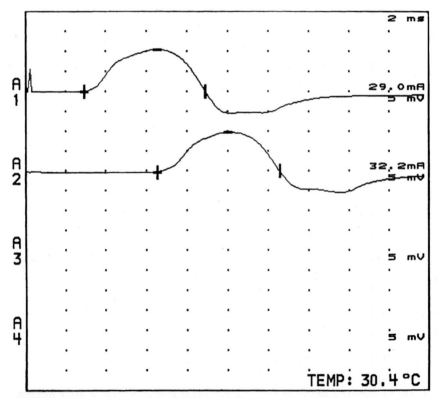

FIGURE 36.12 CMAPs recorded from the thenar muscles with stimulation of the left median nerve at the wrist (*upper potential at A1*) and forearm (*lower potential at A2*). CMAPs, compound muscle action potentials.

   e. To detect disease prior to the development of significant clinical signs (e.g., familial neuropathies)

3. Diseases of the neuromuscular junction [e.g., myasthenia gravis (MG), Lambert–Eaton myasthenic syndrome (LEMS)] can be assessed by **repetitive stimulation of motor nerves.** With postsynaptic fatigability of the neuromuscular junction, if a CMAP is recorded and compared with subsequent CMAPs, a decline in the amplitude of the potential may be observed as progressively fewer muscle fibers respond to the stimuli, even though the nerve is stimulated at rates that a normal muscle could endure for long periods (Fig. 36.13). The hallmark of presynaptic disorders is a significant facilitation of CMAP amplitudes with high-frequency repetitive stimulation.

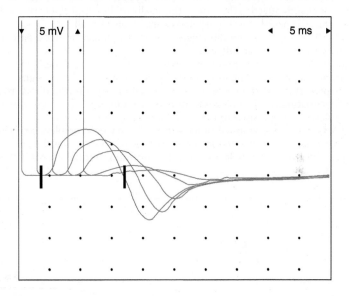

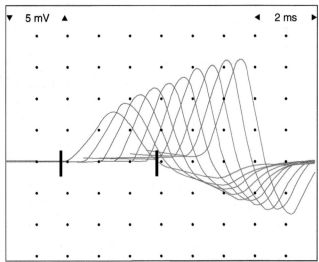

FIGURE 36.13 Decremental response to repetitive stimulation in a patient with generalized MG. **Top:** Decremental response with ulnar nerve stimulation. **Bottom:** Facilitation of CMAP amplitude with high-frequency stimulation, which can be seen in presynaptic disorders of neuromuscular transmission (this specific patient was positive for a P/Q-calcium channel antibody). CMAPs, compound muscle action potentials; MG, myasthenia gravis.

4. **Sensory NCS** are obtained by recording the action potential evoked in a cutaneous nerve by electrical stimulation (Fig. 36.14). Selective sensory NCS can be performed by stimulating nerves that have only sensory components (e.g., the sural nerve) or, alternatively, by selectively stimulating only the sensory components of a mixed nerve. The latter can be done by isolating the sensory components anatomically (i.e., stimulating the digits of the hand and recording over the mixed nerve at the wrist or elbow) or stimulating the mixed nerve and recording over the digits where only sensory axons are present for the most part. Sensory NCS may be valuable for the following purposes.

a. In diffuse disorders affecting the sensory system, for determining which population of sensory nerves is involved (e.g., small fibers carrying pain and temperature sensation or large fibers conveying proprioception), determining whether the disorder is predominantly affecting the axon or the myelin of the peripheral nerve, or determining whether the peripheral sensory nerves are involved at all

b. In focal neuropathies, for demonstrating a site of injury or block, particularly when only sensory nerves are affected

c. For confirmation or quantification when sensory abnormalities appear than motor changes in peripheral neuropathies or before objective clinical signs

d. For predicting whether a lesion is proximal or distal to the dorsal root (e.g., for differentiating brachial plexus from nerve root injury)

e. For determining disease of the dorsal root ganglion

5. The **EMG** is usually performed along with NCS and yields complementary information. A needle electrode is inserted into the muscles of interest and the action potentials generated by groups of muscle fibers (the **motor unit potentials** or **MUPs**) are observed

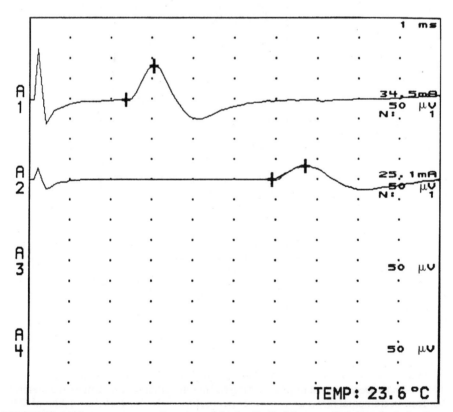

FIGURE 36.14 Sensory nerve action potentials obtained while recording over the index finger with stimulation of the left median nerve at the wrist *(upper response at A1)* and forearm *(lower response at A2).*

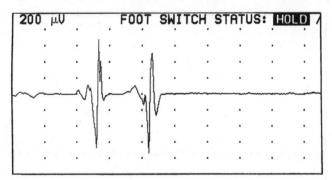

FIGURE 36.15 MUPs recorded with needle insertion into the right biceps muscle during minimal muscle contraction. MUPs, motor unit potentials.

and recorded (Fig. 36.15). The muscle is tested at rest, with slight contraction, and with stronger contraction. Normally, the muscle is silent at rest. In **active neuropathic processes**, as well as in severe or inflammatory myopathies, spontaneous action potentials from single-muscle fibers (fibrillation potentials) may occur (Fig. 36.16). In certain neurogenic processes, especially motor neuron disease and diseases of the proximal root, spontaneous contractions of a single-motor unit (fasciculation potentials) may be observed. Characteristic changes in MUP parameters and recruitment may occur in neurogenic or myopathic processes. In **neuropathic conditions**, the MUPs are often of increased amplitude, duration, and degree of polyphasia with reduced recruitment of fibers with increased effort, whereas in **myopathic processes**, the MUPs may be of decreased amplitude and duration with increased polyphasia and rapid (early) recruitment. Single-muscle fiber action potentials may be studied by a technically more difficult method, **single-fiber EMG** (which is typically used to assess disease of the neuromuscular junction but can be abnormal in neuropathic and myopathic processes).

6. In general, EMG and NCS are used to study and diagnose patients with motor neuron disease (e.g., amyotrophic lateral sclerosis), processes affecting the plexi or nerve roots, entrapment neuropathies, peripheral polyneuropathies, diseases of the neuromuscular junction (e.g., MG), and diseases of the muscle. Because it involves electrical shocks and the insertion of needles into multiple muscles, the EMG/NCS study is uncomfortable. The study is safe as long as electrical safety techniques are applied; a bleeding tendency may limit the EMG study.

B. **EMG/NCS abnormalities.**

1. The EMG/NCS study is essential for evaluation and electrophysiologic diagnosis of **motor neuron disease** (e.g., amyotrophic lateral sclerosis). In general, NCS are normal except perhaps for some decrease in the CMAP amplitudes (because the disease is purely motor, sensory conduction studies are normal). Needle EMG shows diffuse evidence of neurogenic damage from anterior horn cell injury, including abnormal spontaneous activity (fibrillations and fasciculations), abnormal MUP parameters (large, wide, and polyphasic MUPs), and poor recruitment of MUPs with effort. Often the EMG study indicates active neurogenic damage even in muscles or limbs that appear to have little or no clinical involvement. The needle exam may also provide information about prognosis, and the EMG may assist in the diagnosis of other diseases of the anterior horn cells such as the postpolio syndrome and the spinal muscular atrophies.

2. **Radiculopathies** comprise a constellation of symptoms and signs resulting from transient or permanent damage of the nerve at the anatomic level where the nerve exits the spinal canal in the spinal foramina. NCS are generally normal. The EMG shows evidence of neurogenic changes (e.g., fibrillations and MUP changes) in muscles innervated by a specific root, with other muscles innervated by uninvolved roots being spared. The pattern of neurogenic changes depends on the severity of the process, the duration of

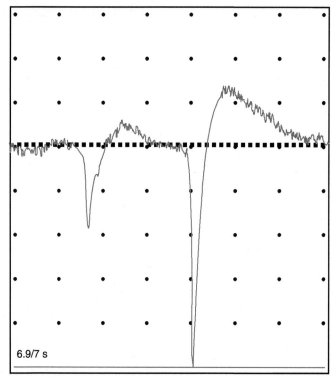

6.9/7 s

FIGURE 36.16 Positive sharp waves in the extensor hallucis longus muscle.

the disease, and the degree of neurogenic repair (reinnervation). The EMG study can be helpful in several ways, as follows.

a. It is useful for confirming disease of the nerve root. In studies of patients with surgically demonstrated cervical or lumbosacral radiculopathies, the EMG is abnormal only about 90% of the time. Thus, a normal study does not preclude the presence of a radiculopathy.

b. It provides further localization by determining which root or roots are affected.

c. It is useful in determining whether there is active denervation (indicated by the presence of fibrillation potentials).

d. It can determine the time elapsed since the onset of the radiculopathy (whether it is acute, subacute, chronic, or old).

e. It may give some information about the severity of the radiculopathy.

f. It may reveal other abnormalities that explain the patient's symptoms.

g. It may help to determine if an abnormality on an MRI scan or myelogram has any physiologic significance.

3. Brachial and lumbosacral **plexopathies** and **entrapment neuropathies** (e.g., carpal tunnel syndrome, ulnar neuropathies at the elbow, and peroneal neuropathies at the fibular head) are localized and diagnosed with EMG/NCS.

4. **Peripheral polyneuropathies** are often investigated by EMG/NCS. The electrophysiologic characteristics of the neuropathic disorder serve as additional sources of information to help characterize the disease and allow a narrowing of the differential diagnostic possibilities. EMG/NCS allow evaluation of the amount of motor and sensory involvement, determines whether the lesion is primarily the result of damage to the myelin sheath or to the axon, indicates whether the lesion is focal or diffuse, determines whether the process is distal or proximal, and gives information concerning the severity and temporal profile of the process. Prolonged distal sensory and motor latencies, slowed conduction velocities, abnormalities of sensory responses and MUPs, and "neurogenic"

EMG changes occur. When abnormal, the study confirms the presence of a neuropathy, but it should be noted that small-fiber sensory neuropathies (i.e., those affecting only sensory nerve fibers conveying pain and temperature sensation) are often associated with normal studies. EMG/NCS can separate a generalized sensorimotor peripheral polyneuropathy from multiple mononeuropathies at sites of common compression (e.g., median and ulnar neuropathies at the wrist). Peripheral polyneuropathies may be divided by electrophysiologic patterns into the following categories:

a. Uniform demyelinating mixed sensorimotor neuropathies, including certain hereditary neuropathies (Fig. 36.17), metachromatic leukodystrophy, Krabbe's disease, and Tangier disease

b. Segmental demyelinating motor sensory polyneuropathies, including inflammatory neuropathies (e.g., Guillain–Barré syndrome also referred as GBS, chronic inflammatory demyelinating polyneuropathy) and neuropathies associated with gammopathies, hypothyroidism, carcinoma or lymphoma, AIDS, Lyme disease, and certain toxins

c. Axonal motor sensory polyneuropathies, including porphyria, certain hereditary neuropathies, lymphomatous neuropathies, and certain toxic neuropathies

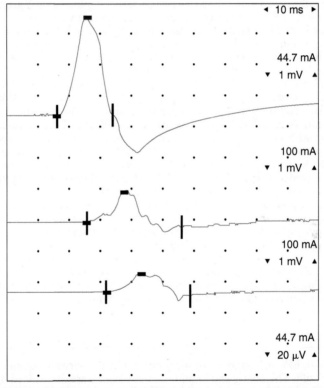

FIGURE 36.17 Motor NCS demonstrating uniform demyelination of the peripheral nerve in a patient with hereditary motor neuropathy (Charcot–Marie–Tooth disease type 1a, CMT). The CMAP amplitude is relatively preserved on proximal as compared with distal nerve stimulation. A diffusely and homogeneously demyelinating process, such as CMT type 1a, will demonstrate relatively preserved CMAP configurations with prolonged latencies and slowed conduction velocities. A nonuniform, segmental demyelinating process (such as acute inflammatory demyelinating peripheral polyneuropathy, that is, GBS) may demonstrate conduction block and variable slowing within the same nerve trunk, resulting in CMAPs with reduced amplitude and dispersed configuration at proximal sites of stimulation (**bottom** image). CMT, Charcot–Marie–Tooth; CMAP, compound muscle action potential; GBS, Guillain–Barré syndrome; NCS, nerve conduction studies.

d. Axonal sensory neuronopathy (disease of the dorsal root ganglion) or neuropathies, including certain hereditary neuropathies, primary amyloidosis, Sjögren's syndrome, paraneoplastic neuropathies, and neuropathies caused by drugs, vitamin B_{12} deficiency, or antidisialosyl ganglioside antibodies (also referred to as "CANOMAD" syndrome)

e. Mixed axonal demyelinating sensorimotor polyneuropathies resulting from uremia or diabetes mellitus

f. Axonal sensorimotor polyneuropathies, including neuropathies caused by nutritional deficiencies, monoclonal gammopathies, alcohol, sarcoidosis, connective tissue diseases, toxins, heavy metals, and drugs

5. **Diseases of the neuromuscular junction** may be diagnosed by repetitive stimulation studies. Repetitive stimulation of motor nerves is used chiefly in the diagnosis of **MG**. In this disease, a characteristic progressive decline in the amplitude of the first few responses to stimulation is revealed at a stimulation rate of 2 per second (Fig. 33.12). The defect may be further characterized by the way it is altered after a brief contraction of the muscle. In some MG patients with normal repetitive stimulation studies, the diagnosis may be assisted by single-fiber EMG. Repetitive stimulation studies are also invaluable in the diagnosis of the LEMS. In the myasthenic syndrome, the initial action potential evoked in the rested muscle by a single-maximal nerve stimulation is greatly reduced in amplitude. A further reduction in the amplitude may occur with repetitive stimulation at low rates, but striking facilitation (enlargement of the MUPs of usually >100%) occurs during stimulation at higher rates. Unusual fatigability of the peripheral neuromuscular system may occasionally be demonstrated in other diseases, such as amyotrophic lateral sclerosis, but this abnormality is of little diagnostic value.

6. Electrodiagnostic studies show a wide variety of abnormalities in patients with **myopathies.** The NCS are essentially normal, except for occasional reductions in CMAP amplitudes. The EMG may reveal fibrillation potentials in severe myopathies or in inflammatory myopathies (e.g., polymyositis). "Myopathic" MUPs are of decreased amplitude and duration with increased polyphasia and rapid recruitment out of proportion to the degree of contraction effort (Fig. 36.18). The EMG studies are usually not sufficient to identify a specific disease, but the pattern of findings can be associated with groups of muscle disorders (Video 36.1). Toxic and endocrine myopathies may produce little or no EMG abnormalities. An EMG/NCS examination can

a. distinguish neurogenic from myopathic disorders as causes of weakness,

b. provide clues to the etiology of a myopathy,

c. provide estimates of the severity and acuteness of the process,

d. assess the activity and course of the disease,

e. provide important information on the distribution of involvement to guide selection of a biopsy site (muscle biopsy must not be performed on a muscle that has been needled but in a corresponding muscle in the opposite extremity), and

f. detect abnormalities even if not clinically apparent.

Evoked Potentials

A. Introduction. EPs are electrical signals generated by the nervous system in response to sensory stimuli. The timing and location of these signals are determined by the sensory system involved and the sequence in which different neural structures are activated. Identical sensory stimuli are presented repeatedly while a computer averages the time-locked low-voltage responses from the brain or spinal cord and unrelated electrical noise and background EEG activity are averaged out.

B. Visual evoked potentials (VEPs).

1. Disorders of central visual pathways are tested by VEPs, which are the cortical responses to visual stimuli. Stroboscopic flashes of light or, more commonly, black-and-white checkerboard patterns evoke potentials over the occipital lobes that are detected by scalp electrodes. The major positive deflection at a latency of approximately 100 ms (the **P100 response**) (Fig. 36.19) is most useful for clinical applications. Delays in this latency suggest damage to visual conducting pathways.

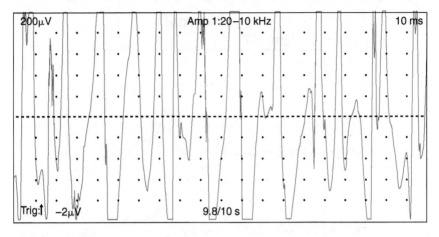

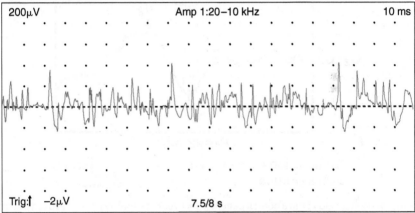

FIGURE 36.18 Top: Typical chronic neurogenic MUAP changes (reduced recruitment, increased amplitude, and duration). **Bottom:** Typical myopathic changes (early recruitment of small, polyphasic units).

2. Unilateral prolongation of the P100 response implies an abnormality anterior to the optic chiasm (usually in the optic nerve) on that side. Bilateral P100 delay can be caused by bilateral lesions either anterior or posterior to the chiasm or by a lesion within the chiasm itself.

3. Uses of VEPs.

a. The VEPs may aid in the detection of a clinically "silent" lesion in a patient suspected of having a demyelinating disease such as multiple sclerosis (MS). It is a sufficiently sensitive indicator of optic nerve demyelination that it can reveal asymptomatic and clinically undetectable lesions. The VEPs reveal abnormalities in 70% to 80% of patients with definite MS who do not have histories of optic neuritis or visual symptoms. Abnormalities are not specific for MS and may be abnormal in a variety of other diseases, including certain ocular diseases, compressive lesions of the optic nerve, nutritional and toxic optic neuropathies, including pernicious anemia, and diffuse CNS diseases such as adrenoleukodystrophy and some spinocerebellar degenerations.

b. The VEP is helpful in distinguishing functional (e.g., psychogenic) visual impairment from true blindness or bilateral optic nerve disease. A normal VEP strongly favors functional illness. It should be mentioned, however, that rare patients have been described with blindness from severe bilateral destruction of the occipital lobes who had essentially normal VEP studies. Also, some patients with functional problems can

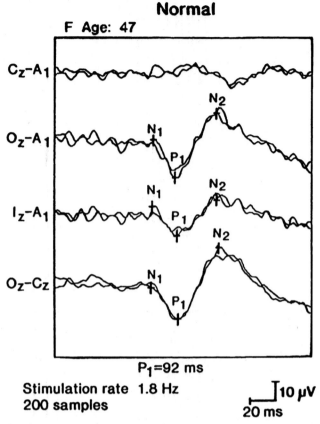

FIGURE 36.19 Full-field VEP in a normal patient *(P1 = P100 response).* VEP, visual evoked potentials.

voluntarily suppress the VEP response by such strategies as transcendental meditation, concentration beyond the plane of the checks, or ocular convergence (see Chapter 33).
  c. The VEPs may be of some assistance in evaluating vision in pediatric patients, for example, in assessing high-risk infants or in the detection of amblyopia.
4. Optical coherence tomography (OCT).
  a. OCT measures retinal nerve fiber thickness and is of increasing interest as an ancillary study in neurologic disease. Its use may eventually eclipse the need for VEPs. It allows for the direct visualization and quantification of unmyelinated axons in the eyes. It may be a useful marker for optic neuritis, as well as for monitoring for the development of macular edema. There are early data suggesting it may be a marker to differentiate neuromyelitis optica from MS, and may be an effective biomarker to track the progression of MS. It may be reasonable to assume that it will one day supplant VEPs, rendering the latter larger obsolete in the management of patients with neurologic disease.
C. Brainstem auditory evoked potentials (BAEPs).
  1. The BAEPs are a series of EPs elicited by auditory clicks and generated by sequential activation of the brainstem auditory pathways. Although five waveforms (I through V) are usually recorded (Fig. 36.20), the most stable and important waveforms are I, III, and V. The I to III interpeak latency is a measure of auditory conduction of the more caudal segment of the brainstem (acoustic nerve to lower pons), whereas the III to V interpeak latency is a measure of conduction in the more rostral pontine and lower midbrain pathways. The I to V interpeak latency is a measure of the total conduction time within the brainstem auditory pathways and auditory nerve.

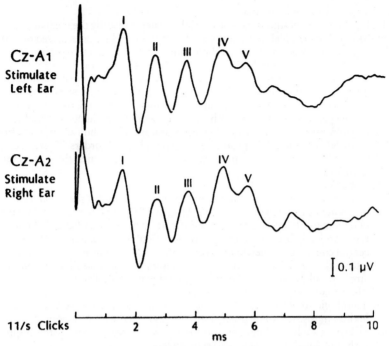

FIGURE 36.20 BAEP study in a normal adult subject with clear identification of waves I, II, and III. BAEP, brainstem auditory evoked potential.

2. A BAEP abnormality is measured by prolongation of interpeak latencies, especially asymmetric prolongations, as well as reduction in amplitude or absence of certain waveforms. A prolonged I-III interpeak latency indicates an acoustic nerve to lower pontine lesion whereas a prolonged III-V interpeak latency indicates a lesion of the upper pons-lower midbrain levels.

3. The BAEPs may be clinically helpful in the following circumstances.
    a. The BAEPs, like VEPs, may be very sensitive to white matter disease and may help confirm or document a lesion within the brainstem, even if there are no brainstem signs or symptoms, when MS is suspected clinically and the patient has a lesion outside the brainstem. Approximately 50% of patients with definite MS exhibit abnormal BAEPs. However, VEPs and somatosensory evoked potentials (SEPs) (see section **D** under Somatosensory Evoked Potentials.) are more sensitive than BAEPs in detecting abnormalities in MS patients. Other demyelinating processes affecting the brainstem, such as central pontine myelinolysis, metachromatic leukodystrophy, and adrenoleukodystrophy, may also cause BAEP abnormalities.
    b. A **posterior fossa tumor** or other mass within or outside of the brainstem can produce abnormal BAEPs by either direct involvement of the brainstem auditory pathways or secondary brainstem compression. The BAEPs are very sensitive screening procedures for acoustic neuromas and other cerebellopontine angle tumors. Monitoring of the BAEPs during such surgeries as acoustic neuroma resections can provide valuable information to the surgeon and help to preserve hearing.
    c. The BAEPs may assist in the determination of **brain death (see Chapter 34).** Preservation of wave I with loss of all subsequent response supports brainstem death in the comatose patient. The BAEP does not, however, provide any information about cortical function in the comatose patient.
    d. The BAEPs may be used to assess **hearing in young children** and in patients otherwise unable to cooperate for standard audiometry. The BAEP testing can estimate hearing threshold and may distinguish conductive hearing loss from sensorineural hearing loss.

D. Somatosensory evoked potentials.
1. Following electrical stimulation of a peripheral nerve (usually the median or ulnar nerve at the wrist or the tibial nerve at the ankle), recording electrodes placed over the spine and scalp reveal a series of electrical potentials that correspond to sequential activation of neural structures along the dorsal column–lemniscal pathway. These SEPs are named according to their polarities and their times of occurrence in normal individuals. Because SEP latencies vary significantly with body height and limb length, absolute latency values are of limited use; interpeak latencies, which measure the time intervals between successive peaks in the sensory pathways, are incorporated in clinical studies.
2. SEPs yield information concerning PNS abnormalities but are not as effective as standard NCS in identifying and localizing peripheral disorders. Therefore, although SEPs have been used to study plexopathies and radiculopathies, their use is limited for these conditions.
3. Uses of SEPs.
   a. SEPs can be used to confirm the presence of a clinically "silent" spinal cord lesion in a patient suspected of having MS. Median SEPs are abnormal in about two-thirds of patients with definite MS; lower-limb SEPs have somewhat greater abnormality rates, probably because of the greater length of white matter traversed. Prolonged central conduction times do not necessarily indicate demyelination because abnormal interpeak latencies may occur with hereditary spastic paraplegia, olivopontocerebellar atrophy, and subacute combined degeneration resulting from vitamin B_{12} deficiency.
   b. Abnormally large (giant) cortical SEPs are characteristic of some relatively rare neurologic conditions, such as progressive myoclonic epilepsy, late infantile ceroid lipofuscinosis, and some other disorders associated with myoclonus.
   c. SEPs may be helpful in demonstrating intact central sensory pathways in patients with functional (e.g., hysterical) sensory loss.
   d. SEPs have been especially helpful in monitoring spinal cord function during surgery (e.g., surgery for correction of spinal scoliosis).

OTHER ANCILLARY NEUROLOGIC STUDIES

A. Polysomnography.
1. Polysomnography consists of continuous monitoring of multiple biologic variables during nocturnal sleep. Eye movements (electrooculography), EEG activity, submental EMG, the electrocardiogram (ECG), and limb movements are routinely monitored. Respiration is monitored with intraesophageal pressure gauges, intercostal surface EMG, rib cage and abdominal strain gauges, oronasal thermistors or CO_2 detectors, ear or finger oximetry, and other means of determining the presence of central, peripheral, or mixed apnea syndromes. A microphone attached to the throat may detect snoring. Each 30-second epoch of the polysomnogram is scored as awake, stage I to IV non–rapid eye movement (REM) sleep, or REM sleep.
2. Polysomnography is used to investigate two types of problems: sleep complaints (i.e., too much or too little sleep) and risk factors or specific syndromes induced by or linked to sleep or specific sleep states. These disorders include the following:
   a. Sleep apnea syndromes, which may be obstructive, central, or mixed
   b. Narcolepsy
   c. Idiopathic CNS hypersomnia
   d. Periodic movements of sleep and sleep-related myoclonus
   e. REM behavioral disorder
   f. Disorders of the sleep–wake cycle
   g. Parasomnias such as sleepwalking, nightmares, night terrors, and head banging
B. Multiple sleep latency test (MSLT).
1. The MSLT consists of five 20-minute attempts, once every 2 hours, to fall asleep throughout the day. The aim is to determine the sleep latency and whether or not REM sleep episodes are recorded during the nap. Patients should be withdrawn from sleep-related medications for 10 to 15 days. The study usually follows polysomnography because knowledge of the patient's previous night's sleep is required for appropriate interpretation. During the study, the EEG, submental EMG, ECG, and eye movements

are monitored. Normal patients have mean sleep latencies >10 minutes and fewer than two sleep-onset REM periods during the study.

2. The MSLT is designed to evaluate the following:
   a. The complaint of **excessive daytime somnolence** by quantifying the time required to fall asleep. Pathologic sleepiness is manifested by a mean sleep latency of <5 minutes.
   b. The possibility of **narcolepsy** by checking for abnormally short latencies to REM sleep. The occurrence of two or more sleep-onset REM periods during the study is strong evidence for narcolepsy, as long as sleep apnea and withdrawal from stimulants and alcohol have been ruled out.

LUMBAR PUNCTURE

A. Introduction. An LP should be considered only after a thorough evaluation of the patient and serious consideration of the potential value and hazards of the procedure (Table 36.1).
B. Indications for CSF examination and LP are as follows.
   1. The CSF examination is a key to the diagnosis and management of various CNS infections, including acute and chronic meningitis and encephalitis. In many patients with fever of unknown origin, even in the absence of meningeal signs, an early LP is commonly of value, especially because meningeal signs may be minimal or absent in very young or elderly patients. Meningeal infection should especially be sought in patients with fever and impaired sensorium or an immunocompromised state (e.g., AIDS patients). If a patient presents with unexplained acute confusion, stupor, or coma, even if afebrile, a CSF examination is necessary for the evaluation of meningoencephalitis. In most clinical settings, a CT scan of the brain or other neuroimaging should be performed before the LP to rule out a possible intracranial mass (e.g., hemorrhage or abscess), which would make LP a potentially lethal procedure. However, in an extremely ill patient in whom acute meningitis, such as meningococcal meningitis, is suspected, treatment should not be delayed while arranging appropriate ancillary testing.
   2. In patients with suspected SAH, an urgent CT scan is indicated to evaluate for the presence of blood. However, in approximately 5% to 10% of patients with **SAH**, CT fails to reveal blood, and a spinal tap is indicated. If the diagnostic LP shows subarachnoid blood or xanthochromia, a cerebral angiogram is needed to determine the source of the hemorrhage.
   3. In patients with **unexplained dementia,** CSF examination may be necessary to evaluate for CNS vasculitis, infection, or granulomatous disease. The CSF should always be examined in a patient with dementia and a positive fluorescent treponemal antibody absorption study. Also, patients with radiographic hydrocephalus may require a CSF study to exclude chronic meningitis as an etiology for the symptomatic hydrocephalus.

TABLE 36.1 **Lumbar Puncture Checklist**

Indication
Herniation risk assessed (normal head CT and/or funduscopic examination)
INR <1.4
Normal activated partial thromboplastin time
Platelet count >70,000
No clopidogrel use within 7 d
No novel oral anticoagulant use within 48 hr
No treatment dose of low-molecular-weight heparin (LMWH) within 24 hr
No VTE prophylaxis dose of LMWH within 12 hr
No GP IIb/IIIa inhibitors (within 8 hr for tirofiban and eptifibatide, and 48 hr for Abciximab)
No evidence of infection at the LP site
Consent form discussed and signed
Hand hygiene

Abbreviations: CT, computed tomography; INR, international normalized ratio; LP, lumbar puncture; VTE, venous thromboembolism.

In patients with suspected sporadic transmissible spongiform encephalopathy (sTSE), a positive radioimmunoassay of the CSF for "prion protein" (14-3-3 protein) is included in the World Health Organization criterion for "probable sporadic TSE." However, there is some doubt as to the effectiveness of 14-3-3 testing because of false positives, lack of laboratory standardization, and clinical variability of sTSE. Other markers [such as neuron-specific enolase (NSE), tau protein, astrocytic (S100b) proteins and amyloid β] have been investigated. Testing for a combination of factors, timing of testing, and serial studies may increase sensitivity. CSF biomarkers may also be used as an early indicator of Alzheimer's dementia. The combination of a reduced concentration of CSF amyloid β, increased total tau, and increased phospho-tau may be highly sensitive and specific for Alzheimer's disease.

4. CSF examination is usually not warranted and may be dangerous in most patients with stroke. However, CSF analysis may assist in the etiologic diagnosis of **unexplained stroke in young or middle-aged patients** who lack atherosclerotic risk factors. Such etiologies as CNS vasculitis, meningovascular syphilis, and AIDS may be diagnosed. Sustained elevation in CSF biomarkers including NSE and S100b are associated with poor outcome following cardiac arrest.

5. CSF studies may aid in the diagnosis of **MS**, although there is no specific CSF marker for this disease. The CSF white blood cell (WBC) counts are typically normal, as are protein and glucose. Elevated CSF immunoglobulin G (IgG) levels, with normal serum IgG levels, and the presence of oligoclonal bands in the CSF are considered characteristic for MS. However, CSF analysis for oligoclonal bands was not included in the Revised 2010 "McDonald Criteria" for the diagnosis of MS. The elevated CSF gamma globulin may also occur in neurosyphilis, viral meningoencephalitis, and SSPE.

6. The CSF analysis can be considered in the evaluation of patients admitted with an **initial tonic–clonic seizure or status epilepticus**, after appropriate neuroimaging, to exclude an active CNS infection or hemorrhage.

7. An LP is necessary to confirm the clinical suspicion of **carcinomatous or leukemic meningitis**. The typical CSF pattern is a pleocytosis with mildly elevated protein content, low glucose, and a positive cytology for malignancy. Multiple LPs may be necessary as though cytology has a high specificity (>95%), and it carries a low sensitivity (<50%). CSF flow cytometry may help increase the diagnostic yield.

8. CSF studies may aid in the diagnosis of certain **inflammatory or demyelinating neuropathies**, such as the GBS or chronic idiopathic demyelinating polyradiculoneuropathy. The CSF protein level is often elevated without an abnormal cellular response. A WBC count >10 per mm^3 should raise suspicion for disorders such as Lyme disease, sarcoidosis, and HIV.

9. Although an LP is generally contraindicated in patients with papilledema, it is indicated to document increased intracranial pressure in a patient suspected of having **idiopathic intracranial hypertension** after neuroimaging studies have been proven to be normal. The CSF is under increased pressure but is otherwise normal in this entity, except for occasional decreased CSF protein levels. Also, an LP is required to document low CSF pressure in rare low-pressure syndromes in a patient whose headaches occur on standing and are relieved by lying down.

10. An LP can be used to deliver **intrathecal antibiotics and chemotherapy** in the treatment for certain CNS infections and meningeal malignancies, respectively. Also, it is required in certain diagnostic procedures such as CT myelography or cisternography.

C. Contraindications for LP.

1. An LP is contraindicated in any patient with **increased intracranial pressure**, except idiopathic intracranial hypertension because of the real danger of cerebral herniation and death.

2. An LP is contraindicated if there is suppuration in the skin or deeper tissues overlying the spinal canal because of the danger of inducing a purulent meningitis.

3. An LP is dangerous in the presence of **anticoagulation therapy or a bleeding diathesis**. Also, heparin should not be reinstituted for a minimum of 2 hours after an LP is performed. In general, an LP is hazardous if the platelet count is below 70,000, or especially if it is below 20,000. In such cases, platelet transfusions should be initiated if possible before the LP. Patients should be assessed for recent use of antiplatelet agents including aspirin and clopidogrel, novel oral anticoagulants, low-molecular-weight heparins, and GP IIb/IIIa inhibitors (see Table 36.1).

4. An LP should not be performed when a **spinal mass** is suspected unless the procedure is part of a myelogram with neurosurgical assistance readily available. A dramatic deterioration in spinal cord or cauda equina function can occur after LP.

D. **Complications of LP.**

1. **Brain herniation and death** may occur if an LP is performed on a patient with an increased intracranial pressure from a cerebral mass lesion. An LP is contraindicated in any patient suspected of having an intracranial mass.

2. **Headache of low-pressure type** may occur in up to 10% of patients after an LP (spinal headache). This type of headache occurs only on standing and is relieved by lying down. It is usually self-limiting but may require an epidural autologous blood patch for relief. Post-LP headache is most common in young women with lower body mass. Higher-gauge (smaller diameter) needle, needle insertion parallel to dural fibers (bevel up with patient on side), and replacing the stylet prior to needle removal are negatively associated with post-LP headache. The occurrence of post-LP headache is unrelated to CSF opening pressure, cells, and protein; patient position during LP; duration of recumbency after LP; amount of CSF removed; or hydration following LP.

3. **Diplopia,** which usually results from unilateral or bilateral cranial nerve VI palsies, may occur rarely and is usually self-limiting.

4. **Aseptic meningitis** may occur rarely and is characterized by posterior neck pain, headache, and neck stiffness. This process is usually self-limiting.

5. **Spinal epidural, subdural, and subarachnoid hematomas** may occur, especially in patients on anticoagulants or with bleeding diatheses. Such hematomas are usually self-limiting and may cause local pain and meningeal irritation. However, epidural hematoma may rarely cause a flaccid and potentially irreversible paraplegia that requires an emergency surgical evacuation.

E. **General comments on the evaluation of LP results.**

1. The normal **CSF pressure** is 70 to 180 mm of water in the lateral recumbent position. Pressures should be >200 mm of water to be considered elevated. In an obese patient with possible idiopathic intracranial hypertension, the pressure should be >250 mm of water to establish this diagnosis.

2. The normal **CSF glucose** content is approximately two-thirds of the serum glucose level, which must be drawn at the time of the LP. Hypoglycorrhachia (low CSF glucose) with few white cells suggests a fungal infection, with many white cells a bacterial infection, and with abnormal (malignant) cells a meningeal malignancy.

3. The **CSF protein** content may be increased (>100 mg/dL) in many CNS infectious, inflammatory, and malignant processes. Causes of elevated CSF protein with normal neuroimaging studies include myxedema, inflammatory demyelinating polyneuropathies, diabetic polyneuropathy, neurofibromas within the CSF pathways, resolving SAHs, gliomatosis cerebri, CNS vasculitis, and any process that causes spinal compression or obstruction of CSF flow.

4. Normally, the CSF can contain up to five lymphocytes or mononuclear cells per cubic centimeter. A **pleocytosis** causes CSF clouding when there are at least 200 cells per cubic centimeter. An increased WBC count occurs with subarachnoid infections, hemorrhages, chemical meningitis, or meningeal neoplasms. Also, it should be noted that a pleocytosis may occur for approximately 24 hours after a generalized seizure episode.

5. If initial spinal fluid appears bloody, one must attempt to determine whether the source of the blood is a traumatic tap or an SAH. If the initial tube of fluid is bloody and subsequent tubes are progressively clear, it is most likely that the tap was traumatic. One should then immediately centrifuge the fluid to see if the supernatant is clear, which suggests a traumatic tap. If the supernatant fluid is xanthochromic (yellow-tinged), it is likely that the blood has been present in the CSF for a few hours. Xanthochromia occurs approximately several hours after a SAH, reaches its greatest intensity at the end of 1 week, and clears in approximately 2 to 4 weeks. It can also be observed in jaundice and hypercarotenemia.

6. The polymerase chain reaction of the CSF has been found to have great utility in the diagnosis of several CNS infections. These include the following:

   a. Herpes simplex virus type 1 (HSE)

   b. Herpes simplex type 2 (HSE in neonates, recurrent meningitis)

c. JC virus (progressive multifocal leukoencephalopathy)
d. Cytomegalovirus (CMV ependymitis and polyradiculopathy associated with AIDS)
e. *Borrellia burgdorferi* (Lyme disease)
f. *Tropheryma whippelii* (CNS Whipple's disease)
g. Toxoplasmosis (CNS toxoplasmosis in AIDS)
h. *Mycobacterium tuberculosis* (TB meningitis)
i. Other viruses causing encephalitis, including enteroviruses, varicella–zoster virus, Epstein–Barr virus, West Nile virus, and herpesvirus type 6 (HSV6).

REFERRALS

All clinical neurophysiologic tests should be performed and interpreted by clinicians with expertise and special training in clinical neurophysiology. Laboratories performing these studies must follow the clinical and technical guidelines that have been published by neurophysiologic societies, the American Academy of Neurology, and other organizations. Strict adherence to these guidelines is mandatory to ensure patient safety and meaningful clinical interpretation. Neurology consultation is suggested whenever LP reveals abnormalities suggesting CNS infection, increased or decreased intracranial pressure, or SAH.

Key Points

- The diagnosis of epilepsy is not made based on the EEG alone but with the entire clinical presentation.
- A normal EEG does not imply that the patient does not have epilepsy.
  - EMG/NCS is an extension of the history and physical examination; if the findings on the ancillary study are not consistent with the clinical information, one or the other is inaccurate.
- EP signals are small and must be averaged from multiple trials in order to produce a robust measurable response.
- Evaluation for narcolepsy involves a specialized sleep study called the MSLT and cannot be determined clearly from a routine sleep study.

Recommended Readings

Aminoff MJ, ed. *Electrodiagnosis in Clinical Neurology*. 6th ed. New York, NY: Churchill Livingstone; 2012.
Berg AT, Scheffer IE. New concepts in classification of the epilepsies: entering the 21st century. *Epilepsia*. 2011;52(6):1058–1062.
Brenner RP, Hirsch LJ, eds. *Atlas of EEG in Critical Care*. 1st ed. Chichester: John Wiley & Sons; 2010.
Daube JR, Rubin DI, eds. *Clinical Neurophysiology*. 3rd ed. New York, NY: Oxford University Press; 2009.
De Meyer G, Shapiro F, Vanderstichele H, et al. Diagnosis-independent Alzheimer's disease biomarker signature in cognitively normal elderly people. *Arch Neurol*. 2010;67(8):949–956.
Donofrio PD, Albers JW. Polyneuropathy: classification by nerve conduction studies and EMG. *Muscle Nerve*. 1990;13:889–903.
DuBois B, Feldman HH, Jacova C, et al. Research criteria for the diagnosis of Alzheimer's disease: revising the NINCDS-ADRDA criteria. *Lancet Neurol*. 2007;6:734–746.
DuBois B, Feldman HH, Jacova C, et al. Revising the definition of Alzheimer's disease: a new lexicon. *Lancet Neurol*. 2010;9:1118–1127.
Dumitru D, Amato AA, Zwarts MJ, eds. *Electrodiagnostic Medicine*. 2nd ed. Philadelphia, PA: Hanley and Belfus; 2002.
Ebersole JS, Husain AM, Nordli DR, eds. *Current Practice of Clinical Electroencephalography*. 4th ed. Philadelphia, PA: Lippincott Williams & Wilkins; 2014.
Hirsh LJ, LaRoche SM, Gaspard N, et al. American Clinical Neurophysiology Society's Standardized Critical Care EEG Terminology: 2012 version. *J Clin Neurophysiol*. 2013;30:1–27.
Kimura J. *Electrodiagnosis in Diseases of Nerve and Muscle*. 4th ed. New York, NY: Oxford University Press; 2013.
Kimura J, Kohara N. Electrodiagnosis of neuromuscular disorders. In: Bradley WG, Daroff RB, Fenichel GM, et al. eds. *Neurology in Clinical Practice*. 3rd ed. Boston, MA: Butterworth-Heineman; 2000:497–519.

Kuntz KM, Kokmen E, Stevens JC, et al. Post-lumbar puncture headaches: experience in 501 consecutive procedures. *Neurology*. 1992;42:1884–1887.

Polman CH, Reingold SC, Banwell B, et al. Diagnostic criteria for multiple sclerosis: 2010 Revisions to the McDonald criteria. *Ann Neurol*. 2011;69(2):292–302.

Preston DC, Shapiro BE. *Electromyography and Neuromuscular Disorders*. 3rd ed. Philadelphia, PA: Elsevier Saunders; 2013.

Schmitt SE, Pargeon K, Frechette ES. Extreme delta brush: a unique EEG pattern in adults with anti-NMDA receptor encephalitis. *Neurology*. 2012;79(11):1094–1100.

Schomer DL, Lopes da Silva FH, eds. *Niedermeyer's Electroencephalography—Basic Principles, Clinical Applications, and Related Fields*. 6th ed. Philadelphia, PA: Wolters Kluwer/Lippincott Williams & Wilkins; 2011.

Whiteley W, Al-Shahi R, Warlow CP, et al. CSF opening pressure: reference interval and the effect of body mass index. *Neurology*. 2006;67:1690–1691.

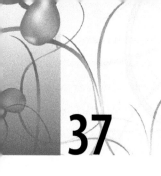

37

Approach to Common Office Problems of Pediatric Neurology

Eugene R. Schnitzler and Nikolas Mata-Machado

Currently, the majority of pediatric neurology consultations are provided in an outpatient clinic or office-based setting. The neurologist who sees children and adolescents may either be a formally trained pediatric neurologist or an adult neurologist with experience and interest in child neurology. In either case, it is important that the physician be able to develop and maintain a rapport with children and their parents. The physician and office staff should provide a gentle and friendly environment for pediatric patients including a waiting area with developmentally appropriate toys and reading materials. It is important that the office be punctual about appointments, and waiting times should be minimized.

Most childhood neurologic disorders are chronic, resulting in the opportunity to form long-term trusting physician–patient/parent relationships. The success of these relationships often hinges on the neurologist's ability to demonstrate empathy, optimism, and encouragement despite the realities of the patient's condition. Finally, pediatric neurology consultation requires a harmonious working relationship with the child's pediatrician or family practice physician. The primary care physician is usually the first provider to screen for neurologic and developmental disorders. It is crucial to promptly inform the primary care provider regarding the outcome of the child's consultation and the resultant diagnostic and treatment recommendations.

Many neurologic conditions seen in children are also encountered in adults. Refer to the appropriate chapters in this book for further review of these topics. This chapter will focus on the more common diagnoses seen in office pediatric neurology. The current national shortage of pediatric neurologists suggests that adult neurologists should familiarize themselves with these disorders and become more accustomed to working with children. Similarly, primary care physicians should become more knowledgeable about pediatric neurology in an effort to optimize healthcare resources. Telemedicine will also provide increasing opportunities for collaboration between primary care providers and pediatric neurologists, particularly in underserved areas.

ATTENTION-DEFICIT/HYPERACTIVITY DISORDER

A. Introduction. Attention-deficit/hyperactivity disorder (ADHD) is usually first diagnosed in elementary school-aged children, but diagnosis can be delayed until adolescence or adulthood. The incidence in childhood is estimated at 11% with boys affected twice as often as girls. Attention is regulated by complex associations between the prefrontal cortex and the striatum. These circuits are thought to be mediated by dopamine and norepinephrine. Decreased regulation results in hyperactivity, impulsivity, distractibility, and impaired attention span.
B. Typically, there are three main ADHD presentations:
  1. **ADHD—predominately hyperactive–impulsive type**
  2. **ADHD—predominately inattentive type**
  3. **ADHD—combined type**
     Although boys usually present with hyperactive–impulsive or combined type ADHD, it is common for girls to present with the inattentive type. Inattentiveness can be manifested by prolonged staring spells because of daydreaming, which may be confused with absence epilepsy by the naïve observer. Hyperactivity and impulsivity are characterized by excessive motoric behavior, fidgeting, and inability to stay seated. The child refuses to take turns, blurts out answers, and interrupts or disrupts the

classroom. Organizational skills are particularly lacking and the child often fails to turn in homework assignments. ADHD may also be accompanied by comorbid conditions such as anxiety, depression, oppositional defiant disorder, obsessive compulsive disorder, learning disabilities, tics, Tourette's syndrome, and autism spectrum disorder. Some of these disorders are discussed further in Chapter 28.

C. **Evaluation.** The history should focus on the child's development and behavioral patterns. Family history of ADHD symptoms in a parent or sibling is very common. Developmental delays in speech and language should raise concern about autism spectrum disorder or cognitive impairment. Inquiries should also be directed to cardiac problems or arrhythmias, which may be a contraindication to pharmacologic management.

Most children with ADHD have normal neurologic examinations. Some may have neurologic soft signs such as mirror movements. However, the child with ADHD hyperactive–impulsive type is easily diagnosed by direct observation of excessive motoric and impulsive behavior in the office. The parent may be embarrassed or oblivious to the situation and unable to control the child. On the other hand, the child with ADHD inattentive type may be well behaved and asymptomatic in the office setting.

It is imperative to auscultate the heart and check resting pulse and blood pressure. If a heart murmur or arrhythmia is detected, consideration should be given to obtaining an electrocardiography (ECG) and cardiology consultation before initiating medications. A history of tics or observation of tics on examination suggests a transient tic disorder or Tourette's syndrome. Imaging studies are not routinely indicated despite some reports of abnormalities on positron emission tomography scans. Electroencephalogram (EEG) is also not routinely required but may be necessary to differentiate inattentive staring from absence seizures. Children with dysmorphic features may warrant chromosome analysis. Screening for thyroid diseases, anemia, or lead toxicity may be indicated in selected cases. Diagnosis is enhanced by psychological testing including standardized behavioral questionnaires and continuous performance testing by computer.

Although once thought to be exclusive to childhood, ADHD is now recognized in adolescents and adults. The diagnosis is not "outgrown," although the more visible features of hyperactivity and impulsivity may be less obvious after puberty. It is not uncommon for parents of children diagnosed with ADHD to recognize similar symptoms in themselves and to seek out medical advice.

Children with ADHD should be managed with the so-called multimodal treatment including an individual education plan or 504 plan provided by the local school district. In addition, parent training in behavioral management and counseling for the child and family may be beneficial. Stimulant medications are also an essential component for successful management of ADHD and have been shown to improve long-term outcomes. These are primarily methylphenidate and amphetamine salt combinations. Both are available in extended-release formulations that reduce the need for medication administration in school. Nonstimulant medications including atomoxetine, clonidine, and guanfacine are other options.

DEVELOPMENTAL DELAY

Developmental delay is defined as the failure to achieve an anticipated milestone at the age-appropriate time. Delays can occur in a distinct area such as gross motor, fine motor, language, or cognitive skills. When more than one area of development is affected, the term *global developmental delay* (GDD) is used. GDD is seen commonly by developmental pediatricians and pediatric neurologists and is estimated to affect 5% to 10% of the pediatric population.

A. **Static encephalopathy.** Infants and toddlers with static encephalopathy fail to achieve motor and/or speech and language milestones on time. The milestone may subsequently be attained, but at a later than expected time or with abnormalities. Once the milestone is achieved, it is generally not lost.

Static encephalopathies can be caused by numerous conditions. These include chromosomal and genetic disorders, cerebral malformations, intrauterine infections, meningitis, encephalitis, trauma, intraventricular hemorrhage, and hypoxic–ischemic encephalopathy. Nevertheless, a substantial percentage of static encephalopathies are idiopathic with regard to etiology. Although most cases of static encephalopathy will result in GDD, milder or more localized cases may result in distinct neurologic or developmental disorders. Examples include cerebral palsy (CP) and autistic spectrum disorders (ASDs).

B. **CP.** Static encephalopathies that primarily affect motor control areas of the brain are described by the term CP. CP occurs with a prevalence of 2.5 per 1,000 live births. A higher prevalence may be seen in premature and low-birth-weight infants. It is further classified based on severity and distribution of spasticity. The most severe variant, spastic quadriplegia, results in spasticity in all four extremities. There is marked delay in motor milestones, accompanied by increased tone, brisk muscle stretch reflexes (MSRs), and Babinski signs. Seizures, microcephaly, feeding difficulties, and psychomotor retardation are common features. Milder variants of CP such as spastic diplegia are common in premature infants following intraventricular hemorrhage and periventricular leukomalacia. Infants with spastic diplegia show spasticity and weakness primarily in the lower extremities with relative sparing of the arms. Infants with hemiplegic CP present with unilateral weakness and spasticity. Intrauterine arterial infarctions, periventricular hemorrhages, and cerebral malformations are the most common etiologies. CP can also be acquired after birth following meningitis, encephalitis, head injuries, and congenital heart disease.

Treatment of CP is a coordinated multidisciplinary effort involving pediatric neurology, orthopedics, physical therapy (PT), occupational therapy (OT), and speech therapy. Patients with CP often have epilepsy and require antiepileptic drugs. Spasticity may be treated with baclofen, diazepam, dantrolene, or botulinum toxin. Orthopedic management includes tendon lengthening, release of contractures, and reduction of joint dislocations. OT and PT are involved in design of orthoses, muscle stretching exercises, gait training, and fine motor rehabilitation.

C. **ASD.** The revisions introduced by *DSM5* (*Diagnostic and Statistical Manual of Mental Disorders*, Fifth Edition) have dramatically changed the definition and scope of autism and developmental language disorders. However, these conditions can still be viewed as static encephalopathies, which primarily affect language and socialization. *DSM5* has rendered the terms pervasive developmental disorder (PDD) and Asperger's syndrome obsolete. The category social (pragmatic) communication disorder (SCD) will now replace these terms.

Symptoms of autism usually begin in the second year of life. Parents often report that early motor milestones developed normally. However, there is marked delay in the acquisition of speech and language. Echolalia is frequently present with the child simply repeating or parroting phrases. It is typical for the child not to respond to his or her name and to appear socially withdrawn or aloof. Stereotypic behaviors, such as spinning, rocking, or hand flapping, are commonly observed. Children and adults with SCD may have normal speech and cognition but lack age-appropriate understanding of language nuances and socialization skills. They tend to be loners with a narrow range of interests, mechanical speech patterns, and stereotypic behaviors.

The prevalence of ASD appears to be continually rising in the United States and more than doubled between 2000 (1 in 150) and 2010 (1 in 68). This increase remains unexplained but may reflect enhanced public awareness and a broadening of the definition of ASD. The etiology of autism is unknown but appears to be multifactorial. In the past two decades, several alternative hypotheses including measles immunization, thimerosal toxicity, and gluten–casein sensitivity have been promulgated and subsequently refuted. Genetic predisposition clearly plays an important role, as indicated by concordance in twins and siblings. Autism has been linked to tuberous sclerosis complex (TSC), fragile X syndrome, Rett's syndrome, and Angelman's syndrome. In addition, numerous suspicious genetic duplications and deletions, as well as copy-number variations, are being identified by chromosome microarray analysis.

Management of ASD is multidisciplinary, but the physician is often requested to coordinate and oversee care. Speech therapy, OT, and applied behavioral analysis therapy are considered beneficial interventions. The amount of each therapy prescribed must be individualized to the developmental level and needs of the patient. Medications may be required to manage hyperactivity, agitation, aggression, and self-injurious behaviors. Stimulant drugs, atypical antipsychotics, SSRIs, as well as clonidine, guanfacine, and naltrexone, have all been studied and utilized in children with ASD.

D. **Progressive cognitive impairment.** In progressive cognitive impairment, acquisition of milestones initially decelerates. Subsequently, there is a loss of previously achieved skills. There may be a combined loss of motor, coordination, and sensory and cognitive functions. Alternatively, loss of skills and functions in one area may precede losses in other areas. The pattern and sequence of regression may yield clues to the diagnosis.

E. **Disorders of white matter (leukodystrophies)** initially present with loss of motor milestones and increasing spasticity. There may also be a loss of vision. Magnetic resonance imaging (MRI) scans demonstrate white matter demyelination. Peripheral neuropathy is often a characteristic feature as well. This can be demonstrated by slowing of peripheral nerve conduction velocities (NCVs). Visual and auditory evoked potential may also demonstrate slowing. Some examples of leukodystrophies include globoid cell leukodystrophy, metachromatic leukodystrophy, Alexander's disease, Canavan's disease, Pelizaeus–Merzbacher disease, and adrenoleukodystrophy. Age of onset, patterns of loss of function, genetic testing, and MRI findings can help to distinguish the various leukodystrophies.

F. **Disorders of gray matter** often present with seizures and loss of cognitive skills. These include amino and organic acidurias, Tay–Sachs disease, ceroid lipofuscinosis, Rett's syndrome, and AIDS encephalopathy.

G. **Disorders with prominent movement disorder** include Wilson's disease (hepatolenticular degeneration), pantothenate kinase-associated neurodegeneration, and Niemann–Pick disease. These may present with dysarthria, dysphagia, dystonia, chorea, and spasticity. Juvenile Huntington's disease and Parkinson's disease may present with chorea, rigidity, and tremor. Ataxia is a prominent feature of ataxia telangiectasia, Refsum's disease, abetalipoproteinemia, and Friedreich ataxia.

H. **Neurocutaneous disorders.** These are genetic conditions characterized by skin lesions and central nervous system (CNS) findings. Neurofibromatosis type 1 (NF1) has autosomal-dominant transmission through the *neurofibromin 1* gene located at 17q.11.z. The National Institute of Health (NIH) lists seven cardinal clinical features of NF1 (Video 37.1). These include six or more café au lait spots (Fig. 37.1), two or more neurofibromas, café au lait freckles in the axillary or inguinal regions (Crowe sign) (Fig. 37.2), optic nerve glioma, two or more Lisch nodules (pigmented iris hamartomas), sphenoid bone dysplasia or thinning of long bone cortex, and a first-degree relative with NF1. Due to the increased incidence of CNS tumors and optic gliomas, periodic imaging of the brain and orbits is recommended.

Neurofibromatosis type 2 (NF2) is much less common and clinical manifestations arise predominantly in early adulthood. The hallmark lesion of NF2 is bilateral vestibular schwannomas (BVS). These typically occur in early adulthood, but are occasionally seen in

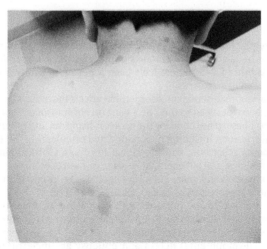

FIGURE 37.1 Café-au-lait spots in a child with NF1. (See color plates.)

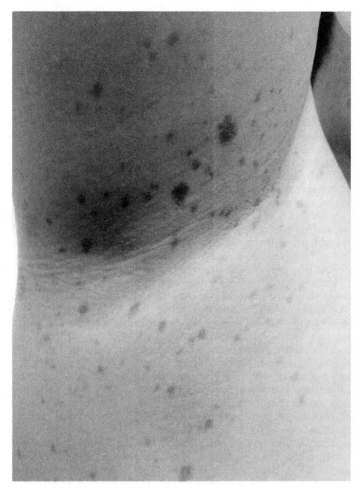

FIGURE 37.2 Axillary freckling in a child with NF1. (See color plates.)

adolescence or even childhood (Fig. 37.3). BVS eventually cause progressive hearing loss, tinnitus, and loss of balance. Schwannomas of the trigeminal nerve, spine, and peripheral nerves as well as other CNS tumors have been reported in adults. Eye findings include cataracts and retinal hamartomas.

TSC is an autosomal-dominant disorder that affects the brain, skin, kidneys, and heart. Mutations have been localized to the *TSC1* gene on chromosome 9 and the *TSC2* gene on chromosome 16. These genes code for the proteins hamartin and tuberin. TSC has several characteristic skin lesions, including hypopigmented macules (Fig. 37.4), shagreen patches (Fig. 37.5), adnoma sebaceum, and subungual fibromas. Cortical hamartomas (tubers), subependymal nodules, and subependymal giant cell astrocytomas are seen in the brain. Cardiac rhabdomyomas and renal angiomyolipomas also occur. Children with TSC are at risk for infantile spasms, partial seizures, ASD, and GDD.

Sturge–Weber syndrome presents with port wine birthmarks in the trigeminal nerve distribution and ipsilateral brain hemangiomas. Affected children also have contralateral focal motor seizures and hemiparesis. Other rare neurocutaneous syndromes associated with developmental delays and epilepsy are incontinentia pigmenti and hypomelanosis of Ito.

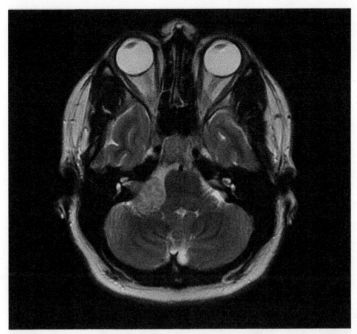

FIGURE 37.3 Brain MRI showing a right vestibular schwannoma in a child with NF2.

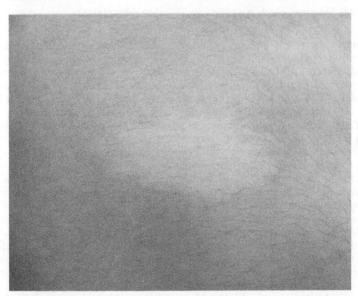

FIGURE 37.4 Hypopigmented macule (ash leaf spot) in a child with TSC. (See color plates.)

I. Evaluation. Children referred for specialty evaluation of developmental delay should have already been screened by their pediatricians. The American Academy of Pediatrics (AAP) recommends such screening utilizing a standardized test at the 9-month, 18-month, and 24- or 30-month well-child care visits. In the absence of such screening, the neurologist should consider administering a standardized general developmental screening test as a

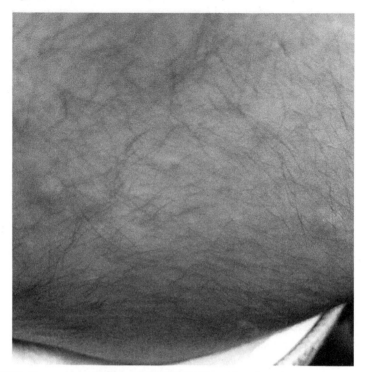

FIGURE 37.5 Shagreen patch in a child with TSC. (See color plates.)

preliminary assessment. Examples of validated developmental screening tests include the Ages and Stages Questionnaires, Child Development Inventory, and the Bayley Infant Neurodevelopmental Screen. When screening for autism, consider more specific inventories such as the Childhood Autism Rating Scale (CARS) and the modified checklist for autism in toddlers (M-CHAT). For higher functioning older children, the Autism Spectrum Screening Questionnaire (ASSQ) may be more appropriate.

A complete examination should be done with particular attention to the nervous system. It is especially important to observe and record somatic growth, head circumference, dysmorphic features, birthmarks, and developmental milestones. Audiologic assessment should routinely be obtained in cases of speech and language delays. Referral to a pediatric ophthalmologist is particularly relevant if lack of eye contact, impaired visual tracking, strabismus, and corneal opacities are noted. Most states now routinely screen newborn infants for congenital hypothyroidism and numerous metabolic disorders including phenylketonuria, galactosemia, biotinidase deficiency, and amino acid/urea cycle disorders. However, these should be repeated if warranted by the patient's presenting signs and symptoms. Screening for lead exposure should be considered if environmental risk factors are identified.

If there is a positive family history of developmental delays or if autism is suspected, genetic testing is indicated. Autistic children should be routinely screened for fragile X syndrome. In addition, chromosome microarray analysis should be obtained with particular attention to duplication at the 15q11–q13 and deletion of 22q11.2 regions. If Rett's syndrome is a consideration, screening for *MeCP2* is recommended.

EEG and MRI are not routinely indicated in cases of static encephalopathies. However, an EEG should be obtained in patients with suspicion of seizures. An EEG should also be considered in patients with regression of language skills to rule out epileptogenic encephalopathies such as Landau–Kleffner syndrome.

Computed tomography (CT) and MRI require sedation and are reserved for patients with abnormalities of head circumference, particularly progressive macrocephaly or microcephaly. Focal or lateralizing neurologic signs (e.g., hemiparesis) are also an indication for imaging studies. Progressive encephalopathies also warrant an MRI to assess for degenerative or structural abnormalities. Periodic neuroimaging is indicated to monitor the progress of children with neurocutaneous syndromes.

MOTOR DISORDERS

Normal motor development follows a defined sequence of milestones. By 2 months of age, the infant lifts the head from prone. Rolling over and transferring objects is accomplished by 5 to 6 months. Sitting independently occurs by 8 to 9 months and walking independently between 12 and 15 months. Delays in the acquisition of milestones are seen in children with hypotonia and weakness. This condition is also described as floppy infant syndrome.

Neuroimaging is indicated if cerebral dysgenesis is suspected. Workup for lower-motor unit disorders includes measurement of creatine kinase level, electromyography/NCV, and muscle biopsy. The edrophonium chloride test can confirm myasthenia gravis (MG). There are now specific DNA probes available for the spinal muscular atrophies, myotonic dystrophy congenital muscular dystrophy, and Prader–Willi syndrome.

A. **Central or cerebral hypotonia.** Hypotonia may be the initial manifestation of CP. These infants may have a history of hypoxic–ischemic encephalopathy, intraventricular hemorrhage, and/or neonatal seizures. Cerebral dysgenesis should be suspected if there are dysmorphic features or other congenital malformations. Although these infants may initially be hypotonic, over time muscle tone increases accompanied by spasticity, weakness, hyperreflexia, and positive Babinski signs.

Children with chromosome abnormalities and genetic syndromes are also typically hypotonic. Examples include Down's syndrome, Lowe's syndrome (oculocerebrorenal syndrome), familial dysautonomia (Riley–Day syndrome), and Prader–Willi syndrome. Prader–Willi syndrome is further characterized by poor feeding in the neonatal period and hypogonadism.

Benign congenital hypotonia may be a mild variant of cerebral hypotonia. Infants with this condition are hypotonic in infancy but gradually recover muscle tone and motor milestones. However, mild developmental delays and learning problems may later be noted in such children.

B. **Spinal cord injuries.** Stretching of the spinal cord may result from traction during delivery, particularly with breech presentation. The infant is often comatose and flaccid at birth and may not survive. Milder cervical cord injuries present with residual hypotonia and must be distinguished from cerebral and lower-motor unit disorders.

C. **Lower-motor unit disorders.**
   4. **Anterior horn cell disorders.** Spinal muscular atrophy (SMA) is caused by degeneration of anterior horn cells in the spinal cord and brainstem. SMA type 1 (Werdnig–Hoffman disease) results in severe hypotonia, weakness, absent MSRs, and tongue fasciculations. Affected children usually die from respiratory complications by 1 year of age. Milder variants (SMA types 2 and 3) present later in infancy or childhood; affected children survive longer, but also have weakness, hypotonia, areflexia, muscle fasciculations, and arthrogryposis.
   5. **Neuropathies.** Hereditary neuropathies generally present beyond infancy. They are divided into hereditary motor sensory neuropathy (HMSN), hereditary motor, and hereditary sensory and autonomic subtypes. Charcot–Marie–Tooth, the most common HMSN, presents in childhood with peroneal muscle atrophy foot-drop, pes cavus, and absent MSRs. Neuropathy may also be a manifestation of systemic diseases such as diabetes and autoimmune disorders as well as leukodystrophies and hereditary ataxia. A number of medications including vincristine, isoniazid, phenytoin, and pyridoxine can cause neuropathy (see Chapter 51).
   6. **Neuromuscular junction disorders.** Transient neonatal myasthenia syndrome may be seen in infants born to mothers with MG. Feeding problems, weak cry, facial weakness, and hypotonia are common features. Genetic myasthenic syndromes are rarer and are characterized by respiratory difficulties, poor feeding, weakness, ptosis, and ophthalmoplegia. Infantile botulism mimics MG, but affected infants also show pupillary dilatation and constipation (see Chapter 53).

7. **Myopathy.** Congenital myopathies present in infancy with hypotonia, motor delays, and proximal muscle weakness. Numerous variants have been described, each with unique findings on muscle biopsy. These include nemaline myopathy, myotubular myopathy, congenital fiber-type disproportion, and central core disease. Metabolic myopathies include lysosomal enzyme deficiencies such as Pompe's disease (acid maltase deficiency). This disorder presents in infancy with weakness, hypotonia, and cardiomyopathy resulting in heart failure. Rare mitochondrial myopathies can also be accompanied by hypotonia and lactic acidosis. Congenital muscular dystrophy presents with hypotonia and arthrogryposis at birth and may also show CNS involvement. Congenital myotonic dystrophy occurs in infants of mothers with the disease. Hypotonia, facial diplegia, arthrogryphosis, and gastroparesis are the common presenting signs. Childhood-onset muscular dystrophy is reviewed in Chapter 52.

D. **Evaluation.** Neurologic and general examination helps to distinguish central hypotonia from lower-motor unit disorders. MSRs are present and may be brisk in central hypotonia but are absent or diminished in lower-motor unit disorders. Tongue fasciculations are seen in SMA. Congenital malformations, dysmorphic features, and abnormalities of head size and shape suggest cerebral dysgenesis. Arthrogryposis suggests an SMA or CMD variant.

ATAXIA

A. **Definition.** Ataxia refers to lack of coordination and impaired control of voluntary movements and balance. The cerebellum controls these functions in conjunction with the sensory input from the vestibular system, basal ganglia, and spinal cord (see Chapter 29).

B. **Acute ataxia.** Intoxication, particularly from alcohol, sedatives, antihistamines, and anticonvulsants, may cause ataxia. Acute postviral cerebellar ataxia usually occurs in preschool children. The onset often coincides with the end of a viral illness, particularly varicella. The onset is very dramatic with the child suddenly becoming unable to walk. Nystagmus may also occur. Recovery is usually complete but may take up to several months. Viral encephalitis with cerebellar and/or brainstem involvement can also present with acute ataxia. There may be accompanying cranial nerve deficits. GBS (Fisher variant) may present with similar findings. Kinsbourne's syndrome, characterized by acute ataxia accompanied by opsoclonus and myoclonus, is thought to be a paraneoplastic condition secondary to occult neuroblastoma.

C. **Chronic progressive ataxia.** Posterior fossa tumors are the most common brain tumors in childhood. Medulloblastoma, ependymoma, cerebellar astrocytoma, and brainstem glioma can all present with slowly progressive ataxia (see Chapter 57). The most common recessive genetic disorder presenting with childhood-onset progressive ataxia is Friedreich ataxia. In addition to ataxia, patients develop scoliosis, cardiomyopathy, retinitis pigmentosa, cataracts, and hearing loss. Absent MSRs and Babinski signs are typically noted. Friedreich ataxia has been localized to an unstable GAA triplet repeat of the *frataxin* gene on chromosome 9q13. Other rare degenerative and metabolic causes of chronic progressive ataxia include ataxia telangiectasia, abetalipoproteinemia, Refsum's disease, vitamin E deficiency, biotinidase deficiency, and a multiple carboxylase deficiency. In addition, more than 20 variants of autosomal-dominant spinocerebellar atrophy have been described with ages of onset ranging from childhood to late adulthood.

D. **Chronic nonprogressive ataxia.** This is typically associated with malformations of the cerebellum and posterior fossa such as Dandy–Walker syndrome, Chiari malformation, and Joubert's syndrome.

E. **Intermittent ataxia.** This may accompany concussion and may also be seen as an ictal or postictal feature of epilepsy. Basilar migraine often presents with ataxia and vertigo followed by occipital headache. Benign paroxysmal vertigo presents in early childhood with sudden brief episodes of pallor, nystagmus, and inability to walk. Ataxia presenting acutely or intermittently may also be a feature of childhood-onset multiple sclerosis.

F. Rare genetic causes of episodic ataxia include urea cycle disorders, intermittent maple syrup urine disease, and Hartnup disease. Episodic ataxia type 1 is caused by a dominantly inherited mutation of the voltage-gated K^+ channel gene (*KCNA1*) located at chromosome 12p13. Affected patients present with brief episodes of ataxia sometimes provoked by startle.

Myokymia and large calves are associated features. Episodic ataxia type 2 has been linked to a calcium-channel gene (*CACNA1A*) at chromosome 19p13. Attacks of ataxia begin in childhood. Some are prolonged and resemble basilar migraine.

G. Evaluation. Because ataxia may be congenital, acute, chronic progressive, chronic nonprogressive, or intermittent, it is important to establish the duration and pattern. Inquiry should be made regarding possible antecedent trauma, toxin exposure, medications, infections, and seizure disorder. Developmental delays and/or regression may also accompany ataxia because of many of these disorders.

H. Examination. Truncal ataxia is assessed by checking gait, station, tandem gait, and Romberg sign. Limb ataxia is tested by evaluating finger-to-nose, heel-to-shin, and rapid alternating movements. Ability to perform tests of coordination is age-dependent and also requires the cognitive understanding of the child. In preverbal children, assessment of gait and coordination is done by observation of the child's movements and activities.

I. Diagnostic studies. Neuroimaging (CT or MRI) is required for most acute ataxias unless intoxication or acute postviral ataxia is determined to be the cause. For acute ataxias, obtain toxicology screening, particularly for alcohol and anticonvulsant drugs, and urine catecholamines. Chronic ataxias also require neuroimaging as well as selective laboratory studies such as urine amino acids, ammonia, phytanic acid, biotin, cholesterol, and cholestanol levels. For the intermittent ataxias, consider selective testing as appropriate for metabolic and genetic disorders (see Chapters 29 and 49).

HEADACHE

A. Acute headache. Headache is a common feature of systemic febrile illnesses and viral syndromes in children. Bacterial illnesses such as otitis media, sinusitis, and meningitis are also accompanied by headaches. Sinusitis may result in facial, frontal, or retro-orbital pain. The pain of otitis media may localize to the temporal region. Meningitis may manifest with diffuse headache, fever, nuchal rigidity, altered mental status, and seizures.

B. The child who presents with acute headache and is afebrile may still have an infectious illness. However, it is more likely that the etiology is the first tension or migraine headache. Head injuries with subarachnoid, subdural, or epidural hemorrhage must be ruled out. Concussions are also typically followed by acute and sometimes chronic headaches. Idiopathic intracranial hypertension (IIH), arterial hypertension, and medication side effects are also considerations.

C. Chronic headache.

1. **Migraine** is common in childhood affecting up to 5% of preadolescent children and 10% of teenagers. The gender ratio is even in children but females predominate in puberty and adolescence. Family history in a first-degree relative is very common and helps to make the diagnosis. Migraine may appear in early childhood. In such cases, migraine equivalents such as cyclic vomiting, benign paroxysmal torticollis, and benign paroxysmal vertigo are the more likely manifestations. Ophthalmoplegic migraine has also been reported in infancy.

   In children, migraines without aura are much more frequent than migraines with aura. The child complains of a moderate to severe diffuse or bifrontal headache accompanied by nausea, vomiting, pallor, and irritability. Older children may be able to better localize the headaches and will describe a throbbing or pulsating quality. The headache may occur at random times and may on occasion awaken the child from sleep. Migraines in children are typically relieved within a few hours by sleep in a darkened room and minor analgesics. Caffeine withdrawal, nitrates, chocolate, monosodium glutamate, alcohol, dairy products, and numerous other foods are thought to trigger migraines. Environmental factors such as secondhand smoke, automobile emissions, perfumes, and atmospheric pressure changes have also been implicated.

   Complicated migraines are also seen in childhood and may require further investigations including neuroimaging. Ophthalmoplegic migraine presents with headache and irritability, followed by unilateral third-nerve palsy. This is manifested by ptosis, mydriasis, and eversion of the affected eye, which may last hours to days.

Basilar migraine presents with posterior headache, nausea, vomiting, ataxia, vertigo, and on occasion, loss of consciousness. Hemiplegic migraine may mimic stroke with unilateral hemisensory, hemiparetic, and aphasic symptoms followed by a severe contralateral headache.

2. **Tension headache.** These headaches occur in children as well as adults. The headaches are frontal or occipital or may have a "hatband" distribution. They tend to occur in the afternoon or evening and have been associated with stress or anxiety. When these headaches occur on a daily basis, school avoidance should be suspected. Chronic daily headache is typically seen in adolescent girls and is defined by more than 15 headaches per month. This condition is also sometimes described as "chronic migraine." Sleep deprivation, skipping meals, excessive gum chewing, smoking, and caffeine withdrawal may exacerbate the headaches. Overuse of analgesics can complicate the situation and result in so-called "rebound" headaches. Biofeedback and/or psychological counseling may be required to treat underlying comorbid conditions such as anxiety, depression, ADHD, and conduct disorders.

Chronic daily headaches caused by mass lesions are associated with increasing intracranial pressure. Abnormalities on neurologic examination appear in the great majority of such children within 4 months of the onset of headaches. These may include papilledema, cranial nerve abnormalities, ataxia, dysmetria, hemiparesis, or focal sensory signs. Reflex asymmetries and a unilateral Babinski sign may also be present.

IIH presents with acute or chronic headaches, vomiting, and double vision accompanied by papilledema. It is commonly seen in obese adolescent girls. A sixth nerve paresis may also be noted. Lumbar puncture (LP) demonstrates elevated cerebrospinal fluid opening pressure and may partially relieve the condition. The mechanism of action is unknown, but IIH has been associated with use of corticosteroids, vitamin A, and tetracyclines. Cerebral venous thrombosis and mastoiditis have also been linked to the condition.

D. **Evaluation.** It is important to assess the frequency, severity, location, and time of day of the headaches. Severity can be assessed by asking the child or parent to grade the headache from 1 to 10. The history should include inquiry regarding development, head injuries, seizures, learning or attention problems, and family members with recurrent headaches. Information should be requested regarding lifestyle factors including caffeine consumption, sleep habits, meal patterns, excessive gum chewing, and exposure to secondhand smoke. In girls, the onset of menarche should be noted because it may be heralded by migraine headaches.

Blood pressure and pulse should be checked personally by the physician or a reliable assistant. A complete general and neurologic examination is required for every child who presents with headaches. The head circumference should be measured. The skull and neck should be auscultated for bruits. The eyes, ears, nose, and throat should be examined including palpation for cervical nodes and sinus tenderness. The temporomandibular joint should be palpated and auscultated for misalignments and clicks. The teeth should be checked for caries, malocclusions, and newly installed braces or appliances.

Most children with headaches do not require neuroimaging provided rapport is established with the parents and timely follow-up can be arranged. If the history and examination suggest acute CNS infection or IIH, an LP should be considered. Acute hypertension may require hospitalization and workup for renal or cardiac diseases. If acute head injury or concussion is suspected, an emergency noncontrast CT scan should be obtained to check for intracranial hemorrhage. Chronic recurrent headaches with typical migrainous or tension features do not require imaging unless they remain refractory to treatment. An MRI should be obtained in children with complicated migraine and IIH or if abnormalities are present on neurologic examination. On occasion, an anxious parent may insist on neuroimaging for the child despite the reassurance that such a procedure is unnecessary. In such instances, it is usually prudent to acquiesce to the parent's request provided there is no obvious contraindication to the neuroimaging procedure. The reader is referred to Chapters 20, 21, and 54 for further information on the approach to patients with acute and chronic headaches.

NONEPILEPTIC PAROXYSMAL DISORDERS

Nonepileptic paroxysmal disorders are defined by their intermittent, recurrent, and abrupt presentation. Between episodes the patient feels well and has no complaints. It is particularly important to distinguish these episodic conditions from epilepsy. Childhood epilepsies are discussed in detail in Chapter 42.

A. Evaluation. A detailed description of the event by a reliable observer is essential for proper classification and diagnosis. Older children can also contribute their personal recollections. Inquiry should be particularly directed toward triggering events or precipitating factors. A videotape of the episode may be particularly useful. Examination is normal in most cases. Diagnostic studies are generally not required. On occasions, EEG and video EEG may be necessary to rule out epilepsy.

B. Breath-holding spells. These are benign, but frightening, paroxysmal episodes that may result in a brief loss of consciousness. Cyanotic syncope occurs in infants and children between 6 months and 4 years of age. The family history is often positive. The child first cries because of anxiety, frustration, or pain. Following prolonged expiration, breathing ceases and the child becomes cyanotic, hypotonic, and briefly unresponsive. Recovery usually occurs quickly but on occasion some brief tonic–clonic movements followed by sleep may occur.

Another variant of breath-holding is pallid syncope. This is usually initiated by a minor head injury, which is thought to trigger a brief reflex asystole. The child becomes pale, limp, and is briefly unconscious.

Breath-holding spells can be diagnosed clinically by the stereotypic sequence of events preceding each episode. On rare occasions or to lessen parental anxiety, an EEG can be done to distinguish these episodes from epileptic seizures.

C. Syncope (fainting). Syncope is common in children, especially during adolescence. It is induced by a transient decrease in blood flow to the brain secondary to a vasovagal reflex. It is almost always precipitated by triggering stimuli such as change of position, pain, or extreme fear or anxiety.

The syncopal event may be preceded by an "aura" of blurry vision, dizziness, and/ or tinnitus. The child then becomes pale and clammy and loses consciousness with an accompanying fall. Brief stiffening, upward eye rolling, vocalizations, and tremulous movements are not uncommon. Tongue biting is unusual in syncope. Recovery of consciousness usually occurs within a minute. In most instances, syncope is considered to be a common benign occurrence that does not warrant extensive neurodiagnostic testing. If syncope is prolonged or recurrent, a cardiology referral with ECG monitoring may be necessary. Syncope is reviewed in more detail in Chapter 7.

D. Other. Episodic weakness, ataxia, tremor, chorea, vertigo, and sensory disturbances are reviewed elsewhere in this chapter or in other chapters under the appropriate headings. However, several other paroxysmal neurologic disorders are unique to infants and young children.

1. **Spasmus nutans** begins in infancy and resolves spontaneously in early childhood. It consists of three cardinal features: head bobbing, torticollis, and nystagmus. Diagnosis may warrant neuroimaging of the brain and orbits to rule out neoplasms, which can rarely present with similar signs.

2. **Sandifer's syndrome** is seen in infancy and consists of paroxysmal opisthotonic posturing sometimes accompanied by vomiting and apnea. The underlying etiology is gastroesophageal reflux, which requires pediatric gastrointestinal consultation.

3. **Paroxysmal infant shuddering** or shivering occurs during wakefulness and may raise concerns about seizures. The child appears to momentarily shiver as if having a chill. Such episodes often occur frequently enough to be captured on videotape in which case they are easily distinguishable from clinical seizures. Later in life, essential tremor may be associated with a history of infant shuddering.

4. **Gratification syndrome (masturbation)** is occasionally seen in infants and young children and may be confused with seizures. These episodes consist of prolonged rocking movements of the pelvis and thighs. Altered breathing, flushing, sweating, and staring are typically seen. These episodes resolve over time with parental reassurance.

ABNORMALITIES OF HEAD SIZE

A. **Normocephaly** is defined as a head circumference measurement between the 2nd and 98th percentile. A head circumference greater than the 98th percentile is macrocephaly, and a head circumference less than the 2nd percentile is microcephaly. Normally the head should grow on a specific percentile. Deviation of growth from the expected percentile should prompt further evaluation and investigations. Macrocephaly and microcephaly are both associated with higher incidences of CNS pathology and developmental delays.

B. **Macrocephaly** may be familial, in which case at least one parent's head will also be large. Differential diagnosis also includes hydrocephalus, which may be communicating or obstructive. Rare metabolic disorders including galactosemia, maple syrup urine disease, mucopolysaccharidoses, and Canavan's disease are associated with macrocephaly. Children with genetic conditions including achondroplasia, fragile X syndrome, cerebral gigantism (Sotos syndrome), and the neurocutaneous disorders commonly have large heads. Benign subdural collections present with progressive enlargement of head circumference, but without signs of increased intracranial pressure.

C. **Microcephaly** may be secondary to genetic causes or cerebral dysgenesis and is commonly associated with congenital syndromes. It is also frequently seen following hypoxic–ischemic encephalopathy, intrauterine infections, and postnatal infection. Craniosynostosis can cause progressive microcephaly when more than one suture is affected. Rett's syndrome also presents with progressive microcephaly.

D. Evaluation. The history may reveal developmental delay or regression. Symptoms of increased intracranial pressure include emesis, irritability, and somnolence. Examination may demonstrate signs of increased intracranial pressure including bulging fontanelle, sunsetting of the eyes, papilledema, or a sixth nerve palsy. The head circumference should be plotted on a standardized growth chart and serial measurements should be obtained. Neuroimaging is indicated in most cases of abnormal head size. Exceptions include familial macrocephaly and possibly benign subdural collections. Genetic and metabolic studies are also considerations if cerebral dysgenesis or storage diseases are suspected.

POSTCONCUSSION SYNDROME

Concussions are biomechanical brain injuries that occur following low-velocity impacts to the head, face, and neck. They are common in children and adolescents who participate in contact sports. In the United States about 300,000 athletic concussions occur each year. Concussions are most commonly seen in football, but also in girls' soccer and basketball and boys' wrestling and hockey. All 50 states have passed legislation mandating education, prevention, and medical supervision of sports-related concussions (SRC). The American Academy of Neurology (AAN), AAP, and American Medical Association (AMA) have all issued position statements regarding management of SRC and return-to-play (RTP) guidelines.

Symptoms of postconcussion syndrome include headache, memory problems, nausea, vomiting, altered sensorium, emotional lability, impaired concentration, and sleep disturbances. Fewer than 10% of SRC are associated with an immediate loss of consciousness. If a concussion is suspected, the athlete should be immediately removed from play and evaluated on the side line by medically trained personnel utilizing a standardized symptom checklist. Loss of consciousness, retrograde amnesia, a post-traumatic seizure, or a Glasgow Coma Scale score <15 warrants immediate physician evaluation.

Neurologic consultation is appropriate in determining the initial severity a concussion and whether neuroimaging is required. Subsequent management of postconcussion syndrome consists mainly of closely monitored physical and cognitive rest until all symptoms have resolved. Extra caution is required if the patient has a history of multiple concussions or if symptoms persist for longer than 10 days. Neuropsychological testing may be indicated in these situations. Alternatively, serial computerized neurocognitive testing programs may be utilized. RTP should be stepwise and carefully supervised by the physician in cooperation with coaches and trainers. Persistent headaches, vertigo, or concentration problems may require long-term neurologic follow-up.

Key Points

- ADHD has an incidence of 11% in childhood. ADHD, predominantly hyperactive-impulsive, ADHD, predominantly inattentive, and ADHD combined are the three main types.
- Developmental delay affects 5% to 10% of children and is frequently caused by static encephalopathies including CP and ASDs.
- The definition of ASDs has been dramatically revised by *DSM5*. Social-pragmatic communication disorder is a new diagnostic category and pervasive developmental disorder and Asperger's syndrome have been eliminated from *DSM5*.
- Neurocutaneous syndromes are neurologic disorders with skin lesions and CNS findings. NF1 and TSC are two types that can present with CNS tumors.
- Headaches are not uncommon in children. Pediatric migraines typically present without aura. There are also migraine variants unique to children including cyclic vomiting and benign paroxysmal torticollis.
- Nonepileptic paroxysmal disorders are characterized by their intermittent recurrent and abrupt presentation. Examples include breath-holding spells, spasms nutans, and Sandifer's syndrome.
- In the United States, about 300,000 athletic concussions occur annually. Guidelines for management and RTP have been issued by the AAN, AAP, and AMA.

Recommended Readings

American Psychiatric Association. *Diagnostic and Statistical Manual of Mental Disorders (DSM-5)*. 5th ed. Arlington, VA: American Psychiatric Association; 2013.

Council on Children with Developmental Disabilities, Section on Developmental Behavioral Pediatrics, Bright Futures Steering Committee, et al. Identifying infants and young children with developmental disorders in the medical home: an algorithm for developmental surveillance and screening (American Academy of Pediatrics Policy Statement). *Pediatrics*. 2006;118:405–420.

DiMario, FJ. *Non-Epileptic Childhood Paroxysmal Disorders*. New York, NY: Oxford University Press; 2009.

Espay AJ, Biller J. *Concise Neurology*. Philadelphia, PA: Wolters Kluwer; 2011.

Fenichel GM. *Clinical Pediatric Neurology: A Signs and Symptoms Approach*. 5th ed. Philadelphia, PA: Elsevier Saunders; 2005.

Giza CC, Kutcher JS, Ashwal S, et al. Summary of evidence-based guideline for clinicians. Update: evaluation and management of concussion in sports. *Am Acad Neurol*. 2013;80(24):2250–2257.

Klein O, Pierre-Kahn A, Boddaert N, et al. Dandy-Walker malformation: prenatal diagnosis and prognosis. *Childs Nerv Syst*. 2003;19:484–489.

Lewis M. *Child and Adolescent Psychiatry: A Comprehensive Textbook*. 3rd ed. Philadelphia, PA: Lippincott Williams & Wilkins; 2002.

Maria BL. *Current Management in Child Neurology*. 3rd ed. Hamilton, ON: BC Decker Inc; 2005.

Reiff M. *ADHD: A Complete and Authoritative Guide*. Elk Grove Village, IL: American Academy of Pediatrics; 2004.

Robertson WC, Schnitzler ER. Ophthalmoplegic migraine in infancy. *Pediatrics*. 1978;61:886–888.

Silberstein SD, Lipton RB, Goadsby, PJ. *Headache in Clinical Practice*. 2nd ed. London, England: Martin Dunitz; 2002.

Tervo RC. Identifying patterns of developmental delays can help diagnose neurodevelopmental disorders. *Clin Pediatr (Phila)*. 2006;45:509–517.

Wyllie E. *The Treatment of Epilepsy: Principles and Practice*. 3rd ed. Philadelphia, PA: Lippincott Williams & Wilkins; 2001.

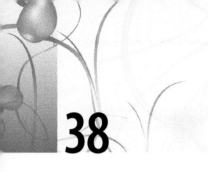

38

Approach to Common Emergencies in Pediatric Neurology

Melissa G. Chung and E. Steve Roach

Traditionally, the field of pediatric neurology has been primarily office based. Over the last decade, pediatric neurocritical care has emerged as a budding subspecialty that focuses upon the acute and emergent management of pediatric neurologic disease. In this chapter, we will address some of the most common pediatric neurocritical care emergencies.

ACUTE NEUROLOGIC WEAKNESS

The differential diagnosis and evaluation of weakness is discussed at length in other chapters. This section focuses on common pediatric neurologic disorders that have a fulminant onset and require prompt recognition, not just for treatment but also because of high likelihood that the child may require cardiorespiratory support in an intensive care setting.

A. **Infant botulism.**

1. **Introduction.** Infant botulism is caused by ingestion of spores of *Clostridium botulinum* in honey or more commonly in dirt. Only children under the age of 1 tend to acquire botulism via this mechanism because their intestinal bacterial flora is immature. The spores germinate in the gastrointestinal tract and they release neurotoxin. This neurotoxin cleaves the soluble *N*-ethylmaleimide-sensitive factor attachment protein receptor proteins in the presynaptic neuromuscular junction and thus blocks release of acetylcholine. Infants initially present with constipation and then develop lethargy, poor appetite, and progressive, symmetric descending hypotonia and weakness. Patients often have poorly reactive pupils, facial diplegia, ptosis, and a diminished gag reflex. About 50% of patients require mechanical ventilation because of inability to protect their airway or diaphragmatic/respiratory muscle weakness. Some infants also develop autonomic dysfunction with irregular heart rates or urinary retention. Children usually will recover completely in weeks to months.

2. **Evaluation.** A clinical diagnosis can be made based on the neurologic exam and history. Stool can be tested for botulinum toxin for confirmation of the diagnosis. However, the patient's significant constipation usually makes obtainment of a stool sample difficult. The sample cannot be obtained using a glycerin suppository because glycerin inactivates the toxin. If there is uncertainty about the clinical diagnosis, electromyography (EMG) and nerve conduction studies (NCS) can be used to help confirm the diagnosis. Expected findings on testing include the following: compound motor unit action potentials with decreased amplitude, tetanic and post-tetanic facilitation, brief small-amplitude motor action potentials with muscle stimulation, and fibrillation potentials or positive sharp waves on EMG.

3. **Treatment.** The most important treatment is supportive care, particularly prompt recognition of impending respiratory failure. Patients are at risk for silent aspiration, so alternative means of nutrition, such as nasogastric or naso-jejunal feedings, are usually indicated in the acute setting. Administration of intravenous (IV) botulism immunoglobulin (BabyBIG) decreases the duration of symptoms. The drug is more effective when given early in the course of illness so it should be administered as soon as possible if infant botulism is strongly suspected, even if the diagnosis has not been confirmed. BabyBIG is available through the Infant Botulism Treatment and Prevention Program.

B. **Myasthenic crisis.**

1. **Introduction.** Myasthenia gravis (MG) is a neuromuscular disorder caused by auto-antibodies to the neuromuscular endplate. Clinically, the disease is characterized by fatigable muscle

weakness. A myasthenic crisis is defined as an acute life-threatening episode that affects the bulbar and/or respiratory muscles and leads to respiratory insufficiency or failure. Approximately 10% to 15% of patients with MG will have at least one myasthenic crisis. A crisis can be triggered by medications, infection, or be unprovoked.

2. **Evaluation.** Respiratory function should be urgently evaluated, including measurement of negative inspiratory force (NIF) and forced vital capacity (FVC). A blood gas can be obtained to assess for hypercapnia that indicates impending respiratory failure. A careful review of changes in medications should be done, especially for new medications (such as magnesium or aminoglycosides) that can worsen MG. Patients also need to be carefully evaluated for signs/symptoms of an infection that provoked the exacerbation.

3. **Treatment.** Early intubation should be strongly considered in patients who are unable to handle their secretions (poor cough or gag reflex), have an FVC with good effort that is <15 mL/kg or drops more than 20% to 30% from their baseline, or NIF is less than –30. Noninvasive positive pressure ventilation can be used in patients with borderline respiratory function but intubation is necessary in patients who lose their ability to protect their airway. Medications that can worsen neuromuscular function should be eliminated/avoided if possible. Any identified infections should be treated. Anticholinesterase dose should be optimized; conversely, anticholinesterase should be stopped if there are any concerns about anticholinergic toxicity. Plasma exchange (PLEX) or intravenous immunoglobulin (IVIG) can be initiated to hasten recovery.

C. **Guillain–Barré syndrome (GBS).**

1. **Introduction.** GBS is a common cause of acute neuromuscular weakness in children. It classically presents with rapidly progressive ascending weakness (usually symmetric) and is usually accompanied by sensory symptoms such as paresthesias, hyperesthesia, tingling, or numbness. A small subset of patients have cranial neuropathies. Patients may develop autonomic dysfunction or respiratory insufficiency/failure from weakness of their respiratory muscles or loss of airway protective reflexes. About 2/3 of patients report an antecedent illness in the preceding 3 weeks. Symptoms progress over a period of days to weeks; most patients reach their maximal weakness by approximately 2 weeks. On examination, patients are areflexic or hyporeflexic in the involved limbs.

2. **Evaluation.** Clinical examination findings and history may strongly suggest a diagnosis of GBS. Many clinicians do a lumbar puncture (LP) to look for albuminocytologic dissociation. However, one must not be overly dependent upon this finding to make a diagnosis of GBS; cerebrospinal fluid (CSF) protein levels are normal still in a significant number of patients during the first week of symptoms, especially patients with a Miller-Fisher variant. About 15% of patients also have a CSF mild pleocytosis; alternative diagnoses should be explored if the CSF white blood cell count is above 50 cells/μL. Magnetic resonance imaging (MRI) of the spine with contrast is not necessary, but it can provide further supporting evidence if the MRI shows enhancement and/or thickening of the thoracolumbar nerve roots and cauda equine. EMG/NCS also are not necessary to make the diagnosis and may be normal early on. EMG/NCS findings that are consistent with a diagnosis of GBS include the following: delayed distal latencies, conduction block, prolonged or absent F waves or H reflexes, or temporal dispersion of waveforms. For prognosis, EMG/NCS can be done/repeated several weeks after onset of symptoms to look for evidence of axonal injury versus demyelination. While symptoms are still progressive, all patients also should have serial pulmonary function testing (FVC and NIF) and cardiovascular monitoring because of the risk of dysautonomia.

3. **Treatment.** Strongly consider early intubation for patients who are unable to handle their secretions (poor cough or gag), have an FVC with good effort that is <15 mL/kg or drops more than 20% to 30% from their baseline, or NIF is less than –30. Patients with neck flexor/extensor or facial weakness also should be considered at high risk for respiratory failure. One should avoid treatment of abnormal vital signs, particularly hypertension, with long-acting medications, as these changes may be due to dysautonomia and thus short-lived. Foley catheterization or intermittent straight catheterization may be necessary because of neurogenic bladder. Some patients develop significant hyperesthesia or neuropathic pain; medications such as gabapentin, pregabalin, or tricyclic antidepressants can reduce discomfort. In adults, treatment of severe GBS with IVIG

or PLEX speeds recovery versus supportive care alone. Less robust pediatric data are available but trials also suggest that IVIG may hasten recovery in children.

D. **Idiopathic transverse myelitis.**

1. **Introduction.** Acute transverse myelitis (TM) is characterized by progressive development of neurologic signs/symptoms referable to the spinal cord (usually bilateral weakness, sensory level, and/or bowel/bladder dysfunction). Patients may complain of nonspecific myalgias or fevers prior to the onset of neurologic symptoms. The initial neurologic complaint is usually ascending paresthesias, followed by sensory loss with a spinal level, (initially) flaccid paralysis, and bladder/bowel dysfunction. Autonomic dysfunction and respiratory compromise also may occur depending on the level of spinal cord involvement. Symptoms usually reach their maximum between 4 hours and 21 days after onset. Idiopathic TM is secondary to focal immune-mediated inflammation of the spinal cord.

2. **Evaluation.** An MRI of the spine with contrast should be done to look for swelling and contrast-enhanced T2 lesions usually over multiple segments in the spinal cord. MRI of the brain also can be considered as concurrent brain lesions might suggest an alternative diagnosis. Testing for neuromyelitis optica should be sent if a patient has longitudinally extensive lesions (>3 vertebral segments) or a history/examination suggestive of optic neuritis. CSF and serum studies also can be helpful to rule out other causes of TM, such as infectious or rheumatologic, as indicated by the patient's clinical history. Testing for reversible causes of myelopathy, such as vitamin B_{12} deficiency and thyroid dysfunction, should be strongly considered as well. In patients with idiopathic TM, CSF studies may show evidence of inflammation with moderate pleocytosis (50 to 100 cells/μL) and elevated protein. Oligoclonal bands are usually negative in cases of idiopathic TM.

3. **Treatment.** High-dose IV methylprednisolone should be initiated as early as possible for treatment of idiopathic TM. Patients who fail to improve after treatment with steroids may benefit from plasmapheresis. Supportive care for respiratory insufficiency, autonomic dysfunction, bowel/bladder dysfunction, gastroparesis, and spasticity may be required depending upon the level of the spinal cord lesion.

E. **Acute disseminated encephalomyelitis (ADEM).**

1. **Introduction.** ADEM is an immune-mediated demyelinating disease that affects the central nervous system (CNS), predominantly the white matter. ADEM occurs more frequently in children than adults and tends to be a monophasic disease. Children typically present with headache, nausea, fatigue, and/or fevers prior to development of encephalopathy and focal neurologic symptoms. The neurologic symptoms are referable to multifocal lesions in the brain and may include weakness, ataxia, cranial neuropathies, or changes in vision. Seizures are common in patients with ADEM. It is commonly considered a postinfectious or postvaccination phenomenon. However, the definition proposed by the International Pediatric Multiple Sclerosis Study group in 2007 does not require an antecedent illness; instead the definition only requires that the child have encephalopathy and multifocal neurologic symptoms.

2. **Evaluation.** MRI brain with and without contrast reveals multiple fluid-attenuated inversion recovery (FLAIR) or T2-weighted lesions in the brain and spinal cord, primarily within the white matter. Deep gray matter involvement also has been reported. Lesions tend to be larger and more confluent than the lesions typically seen with multiple sclerosis; most lesions are also expected to enhance with ADEM because it is usually a monophasic disease. CSF studies are also helpful for ruling out infectious mimickers of ADEM. If an LP is done, then the CSF protein and white blood cell count are usually elevated with a lymphocytic predominance in patients with ADEM. The presence of oligoclonal bands is variable.

3. **Treatment.** Patients may require admission to the intensive care unit for supportive care, including intubation, depending upon the degree of encephalopathy and brainstem involvement. Seizures should be managed as needed with antiepileptic medications. Some patients develop malignant cerebral edema and may require aggressive intracranial pressure (ICP) management; decompressive craniectomy can be considered in cases with refractory intracranial hypertension due to tumefactive lesions. High-dose IV methylprednisolone, usually followed by an oral taper of steroids over several weeks, is the first-line treatment for ADEM. If steroids fail, then second-line treatment is PLEX. Some studies have reported that IVIG can be used as a second-line agent if steroids fail.

ACUTE VASCULAR LESIONS

Cerebrovascular disorders are described in detail in Chapters 40 and 41. As children have different risk factor and etiology for stroke, a brief overview of pediatric stroke is provided below.

A. **Intracranial hemorrhage.**

1. **Introduction.** The most common causes of intracranial hemorrhage (ICH) in children are trauma, coagulopathies, neoplasm, infection, or vascular malformations. In infants and children, abusive head trauma is a relatively frequent cause of ICH and is a diagnosis that must be not be missed. Premature infants are predisposed to develop intraventricular hemorrhage (IVH) because of the immaturity of their germinal matrix. In late-preterm infants or term infants, IVH is secondary to deep venous thromboses. The clinical presentation of ICH in children varies depending upon the location of the hemorrhage and age of the patient. Infants may simply present with irritability or lethargy and fussiness; an enlarged or bulging fontanel in an infant indicates underlying cerebral edema or increased pressure. Seizures occur frequently in children of all ages with ICH.

2. **Evaluation.** A full coagulation panel, including fibrinogen, complete blood count, and liver function testing should promptly be sent. Head computerized tomography (CT) can quickly confirm and define the extent of the hemorrhage and associated edema. An MRI brain is useful for further evaluation, particularly to assess for underlying lesions or focal ischemia. Vascular imaging (MR or CT angiography) should be done to evaluate for an underlying vascular lesion if there is not an obvious cause for an intraparenchymal hemorrhage. However, the imaging may not be revealing until after the blood is reabsorbed. Thus, many patients need repeat imaging after a few months. If repeat CTA and MRA are negative and there is a high suspicion for a CNS vascular malformation, then a catheter cerebral angiogram is indicated. Nonaccidental trauma also should be considered as possible cause for ICH, particularly in cases where the provided history is incongruent with the child's injuries; a dilated ophthalmologic examination and a skeletal survey should be done if NAT is suspected.

3. **Treatment.** Coagulopathies should be corrected. Vitamin K should be given to patients with liver failure. General neuroprotective measures include maintaining relative normotension (avoiding both extreme hypertension and hypotension), normoglycemia, normocarbia, and avoidance of hypoxia, hyponatremia, or hyperthermia. Seizures should be aggressively treated. Consider long-term EEG monitoring particularly in young children under 2 years of age and those with abusive head trauma because of the high risk of nonconvulsive seizures in these patient populations. Edema usually peaks about 48 to 72 hours and patients should be monitored carefully for evidence of malignant cerebral edema. Neurosurgical intervention (evacuation of hematoma, craniectomy, extraventricular drain placement, and so on) is indicated in specific circumstances and should be considered on a case-to-case basis.

B. **Arterial ischemic stroke (AIS).**

1. **Introduction.** AIS occurs in approximately 1:3,000 neonates and 3.5 to 4.5 per 100,000 children. Common causes of AIS in children include sickle cell anemia, congenital heart disease, infection, arteriopathy, and hypercoagulable states. Children with certain genetic disorders including Trisomy 21, neurofibromatosis type 1, Fabry's disease, Marfan's, Ehlers-Danlos, and dwarfism are at increased risk for stroke. Approximately 25% of pediatric AIS are classified as "idiopathic" after a complete evaluation. Like adults, some children with AIS present with acute onset of focal neurologic symptoms; however, children, unlike adults, may have stuttering symptoms and frequently have acute symptomatic seizures around the time of their stroke. The challenge to diagnosing pediatric AIS is that stroke mimics, such as complex migraines or Todd's paralysis, are more common than AIS.

2. **Evaluation.** Recognition of pediatric AIS is often delayed with an average time from symptom onset to diagnosis of over 20 hours; thus, the first step in diagnosis is inclusion of AIS in the differential diagnosis for acute neurologic symptoms in children. The acute infarct may not be visible initially on CT scan. MRI of the brain with diffusion-weighted imaging can define the area of infarction. Vascular imaging (MR or CT angiography or in some cases a formal cerebral angiogram) should be done to evaluate for evidence

of arteriopathy or thrombus. A complete blood count and coagulation panel should be sent. Hypercoagulable testing can be considered; consultation with a hematologist may be helpful. An echocardiogram with a bubble study can be done to look for a shunting lesion or cardiac thrombus. Characteristics of the individual patient guides further diagnostic evaluation.

3. **Treatment.** Patients with sickle cell disease and AIS should be exchange transfused with goal of hemoglobin S <30%. Hyperacute therapy with tissue plasminogen activator (tPA) has not been approved for pediatric use but can be considered with informed consent, particularly in the adolescent patient. The Thrombolysis in Pediatric Stroke (TIPS) study protocol can be used as a reference for tPA administration in children. Anticoagulation is reasonable if AIS is secondary to cardiac emboli or dissection. If anticoagulation is not indicated, then therapy with an antiplatelet agent is reasonable. Underlying infection or cardiac dysfunction should be treated. Avoid dehydration. Patients with a severely depressed mental status or significant cranial neuropathies may require intubation for airway protection. Patients with large hemispheric infarctions are at risk for malignant cerebral edema and early involvement of neurosurgery can be considered. However, the benefit of decompressive craniectomy in children with AIS is unclear and should be evaluated on a case-by-case basis. Early therapies should be initiated. If a child has facial or bulbar weakness, then a swallow evaluation must be done before allowing oral intake because of the high risk of silent aspiration.

C. **Cerebral venous sinus thrombosis (CVST).**

1. **Introduction.** Symptomatic CVST occurs in about 2.6 per 100,000 neonates per year and 0.4 to 0.7 per 100,000 children per year. Neonates may present with seizures or vague symptoms such as irritability, lethargy, or emesis. Older children may complain of headaches, vision changes, or focal neurologic symptoms. Seizures are common across all age groups. Important risk factors for CVST include dehydration, infection, iron deficiency anemia, cancer, medications (such as estrogen-containing contraceptives), acquired or congenital prothrombotic states, thyroid dysfunction, trauma, or rheumatologic disease. CVST may result in venous infarction, and intraventricular or intraparenchymal hemorrhage.

2. **Evaluation.** CNS imaging (usually CT or MR brain combined with venography) is required for diagnosis of a CVST. A complete blood count and baseline coagulation studies should be done. Careful review of the patient history, including their medication history, may reveal an obvious cause for the CVST. If the patient history does not reveal a predisposing factor for CVST, then a hypercoagulable evaluation should be done in the subacute setting. A careful visual examination, including a funduscopic examination and visual field testing, is important because of the risk of vision loss from increased ICP.

3. **Treatment.** Treatment of CVST with anticoagulation is reasonable. Antiplatelet therapy can be considered as an alternative therapy if anticoagulation is contraindicated. In refractory and symptomatic cases of CVST, endovascular intervention may be an option for treatment. Supportive care for CVST includes adequate hydration, treatment of seizures, and treatment of infection. If a patient has unrelenting headaches, visual symptoms, and/or papilledema, then a diagnostic and therapeutic LP is indicated to evaluate for increased ICP (similar to idiopathic intracranial hypertension). Highly symptomatic patients or those with visual changes may require ongoing therapy with acetazolamide.

ALTERED MENTAL STATUS/ENCEPHALOPATHY

Chapter 1 in this book presents a broad differential diagnosis for encephalopathy. The section below highlights common causes for altered mental status in children, particularly in the pediatric intensive care unit.

A. **Infectious meningitis and encephalitis.**

1. **Introduction.** A wide range of bacterial, parasitic, and viral infections can cause infectious meningitis and or encephalitis in children. With meningitis, parents usually have high fever, neck stiffness/"meningeal signs" and headaches. They may or may not have encephalopathy, whereas patients with encephalitis are invariably encephalopathic.

Common complications of CNS infection include empyema, arterial or venous infarctions, septic aneurysms, or seizures.

2. **Evaluation.** Diagnosis is usually established via LP. Opening pressure should be measured with the LP along with the typical studies (cell count, protein, glucose, bacterial culture). Polymerase chain reaction (PCR) testing for common bacteria, such as *Streptococcus Pneumoniae*, can be done if the patient received antibiotics before obtaining a CSF culture. Viral PCR testing also should be tailored to the patient. For encephalopathic patients, herpes simplex virus PCR and empiric treatment with acyclovir pending results should be considered especially if the child is immunosuppressed or has fulminant onset of temporal lobe seizures and encephalopathy. Immunosuppressed patients are at risk for atypical causes of CNS infection such as Cryptococcus or amebiasis and require more thorough laboratory testing than the otherwise healthy child. MRI brain with and without contrast can be done to evaluate for CNS injury or inflammation and acute cerebrovascular injury. For patients with waxing and waning mental status or those with profound encephalopathy, especially after a clinical seizure, consider continuous EEG monitoring for evaluation of nonconvulsive seizures.

3. **Treatment.** Start appropriate antimicrobials without delay. Antibiotics should not be withheld if CSF cannot be obtained in a timely fashion. Seizures should be aggressively treated. Dehydration should be avoided. See above for treatment of CVST. Septic emboli do not require anticoagulation; however, follow-up imaging should be done to look for development of an abscess or an aneurysm. Neuropsychological testing also may be helpful to facilitate return to school during the recovery phase.

B. **Posterior reversible encephalopathy syndrome (PRES).**

1. **Introduction.** PRES is a clinical and radiologic syndrome thought to be secondary to endothelial dysfunction and failure of the normal cerebrovascular autoregulation. Risk factors for PRES include hypertension or fluctuating blood pressures, immunosuppressive/ transplant medications, especially tacrolimus, cyclosporine, or high-dose steroids, bone marrow transplantation, renal failure, preeclampsia, and autoimmune disorders. Patients classically present with encephalopathy, changes in vision, and headaches over a period of hours to days. Seizures occur frequently in children with PRES. About 5% to 15% of patients have focal neurologic deficits depending upon the specific areas of the brain that are affected. Most patients recover completely but PRES is not always completely reversible.

2. **Evaluation.** Classically, the patient has bilateral subcortical white matter lesions with vasogenic edema "posteriorly" in the parietal and occipital lobes on CNS imaging. However, patients also may have frontal or temporal lobe, brainstem, cerebellar, or rarely spinal cord involvement. CT of the brain may show the characteristic areas of vasogenic edema but MRI brain more definitively shows the T2/FLAIR lesions. Some lesions may enhance with contrast. Up to a third of cases also may have areas of restricted diffusion on MRI. Repeat brain imaging should be considered if a patient with PRES acutely deteriorates because up to a quarter of patients will have ICH. Coagulation panels and a complete blood count should be done if the patient does have an ICH. LP can be considered if the clinical presentation also is concerning for infection, especially because many of the patients who are at risk for PRES are also at risk for opportunistic CNS infections. Continuous EEG monitoring should be strongly considered in patients with ongoing encephalopathy because of high prevalence of seizures (including nonconvulsive seizures) in patients with PRES.

3. **Treatment.** Primary treatment is control of blood pressure and discontinuation of the inciting drug if feasible. In general, if the patient has severe hypertension, then the blood pressure should be lowered only by about 25% in the first few hours; rapid or overly aggressive lowering of the blood pressure may result in cerebral ischemia. Supportive care should include seizure control and correction of coagulopathy in patients with an ICH. Patients with a severely depressed mental status may require intubation for airway protection.

C. **Methotrexate toxicity.**

1. **Introduction.** About 5 days to 2 weeks after treatment with high-dose methotrexate or intrathecal methotrexate, some patients develop acute encephalopathy along with headache, seizures, and/or stroke-like symptoms, such as a focal hemiparesis or aphasia.

Symptoms may develop slowly over hours and wax and wane. Patients usually recover within a week to a month. The pathophysiology of methotrexate toxicity is unclear but methotrexate-mediated release of adenosine has been implicated.

2. **Evaluation.** Given the broad differential diagnosis for encephalopathy, seizures, and new neurologic symptoms in immunosuppressed patients, consider doing an LP to evaluate for infection and an MRI brain with and without contrast. In a patient with stroke-like symptoms, the MRI brain with diffusion-weighted imaging must be done to rule out an acute cerebrovascular event. The MRI in patients with methotrexate toxicity may show areas of restricted diffusion in a nonvascular distribution. The centrum semiovale is frequently affected. There is no role for measurement of methotrexate levels.

3. **Treatment.** Most patients recover without any intervention. However, acutely, they may require supportive care including seizure control and/or airway support. Small case reports suggest that aminophylline (an adenosine antagonist), leucovorin, or dextromethorphan [N-methyl-D-aspartate (NMDA) receptor antagonist] may help with the encephalopathy. If the patient requires repeat treatment with methotrexate, then he is at risk for recurrent methotrexate toxicity and planned leucovorin rescue should be considered.

D. **Autoimmune encephalitis.**

1. **Introduction.** Patients with encephalitis present with altered mental status and possibly headaches, seizures, focal neurologic symptoms, and/or persistent low-grade fevers. Previously, a large number of cases of encephalitis did not have an identifiable infectious etiology; an estimated 63% of patients in the California encephalitis project did not have an infectious etiology. Over the last few decades, a number of immune-mediated encephalitides have been described that likely account for these "cryptogenic" cases of encephalitis. In adults, autoimmune encephalitis, especially limbic encephalitis, is frequently thought of as a paraneoplastic phenomenon. Most children do not have a clear trigger or identifiable reason as to why they developed autoimmune encephalitis. Patients can present with vague symptoms of encephalitis but a few of the antibody-mediated encephalitides have very well-defined clinical presentations. For instance, anti-NMDA receptor encephalitis presents with significant psychiatric features, memory problems, speech difficulties, dyskinesias (particularly orofacial), seizures, and autonomic instability.

2. **Evaluation.** Systemic inflammatory markers may be normal. LP may support the diagnosis of an autoimmune encephalopathy if there is a mild CSF pleocytosis (usually <100 white blood cells/μL) or elevated protein. MR brain also may show evidence of T2-weighted signal abnormalities in the temporal lobes, which supports a diagnosis of limbic encephalitis. Specific auto-antibodies, such as anti-NMDA, can be sent from the CSF and serum. Autoimmune antibody panels are commercially available via laboratories such as ARUP or Mayo Clinic. The significance in childhood disease of some of the known autoimmune antibodies, such as anti-glutamic acid decarboxylase antibodies or voltage-gated potassium channel antibodies, remains unclear; some studies have proposed that these antibodies may be markers of an immune-mediated process rather than the disease-causing antibody. Seizures are common in patients with autoimmune encephalitis, so consider EEG monitoring to rule out nonconvulsive seizures in persistently encephalopathic patients. Imaging to look for an occult malignancy (such as CT of the chest, abdomen, and pelvis or at least a pelvic ultrasound) is reasonable, especially in syndromes that may be paraneoplastic. If the patient has severe chorea and/or dystonia, then serial creatinine kinase (CK) levels should be followed because of the risk of rhabdomyolysis.

3. **Treatment.** First-line treatments include IVIG, a burst of high-dose steroids, or PLEX. Second-tier treatment is rituximab or cyclophosphamide. Patients may require ongoing immunotherapy after the initial episode resolves. Very little high-level data exist about the ideal treatment regimen and timing of immunosuppressive therapy in these patients. For patients with paraneoplastic syndromes, such as anti-NMDA receptor encephalitis caused by an ovarian teratoma, the underlying malignancy must be treated. Meanwhile, supportive care includes seizure control and atypical antipsychotic medications for patients with severe agitation/delirium. Patients with severe encephalopathy or refractory status epilepticus (RSE) may require intubation for airway protection. Many children with autoimmune encephalitis will require aggressive therapies and rehabilitation during the recovery phase.

E. **Hypoxic ischemic encephalopathy (HIE).**

1. **Introduction.** HIE is caused by a global decrease in oxygen to the brain. The extent and severity of injury depend upon the duration and severity of oxygen deprivation. Injury tends to be most severe in areas of the brain that have a high metabolic demand; thus, the deep gray matter is one of the first areas of the brain that is injured. The patient's neurologic deficits and prognosis depend upon the degree and location of CNS injury. HIE may lead to lifelong static encephalopathy, weakness and spasticity, and epilepsy. In more severe cases, patients develop paroxysmal autonomic instability and dystonia syndrome, which is quite challenging to control.

2. **Evaluation.** The extent of HIE is best characterized by MRI brain including diffusion-weighted imaging. MR spectroscopy is also a sensitive marker for mild brain injury in neonatal HIE. In neonates, metabolic disorders can mimic the MRI pattern of HIE so the newborn screen and patient must be carefully reviewed.

3. **Treatment.** Newborn infants over 35 weeks of age with perinatal asphyxia and evidence of encephalopathy (moderate to severe HIE) should be cooled. Eleven randomized control studies have shown that therapeutic hypothermia decreases death and neurodevelopmental disability from neonatal asphyxia. There is also level one data that hypothermia improves outcome after adult cardiopulmonary arrest, especially if due to ventricular fibrillation or tachycardia. However, current data does not support the routine use of therapeutic hypothermia in children after cardiac arrest. The recent Therapeutic Hypothermia After Out of Hospital Cardiac Arrest in Children study showed no benefit to cooling pediatric patients after cardiac arrest; notably, though, only 40% of patients in the cooling arm completed the protocol. General postarrest care focuses on prevention of secondary injury by aggressive control of seizures (including considering prolonged EEG monitoring for nonconvulsive seizures), airway/ventilator support as needed, and avoidance of fever, hypoxia, hypotension, or hyponatremia. There is no data to support use of steroids, ICP monitoring, strict ICP-driven management, or decompressive craniectomy in pediatric HIE.

F. **Acute liver failure (ALF) and neurologic sequelae.**

1. **Introduction.** Hepatic encephalopathy from ALF is characterized by changes in personality, sleep, concentration, asterixis, or ultimately coma. Patients may develop severe cerebral edema and ultimately herniation. The pathophysiology of hepatic encephalopathy is not fully understand but may be related to microglia-driven inflammation and hyperammonemia-induced increase in glutamine production in astrocytes. With severe hepatic encephalopathy, cerebral autoregulation fails and contributes to the development of cerebral edema. Patients with ALF are also at risk for life-threatening ICH because of inadequate synthesis of coagulation factors.

2. **Evaluation.** The West Haven classification system is used to grade the severity of hepatic encephalopathy. The scale ranges from Grade 0 (subtle changes in memory, concentration, intelligence, and coordination) to Grade 5 (coma). An ammonia level should be sent; however, the absolute value does not strictly correlate with the degree of encephalopathy. Head CT should be considered in patients with significant or worsening encephalopathy to look for cerebral edema. Abrupt worsening in the neurologic exam, new seizures, and/or severe headaches also should trigger imaging to look for an ICH. EEG may be helpful to establish a patient's baseline EEG background and can be followed serially to look for worsening signs of encephalopathy. Investigation for the cause of ALF is usually driven by the Hepatology Service but a thorough neurologic history and examination may point toward testing that is not routinely done. For instance, consider testing for the polymerase gamma mutation in a patient with a prior history of seizures, myoclonus, cognitive impairment, and new-onset ALF.

3. **Treatment.** The definitive treatment for hepatic encephalopathy is recovery of liver function, which may require liver transplantation. While liver function is being addressed, lactulose can be used to help lower the ammonia levels but this medication only works if the patient is stooling. Hemodialysis may be required for ammonia clearance; however, in patients with hepatorenal syndrome, blood urea nitrogen should be lowered slowly to avoid an abrupt decrease in serum osmolality and worsening of cerebral edema. See above regarding management of ICH.

MOVEMENT DISORDERS

The differential diagnosis of patients with movement disorders includes hyperkinetic movements (Chapter 28), hypokinetic movements (Chapter 30), or ataxia (Chapter 29). We have selected a few key pediatric movement disorders that must be quickly recognized because delay in treatment can lead to significant morbidity and mortality.

A. Opsoclonus myoclonus syndrome (OMS).
  1. Introduction. OMS or "dancing eyes" syndrome is an autoimmune movement disorder typically characterized by ataxia, myoclonus, opsoclonus, and behavioral changes (Video 38.1). The onset of symptoms may be acute or subacute. The most common age of onset is 2 years. Prompt diagnosis of OMS is important because there is a strong association between OMS and neuroblastoma (NB). The reported percentage of patients with children with OMS and NB varies widely in the literature from 2% to 3% to 100%. Approximately 2% to 3% of children with an NB develop OMS. The minority of patients will recover completely with treatment. However, the majority of patients have lasting motor and cognitive disabilities despite aggressive immunomodulatory treatment.

  2. Evaluation. The diagnosis is made clinically. A proposed international definition for OMS requires a patient to have at least three of the following: (1) myoclonus and/or ataxia; (2) opsoclonus or ocular flutter; (3) behavioral and/or sleep disturbance; and (4) NB. However, once the diagnosis of OMS is made, the patient needs a thorough evaluation for an occult NB including MRI or CT scan of the chest, abdomen, and pelvis and measurement of urine catecholamines. If these studies are not fruitful, then a radiolabeled iodine scintigraphy scan should be considered.

  3. Treatment. Oncology should be consulted for management if the patient is found to have an NB and some patients may improve with treatment of the NB alone. However, many patients require immunomodulatory treatment. The literature does not support one specific regimen. Patients can be treated with steroids (e.g., prednisone or prednisolone, dexamethasone, or adrenocorticotropic hormone). Alternatively, steroid-sparing regimens with IVIG, azathioprine, rituximab, or cyclophosphamide are options.

B. Baclofen withdrawal.
  1. Introduction. Baclofen is used frequently to treat spasticity, either orally or via an intrathecal pump. Intrathecal delivery of the drug is much more potent. Unfortunately, mechanical problems with the pump or failure to refill the reservoir may disrupt intrathecal administration of the drug. Abrupt withdrawal of baclofen can be fatal and is characterized by increased spasticity, hyperthermia, agitation, or loss of consciousness. Eventually, patients develop rhabdomyolysis, seizures, metabolic acidosis, hypotension, arrhythmias, and ultimately death.

  2. Evaluation. The signs and symptoms of baclofen withdrawal mimic septic shock, which is a much more common diagnosis; thus, the first step toward effective treatment is consideration of the diagnosis. The baclofen pump should be interrogated to look for any anomalies in drug delivery and to ensure that the reservoir is not dry. Plain films should be done to look for fractures or displacement of the catheter. If these first two steps are not helpful and baclofen withdrawal is suspected, then a dye study can be done to further investigate the catheter. Serial CK levels need to be followed given the risk of rhabdomyolysis. For severe cases, chemistries/renal function and urine output must be followed and patients require close temperature and cardiovascular monitoring.

  3. Treatment. As soon as a diagnosis is made, the problem with drug delivery should be corrected urgently. In the interim, fevers should be aggressively managed with antipyretics and external cooling devices. Insensible fluid losses are high so patients may need aggressive fluid resuscitation, especially if CK is elevated. If intrathecal drug delivery cannot be reestablished quickly, then high-dose systemic baclofen, diazepam, or other benzodiazepines such as a midazoalam drip may blunt the withdrawal. Much higher doses of enteral baclofen is needed to achieve the same effect and also will have more systemic side effects. Case reports also suggest that dantrolene might be an effective treatment.

C. Status dystonicus.
   1. Introduction. Status dystonicus is an uncommon movement disorder emergency but it can lead to significant morbidity and mortality if it is not quickly recognized and treated. As the name implies, status dystonicus is development of severe and unrelenting dystonia. Similar to baclofen withdrawal, which is discussed above, patients can develop severe hyperthermia, dehydration, and rhabdomyolysis with resulting metabolic acidosis, acute renal failure, and electrolyte derangements, especially life-threatening hyperkalemia. Dystonia of the respiratory muscles can lead to respiratory failure. Status dystonicus may occur secondary to an exacerbation of a patient's baseline dystonia triggered by pain, stress, or infection. Certain medications, such as dopamine antagonists, also may trigger an attack. Patients with aristaless homeobox (ARX) gene mutations seem to be particularly prone to developing recurrent episodes of status dystonicus.
   2. Evaluation. Diagnosis is made clinically. Mimickers such as malignant hyperthermia, baclofen withdrawal, or neuroleptic malignant syndrome should be considered, although therapy is similar for many of these diagnoses. Temperature and vital signs must be carefully monitored. Blood gas, chemistries (including renal function), and CK should be carefully followed. Because of the risk of acute renal failure, urine output also should be monitored carefully.
   3. Treatment. If the patient is having increasing dystonia but is not yet in status, then analgesic and sedation medications should be trialed. Chloral hydrate may help the patient sleep and break the cycle of dystonia. Benzodiazepines also have been reported to be efficacious. Clonidine, which is an alpha agonist, is an option for treatment, particularly if the patient has significant hypertension and tachycardia. If a trigger can be identified, such as a source of pain, then it should be eliminated. If severe hyperthermia, metabolic derangements, or rhabdomyolysis already have begun, then patients must be treated quickly and aggressively and should be monitored in a critical care setting. Patients with dystonia of the neck or respiratory muscle may require intubation because of upper airway obstruction. Aggressive rehydration, antipyretics, and mechanical cooling should be initiated. If frequent intermittent doses of sedation/pain medication are not effective, then continuous infusions of medication, such as midazolam or dexmedtomidine, should be initiated and elective intubation may be required. Propofol has been used in adults but prolonged infusions should not be used in children because of the increased risk of propofol infusion syndrome. If continuous sedative medications fail to control the life-threatening symptoms, then the next step is paralysis. Once temporizing measures are in place, long-term dystonia-specific interventions can be started that will help reverse the process. Trihexyphenidyl, baclofen, gabapentin, and tetrabenazine are some pharmacologic options. Ultimately for severe, refractory cases, invasive interventions such as intrathecal baclofen pump placement, deep brain stimulation, and/or pallidotomy may be necessary.

EPILEPSY

There are several types of epilepsy that require urgent recognition, such as infantile spasms, in children. These are described in detail elsewhere in this book. We would refer the reader to Chapter 42.

A. RSE or super-refractory status epilepticus.
   1. Introduction. RSE describes ongoing seizure activity despite administration of two or three appropriate drugs. As the seizure continues, it becomes less responsive to drugs, likely due to internalization of gamma amino-butyric acid receptors and upregulation of NMDA receptors. Prolonged seizures eventually result in cerebral injury and potentially cerebral edema. Unchecked status epilepticus also has direct detrimental effects on multiple organ systems including the cardiac and respiratory systems. Recent data suggest that a higher seizure burden in critically ill children is associated with worse outcomes even after controlling for severity of illness. Thus, RSE is a true neurologic emergency.
   2. Evaluation. For a child with no prior history of seizures, one must ensure that reversible causes of seizures, such as hyponatremia, hypoglycemia, or hypocalcemia, are ruled out or effectively treated. After reversible causes of status epilepticus are eliminated, the

evaluation for an underlying cause for new-onset seizure/status epilepticus is guided by individual patient characteristics. Continuous EEG monitoring is important for ongoing management of RSE. Over time, clinical monitoring for seizures becomes less reliable because patients develop electroclinical dissociation. Adult studies have shown that there is a high incidence of nonconvulsive seizures after convulsive status epilepticus; smaller studies suggest that this phenomenon also occurs in children.

3. Treatment. The goal of treatment can be either cessation of electrical evidence of seizures or achieving suppression burst pattern on EEG. RSE treatment requires timely administration of antiepileptics and rapid escalation to continuous infusions of medication. Most patients need blood pressure and respiratory support as medications are titrated upwards so these children should be monitored in a critical care setting. Multiple different treatment pathways exist. Second-line medications after benzodiazepines include fosphenytoin or phenytoin, valproic acid, levetiracetam, phenobarbital, and lacosamide. Third-line medications are generally continuous infusions such as midazolam, pentobarbital, ketamine, or inhaled anesthetics. A trial of pyridoxine should be considered in neonates. Hypothermia is being studied as a possible therapy for super-refractory status epilepticus but is not a well-established treatment. A proposed algorithm for management of adult generalized status epilepticus can be found in Chapter 63. Of note, though, propofol is frequently used in adults but should not be routinely used in children because of the increased risk of propofol infusion syndrome. Once seizure control or suppression burst is achieved, general practice is to allow 24 to 48 hours of "brain rest" before attempting to wean the continuous infusions.

Key Points

- Although the manifestations and etiology of cerebrovascular dysfunction in children differ from those of adults, vascular lesions are far more common among children than once suspected. Prompt diagnosis and treatment of these children can minimize the likelihood of recurrent stroke and promote functional recovery.
- Immune-mediated encephalopathies often lead to devastating, sometimes permanent, neurologic dysfunction. In contrast to adults with these conditions, underlying malignancy is relatively uncommon among children with immune-mediated encephalopathy. Immunomodulation with IVIG, burst of high-dose steroids, PLEX, or other therapies is often effective.
- Therapeutic hypothermia minimizes the severity of permanent neurologic impairment in neonates with hypoxia and ischemia, but there is no evidence that hypothermia offers the same benefit in older children.
- It is important to recognize opsoclonus in children, because it often constitutes a paraneoplastic syndrome. The most common underlying tumor in children with opsoclonus is NB, and recognition of the opsoclonus in these individuals often initiates a systematic search for the tumor and earlier removal. In some instances, opsoclonus may improve following tumor removal, while other children require immune modulation therapy in addition.
- Children with acute or rapidly progressive neuromuscular weakness from whatever cause are at high risk for respiratory failure and may need to be intubated because of respiratory muscle weakness and/or loss of an effective cough and gag. It is preferable to anticipate this problem and electively intubate rather than awaiting the occurrence of frank respiratory failure.

Recommended Readings

Abend NS, Dlugos DJ. Treatment of refractory status epilepticus: literature review and a proposed protocol. *Pediatr Neurol.* 2008;38(6):377–390.

Afshar M, Birnbaum D, Golden C. Review of dextromethorphan administration in 18 patients with subacute methotrexate central nervous system toxicity. *Pediatr Neurol.* 2014;50(6):625–629.

Alderliesten T, de Vries LS, Benders MJ, et al. MR imaging and outcome of term neonates with perinatal asphyxia: value of diffusion-weighted MR imaging and ^{1}H MR spectroscopy. *Radiology.* 2011;261(1):235–242.

Allen NM, Lin JP, Lynch T, et al. Status dystonicus: a practice guide. *Dev Med Child Neurol.* 2014;56(2):105–112.

Amlie-Lefond C, Chan AK, Kirton A, et al. Thrombolysis in acute childhood stroke: design and challenges of the thrombolysis in pediatric stroke clinical trial. *Neuroepidemiology.* 2009;32(4):279–286.

Armangue T, Leypoldt F, Dalmau J. Autoimmune encephalitis as differential diagnosis of infectious encephalitis. *Curr Opin Neurol.* 2014;27(3):361–368.

Armangue T, Petit-Pedrol M, Dalmau J. Autoimmune encephalitis in children. *J Child Neurol.* 2012;27(11):1460–1469.

Arnon SS, Schechter R, Maslanka SE, et al. Human botulism immune globulin for the treatment of infant botulism. *N Engl J Med.* 2006;354(5):462–471.

Arya R, Gulati S, Deopujari S. Management of hepatic encephalopathy in children. *Postgrad Med J.* 2010;86(1011):34–41; quiz 40.

Chevret L, Durand P, Lambert J, et al. High-volume hemofiltration in children with acute liver failure*. *Pediatr Crit Care Med.* 2014;15(7):e300–e305.

Coffey RJ, Edgar TS, Francisco GE, et al. Abrupt withdrawal from intrathecal baclofen: recognition and management of a potentially life-threatening syndrome. *Arch Phys Med Rehabil.* 2002;83(6):735–741.

Coffey RJ, Ridgely PM. Abrupt intrathecal baclofen withdrawal: management of potentially life-threatening sequelae. *Neuromodulation.* 2001;4(4):142–146.

Dale RC, de Sousa C, Chong WK, et al. Acute disseminated encephalomyelitis, multiphasic disseminated encephalomyelitis and multiple sclerosis in children. *Brain.* 2000;123(pt 12):2407–2422.

Defresne P, Hollenberg H, Husson B, et al. Acute transverse myelitis in children: clinical course and prognostic factors. *J Child Neurol.* 2003;18(6):401–406.

Fokke C, van den Berg B, Drenthen J, et al. Diagnosis of Guillain-Barré syndrome and validation of Brighton criteria. *Brain.* 2014;137(pt 1):33–43.

Green LB, Nelson VS. Death after acute withdrawal of intrathecal baclofen: case report and literature review. *Arch Phys Med Rehabil.* 1999;80(12):1600–1604.

Hacohen Y, Singh R, Rossi M, et al. Clinical relevance of voltage-gated potassium channel–complex antibodies in children. *Neurology.* 2015;85(11):967–975.

Hacohen Y, Wright S, Waters P, et al. Pediatric autoimmune encephalopathies: clinical features, laboratory investigations and outcomes in patients with or without antibodies to known central nervous system autoantigens. *J Neurol Neurosurg Psychiatry.* 2013;84(7):748–755.

Hughes RA, Swan AV, van Doorn PA. Intravenous immunoglobulin for Guillain-Barré syndrome. *Cochrane Database Syst Rev.* 2014;9:CD002063.

Hynson JL, Kornberg AJ, Coleman LT, et al. Clinical and neuroradiologic features of acute disseminated encephalomyelitis in children. *Neurology.* 2001;56(10):1308–1312.

Inaba H, Khan RB, Laningham FH, et al. Clinical and radiological characteristics of methotrexate-induced acute encephalopathy in pediatric patients with cancer. *Ann Oncol.* 2008;19(1):178–184.

Jacobs SE, Berg M, Hunt R, et al. Cooling for newborns with hypoxic ischaemic encephalopathy. *Cochrane Database Syst Rev.* 2013;1:CD003311.

Jones CT. Childhood autoimmune neurologic diseases of the central nervous system. *Neurol Clin.* 2003;21(4):745–764.

Juel VC. Myasthenia gravis: management of myasthenic crisis and perioperative care. *Semin Neurol.* 2004;24(1):75–81.

Kellie SJ, Chaku J, Lockwood LR, et al. Late magnetic resonance imaging features of leukoencephalopathy in children with central nervous system tumors following high-dose methotrexate and neuraxis radiation therapy. *Eur J Cancer.* 2005;41(11):1588–1596.

Li Y, Gor D, Walicki D, et al. Spectrum and potential pathogenesis of reversible posterior leukoencephalopathy syndrome. *J Stroke Cerebrovasc Dis.* 2012;21(8):873–882.

Miyazawa R, Hikima A, Takano Y, et al. Plasmapheresis in fulminant acute disseminated encephalomyelitis. *Brain Dev.* 2001;23(6):424–426.

Moler FW, Silverstein FS, Holubkov R, et al. Therapeutic hypothermia after out-of-hospital cardiac arrest in children. *N Engl J Med.* 2015;372(20):1898–1908.

Nachulewicz P, Kaminski A, Kaliciński P, et al. Analysis of neurological complications in children transplanted due to fulminant liver failure. *Transplant Proc.* 2006;38(1):253–254.

Pang KK, de Sousa C, Lang B, et al. A prospective study of the presentation and management of dancing eye syndrome/opsoclonus-myoclonus syndrome in the United Kingdom. *Eur J Paediatr Neurol.* 2010;14(2):156–161.

Patwa HS, Chaudhry V, Katzberg H, et al. Evidence-based guideline: intravenous immunoglobulin in the treatment of neuromuscular disorders: report of the Therapeutics and Technology Assessment Subcommittee of the American Academy of Neurology. *Neurology.* 2012;78(13):1009–1015.

Pranzatelli MR, Tate ED, Travelstead AL, et al. Immunologic and clinical responses to rituximab in a child with opsoclonus-myoclonus syndrome. *Pediatrics.* 2005;115(1):e115–e119.

Pranzatelli MR, Tate ED, Travelstead AL, et al. Insights on chronic-relapsing opsoclonus-myoclonus from a pilot study of mycophenolate mofetil. *J Child Neurol.* 2009;24(3):316–322.

Qureshi AI, Choudhry MA, Akbar MS, et al. Plasma exchange versus intravenous immunoglobulin treatment in myasthenic crisis. *Neurology.* 1999;52(3):629–632.

Rabinstein AA, Wijdicks EF. Warning signs of imminent respiratory failure in neurological patients. *Semin Neurol.* 2003;23(1):97–104.

Raj S, Overby P, Erdfarb A, et al. Posterior reversible encephalopathy syndrome: incidence and associated factors in a pediatric critical care population. *Pediatr Neurol.* 2013;49(5):335–339.

Rao S, Elkon B, Flett KB, et al. Long-term outcomes and risk factors associated with acute encephalitis in children. *J Pediatric Infect Dis Soc.* 2015;pii:piv075.

Roach ES, Golomb MR, Adams R, et al. Management of stroke in infants and children: a scientific statement from a Special Writing Group of the American Heart Association Stroke Council and the Council on Cardiovascular Disease in the Young. *Stroke.* 2008;39(9):2644–2691.

Roodbol J, de Wit MC, Aarsen FK, et al. Long-term outcome of Guillain-Barré syndrome in children. *J Peripher Nerv Syst.* 2014;19(2):121–126.

Rosow LK, Strober JB. Infant botulism: review and clinical update. *Pediatr Neurol.* 2015;52(5):487–492.

Sahlas DJ, Miller SP, Guerin M, et al. Treatment of acute disseminated encephalomyelitis with intravenous immunoglobulin. *Neurology.* 2000;54(6):1370–1372.

Sébire G, Tabarki B, Saunders DE, et al. Cerebral venous sinus thrombosis in children: risk factors, presentation, diagnosis and outcome. *Brain.* 2005;128(pt 3):477–489.

Suleiman J, Brilot F, Lang B, et al. Autoimmune epilepsy in children: case series and proposed guidelines for identification. *Epilepsia.* 2013;54(6):1036–1045.

Suleiman J, Dale RC. The recognition and treatment of autoimmune epilepsy in children. *Dev Med Child Neurol.* 2015;57(5):431–440.

Tan WF, Steadman RH, Farmer DG, et al. Pretransplant neurological presentation and severe posttransplant brain injury in patients with acute liver failure. *Transplantation.* 2012;94(7):768–774.

Winick NJ, Bowman WP, Kamen BA, et al. Unexpected acute neurologic toxicity in the treatment of children with acute lymphoblastic leukemia. *J Natl Cancer Inst.* 1992;84(4):252–256.

39 Approach to Ethical Issues in Neurology

Bhupendra O. Khatri and Michael P. McQuillen

Neurologists deal with ethical issues, far more than other medical specialists do. Rapidly advancing neuroscience research and therapies bring ethical implications to the forefront. Today's neurologist has to embrace the science of ethics as well as stay in sync with emerging technologies, third-party healthcare payers, genetic modifications, and government regulatory laws, while keeping their patient's best interests in mind.

ETHICS IN THE 21ST CENTURY

Major forces that determined the shape of ethics in the last century have changed. For example, conflict of interest in medicine and the passage of the Sunshine Act (in 2010 as part of the Affordable Care Act) require applicable manufacturers of covered drugs, devices, biologicals, and medical supplies to report annually all payments and other transfers of value to physicians and teaching hospitals; these matters require some discussion. Transparency in science is necessary, but the restrictions imposed by the Sunshine Act may deter physicians from working closely with industry to bring new drugs and devices to market. The 21st century also ushered in many changes in the way medicine is practiced. The cost of health care has risen drastically over the past few decades. Hospitals and healthcare systems are rapidly buying up physician practices, nationally. These organizations control every aspect of the medical pipeline, dictating which tests and procedures to perform; how much to charge; and which patients to admit. Insurance carriers are canceling contracts with physicians deemed "financial drainers." "Independent" physician practices are becoming rare. A fundamental question is whether today's physicians are able to practice in an ethical manner without being coerced by so many external forces that control them. The medical fiduciary role that physicians once held is now controlled by other parties. Should third-party payers, healthcare systems, and legislatures also be regulated for conflicts of interest in medicine? Should they be the ethical guardians of health care? To answer these questions, let us first look at the history of clinical ethics.

HISTORICAL BACKGROUND AND IMPLICATIONS OF CLINICAL ETHICS

Clinical ethics—The business of being human in the interchange between physician and patient has been an integral part of that interchange for as long as there has been a profession of medicine. Until the past several decades, however, it was assumed that being a physician meant being ethical; that everyone's ethics were the same (or at least of equivalent worth); and that there was no underlying theory or set of standards necessary for ethical decision making. In part, this state of affairs was a reflection of the simplicity of life in general, and of medicine in particular. With advances in technology, more options became possible—options to evaluate new forms of treatment (clinical research) as well as to utilize proven diagnostic and therapeutic modalities (with their inherent risk–benefit calculus). In today's world, questions of *who* should make *which* decisions in *what* circumstances, as well as who could and should *pay* for the costs of implementing those decisions are being asked. As these changes have taken place, particular judgments no longer stood in isolation, but rather led to the formulation of rules that could govern in similar situations; a recognition of the **principles** upon which such rules might be based; and the development of **theories** underlying the principles—much as an understanding of anatomy, biochemistry, pathophysiology, and other basic sciences made it possible to clarify approaches to the complicated medical problems of stroke (for example). Some theorists appealed directly to **conscience,** developed and refined in reflection on individual cases without the formality of the process just described. Underlying it all, however, was the realization that ethical problems arise in almost any clinical situation, and that such problems should be addressed just as systematically as any dimension of the given clinical situation. This realization called forth a new academic discipline (**biomedical** or **clinical ethics**) out of what previously had been purely philosophical and, in a sense, impractical thought (**theoretical ethics**). From this generic discipline, there has evolved a particular focus on neurologic ethical dilemmas (**neuroethics).**

In reality and from the start, the discipline of ethics found fertile ground in neurology, where ethical theory met real-life problems such as **brain death;** the **vegetative state** and other conditions of incapacity; **neurogenetic diseases;** and a whole gamut of **issues at the end of life.** More recently, questions relating to **neuroenhancement, stem cell research,** and other matters have been added to the stew. Early on, this meeting generated encounters with the law and the recognition that what is ethical may not be legal, and *vice versa.* To plow the field, one must first understand the background of ethical theories; develop a structured approach to the recognition and solution of ethical problems; and understand how that approach helps to deal with particular problems, as well as developing an effective interface with the law.

ETHICAL THEORIES

Before accepting any ethical theory as a basis upon which practical judgments can be made, ultimately and validly, one should inquire as to whether the basis of theory is adequate to the task by virtue of its satisfying certain criteria, and then look to the basis of the theory to determine its usefulness and applicability. No one theory satisfies every clinical situation. Some are better adapted to one circumstance and others to another, while yet additional circumstances demand a hybrid of complementing theories.

A. Criteria of an adequate theory. Beauchamp and Childress set forth a series of questions that should be answered in the affirmative with regard to any particular theory, if that theory is to be regarded as adequate and helpful in a given clinical situation. Their questions are as follows:

1. Is it clear? Or is the language by which the theory is formulated so complex as to muddle the situation?

2. Is it coherent? Coherence is a necessary (although not sufficient) criterion of an adequate theory. It is missing when theory elements are in contradiction, one with another.

3. Is it complete, or at least comprehensive? Does the theory deal with all of the major questions raised in diverse clinical circumstances, or are there serious concerns on which the theory is silent?

4. Is it simple? Are there enough norms so that the theory can be used without confusion by clinicians, or are there so many that the answer becomes lost in practice?

5. Can it explain and justify the conclusions reached with its help? Or does it simply set forth in other words a preexistent, intuitive belief?

6. Does it yield new insights? Or does it only serve to repeat old convictions?

7. Is it practical? In short, does it provide a useful answer to the clinical problem or one that is attractive in theory only?

B. Types of ethical theory.

1. Utilitarianism. This theory looks to the **consequences** of acts and holds that an action is good if it produces more benefit than harm. It is the basis of the **risk–benefit analysis,** regularly used by clinicians in deciding and discussing with patients a recommended course of action in a given clinical circumstance. Problems arise when one looks for definitions of *risk* of harm and *benefit* (to or for whom?); to the relation between the individual acting or deciding and the society of which that individual is a member; and at single actions, each in isolation, or at classes of actions governed by rules that appeal to the principle of utility.

2. Obligation-based theory. The test of this theory is the **categorical imperative** of Immanuel Kant: the reason for an action should apply to everyone, and in all situations; moral rules are absolute. Problems arise when such rules—often abstract and legalistic, rather than relational—are found to be in conflict with each other in a particular circumstance.

3. Virtue-based, or character, ethics. This approach looks to the person acting and to the motives and desires that propel that person's actions. Because even the most virtuous person can act wrongly—even for the best of reasons—a viable ethical theory cannot rest on character alone.

4. Rights-based ethics, or liberal individualism. Rights are justified claims that an individual or group is entitled to make upon a society at large. Such claims, while protecting the interests of an individual, at the same time may impose a corresponding obligation upon others. Rights may be *positive* (requiring an action by others) or *negative* (precluding such action). Overemphasis on rights may neglect the legitimate demands of the society at large.

5. Communitarian ethics. Rather than the rights of the individual, communitarians look to the needs of society at large. Although different communitarians may state the needs of society in different ways, an overemphasis on this aspect of morality may neglect the legitimate interests of individuals in that society.

6. An ethics of care. Sometimes referred to as **feminist** ethics, the focus of this approach is on a caring, attached relationship between persons and on the implications of such a relationship. Impartiality and balance may suffer as a consequence, the result being a less complete and practical system than obtained with other theories.

7. Casuistry. This term invokes an image of Jesuitical sophistry, but really refers to the need to make decisions according to the particulars of any given situation. In reality, it was St. Thomas Aquinas who first described "situation ethics," a much (and properly) maligned theory when reduced to the proposition that all morality is relative, dependent *solely* on the circumstances of an action. Every detail of the case is examined and weighed, and a judgment reached, often by analogy to similar cases. The connection between cases provides a maxim to rule the case—but which maxim is given most credence in any particular situation, and why?

8. Ethics based on principles, or "common morality." A "bottom up" approach to validating particular judgments looks to rules that govern such judgments, and from rules to the principles from which they are derived. Four such principles are woven into "commonsense" morality—an ethics that grows out of the nature of human beings, one that is simply put as "do good and avoid evil." The principles in question are as follows:

   a. Respect for the autonomous choices of other persons (**autonomy**)
   b. The obligation not to inflict harm intentionally (**nonmaleficence**)
   c. Actions taken for the benefit of others (**beneficence**)
   d. A fair, equitable, and appropriate distribution of goods in society (**justice**).

   Critics of the principlist approach refer to its elements as a mantra (specifically, the *Georgetown Mantra*, because its authors—Robert Beauchamp and James Childers—were at Georgetown University when they articulated it) without substance; one that does not offer a schema for resolving conflict when more than one principle applies; a ritualistic incantation without a unifying, overriding theory to govern its use. When all is said and done, similar objections can be leveled against *any* ethical theory. The heart of the matter is to recognize the (ethical) problem and to admit with honesty which approach to solving it is used and why. In today's medical climate, however—when physicians have become *providers*, patients are now *clients*, and *any* cost is a *medical loss* to the insurance company (or governmental agency) that funds a *managed care* plan (see Section **C** under Ethical Decision Making in General)—*any* of these theories, meant to guide ethical decision making in the practice of medicine, comes in conflict with the principles of *business* ethics. Those for whom the principles of business ethics are paramount have a primary fiduciary duty to the providers of capital—taxpayers, investors, and society at large—whose goals may be vastly different than those of traditional medicine. In a certain sense, the principle of justice comes to the fore in resolving these conflicts. Practical solutions (see Section **C** under Ethical Decision Making in General) that preserve the essentials of the theory on which the physician's judgment and actions are based in any particular situation must be sought as a way out of such dilemmas.

Case Method Approach to Clinical Ethics

John Fletcher and his associates developed a *case method approach* to the recognition and solution of ethical dilemmas that mimics standard decision making in medicine. The elements of the method are as follows:

A. Assessment. What is the nature of the medical problem and the relevant context in which that problem occurs? What are the options for therapy, their foreseeable risks and benefits, their short- and long-term prognoses, and the costs and resources (or mechanisms for payment) that are available? What do the patient, family, and surrogate decision makers *want*? What does the patient *need*, and what other needs may compete with that need? Are there any institutional, societal, or legal factors impinging on the patient or problem? What are the ethnic, cultural, and religious backgrounds from which the problems have arisen?

B. Identification of ethical problem(s). Which ethical problems, ranked in order of importance, are self-evident, and which are hidden? Which ethical theories are most relevant to such problems? Are there analogous cases in medicine or law—and, if so, how do they apply? Which guidelines are most appropriate?

C. Decision making and implementation. What are the ethically acceptable options for solving the problems, and which are *most* acceptable? What justifications can be given for the preferred resolution of the problems? How can the preferred resolutions of the problem be accomplished? Is ethics consultation necessary or desirable? Is judicial review necessary or desirable?

D. Evaluation. This is an ongoing process that seeks to recognize missed opportunities and correct unworkable solutions. The process carries a preventive dimension that may propose changes in policy or provide educational opportunities to minimize the chance that similar problems will occur.

Ethical Decision Making in General

At the heart of any interaction between physician and patient is the matter of *who* decides *what* shall be done *when*. The physician brings to this interaction experience, knowledge, skill, and a set of personal values that may or may not be the same as, or even compatible with, those of the patient. In years past, the physician's judgment ruled supreme. Today, that judgment is tempered not only by a primacy of respect for the wishes of the patient, but also by the rules and regulations of various healthcare plans as well as by statutory and case law.

A. The primacy of the patient. A competent patient with the capacity for decision making can and should decide—even before the fact, anticipating the future through **advance directives** [e.g., a "living will" and a durable power of attorney for healthcare decisions ("health care proxies")]. Because many neurologic illnesses are chronic and inexorably disabling, often leaving the person without the capacity to decide, it is wise to introduce discussion of advance directives early in the course of caring for such a patient. Indeed, federal directives now *require* patients to be asked, on admission to hospital, whether they have executed, or wish to execute, an advance directive. A **bond of trust** should first be established, so that the patient does not interpret such discussions as a plan to abandon them at the end of life—an element of ethical decision making missing from the federal requirement. It is important to emphasize that decisions may change as a situation evolves.

B. Surrogate decision making. When capacity is lost, surrogates may be called upon to decide for the patient. Unless previously identified and appointed (in a healthcare proxy), the appropriate surrogate may be selected according to a hierarchy spelled out in state law. In extreme circumstances, a court-appointed surrogate may be necessary. Surrogates may strive to determine what the patient would have wanted (**substituted judgment standard**) or may try to decide what is best for the patient (**best interests standard**). The former standard is generally thought to be better, avoiding as it does conclusions made by one person (the surrogate) about another's (the patient's) "quality of life." Courts may require "clear and convincing evidence" of what it is the patient would have wanted under the circumstances in question. However, because such a scenario rarely exists in fact, and people often change their minds, requirements of this sort are most impractical. In all instances, it is wise to seek consensus and to continue to act in favor of life until that consensus is reached. It may take time to develop consensus, even when a surrogate has previously been appointed, especially when capacity is lost suddenly and without warning (e.g., after stroke). Physicians should be sensitive to the possibility of ulterior motives on the part of surrogates, fiscal, or otherwise.

C. **"Managed care" plans.** The spiraling cost of health care, among many contributing factors, has fueled an ongoing process of "healthcare reform"—much of which is basically about money. Because an immediate effect of healthcare decisions is the expenditure of money, a feature common to many proposals for such reform is a process requiring approval before decisions can be implemented. Sometimes the process has at its center a "gatekeeper"—often a primary care physician, who may be guided by situation-specific protocols. The rewards built into the system are keys to its ethical dimension. Under traditional fee-for-service medicine, the more a physician did, the more that physician was paid. Often under "managed care," the *less* a physician does, the *more* that physician is paid. The concept of "managed care" emphasizes the physician's obligation to *all* patients covered by a given plan—indeed, to society at large (i.e., putting the principle of **justice** foremost). If a physician hews to the primacy of the patient (the principle of **autonomy**) as the guiding principle in ethical decision making (see Section **A** under Ethical Decision Making in General), *any* decision suggested by a physician and made by a patient should be made in the particular *patient's* best interest. No tests should be done and no treatment instituted, without that interest in the forefront of the physician's mind. If the system stands in the way of such decisions, physicians should oppose the system on behalf of their patients, vigorously—but fairly as well, not "gaming" the system with fabrications and the like. "Managed care" plans that reward physicians with incentives that limit or compromise care (e.g., by restricting the time that can be spent with a patient; denying access to appropriate consultants; requiring the use of generic drugs when they may be less effective or more toxic; and the like) should be avoided.

To guide the physician through this narrow maze of ever-diminishing resources at a time of ever more complex and expensive options for diagnosis and therapy, the field of **evidence-based medicine** has developed. **Practice guidelines, critical pathways,** and similar approaches are being articulated from a wide range of sources. Physicians are well advised to listen to and follow such approaches *unless* the approach is of the *gobsat* ("**g**ood **o**ld **b**oys **s**itting **a**round a **t**able") variety.

APPROACHES TO PARTICULAR PROBLEMS

A. **"Brain death."** An unwanted consequence of the development of more effective intensive care was the recognition that patients whose brains had suffered complete and irreversible loss of all brain function could continue to manifest adequate cardiovascular, renal, and gastrointestinal functions, as long as pulmonary function was supported by a ventilator. The *presence* of death—previously identified by the absence of heart action and breathing—could no longer be affirmed in such patients. This state of affairs called for the development of a new set of *criteria* by which the *presence* of death could be recognized—**not** for a new *definition* of death. Once those criteria are satisfied, the patient **is** dead—an unsettling conclusion for many to whom a warm body with a strong pulse and a chest moving in rhythm with a machine *cannot* be dead, *must* be asleep.

1. **"Whole brain" criteria.** Death of the *whole* brain is recognized in a normothermic body when loss of brain function results from an identifiable, irreversible, structural lesion, in the absence of sedative–hypnotic drugs or other, potentially reversible, metabolic conditions. Clinical examination for death of the whole brain requires the absence of brainstem reflexes (e.g., oculocephalic and ice water caloric stimulation evokes no eye movement; pupils are dilated and fixed to light; corneal responses are not present) and no ventilatory movement when the ventilator is stopped after a period of ventilation with 100% oxygen, even though the Pco_2 increases above 60 torr without ventilation. Recognition must be affirmed with a second examination, separated in time from the first by a variable interval, dependent on factors such as age and clinical cause. The interval may be specified by local statute or hospital policy. As with the use of cardiorespiratory criteria to recognize the presence of death, the patient is dead when the criteria are

satisfied—that is, when the second examination affirms the findings of the first. A number of **confirmatory tests** are helpful when the clinical condition is compromised (e.g., when a patient has been in barbiturate coma after head injury) and may be **required** in certain circumstances (e.g., the patient is a child younger than 1 year). However, such tests are neither necessary nor sufficient to affirm the presence of death by themselves.

2. **"Brainstem" criteria.** In the UK, emphasis has been placed on the fact that the clinical examination on which the criterion of "brain death" is based looks only at the functions of the brainstem and not at whole-brain function. Higher cortical function is irrelevant in UK practice. This means that a person whose brainstem has irreversibly ceased to function but whose cerebral hemispheres are still working—a person with the so-called "locked in" syndrome—can be declared dead in the UK, even though their cerebral hemispheres are still functioning. To the astute clinician, evidence of a working brain (in the form of eye movement, eyelid blinking, and the like) can usually be recognized, if one takes the time to look for it. However, in part because of this dilemma, many "brain death" policies and procedures in the US require a confirmatory test (e.g., isoelectric electroencephalography or cerebral angiography showing no flow within the cranium) to demonstrate that higher brain function is or must be absent to affirm the presence of "brain death."

3. **"Higher brain" death.** Certain philosophers (e.g., Robert Veatch) have called for a new *definition* of death, one holding that death is the permanent loss of that which is essential to the nature of a human being—consciousness and cognition. Prescinding from the difficulty of establishing the *criteria* by which death, so defined, might be recognized, certain practical problems arise when one considers the implementation of such a definition (e.g., can someone in the end stages of Alzheimer's disease, still breathing with normal vegetative function, be buried?).

4. **Ethical considerations.**

   a. *Telling the family.* Once a physician has recognized the presence of death using "brain death" criteria, the fact of that recognition should be conveyed to the family and others with ethical standing in those circumstances. The physician should be aware that statutory law (as in New Jersey) or Department of Health regulations (as in New York) may make allowance for the family to reject the use of "brain death" criteria on religious grounds—in which case the physician may be required to rely on traditional (e.g., cardiorespiratory) criteria in identifying the fact that death has occurred. As in every interchange between physician and patient (including the extended patient-family and others), the physician should convey the fact gently, with compassion, and repeatedly until the fact is understood and accepted, if necessary. Although the family and others should not be burdened by being asked for permission to discontinue the ventilator (and thus, to allow cardiovascular death to ensue within a short time), the physician should be sensitive to reactions of denial and the like. The family should be given time to assimilate and accept the sorrowful fact of death. The physician should be sensitive to different ethnic and cultural heritages and to unresolved issues from the past, which can determine how long it will take for acceptance of that fact to occur. Terms such as *brain death* and *life support* should be avoided because they convey erroneous information. When someone *is* dead, the *person* is dead—not just the brain—and there is no longer any *human* life to support.

   b. *After "brain death."* In addition to solving the problem of inappropriate and theoretically indeterminable use of a scarce resource (e.g., an intensive care bed), recognizing the death of a person whose body can continue to be kept "alive" permits a utilitarian calculus for the benefit of others. This is true in two instances—organ donation and the continued nurturing of an unborn child beyond the point of viability inside the body of a mother who has died. Permission for either action must be sought in the standard manner (see Section **A** and **B** under Ethical Decision Making in General). Considerations of **justice** weigh heavily in these situations. Different ethical theories come to different conclusions with regard to either action.

B. **The "vegetative state."** Although the condition is regarded by some as a "fate worse than death," a certain proportion of patients who have incurred overwhelming damage to their cerebral hemispheres (e.g., from anoxia after cardiac arrest or from massive traumatic brain damage or stroke) may—after a period of coma—evolve into a state of "wakefulness without awareness" accompanied by sleep–wake cycles and essentially intact brainstem and autonomic functions. Other patients may reach this state at the end of a chronic degenerative process. In 1994, a multisociety task force published its consensus on the clinical, diagnostic, and prognostic features of this condition—a consensus with the particulars of which some physicians disagree, particularly because the task force did not acknowledge the concept of a **"minimally conscious state"** or deal with implications of the "locked-in" syndrome and other stops along the way from coma to full consciousness. At the heart of the matter is the issue of whether a patient in a "vegetative" (or any related) state is *truly unaware* of *all* stimuli and has no *conscious* thought; *when* the condition can rightly be regarded as *persistent* or *permanent*; and what, if any, impact may be had by a variety of therapeutic efforts, and at what cost. Some regard these issues as incapable of anything but an arbitrary resolution. The task force deemed that *any* motor response of a patient in a "vegetative state" was primitive, random, or reflex and, as such, could not be interpreted as evidence of cognition. Further, the task force relied on imaging and pathologic studies, using modalities available at the time, as excluding any anatomic substrate for consciousness. Techniques such as functional magnetic resonance imaging, single-photon emission computed tomography, and so forth have called these judgments to question.

1. Withholding/withdrawing. It is generally accepted that patients with the capacity to decide for themselves are *not* obliged to accept *all* treatments, diagnostic studies, and the like, and may reject these even if one of the results of such rejection is death. With patients in the "vegetative state," such decisions devolve upon surrogates, duly identified (see Section **B** under Ethical Decision Making in General). Most commonly, a burdens–benefit calculus is used to make a decision to reject. Such decisions should *never* be made with the *intent* of *causing* death but *may* be made even when the probability is that death will ensue. The obligations of the physician in this process are 3-fold: to reach medical certainty, as far as that is possible; to convey that certainty to the decision makers, as gently and as often as is necessary to ensure understanding and acceptance; and to respect and implement their decision, as long as that does not violate the conscience of the physician. From an ethical point of view, *withholding* is more problematic than *withdrawing*. Withholding does not give the patient the benefit of a therapeutic trial, even a time-limited trial. The physician does not know whether what might have been proposed would have helped the patient if it is not tried. It is imperative that all involved recognize (and behave accordingly with such recognition) that it is not *care* that is being withheld or withdrawn but rather a *burdensome* treatment or diagnostic study without *sufficient* benefit for the patient. The natural tendency to avoid such patients, visit them less often, even not to speak (as though they might understand), should be steadfastly eschewed.

2. Nutrition and hydration. Given the deep meaning of food and water in human society, it is no wonder that some have balked at the withholding or withdrawing of these as symbolic of abandonment of the patient. Others have equated the food and water given to a patient in the "vegetative state"—generally through a gastrostomy tube, with all of its attendant paraphernalia and cost—with any other therapy that may be rejected (for reasons previously given), making such a decision to take that action more acceptable by use of the terms "artificial nutrition and hydration." Clearly, it is licit to reject such measures for the *benefit* of the patient—as when the *intent* is to minimize excess gastric or pulmonary secretions, incontinence, and the like. However, when the *intent* is to *cause* death, some regard that not as a benefit for the patient, but rather as the beginning of a "slippery slope" that would lead inexorably to the elimination of "absolutely worthless human beings." (Recall that intellectual disability children were referred to as "absolutely worthless human beings" in Nazi Germany.)

3. Other considerations. In making judgments about *level of care* of patients in the "vegetative state" or with other devastating, irremediable neurologic conditions, the physician is increasingly called upon to consider questions of **distributive justice.** These arise in such matters as access to intensive care, "managed care" decisions, and even conservation of individual and group resources. *Ethical* physicians owe *primary responsibility* to their patients, unless both have knowingly entered into a contract with each other that permits limitation of care on such bases. That is not to demean the need to be in constant dialogue with the patient or surrogate, in a gentle yet persistent effort to convince them of the reason of a considered position that may be different from theirs.

C. **Neurogenetic diseases.**

Currently available technology to raise "designer babies" and the various potentials of stem cell therapy raise important ethical and moral issues. Designer babies are generally made through *in vitro* fertilization, where the embryo is removed from a woman and is manipulated to have certain desired qualities, and then returned to the womb to finish development. Parents may (for example) decide to "design" the new baby in a manner that it can be an organ donor for a sibling who has an illness requiring such a need. Should parents be allowed to *design* their babies? Is it unethical to restrict the kind of children people have? Should it be allowed, unless the genetic engineering causes harm to the baby or society? At what point do the inherent risks of genetic manipulation outweigh parental concerns for their children? These are just some of the ethical and moral issues the public, researchers, and policy makers must consider.

1. **Genetic testing.**

There has been an explosion in the disorders since 1983, when a marker for the gene for Huntington's disease was identified on chromosome 4.

2. **Diagnostic testing.** Research and commercial laboratories can provide the physician with DNA and non-DNA information helpful in the diagnosis of more than two dozen disorders of the central and peripheral nervous system (including various genetic forms of myopathy) with the likelihood that information about more diseases—and even such considerations as behavioral traits—will be available in the near future. Such testing may yield information pertinent not only to the diagnosis of an existing condition but also in the presymptomatic—even prenatal—situation, as well as with regard to carrier detection. Some—but by no means all—institutions use an extensive counseling system before and after testing, to ensure thorough, informed decision making for testing and appropriate support after results are made known to the patient, or the guardian or surrogate.

a. *Ethical considerations.* Because the information garnered through diagnostic testing for neurogenetic disease in essence belongs to the person(s) being tested, it is important to their decision making that they understand all of the implications of testing and are prepared—with support from the physician—to deal with those implications. For example, knowledge that one is a carrier of a neurogenetic disease may allow for more responsible parenthood. Prenatal recognition that a neurogenetic disease is present in a developing infant may allow that infant's parents to prepare to shoulder the burden of that disease or to elect termination of the pregnancy. Because certain neurogenetic diseases (e.g., Huntington's disease) are associated with a higher rate of suicide than obtained in the population at large, presymptomatic diagnosis may enhance the risk of suicide, especially in a person who has experienced the ravages of the disease in an affected family member. Confirmation of the diagnosis of a neurogenetic disease may help the patient to cope with that disease because certainty is always easier to deal with than uncertainty. Caution must be expressed over the misuse of information from diagnostic testing—by employers and insurers (especially healthcare insurers), who might arbitrarily exclude persons with proven disease without reference to the impact (present or future) of the particular disease on specific job performance or to its call on pooled healthcare resources. With regard to the latter issue, competing considerations of **justice** may enter in and may require the person being tested to disclose the results of testing. In the last analysis, the physician requesting the test as well as the person being tested should be aware of and informed about the various aspects of testing before proceeding with it. Genetic testing should never be done as part of the "routine" evaluation of a patient without such considerations being taken into account and explored.

b. *Gene therapy.* A promise for the future in neurogenetic disease is the hoped-for ability to insert or replace missing or defective genes in the cells of persons affected by such diseases. When the manipulation is directed at the affected cells, the procedure is termed **somatic cell therapy;** when it is directed at the initial fusion of sperm or ovum (or at those precursors of new human life themselves), it is termed **germ cell therapy.** Somatic cell therapy raises issues common to research (see Section **F** under Approaches to Particular Problems). Germ cell therapy, with its implications for future generations, raises other considerations beyond the scope of this chapter.

Mention should be made, however, of the proposed role of **stem cells** in this line of research. Stem cells, as the name implies, have the capacity of developing into any tissue (*totipotential*); many but not all tissues (*pluripotential*); or only some tissues (*unipotential*). They differ in *source* of derivation. Totipotential stem cells come from an embryo at the very earliest stage of development; pluripotential cells come from fetal tissue; and unipotential cells from adult tissue (e.g., bone marrow). The embryo and fetus do not survive harvesting of stem cells, so although the *goal* of stem cell development (e.g., cure of neurodegenerative diseases; repair of traumatic brain and spinal cord injury; cure of stroke; and so on) may be understandably laudable, the moral status of the *source* of stem cells cannot be ignored.

D. **Static or progressive disorders with intact cognition.** A spectrum of neuromuscular or spinal cord diseases have in common absence or loss of varying degrees of motor function (and hence—basically—of independence) with intact higher cortical function. Examples include spinal muscular atrophy, muscular dystrophy, spinal cord dysraphisms (e.g., meningomyelocele), injuries, and other illnesses [e.g., multiple sclerosis (although mental functions may be impaired in multiple sclerosis)].

1. **Truth-telling.** Truth-telling becomes exceptionally painful for a physician when confronted with a healthy mind in a body now or predictably about-to-be robbed of its normal function. Maintaining hope and thwarting inevitable depression without making false and empty promises is an art not easily learned—and yet one whose reward is 100-fold from the patient and family, for whom life does, indeed, go on. Truth—though painful for physician and patient alike—is a reliable ally in the practice of this art. Physicians must be exceedingly sensitive to, and take time to care for, the emotional dimensions of the state in which their patients find themselves. As difficult as it may be not to do so, one must never abandon patients in this state. This is especially true in circumstances in which breathing becomes progressively more difficult.

2. **Problems at the end of life.** Despite all attempts at describing life on a ventilator, the patient may not be able to decide what that life might be like unless a trial of assisted ventilation is undertaken. After this point, the problem of withdrawing such assistance enters the scene. Minimizing suffering during withdrawal (e.g., with sedative–analgesic medications) runs the risk of suppressing what ventilatory function the patient still has. However, as long as the *intent* is the relief of that suffering and *not* to *cause* a more rapid demise, the use of such medication is appropriate (see Section **G** under Approaches to Particular Problems). In all such circumstances, physicians should call upon colleagues with complementing skills (such as nurses, social workers, physiotherapists, hospice workers, and the like) to help them implement the healthcare decisions reached by their patients, properly informed.

E. **Static or progressive disorders with impaired cognition.** Absence or loss of that which makes us uniquely human—consciousness and related higher neurologic functions—poses a number of dilemmas for the physician, who must deal with surrogates or even the courts in attempting to resolve those dilemmas. The paradigm clinical conditions range from anencephaly at one end of life to end-stage Alzheimer's disease at the other, with varying degrees of mental retardation and behavioral disorders—all of diverse causation—in between.

1. **Limiting medical interventions.** Until a new definition of death (see Section **A.3** under Approaches to Particular Problems) is accepted, persons with these conditions remain human beings—as difficult as it may be to recognize that fact at any given moment. One may argue whether some human beings have more of a right to use healthcare resources than others, but that is a societal decision that must not be invoked at the bedside of a given patient by that patient's physician, absent agreement by the decision maker for that patient. On the other hand, the focus of decision making should properly be on compassionate *care*, not high-technology *cure*, once it is clear that one is dealing with a definitive, irreversible, process.

2. **Making decisions.** Surrogate decision making according to a **substituted judgment** standard (see Section **B** under Ethical Decision Making in General) is particularly problematic when the person has never had the capacity for independent judgment (e.g., an infant with anencephaly, or a person of any age with severe mental retardation). A sorry chapter in US jurisprudence in this regard dealt with involuntary sterilization—justified by the alternate, more subjective, **best interests** standard. The latter standard

is often used in dealing with unwanted, sometimes self-injurious, behavior by means of medication, restraints, institutionalization, and the like—even "psychosurgery." Extreme caution must be the rule, and compassion the guide. The use of **advance directives**—particularly the appointment of someone to hold a **durable power of attorney for healthcare decisions**—is critical to the goal of making decisions when patients can no longer articulate their own decisions. Physicians who care for patients with neurodegenerative disorders (in particular) are well advised to encourage their patients to consider and implement advance directives earlier rather than later, involving friends and family in discussions that will make possible valid substituted judgments, when and if those become necessary, well *before* their patients lose the capacity for truly informed decision making.

3. Involvement of family. Family members and others bearing responsibility for the care of persons without the capacity to decide for themselves should be intimately involved with decision making in this category, unless there is a valid reason for them not to be involved. When capacity has been present and is now lost (as in the end stages of Alzheimer's disease), attention should be paid to healthcare proxies, if previously executed. It must be borne in mind that people change their minds, especially as circumstances change. Few of us can *truly* be aware of what it is like to become demented, nor can we truly know what it is we would decide for ourselves if and when we were to reach such a state. The burden of dementia is on those who care for the demented, not on the demented themselves.

F. Research in neurology. Dr. Labe Scheinberg once described the practice of neurology with the aphorism, "diagnose—then adios!" at a time when there were few, if any, effective treatments for neurologic disease. The last decade of the 20th century was deemed the "Decade of the Brain" because of the remarkable advances in the understanding and management of neurologic disease that began to come forward during that time. The move from Dr. Scheinberg's aphorism to a brave and wonderful new world occurred in large measure because of research—often involving human subjects early (because no appropriate animal model existed), often with great risk (in searching for an elusive benefit), and often raising the spectra of a conflict of interest (between physicians caring for patients and conducting meaningful research by enrolling those patients in controlled clinical trials).

1. Valid versus invalid research. The *sine qua non* of valid research is peer review—approval of a research proposal by a thoughtful, responsible, knowledgeable group of peers to judge the question as worthy of being asked; the answer as likely to be forthcoming; and the hoped-for benefit as worth the predicted risk. The availability of external funding makes it possible to conduct approved research honestly and openly, without employing the subterfuge of paying for research under the guise of acceptable patient care. The process that affects valid research involves institutional review boards and other oversight bodies to ensure validity at every step along the way.

2. Consent issues. Persons with devastating illnesses (e.g., most neurologic diseases) are particularly vulnerable to any offer of hope, even when that offer wears the cloak of a research hypothesis. The offer of hope may come in the form of a controlled clinical trial, in which the decision as to which treatment (e.g., active treatment or placebo) the patient is to receive is made by the parameters of the trial, *not* by the patient's physician. Physicians who refer their patients for enrollment in such a trial must do that with **clinical equipoise**—meaning that they must agree that the trial is necessary; that there is not, as yet, any proven approach that would guarantee benefit to their patient (for if there is, their patient cannot be denied access to that—which may mean a more cumbersome, likely less valid, trial of the unproven therapy); and that the risks of the trial are balanced by the benefits their patient can expect. If there is no expected benefit to patients, then—at the very least—society should benefit from the expected gain in knowledge that will come from the trial. Consent is especially problematic for children and for others without the capacity to give their own consent. Some have gone so far as to take the position that nontherapeutic research involving patients should *never* be done, whereas others emphasize a broader debt to society that can *only* be paid by advancing knowledge through valid clinical research.

G. Chronic pain. Diverse neurologic conditions are commonly associated with pain, often requiring hefty doses of potent analgesics for relief—doses of medications that may suppress respiration, lower blood pressure to dangerous levels, and have other unwanted effects. The ruling principle here is that of the **double effect**—the unwanted (indirect, merely permitted) effects (in this instance, possible aspiration or even death) are allowed, as long as the primary (direct, intended) effect (in this instance, relief of pain and suffering) is desirable, and cannot be achieved in any other way. It is important to remember that pain can be physical and identifiable, or metaphysical and existential. Adequate relief of both kinds of pain is at the heart of **comfort care,** which can be chosen by patients at any stage of their lives, especially at the end of a terminal illness. In this regard, **hospice** may be an ideal setting in which to provide such care (although the trajectory of neurologic illness often exceeds the arbitrary limits set by Medicare and other funding agencies for the provision of hospice care).

INTERFACE WITH THE LAW

Many of the most notable, landmark legal decisions involving patient decision making have dealt with patients with neurologic problems. In the matter of surrogate decision making with regard to the withholding or withdrawal of medical treatment, *Quinlan* and *Saikewicz* set the standard of substituted judgment for once-competent and never-competent patients, respectively. *Conroy* affirmed the fact that autonomy remains intact, even when a person is no longer able to assert that right or even appreciate its effectuation. *Cruzan* acknowledged the right of states to require stringent ("clear and convincing") evidence of the prior wishes of a once-competent person as applicable to his or her current status. The physician should be aware of such cases and should try to discern their relevance to the situation at hand (see Section **B** under Case Method Approach to Clinical Ethics). The physician should recognize that the impact of such cases (in terms of setting precedent) is limited to the jurisdiction in which the decision was rendered but may (in terms of argument) be of probative value in other jurisdictions.

THE MEDICAL PROFESSION AND THE DRUG INDUSTRY

The medical profession and the drug industry have had a symbiotic relationship for hundreds of years. The pharmaceutical companies cannot sell their products directly to patients. They need healthcare providers to prescribe the use of their products once they have passed the rigorous regulatory criteria set forth by the Food and Drug Administration (FDA). Likewise, doctors depend on the pharmaceutical industry to provide drugs to treat their patients. The decision to pick a particular drug therapy should be based exclusively on what is *best* for a given patient, without any potential conflict of interest. However, as in all partnerships, a conflict between the partners is to be expected. Much has been written about the influence pharmaceutical industry has on healthcare providers. The industry markets directly to healthcare providers through medical representatives and also by contracting with the providers to act as their "consultants" who give promotional talks. In a recent year the industry spent over $600 million on such promotional talks. However, the drug companies' recent commitment to mandatory compliance and ethical training for all their employees and speakers (consultants) ensures that only appropriate and FDA-approved information is disseminated. All materials used in advertising and promotion of a product now have to be approved in accordance with the FDA guidelines. Consultants who speak for companies have to undergo mandatory "compliance and regulatory" training. Penalties to physicians and drug companies are heavy when rules are broken. Meals and value of "gifts" (now regulated and restricted to educational material *only*) are reported and available to the public (by means of the Sunshine Act, passed in 2010) for transparency and to declare any conflict of interest.

Direct-to-consumer (DTC) advertising is legal in the United States and is regulated by the FDA. In 2014, the industry spent over US $5 billion in DTC advertising. Consumers receive a biased message and are unduly influenced to seek the medication they want (in some instances demanding the drug or else seek out a physician who will). All of these raise ethical concerns regarding DTC advertising—which is banned in all countries of the world, except the United States and New Zealand. Surveys carried out in New Zealand and in the United States show that, when a patient asks for a specific drug by name, they receive it more often than not. DTC has an impact on the patient/physician relationship. The most logical and ethical question is: as it is legal to advertise prescription drugs in the United States, and recognizing that the drug companies need to make money in order to be able to develop more and better drugs, is it in the best interest of patients to have physicians give talks (the content of which is strictly regulated by FDA guidelines) to consumers and healthcare workers, and be paid by drug companies for giving such talks, or would it be better—and more ethical—for those companies to spend five times more money on DTC advertising?

Delivery of health care in the 21st century is heavily influenced by various industries such as insurance companies (who dictate which patient should get what drug—often based on the kickback they receive from the pharmaceutical companies); hospitals and corporations [who are now increasingly hiring physicians and "punish" healthcare providers for ordering too many tests or prescribing expensive therapies (and rewarding them, financially, if their practice is lucrative)]; digital media [which allow for patients to share publicly their interpretation of care (and the consequences of it) they receive from a particular physician]; and various government regulatory agencies [which have put an ever-increasing demand on physicians (e.g., mandatory electronic health records; federally mandated conversion to ever-changing ICD codes; and the like)]. The ethical consequences of all these challenges cannot be ignored, if physicians are to play a central role in their patients' welfare. A recent example of how patients' health and welfare are manipulated (for better or worse) is evidenced by hundreds of millions of dollars received by politicians from America's healthcare industry to block the introduction of Affordable Care Act. The largest contribution, totaling close to $1.5 million, went to Max Baucus, the chairman of the senate committee drafting the new law. From 2003 to 2008, Baucus received $3,973,485 from the health sector, including $852,813 from pharmaceutical companies, $851,141 from health professionals, $784,185 from the insurance industry, and $465,750 from HMOs/health services, according to the Center for Responsive Politics. A 2006 study by Public Citizen found that, between 1999 and 2005, Baucus, along with former Senate majority leader Bill Frist, took in the most special-interest money of any senator.

Do millions of dollars in campaign contributions received by politicians who make healthcare laws and regulations each year affect how a physician can treat his or her patient?

These are but some of the ethical dilemmas, above and beyond those that arise in the physician–patient relationship, facing the medical profession today.

REFERRALS

Most ethical dilemmas can (and should) be dealt with by physicians with colleagues (nurses, social workers, clergy, and the like) in the care of their patients—perhaps with the help of ethics consultation and the awareness of hospital administration and attorneys. In solving such dilemmas, physicians should keep the general principles of decision making, truth-telling, and involvement of family (see Sections A under Ethical Decision Making in General and F under Approaches to Particular Problems in particular) in mind at all times. Physicians should not hesitate to seek the guidance and assistance of senior, more experienced clinicians in dealing with these issues at a practical level. Generally, recourse to the courts should be a last resort, because the legal process takes an interminable length of time and is often not sensitive to the important nuances of a particular situation.

CASE STUDIES/VIDEOS

A. Maria.

Maria is a 94-year-old lady with chronic headaches and dementia for more than 10 years. She was born and raised in Latin America, speaks very little English, and has been residing in a nursing home for the past 2 years. She is confined to a wheelchair, needs help with transfers, and has been incontinent of bowel and bladder. She feeds herself, and gets slightly agitated in the evening. During clinic visits she is always pleasant, speaking only in Spanish. She always asks her neurologist if he has any children, wants to meet his family, and complains about the food she gets at the nursing home. She will write her husband's and children's names but does not always recognize her daughter (who always accompanies her to the clinic). Maria always asks me to do a brain scan for her headaches and complains that the medicine I give her does not help. When I tell her that I would prescribe another medicine, she thanks him profusely and kisses his hand. Sometimes she laughs when he asks her why she has no gray hair, pointing to her daughter and telling him that she puts color in her hair. This has been her baseline for a number of years.

Six months ago, her daughter received a call from the nursing home. The nurse told her that her mother was "terminal"—but not to worry, because they would not let her "suffer." She would be given intravenous (IV) morphine. At the most she would live for only a week. The social worker then called to inquire if the family had made funeral arrangements. Shocked to hear all of these, her daughter rushed to the nursing home—only to find that her mother was not critically ill at all! She was her "usual" self. She immediately called her siblings (who live out of state). Collectively, they all protested and actually had to argue with the nursing home "team" to not to put her on morphine.

With the consent of her daughters, her neurologist did an hour-long video interview of Maria, 6 months after the nursing home had decided that she was "terminal" and needed to be placed on morphine drip to ease her death. When he questioned her daughter as to actually what reason they gave her for wanting to put her on morphine drip, she said, they had upgraded her stay at the nursing home to hospice—so that she could qualify for more help. The family agreed with this decision. They liked the fact that their mother would now get a Spanish-speaking caregiver for a couple of hours each day. After 6 months in hospice care, the nursing home decided that her quality of life was becoming extremely poor. She was not eating well, and complained of headaches. High-dose morphine and Ativan were ordered. *Per* the family's request, this was not allowed. In fact, she was taken off all her other meds (except for antihypertensive medication and folic acid), and was given low-dose oxycodone as needed.

A short video (Video 39.1) of the neurologist's interview with Maria, 6 months after the above incident, is attached.

Do you believe that the decision to treat Maria with IV morphine 6 months earlier was to hasten her death? Is this an "acceptable" outcome for someone who is 94 years old and in hospice care, or do you feel that the decision was unethical? Can the decision be justified based on the fact that an increasing number of people with chronic, nontreatable diseases are living longer, raising the cost of medical care and drawing on restricted resources which may otherwise be available for those who are "not as bad?"

B. Dan.

Dan wants to die, but his doctors and the ethics committee at a hospital to which he was recently admitted for treatment of pneumonia does not support his decision. Dan is 32 years old, totally paralyzed from the neck down, and has been respirator-dependent since the age of 3. A car accident had caused severe and irreversible damage to the spinal cord in his neck. Dan cannot remember life without a respirator. Even when he dreams, he sees himself as totally helpless and dependent on his caregivers for all his activities of daily living. It drives him insane when he has an itch and there is no one around to scratch it. His mother inserts a catheter through his penis several times a day to empty his bladder. He has no control over his bowels. However, he can see, talk, and take food by mouth. Most importantly, he can think, but thinking has become his worst enemy. He spends a lot of his time thinking about the state of his life—where his life is heading and the quality of that life. He feels trapped in his body, 24 hours a day, 7 days a week.

He wants to die, but his physicians and the ethics committee will not support his decision. His mother supports his decision, but his father (divorced when Dan was 5 years old) does not agree, citing his own faith for that reasoning.

A part of a video interview (Video 39.2) with Dan is attached. What ethical decision would you arrive at, and how would you justify that decision?

Key Points

- Exploring ethical considerations in the 21st century:
  - ethical theories on which to base your practical judgments
  - ethical considerations for patients with altered mental status, or in coma or the vegetative state
- Examining important elements of informed consent, including comprehension, decision-making capacity, full disclosure of risks and benefits, and the ability to grant, withhold, or withdraw consent.
- Approaching brain death from clinical, ethical, and legal standpoints.
- Exploring moral and ethical issues related to advances in genetic testing, gene and stem cell therapy.
- Examining end-of-life situations.
- Understanding the ethical implications of the long and symbiotic relationship that exists between the medical profession and the drug industry.

Recommended Readings

American Academy of Neurology Code of Professional Conduct. *Neurology*. 1993;43:1257 (revisions available on the AAN website).

American Medical Association Council on Ethical and Judicial Affairs. *Code of Medical Ethics: Current Opinions and Annotations, 2010–2011*. Chicago, IL: American Medical Association; 2010.

Beauchamp TL, Childress JF. *Principles of Biomedical Ethics*. 7th ed. New York, NY: Oxford University Press; 2012.

Bernat JL. *Ethical Issues in Neurology*. 3rd ed. Boston, MA: Butterworth-Heinemann; 2008.

Fletcher JC, Lombardo PA, Spencer E. *Fletcher's Introduction to Clinical Ethics*. 3rd ed. Frederick, MD: University Publishing Group; 2005.

Gariner D, Shemie S, Manara A, et al. International perspective on the diagnosis of death. *Brit J Anaesth*. 2012;108(suppl 1):114–128.

Giordano JJ, Gordijn B, eds. *Scientific and Philosophical Perspectives in Neuroethics*. New York, NY: Cambridge University Press; 2010.

In re Quinlan, 70 N.J. 10, 355 A.2d 647, *cert. denied sub nom. Garger v. New Jersey*, 429 U.U. 922, 1976.

Jennett B. *The Vegetative State: Medical Facts, Ethical and Legal Dilemmas*. New York, NY: Cambridge University Press; 2002.

Lo B. *Resolving Ethical Dilemmas: A Guide for Clinicians*. 5th ed. Philadelphia, PA: Lippincott Williams & Wilkins; 2013.

Rosenbaum L. Reconnecting the dots — reinterpreting industry–physician relations. Conflict of interest [3 part series]. *N Engl J Med*. 2015;(1)1860–1864;(2)1959–1963;(3)2064–2068.

Wachter R. *The Digital Doctor: Hope, Hype, and Harm at the Dawn of Medicine's Computer Age*. New York, NY: McGraw-Hill; 2015:320.

Wijdicks EFM, ed. *Brain Death*. 2nd ed. Philadelphia, PA: Lippincott Williams & Wilkins; 2013.

40 Ischemic Cerebrovascular Disease

José Biller and Rochelle Sweis

Cerebrovascular disease comprises a heterogeneous group of disorders that herald their presence by producing symptoms and signs resulting from either **ischemia** or **hemorrhage** within the central nervous system (CNS). The term **stroke** is most commonly used by both physicians and the general public to refer to any one of this diverse group of disorders. It connotes the notion that onset of symptoms is abrupt and leaves a lasting physical or cognitive disability. An ischemic stroke is an acute **brain attack** caused by the interruption of blood flow within one or more arterial territories of the brain.

Stroke is currently the second most common cause of death worldwide, and a primary cause of long-term disability in much of the industrialized world. Cerebrovascular disease is also the most common neurologic condition necessitating hospitalization. Patients surviving a transient ischemic attack (TIA) or ischemic stroke are at increased risks of recurrent ischemic events and have a reduced life expectancy.

There are two main types of strokes—ischemic and hemorrhagic. The focus of this chapter is to outline the general approach to the diagnosis and management of ischemic stroke.

Of the 795,000 new or recurrent strokes in the United States each year, approximately 87% result from **cerebral infarction.** On average, someone in the United States has a stroke every 40 seconds, and someone dies of a stroke every 4 minutes. Ischemic stroke may result from (1) large-artery atherosclerotic disease, (2) small-artery disease (lacunes), (3) cardioembolism, (4) hemodynamic (watershed) infarction, (5) nonatherosclerotic vasculopathies, (6) hypercoagulable disorders, or (7) cryptogenic or infarction of undetermined causation (aka: embolic strokes of undetermined source).

Ischemia sets in motion a cascade of biochemical alterations leading to lactic acidosis, influx of calcium and sodium, and efflux of potassium that culminates in cell death. The pathogenesis of ischemic strokes can be conceptualized as a permanent lack of blood flow to a focal region of the brain, depriving it of needed glucose and oxygen. Normal **cerebral blood flow (CBF)** to the adult brain is 50 to 55 mL/100 g/minute. The threshold for synaptic transmission failure occurs when CBF decreases to approximately 8 to 10 mL/100 g/minute. At this level, neuronal death can occur. The brain region with a CBF level from 8 to 18 mL/100 g/minute sometimes is called the **ischemic penumbra.** Rational treatment of patients with ischemic cerebrovascular disease depends on accurate diagnosis. Most interventional strategies aim to promote rapid perfusion of brain tissue and to treat the complications of **brain swelling** postischemic stroke.

The cause of an ischemic stroke must first be established through an expeditious but careful history-taking, detailed physical examination, and paraclinical investigations. A basic evaluation, to be performed for all patients with ischemic stroke, includes complete blood cell count (CBC) with differential and platelet count, erythrocyte sedimentation rate, prothrombin time (PT), activated partial thromboplastin time (aPTT), plasma glucose level, blood urea nitrogen, serum creatinine, lipid analysis, urinalysis, chest radiography, and electrocardiography. Creatine kinase (CK) and CK-MB fraction and cardiac troponins provide evidence of a concurrent myocardial infarction (MI).

Computed tomography (CT) should also be performed on all patients because it may depict hemorrhagic lesions that can mimic an ischemic stroke. If cerebellar or brainstem symptoms are present, imaging should include thin cuts through the posterior fossa. Magnetic resonance imaging (MRI) is superior to CT in evaluation for cerebral ischemia (Fig. 40.1). MRI with diffusion-weighted imaging (DWI) is useful to delineate ischemic strokes. MRI with DWI or perfusion-weighted imaging is useful to visualize the **ischemic penumbra** (Fig. 40.2). Computed

CT	FLAIR	DWI	ADC

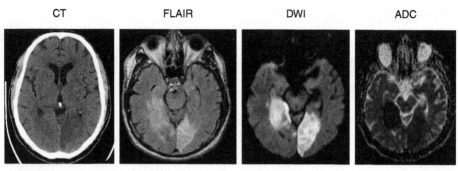

FIGURE 40.1 A 69-year-old man had new onset of right-sided visual blurring and right-sided numbness. Neuroimaging studies demonstrate left occipital and right medial temporal infarcts; the right side temporal infarct was harder to be visualized on CT. (Courtesy of Dr. Lotfi Hacein-Bey.). ADC, apparent diffusion coefficient; CT, computed tomography; DWI, diffusion-weighted imaging; FLAIR, fluid attenuated inversion recovery.

DWI	ADC	Contrast MR	Perfusion MRI

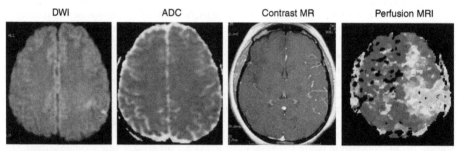

FIGURE 40.2 Perfusion/diffusion mismatch. Acute left ICA occlusion in a 29-year-old woman. There are very small diffusion defects in the left posterior frontal lobe. Perfusion MRI shows that the full left MCA territory is at risk. (Courtesy of Dr. Lotfi Hacein-Bey.). ADC, apparent diffusion coefficient; DWI, diffusion-weighted imaging; ICA, internal carotid artery; MCA, middle cerebral artery; MRI, magnetic resonance imaging. (See color plates.)

tomographic angiography (CTA) or magnetic resonance angiography (MRA) complements the information obtained with MRI and frequently delineates the pathoanatomic substrate of the stroke. Gadolinium-enhanced multicontrast-weighted MRI may also allow accurate quantification of carotid artery plaque instability. CT perfusion is also useful to visualize the ischemic penumbra. The emphasis in screening should be on noninvasive testing including carotid duplex ultrasound and transcranial Doppler (TCD) ultrasound. Carotid duplex ultrasound is often obtained when clinical manifestations could be attributed to carotid artery disease. Increased plaque echolucency has been associated with higher risks of stroke and TIA. TCD ultrasound identifies high-risk patients with sickle cell anemia, indirectly assesses cerebral perfusion reserve, and may also enhance the effect of ultrasound on thrombolysis.

Cardiac investigations to determine whether emboli have cardiac sources are advised in selected circumstances. Two-dimensional echocardiography for older patients with ischemic stroke is limited to patients with clinical clues of heart disease. Two-dimensional echocardiography should be considered for all patients younger than 45 years with otherwise unexplained ischemic stroke. Transesophageal echocardiography should be used for selected individuals, particularly for evaluation of mitral and aortic prosthetic valves or vegetations, whenever there is a need for better visualization of the left atrial appendage or interatrial septum, or when a right-to-left shunt is suspected.

Most patients with ischemic stroke have extracranial (EC) or intracranial (IC) **cerebrovascular atherosclerosis.** Cerebrovascular atherosclerosis primarily affects the carotid bulb, carotid siphon, middle cerebral artery (MCA) stem, origin, and IC segments of the vertebral arteries, and basilar artery. Ischemia results from thrombotic vascular occlusion, embolization of atherosclerotic debris, or hemodynamic disturbances causing focal hypoperfusion in areas in which the circulation is inadequate.

Natural History and Prognosis

A. **Ischemic stroke resulting from large-artery atherosclerotic disease.** Large-artery atherothrombotic infarctions almost always occur in patients who already have significant risk factors for cerebrovascular atherosclerosis, such as arterial hypertension, cigarette smoking, diabetes mellitus, dyslipidemia, asymptomatic carotid bruits, asymptomatic carotid stenosis, and TIAs.

1. A **TIA** is defined as a transient episode of neurologic dysfunction caused by focal brain or retinal ischemia without infarction. The conventional boundary in differentiating between a TIA and stroke has been 24 hours. Yet, most TIAs last only a few minutes. As TIAs may be associated with variable rates of infarction on diffusion-weighted MRI, a new "tissue based definition" of TIA is now commonly used: brief episodes of neurologic dysfunction caused by focal retinal or brain ischemia with symptoms typically lasting <60 minutes, and without evidence of acute infarction.

   TIAs are most often caused by thromboembolism associated with large-artery atherosclerosis, cardioembolism, or small-vessel (lacunar) disease. TIAs are important harbingers of subsequent stroke and are often associated with lesions on brain imaging. TIAs involving the anterior or carotid circulation should be distinguished from those involving the posterior or vertebrobasilar circulation.

   a. The following symptoms are considered typical of TIAs in the **carotid circulation:** ipsilateral amaurosis fugax, contralateral sensory or motor dysfunction limited to one side of the body, aphasia, contralateral homonymous hemianopia, or any combination thereof.

   b. The following symptoms represent typical TIAs in the **vertebrobasilar system:** bilateral or shifting motor or sensory dysfunction, complete or partial loss of vision in both homonymous fields, or any combination of these symptoms. Isolated diplopia, vertigo, dysarthria, and dysphagia should not be considered TIAs, but in combination with one another or with any of the symptoms just listed, they should be considered vertebrobasilar TIAs.

   c. Preceding TIAs occur in approximately 30% to 50% of patients with atherothrombotic brain infarction, in 15% to 25% of lacunar infarctions, and in 10% of cardioembolic infarctions.

   d. A TIA is a risk factor for stroke. The independent risk of a subsequent stroke is at least three times greater for patients with histories of TIAs than for those who have not had TIAs. The **ABCD2** score is useful for stroke risk stratification in patients with TIAs: **A**ge >60 years = 1 point; **B**lood pressure >140/90 mm Hg = 1 point; **C**linical unilateral weakness = 2 points; speech-only impairment = 1 point; **D**uration >60 minutes = 2 points, <60 minutes = 1 point; **D**iabetes = 1 point. Scores of 4 or greater in the **ABCD2** score indicate moderate to high stroke risk.

2. **Atherosclerosis** tends to occur in areas of reduced flow shear such as the posterior aspect of the carotid artery bulb. It primarily affects the larger EC and IC vessels. Approximately 80% of ischemic strokes occur in the **carotid or anterior circulation,** and 20% in the **vertebrobasilar or posterior circulation** (Fig. 40.3).

3. The mechanism of large-artery atherothrombotic infarction is either **artery-to-artery embolization** or **in situ formation of a thrombus** in the setting of preexisting arterial stenosis. Artery-to-artery embolism or low CBF is a common mechanism of cerebral ischemic events. Embolism from ulcerated carotid atherosclerotic plaques is the most common cause of cerebral infarction. In situ thrombosis occurs in the proximal carotid, distal vertebral, and basilar arteries. Such a circumstance may arise in association with hypercoagulable states. When the internal carotid artery (ICA) occludes, it can also cause low-flow ischemic events depending on status of the collateral circulation.

B. **Ischemic strokes resulting from small-vessel or penetrating artery disease (lacunes).** Long-standing arterial hypertension affects primarily the smaller penetrating IC vessels. It induces hypertrophy of the media and deposition of fibrinoid material into the vessel

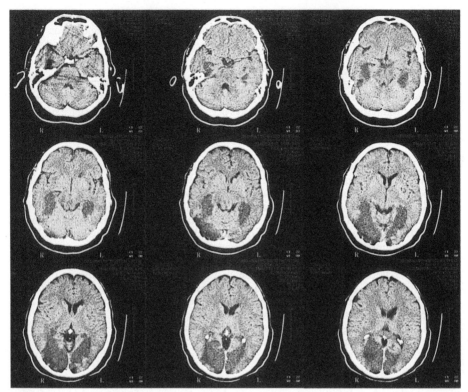

FIGURE 40.3 Axial unenhanced CT shows areas of low attenuation involving the medial aspects of both temporal lobes, both occipital lobes, the midbrain, and the pons in a patient with a diagnosis of basilar arterial occlusion. CT, computed tomography.

wall (fibrinoid necrosis), which eventually leads to occlusion. **Lacunes** are small ischemic infarcts in the deep regions of the brain or brainstem ranging in diameter from 0.5 to 15.0 mm resulting mainly from lipohyalinosis of penetrating arteries or branches related to long-standing arterial hypertension—chiefly the anterior choroidal, middle cerebral, posterior cerebral, and basilar arteries. Diabetes mellitus and EC arterial and cardiac sources of embolism are found less frequently.

C. **Ischemic stroke resulting from cardioembolism.** Cardioembolic strokes are associated with substantial morbidity and mortality. Embolism of cardiac origin accounts for approximately 15% to 20% of all ischemic strokes. Emboli from cardiac sources frequently lodge in the MCA territory, are often large, and often have the worst outcomes. Although most types of heart disease can produce cerebral embolism, certain cardiac disorders are more likely to be associated with emboli (Table 40.1). Low or uncertain embolic risk disorders include mitral valve prolapse, mitral annulus calcification, aortic valve calcification, calcific aortic stenosis, bicuspid aortic valve, atrial flutter, patent foramen ovale, atrial septal aneurysms, valvular strands, and a Chiari network. Identification of a cardiac source of potential embolism is helpful for management. However, finding a potential cardiac embolic source is not by itself sufficient to diagnose cardio embolic cerebral infarction because many cardiac problems can coexist with cerebrovascular atherosclerosis.

D. **Ischemic stroke resulting from hemodynamic mechanisms.** Another mechanism of ischemic CNS damage is decreased systemic perfusion pressure that causes diminished blood flow to the brain in a diffuse manner. This occurs most commonly in the setting of cardiac pump failure or systemic hypotension. **Border-zone** ischemia is often explained by the combination of two frequently interrelated processes—hypoperfusion and embolization. This type of insult is most critical in border-zone territories, or so-called watershed areas,

TABLE 40.1 Cardiac Sources with High-Risk Embolic Potential

AF
Acute MI
Mechanical prosthetic heart valves
Rheumatic mitral stenosis
Dilated cardiomyopathies
Infective endocarditis
Atrial myxomas

Abbreviations: AF, atrial fibrillation; MI, myocardial infarction.

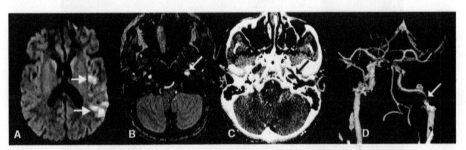

FIGURE 40.4 A 47-year-old man with acute onset of aphasia and right upper extremity weakness from left hemispheric ischemic injuries demonstrated on DWI MRI **(A,** *arrowheads***).** Source image from MRA shows enlargement of the left ICA immediately inferior to the petrous canal **(B,** *arrow***)** because of aneurysmal dilatation of the false lumen by an intimal flap. CTA, axial image **(C)** and three-dimensional reconstruction **(D)** show the same findings. CTA, computed tomographic angiography; DWI, diffusion-weighted imaging; ICA, internal carotid artery; MRA, magnetic resonance angiography; MRI, magnetic resonance imaging. (See color plates.)

in the most distal regions of supply of the major arterial territories. Border-zone ischemia can result in several characteristic syndromes depending on whether the ischemia is in the border-zone territory of all three major arterial systems (anterior, middle, and posterior cerebral arteries), the territory between the anterior and middle cerebral arteries, or the territory between the middle and posterior cerebral arteries. **Watershed infarcts** are often bilateral, but can be unilateral when preexisting ipsilateral vascular disease causes focal hypoperfusion in the most distal territory. Other mechanisms whereby watershed infarcts develop include microemboli and hematologic abnormalities.

E. Ischemic stroke resulting from nonatherosclerotic vasculopathies. Several nonatherosclerotic forms of vasculopathy are predisposing factors for ischemic stroke. These vasculopathies include, among others, cervicocephalic arterial dissection (Figs. 40.4 and 40.5A–C), Moyamoya, fibromuscular dysplasia, and cerebral vasculitis. Together, these uncommon conditions represent 5% of all ischemic strokes. They are relatively more common among children and young adults.

F. Ischemic stroke resulting from hypercoagulable disorders. Alterations in hemostasis have been associated with an increased risk of ischemic stroke. These conditions include deficiencies in the anticoagulant proteins such as antithrombin, protein C, protein S, activated protein C resistance, factor V Leiden mutation, prothrombin gene (*G20210A*) mutation, and heparin cofactor II; disorders of fibrinogen or the fibrinolytic system; methylene-tetrahydrofolate reductase gene mutation; lipoprotein (a) disorders; and secondary hypercoagulable states encountered in patients with malignancies, pregnancy/puerperium, the antiphospholipid antibody syndrome, nephrotic syndrome, polycythemia vera, sickle cell disease, thrombotic thrombocytopenic purpura (TTP), and paroxysmal nocturnal hemoglobinuria. These disorders account for 1% of all strokes and for 2% to 7% of ischemic strokes in young patients.

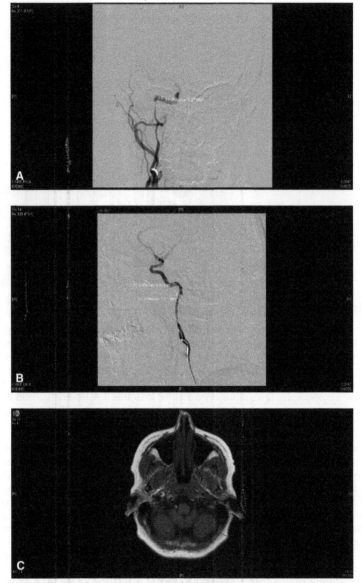

FIGURE 40.5 A: Angiogram of a 51-year-old woman with prior history of head trauma depicts a right ICA chronic dissection with luminal irregularities, severe stenosis, and delayed IC flow. **B:** Angiogram of acute on chronic left ICA dissection with luminal irregularities, severe stenosis, and small elevated flap predisposing patient to thrombus formation and ischemic stroke, treated with anticoagulation. **C:** Axial T1 weighted fat saturated MRI image shows right ICA high signal crescent sign, characteristic for arterial dissection. IC, intracranial; ICA, internal carotid artery; MRI, magnetic resonance imaging.

G. **Ischemic stroke of undetermined causation.** Despite extensive evaluation, in as many as one-third of ischemic strokes, a cause cannot be determined. This percentage is possibly higher among patients younger than 45 years (Video 40.1). It is possible that some of these strokes are caused by cardioembolic or hematologic events not readily demonstrable.

1. If no cause of ischemic stroke is discovered, patients should undergo prolonged ambulatory cardiac monitoring in an attempt to uncover paroxysmal atrial fibrillation (PAF). Studies in patients with pacemakers or cardioverter-defibrillators revealed PAF is more prevalent than persistent atrial fibrillation and carries the same stroke risk as persistent atrial fibrillation (AF). Technologic advances have made it possible to monitor for PAF episodes for months and even years and quantitate the duration and frequency of PAF. Modes of prolonged cardiac monitoring are either noninvasive relying on surface electrodes (Holter-sensitive and specific for PAF detection), external loop recorder, ambulatory telemetry, or invasive (implantable loop recorder, dual-chamber pacemaker/defibrillator). Yield of detecting PAF increases with duration, device sensitivity, PAF definition, and strict patient selection, specifically targeting those patients who have suffered cryptogenic ischemic strokes. Patient risk factors for PAF include older age, cryptogenic stroke, vascular risk factors based on CHADS2 or CHA2DS2-VASC score or vascular disease, left atrial enlargement, left atrial appendage dysfunction, premature atrial complexes on electrocardiography (ECG), and single or multiple cortical and subcortical areas of restricted diffusion on MRI. Oral anticoagulation would be the treatment of choice for PAF but the decision should be made based on risk stratification scores assessing risk of stroke (CHADS2, CHA2DS2-VASC scores) and hemorrhage (HAS-BLED and HEMORRHAGES scores). Questions that remain uncertain mandating further research include which is the best monitoring device to use, duration of monitoring, patient selection, and risk of stroke associated with brief (seconds) episodes of PAF.

PREVENTION

The prevention of strokes follows three main avenues—control of modifiable risk factors, pharmacologic therapy, and surgical intervention. Knowledge and control of modifiable risk factors are paramount in prevention of primary and secondary strokes. Treatable or modifiable risk factors include arterial hypertension, diabetes mellitus, cigarette smoking, hyperlipidemia, excessive alcohol intake, obesity, and physical inactivity. Other risk factors include age and gender, cardiac disease, TIAs, previous strokes, asymptomatic carotid bruit or stenosis, high hemoglobin level or hematocrit, increased fibrinogen level, use of oral contraceptives, and possibly race and ethnicity.

A. **Hypertension** predisposes to ischemic stroke by aggravating atherosclerosis and accelerating heart disease. Approximately, 60 million Americans have arterial hypertension. Arterial hypertension is the most important modifiable risk factor for stroke, increasing the relative risk 3- to 4-fold. Blood pressure lowering also reduces the risk of stroke in individuals with isolated systolic hypertension and in elderly subjects. Blood pressure treatment resulting in a decrease in mean diastolic blood pressure of 5 mm Hg over 2 to 3 years is associated with a 40% reduction in risk of stroke. Blood pressure targets are individualized according to age, ethnicity, and coexisting comorbidities. Reduction of blood pressure is more important than the specific antihypertensive agent or modality use.

B. **Diabetes mellitus** increases the risk of ischemic cerebrovascular disease 2- to 4-fold compared with the risk among persons without diabetes. In addition, diabetes increases morbidity and mortality after stroke. Most persons with diabetes die of atherosclerotic cardiovascular complications, and atherosclerosis causing blockage to the arteries in the heart and brain accounts for >80% of all deaths in diabetes. Rigorous blood pressure control is particularly recommended for diabetic patients. Patients with diabetes who have concomitant hypertension should be treated with a regimen that includes an angiotensin-converting-enzyme (ACE) inhibitor or an angiotensin receptor blocker. There is presently no evidence to suggest that tighter diabetic control decreases the risk of stroke or recurrent stroke.

C. **Cigarette smoking** is an independent risk factor for ischemic stroke among men and women of all ages. More than 5 years may be required before a reduction in stroke risk is observed after cessation of smoking.

D. Hyperlipidemia. There is a positive association between serum cholesterol and risk of ischemic stroke. Patients with TIAs or ischemic stroke with elevated cholesterol, comorbid coronary artery disease, or evidence of an atherosclerotic lesion should be managed with 3-hydroxy-3-methylglutaryl-coenzyme A (HMG CoA) reductase inhibitors (statins). The

TABLE 40.2 Stroke Evaluation Targets for Potential Thrombolysis Candidates: NINDS Guideline Recommendations

Time Interval	Time Target
EMS transport from home ED	10 min
Time from arrival in ED to availability of neurologic expertise	15 min (phone or physical presence)
Time from arrival in ED to completion of head CT	25 min
Time from arrival in ED to completion of CT interpretation	45 min
Time from arrival in ED to treatment with thrombolytics	60 min
Time from arrival in ED to admission in monitored bed	3 hr

Abbreviation: CT, computed tomography; ED, emergency department.

statins block the rate-limiting step in cholesterol biosynthesis. These agents not only effectively lower the rate of cholesterol biosynthesis, but a number of cholesterol-independent or pleiotrophic effects allow statins to exert important influences on a number of critical cellular signaling mechanisms. Meta-analysis of randomized trials of statins in primary or secondary preventions has shown a relative stroke risk reduction of approximately one-fifth. In the Stroke Prevention by Aggressive Reduction in Cholesterol Levels, treatment with atorvastatin 80 mg daily significantly reduced the risk of nonfatal or fatal stroke, and the risk of stroke or TIA compared with placebo. A reduction in major cardiovascular events was also observed. Although atorvastatin was associated with fewer ischemic strokes than placebo, hemorrhagic strokes were more frequent in the atorvastatin-treated group. Further data are needed regarding the effective range of HMG CoA reductase inhibitor doses in these patients.

E. **Excessive alcohol use.** There is a J-shaped association between alcohol consumption and ischemic stroke. Lower doses (upto two drinks a day) offer reduced risk and higher doses elevate the risk. Moderate alcohol intake may elevate high-density lipoprotein concentration.

F. **Obesity and physical inactivity.** Obesity exerts an independent increase in risk of stroke among men younger than 63 years. This increase is greater among cigarette smokers and patients with hypertension, elevated blood glucose, or hyperlipidemia. There is some evidence that physical activity can reduce the risk of stroke.

TREATMENT

Ischemic stroke is a medical emergency. Any patient with acute ischemic stroke should be admitted to hospital for prompt evaluation (Table 40.2) and treatment. This is best accomplished in an intensive care unit or stroke unit. Management must be individualized according to the pathophysiologic process.

A. **General measures.** Particular attention should be paid to the following parameters (Table 40.3).
  1. **Medical measures.**
     a. **Respiratory tract protection and infection.** The airway of an obtunded patient should be protected. Some critically ill patients need ventilatory assistance. Aspiration and atelectasis should be prevented. **Nosocomial pneumonia** frequently complicates

TABLE 40.3 Areas of Emphasis in General Medical Measures

Respiration	Hospital-Acquired Infection
Blood pressure	VTE
Fluids and electrolytes	Seizures
Skin care	Spasticity
Dysphagia, aspiration	Depression
Urinary dysfunction	

Abbreviation: VTE, venous thromboembolism.

stroke and is a leading cause of mortality in the second to fourth weeks following cerebral infarction. Risk factors for nosocomial pneumonia include advanced age, prolonged hospitalization, serious medical comorbidity, immunosuppression, and endotracheal intubation.

Dysphagia is common after stroke. Failure of the swallowing process increases the risks of aspiration, malnutrition, and dehydration. The risk of pneumonia is increased by aspiration, which occurs in as many as 25% of unilateral hemispheric strokes and 70% of bilateral hemispheric or brainstem strokes. A meticulous history and examination of the oral, pharyngeal, and esophageal stages with a modified barium swallow using videofluorography are recommended. Oral ingestion of food or liquids is often precluded in the first 24 to 48 hours. Nasogastric feedings are often necessary. Some patients may need a gastrostomy to maintain adequate nutritional intake.

b. Urinary tract infections. Urinary bladder dysfunction can complicate stroke, particularly basal ganglia, frontoparietal, and bilateral hemispheric strokes. Urinary tract infections are an important cause of hyperpyrexia following stroke. They contribute to almost one-third of stroke-related deaths and are present in almost one-half of patients in autopsy series. Incontinent or comatose patients should be catheterized, preferably with a condom catheter for men or a closed Foley's catheter for women. Many patients need an indwelling catheter, which is associated with a risk of infection. In addition, even continent patients can have postvoiding residuals that also increase the likelihood of urinary tract infections.

c. Electrolytic and metabolic disturbances.

(1) **Electrolytic disturbances.** Stroke patients are at risk of electrolyte disturbances resulting from reduced oral intake, potentially increased gastric and skin losses, and derangements in secretion of antidiuretic hormone (ADH). Levels of ADH increase after stroke. In some cases, inappropriate secretion of ADH places the patient at risk of hyponatremia. Possible mechanisms include damage to the anterior hypothalamus and a prolonged recumbent position. In most cases, these alterations do not persist beyond the first week after a stroke.

(2) **Hyperglycemia** in acute stroke is a common phenomenon and correlates with a poor outcome. Hyperglycemia increases the extent of ischemic brain damage. High-serum glucose levels increase anaerobic metabolism, increase lactic acid production in ischemic brain tissue, and cause cellular acidosis. Hypotonic solutions or fluids containing glucose should be avoided.

d. **Venous thromboembolism** (VTE) is a common complication among patients with acute ischemic stroke. The risk is highest in the early weeks after ictus, but remains significant in the chronic phase. The frequency of **deep venous thrombosis** (DVT) ranges from 20% to 40% in hospitalized stroke patients, and approximately 75% of stroke patients may develop DVT without prophylaxis. Moreover, lethal pulmonary embolism may account for upto 25% of the early poststroke deaths. Prophylaxis of VTE is an essential component of stroke center protocols. Prevention includes the use of pressure gradient stockings, pneumatic compression stockings, low-dosage subcutaneous unfractionated heparin (UFH) (5,000 units every 8 to 12 hours), or low-molecular-weight heparin (enoxaparin 40 mg once daily, dalteparin 5,000 units once daily, or tinzaparin 4,500 units once daily).

e. **Cardiac events** constitute an important cause of death after acute stroke because 40% to 70% of these patients have baseline **coronary artery disease.** Cardiac manifestations that can occur after acute ischemic stroke include ECG abnormalities, cardiac arrhythmias, elevation of CK-MB or cardiac selective troponin levels, left ventricular dysfunction, and MI. Approximately 15% of deaths following ischemic stroke are from fatal arrhythmia or MI. As many as 30% of patients have ST segment depression on an ECG in the first 48 hours after the event, and 35% have ventricular couplets or tachycardia. Other changes include QT interval prolongation, T-wave inversion, or increases in duration and amplitude of T waves. Strokes restricted to the insular cortex have been associated with arterial hypertension, cardiac arrhythmias, increased risk of myocardial injury, raised catecholamine levels, and an increased susceptibility to sudden death.

f. **Cerebral autoregulation** is lost during acute ischemic stroke. The blood pressure should be measured frequently during the first few days after ischemic stroke. Transient blood pressure elevation following acute cerebral infarction and normalization over days without treatment are common. Mild to moderate hypertension may be compensatory, and rapid lowering of the blood pressure is generally not recommended. Exceptions to this rule include patients with hypertensive encephalopathy and cerebral ischemia secondary to aortic dissection.

g. Pressure sores. Stroke patients, like other patients with reduced mobility, are at increased risk of having pressure sores. Altered level of consciousness, peripheral vascular disease, and malnourishment are contributing factors. Pressure sores develop most often over bony prominences—sacrum, ischium, trochanters, and the areas around the ankles and heels. The patient's position should be changed frequently to reduce pressure and shear forces. Flotation beds help reduce the risk. Treatment includes debridement and moist dressing. Surgical treatment is sometimes necessary. Cellulitis in the surrounding skin and systemic infection necessitate antibiotic therapy.

h. Depression. Depression occurs in the first few weeks after stroke, but is maximal between 6 and 24 months afterward. Patients with left frontal strokes appear to be more susceptible than are those with right hemisphere or brainstem strokes, but this remains debatable. Depression also correlates with severity of neurologic deficit and quality of available social support. Therapy for poststroke depression is the same as that for endogenous depression.

2. Neurologic measures. Approximately 30% of patients with acute ischemic strokes worsen after the initial event, but deterioration after stroke or "stroke in evolution" does not necessarily equate to propagating thrombus or recurrent embolism (Table 40.4). Massive hemispheric infarctions have a high mortality. Large (malignant) MCA territory strokes (5% of all strokes) are associated with poor prognosis. The underlying mechanism of malignant MCA infarction is often either a carotid terminus occlusion or a proximal MCA occlusion. Acute cerebellar infarction may cause brainstem compression with hydrocephalus.

a. **Brain edema** is the most common cause of deterioration and early death during the first week after acute cerebral infarction. Risk factors for malignant cerebral edema include National Institute of Health Stroke Scale (NIHSS) >20 in left hemispheric strokes (>15 for right hemispheric strokes), carotid terminus thrombus, nausea and vomiting, elevated white blood cells, >50% MCA territory involvement, and additional involvement of anterior cerebral artery (ACA) and posterior cerebral artery territories. Young patients and patients with large infarcts are most affected.

TABLE 40.4 Causes of "Stroke in Evolution"

Thrombosis of a stenotic artery
Thrombus propagation
Recurrent embolism
Collateral failure
Hypoperfusion resulting from hypovolemia, decreased systemic pressure, or decreased cardiac output
Hypoxia
Brain edema
Seizures
Metabolic evolution of ischemic insult
Pneumonia
Urosepsis
Electrolyte abnormalities
Medication effects
Herniation syndromes
Brainstem compression
Hydrocephalus
Hemorrhagic transformation

Massive **cerebral edema** complicates approximately 10% of large hemispheric strokes. Edema develops within several hours after an acute ischemic brain insult and peaks around 3 to 5 days. **Ischemic brain edema** is initially **cytotoxic** and later **vasogenic.** Cytotoxic edema involves predominantly the gray matter, whereas vasogenic edema involves predominantly the white matter. No specific pharmacologic agent has been proved effective against ischemic cerebral edema. Corticosteroids have not been proved useful in the management of ischemic cerebral edema and may even be detrimental. Mannitol does not cross the **blood–brain barrier** and may accentuate compartmentalized pressure gradients between abnormal and normal brain regions. Hypernatremia, hypokalemia, and hypocalcemia can result from excessive osmotherapy. Excessive osmotherapy can also result in intravascular volume depletion and arterial hypotension. Normal saline solution is administered to prevent intravascular depletion. In appreciation of the role of brain tissue shifts, hypertonic saline administration or surgical evacuation of life-threatening supratentorial infarctions by means of hemicraniectomy and duroplasty may have to be considered (see section **B.2** under Treatment).

   b. **Hemorrhagic transformation** occurs in approximately 40% of all ischemic infarcts, and of these, 10% show secondary clinical deterioration. Hemorrhagic transformation often occurs in the first few weeks following stroke, most often in the first 2 weeks. Risk factors for hemorrhagic transformation include large strokes with mass effect, enhancement on contrast CT scans, and severe initial neurologic deficits.

   c. **Seizures** occur in 4% to 6% of cases of ischemic infarction, mostly in carotid territory cortical infarcts. Infarcts in the posterior circulation are infrequently associated with seizures. Cardioembolic strokes have been found to be more epileptogenic than atherothrombotic strokes, but several studies have found no significant difference. Seizures associated with lacunar infarcts are extremely rare. Partial seizures are more common than are generalized tonic–clonic seizures. Many seizures occur within 48 hours of onset of symptoms. In general, seizures are self-limited and respond well to antiepileptic drugs. Patients with seizures that occur in the first few days after the ischemic event do not have increased mortality. Status epilepticus is unusual.

3. **Rehabilitation.** Prevention of complications is the first stage of rehabilitation. Patients who need inpatient rehabilitation are transferred to the appropriate rehabilitation facility. The long-term prognosis for stroke depends on severity and type of neurologic deficit, the cause of the stroke, medical comorbidity, premorbid personality, family constellation, home environment, type of community and available services, and the rehabilitation team. Approximately, 50% to 85% of long-term survivors of stroke are able to walk independently, most of the recovery taking place in the first 3 months. Approximately, two-thirds of long-term survivors eventually become independent for activities of daily living, and approximately 85% of surviving patients eventually return home.

B. **Specific measures.**

1. **Medical therapy.** General measures and use of antithrombotic agents (antiplatelet agents or anticoagulants) and thrombolytic agents remain the mainstays of medical therapy for acute ischemic stroke.

   a. **Antiplatelet agents.** Antiplatelet agents such as aspirin, the combination of extended-release dipyridamole plus aspirin, and clopidogrel play a critical role in the secondary prevention of atherothrombotic events. Antiplatelet therapy is highly effective in reducing the risk of recurrent vascular events and is recommended over warfarin for noncardioembolic ischemic strokes. Antiplatelet therapy should be avoided in the first 24 hours following the administration of intravenous (IV) tissue plasminogen activator (tPA) for acute ischemic stroke.

      (1) **Aspirin.** The mechanism of action of aspirin is irreversible inhibition of platelet function through inactivation of cyclooxygenase. Aspirin reduces the combined risk of stroke, MI, and vascular death by approximately 25%. Early (within the first 48 hours) aspirin therapy (160 to 325 mg/day) is recommended in patients with ischemic stroke who are not receiving thrombolytic therapy. The US Food and Drug Administration (FDA) recommends a dose of 50 to 325 mg/day of aspirin in the secondary prevention of noncardioembolic ischemic stroke. The

main side effect is gastric discomfort. A subpopulation of patients may be resistant to the antiplatelet effects of aspirin.

(2) **Dipyridamole plus aspirin.** Dipyridamole is a cyclic nucleotide phosphodiesterase inhibitor. The Second European Stroke Prevention Study (ESPS-2) randomized 6,602 patients with previous TIA or stroke to treatment with aspirin alone (25 mg twice per day), modified-release dipyridamole (200 mg twice per day), the two agents in combination, or placebo. The investigators reported an additive effect of dipyridamole (37%) when coprescribed with aspirin. There was a decrease in stroke rate with combined treatment versus either agent alone (aspirin, 18%; dipyridamole, 16%). Both low-dose aspirin and high-dose dipyridamole in a modified-release form alone were better than placebo. The combination of aspirin and dipyridamole was effective in reducing the rate of nonfatal stroke, but had little effect on the rate of MI or fatal stroke. Addition of the European and Australian Stroke Prevention Reversible Ischemia Trial data to the meta-analysis of previous trials results in an overall risk ratio for the composite of vascular death, stroke, or MI of 0.82 (95% CI 0.74 to 0.91) in favor of the dipyridamole plus aspirin regimen. A randomized clinical trial comparing aspirin plus extended-release dipyridamole versus clopidogrel in more than 20,000 patients found no difference in recurrent stroke or a composite outcome of stroke, MI, or death after 2.5 years of follow-up. The main side effects of dipyridamole are gastrointestinal (GI) distress and headaches.

(3) **Clopidogrel.** Clopidogrel is a platelet adenosine diphosphate receptor antagonist. In a study enrolling more than 19,000 patients with atherosclerotic vascular disease manifested as either recent ischemic stroke, recent MI, or symptomatic peripheral arterial disease, 75 mg of clopidogrel was modestly more effective (8.7% relative risk reduction) than 325 mg of aspirin in reducing the combined risk of ischemic stroke, MI, or vascular death. The side-effect profile was thought to be relatively benign, with no increased incidence of neutropenia, although a report associated the use of clopidogrel with TTP in 11 patients. Several of these patients were taking concomitant medications. Clopidogrel is a reasonable alternative in patients allergic to aspirin. The addition of aspirin to clopidogrel increases the risk of hemorrhage and is not routinely recommended in patients with ischemic stroke or TIA. However, a recent Chinese study determined the safety and superiority of combination therapy with clopidogrel and aspirin to aspirin monotherapy for reducing the risk of stroke in the first 90 days when administered within 24 hours after onset of minor stroke or TIA. Functional variants in the cytochrome P450 genes can alter the effectiveness of clopidogrel.

(4) **Other agents.** Cilostazol, a phosphodiesterase III inhibitor, is often used for stroke prevention in Japan and other East Asian countries. Triflusal, which is chemically related to aspirin, is considered to be an acceptable first-line antiplatelet agent in some European countries.

(5) **Summary.** Aspirin at doses of 50 to 325 mg/day extended-release dipyridamole 200 mg plus aspirin 25 mg twice daily, or clopidogrel 75 mg/day, are all acceptable alternatives for initial therapy.

b. **Anticoagulants.**

(1) **Prevention.**

(a) **Warfarin.** Warfarin inhibits the **vitamin K-dependent gamma-carboxylation** of factors II, VII, IX, and X. Warfarin is indicated for primary and secondary prevention of stroke among patients with nonvalvular atrial fibrillation (NVAF). Data from a series of AF trials demonstrate an approximate two-third risk reduction in the rate of stroke occurrence when patients are treated to a goal international normalized ratio (INR) range of 2.0 to 3.0. The risk of stroke is the same for patients with chronic or PAF. Warfarin is also indicated for prevention of stroke in patients with rheumatic AF, mechanical prosthetic heart valves, or other selected subgroup of patients with other high-risk cardiac sources of embolism.

(b) **New Oral Anticoagulants (NOACS).** Dabigatran, a reversible oral direct thrombin inhibitor, and the anti-Xa agents (rivaroxaban, apixaban, edoxaban) are used as alternative agents for adjusted-dose warfarin in the prevention of stroke in patients with NVAF. The RE-LY study was a phase III, prospective, randomized, open-label trial comparing dabigatran (110 or 150 mg twice daily) with warfarin. Dabigatran was the first NOAC approved by the US FDA, has a rapid onset of action (1 to 2 hours), is 80% renally excreted, and contraindicated with concurrent administration of P-glycoprotein inducers. Dabigatran 150 mg twice daily was superior to warfarin for the primary efficacy endpoint of stroke and systemic embolism without significant differences in major bleeding; GI bleeding was more frequent with Dabigatran. Dabigatran 110 mg twice daily was noninferior to warfarin for the primary endpoint and had a 20% reduction in major bleeding. Results were confirmed by the RELY-ABLE study, which assessed the long-term effects of the two doses of Dabigatran at 2 year follow-up. Rivaroxaban, the second NOAC approved by the FDA, was studied in the ROCKET AF trial; Rivaroxaban also has a rapid onset of action (2 to 4 hours), has a renal excretion of 35%, and is contraindicated with cytochrome P450 isoenzymes and P-glycoprotein inhibitors because of increased risk of bleeding. Rivaroxaban was shown to be noninferior to warfarin but failed to show superiority for prevention of stroke or systemic embolism. There was greater GI bleeding in the Rivaroxaban group but less frequent IC and fatal bleeding. Apixaban and edoxaban were the last NOACs approved by the FDA. The ARISTOTLE trial demonstrated superiority of apixaban over warfarin with fewer primary outcomes of both ischemic and hemorrhagic stroke and systemic emboli, but the overall rate of ischemic strokes was similar. GI bleeding was similar among both groups, but apixaban had significantly fewer IC bleeds. All-cause mortality was significantly lower in the apixaban group. Apixaban was also compared to aspirin in the AVERROES, which was prematurely stopped because of a clear benefit of Apxiaban for prevention of ischemic stroke and systemic embolism; major and IC bleeding was similar between both groups. Finally, edoxaban at higher dosing (60 mg once daily) was noninferior to warfarin in stroke prevention but inferior at lower dosing (30 mg once daily); major and IC bleeding was less with edoxaban except for GI bleeding. No trial has been completed comparing the NOACs. Dabigatran 150 mg twice daily is the only NOAC shown to decrease ischemic stroke compared to warfarin. Aside from apixaban, all NOACs were associated with more GI bleeding than warfarin. Dabigatran is renally excreted but apixaban and Rivaroxaban are less dependent on renal elimination. Rivaroxaban and edoxaban are dosed once daily, which may be attractive noncompliant patients. NOACs remain contraindicated in patients with mechanical heart valves, rheumatic heart disease, or severe renal insufficiency.

(2) Treatment.

(a) Thrombolytics. Thrombolytic therapy has been a major milestone in the management of acute ischemic stroke. In June 1996, the US FDA approved the use of IV tPA (Alteplase) for ischemic stroke within 3 hours of symptom onset. IV tPA initiated within 3 hours of symptom presentation is a first-line treatment for acute ischemic stroke in selected patients (Table 40.5). Patients are given 0.9 mg/kg/dose (maximum 90 mg dose); 10% of the total dose is administered as a loading dose over 1 minute with the remainder administered over 60 minutes. In the NINDS rt-PA Stroke Trial, favorable outcome was achieved in 31% to 50% compared with 20% to 38% of patients given placebo. Overall, for every 100 patients with acute ischemic stroke treated with IV tPA in the 0- to 3-hour window, 32 patients are benefitted and 3 patients are harmed. The major risk of treatment is symptomatic intracerebral hemorrhage that occurred in 6.4% of patients treated with IV tPA compared to 0.6% of patients given placebo in the NINDS rt-PA Stroke Trial. Predictors of favorable outcome associated with thrombolytic therapy include treatment within 90 minutes, normal baseline CT scan, milder baseline stroke severity, no history of diabetes mellitus, normal pretreatment blood glucose level, and normal pretreatment blood

TABLE 40.5 Exclusion Criteria for Intravenous Thrombolytic Therapy within 3 Hours of Ischemic Stroke Onset

Minor or rapidly improving neurologic deficits (relative contraindication)

Seizure at the onset of symptoms (if residual impairments are postictal)

Symptoms suggestive of subarachnoid hemorrhage

Systolic blood pressure ≥185 mm Hg or diastolic blood pressure ≥110 mm Hg after two attempts to reduce blood pressure

Stroke or serious head trauma in the previous 3 mo

Major surgery in the previous 14 d

History of IC hemorrhage

GI or genitourinary bleeding in the last 21 d

Arterial puncture at a noncompressible site in the previous 7 d

Received heparin therapy within the preceding 48 hr and the aPTT is elevated INR >1.7 or PT >15 s

Platelet count < 100,000 μL

Glucose level <50 mg/dL (<2.7 mmol/L)

MI in the previous 3 mo

Abbreviations: aPTT, activated partial thromboplastin time; GI, gastrointestinal; IC, intracranial; MI, myocardial infarction; PT, prothrombin time.

pressure. Predictors of less favorable outcome and/or cerebral hemorrhage include increasing age, hypoattenuation with mass effect or hypoattenuation in ≥one-third of the MCA territory, diabetes mellitus, pretreatment blood glucose >11 mmol/L, hypertension before, during, and after treatment or requiring postrandomization treatment, severe pretreatment neurologic deficit.

Data by the investigators of the ECASS 3 trial show that IV thrombolytic therapy is also beneficial when initiated within 3 to 4.5 hours of onset of acute ischemic stroke. The ECASS 3 study had strict exclusion criteria such as age over 80 years, combination of previous stroke and diabetes mellitus, oral anticoagulant therapy (regardless of INR values), an NIHSS score of >25, and evidence of major infarct on CT scan with compromise of >one-third of the MCA territory.

NINDS time target recommendations for potential thrombolysis candidates are as follows: Door to door: 10 minutes, Access to neurologic expertise: 15 minutes, Door to CT completion: 25 minutes, Door to CT interpretation: 45 minutes, **Door to treatment: 60 minutes**, Door to monitored bed: 3 hours.

If IC hemorrhage occurs after thrombolytic therapy, stop tPA if still infusing, obtain emergent nonenhanced head CT, check CBC, PT (INR), aPTT, fibrinogen, type, and screen. Transfuse 10 units of cryoprecipitate, 6 to 8 units platelets, 2 units fresh frozen plasma (FFP) every 6 hours; hematology and neurosurgery should be consulted.

If orolingual edema occurs, administer IV solumedrol, Benadryl, and an H2 blocker; hold ACE inhibitor. Awake fiberoptic intubation may be necessary if symptoms progress.

(b) **Endovascular treatment.** Certain patients, deemed unsuitable for IV thrombolytic therapy, may be candidates for mechanical thrombectomy that is recommended over intra-arterial thrombolysis. Patients deemed suitable for IV thrombolysis should still receive IV rtPA even if endovascular treatment is being considered. Inclusion criteria include prestroke modified Rankin Scale (mRS) score 0 to 1, IV tPA administered within 4.5 hours, age 18 years or older, NIHSS ≥6, occlusion of ICA terminus or proximal MCA (M1), and Alberta Stroke Program Early CT Score (ASPECTS) ≥6, and groin puncture can be achieved within 6 hours of symptom onset. Initial imaging should consist of nonenhanced CT head and noninvasive IC vascular study (CT angiogram). Benefit of perfusion imaging is uncertain and may delay time to groin puncture and reperfusion (Fig. 40.6).

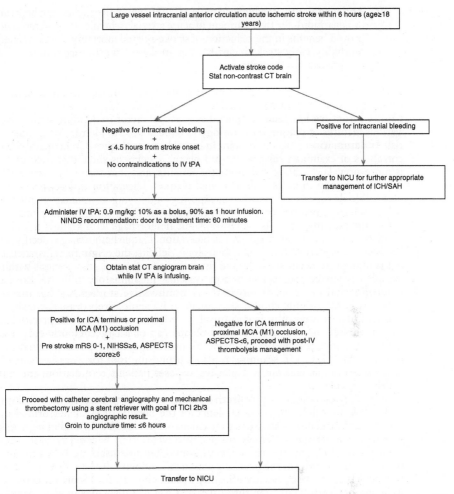

FIGURE 40.6 ASPECTS, Alberta stroke program early CT score; CT, computed tomography; ICA, internal carotid artery; MCA, middle cerebral artery.

Endovascular treatment within 6 hours may also be reasonable for carefully selected patients with occlusion of the M2 or M3 portions of the MCA, anterior, or posterior circulation. Conscious sedation is recommended over general anesthesia. The usefulness of mechanical thrombectomy devices other than stent retrievers is not well established; stent retrievers are therefore indicated in preference to other devices. The goal of thrombectomy should be a TICI 2b/3 angiographic result as soon as possible and within 6 hours in order to maximize functional outcome. Additional use of IA tPA to endovascular therapy may be reasonable if completed within 6 hours of symptom onset. The use of a proximal balloon guide catheter or a large-bore distal access catheter in conjunction with a stent retriever may be beneficial. Although benefits remain uncertain, endovascular treatment may be used in patients younger than 18 years with large-vessel occlusion if initiated within 6 hours, those with prestroke mRS >1, ASPECTS score <6, and NIHSS <6 with occlusion of ICA or proximal MCA. At the time of thrombectomy, angioplasty and stenting of proximal cervical ICA stenosis or occlusion may be considered but utility is unknown.

(c) Anticoagulants. Randomized trials of UFH, low-molecular-weight heparin, or heparinoids for the treatment of acute arterial ischemic stroke showed no proven benefits in the reduction of stroke-related mortality, stroke-related morbidity, early stroke recurrence, or stroke prognosis, except in cases of cerebral venous thrombosis.

2. Surgical therapy.
   a. Carotid endarterectomy (CEA). Approximately, 15% of ischemic strokes are caused by EC ICA stenosis. In addition to the degree of carotid artery stenosis, **plaque structure** has been postulated as a critical factor in defining stroke risk. Various features of **plaque morphology** have been used to identify symptomatic risk. **Inflammation** is also important in carotid artery plaques. Clinicopathologic correlates of examined surgical carotid plaque specimens show that **ulceration** is more prevalent among symptomatic patients, and that thrombus formation is more common in cases with ulcerated plaques. Ulceration is described as an observable disruption of the intima, exposing underlying atheromatous plaque. Atherosclerotic plaques prone to rupture consist of an inflammatory process within the cap, angiogenesis, and intraplaque hemorrhage with gradual thinning of the fibrous cap, loss of integrity, and ulceration. Plaque hemorrhage specifically has been associated with ischemic neurologic deficits; the origin remains unclear but is thought to occur secondary to fissures within the cap, angiogenesis within the atherosclerotic plaque, and/or a perivascular inflammatory infiltrate. Precise determination of vessel **stenosis** using noninvasive studies has significant potential in the routine clinical assessment of ischemic cerebrovascular disease. Carotid ultrasonography is commonly used, but MRI is now a promising tool, accurately identifying ulcerated plaque cap or a large necrotic core and quantifying intraplaque hemorrhage. Fluorodeoxyglucose positron emission tomography (PET) CT scanning is also a promising tool for assessing carotid atherosclerotic plaques but is expensive, exposes patients to radiation, and not widely available.

   Results from landmark prospective studies comparing best medical therapy with **CEA** provide compelling evidence of the benefit of CEA performed by experienced surgeons in improving the chance of stroke-free survival in high-risk **symptomatic patients.** Timely surgical intervention in selected patients with hemispheric TIAs, amaurosis fugax, or completed nondisabling ICA territory ischemic strokes within the previous 6 months, and with 70% to 99% diameter reducing ICA stenosis, can significantly reduce the risk for recurrent cerebral ischemia or death. With low surgical risk, CEA also provides modest benefit in symptomatic patients with ICA stenosis of 50% to 69%, especially among men with hemispheric ischemia who are not diabetic. The procedure's benefit is greatest if done within the first 2 weeks from the ischemic event. There is no evidence that CEA provides any benefit over medical therapy if the degree of stenosis is <50%.

   Controversy still surrounds the selection of **asymptomatic patients** (60% to 99% stenosis) for CEA. Based on combined data from the Asymptomatic Carotid Atherosclerosis Study and the Asymptomatic Carotid Surgery Trial Collaborators, the 5-year risk of stroke in these patients randomized to best medical therapy was around 12%, falling to approximately 6% with CEA. This modest benefit favoring CEA assumes that operative complications are below 3%. Postoperatively, patients should be monitored closely for development of hyperperfusion syndrome and IC hemorrhage.

   It is not known when CEA can be performed safely after thrombolysis; some studies have reported no major complications when CEA was performed a median of 8 days with close monitoring of blood pressure in the pre-, peri-, and postoperative period.
   b. Carotid angioplasty and stenting (CAS). Preliminary data of CAS suggest that CAS may have comparable efficacy to CEA. The Carotid Revascularization Endarterectomy versus Stenting Trial (CREST) showed no significant difference in the composite of any stroke, MI, or death between symptomatic and asymptomatic

patients receiving carotid artery stenting or CEA. In contrast to CREST, other studies have reported an excess risk of new ischemic lesions in patients who underwent CAS. Thus, the relative merit of CEA versus CAS remains a matter of intense debate.

c. **EC/IC bypass surgery.** An early randomized study of medical therapy versus EC/IC bypass surgery failed to show a benefit for surgery. The measurement of oxygen extraction fraction (OEF) by PET has allowed investigators to identify particular high-risk patients who might benefit from EC/IC bypass. However, preliminary data showed no benefit in the reduction of ipsilateral ischemic stroke in patients with symptomatic ICA occlusion and increased OEF on PET.

d. **Decompressive surgery.** In some circumstances of malignant cerebral edema (malignant MCA infarction), early (<48 hours) decompressive surgery with hemicraniectomy and durotomy may be lifesaving (Fig. 40.7A–F). A fronto-temporo-parietal decompressive hemicraniectomy and durotomy should be at least 12 cm in diameter with extension to the floor of the middle cranial fossa with preservation of the superficial temporal artery and facial nerve branches. Mortality and functional

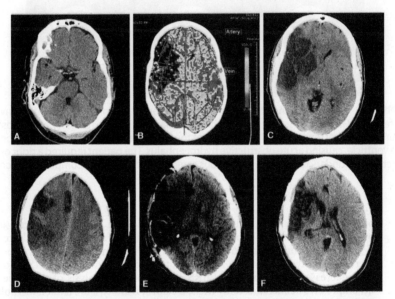

FIGURE 40.7 A: Noncontrast CT of the brain shows hyperdensity in the expected location of the right MCA suggestive of thrombus. There was also loss of the normal gray–white differentiation involving the right frontal and temporal lobes in the territory of the MCA. **B:** CT perfusion demonstrates decreased CBF. There was also decreased cerebral blood volume with associated increased mean transit time (not shown in this composite) in the right frontal and temporal lobes compatible with infarct. **C:** Large area of ischemic change involving the distribution of the right MCA. There is mass effect with midline shift to the left approximately 1.1 cm. There is no evidence of hemorrhagic transformation. **D:** Large area of ischemic change involving the distribution of the right MCA as well as a smaller focus involving the distal right ACA territory. **E:** Postoperative changes from a large right hemicraniectomy and duraplasty. A previously noted subfalcine herniation to the left has decreased from 8 to 4 mm. **F:** Postsurgical change of recent large right convexity cranioplasty. There is abnormal low density and focal volume loss involving the cortex and subcortical white matter of the right cerebral hemisphere, predominately in the right MCA distribution including the right basil ganglia as well as portions of the right ACA territory. These findings are consistent with encephalomalacia at the sites of chronic infarct. There is ex vacuo dilatation of the frontal horn of the right lateral ventricle. ACA, anterior cerebral artery; CBF, cerebral blood flow; CT, computed tomography; MCA, middle cerebral artery. (See color plates.)

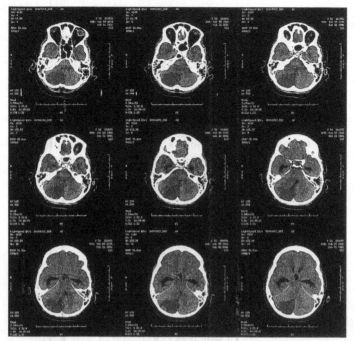

FIGURE 40.8 Axial unenhanced CT demonstrates a large area of low attenuation involving the inferior and posterior aspects of the right cerebellar hemisphere (territory of the posterior–inferior cerebellar artery) causing effacement of the brainstem cisterns and compression of the fourth ventricle, causing acute obstructive hydrocephalus. The patient required a right occipital craniectomy secondary to her large edematous cerebellar infarction. CT, computed tomography.

outcome are improved in patients 18 to 60 years old with NIHSS ≥15, decreased level of consciousness, intact pupil reactivity, and infarct of at least 50% MCA territory (Video 40.2). For patients 61 to 82 years old, decompressive hemicraniectomy increases survival but has no impact on functional outcome of mRS 0 to 2, but does decrease severe disability (mRS 3–4). A pooled analysis of the three major decompressive hemicraniectomy trials, Decimal, Destiny, and Hamlet, was published in the *Lancet* in 2007 looking at primary outcome measure of mRS ≤4 in patients 18 to 60 years old, <45 hours from symptom onset, NIHSS >15, infarct volume >145 cm³, and CT with at least 50% infarction of the MCA territory. Although decompressive hemicraniectomy improved survival, 78% versus 28% (NNT 2), it also resulted in a 15-fold increase in patients with mRS of 4 at 1 year compared to the conservative group (75% surgical vs 24% conservative, NNT 2). In cases of cerebellar infarction with mass effect, when fourth ventricular compression and hydrocephalus are the primary concerns, some neurosurgeons prefer to perform a ventriculostomy. This procedure may be associated with a risk of upward cerebellar herniation through the free edge of the tentorial incisura (Fig. 40.8). For this reason, other neurosurgeons favor posterior fossa decompressive surgery for such patients.

Key Points

- Ischemic stroke can be caused by large-artery atherosclerotic disease, small-artery disease (lacunes), cardioembolism, hemodynamic (watershed) infarction, non-atherosclerotic vasculopathies, hypercoagulable disorders, or cryptogenic or infarction of undetermined causation.
- Prevention of ischemic stroke entails control of modifiable risk factors (arterial hypertension, diabetes mellitus, dyslipidemia, cigarette smoking, obesity, excessive alcohol intake), pharmacologic therapy, and surgical intervention.
- Antithrombotic agents (antiplatelet agents or anticoagulants) and thrombolytic agents are the mainstays of medical therapy for acute ischemic stroke.
- IV tPA initiated up to 4.5 hours of symptom onset is a first-line treatment for acute ischemic stroke in selected patients.
- Endovascular mechanical thrombectomy should be pursued for patients with an occlusion of the ICA terminus or proximal MCA (M1) with groin puncture achieved within 6 hours of symptom onset. Patients deemed suitable for IV thrombolysis should still receive IV tPA even if endovascular treatment will be pursued.
- Endovascular treatment within 6 hours is also reasonable for patients with occlusion of the M2 or M3 portions of the MCA, anterior, or posterior circulation.
- CEA performed by experienced surgeons improves survival in high-risk symptomatic patients. The benefit of carotid artery angioplasty and stenting over CEA remains uncertain.
- In patients with malignant cerebral edema, early (<48 hours) decompressive surgery with hemicraniectomy and durotomy may be lifesaving.

Recommended Readings

Adams HP Jr, Adams RJ, Del Zoppo G, et al. Guidelines for the early management of patients with ischemic stroke: guidelines update. *Stroke.* 2005;36:916–923.

Amarenco P, Bogousslavsky J, Callahan A, et al. High-dose atorvastatin after stroke or transient ischemic attack. *N Engl J Med.* 2006;355:549–559.

Asymptomatic Carotid Surgery Trial Collaborators. The MRC Asymptomatic Carotid Surgery Trial (ACST): carotid endarterectomy prevents disabling and fatal carotid territory strokes. *Lancet.* 2004;363:1491–1502.

Baigent C, Keech A, Kearney PM, et al. Efficacy and safety of cholesterol-lowering treatment: prospective meta-analysis of data from 90,056 participants in 14 randomized trials of statins. *Lancet.* 2005;366:1267–1278.

Berkhemer OA, Puck FSS, Beumer D, et al; MR CLEAN investigators. A randomized trial of intraarterial treatment of acute ischemic stroke. *N Engl J Med.* 2015;372:11–20.

Bhogal SK, Teasell R, Folley N, et al. Lesion location and post-stroke depression: systematic review of the methodological limitations in the literature. *Stroke.* 2004;35:794–802.

Brott TG, Hobson RW 2nd, Howard G, et al; CREST Investigators. Stenting versus endarterectomy for treatment of carotid artery stenosis. *N Engl J Med.* 2010;363:11–23.

Campbell BC, Mitchell PJ, Kleinig TJ, et al; EXTEND-IA Investigators. Endovascular therapy for ischemic stroke with perfusion-imaging selection. *N Engl J Med.* 2015;372:1009–1018.

CAPRIE Steering Committee. A randomized, blinded, trial of clopidogrel versus aspirin in patients at risk of ischemic events (CAPRIE). *Lancet.* 1996;348:1329–1339.

Donnan GA, Fisher M, Macleod M, et al. Stroke. *Lancet.* 2008;371:1612–1623.

Easton JD, Saver JL, Albers GW, et al. Definition and evaluation of transient ischemic attack: a scientific statement of healthcare professionals from the American Heart Association/American Stroke Association Stroke Council; Council on Cardiovascular Surgery and Anesthesia; Council on Cardiovascular Radiology and Intervention; Council on Cardiovascular Nursing; and the Interdisciplinary Council on Peripheral Vascular Disease. *Stroke.* 2009;40:2276–2293.

European Carotid Surgery Trialists' Collaborative Group. MRC European Carotid Surgery Trial: interim results for symptomatic patients with severe (70–99%) or with mild (0–29%) stenosis. *Lancet.* 1991;337:1235–1243.

European Stroke Prevention Study (ESPS-2) Working Group. ASA/dipyridamole is superior to either agent alone and to placebo. *Stroke.* 1996;27:195.

Executive Committee for the Asymptomatic Carotid Atherosclerosis Study. Endarterectomy for asymptomatic carotid artery stenosis. *JAMA.* 1995;273:1421–1428.

Expert Panel on Detection, Evaluation, and Treatment of High Blood Cholesterol in Adults (Adult Treatment Panel III). Executive summary of the third report of the National Cholesterol Education Program (NCEP). *JAMA.* 2001;285:2486–2497.

Goyal M, Demchuk AM, Menon BK, et al; ESCAPE Trial Investigators. Randomized assessment of rapid endovascular treatment of ischemic stroke. *N Engl J Med.* 2015;372:1019–1030.

Grubb RL Jr, Powers WJ, Derdeyn CP, et al. The carotid occlusion surgery study. *Neurosurg Focus.* 2003;14:1–7.

Hacke W, Kaste M, Bluhmki E, et al; ECASS Investigators. Thrombolysis with alteplase 3 to 4.5 hours after acute ischemic stroke. *N Engl J Med.* 2008;359:1317–1329.

Halkes PH, van Gijn J, Kappelle LJ, et al. Aspirin plus dipyridamole versus aspirin alone after cerebral ischaemia of arterial origin (ESPRIT): randomized controlled trial. *Lancet.* 2006;367:1665–1673.

Hankey GJ, Counsell C, Sandercock P. Low-molecular-weight heparins or heparinoids versus standard unfractionated heparin for acute ischemic stroke (Cochrane review). *The Cochrane Library* (Oxford: Systemic Reviews). 2005(3). Update Software.

Hart RG, Diener HS, Coutts SB, et al. Embolic strokes of undetermined source: the case for a new clinical construct. *Lancet Neurol.* 2014;13:429–438.

Hart RG, Halperin JL, Pearce LA, et al. Lessons from the stroke prevention in atrial fibrillation trials. *Ann Intern Med.* 2003;138:831–838.

Hinojar R, Jimenez-Natcher JJ, Fernandez-Golfin C, et al. New oral anticoagulants: a practical guide for physicians. *Eur Heart J.* 2015;1:134–145.

International Stroke Trial Collaborative Group. The International Stroke Trial (IST): a randomized trial of aspirin, subcutaneous heparin, both, or neither among 19435 patients with acute ischaemic stroke. *Lancet.* 1997;349:1569–1581.

Johnston SC, Rothwell PM, Nguyen-Huynh MN, et al. Validation and refinement of scores to predict very early stroke risk after transient ischemic attack. *Lancet.* 2007;369:283–292.

Kase CS, Albers GW, Bladin C, et al. Neurological outcome in patients with ischemic stroke receiving enoxaparin or heparin for venous thromboembolism prophylaxis: sub-analysis of the prevention of VTE after acute ischemic stroke with LMWH (PREVAIL) study. *Stroke.* 2009;40:3532–3540.

Katayoun, V, Hofmeijer J, Juettler E, et al. Early decompressive surgery in malignant infarction of the middle cerebral artery: a pooled analysis of three randomized controlled trials. *Lancet.* 2007;6(3):215–222.

Kidwell CS, Jahan R, Gornbein J, et al; MR RESCUE Investigators. A trial of imaging selection and endovascular treatment for ischemic stroke. *N Engl J Med.* 2013;368:914–923.

Lawes CM, Bennett DA, Feigin VL, et al. Blood pressure and stroke: an overview of published studies. *Stroke.* 2004;35:776–781.

Meier P, Knapp G, Tamhane U, et al. Short-term and intermediate term comparison of endarterectomy versus stenting for carotid artery stenosis: systematic review and meta-analysis of randomized controlled clinical trials. *BMJ.* 2010;340:c467.

Mofidi R, Green BR. Carotid plaque morphology: plaque instability and correlation with development of ischemic neurologic events. In: Rezzani R, ed. *Carotid Artery Disease – From Bench to Bedside and Beyond* [Chapter 4]; 2014:85–104. Available at http://www.intechopen.com/books/carotid-artery-disease-from-bench-to-bedside-and-beyond/carotid-plaque-morphology-plaque-instability-and-correlation-with-development-of-ischaemic-neurologi.

Mohr JP, Thompson JLP, Lazar RM, et al. Comparison of warfarin and aspirin in the prevention of recurrent ischemic stroke. *N Engl J Med.* 2001;345:1444–1451.

Molina CA, Chamorro A, Rovira A, et al. REVASCAT: a randomized trial of revascularization with SOLITAIRE FR device vs. best medical therapy in the treatment of acute stroke due to anterior circulation large-vessel occlusion presenting within eight-hours of symptom onset. *Int J Stroke.* 2013;10:619–626.

National Institute of Neurological Disorders and Stroke rt-PA Stroke Study Group. Tissue plasminogen activator for acute ischemic stroke. *N Engl J Med.* 1995;333:1581–1587.

NINDS. In: Proceedings of a National Symposium on Rapid Identification and Treatment of Acute Stroke. Bethesda, MD: NINDS; 1997. NIH publication 97–4239.

North American Symptomatic Carotid Endarterectomy Trial Collaborators. Beneficial effect of carotid endarterectomy in symptomatic patients with high-grade carotid stenosis. *N Engl J Med.* 1991;325:445–453.

Powers WJ, Derdeyn CP, Biller J, et al. 2015 AHA/ASA focused update of the 2013 guidelines for the early treatment of patients with acute ischemic stroke regarding endovascular treatment. *Stroke.* 2015;46:1–47.

Publication Committee for the Trial of ORG 10172 in Acute Stroke Treatment (TOAST) Investigators. Low molecular weight heparinoid ORG 10172 (danaparoid), and outcome after acute ischemic stroke: a randomized controlled trial. *JAMA.* 1998;279:1265–1272.

Rabinstein AA. Prolonged cardiac monitoring for detection of paroxysmal atrial fibrillation after cerebral ischemia. *Stroke.* 2014;45:1208–1214.

Rothwell PM, Eliasziw M, Gutnikov WCP, et al; Carotid Endarterectomy Trialists Collaboration. Endarterectomy for symptomatic carotid stenosis in relation to clinical subgroups and timing of surgery. *Lancet.* 2004;363:915–924.

Ruiz-Irastorza G, Crowther M, Branch W, et al. Antiphospholipid syndrome. *Lancet*. 2010;376:1498–1509.

Sacco RL, Adams R, Alpas G, et al. Guidelines for prevention of stroke in patients with ischemic stroke or transient ischemic attack: a statement for healthcare professionals from the American Heart Association, American Stroke Association, Council on Stroke: co-sponsored by the Council on Cardiovascular Radiology and Intervention. *Stroke*. 2006;37:577–617.

Saver J, Goyal M, Bonafe A, et al; SWIFT PRIME Investigators. Solitaire with the intention for thrombectomy as primary endovascular treatment for acute ischemic stroke (SWIFT PRIME) trial: protocol for a randomized, controlled, multicenter study comparing the Solitaire revascularization device with IV tPA and IV tPA alone in acute ischemic stroke. *Int J Stroke*. 2015;10:439–448.

Staessen JA, Gasowski J, Wang JF, et al. Risks of untreated and treated isolated systolic hypertension in the elderly: meta-analysis of outcome trials. *Lancet*. 2000;355:865–872.

Vahedi K, Hofmeijer J, Juettler E, et al. Early decompressive surgery in malignant infarction of the cerebral artery: a pooled analysis of three randomized controlled trials. *Lancet Neurol*. 2007;6:215–222.

Wang Y, Wang Y, Zhao X, et al. Clopidogrel with aspirin in acute minor stroke or transient ischemic attack. *N Engl Med*. 2013;369:11–19.

Warlow C, Sudlow C, Dennis M, et al. Stroke. *Lancet*. 2003;362:1211–1224.

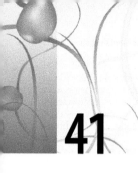

41 Hemorrhagic Cerebrovascular Disease

Harold P. Adams, Jr.

Hemorrhagic cerebrovascular disease includes nontraumatic bleeding that occurs primarily in the brain [intracerebral hemorrhage (ICH)], the ventricles [intraventricular hemorrhage (IVH)], the subarachnoid space [subarachnoid hemorrhage (SAH)], or the subdural space [subdural hematoma (SDH)]. Bleeding often simultaneously involves the brain, ventricles, and the subarachnoid space. Hemorrhagic diseases of the spinal cord are much less common. Most cases of SDH and epidural hemorrhage are related to trauma and are not included in this discussion.

Nontraumatic intracranial hemorrhages (hemorrhagic strokes) annually affect approximately 75,000 Americans, accounting for approximately 20% of all strokes. The 1-month mortality of intracranial hemorrhage approaches 35% to 50%; most of the deaths occur within the first 24 to 48 hours of the onset of the illness. Approximately 10% of cases do not survive long enough to reach a hospital or they die shortly after arriving in an emergency department. Mortality is highest among persons older than 60, those with secondary IVH, and those with severe neurologic impairments (in particular, coma). Only 20% of survivors of intracranial hemorrhage achieve functional independence.

Although the incidence of stroke, including hypertensive hemorrhage, has declined, the rate of SAH, largely due to ruptured intracranial saccular aneurysms, remains stable. The frequency of hemorrhagic stroke may increase in the future as the result of the aging of the American population, an increase in the prevalence of cerebral amyloid angiopathy, increased abuse of drugs that cause hypertensive crises, and the widespread prescription of medications that affect coagulation, in particular agents to prevent stroke among high-risk patients. Although the likelihood of hemorrhagic stroke increases with advancing age, intracranial bleeding also occurs in children and young adults. Because ischemic strokes are relatively uncommon in persons younger than 45, the relative proportion of hemorrhagic events is very prominent in these age groups. The patient's age also affects the diagnosis of the most likely cause of the intracranial hemorrhage. For example, cerebral amyloid angiopathy and hypertension are leading causes of bleeding in the elderly, whereas the average age of patient with a ruptured vascular malformation is approximately 30. Even when trauma is excluded, the risk of hemorrhagic stroke is greater among men than women. The incidence of hemorrhagic stroke is higher among Americans of African or Asian heritage than among those with European ancestry. Intracranial hemorrhage is an especially important cause of death among young African Americans.

CAUSES OF HEMORRHAGIC STROKE

Intracranial hemorrhage is secondary to a large variety of diseases (Table 41.1). In most cases, the most likely explanation for the hemorrhage can be determined.

A. **Occult craniocerebral trauma.** Trauma is the most common cause of intracranial bleeding. The most typical patterns of bleeding are SDH, epidural hematoma, or cortical parenchymal contusions, most commonly at the temporal, frontal, or occipital tips. A history of injury may be lacking if a patient is found unconscious and other clues should be sought such as lacerations, Battle's sign, or soft tissue swelling. While trauma remains in the differential diagnosis, the scenario of a patient with a primary hemorrhage suffering secondary trauma should be considered.

B. **Arterial hypertension.** ICH may be a complication of either acute or chronic arterial hypertension. Sustained chronic hypertension leads to degenerative changes in small

TABLE 41.1 Causes of Hemorrhagic Stroke

Occult craniocerebral trauma
Aneurysms
   Saccular (berry)
   Nonsaccular
      Infective
      Neoplastic
      Posttraumatic
      Dolichoectatic (fusiform)
      Dissection
Vascular malformation
   AVM
   Cavernous malformation
   Developmental venous anomaly
   Telangiectasis
Dural arteriovenous fistula
Arterial hypertension
   Chronic hypertension (Charcot–Bouchard aneurysm)
   Acute hypertension
      Eclampsia
      Stress-related
      Glomerulonephritis
Postoperative hyperperfusion
   After carotid endarterectomy
   After carotid artery angioplasty/stenting
Moyamoya disease/syndrome
Drug abuse
   Amphetamines/methamphetamine
   Cocaine
Tumors
   Primary
   Metastatic
Cerebral amyloid angiopathy
Vasculitis
   Multisystem necrotizing vasculitis
   PACNS
Bleeding disorders
   Hereditary
      Hemophilia
      Sickle cell disease
   Acquired
      Thrombocytopenia
      Leukemia
   Iatrogenic
      Thrombolytic agents
      Anticoagulants
      Antiplatelet agents
Venous thrombosis
Hemorrhagic transformation of an infarction

Abbreviations: AVM, arteriovenous malformation; PACNS, primary angiitis of the central nervous system.

penetrating arteries in the deep structures of the brain. Sudden, severe hypertension may overwhelm the autoregulatory responses of the cerebral vasculature and an arteriole may rupture. Acute, severe arterial hypertension may be secondary to acute glomerulonephritis, eclampsia, severe emotional stress, or the use of a sympathomimetic agent. The most common sites for hypertensive hemorrhage are the basal ganglia (putamen in particular), thalamus, pons, cerebellum, or deep lobar white matter. Hypertension should be considered as the likely cause of a hematoma located in deep gray matter structures of the cerebral hemisphere if the patient has a history of hypertension. Other features of chronic hypertension, such as retinopathy, left ventricular hypertrophy, or renal dysfunction, are supportive of the diagnosis. The magnetic resonance imaging (MRI) finding of asymptomatic microhemorrhages located in deep structures also points to chronic hypertension. Hemorrhagic stroke may be attributed to hypertension because of the presence of an elevated blood pressure measured upon arrival to an emergency department. However, arterial hypertension is common among acutely ill patients with intracranial hemorrhage of many causes and the finding of an elevated blood pressure should not automatically lead to the diagnosis of hypertensive hemorrhage. Acute hypertensive crises (hypertensive encephalopathy) may be associated with SAH that is most commonly located over the convexity of the cerebral hemisphere.

C. Saccular aneurysm. Rupture of a saccular aneurysm is the most common cause of nontraumatic SAH and it is an important cause of ICH. Annually, approximately 30,000 Americans will have aneurysmal SAH. Approximately 1% to 5% of adults harbor intracranial aneurysms but a minority of these lesions actually rupture. In general, the risk for rupture is correlated with the size of the aneurysm, with the highest risk found with aneurysms larger than 6 mm in diameter. Aneurysms in the posterior circulation are associated with a higher risk of bleeding than similarly sized aneurysms in the carotid circulation. Approximately 85% of saccular aneurysms are in the carotid circulation with the most common sites being the junction of the internal carotid artery–posterior communicating artery, the bifurcation of the middle cerebral artery, and the anterior communicating artery. The most common sites in the posterior circulation are the bifurcation of the basilar artery and the origin of the posterior inferior cerebellar artery. Patients with autosomal-dominant polycystic kidney disease have a high prevalence of intracranial aneurysms. Approximately 10% of patients have a family history of cerebral aneurysms.

D. Other aneurysms. Infective, neoplastic, and traumatic aneurysms are rare causes of intracranial hemorrhage. These lesions are usually located in peripheral branch pial arteries on the cortical surface of the cerebral hemispheres. They are smaller than saccular aneurysms, but they have a relatively high risk of hemorrhage. Dolichoectatic (fusiform) aneurysms are tortuous, elongated arterial enlargements most commonly found in the basilar arteries of patients with extensive atherosclerosis or Fabry's disease. Hemorrhage is an uncommon complication. Spontaneous or traumatic dissecting aneurysms of intracranial arteries, particularly of the basilar or distal vertebral arteries, are potential causes of atypical SAH.

E. Vascular malformations. Vascular malformations are classified as arteriovenous malformation (AVM), developmental venous anomaly, cavernous malformation, and telangiectasia. They may be located in any part of the brain. Although familial cases, as with hereditary hemorrhagic telangiectasia (HHT) or familial cavernous malformations may occur, most are sporadic. The rate of bleeding is especially high among persons with HHT. The prevalence of vascular malformations is less than that of saccular aneurysms and most affected persons never have a hemorrhage. ICH is the presenting symptom in approximately 50% of cases. Nonhemorrhagic symptoms include recurrent and stereotypic headache, seizures, or progressive neurologic impairments. Patients with a large AVM that causes turbulent flow may have pulsatile tinnitus and a cranial bruit may be auscultated. A dural arteriovenous fistula also may cause a hemorrhage and may mimic a vascular malformation.

F. Cerebral amyloid angiopathy. Cerebral amyloid angiopathy (congophilic angiopathy) is a leading cause of lobar hemorrhage in older persons. With aging, amyloid is deposited in the walls of cortical and leptomeningeal arterioles. Presumably, the protein accumulation leads to vascular fragility and bleeding. The hemorrhages, which are most commonly located in the frontal and parietal lobes, usually arise at the junction of the cerebral cortex and adjacent white matter. Multiple or recurrent hemorrhages are common and cerebellar hemorrhages may develop. Cerebral amyloid angiopathy should be considered as the likely cause of lobar ICH in persons older than 75. Because approximately 70% of affected patients also have a history of Alzheimer's disease, a past history of dementia or cognitive decline increases the likelihood that an ICH in an elderly patient is due to amyloid angiopathy. The presence of microhemorrhages at the cortical/white matter junction seen by MRI is also supportive of the diagnosis.

G. **Vasculitis.** Multisystem or primary angiitis of the CNS (PACNS) vasculitis is a rare cause of intracranial hemorrhage. Bleeding is most commonly associated with a necrotizing vasculitis, such as periarteritis nodosa. Vasculitis may be the cause of bleeding among some young patients who have hemorrhagic stroke following the use of a sympathomimetic agent. An association between ICH and vasculitis secondary to varicella-zoster virus has been reported and the risk of ICH also is increased among persons who have human immunodeficiency virus.

H. **Bleeding disorders.** Intracranial hemorrhage is a potential complication of several inherited or acquired bleeding diatheses including hemophilia, sickle cell disease, thrombocytopenia, and leukemia. Intracranial bleeding also may complicate the use of thrombolytic or antithrombotic agents. The medications may not be the sole cause of bleeding in some cases; rather, the agents may exacerbate hemorrhage from another cause. Still, the severity of bleeding is worse and the prognosis is poorer among patients with hemorrhage secondary to a coagulation disorder than among other causes of intracranial hemorrhage. Intracranial hemorrhage is a potential complication of use of warfarin; it is associated with a higher likelihood of mortality than with bleeding of other causes. This complication should be considered whenever a patient has acute neurologic symptoms while taking oral anticoagulants, even if there is no other evidence of bleeding. The risk of ICH is increased among the elderly and those who have leukoaraiosis present of brain imaging studies. Persons with a past history of stroke or poorly controlled hypertension also have a high risk of hemorrhage. The risk of intracranial bleeding increases when the international normalized ratio (INR) exceeds 3 to 4. One of the advantages of the new oral anticoagulants (dabigatran, rivaroxaban, apixaban, and edoxaban) for treatment of patients with nonvalvular atrial fibrillation is a lower risk of intracranial hemorrhage than that associated with warfarin. The risk of hemorrhagic stroke is lower with the use of antiplatelet agents. The combination of aspirin and clopidogrel does have a higher risk of serious bleeding than the use of either medication alone. The combination of warfarin and aspirin also is associated with an increased risk of bleeding.

I. **Drug abuse.** The abuse of drugs such as cocaine or methamphetamine has been associated with intracranial hemorrhage. These drugs may lead to bleeding because of sudden surges in blood pressure or because of the development of a vasculitis. In addition, a secondary increase in blood pressure may lead to rupture of a vascular malformation or aneurysm. Intracranial hemorrhage also has been associated with heavy alcohol use.

J. **Moyamoya.** Moyamoya is an uncommon cause of hemorrhagic stroke in children and young adults (Video 41.1). The arteriographic hallmarks of moyamoya are occlusions of the major arteries of the anterior circulation and the appearance of a network of fine blood vessels at the base of the brain. Moyamoya disease appears to be inherited on an autosomal-dominant basis and is most common among persons of northeastern Asian ancestry. Moyamoya syndrome is diagnosed when similar arteriographic findings occur among patients with a number of acquired disorders. Hemorrhage may be secondary to rupture of an aneurysm, most commonly in the posterior circulation, or rupture of a small collateral vessel.

K. **Venous thrombosis.** Occlusion of a cortical vein (cortical vein thrombosis) or cerebral venous sinus (sinus thrombosis) is an uncommon etiology of hemorrhagic stroke. Bleeding is most common among patients with thrombosis of the superior sagittal sinus. In this situation, the areas of bilateral bleeding are parasagittal in location and in a thumbprint pattern. The clinical course of cerebral venous sinus thrombosis differs from that of most other hemorrhagic strokes. Most patients have worsening headache, seizures, altered consciousness, and focal neurologic signs that evolve over a few days. Cerebral venous sinus thrombosis is more common among women and is often correlated with the peripartum state or the use of oral contraceptives. It may also occur among persons who are dehydrated, have malignancies, have undergone a recent cranial operation, or have an otolaryngologic infection.

L. **Brain tumors.** Hemorrhage may be the initial symptom of a highly vascular metastatic brain tumor including choriocarcinoma, melanoma, or carcinoma of the kidney, thyroid, breast, or lung. The most common primary tumors associated with bleeding are glioblastoma and pilocytic astrocytoma. Patients may have a history of evolving neurologic symptoms such as headache or personality change prior to the bleeding event. The presence of extensive brain edema detected by brain imaging during the first hours after the hemorrhage or multiple hemorrhagic lesions should prompt consideration of an underlying brain tumor.

M. **Hemorrhagic transformation of an ischemic stroke.** Modern brain imaging allows for discovery of hemorrhagic changes in the ischemic lesions in a sizable proportion of patients with a recent stroke. A smaller percentage has neurologic worsening secondary to hemorrhagic transformation of the infarction. The risk of this complication increases with the use of thrombolytic agents, anticoagulants, or endovascular interventions within the first hours after stroke.

N. **Reperfusion hemorrhage.** Hemorrhage is a potential subacute complication of surgical interventions (carotid endarterectomy or angioplasty/stenting) used to treat severe stenoses of extracranial arteries. The hemorrhage is attributed to an increase in perfusion to an area of the brain in which autoregulation has been disturbed by the severe stenosis of the parent vessel. The bleeding, which is in the hemisphere ipsilateral to the treated artery, usually occurs 2 to 3 days after the surgical procedure and presents with headache, seizures, and new focal neurologic signs.

MANIFESTATIONS OF HEMORRHAGIC STROKE

The clinical features of hemorrhagic stroke are generally the same in children and adults. The symptoms and signs of primary IVH and SAH may differ from those of ICH in that focal neurologic signs are usually absent or subtle. Because of the absence of prominent focal neurologic signs, errors in diagnosis are more likely to occur among patients with SAH than among patients with bleeding primarily in the brain.

A. **Clinical presentation.** Hemorrhagic stroke is usually a sudden and dramatic event. The patient or observers often relate the circumstances surrounding the onset of symptoms. A headache, of any quality and location, usually described as intense and often is pronounced as the "worst headache of my life." The term thunderclap is often used to describe these headaches. A severe headache accompanied by a transient loss of consciousness or one that is cataclysmic in onset is a premier symptom of aneurysmal SAH. Approximately 40% of patients with ICH will have severe headache. Other symptoms include nausea, vomiting, prostration, photophobia, phonophobia, and nuchal rigidity. The presence of nausea and vomiting and focal signs suggestive of a lesion in a cerebral hemisphere is predictive of a hemorrhage event. The exception to the rule of sudden onset of headache is the course of venous sinus thrombosis, in which the headache may slowly worsen over hours to days.

Disturbances in consciousness are common. Prolonged unresponsiveness, including coma, occurs among patients with major hemorrhages. Transient alteration in alertness, which may mimic syncope, may be present at the time of the hemorrhage. Disorientation, confusion, or delirium also may occur. Although focal or generalized seizures may develop, recurrent seizures or status epilepticus are uncommon.

Focal neurologic symptoms/signs reflect the location of the hematoma. The most common pattern is a contralateral hemiparesis and sensory loss secondary to a hematoma in the basal ganglia. Patients with cerebellar hemorrhages may have a subacute course. They report headache, vertigo, disturbed balance, nausea, and vomiting. Signs of increased intracranial pressure (ICP) or brainstem compression subsequently appear, including declines in consciousness, cranial nerve palsies, and motor impairments. Although most patients with SAH or primary IVH do not have focal neurologic signs, some patients with aneurysms will have focal impairments. The most common is a third nerve palsy secondary to a ruptured aneurysm located on the posterior communicating artery.

B. **General examination.** Assessment of the vital signs, airway, breathing, and circulation (ABCs) of emergency care is the first step in the examination of the critically ill person with a suspected intracranial hemorrhage (Table 41.2). Vital signs are measured closely and neurologic assessments are done frequently to monitor for evidence of neurologic worsening or improvement. Securing the airway, most commonly with intubation, should be used for treatment of those patients with impaired consciousness, seizures, vomiting, or evidence of brainstem dysfunction. Patients with severe bleeding may have respiratory abnormalities that lead to hypoxia, hypercapnia, or acidosis. Fever is relatively common especially among patients with IVH and SAH. Electrocardiographic abnormalities and cardiac arrhythmias

TABLE 41.2 Examination of a Patient with Suspected Intracranial Hemorrhage

Vital signs
  Airway
  Breathing and respiratory pattern
  Temperature
  Cardiovascular assessment
    Heart rate and rhythm
    Blood pressure
Screening for bleeding elsewhere
  Petechiae and ecchymosis
Signs of craniocerebral trauma
  Battle's sign
  Raccoon eyes
  Ocular hemorrhage
  Scalp laceration or hematoma
Signs of meningeal irritation
  Brudzinski's sign
  Kernig's sign
Ocular signs
  Subhyaloid, retinal, or conjunctival hemorrhages
  Papilledema
Neurologic examination
  Level of consciousness—GCS
  Cognition and language
  Articulation
  Motor
  Sensory
  Visual fields
  Cranial nerves

Abbreviation: GCS, Glasgow Coma Scale.

may also be detected. Some of the cardiac arrhythmias may be life-threatening and require emergency treatment. Most patients will have an elevated blood pressure. Neurogenic pulmonary edema also is a potential complication of severe hemorrhages.

Detection of a bruit over the head may point to an AVM. Multiple areas of ecchymosis or petechiae may suggest infective endocarditis, recent trauma, or an underlying coagulation disorder. Evidence of cervical spine, facial, or cranial injury should be sought. Neck pain or tenderness may represent an associated cervical spine injury in a patient with cranial trauma that may be secondary to the hemorrhage. The neck should not be flexed to screen for signs of meningeal irritation until a cervical spine fracture has been excluded. Meningeal irritation may result from blood in the subarachnoid space. Nuchal rigidity (Brudzinski's sign) may not be present in patients with a hematoma restricted to the brain or in those who are comatose. A stiff neck is prominent among patients with SAH but this sign may take several hours to appear. Ocular hemorrhages (subhyaloid, conjunctival, or retinal) may be detected in approximately 20% of patients, especially among those with impaired consciousness. Because the course of the illness is short, papilledema is not commonly found in the first hours of the illness. The exception to this rule is patients who have bleeding secondary to venous sinus thrombosis or in some patients with brain tumors.

C. Assessment of consciousness. The most important component of the neurologic examination is the examination of the patient's level of consciousness because it strongly correlates with the severity of the hemorrhage and prognosis. While the easily calculated Glasgow Coma Scale (GCS) was originally developed to assess patients with head injuries, it is directly applicable to persons with nontraumatic brain hemorrhages. In general, score of 8 or less on the GCS correlates with a very poor prognosis. The score on the GCS is also one of

TABLE 41.3 The Intracerebral Hemorrhage Scale and the Hunt–Hess Scale

Intracerebral Hemorrhage Scale	Points (Score Ranges from 0 to 6 Points)
GCS Score	
3–4 points	2
5–12 points	1
13–15 points	0
Volume of ICH on CT (cm3)	
30 cm or greater	1
Less than 30 cm	0
IVH	
Present	1
Absent	0
Hemorrhage Infratentorial in Location	
Yes	1
No	0
Age	
80 years or older	1
Younger than 80	0
Hunt and Hess Scale for Subarachnoid Hemorrhage	
Grade	**Findings**
1	Asymptomatic, mild headache, slight nuchal rigidity
2	Moderate to severe headache, nuchal rigidity, cranial nerve palsy but no other neurologic deficit
3	Drowsiness, confusion, mild focal neurologic deficit
4	Stupor, moderate to severe hemiparesis
5	Coma, decerebrate posturing

Abbreviations: CT, computed tomography; GCS, Glasgow Coma Scale; ICH, intracerebral hemorrhage; IVH, intraventricular hemorrhage.

the major components of the Intracerebral Hemorrhage Score (Table 41.3). The level of consciousness is also a major contributor to scoring the Hunt–Hess scale to determine the severity of SAH.

D. Neurologic examination. The remainder of the neurologic examination is aimed at detecting abnormalities that reflect the location of the hemorrhage within the brain. Depending upon the site of the bleeding, motor, sensory, language, or cranial nerve impairments are found.

DIFFERENTIAL DIAGNOSIS OF HEMORRHAGIC STROKE

The differential diagnosis of an intracranial hemorrhage is not extensive. The brief course, clinical severity, and the prominent focal neurologic signs are relatively specific.

A. Ischemic stroke. The leading alternative diagnosis is acute ischemic stroke. Although there are no unique features, patients with hemorrhagic stroke are generally more seriously ill than those with ischemic events. Headaches, an early decline in consciousness, nausea, vomiting, photophobia, and phonophobia are more prominent with hemorrhagic lesions.

B. Craniocerebral trauma. Differentiation of traumatic from spontaneous intracranial hemorrhage may be difficult when a patient is comatose and no history is available. In general, deep hemorrhages within the brain are not secondary to trauma.

C. Subarachnoid and primary intraventricular hemorrhage. In contradistinction to ICH, the differential diagnosis of SAH and primary IVH is broad (Table 41.4). Although these patients usually seek medical attention because of the severity of their symptoms, physicians may be misled because of the absence of focal neurologic signs or disturbances in consciousness. The

TABLE 41.4 Differential Diagnosis of Subarachnoid Hemorrhage

Migraine headache
Tension headache
Sinusitis
Viral meningitis
Influenza or systemic illness
Hypertensive crisis including eclampsia
Head or cervical spine injury
Herniated cervical disk
Alcohol or drug intoxication

diagnosis of SAH is missed in approximately 15% of cases, a scenario that most commonly occurs in the least seriously ill patients. Failure to recognize a ruptured aneurysm has serious implications because of the high risk of a potentially fatal recurrent hemorrhage and because of the availability of effective therapies that can be administered. The only way to avoid missing an SAH or primary IVH is to maintain a high index of suspicion. Patients who have a sudden onset of an exceptionally severe headache or a headache associated with loss of consciousness need to be screened. The absence of focal neurologic signs or meningeal irritation does not preclude the diagnosis. Atypical symptoms of SAH include severe neck, face, shoulder, eye, or ear pain. A ruptured aneurysm in the posterior fossa may produce neck or back pain as a primary symptom.

DIAGNOSTIC STUDIES

The goals of the emergency evaluation are (1) to confirm hemorrhage as the cause of the neurologic symptoms, (2) to screen for acute neurologic or medical complications, and (3) to determine the most likely explanation for the bleeding event (Table 41.5). These persons are at high risk for a variety of serious neurologic complications including brain edema, increased ICP, hydrocephalus, and seizures. Medical complications include myocardial ischemia, cardiac arrhythmias, neurogenic pulmonary edema, respiratory abnormalities, gastrointestinal bleeding, and fluid and electrolyte disturbances. Before they are moved, patients with possible craniocerebral trauma should have imaging of the cervical spine.

A. Computed tomography (CT) of the brain (Fig. 41.1). The single most important diagnostic study is CT of the brain. It is relatively inexpensive, noninvasive, quick, easy to perform, and available at most hospitals. The yield of CT is extraordinarily high. When it is performed within 24 hours of onset, blood density can be detected in almost 100% of patients with ICH and approximately 95% of patients with SAH. The presence of a "spot sign" on an early, contrast-enhanced CT study/computed tomographic angiography (CTA) predicts those patients who are likely to have enlargement of their hematoma. Sequential CT studies obtained during the first hours of the illness often show enlargement of a hematoma presumably as a result of continued bleeding. Besides detecting the blood in the subarachnoid space in most cases of SAH, the pattern and severity of the bleeding seen on CT help predict subsequent complications including vasospasm. With aneurysmal SAH, CT will demonstrate subarachnoid blood primarily in the basal cisterns near the Circle of Willis. The location of the bleeding also points to the likely site of the ruptured aneurysm. Isolated subarachnoid blood found over the convexity may represent a hypertensive crisis associated with cerebral vasoconstriction syndrome or hypertensive encephalopathy. Blood located around the brainstem is a feature of perimesencephalic SAH. CT may miss a small collection of subarachnoid blood in a patient with a mild hemorrhage or if the bleeding is in the posterior fossa. If the CT is performed several days after the event, the yield of the test in detecting the bleeding decreases considerably because the blood may have been reabsorbed. CT also detects early complications of hemorrhage including hydrocephalus, mass effect, brain edema, and herniation. Contrast-enhanced CT may detect an underlying vascular malformation or aneurysm. CTA is a valuable method to image the vasculature at

TABLE 41.5 Diagnostic Studies of Patients with Hemorrhagic Stroke

Initial Emergency Studies
CT of the brain
Cervical spine films (if neck injury is being considered)
Electrocardiogram
Pulse oximetry
Complete blood count including platelets
Activated partial thromboplastin time
Prothrombin time/INR
Serum electrolytes
Blood glucose
CSF examination (if SAH is suspected and CT is negative)

Subsequent Emergency Studies
CTA
MRI and MRA
Arteriography

Additional Studies
TCD
Blood cultures (if infective endocarditis is suspected)
Fibrinogen
Sickle cell screen
Erythrocyte sedimentation rate
C-reactive protein
Urine and blood screens for illicit drugs
Brain and meningeal biopsy

Abbreviations: CT, computed tomography; CSF, cerebrospinal fluid; CTA, computed tomographic angiography; INR, international normalized ratio; MRI, magnetic resonance imaging; MRA, magnetic resonance angiography; SAH, subarachnoid hemorrhage; TCD, transcranial Doppler.

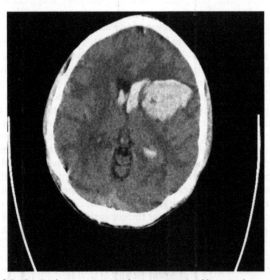

FIGURE 41.1 CT of the brain demonstrates a large putaminal hemorrhage with secondary IVH and shift of midline structures. In addition, the sulci are obliterated, which provides indirect evidence of mass effect and increased ICP. CT, computed tomography; ICP, intracranial pressure; IVH, intraventricular hemorrhage.

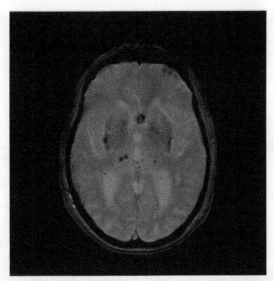

FIGURE 41.2 Gradient echo sequence MRI of the brain reveals several small microhemorrhages in the basal ganglia and the thalamus bilaterally. In addition, an aneurysm of the anterior cerebral artery is also visualized. MRI, magnetic resonance imaging.

the base of the brain, and, in particular, to examine the anatomic relationships of saccular aneurysms. CTA also may be used to monitor for the development of vasospasm that complicates SAH.

B. **MRI.** Multisequence MRI is as sensitive as CT in the detection of intracranial bleeding (Fig. 41.2). It also provides additional data about the most likely cause of bleeding. Although more expensive and not as widely available as CT, MRI does have advantages. Because of time-linked changes in the responses of iron in the hematomas of varying ages, MRI provides information about the age of the hemorrhagic lesion. A gradient echo sequence is useful in detecting microhemorrhages, which are often found among patients with amyloid angiopathy or long-standing hypertension. Abnormal flow voids may be found with vascular malformations. MRI is also useful in screening for tumors or cerebral venous sinus thrombosis. Magnetic resonance venography is used to screen for venous sinus thrombosis and magnetic resonance angiography (MRA) also may be performed to detect aneurysms or vascular malformations.

C. **Examination of the cerebrospinal fluid.** The role of the examination of the cerebrospinal fluid (CSF) has declined with the advent of modern brain imaging. If CT or MRI shows a hemorrhage, there is little reason to evaluate the CSF for the presence of blood. Conversely, CSF examination remains important if SAH is suspected and CT does not show blood. The most common situation is among alert patients with mild signs. The risk of neurologic complications, including herniation, following lumbar puncture (LP) is low in an alert patient who does not have focal signs and has no mass found on CT. Determining whether the source of blood in the CSF is from an intracranial hemorrhage or is secondary to the procedure itself (blood tap) may be difficult. Bloody CSF from SAH usually does not clear in sequentially collected tubes. Xanthochromia (yellowing) of the CSF supernatant after centrifugation is the most reliable sign that the blood truly represents SAH but it can take up to 12 hours to appear. A physician should immediately centrifuge a blood CSF specimen to check for xanthochromia because a delay of several hours may give a false-positive result. The CSF findings evolve over subsequent days and if the LP is delayed, only slightly yellow fluid, an elevated CSF protein, or an inflammatory response that mimics viral meningitis may be found.

D. **Arteriography.** The role of catheter cerebral arteriography has changed with the increased use of CTA and MRA to detect vascular malformations or aneurysms (Fig. 41.3). It is

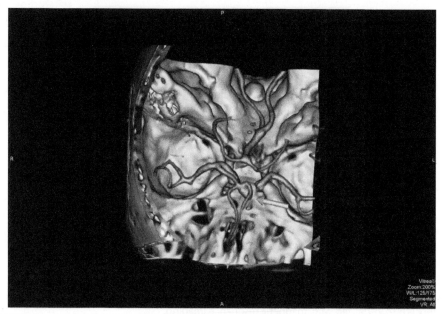

FIGURE 41.3 CTA visualizes an anterior communicating artery aneurysm (*arrow*) in a patient with an SAH. CTA, computed tomographic angiography; SAH, subarachnoid hemorrhage. (See color plates.)

usually not needed for evaluation of older patients with a history of hypertension and a hemorrhage located in the thalamus or basal ganglia. It may be useful in detecting small aneurysms or vasculitis. It may be used to screen for vasospasm after SAH. Currently, the most common scenario for arteriography is its performance as a preliminary step for endovascular treatment of an aneurysm or vascular malformation. It also may be combined with interventions to treat vasospasm.

E. **Other diagnostic studies.** Patients should have coagulation studies to screen for a possible explanation for the hemorrhage. In addition, the results of these tests will influence acute surgical management decisions. Electrocardiography and hematologic and biochemistry studies are part of the evaluation to screen for medical complications or comorbid illnesses. Transcranial Doppler (TCD) has been used to monitor for the development of cerebral vasospasm following SAH.

TREATMENT

A. **Prevention.** Prevention is the most cost-effective strategy for treatment of patients at high risk for hemorrhagic stroke. Administration of antihypertensive agents to patients with acute or chronic elevations of blood pressure may lower the risk of an ICH. Abstinence from use of vasoconstricting drugs of abuse also lessens the risk of hemorrhage. Careful administration of thrombolytic, anticoagulant, and antiplatelet agents also decreases the risk of an intracranial hemorrhage. Management of inherited or acquired disorders of coagulation, including, when appropriate, the administration of clotting factors, is also effective in lowering the risk of a hemorrhagic stroke. Management of an unruptured vascular malformation or aneurysm is often recommended. Choices include endovascular or direct surgical occlusion of larger aneurysms. Surgical resection, focused irradiation, or endovascular therapies alone or in combination are potential therapies for treatment of an AVM. However, recent evidence suggests that in some cases the risks of the interventions, which include stroke, may be greater than the likelihood of a hemorrhage. Unfortunately, in many cases, the initial presentation of the underlying disease is the hemorrhagic stroke and no specific preventive therapy could have been done.

TABLE 41.6 Emergency Management of Hemorrhagic Stroke

ABC of life support—intubation if airway is compromised
Frequent measurements of vital signs and blood pressure
Frequent assessments of neurologic status
Cardiac monitoring, treat serious arrhythmias
Treat fever
Supplemental oxygen—only if hypoxia is present
Intravenous access with slow infusion of normal saline
Treat pain, nausea, vomiting, and seizures

B. **Referral and admission.** Patients with hemorrhagic stroke are critically ill. Inpatient care is warranted because of the life-threatening nature of the illness and because of the high risk of serious neurologic and medical complications. The facilities and personnel required for successful management of these patients are not usually available in most community hospitals. Admission to a specialized treatment facility that has monitoring capabilities and intensive unit level care is needed. The high-risk nature of hemorrhagic stroke means that most patients are referred to comprehensive stroke centers that have critical care, vascular neurology, and neurosurgical expertise.

C. **General management.** Measures to control or prevent acute medical and neurologic complications are part of emergency general management (Table 41.6). Endotracheal intubation and ventilatory assistance may be needed. Cardiac monitoring to detect arrhythmias and frequent measurements of vital signs and the neurologic status should be performed. Hypoxic patients receive supplemental oxygen. Fever should be addressed. Access for intravenous administration of medications and fluids is needed and normal saline is infused slowly. Hypotonic solutions are generally avoided because of their potential effects on the formation of brain edema and because patients may have hyponatremia. Hypoglycemia and hyperglycemia should be promptly managed. Symptoms such as headache, nausea, vomiting, or agitation warrant treatment. Patients who have had seizures receive antiepileptic drugs but the prophylactic use of these agents to patients who have not had seizures is controversial. Because of concerns that the stress of a seizure may induce rebleeding, many physicians prophylactically prescribe anticonvulsants to patients with ruptured aneurysms.

D. **Treatment of arterial hypertension.** Elevations in blood pressure may worsen intracranial bleeding, promote brain edema formation, or induce recurrent rupture of an aneurysm. Most patients' blood pressures decline as pain, agitation, seizures, and vomiting are controlled. The level of blood pressure that mandates medical management is not known but the usual goal is a systolic blood pressure <160 mm Hg. Because elevations in ICP may induce compensatory increases in blood pressure, special caution is exercised when lowering the blood pressure among patients with intracranial hypertension. Responses to antihypertensive agents may be exaggerated. Short-acting parenteral medications are preferred because the dosages may be titrated in response to the patient's blood pressure and neurologic status (Table 41.7). In addition, caution should be exercised when using sodium nitroprusside because its secondary cerebral vasodilatory actions may worsen ICP.

E. **Halting continued bleeding.** Many patients have growth of the hematoma during the first few hours of the illness. This is particularly true for patients who have hemorrhages complicating the use of oral antithrombotic agents. Recombinant factor VIIa did not improve outcomes among patients with spontaneous hemorrhages. Patients with bleeding secondary to warfarin are being treated with four-factor prothrombin complex concentrates; the INR can be reversed in a manner of minutes. These patients also receive vitamin K. There is no specific agent to reverse the anticoagulant effects of the new oral factor-X inhibitors although antidotes are being developed. A recent study demonstrated the utility of the monoclonal antibody, idarucizumab, in reversing the effects of dabigatran in patients with serious bleeding or who needed emergency surgical interventions.

F. **Increased ICP and brain edema.** Increased ICP is an important complication of major intracranial hemorrhages; it results from the mass effect of the hematoma, brain edema, or

TABLE 41.7 Emergency Management of Arterial Hypertension

If systolic blood pressure is >200 mm Hg/mean blood pressure is >150 mm Hg
  Aggressive lowering of blood pressure with intravenous infusion
  Monitor blood pressure every 5 min
If systolic blood pressure is >180 mm Hg/mean blood pressure is >130 mm Hg and evidence of increased ICP
  Reduce blood pressure with intermittent or continuous infusion of medications
  Goal to keep cerebral perfusion pressure >80 mm Hg
If systolic blood pressure is >180 mm Hg/mean arterial blood pressure is >130 mm Hg and no evidence of increased ICP
  Modest reduction of blood pressure with intermittent or continuous infusion of medications
Choices of medications
  Labetalol
    Intermittent doses: 5–20 mg every 15 min
    Continuous infusion: 2 mg/min (maximum 300 mg in 1 d)
  Nicardipine
    Continuous infusion: 5–15 mg/hr
  Esmolol
    Intermittent doses: 250 μg/kg push loading dose
    Continuous infusion: 25–300 μg/kg/min
  Enalapril
    Intermittent doses: 1.25–5 mg every 6 hr
  Hydralazine
    Intermittent doses: 5–20 mg every 30 min
    Continuous infusion: 1.5–5 μg/kg/min
  Nitroprusside
    Continuous infusion: 0.1–10 μg/kg/min
  Nitroglycerine
    Continuous infusion: 20–400 μg/min

Abbreviation: ICP, intracranial pressure.

acute hydrocephalus. Monitoring for ICP may be used to guide treatment; most commonly, this involves placement of an intraventricular catheter. Impaired venous return, fever, agitation, hypoxia, hypercapnia, and hypoventilation may exacerbate ICP and should be managed. Early measures include elevation of the head of the bed, modest fluid restriction, and avoidance of potentially hypo-osmolar fluids. Corticosteroids are not useful. Intubation and hyperventilation are instituted if a patient's condition is deteriorating. Hyperosmolar therapies, most commonly hypertonic saline or mannitol, are prescribed to treat seriously elevated ICP.

G. **Emergency surgical management.** An early decision involves the need for surgical evacuation of a hematoma that is causing mass effects or increased ICP. A ventricular catheter may be used to drain CSF if the patient has secondary hydrocephalus; it can be used to lower ICP and may forestall the need for a craniectomy. Removal of a large, mass-producing hematoma may be a life-saving procedure. Choices include an open craniotomy, minimally invasive surgery, or endoscopic aspiration. Administration of thrombolytic agents to aspiration of an IVH or ICH appears promising. The location and size of the hematoma and the patient's neurologic status, course, and general health affect a decision about surgery (Table 41.8). In general, surgery is recommended for the treatment of a large cerebellar hematoma that is compressing the brainstem or obstructing CSF outflow. Patients with lobar hematomas within 1 cm of the cortical surface may be considered for surgery. However, patients with small-to-moderate-sized hematomas of the cerebral hemisphere do not need surgery. Patients with hemorrhages arising in the thalamus or basal ganglia are not usually surgically treated. There is no evidence that surgical evacuation of such hematomas improves outcomes. There

TABLE 41.8 Indications for Emergency Surgical Evacuation of Hematoma

Surgery Indicated
Cerebellar hematoma >3 cm in diameter with compression of brainstem or development of hydrocephalus (often in conjunction with ventricular drainage)
Hemorrhage with a structural lesion (aneurysm or vascular malformation) that needs to be managed surgically
Moderate-to-large lobar hematoma close to the cortical surface
Surgery not Indicated
Small hematoma or minimal impairment
Large, deep hematoma (thalamus or basal ganglia)
Patient with large hematoma with severe impairments

are no data about the utility of decompressive craniectomy in improving outcomes after intracranial hemorrhage. Administration of rtPA into an intracerebral hematoma or IVH is being studied. The rationale for the use of the thrombolytic agent is that it may promote resolution of the thrombus, which in turn augments aspiration of the hematoma. The doses of recombinant tissue plasminogen activator (rtPA) used in this situation are very low.

H. **General inpatient care.** The components of emergency management are continued after admission to the hospital. Given the seriousness of the illness, most patients are admitted to an intensive care unit setting for monitoring and treatment. Careful nursing care and regular assessments of the patient's condition and vital signs are continued. To decrease the risk of aspiration and pneumonia, liquids and food are not given by mouth until the patient's ability to swallow safely has been confirmed. If the patient cannot take fluids by mouth, a nasogastric tube should be placed. Care in avoiding pulmonary complications is part of general management. Modest fluid restriction is continued for patients who have a large hematoma. Management of intravenous fluids should emphasize maintaining normal electrolyte levels. Some patients will have hyponatremia secondary to cerebral salt wasting and these patients will need hypertonic fluids. Incontinence often mandates placement of an indwelling bladder catheter. Because of the risk of urinary tract infection, the catheter should be removed as quickly as possible. Because bedridden patients have a high risk of deep venous thrombosis that may lead to pulmonary embolism, they may be given enoxaparin or heparin after the risk of continued bleeding has been abated. If a risk for recurrent bleeding is high and the patient has deep vein thrombosis, a filter can be placed in the inferior vena cava. When the patient's condition has stabilized, increased activity, mobilization, and rehabilitation may begin.

CAUSE-SPECIFIC TREATMENT

Management of the cause of bleeding is a key component of the overall treatment for patients with intracranial hemorrhage. Treatment of bleeding diatheses and arterial hypertension already has been discussed.

A. **Vascular malformations.** Patients with a ruptured vascular malformation, most commonly an AVM, may be treated to prevent a second hemorrhage. Because the risk of early recurrent bleeding is relatively low, treatment is usually delayed until the hematoma has reabsorbed. Options for treatment include surgical resection, endovascular administration of vascular occlusive materials, and focused irradiation; these interventions may be done alone or in combination. Decisions for treatment are influenced by the size and location of the malformation and the number and caliber of feeding arteries. Lesions in neurologically eloquent areas and those that are deep in the brain may not be surgically approachable. A high-flow malformation is also a problem because a postoperative state of hyperperfusion leading to hemorrhage or severe brain edema that may follow resection. A staged series including both endovascular and surgical procedures may be performed. Small and deep vascular malformations may be treated with focused, high-intensity radiation that leads

TABLE 41.9 Management of Patients with Aneurysmal Subarachnoid Hemorrhage

Prevention of Recurrent Hemorrhage
Surgical clipping of aneurysm
Endovascular obliteration of aneurysm
Antihypertensive agents
Brief course of antifibrinolytic therapy
Prevention of Vasospasm and Ischemic Stroke
Avoidance of dehydration, hyponatremia, and hypotension
Avoidance of antifibrinolytic agents
Reduction of increased ICP
Nimodipine—dose of 60 mg orally or by nasogastric tube every 4 hr
Drug-induced hypertension
Intra-arterial administration of vasodilator medications
Angioplasty

Abbreviation: ICP, intracranial pressure.

to secondary fibrosis and gradual occlusion of the vessels. Some patients with very large vascular malformations may not be treatable with any of the currently available modalities.

B. Saccular aneurysms. Patients with ruptured saccular aneurysms are vulnerable to both recurrent hemorrhage and ischemic stroke (Table 41.9). Rebleeding is a largely fatal event that peaks during the first 24 hours, when the risk is approximately 4%. The overall risk of recurrent hemorrhage during the first 10 days approaches 20%. The symptoms of rebleeding are similar to those of the initial hemorrhage; another CT will show increased intracranial hemorrhage. The most effective measures to forestall rebleeding are direct surgical obliteration of the aneurysm by clipping or endovascular occlusion of the aneurysm by inserting coils. In general, the goal is to treat the patient as quickly as possible. The selection of endovascular or direct surgical treatment is influenced by the patient's condition, the location of the aneurysm, the presence of serious comorbid diseases, and the presence of vasospasm. Because the morbidity of endovascular treatment is less than that accompanying surgical clipping, the use of endovascular procedures has expanded. Lowering blood pressure or the administration of antifibrinolytic agents to prevent recurrent bleeding can be prescribed but they may be associated with an increased risk of ischemia. Vasospasm is an arterial process that occurs almost exclusively in association with aneurysmal SAH. It is most likely to occur among patients with extensive subarachnoid blood found on CT. The progressive arterial narrowing peaks at 7 to 10 days after SAH and thereafter gradually abates. The arterial narrowing leads to hypoperfusion, which causes brain ischemia. The symptoms of vasospasm are worsening headache, altered consciousness, and focal neurologic signs that may wax and wane. TCD ultrasonography may detect alterations in flow velocities in major arteries before the clinical signs appear. The arterial narrowing also may be detected on sequential CTA studies. Nimodipine is initiated after the diagnosis of SAH because it does improve outcomes. The medication presumably lessens the ischemic effects of the vasospasm; it is unclear whether the medication has any effect on the arterial process. Drug-induced hypertension is prescribed to patients in whom ischemic symptoms develop. Although no controlled trials have shown efficacy of this regimen, several studies report success. The regimen is rigorous and requires monitoring. Besides inducing myocardial ischemia, the regimen could promote recurrent aneurysmal rupture if the aneurysm has not been treated. Hypervolemic hemodilution, which was combined with the hypertension, is no longer used. Arteriography, which may be used to confirm the vasospasm, may be complemented by angioplasty or endovascular administration of medications to treat the arteriopathy.

Key Points

- ICH accounts for approximately 20% of all strokes. It is the primary alternative diagnosis to ischemic stroke.
- ICH remains a highly fatal disease with death commonly because of brain injury itself or secondary to increased ICP.
- A broad spectrum of diseases cause intracranial hemorrhage. The most common are hypertension, saccular aneurysms, vascular malformations, and bleeding disorders. Determination of the cause of the hemorrhage is crucial in both prognosis and treatment.
- With the use of modern brain imaging, the diagnosis of ICH is becoming easier. In addition, vascular imaging is performed to look for the underlying blood vessel disease.
- Initial management involves general emergency care, treatment of the increased ICP, and measures aimed at the hematoma, including surgery. Other surgical procedures are done to treat the causes of hemorrhage such as intracranial aneurysms or vascular malformations.

Recommended Readings

Anderson CS, Qureshi AI. Implications of INTERACT2 and other clinical trials: blood pressure management in acute intracerebral hemorrhage. *Stroke*. 2015;46:291–295.

Andrews CM, Jauch EC, Hemphill JC 3rd, et al. Emergency neurological life support: intracerebral hemorrhage. *Neurocrit Care*. 2012;17(suppl 1):S37–S46.

Connolly ES Jr, Rabinstein AA, Charhuapoma JR, et al. Guidelines for the management of aneurysmal subarachnoid hemorrhage: a guideline for healthcare professionals from the American Heart Association/American Stroke Association. *Stroke*. 2012;43:1711–1737.

Dusick JR, Gonzalez NR. Management of arterial vasospasm following aneurysmal subarachnoid hemorrhage. *Semin Neurol*. 2013;33:488–497.

Grise EM, Adeoye O. Blood pressure control for acute ischemic and hemorrhagic stroke. *Curr Opin Crit Care*. 2012;18:132–138.

Hanger HC, Geddes JA, Wilkinson TJ, et al. Warfarin-related intracerebral hemorrhage: better outcomes when reversal include prothrombin complex concentrates. *Intern Med J*. 2013;43:408–416.

Hemphill JC, Greenberg SM, Anderson CS, et al. Guidelines for the management of spontaneous intracerebral hemorrhage: a guideline for health care professionals from the American Heart Association/American Stroke Association. *Stroke*. 2015;46:2032–2060.

Kowalski RG, Claasen J, Kreiter KT, et al. Initial misdiagnosis and outcome after subarachnoid hemorrhage. *JAMA*. 2004;291:866–869.

Mendelow AD, Gregson BA, Rowan EN, et al. Early surgery versus initial conservative treatment in patients with spontaneous supratentorial intracerebral haematomas (STICH II): a randomised trial. *Lancet*. 2013;382:397–408.

Molyneus AJ, Kerr RS, Yu LM, et al; International Subarachnoid Aneurysm Trial (ISAT) Collaborative Group. International subarachnoid aneurysm trial (ISAT) of neurosurgical clipping versus endovascular coiling in 2143 patients with ruptured aneurysms: a randomised trial. *Lancet*. 2001;36:1267–1274.

Pollack CV Jr, Reilly PA, Eikelboom J, et al. Idarucizumab for dabigatran reversal. *N Engl J Med*. 2015;373:511.

Shivashankar R, Miller TR, Jindal G, et al. Treatment of cerebral aneurysms – surgical clipping or endovascular coiling: the guiding principles. *Semin Neurol*. 2013;33:476–487.

Steiner T, Juvela S, Unterberg A, et al; European Stroke Organization. European Stroke Organization guidelines for the management of intracranial aneurysms and subarachnoid haemorrhage. *Cerebrovasc Dis*. 2013;35:93–112.

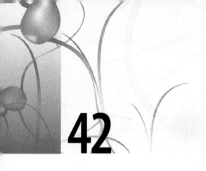

42

Epilepsies in Children

Hema Patel and David W. Dunn

Approximately 3% of the population of the United States is expected to have epilepsy at some time during their lives. Among children, 2% to 5% have a febrile seizure during the first 5 years of life, 2% have a single afebrile seizure, and 0.5% have recurrent afebrile seizures.

CLASSIFICATION

Accurate characterization of epilepsy has practical significance. Differentiation between partial and generalized seizures is important for the appropriate choice of antiepileptic drug (AED) therapy and determination of possible etiology and prognosis. Epileptic syndromes are classified with particular reference to age at onset, etiologic factor, site of seizure onset, and prognosis. Chapter 6 provides clinical descriptions of the different types of seizures.

LOCALIZATION-RELATED (FOCAL, PARTIAL) EPILEPSIES AND EPILEPTIC SYNDROMES

Localization-related (focal, partial) epilepsies and syndromes are characterized by partial seizures (simple or complex partial) arising from a focal cortical area with occasional progression to a secondarily generalized tonic–clonic seizure (GTCS). If this progression is rapid, the initial focal nature may be masked. A simple partial seizure is associated with intact consciousness, whereas during a complex partial seizure, consciousness is impaired. Electroencephalography (EEG) shows focal epileptiform discharges overlying the epileptogenic region.

A. **Idiopathic localization-related epilepsy with age-related onset** represents a group of epileptic syndromes that constitute approximately one-fifth of all cases of epilepsy with onset before 13 years of age. Idiopathic epilepsy is characterized by genetic predisposition, focal (localization-related) seizures and EEG abnormalities, normal intellect and normal findings at neurologic examination and neuroimaging studies, and an excellent prognosis. Currently, the following syndromes are recognized by the International League Against Epilepsy.

  1. **Benign epilepsy of childhood with centrotemporal spikes (BECTS).** Previously known as *benign rolandic epilepsy*, this disorder is the most frequent epilepsy syndrome in childhood.
     a. BECTS accounts for 13% to 23% of all childhood epilepsies and 75% of all benign focal childhood epilepsy.
     b. **Age at onset** is between 3 and 13 years; peak age is 7 to 8 years. Boys are more commonly affected.
     c. **Clinical features** include unilateral paresthesias and clonic activity of the tongue, lip, and cheek, dysarthria or speech arrest, excess salivation, and occasional progression to a GTCS. Seizures are usually nocturnal, during sleep, though 20% to 30% have seizures only during wakefulness.
     d. **EEG** shows frequent, unilateral or bilateral, high-amplitude centrotemporal spike–slow-wave discharges with a horizontal dipole that are activated by sleep, superimposed on a normal background. Thirty percent have spikes only during sleep. Therefore, a sleep-deprived EEG to include sleep should be obtained if this diagnosis is suspected. Approximately 50% of close relatives may also have EEG

abnormalities between ages 5 and 15 years. Only 12% of patients who inherit the EEG abnormality have seizures.

e. **Treatment** is usually unnecessary after the first or even the second seizure. AED therapy can be initiated if seizures are frequent or if they are sufficiently disturbing to the patient or family. All major AEDs prescribed for partial seizures have been reported to be successful even in small doses, such as carbamazepine, oxcarbazepine, valproic acid, gabapentin, phenobarbital, and phenytoin.

f. **Prognosis** is excellent. Approximately 13% to 20% of patients have only a single seizure. Seizures usually resolve within 1 to 3 years of onset and almost always by 14 to 16 years of age. Approximately 1% to 2% persist into adult life.

2. **Benign occipital epilepsy (BOE).** Two forms include the more common early-onset type (Panayiotopoulos type) and rare late-onset type (Gastaut type).

a. **BOE** occurs less frequently than BECTS.

b. **Age at onset.** Early-onset type—4 to 5 years, with female preponderance; late-onset type—8 to 9 years, with both sexes equally affected.

c. **Clinical features.** Early-onset type is characterized by ictal vomiting, tonic eye deviation, only occasionally progressing to GTCS seizures. The seizures are infrequent, often prolonged and usually nocturnal. The late-onset type is characterized by frequent, brief (a few seconds to 2 to 3 minutes), usually diurnal seizures with mainly visual illusions or hallucinations (multicolored circles or spots) or blindness, followed by hemiclonic convulsions and postictal headaches. Consciousness may be preserved, but it is impaired if the seizure secondarily generalizes. BOE is often misinterpreted as basilar migraine (Bickerstaff).

d. **EEG** shows occipital paroxysms of high amplitude, often bilateral sharp or spike–slow-wave complexes attenuating with eye opening and activated by sleep. Generalized or centrotemporal spike waves are found in one-third of all cases.

e. **Treatment** is similar to that of patients with BECTS.

f. **Prognosis.** BOE carries a good prognosis, although it is not as benign as BECTS.

g. Clinical remission rates vary from 60% to 90%.

Two syndromes have been recognized among adult patients—autosomal-dominant nocturnal frontal lobe epilepsy and benign familial temporal lobe epilepsy.

B. **Symptomatic localization-related epilepsy.** Most forms of localization-related epilepsy are symptomatic or acquired. Clinical manifestations depend on the anatomic location of the epileptogenic focus. Temporal lobe seizures (complex partial seizures) are the most common type of symptomatic partial seizures (see Chapter 6).

GENERALIZED EPILEPSIES AND EPILEPTIC SYNDROMES

Generalized epilepsies and syndromes are characterized by seizures that are generalized from onset, usually associated with impairment of consciousness and generalized epileptiform discharges on EEG reflecting involvement of both hemispheres. They include absence seizures, atypical absence seizures, myoclonic seizures, GTCS, atonic seizures, tonic seizures, clonic seizures, and infantile spasms.

A. **Idiopathic generalized epilepsy with age-related onset.** In these disorders, which are listed in the order of age of appearance, the seizures and EEG abnormalities are generalized from the onset. Intellect and findings at neurologic examination and neuroimaging are normal (idiopathic). There is a genetic predisposition with no other identifiable etiologic factor.

1. **Benign familial neonatal seizures (BFNS).** This is a rare, autosomal-dominant form of epilepsy with a genetic defect localized to chromosome 20q and 8q. The genes encode voltage-gated K^+ channels expressed in the brain (*KCNQ2 and KCNQ3*). Seizures occur during the first week of life, usually the second or third day. Diagnosis requires family history of neonatal seizures and exclusion of other causes such as infection, metabolic, toxic, or structural abnormalities. Approximately 10% to 15% develop subsequent nonfebrile seizures.

2. **Benign idiopathic neonatal seizures (fifth-day fits).** Partial clonic or apneic seizures occur on the fifth day of life without known cause and generally cease within 15 days.

3. The neonate is neurologically normal, and prognosis is good with no seizure recurrence. Subsequent psychomotor development is normal.

4. Benign myoclonic epilepsy in infancy. This is a rare syndrome accounting for less than 1% of childhood epilepsies.

   a. **Age at onset** is 4 months to 3 years, typically within the first year.

   b. Clinical features. Brief, generalized myoclonic seizures usually involving the head and upper extremities occur several times daily in an otherwise normal child, usually with a family history of epilepsy.

   c. **EEG** shows brief, generalized bursts of spike–polyspike wave activity, with a normal background.

   d. Treatment. Valproic acid is the drug of choice. Lamotrigine, ethosuximide, and clonazepam can be used if valproic acid is ineffective.

   e. Prognosis. Response to treatment is good. Occasionally, some psychomotor delay and behavioral abnormalities may persist, with progression to GTCS in adolescence questioning the term benign.

5. **Childhood absence epilepsy (pyknolepsy) (see Video 42.1; see Chapter 6).**

6. **Juvenile absence epilepsy (see Chapter 6).**

7. **Juvenile myoclonic epilepsy (impulsive petit mal) of Janz (see Chapter 6).**

8. **Epilepsy with GTCS on awakening (see Chapter 6).**

9. **Generalized epilepsy with febrile seizures plus (GEFS+).**

   Autosomal-dominant disorder manifesting with febrile seizures in children <1 year of age, which persist beyond 5 to 6 years, when nonfebrile seizures, usually GTCS, also occur. Seizures may persist into adolescence or longer. Family history of febrile seizures is necessary to the diagnosis. It has been linked to a number of gene loci (*SCN1B*, *SCN1A*, and *GABRG2*). GEFS+ occurs with inherited missense mutations of *SCN1A*, while de novo truncating mutations result in severe myoclonic epilepsy of infancy (SMEI; Dravet's syndrome).

B. Symptomatic or cryptogenic generalized epilepsy. These disorders, which are listed in order of age of appearance, include generalized epilepsy syndromes secondary to known or suspected disorders of the central nervous system (CNS; symptomatic) or to disorders, the causes of which are hidden or occult (cryptogenic).

   1. **Infantile spasms (West's syndrome) (see Video 42.2).**

      a. Etiology. With the availability of newer neuroimaging techniques, only 10% to 15% of cases are cryptogenic. In symptomatic cases, there is evidence of previous brain damage (mental retardation, neurologic and radiologic evidence, or a known etiologic factor) (Table 42.1).

      b. Age at onset. Onset occurs in infancy (peak 4 to 8 months).

TABLE 42.1 Causes of Secondary Generalized Epilepsy Syndromes (Infantile Spasms and LGS)

Idiopathic, Cryptogenic
Symptomatic
Perinatal factors: hypoxic-ischemic encephalopathy, hypoglycemia, and hypocalcemia
Infection: intrauterine infection (toxoplasmosis, rubella, and cytomegalovirus, herpes), meningoencephalitis
Cerebral malformation: holoprosencephaly, lissencephaly, polymicrogyria, Aicardi's syndrome
Vascular: infarction, hemorrhage, porencephaly
Neurocutaneous syndromes: tuberous sclerosis complex, Sturge–Weber syndrome, and others (e.g., neurofibromatosis type 1)
Metabolic disease: nonketotic hyperglycinemia, pyridoxine deficiency, aminoacidopathy (phenylketonuria, maple syrup urine disease)
Chromosomal disorders: Down's syndrome, Angelman's syndrome (happy puppet syndrome: abnormality in chromosome 15q11–13, seizures, developmental delay, dysmorphic features, and paroxysms of inappropriate laughter)

Abbreviation: LGS, Lennox–Gastaut syndrome.

c. **Clinical features** compose the triad of infantile spasms, mental retardation, and hypsarrhythmia. Infantile spasms occur in clusters, frequently during drowsiness and on awakening, characterized by brief nodding of the head associated with extension or flexion of the trunk, and often of the extremities. They occur rapidly, suggestive of a startle reaction. They can be flexor (salaam attacks), extensor, or most commonly, mixed spasms. They are almost always associated with arrested development.

d. **EEG** shows hypsarrhythmia—chaotic, high-amplitude, disorganized background with multifocal independent spike-and-wave discharges and electrodecremental periods. Intravenous (IV) pyridoxine (vitamin B_6) should be administered in a dose of 100 mg during the EEG to exclude pyridoxine-dependent infantile spasms.

e. **Treatment.**

(1) Underlying conditions are managed as identified. Adrenocorticotropic hormone (ACTH) and vigabatrin are the initial drugs of choice.

(2) **ACTH.** Opinions vary regarding dosage and duration of ACTH therapy, ranging from high-dose therapy (150 IU/m^2/day) to low-dose therapy (20 to 40 IU/day). We recommend starting at 40 to 80 IU/day administered intramuscularly and continuing for 3 to 4 weeks, or for a shorter period if an early positive clinical response is observed. The dosage is then slowly decreased approximately 20% per week over 6 to 9 weeks. If seizures recur during withdrawal, the dosage should be increased to the previous effective level. ACTH therapy is initiated in the hospital under the guidance of a pediatric neurologist. Parents should be taught the injection technique with systematic rotation of the injection site.

(3) **Side effects of ACTH therapy** are irritability, hyperglycemia, hypertension, sodium and water retention, potassium depletion, weight gain, gastric ulcers, occult gastrointestinal bleeding, suppression of the immune system, infection, cardiomyopathy, congestive heart failure, and diabetic ketoacidosis.

(4) **Laboratory tests before initiation of ACTH therapy** include baseline EEG, serum electrolytes, blood urea nitrogen (BUN), serum creatinine, glucose, urinalysis, complete blood count (CBC), chest radiograph, and tuberculin skin test when appropriate.

(5) **Laboratory tests performed weekly during ACTH therapy** include serum electrolytes, blood glucose, stool guaiac, and monitoring of weight and blood pressure.

(6) **Concomitant management.** An antacid or a histamine H_2 receptor antagonist (ranitidine) should be administered during ACTH therapy.

f. **Alternative treatment.**

(1) **Prednisone** may be substituted when ACTH cannot be administered because parents cannot or will not learn to give injections. It is administered orally at 2 to 3 mg/kg/day for 3 to 4 weeks and gradually withdrawn in a schedule similar to ACTH withdrawal.

(2) **Other AEDs.** Vigabatrin (100 to 150 mg/kg/day) has the best response rates in patients with tuberous sclerosis. However, irreversible constriction of peripheral vision may occur in 30% to 50% of patients. It is therefore administered for not more than 6 months, and discontinued in 3 weeks if no response is noted. Valproic acid (usually at high therapeutic levels of 75 to 125 μg/mL) is used cautiously because of a higher risk of liver dysfunction in children younger than 2 years of age. Topiramate, zonisamide, and clonazepam have also been reported to be effective. Nitrazepam and clobazam have also been tried.

(3) **Excisional surgery** of the region of cortical abnormality defined at EEG, magnetic resonance imaging (MRI), and positron emission tomography (PET) is being performed on children with infantile spasms intractable to medical therapy, but only in specialized centers.

g. **Prognosis.** West's syndrome has a high morbidity, with a 90% incidence of mental retardation. From 25% to 50% of cases evolve into other type of epilepsies such as Lennox–Gastaut syndrome (LGS), with the infantile spasms transforming to other seizure types (GTCS, myoclonic, and tonic seizures) over subsequent years. Favorable prognostic indicators are as follows:

(1) Cryptogenic spasms have a better prognosis than symptomatic cases.

(2) Normal development before the onset of spasms and normal brain MRI

(3) Short duration of seizures before control

2. **LGS.**
   a. Etiology. A large number of patients have a history of infantile spasms. About 10% to 40% of cases are cryptogenic. In the 60% to 90% of symptomatic cases, a specific cause, usually perinatal insult, is found (Table 42.1).
   b. **Age at onset** is 1 to 8 years of age, with peak between 3 and 5 years.
   c. **Clinical features** are seizures of multiple types, typically tonic, atypical absence, and also atonic, and myoclonic seizures. GTCS and partial seizures may also be seen. Seizures are often frequent and intractable to medical treatment. Most patients have cognitive dysfunction.
   d. **EEG** shows slow background activity, generalized, bisynchronous, 2 to 2.5 Hz spike and sharp–slow-wave discharges activated by sleep, generalized paroxysmal fast spike activity (10 Hz), and other multifocal epileptiform abnormalities.
   e. Treatment.
      (1) **AEDs.** Broad-spectrum AEDs such as valproic acid are required for treatment against all the different types of seizures associated with LGS. However, these seizures are often intractable, and valproic acid may have to be used in combination with other broad-spectrum AEDs. Ethosuximide, **lamotrigine, and topiramate** have successfully demonstrated efficacy as adjunctive therapy in LGS. Rufinamide, zonisamide, and levetiracetam have also been reported to be effective. Felbamate, though effective, is infrequently used because of severe side effects such as aplastic anemia and acute liver failure. Phenytoin and phenobarbital may be helpful in controlling the associated GTCS. Benzodiazepines (clonazepam, nitrazepam, and clobazam) can be used, but may be associated with side effects of decreased alertness and drowsiness, which are associated with increased seizure frequency. IV diazepam or lorazepam may induce tonic seizures, and carbamazepine can exacerbate absence seizures.
      (2) **Ketogenic diet** may be effective for patients with otherwise intractable seizures. Benefits include fewer seizures, less drowsiness, and fewer concomitant AEDs.
      (3) **ACTH** has been found to be effective in the treatment of some patients.
      (4) **Psychological support** for the child and family. A prescription for protective helmets to prevent head injuries in patients with drop attacks is helpful.
      (5) **Surgical procedures** such as corpus callosotomy, hemispherectomy, and rarely resection of a localized lesion have been tried with variable results. Vagal nerve stimulation is also effective with at least 50% reduction in seizure frequency in follow-up periods as long as 5 years.
3. Myoclonic astatic epilepsy (MAE)—Doose's syndrome.
   a. **Age at onset** is from 6 months to 6 years with a peak at 3 years, with male preponderance.
   b. Clinical features. GTCS are seen at onset, progressing to the characteristic myoclonic or myoclonic astatic seizures characterized by a myoclonic jerk followed by loss of muscle tone, which may result in a sudden fall. Absence seizures are seen as well, often associated with a clonic component. Seizures occur frequently on awakening. Tonic seizures are less common in contrast to LGS.
   c. **EEG** may be initially normal except for brief bursts of parietal 4 to 7 Hz theta activity. Brief bursts of generalized spike and polyspike wave discharges are seen later.
   d. Treatment. Valproic acid is the drug of choice. Ethosuximide and ketogenic diet are also effective.
   e. **Prognosis** ranges from remission of seizures with normal development to intractable epilepsy with severe cognitive impairment.
4. Symptomatic seizures. Myoclonic seizures are difficult to differentiate from nonepileptic myoclonus. However, characteristic epileptiform discharges associated with myoclonic jerks in myoclonic epilepsy help differentiate the two.
   a. **Early myoclonic encephalopathy** is characterized by the onset of medically intractable myoclonic seizures and partial seizures in early infancy before 3 months of age, burst suppression on EEG, and very poor prognosis including profound neurologic impairment or death in the first year of life. Multiple causes include inborn errors of metabolism such as nonketotic hyperglycinemia, methymalonic acidemia, and proprionic acidemia.

b. **Early infantile epileptic encephalopathy (Ohtahara's syndrome)** is characterized by an early onset of tonic spasms within the first few months of life, which are medically intractable. Myoclonic seizures are rare. The burst-suppression pattern on EEG is present during waking and sleep states. MRI demonstrates severe developmental anomalies such as hemimegalencephaly, porencephaly, and Aicardi's syndrome. The prognosis is very poor. Mutations in the gene encoding syntaxin binding protein 1 (*STXBP1*) have been reported.

c. **Severe Myoclonic Epilepsy in Infancy (Dravet's syndrome)** represents 3% to 5% of all epilepsies starting in the first year of life. The disorder begins in the first year of life as febrile seizures, followed by myoclonic seizures, atypical absences, and convulsive seizures between 1 and 4 years of age. The seizures are often triggered by fever, hot baths, or hot weather. The child is initially normal, but cognition becomes progressively impaired. EEG shows generalized spike and polyspike–slow wave activity, focal or multifocal spikes. Photosensitivity is seen in 40%. Sodium-channel blockers such as carbamazepine, oxcarbazepine, phenytoin, and lamotrigine may induce worsening of seizures. The seizures are medically intractable, but may respond to valproic acid, topiramate, and clobazam. Stiripentol has also proved to be effective as is ketogenic diet. A link between SMEI and GEFS+ has been identified in several families. *SCN1A* gene mutations (both truncating and missense) on chromosome 2p24 in coding for the neuronal voltage-gated sodium channel α1 subunit have been found in 80% of patents with SMEI, and 95% of these are de novo. Prognosis is poor with persistent severe developmental delay and intractable seizures.

d. **Symptomatic myoclonic epilepsy** is associated with specific progressive neurologic diseases such as Lafora's disease, Baltic myoclonus (Unverricht–Lundborg disease), neuronal ceroid lipofuscinosis (Batten's disease), sialidosis, mitochondrial encephalomyopathy, and Ramsay–Hunt syndrome.

EPILEPSIES AND SYNDROMES UNDETERMINED WHETHER FOCAL OR GENERALIZED

A. **Neonatal seizures.** Seizures occur most frequently in the neonatal period than at any other time in life, with an incidence of 1.5 to 5.5 per 1,000 live births.

1. **Clinical features.** Neonatal seizures (occurring between birth and 2 months) are more fragmentary than are seizures among older children. GTCS do not occur in neonates. Common causes are outlined in Table 42.2. Neonatal seizures are classified as follows:

   a. **Seizures associated with electrographic signatures** include focal and multifocal clonic seizures, focal tonic seizures, generalized myoclonic seizures, and, rarely,

---

TABLE 42.2 Common Causes of Neonatal Seizures

Hypoxic-Ischemic Encephalopathy
Metabolic: hypocalcemia, hypoglycemia, hyponatremia, hypernatremia, hypomagnesemia
Trauma: subdural hematoma, intracerebral hemorrhage
Vascular: ischemic stroke, sinovenous thrombosis
Infection: sepsis, meningitis (group B β-hemolytic Streptococcus), encephalitis, TORCH, HIV
Congenital abnormalities: lissencephaly, holoprosencephaly, other migrational disorders
Inborn errors of metabolism: amino acid disturbances (urea cycle disorder and nonketotic hyperglycinemia), pyridoxine dependency, phenylketonuria, galactosemia
Drug withdrawal: heroin, barbiturate, methadone
Neurocutaneous and genetic syndromes: tuberous sclerosis complex, ARX (Aristaless-related homeobox) mutations that are associated with congenital malformations such as lissencephaly
BFNS, fifth-day fits

Abbreviations: BFNS, benign familial neonatal seizures; HIV, human immunodeficiency virus; TORCH, toxoplasmosis, rubella, cytomegalovirus, herpes.

apnea. These seizures are usually associated with focal structural lesions (infarction or hemorrhage), infection, or metabolic abnormalities (hypoglycemia or hypocalcemia).

b. **Seizures not associated with electrographic signatures** include generalized tonic seizures, focal and multifocal myoclonic seizures, and subtle seizures (oral–buccal–lingual movements, bicycling movements, and some rhythmic ocular movements such as horizontal eye deviation). These seizures are usually observed among lethargic, comatose neonates with poor prognoses, such as those with severe hypoxic-ischemic encephalopathy.

2. Evaluation. Neonatal seizures should be managed in a neonatal intensive care unit by experienced personnel, including a pediatric neurologist and a neonatologist.

a. History and examination. History of maternal illness, infection, or drug and alcohol abuse during pregnancy should be obtained. Family history of neonatal seizures is suggestive of BFNS. Evaluation of the skin, anterior fontanel, and neurologic and ophthalmologic examinations should be performed. Presence of skin rash and chorioretinitis may suggest toxoplasmosis.

b. **Laboratory data** include CBC, serum glucose, electrolytes, BUN, serum creatinine, liver function tests, magnesium, calcium, phosphate, ammonia, lactate, pyruvate, biotinidase, lumbar puncture (LP) to rule out CNS infection and subarachnoid hemorrhage (SAH), titers for toxoplasmosis, rubella, cytomegalovirus, herpes (TORCH), and HIV. Additional studies such as plasma amino acids and very-long-chain fatty acids, urinalysis for amino acids and organic acids, cerebrospinal fluid (CSF) lactate, and neurotransmitters may be indicated if metabolic disorders are suspected. Ultrasonography of the head at bedside to rule out intracranial hemorrhage and a non-contrast-enhanced computed tomography (CT) or MRI of the head can be performed when the neonate's condition is stable. EEG is useful for the diagnosis of subclinical seizures and assessment of prognosis. EEGs with low-voltage, burst-suppression, or isoelectric patterns suggest poor prognosis.

3. Treatment.

a. **Management of underlying cause** such as CNS infection or specific metabolic abnormality (hypoglycemia, hypocalcemia, or hypomagnesemia)

b. **Phenobarbital,** the initial drug of choice, is administered IV as a loading dose of 20 mg/kg followed by additional 5 to 10 mg/kg boluses as required to achieve serum levels between 20 and 40 μg/mL and to control clinical seizures. Maintenance dose of 3 to 4 mg/kg/day is usually sufficient because phenobarbital has a relatively long half-life in neonates. Cardiorespiratory monitoring is important because IV administration can be associated with respiratory depression and hypotension.

c. **Fosphenytoin** is added if a phenobarbital level of 40 μg/mL is not sufficient to control seizures. An IV loading dose of 20 mg/kg phenytoin equivalent (PE) results in serum levels ranging from 15 to 20 μg/mL, followed by a maintenance dose of 3 to 4 mg/kg/day. Phenytoin is no longer used because it has to be infused slowly at 1 mg/kg/minute with cardiac monitoring, as it can cause cardiac arrhythmias and hypotension. It is alkalotic and may lead to local venous thrombosis or tissue irritation. Use of fosphenytoin is preferred because it reduces these risks.

d. **Benzodiazepines** are third-line treatments. Midazolam is usually the benzodiazepine of choice. It is administered IV at a loading dose of 0.15 mg/kg followed by 0.04 to 0.4 mg/kg/hour infusion. Lorazepam 0.05 to 0.1 mg/kg administered IV enters the brain rapidly, being effective in <5 minutes. Being less lipophilic, it does not redistribute from the brain as rapidly as does diazepam, so the duration of action is longer, being 6 to 24 hours. Lorazepam is less likely to produce respiratory depression or hypotension than diazepam.

e. **Newer AEDS**. Levetiracetam and topiramate are also used for refractory neonatal seizures. IV levetiracetam has been advocated by some, as a second line of treatment instead of fosphenytoin, if phenobarbital is ineffective.

f. **Pyridoxine** (100 mg IV) administered during EEG monitoring stops seizures and normalizes the EEG within minutes in the rare patient with pyridoxine-dependent seizures.

B. **Acquired epileptic aphasia (Landau–Kleffner syndrome)** is characterized by acquired aphasia, with onset between 3 and 7 years, including verbal auditory agnosia, rapid reduction of spontaneous speech, and behavioral and psychomotor disturbances, during the first decade of life. Seizures (generalized and focal) and EEG abnormalities, including multifocal spikes and spike–wave discharges commonly in the temporal or parieto-occipital regions, are activated by sleep. The ultimate outcome is still unclear.

SPECIAL SYNDROMES

A. Situation-related seizures.

  1. Febrile seizures.

   a. Incidence. Febrile seizures occur in 2% to 5% of young children.

   b. Age at onset ranges from 3 months to 5 years (peak 18 months to 2 years). The disorder is familial.

   c. Clinical features manifest within the first few hours of acute infection, usually associated with the rising phase of the temperature curve. They are typically associated with viral upper respiratory tract, gastrointestinal, and middle ear infections. Bacterial infection is rarely associated with febrile seizures. Intracranial infection and other defined causes such as dehydration and electrolyte imbalance should be excluded.

   (1) Simple febrile seizures present as single, brief (<15 minutes), GTCS. They represent 80% to 90% of all febrile seizures, and are usually seen in neurologically normal children.

   (2) Complex febrile seizures are prolonged (>15 minutes), have focal features (focal onset or postictal Todd's paralysis), and more than one seizure occurs within 24 hours.

   d. Evaluation. LP is indicated unless the possibility of meningitis can be confidently eliminated clinically. It should be performed for all children younger than 18 months with the first febrile seizure. If in doubt, err on the side of performing LP. It should be strongly considered in the evaluation of infants and children who have received antibiotic treatment because such treatment can mask evidence of meningitis. Neuroimaging and EEG are indicated if there are focal deficits or CNS infection is suspected.

   e. Acute management of seizures.

   (1) Prolonged febrile seizures can be treated with IV lorazepam, diazepam, or phenobarbital.

   (2) Rectal diazepam gel (Diastat 0.2 to 0.5 mg/kg) can be administered at the onset of a seizure in children with history of prolonged seizures.

   (3) Any underlying infection or fever should be controlled.

   f. Long-term management of seizures. No treatment is necessary if the patient has isolated simple febrile seizures without major risk factors for recurrence.

   (1) Daily phenobarbital treatment reduces the risk of recurrent febrile seizures and may be used for patients with complex febrile seizures that carry increased risk of later epilepsy. Because 90% of febrile seizures recur within 2 years, treatment should be continued for at least 2 years or for 1 year after the last seizure, whichever is longer. Valproic acid is the second choice because of an increased incidence of side effects, including liver toxicity, in this age group. Carbamazepine and phenytoin do not prevent recurrent febrile seizures.

   (2) Some pediatric neurologists use oral diazepam, administered only when fever is present, and have found it effective in reducing the risk of recurrent febrile seizures. Side effects include lethargy, irritability, and ataxia.

   g. Prognosis. Approximately 33% of children with febrile seizures have at least one recurrence, and 9% have three or more seizures. Remission occurs by 6 years of age in approximately 90% of children.

   (1) Risk factors for recurrence include young age (<1 year) at initial seizure, seizures occurring with low-grade fever, and a family history of febrile seizures.

   (2) Risk factors for the development of epilepsy include complex febrile seizures, underlying developmental or neurologic abnormalities, and family history of nonfebrile seizures. Three percent to six percent of children with febrile seizures will develop epilepsy. Prolonged febrile seizures may lead to temporal lobe epilepsy with hippocampal sclerosis. Patients with two risk factors have approximately 13% chance of developing epilepsy, whereas the risk is only 0.9% if risk factors are absent.

2. **Seizures related to identifiable situations** such as use of drugs (stimulants or neuroleptics) or alcohol, and sleep deprivation.

B. Isolated, apparently unprovoked epileptic events. Treatment is not indicated unless there are significant risk factors for recurrence.

C. **Epilepsy characterized by specific modes of seizure precipitation** includes seizures occurring in response to discrete or specific stimuli (reflex epilepsy), such as reading epilepsy, hot water epilepsy, and arithmetic epilepsy.

D. **Chronic progressive epilepsia partialis continua of childhood (Kojewnikoff's syndrome)** is thought to be a result of chronic encephalitis (Rasmussen's encephalitis). The cause is unknown. It is characterized by partial motor seizures, often associated with myoclonus, which are resistant to treatment. This condition results in progressive hemiplegia with unilateral brain atrophy and mental retardation.

EVALUATION

Details regarding histories, physical examinations, and studies such as EEG and neuroimaging are discussed in Chapter 6. Important aspects of the evaluation with respect to children follow. Determine whether the paroxysmal events in question are in fact epileptic. They should be differentiated from nonepileptic paroxysmal events in children.

SPECIFIC PREDISPOSING FACTORS FOR CHILDHOOD SEIZURES

A. Birth history.
  1. Prenatal. Prematurity, complications (e.g., toxemia or premature labor), medications, smoking, and alcohol and drug abuse
  2. Perinatal. Low birth weight, low Apgar scores, and complications of labor and delivery
  3. Postnatal. Intensive neonatal respiratory care, complications such as meningitis and intraventricular hemorrhage
B. Developmental history. Learning disabilities, attention deficit, and developmental regression

PHYSICAL EXAMINATION

A. Head circumference. Microcephaly and macrocephaly are associated with various neurologic disorders.
B. **Height and weight** abnormalities
C. **Dysmorphic features** associated with chromosomal anomalies, storage diseases, or brain malformations
D. Skin. Café au lait spots are seen in neurofibromatosis, hypopigmented macules and adenoma sebaceum in tuberous sclerosis, and facial hemangiomas in Sturge–Weber syndrome.
E. Hair. Broken hair and alopecia suggest metabolic disorders (biotinidase deficiency, Menkes' syndrome, and argininosuccinic aciduria).
F. Mental status and developmental milestones. Loss of previously attained milestones may be indicative of a neurodegenerative disease (e.g., Rett's syndrome), whereas delays in achieving developmental milestones reflect static encephalopathies (e.g., cerebral palsy). Presence of anxiety, depression, and stressors such as family conflict may lead to the diagnosis of psychogenic seizures.
G. Systemic exam. Organomegaly may suggest a storage disease or an inborn error of metabolism.

LABORATORY TESTING

In addition to EEG and MRI of the head, other important studies in children include the following:
A. Chemical and metabolic screening. Electrolytes, glucose, calcium, magnesium, hepatic and renal function tests, and toxic screening for possible drug ingestion. Specific metabolic or neurodegenerative disorders may be diagnosed with tests such as thyroid function tests,

urinalysis for amino acids, organic acids, homocysteine (cobablamin G deficiency and methylenetetrahydrofolate reductase deficiency), lysosomal enzymes (mucopolysaccharidosis and Batten's disease), and very-long-chain fatty acids (peroxisomal disorders such as adrenoleukodystrophy). Elevation of serum prolactin levels is seen with GTCS, may be normal with focal seizures, and can help differentiate seizures from nonepileptiform paroxysmal disorders. However, it is not routinely performed because it has to be measured within 30 minutes after an episode and compared with baseline values.

B. **LP** is indicated if there are signs of acute CNS infection or inflammation (e.g., fever or stiff neck). It is indicated for all children younger than 18 months with a history of fever and seizures, because clinical signs of CNS infection may be absent. It should be performed on all febrile patients with new-onset seizures. A low CSF glucose with normal CSF cell count and protein and normal serum glucose suggests glucose transporter 1 deficiency (GLUT 1 deficiency), which can be confirmed with genetic testing of SLC2A1.

C. **Chromosomal analysis** is indicated if dysmorphic features suggest chromosomal abnormalities.

D. **Genetic testing.** Mutations in *SCN1A* have been associated with SMEI and GEFS+, and mutations in *SCN1B*, with GEFS+. Mutations in *KCNQ2* gene have been associated with BFNC. Ohtahara's syndrome has been associated with *STXBP1* and infantile spasms with *ARX*. Children with epileptic encephalopathy (early-onset intractable seizures, developmental delay, cognitive impairment) should have chromosome microarray or targeted sequencing panels of epileptic encephalopathy genes including *SCN1A*, *SCN1B*, *SCN8A*, *KCNQ2*, *STXBP1*, and *PCDH19*.

E. **Simultaneous prolonged video EEG monitoring** in an epilepsy unit can help determine the exact nature of paroxysmal events if they cannot be defined with routine EEG.

TREATMENT

SINGLE SEIZURE

Approximately 9% of the population has a seizure sometime during their lives, and approximately 3% have more than one seizure. The first unprovoked seizure is defined as a single seizure or flurry of seizures within 24 hours in a child older than 1 month without prior history of unprovoked seizures. The risk of recurrence is 27% to 52%. It is highest in the first 6 months after the initial event. It is low if the patient has normal findings at neurologic examination, a single GTCS with a negative family history, normal findings at neuroimaging, and a normal or mildly slow EEG. It is higher if there is underlying structural or metabolic etiology.

A. Indications for treatment.
1. Clear-cut epileptiform abnormalities at EEG
2. Lesions on neuroimaging studies
3. Abnormal findings at neurologic examination that suggest previous brain damage
4. First seizure during sleep
5. Active CNS infection (encephalitis, meningitis, or abscess)
6. Certain types of seizures, including infantile spasms, LGS, and focal seizures
7. Unprovoked or asymptomatic single seizure with history suggesting that one may have occurred earlier

B. **Treatment** is not indicated when seizures are provoked by a correctable metabolic disturbance (glucose or electrolyte abnormalities), sleep deprivation, exposure to drugs or alcohol, febrile illness, or physical or emotional stress. In such cases, the underlying disturbance should be corrected.

GENERAL PRINCIPLES OF TREATMENT

A. **Choice of appropriate drug** should be based on the clinical description of the seizures (Table 42.3). This choice may be influenced by other factors, such as the patient's age, associated medical illnesses, and economic circumstances.

B. **Monotherapy.** Approximately 50% of children should respond to monotherapy with the first drug and another 15% to monotherapy with the second drug. If the first drug is ineffective, start a second AED with a different mechanism of action and low potential for adverse effects and drug interactions. After therapeutic levels are achieved, gradually withdraw the first drug.

C. **Polypharmacy** is indicated only if monotherapy with at least two first-line AEDs fails, and should be initiated only after consultation with a pediatric neurologist. Associated problems include drug interactions, difficulties in acquiring therapeutic levels of either drug despite use of adequate doses, increased risks of toxicity, increased cost, and reduced compliance.

D. **Simplify medication schedule.** Decreasing the number of doses improves compliance.

E. **Avoid sedative anticonvulsants** such as benzodiazepines, especially for patients with secondary generalized epilepsy syndrome, because increased sedation can result in increased seizures.

F. **Maintain a seizure diary.** Record seizure frequency, medication dosages and levels, and occurrence of side effects, if any.

G. **AED level** should be checked, preferably before the morning dose to obtain the lowest (trough) level and at a consistent time to avoid misinterpretation of fluctuations. CBC and aspartate aminotransferase levels are checked every 1 to 2 months initially and then every 6 months after a steady dosage has been established. AED blood level should be checked.

1. After starting a medication, to aid in initial titration of dose to achieve a therapeutic level
2. After making a major change in drug dosage
3. If seizures persist despite "correct therapy"
4. If symptoms of toxicity develop
5. If noncompliance is suspected

H. **Repeat EEG** during therapy if there is a change in the character of the seizures or if the child has been seizure-free for a considerable period to help decide whether medications can be withdrawn.

DRUG THERAPY

The following information serves as a broad guideline for AEDs commonly used to treat children. Indications are listed in Table 42.3. Details regarding their metabolism, side effects, and interactions are discussed in detail in Chapter 43.

TABLE 42.3 Drugs for the Management of Epilepsy

Seizure Type	First-Line Drug	Second-Line Drug
Partial		
Simple partial, complex partial, secondary GTCS	Carbamazepine, oxcarbazepine	Lamotrigine, levetiracetam, valproic acid, phenytoin, phenobarbital
Generalized		
Absence (typical and atypical)	Ethosuximide, valproic acid	Lamotrigine, clonazepam, acetazolamide
Myoclonic	Valproic acid	Levetiracetam, zonisamide, clobazam, clonazepam
Tonic–clonic	Valproic acid	Lamotrigine, topiramate, rufinamide, levetiracetam, phenytoin
Atonic	Valproic acid	Lamotrigine, rufinamide, clobazam, topiramate, levetiracetam, felbamate

Phenobarbital and valproic acid are used for atypical febrile seizures. Fosphenytoin and phenobarbital IV are used for status epilepticus.
Abbreviation: GTCS, generalized tonic–clonic seizure.

A. **Phenytoin (Dilantin; Parke-Davis).**
   1. **Administration (5 to 8 mg/kg/day).** Children have shorter elimination half-lives than adults and should be given two divided doses. Phenytoin has nonlinear elimination kinetics. Therefore, small increases in dose after therapeutic levels of 10 to 20 μg/mL have been achieved resulting in large increases in plasma levels and toxicity.
   2. **Formulation.** Capsules: Dilantin, 30 mg, 100 mg; Infatabs: 50 mg; Phenytoin 100 mg, 200 mg, 300 mg (extended release); suspension: 125 mg/5 mL, 30 mg/5 mL. Dilantin suspension is not recommended for routine use because it is unreliable. Parenteral: injectable sodium phenytoin (Dilantin and generic 50 mg/mL), fosphenytoin [Cerebyx (Pfizer) 50 mg PE/mL].
   3. **Side effects.** Dose-related side effects are nystagmus, ataxia, and drowsiness. Gingival hypertrophy (20% to 50% of patients) requiring more frequent dental cleaning, hirsutism, coarsening of features, blood dyscrasias, Stevens-Johnson syndrome, lymphadenopathy, systemic lupus erythematosus, and megaloblastic anemia can also occur. Long-term administration has been associated with vitamin D, vitamin K, and folic acid deficiency. Fetal hydantoin syndrome is characterized by craniofacial anomalies, hypoplasia of distal phalanges, intrauterine growth retardation, and mental deficiency. The term has been replaced by "fetal anticonvulsant syndrome," because the malformations are also seen in children of mothers who have been exposed to a variety of other AEDs such as valproic acid, carbamazepine, and phenobarbital as well.

B. **Carbamazepine (Tegretol, Tegretol XR; Novartis. Carbatrol, Shire–Richwood).**
   1. **Administration.** Start at 5 mg/kg/day and increase by 5 mg/kg/day every 5 to 7 days to a maximum of 10 to 30 mg/kg/day in bid (for sustained-release preparations) and tid doses to achieve therapeutic blood levels of 4 to 12 μg/mL. Carbamazepine can exacerbate absence, atypical absence, and myoclonic seizures.
   2. **Formulation.** Tablets: 200 mg; chewable tablets: 100 mg; elixir: 100 mg/5 mL; sustained-release preparations: Tegretol XR: 100 mg, 200 mg, 400 mg; Carbatrol extended-release capsules: 200 mg, 300 mg. If oral administration is contraindicated, Tegretol suspension (100 mg/5 mL) can be given rectally, diluted 1:1 with water in an enema at a dose of 10 to 30 mg/kg to attain therapeutic levels.
   3. **Side effects.** Dose-related side effects are sedation, blurred vision, and leukopenia. Agranulocytosis, aplastic anemia, and syndrome of inappropriate antidiuretic hormone secretion also may occur. There is a 0.5% to 1% risk of spina bifida and other anomalies associated with the fetal anticonvulsant syndrome, with first-trimester exposure to carbamazepine.

C. **Oxcarbazepine (Trileptal; Novartis).**
   1. **Administration.** 10 mg/kg/day, to be increased by the same amount weekly to 20 to 40 mg/kg/day, in two divided doses to achieve therapeutic blood level of 10 to 35 mg/L. It has less potential for drug interactions because of lack of auto-induction.
   2. **Formulation.** Tablets: 150 mg, 300 mg, 600 mg; suspension: 300 mg/5 mL.
   3. **Side effects.** Somnolence, dizziness, and headaches. Cross-allergy between carbamazepine and oxcarbazepine occurs in 35% of cases. Hyponatremia is more frequent than with carbamazepine, seen in 2.5% of patients.

D. **Phenobarbital (various generic formulations).**
   1. **Administration.** 3 to 8 mg/kg/day in a single daily dose or two divided doses to achieve therapeutic blood levels of 15 to 40 μg/mL. The serum half-life increases with age. It is 20 to 65 hours for patients younger than 10 years and 64 to 140 hours for those older than 15 years. Therefore, children need higher maintenance dosages of 4 to 8 mg/kg/day; adults need only 1 to 2 mg/kg/day. It can exacerbate absence, atypical absence, and myoclonic seizures, if used for GTCS in patients with generalized epilepsy.
   2. **Formulation.** Tablets: 15 mg, 16.2 mg, 30 mg, 32.4 mg, 60 mg, 64.8 mg, 97.2 mg, 100 mg; elixir: 20 mg/5 mL. Parenteral: injectable sodium phenobarbital (60 mg/mL, 130 mg/mL).
   3. **Side effects.** Hyperactivity, sedation, learning disabilities, personality changes, and Stevens–Johnson syndrome. Long-term administration has been associated with vitamin D, vitamin K, and folic acid deficiency.

E. Valproic acid (Depakene, Depakote, Depacon; Abbott).

1. **Administration.** Start at 10 to 15 mg/kg/day or lower, and gradually increase to a maximum of 60 mg/kg/day in three divided doses to achieve therapeutic blood levels of 40 to 100 μg/mL.

2. **Formulation.** Depakote (divalproex sodium): enteric-coated tablets, 125 mg, 250 mg, 500 mg; sprinkles, 125 mg; extended-release tablets, 250 mg, 500 mg. Depakene (valproic acid): capsules, 250 mg; syrup, 250 mg/5 mL. Parenteral IV preparation: Depacon (100 mg/mL) starting at 10 to 15 mg/kg/day increased 5 to 10 mg/kg/day/week to a maximum of 60 mg/kg/day infused over 60 minutes at a rate not to exceed 20 mg/minute. If oral administration is contraindicated (e.g., paralytic ileus), Depakene elixir (250 mg/5 mL) can be given rectally, diluted 1:1 with water in an enema at a dose of 20 mg/kg to attain therapeutic levels of 40 to 100 μg/mL.

3. **Side effects.** Dose-related side effects include nausea, vomiting, and gastric irritation, minimized with the use of the sprinkle or enteric-coated preparation or administration after meals. Other side effects include weight gain, alopecia, tremor, and thrombocytopenia. Idiosyncratic toxicity includes pancreatitis (0.5%) and liver failure. Liver failure is more common among children younger than 2 years, and with polypharmacy. It can be a fulminant progressive failure or a subacute gradually progressive failure. Valproic acid is therefore contraindicated in the treatment of children with preexisting hepatic damage, organic aciduria, or carnitine deficiency. Carnitine (Carnitor, 10% solution or 330 mg tablet) should be administered 50 mg/kg/day in two or three divided doses in conjunction with valproic acid to children undergoing long-term, high-dose therapy with poor nutrition (e.g., cerebral palsy). Baseline liver function and serum ammonia should be checked before starting valproic acid and at least monthly for the first 4 to 6 months while this medication is being given. It may be associated with increased risk of polycystic ovarian syndrome.

F. Lamotrigine (Lamictal; GlaxoSmithKline).

1. **Administration.** Coadministration of valproic acid increases the elimination half-life of lamotrigine to 60 hours or more. Therefore, the dose needs to be adjusted. Children not taking valproic acid: initial dose of 0.6 mg/kg/day for 2 weeks, increased to 1 mg/kg/day for 2 weeks and thereafter, slowly titrated to a maximum of 5 to 15 mg/kg/day twice a day. Children taking valproic acid: initial dose of 0.15 mg/kg/day for 2 weeks, increased to 0.3 mg/kg/day for 2 weeks and slowly titrated to a maximum of 1 to 5 mg/kg/day twice a day. Therapeutic blood levels are 5 to 15 mg/mL.

2. **Formulation.** Chewable dispersible tablet: 2 mg, 5 mg, 25 mg; tablets: 25 mg, 100 mg, 150 mg, 200 mg.

3. **Side effects.** Common adverse effects among children include somnolence, rash, vomiting, laryngitis, ataxia, and headache. Risk of skin rash in children is 1 in 100 to 200 as compared with 3 in 1,000 in adults and is seen within the first 6 weeks. The incidence of rash increases with higher initial doses and faster rates of dose escalation, especially among children receiving valproic acid.

G. Topiramate (Topamax; Ortho-McNeil).

1. **Administration.** Initiated at 0.5 to 1 mg/kg/day increased slowly to 4 to 9 mg/kg/day, given in two divided doses. Faster titration schedules have resulted in increased CNS side effects. Therapeutic blood levels are 3.4 to 16.6 μg/mL.

2. **Formulation.** Tablets: 25 mg, 50 mg, 100 mg, 200 mg; sprinkle capsule: 15 mg, 25 mg.

3. **Side effects.** Somnolence, dizziness, ataxia, psychomotor slowing, speech disorder, paresthesia, kidney stones (1.5%), and weight loss. Decreased sweating usually with exposure to hot weather occurs more frequently in children. Acute myopia with secondary angle closure glaucoma has been reported, usually within the first month. New data suggest a higher risk of cleft palates in babies born to women taking the drug.

H. Levetiracetam (Keppra; UCB Pharma).

1. **Administration.** Initiated at 10 to 20 mg/kg/day, increased by 20 mg/kg/day every 2 weeks to reach a maximum dose of 40 to 60 mg/kg/day given twice a day. For children younger than 4 years, dose is determined by the doctor.

2. **Formulation.** Tablets: 250 mg, 500 mg, 750 mg, 1,000 mg; oral solution, 100 mg/mL.

3. **Side effects.** Fatigue, coordination problems, sleepiness, mood and behavior changes, such as anger, anxiety, depression, hostility, and irritability.

I. **Zonisamide (Zonegran; Eisai).**
1. **Administration.** 4 to 8 mg/kg/day divided twice a day. Therapeutic blood levels are 10 to 30 μg/mL. May be effective in myoclonic seizures as in progressive myoclonic epilepsies such as Unverricht–Lundborg syndrome (Baltic myoclonus).
2. **Formulation.** Capsule: 25 mg, 50 mg, 100 mg.
3. **Side effects.** Somnolence, dizziness, anorexia, headaches, confusion, cognitive impairment, oligohidrosis hyperthermia, and renal calculi (4%). Contraindicated in care of patients with hypersensitivity to sulfonamides (zonisamide is a sulfonamide).

J. **Felbamate (Felbatol; Wallace).**
1. **Administration.** Begin at 15 mg/kg/day for first week, 30 mg/kg/day for the second week, and 45 mg/kg/day divided three times a day from the third week (maximum 3,600 mg/day). Therapeutic blood levels are 50 to 110 μg/mL.
2. **Formulation.** Tablets: 400 mg, 600 mg; oral suspension 600 mg/5 mL.
3. **Adverse effects.** Gastrointestinal side effects, including weight loss and anorexia, have been most prominent. Insomnia, somnolence, and fatigue also have occurred. Rash may occur if the patient is also taking Depakote. On August 1, 1994, a year after felbamate was approved, several cases of aplastic anemia and hepatotoxicity were reported. Physicians should restrict use of this drug only to children with severe epilepsy, especially LGS, which is refractory to other therapies with close monitoring of blood work according to specific guidelines.

K. **Ethosuximide (Zarontin; Parke-Davis).**
1. **Administration.** 20 to 40 mg/kg/day in two or three divided doses. Therapeutic blood levels are 40 to 100 μg/mL.
2. **Formulation.** Capsules: 250 mg; syrup: 250 mg/5 mL
3. **Side effects.** Gastric irritation, anorexia, nausea, vomiting, drowsiness, and hallucinations

L. **Clonazepam (Klonopin; Roche).**
1. **Administration.** 0.03 to 0.10 mg/kg/day in two or three divided doses. Therapeutic blood levels are 0.02 to 0.08 μg/mL.
2. **Formulation.** Tablets: 0.5 mg, 1 mg, 2 mg
3. **Side effects.** Drowsiness, ataxia, irritability, diplopia, and drooling

M. **Clorazepate (Tranxene; Abbott).**
1. **Administration.** 0.3 mg/kg/day, increased to a maximum of 3 mg/kg/day. Therapeutic blood levels are not established.
2. **Formulation.** Tablets: 3.75 mg, 7.5 mg, 15 mg
3. **Side effects.** Drowsiness, dizziness, ataxia, and drooling

N. **Rufinamide (Banzel; Eisai).**
1. **Administration.** Therapy should be initiated at 10 mg/kg/day in two divided doses, to be increased by 10 mg/kg increments every 2 days to a target dose of 45 mg/kg/day or 3,200 mg/day whichever is less.
2. **Tablets.** 200, 400 mg; suspension: 40 mg/mL
3. **Side effects.** Somnolence, headache, dizziness, fatigue, and somnolence. It is contraindicated in patients with familial short QT syndrome. Multiorgan hypersensitivity syndrome has been reported in association with Banzel therapy, especially in children <12 years of age.

O. **Vigabatrin (Sabril; Lundbeck).**
1. **Administration.** Initial dosing of 50 mg/kg/day in two divided doses is increased by 25 to 50 mg/kg/day every 3 days up to a maximum of 150 mg/kg/day.
2. **Formulation.** 500 mg powder per packet for oral solution; 500 mg tablet
3. **Side effects.** Progressive and permanent bilateral concentric visual field constriction has been noted in 30% or more patients. It can be mild to severe resulting in disability. It should therefore be withdrawn from a pediatric patient treated for infantile spasms who fails to show benefit within 2 to 4 weeks. Abnormal MRI signals have been noted in some, but they generally resolve with discontinuation of therapy. Anemia, somnolence, and weight gain have also been reported.

P. **Clobazam (Onfi; Lundbeck).**
1. **Administration.** Therapy is initiated at a low dose. Dose range is 10 mg to 40 mg/day, and 0.4 to 0.8 mg/kg/day in children <12 years of age, administered in a bid dosing.

2. **Formulation.** Tablet: 10 mg, 20 mg; suspension: 2.5 mg/mL
3. **Side effects.** Common side effects include drowsiness and sedation. Dry mouth, and behavioral problems including restlessness and aggressive outbursts have also been noted.

Q. **Lacosamide (Vimpat; UCB Pharma).**

1. **Administration.** Approved for adults with partial-onset seizures. Start with 50 mg/day increasing to a maintenance of 200 to 400 mg/day. Lower doses are used in children.
2. **Formulation.** Tablet: 50 mg, 100 mg, 150 mg, 200 mg; oral solution 10 mg/mL; IV solution: 200 mg/20 mL.
3. **Side effects.** Prolonged PR interval, multiorgan hypersensitivity reaction, dizziness, ataxia, fatigue, nausea, blurred vision, tremor

R. **Perampanel (Fycompa).**

1. **Administration.** Approved for treatment of partial-onset seizures in patients ≥12 years of age. Start at 2 mg at night increasing to maintenance of 8 to 12 mg/day. If added to enzyme-inducing AEDs such as PHT, CBZ, and OXC, start at 4 mg at night.
2. **Formulation.** Tablets: 2 mg, 4 mg, 6 mg, 8 mg, 10 mg, 12 mg
3. **Side effects.** Anger, aggression, irritability, dizziness, somnolence. Violent thoughts or threatening behavior including homicidal ideation has been observed in a few patients.

S. **Other antiepileptic medications** available in the United States include tiagabine (Gabitril; Abbott), gabapentin (Neurontin; Parke-Davis), and pregabalin (Lyrica; Parke-Davis). Stiripentol used for Dravet's syndrome is currently not approved in the United States.

PSYCHOSOCIAL ISSUES

A. Avoid risk factors such as fatigue and sleep deprivation. Seat belts and bicycle helmets should be worn to prevent head injuries that may lead to seizures.
B. **Seizure precautions.** Bathtubs should be avoided; only showers should be taken. Activities such as climbing of heights, swimming without supervision, driving, contact with heavy machinery and fire, and other activities that could be dangerous in the event of a seizure should be avoided.
C. Parents should guard against overprotection, which can develop out of fear and anxiety. Unnecessary limitations prevent the child from taking the risks necessary for him or her to become an independent person and develop self-confidence.
D. Parents must inform schoolteachers (as well as babysitters) about the child's seizures. This allows teachers to be prepared to deal with seizures in the classroom and the reactions of classmates. Teachers should be expected to provide information about frequency of seizures during school hours, changes in the child's behavior, unexplained changes in school performance, and abnormal behavioral and social problems that may require referral for counseling.
E. If certain activities must be restricted because of poor seizure control, substitute exercise programs must be found.
F. A medication schedule that avoids school hours should be planned because it is often inconvenient and embarrassing for a child to take AEDs at school.
G. Children with epilepsy have an increased risk of learning disabilities, attention-deficit hyperactivity disorder, anxiety, and depression. The Food and Drug Administration (FDA) has warned that AEDs may be associated with suicidal ideation.
H. Referral to services such as the Epilepsy Foundation of America or local support groups for counseling.

STATUS EPILEPTICUS

DEFINITION

One or more seizures lasting for more than 30 minutes without full recovery of consciousness between seizures

TYPES

A. **Generalized convulsive status epilepticus** is characterized by persistent GTCS. In children, it is associated with a higher morbidity and mortality than in adults. We, therefore, focus on the management of this type of status epilepticus.

B. **Nonconvulsive status epilepticus** includes cases of absence status and complex partial status and is often described as "twilight state."

PRECIPITATING FACTORS

A. Abrupt discontinuation, noncompliance, or changes in anticonvulsant therapy

B. Acute intercurrent infections such as meningitis and encephalitis

C. Acute metabolic disturbances, such as electrolyte disturbances and hypoglycemia

D. Acute cerebral insult such as anoxia, hypoxia–ischemia, trauma (SAH, subdural hematoma, and depressed skull fractures)

PROGNOSIS

Approximately 15% of all patients with epilepsy have an episode of status epilepticus at some time in their lives. It is more common in those younger than 2 years of age. Recurrent status epilepticus is more common among children. In the pediatric age group, the mortality rate is approximately 3% to 11%, with higher rates within the first 6 months of life.

TREATMENT

A. **Confirmation of diagnosis of status epilepticus.** The longer the seizure continues, the more difficult it is to control and the greater the possibility of permanent brain damage.

B. **General measures.**

   1. Initiate supportive measures—see Table 42.4.

   2. Place an IV line (preferably two, one with normal saline solution). Blood should be obtained at this time for CBC, electrolytes, calcium, magnesium, phosphorus, glucose, liver function tests, AED levels, toxicology screening, and blood cultures if febrile.

   3. Administer IV 25% glucose at 2 mL/kg.

   4. Identify and treat precipitating factors. For a patient with known seizures in whom status epilepticus may have been caused by AED withdrawal, the treatment of choice is reinstatement of the same drug.

C. **Drug treatment** involves administration of a drug for immediate termination of the seizure and a second drug for maintenance therapy. The initial treatment is similar regardless of the type of seizure. Maintenance treatment varies depending on the type of epilepsy. The protocol is presented in Table 42.4.

   1. **Benzodiazepines.**

      a. **Lorazepam (Ativan; Wyeth-Ayerst)** is recommended as a first-line treatment. The advantages are rapid onset of action, prolonged antiepileptic activity compared with diazepam, less respiratory depression and sedation, and a lower rate of seizure recurrence. **IV diazepam** (0.2 to 0.5 mg/kg/dose, maximum of 5 mg administered over 2 to 5 minutes) is not routinely used because of disadvantages including short duration of action (<30 minutes), high incidence of respiratory depression, and tendency to precipitate tonic status in patients with LGS.

   2. **Fosphenytoin (Cerebyx; Parke-Davis).** After IV lorazepam has been administered, IV fosphenytoin is given to achieve therapeutic levels of 18 to 20 μg/mL. Fosphenytoin is a water-soluble disodium ester prescribed as equimolar amounts of phenytoin called *PEs*. This prodrug is rapidly converted to phenytoin by phosphatase in the blood stream, reaching peak brain levels 15 minutes after administration. The loading and maintenance doses of fosphenytoin in PEs are identical to those of phenytoin. Fosphenytoin can be administered IV and intramuscularly with minimal local tissue damage and at faster rates of administration with fewer adverse effects than with phenytoin. Pruritus and paresthesia can occur. IV phenytoin can also be used. Disadvantages of phenytoin include cardiac

TABLE 42.4 Management of Generalized Tonic–Clonic Status Epilepticus in Children

Time from Start of Treatment	Procedure
0–5 min	Verify diagnosis of status epilepticus. Monitor cardiorespiratory function. Administer oxygen by nasal cannula or mask, obtain vital signs, ECG, pulse oximetry, insert IV line. Draw glucose, electrolytes, calcium, magnesium, phosphorus, CBC, AED levels, and toxicology if applicable. Start IV normal saline solution. Administer 25% glucose at 2 mL/kg
5 min	IV lorazepam, 0.05–0.1 mg/kg, at 1–2 mg/min to maximum of 5 mg, may be repeated in 10 min if needed
10–30 min	If seizures continue, start IV fosphenytoin 20 mg PE/kg infused at 3 mg PE/kg/min, not to exceed 150 mg PE/min (if not available, use IV phenytoin 20 mg/kg, at 1 mg/kg/min, not to exceed 50 mg/min) with ECG and blood pressure monitoring; additional 10 mg/kg may be given if seizures continue
31–60 min	If seizures persist, administer IV phenobarbital 20 mg/kg at a rate of 1 mg/kg/min, not to exceed 50 mg/min; additional 10–20 mg/kg may be given if seizures continue
>60 min	If seizures persist, options include (1) IV pentobarbital—initial loading dose of 5 mg/kg followed by maintenance infusion of 1–3 mg/kg/hr with EEG monitoring to produce burst-suppression pattern. (2) IV midazolam 0.1–0.3 mg/kg loading dose followed by maintenance infusion of 0.05–2 mg/kg/hr. (3) Propofol 1–2 mg/kg loading dose followed by maintenance infusion of 1–10 mg/kg/hr. (4) IV thiopental 5 mg/kg followed by maintenance infusion. If seizures are not controlled, ask an anesthesiologist to institute general anesthesia with halothane and neuromuscular blockade

Abbreviations: AED, antiepileptic drug; CBC, complete blood count; ECG, electrocardiography; EEG, electroencephalography.

arrhythmias and hypotension requiring close electrocardiographic and blood pressure monitoring. Intramuscular administration is avoided because of unpredictable absorption and muscle irritation. IV extravasation can result in phlebitis and tissue necrosis. Poor absorption occurs in children, resulting in difficulty in maintaining steady therapeutic levels, especially when the patient is switched to the oral form for maintenance. Phenytoin should be administered in normal saline solution, because it precipitates in glucose solutions.

3. **IV phenobarbital** is administered if seizures persist. It is often used as the first choice in children under 6 years of age. In the treatment of neonates, this may be administered as a single dose. In the case of older children, it may be divided into aliquots of 10 mg/kg to avoid respiratory depression until seizures stop or a maximum loading dose of 20 mg/kg. Additional 10 to 20 mg/kg may be necessary to achieve therapeutic levels of 35 to 40 μg/mL. Disadvantages of phenobarbital include hypotension and respiratory depression. IV valproate and levetiracetam are not currently FDA approved for treatment of status epilepticus.

4. **A more detailed history interview and neurologic examination** should be performed at this time. Evaluate the initial blood work. Before initiating additional therapies, it is preferable to obtain CT scans without contrast enhancement and to perform LP to look for causes such as intracranial structural lesions or infections. Consider LP for any child with a fever, especially if younger than 18 months, because meningitis can occur without clinical signs of neck stiffness.

5. **Refractory status epilepticus.** If seizures persist for 60 minutes and the patient does not respond to loading doses of fosphenytoin and phenobarbital, anesthetizing agents such as pentobarbital, midazolam, or propofol should be considered. Phenobarbital can be used in additional IV boluses of 5 to 10 mg/kg with EEG monitoring until seizures stop and a burst-suppression pattern is obtained on the EEG. The disadvantage of phenobarbital coma is that because of a longer half-life, the effect takes longer to wear off.

The recommended duration of pharmacologic induced coma is 48 to 72 hours. During this time, the patient is rechecked for seizures by means of decreasing the infusion rate. If seizures persist, the procedure is repeated. If seizures are adequately controlled, medication is slowly withdrawn. Administration of coma requires an intensive care unit setting with controlled mechanical ventilation and close cardiac monitoring.

6. If seizures are still not controlled, general anesthesia with halothane and neuromuscular blockade is recommended.

MEDICATION WITHDRAWAL

Although there is no consensus on how long a patient should remain seizure-free before drug withdrawal is considered, a seizure-free period of 2 to 4 years is recommended. Relapse rates are higher among adults than among children. Approximately 50% of seizure recurrences occur within 6 months of tapering the AED, and 60% to 90% occur within the first year. Children with febrile seizures have a 97% chance of outgrowing them by 6 years of age. There is an 80% to 85% chance of remission among children with only absence seizures.

FAVORABLE FACTORS ASSOCIATED WITH LOWER RELAPSE RATE

A. Reasonable ease of seizure control
B. Normal neurologic examination findings and developmental milestones
C. Normal EEG findings at time of withdrawal
D. Seizure onset between 2 and 12 years of age
E. Certain seizure types—simple febrile seizures, BECTS, childhood absence epilepsy.

UNFAVORABLE FACTORS ASSOCIATED WITH INCREASED CHANCE OF RECURRENCE

RECURRENCE RATE BEING HIGHER IN REMOTE SYMPTOMATIC EPILEPSY (EPILEPSY DUE TO AN IDENTIFIABLE CAUSE)

A. Recurrence rate is higher in remote symptomatic epilepsy (epilepsy due to an identifiable cause)
B. Seizures of long duration before successful establishment of control
C. Abnormal EEG findings at time of medication withdrawal
D. Abnormal neurologic examination findings
E. Seizure onset <2 years of age or after 12 years of age
F. Certain seizure types—focal seizures, infantile spasms, LGS, juvenile myoclonic epilepsy.

VAGAL NERVE STIMULATION

In the United States, FDA approval indicates use of vagal nerve stimulation as adjunctive therapy for refractory partial seizures in the care of adults and children older than 12 years. It has also successfully been used in younger children for other seizure disorders such as LGS. Indications for consideration of the device include medically refractory seizures, adequate trial of at least three AEDs, exclusion of nonepileptic events, and lack of surgery candidacy. Children who have undergone vagotomy (unilateral or bilateral) should not be given implants. Cervical masses should be excluded because cervical MRI may not be performed once the device is implanted. Cardiac arrhythmias, conduction abnormalities, and chronic obstructive pulmonary diseases are also considered as risk factors. Common side effects include voice hoarseness, cough, dyspnea, and rarely left vocal cord paralysis and parasthesias. It is associated with a 50% reduction in seizure activity in 30% to 50% of individuals.

SURGICAL THERAPIES

Procedures that resect or disconnect epileptogenic areas can reduce or eliminate seizures in patients with medically intractable epilepsy. These procedures are performed in specialized epilepsy centers. Extensive preoperative evaluation includes video EEG monitoring to identify seizure focus, neuropsychiatric evaluation, neuroimaging studies (MRI, single-photon emission computed tomography, and PET), intracarotid amobarbital test (Wada's test), and even invasive studies (subdural and depth electrodes), if indicated. The most common types of epilepsy surgery in the care of children are as follows.

RESECTIVE SURGERY

Removal of the epileptogenic area (e.g., temporal lobectomy)

CORPUS CALLOSOTOMY

Interruption of the anterior two-thirds of the corpus callosum, effective for atonic seizures, tonic seizures, and GTCS

HEMISPHERECTOMY

One cerebral hemisphere is disconnected from the rest of the brain, and a limited area is resected. It is performed for early-onset or congenital hemiplegia in which seizures arise from one side of the brain.

Key Points

- Currently, epilepsies are classified as localization-related (focal, partial), generalized epilepsies and epileptic syndromes, epilepsies and syndromes undetermined whether focal or generalized, and situation-related seizures.
- Epileptic encephalopathies often begin early and are characterized by severe cognitive and behavioral impairment and frequently intractable seizures. Examples include Ohtahara's syndrome, Dravet's syndrome, MAE, infantile spasms, and LGS.
- Neonatal seizures are more fragmentary than seizures after 2 months of age and have multiple possible causes including hypoxia-ischemia, metabolic derangements, trauma, vascular lesions, infections, CNS anomalies, inherited metabolic or genetic syndromes, and drug withdrawal.
- Febrile seizures are common, affect 2% to 5% of children, have a peak onset of 18 to 24 months, and typically remit by 6 years of age.
- Beyond basic metabolic studies (glucose, calcium, electrolytes), EEG, and neuroimaging, evaluation of seizures in children may require LP for seizures with fever, assessment for inborn errors of metabolism in children with seizures and regression, and chromosomal microarray for seizures in children with dysmorphic features and in children with epileptic encephalopathy.
- First seizures do not require AEDs unless there are abnormalities on the neurologic examination, epileptic discharges on EEG, abnormalities on neuroimaging, or diagnosis of epilepsies with a high recurrence risk such as infantile spasms, myoclonic or atonic epilepsies, or absence epilepsy.
- After 2 to 4 years of seizure freedom, favorable factors for successful withdrawal of AEDs include ease of seizure control, normal neurologic examination, normal EEG at the time of medication withdrawal, seizure onset between 2 and 12 years of age, and specific seizure types such as benign epilepsy with centrotemporal spikes and childhood absence epilepsy.

Recommended Readings

Berg AT, Berkovic SF, Brodie MJ, et al. Revised terminology and concepts for organization of seizures and epilepsies: report of the ILAE Commission on Classification and Terminology, 2005-2009. *Epilepsia.* 2010;51:676–685.

Commission on Classification and Terminology of the International League against Epilepsy. Proposal for revised classification of epilepsies and epileptic syndromes. *Epilepsia.* 1989;30:389–399.

Cook M, Shorvon S, Guerrino R, eds. *Oxford Textbook of Epilepsy and Epileptic Seizures (Oxford Textbooks in Clinical Neurology).* Oxford, England: Oxford University Press; 2013.

Duchowny M, Cross H, Arzimanoglou A, eds. *Pediatric Epilepsy.* New York, NY: McGraw Hill Education; 2012.

Engel J Jr, Pedley T, eds. *Epilepsy: A Comprehensive Textbook.* 2nd ed. Philadelphia, PA: Wolters Kluwer; 2008.

Mercimek-Mahmutoglu S, Patel J, Cordeiro D, et al. Diagnostic yield of genetic testing in epileptic encephalopathy in childhood. *Epilepsia.* 2015;56:707–716.

Wyllie E, Cascino GD, Gidal BE, et al, eds. *Wyllie's Treatment of Epilepsy: Principles and Practice.* 5th ed. Philadelphia, PA: Lippincott Williams & Wilkins; 2011.

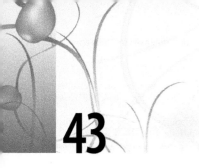

43

Epilepsy in Adults

Omkar N. Markand

Definitions

A. An epileptic seizure is a transient and reversible alteration of behavior caused by a paroxysmal, abnormal, and excessive neuronal discharge.

B. Epilepsy is traditionally defined as two or more recurring unprovoked seizures.

C. International League Against Epilepsy recently provided an operational definition of epilepsy as:

1. At least two unprovoked epileptic seizures occurring more than 24 hours apart
2. One unprovoked seizure and a probability of further seizures similar to general recurrence risk (at least 60%) after two unprovoked seizures, occurring over the next 10 years
3. Diagnosis of an epilepsy syndrome.

Classifications

There are two classifications—one of seizure types and one of epilepsy or epileptic syndromes. Accurate diagnosis of the type of epileptic seizure and the categorization of epilepsy (or epileptic syndrome) for each patient are essential prerequisite for proper medical and surgical management as well as prognosis.

A. **Classification of epileptic seizures (1981).** It is based on the patient's behavior during seizures and on the associated electroencephalography (EEG) characteristics. Epileptic seizures are classified into two main types—partial and generalized.

1. **Partial (focal) seizures** arise at localized areas in the cerebral cortex, and are associated with focal interictal and focal-onset ictal EEG changes. Clinically, a partial seizure can range in intensity from a disorder of sensation without loss of consciousness to a generalized convulsion.

   a. *Simple partial seizures.* Consciousness remains intact. Such seizures can be motor seizures (focal motor twitching or Jacksonian seizures), sensory seizures (numbness or tingling involving parts of the body), autonomic seizures, or seizures with psychic symptoms.

   b. *Complex partial seizures.* Consciousness is impaired. These seizures constitute the most common seizure type in adults (Video 43.1). Approximately 85% have an epileptogenic focus in the temporal lobe, whereas the remaining 15% are of extratemporal origin, usually frontal.

   c. *Secondarily generalized (tonic–clonic) seizures.* During any focal seizure (simple or complex partial), the epileptic excitation can spread widely to bilateral hemispheric regions, resulting in a generalized tonic–clonic convulsion.

2. **Generalized seizures** are characterized by generalized involvement of the brain from the outset without consistent focal areas of ictal onset. There are many subtypes.

   a. **Absence seizures,** also known as petit mal seizures, have a dominant feature of brief loss of consciousness with no or minimal motor manifestations (e.g., twitching of the eyelids). During the seizure, the EEG shows 3-Hz generalized spike–wave discharges. Absence seizures are often divided into typical and atypical absences.

   b. **Myoclonic seizures** are brief jerks involving part of the body or the entire body (Video 43.2).

   c. **Clonic seizures** are rhythmic twitching of the body.

d. **Tonic seizures** are brief attacks of stiffness in part of the body or the entire body.

e. **Atonic seizures** are losses of posture with resultant drop attacks.

f. **Tonic–clonic seizures** are generalized convulsions or grand mal seizures. It is important to emphasize that some of these are generalized from the outset and some are secondarily generalized, that is, they start as focal seizures and then become generalized. The second type is the most common among adults. The presence of an aura, focal manifestations during the seizure, and postictal focal deficits favor a secondarily generalized tonic–clonic seizure.

Confusion can arise in differentiating absence seizures and complex partial seizures. Both can present with a brief loss of awareness or altered responsiveness, and in both there may be automatic activities of various kinds. Diagnosis is aided by EEG findings (generalized spike–wave discharges in absence seizures and focal epileptiform abnormalities in complex partial seizures). Correct diagnosis is critical for instituting proper antiepileptic drug (AED) therapy.

B. **Classification of epilepsy or epileptic syndromes (1989).** Classifying the seizure type, although useful, is of limited value because seizures usually appear as part of a cluster of other symptoms and signs that include etiologic factor, site of seizure onset, age, precipitating factors, response to medication, and prognosis. Hence, the ultimate goal is to diagnose an epileptic syndrome. This is very important. It helps to choose the appropriate AEDs to control seizures and to avoid using an AED, which may not only be ineffective but may even exacerbate seizures.

1. **Localization-related (focal or partial) epilepsy or epileptic syndromes** are disorders in which a localized origin of the seizures can be established. The patient has focal or secondarily generalized tonic–clonic seizures. EEG shows focal epileptiform discharges overlying the epileptogenic focus.

a. Most localization-related epilepsies are **acquired** or **symptomatic.** Temporal lobe epilepsy is the common localization-related epilepsy among adults, and it is often associated with mesial temporal sclerosis on the magnetic resonance imaging (MRI) scan.

b. There are age-related **idiopathic** or **primary** localization-related epileptic syndromes. The best known is benign rolandic epilepsy of childhood.

2. **Generalized epilepsy or epileptic syndromes** are disorders that involve one or more types of generalized seizures. EEG shows generalized epileptiform abnormalities.

a. **Primary (idiopathic) generalized epilepsy (PGE)** is characterized by generalized seizures without any identifiable etiologic factor. Genetic factors predominate. EEG shows generalized spike–wave or polyspike–wave discharges with a normal background activity. Common syndromes include childhood absence epilepsy, juvenile myoclonic epilepsy (JME), juvenile absence epilepsy, and tonic–clonic seizures occurring often in the early morning ("awakening" grand mal).

b. **Secondary (symptomatic) generalized epilepsy** is characterized by various types of generalized seizures resulting from acquired cerebral diseases (e.g., seizures secondary to ischemic–hypoxic encephalopathy or following severe cerebral trauma or intracranial infection) or from inborn errors of metabolism (e.g., lipidosis and progressive myoclonus epilepsy). EEG shows generalized, irregular spike–wave, 2.5 Hz or less in frequency with an abnormally slow background activity. Patients usually have varying degrees of cognitive and neurologic deficits, and the seizures are often drug resistant. Within this category are three commonly recognized age-related syndromes—**West's syndrome** (infancy) and **Lennox–Gastaut syndrome** (childhood) and severe epilepsy with independent multifocal spike discharges occurring in childhood and adults.

C. **Newer ILAE classification of epileptic seizures and epilepsies (2010).**

1. The 2010 **classification of seizures** is still very similar to the previous one of 1981 and continues to separate epileptic seizures into generalized and focal seizures, but emphasizing their origin in neural networks rather than in discrete anatomical regions. The generalized seizures arise in some cortical area with rapid spread to bilaterally distributed neural networks including cortical and subcortical structures, but not necessarily the entire cerebral cortex. The focal seizures are categorized as those arising

in neural networks in one hemisphere remaining discretely localized before spreading more widely. Epileptic spasms have been included under the category without a clear-cut focal or generalized onset.

2. In the 2010 classification, the focal-onset epileptic seizures are not subdivided into simple partial or complex partial seizures as in 1981 classification because alteration of awareness is often difficult to ascertain and that the pathophysiologic mechanism may not be distinctive in the two subtypes.

3. For the epileptic seizures of generalized onset, there is very little change compared to the 1981 classification. Myoclonic seizures are further refined into myoclonic–atonic (jerk followed by decreased muscle tone) and myoclonic–tonic (jerk followed by increased muscle tone). Absences with eyelid myoclonia and myoclonic absences have been added to the typical and atypical absences.

4. The original ILAE classification of epilepsies and epilepsy syndrome (1989) was based on the dichotomy of focal- versus generalized-onset seizures and identifiable etiology (symptomatic with known identifiable etiology and idiopathic without identifiable cause) resulting into four subcategories: symptomatic focal (localization-related) epilepsies, idiopathic focal (localization-related) epilepsies, idiopathic (primary) generalized epilepsies, and symptomatic (secondary) generalized epilepsies. In the 2010 classification, these terms have been largely abandoned. The dividing line between idiopathic and symptomatic generalized epilepsies is often difficult to define with significant overlap. The new proposal recommends **classifying epilepsies** according to distinctive electroclinical syndrome and identifiable causation. The epilepsies are broadly divided into:

   a. Age-related electroclinical syndrome (neonatal period, infancy, childhood, adolescence to adult)
   b. Surgical syndrome (temporal lobe epilepsy with hippocampal sclerosis, Rasmussen syndrome, gelastic seizures with hypothalamic hamartoma)
   c. Epilepsy with structural-metabolic causes
   d. Epilepsies of unknown cause

   Even though the newer classification of epilepsies and epilepsy syndrome is gaining some acceptance, the older classification still remains strongly entrenched into the vocabulary of epilepsy community. The author has, therefore, decided to maintain it in this chapter for the time being until the newer classification gets more widely accepted.

EVALUATION

It is essential to establish that the spells or episodes are indeed epileptic seizures. Nonepileptic physiologic disorders that result in transient, reversible alterations of behavior or function, such as syncope, migraine, breath-holding spells, anxiety episodes, transient ischemic attacks, hypoglycemic episodes, and narcoleptic–cataplectic attacks, must be differentiated from epileptic seizures. Moreover, there are nonepileptic psychogenic seizures or pseudoseizures that are conversion reactions characterized by episodes of motor activity and lack of awareness but not associated with ictal EEG patterns and without an underlying physiologic basis.

A. A **history** of the episodes, obtained not only from the patient but also from one or more observers, is perhaps the most essential element in making the diagnosis of epileptic seizures and differentiating them from nonepileptic disorders.

B. **Physical and neurologic examinations** can help detect the underlying cause of the brain disorder responsible for the epilepsy by uncovering evidence of a focal cerebral lesion or another neurologic disorder, such as tuberous sclerosis or neurofibromatosis.

C. Neuroimaging. Compared to computed tomography of the head with and without contrast, MRI of the brain is the imaging procedure of choice. It is particularly sensitive in detecting hamartoma, cavernous malformation, low-grade glioma and mesial temporal sclerosis.

D. **EEG** is the most informative test for confirming epileptic nature of the episodes, classification of the seizure type, and even the epileptic syndrome. It also aids in initiation, selection, and discontinuation of antiepileptic therapy. Not all patients with epilepsy have interictal epileptiform abnormalities; approximately 50% have such abnormalities in a routine awake-and-asleep EEG study that includes hyperventilation and intermittent photic stimulation. The yield increases with repeated EEG studies with sleep deprivation and extra recording electrodes. On the other hand, 1% to 2% of healthy persons without clinical seizures have epileptiform abnormalities in EEG studies. Hence, an interictal EEG alone can neither prove nor exclude a diagnosis of epilepsy. Similarly, the presence of interictal epileptiform EEG abnormalities does not automatically warrant AED therapy, and the absence of such abnormalities is not sufficient grounds for discontinuing AED treatment.

E. **24-hour video EEG or prolonged EEG.** This is indicated to detect epileptiform abnormalities in those patients who had previously a normal routine EEG (awake and asleep) and in whom the epileptic nature of the episodes needs to be established before starting or changing antiepileptic medication.

F. **Prolonged video EEG monitoring.** Patients with drug-resistant epilepsy or poorly characterized episodes may need prolonged monitoring that consists of simultaneous monitoring of the patient's behavior and EEG to provide detailed clinical and EEG correlation of episodic events. This is an expensive and time-consuming technique and is thus left to the discretion of a consulting neurologist specialized in epilepsy. Only 5% to 10% of patients believed to have epilepsy need this technique to characterize and classify the epileptic episodes. Video EEG is mandatory in the presurgical evaluation of patients to document epileptic seizures prior to surgical resection to treat epilepsy, and even before placing a patient on vagus nerve stimulation (VNS). It is also very helpful in patients who have frequent episodes that are suspected to be of the nonepileptic psychogenic type.

G. **Home video recording.** With the universal availability of "smart phones" the relatives are encouraged to record one or more of the patient's events. This cheapest monitoring can often provide very critical information regarding the nature of the episodes even without the benefit of concomitant EEG as in the formal video EEG monitoring.

GENERAL PRINCIPLES IN TREATING PATIENTS WITH EPILEPSY

A. AED therapy should be initiated only when the diagnosis of epileptic seizures is well established. If the patient's episodes are yet to be clearly defined and there is reasonable doubt of their being epileptic in nature, it is prudent to wait until the diagnosis of epilepsy can be confirmed.

B. **Monotherapy** is preferable to the use of several drugs because it has fewer toxic side effects, less likelihood of drug interactions, and better compliance. The chosen AED (see Table 43.1) should be slowly increased until seizures are controlled or until clinical signs of toxicity develop. If seizures are not adequately controlled at the maximum tolerable dosage, a second AED is slowly introduced. After the second drug attains therapeutic levels, the first drug is gradually withdrawn. Monotherapy adequately controls new-onset epilepsy in about two-thirds of the patients.

C. **Polytherapy** with a combination of two AEDs becomes necessary only if monotherapy trial of two or more first-line AEDs has been unsuccessful. When using two AEDs, select those with different mechanism of action. Avoid using more than two AEDs simultaneously. If a combination of two AEDs in the treatment of a compliant patient with blood levels in the therapeutic range fails to provide adequate control of epileptic seizures, **referral to an epileptologist or comprehensive epilepsy center** is indicated for further evaluation and management.

D. **AEDs with sedative or hypnotic side effects** (e.g., phenobarbital, primidone, and clonazepam) need to be avoided unless first-choice AED does not work. A patient on polytherapy that includes one of the aforementioned sedative AEDs is best served by a gradual withdrawal of the sedative AED while the dosage of the other AED is maximized. Discontinuation of sedative–hypnotic AEDs is followed not only by a reduction in side effects but also by better control of seizures in many instances.

E. **Simplify drug schedules.** With few exceptions, most AEDs have long elimination half-lives (see Table 43.3), and thus can be prescribed in one or two divided daily doses.

F. **Adherence** must be emphasized. Medication is best taken at the time of meals for easy remembrance. For most AEDs, an occasional missed dose can be made up by taking an additional dose within the same 24-hour period. It is also convenient for the patient to put

TABLE 43.1 **AEDs: Year Introduced, Mechanism of Action, and Indications**

AED	Year Introduced	Mechanism of Action	Indications Approved	Indications Off-label
Traditional AEDs				
Phenobarbital	1912	↑ GABA, ↓ Na	(1) Partial and sec. gen. t-c (mono and adj) (2) GTC status	
Primidone	1954	↑ GABA, ↓ Na	Partial and sec. gen. t-c (mono and adj)	
Phenytoin	1938	↓ Na	(1) Partial and sec. gen. t-c (mono and adj) (2) PGE with gen. t-c (3) SE	PGE with gen t-c
Carbamazepine	1962	↓ Na	Partial and sec. gen. t-c (mono and adj)	
Valproate	1978	↓ Na, ↓ Ca (T), ↑ GABA	(1) Partial and sec. gen. t-c (mono and adj) (2) PGE with absences, myoclonic, t-c szs (3) SGE	PGE with gen t-c
Clonazepam	1975	↑ GABA ↓ Na	PGE with absences, myoclonic or t-c szs	Partial epil. with gen. t-c szs
Ethosuximide	1958	↓ Ca (T)	PGE with absences only	
Second-generation AEDs				
Felbamate	1993	↓ Na, ↑ GABA, ↓ Glutamate	Intractable[a] partial epil. (adj, mono), SGE (adj, mono)	
Gabapentin	1993	↓ Ca ($\alpha_2 \delta$ subunit binding)	Partial epil. (adj)	Partial epil. (mono)
Lamotrigine	1994	↓ Na, ↓ Glutamate	Partial epil. (adj), partial epil. (mono conversion)	(a) JME, (b) PGE with absences, (c) newly dx. epil. (mono)
Topiramate	1996	↓ Na, ↑ GABA	Partial epil. (adj), GTC (mono)	(a) PGE with GTC and other seizure types, (b) SGE
Tiagabine	1997	↑ GABA	Partial epil. (adj)	–
Levetiracetam	1999	SV$_2$ binding decreases transmitter release	(1) Partial epil. (adj), (2) myoclonic seizure of JME (adj), (3) PGE with GTC (adj)	(a) JME (mono), (b) PGE with other szs, (c) SGE, (d) newly diagnosed epil. (mono)
Oxcarbazepine	2000	↓ Na	Partial epil. (adj) and (mono)	
Zonisamide	2000	↓ Na, ↓ Ca (T), ↓ Glutamate	Partial epil. (adj)	PGE

534

Third-generation AEDs

Pregabalin	2005	↓ Ca ($\alpha_2\delta$ subunit binding)	Partial epil. (adj)
Lacosamide	2008	↓ Na, slow inactivation	Partial epil. (adj)
Rufinamide	2008	↓ Na	Szs with Lennox–Gastaut syndrome (adj)	Partial epil. (adj)
Vigabatrin	2009	↑ GABA (↓ GABA-T)	Partial epil. (adj), infantile spasm
Ezogabine	2011	↑ K (KCNQ/KU7)	Partial epil. (adj)
Clobazam	2011	↑ GABA	Szs with Lennox–Gastaut syndrome (adj)	SGE, partial epil. (adj)
Perampanel	2012	↓ Glutamate (AMPA antagonist)	Partial epil. (adj), PGE with GTC (adj)
Eslicarbazepine	2013	↓ Na	Partial epil. (adj)

[a]Used only for refractory epilepsy when possible benefits outweigh known serious liver and bone marrow toxicity.

Abbreviations: AED, antiepileptic drug; AMPA, alpha-amino-3-hydroxy-5-methyl-4-isoxazolepropionic acid; adj, adjunctive; Ca, calcium currents; Ca (T), low-threshold T current; GABA, γ-aminobutyric acid transmission; GTC, generalized tonic–clonic; JME, juvenile myoclonic epilepsy; K, potassium current; mono, monotherapy; Na, sodium currents; PGE, primary (idiopathic) generalized epilepsy; SGE, secondary generalized epilepsy; SV₂, synaptic vesicle protein 2; gen. t–c, generalized tonic–clonic seizures; SE, status epilepticus; sec. gen. t–c, secondarily generalized tonic–clonic seizures; ↓, decrease; ↑ increase.

the medication in a plastic pillbox with divided compartments and to make sure at bedtime that the entire day's medication has been taken.

G. Advise the patient to maintain a **seizure diary** and bring it at every office visit to assist in evaluating the effectiveness of the therapy.

H. Emphasize to the patient the need for constant **medical follow-up care.** Once AED therapy is well established and the seizures have been brought under satisfactory control, the patient may be followed every 6 to 12 months. During the follow-up visits, evaluate the patient for evidence of drug toxicity or development of a progressive neurologic disorder. Complete blood count (CBC), liver function tests, and serum electrolytes may need to be performed every 6 to 12 months to detect untoward effects of AEDs on the bone marrow and liver in patients receiving valproate, carbamazepine, and phenytoin. However, routine blood testing at periodic intervals is a controversial issue because serious side effects are rare and, when they occur, they do so over a short period to be detected by periodic monitoring.

I. A patient who achieves good control with drug therapy may have a **"breakthrough" seizure** during periods of physical or mental stress, sleep deprivation, or febrile illness. Appropriate management of such precipitants rather than increases in dose or changes in the AED is indicated.

J. **Generic substitution** for brand-name AEDs can reduce the cost of medication, but the bioavailabilities of generic and proprietary AEDs are not the same. Generic preparations are required by the US Food and Drug Administration (FDA) to provide bioavailabilities within ±20% of those of the corresponding proprietary formulations, but some patients may be sufficiently sensitive to these fluctuations so that replacing one with the other may lead to either loss of seizure control or signs of neurotoxicity. This problem applies primarily to phenytoin and carbamazepine. It is probably prudent to continue brand-name AED if the patient is seizure free on that formulation. If changed to generic AED the patient needs to be warned of the possibility of breakthrough seizures or drug toxicity. When a generic AED is used, the formulation by the same manufacturer is preferred.

K. **Therapeutic drug levels** are rough guides to the ranges that provide best seizure control while avoiding dose-related side effects. The blood should be drawn preferably before the morning dose of AEDs so as to obtain the lowest (trough) levels. The blood levels are not to be followed rigidly for a given patient. Some patients may attain complete seizure control at low "therapeutic" levels, and increasing the dose to attain idealized levels is not indicated. On the other hand, there are patients who need higher than "therapeutic" levels for control of their seizures and tolerate such levels without significant untoward side effects. AED blood levels are indicated under the following circumstances:

1. To determine the baseline plasma dose level
2. When the patient is believed to be noncompliant
3. When the patient does not respond adequately to the usual dosage of an AED
4. When symptoms and signs of clinical toxicity are suspected
5. When there is a question of drug interaction
6. To establish the correct dosage for a pregnant patient or a patient with diseases affecting the pharmacokinetics of the AEDs (hepatic, renal, or gastrointestinal disorders).

   Usually total serum levels of AEDs are obtained. When metabolism of AEDs may be altered or serum protein levels are likely to be low (e.g., hepatic or renal disorders and pregnancy), free levels of highly protein-bound AEDs may become necessary.

L. Emphasize the need to regularize the time and duration of sleep, because **sleep deprivation** tends to potentiate seizures.

M. Concomitant use of other drugs. Alcohol in any form is best avoided or used in small amounts (e.g., one drink) because of possible interactions with most AEDs. Be aware of drugs that lower the seizure threshold (e.g., tricyclic antidepressants, Welbutrin, and phenothiazines) or those that can cause drug interactions (increasing or decreasing the levels of AEDs); they should be used with caution. Some AEDs affect the elimination kinetics of many drugs metabolized in the liver (e.g., birth control pills, corticosteroids, anticoagulants, and cyclosporine), necessitating proper dose adjustment of these comedications.

N. Encourage the patient to make **some life adjustments** necessary to lead a normal life as much as possible. Moderate exercise needs to be encouraged; it does not affect seizure frequency. Participation in highly competitive sports increases the risk of physical injury. Individualize instructions to the patient by considering the risk of a particular sport against the patient's aspirations. Swimming may be permitted under supervision for a patient with good control of seizures. Bathing in a bathtub is to be avoided; instead, a shower is recommended.

O. Most adults who have epilepsy are able to maintain competitive **employment** and should be encouraged to do so. This improves their self-esteem and their acceptance in the mainstream of society. There are, however, some realistic limitations. Occupations, such as working with heavy machines, working above ground level, working close to water or fire, driving trucks or buses, and flying planes, may be off limits for reasons of personal and public safety.

P. **Educate** the family members or caregivers regarding proper care of the patient when a seizure occurs. During a grand mal seizure, the patient should be helped to lie on the ground, a bed, or a couch and should be turned on one side to avoid aspiration. An object such as a spoon or a finger should *never be thrust into the patient's* mouth. Pushing a hard object into the mouth often results in broken teeth. The patient must be closely watched and the sequence of events carefully observed during a seizure, which can help determine the type of seizure.

Q. Hospitalization. For a patient with a known history of seizures, an isolated self-limiting seizure does not constitute a need to call for an ambulance and to rush the patient to an emergency department. However, if the seizure lasts longer than 5 minutes or if the patient has repeated seizures without regaining consciousness between them, prompt transfer to a nearby hospital becomes essential. Medical attention must also be sought if the patient had a fall and sustained bodily injury.

R. Driving. Most states have laws denying driving privileges to patients with uncontrolled epilepsy but permit driving once the seizures have been brought under control with AEDs. In a few states, doctors are required to report cases of epilepsy. The period of time that the patient must remain seizure-free before being permitted to drive varies from 3 months to 2 years, depending on the state. Rare patients who have only nocturnal seizures or who have only simple partial seizures (no loss of consciousness) may be exempted from driving restrictions. Reinstitution of driving privileges may require reapplication, a letter from the treating physician, or a determination made by a state-appointed board. Some states require the treating physician to certify at regular intervals that the patient has continued to remain seizure-free before reissuing the driving permit. Because the laws regarding driving vary widely among different states and are frequently changing, physicians are best advised to obtain their current state registration. In general, patients with frequent seizures with altered consciousness must be advised to refrain from driving until seizures can be satisfactorily controlled. That the patient has been properly advised must be documented in the patient's record. There is no consensus as to how long the patient should be advised not to drive in the case of a breakthrough seizure after being seizure-free for a long period. If such a seizure follows a known precipitant such as infection, mental or physical stress, prolonged sleep deprivation, or poor compliance, observation for at least 3 to 6 months is required before driving is permitted again.

ANTIEPILEPTIC DRUGS

A. Mechanism of action, and efficacy of AEDs. Table 43.1 lists the AEDs presently available in the United States. The table summarizes the mechanism of action, year of introduction in the treatment of epilepsy, and FDA-approved as well as off-label utility of these AEDs.

According to the duration of availability, the AEDs can be divided into **first-generation or traditional AEDs,** which were available before 1993; **second-generation AEDs,** which became available between 1993 and 2004; and **third-generation AEDs,** which became available in the United States in or after 2005. The second- and third-generation AEDs are often grouped as **Newer AEDs** but sufficient clinical experience, side-effect profile, and teratogenic data are available only for the second-generation AEDs.

An **ideal AED** should be effective against multiple seizure types, effective against seizures resistant to traditional AEDs, have low neurologic and systemic toxicity, and should have favorable pharmacokinetics: complete oral absorption, minimal binding to plasma protein, primarily renal elimination, long elimination half-life, linear kinetics, and no enzyme induction or inhibition. Newer AEDs have substantial advantages over traditional AEDs including absence of side effects, none or fewer drug interactions, and

TABLE 43.2 AEDs of Choice for Specific Type of Seizures and Epilepsy Syndromes

Type of Seizure or Syndrome	Recommended AED		
	First Choice	Second Choice	Possibly Useful
Partial (focal) Epilepsy			
Simple partial, complex partial; secondary generalized tonic–clonic seizures	OXC/CBZ/PHT/ LTG/ESC	TPM/LTC/PGL/VPA/ ZNS/LCM	GBP/PB/PRM/EZG/ FBM[c]
PGE			
Primary generalized tonic–clonic seizures	VPA/TPM/LTG[a]	ZNS/OXC//LTC	PRP
Absence epilepsy without motor seizures	ESM/VPA	LTG[a]	CLZ
Absence epilepsy with generalized tonic–clonic seizures	VPA	LTG[a]/TPM/LTC	CLZ
Myoclonic seizures	VPA/LTC[a]	LTG[a]/LTC/ZNS[b]	CLZ
Myoclonic seizures with absence or generalized tonic–clonic seizures	VPA/LTG[a]/LTC[a]	LTG[a]/TPM/LTC/ ZNS	
Secondary Generalized Epilepsy			
Usually multiple seizure types, e.g., tonic, absence, myoclonic, clonic, atonic, tonic–clonic	VPA/LTG/LTC	CLB/TPM/ZNS/RFM	FBM[c], OXC, ketogenic diet

AEDs separated by virgules are roughly equal in efficacy. The choice of specific AED for a given patient should be based on factors such as toxicity and cost. Sedative AEDs are generally considered second-line drugs.
[a]Because of the risk of neural tube defect with VPA, LTG or LTC may be the drug of first choice in treatment of women considering pregnancy.
[b]Particularly useful for progressive myoclonic epilepsy.
[c]High incidence of serious side effects.
Abbreviations: AED, antiepileptic drug; CBZ, carbamazepine; CLZ, clonazepam; CLB, clobazam; ESM, ethosuximide; ESC, eslicarbazepine; EZG, ezogabine; FBM, felbamate; GBP, gabapentin; LTG, lamotrigine; LTC, levetiracetam; LCM, lacosamide; OXC, oxcarbazepine; PHT, phenytoin; PB, phenobarbital; PRM, primidone; PGL, pregabalin; PGE, primary (idiopathic) generalized epilepsy PRP, perampanel; RFM, rufinamide; TPM, topiramate; TGB, tiagabine; VPA, valproic acid; ZNS, zonisamide.

favorable pharmacokinetics. Therefore, the second-generation AEDs have largely replaced the traditional AEDs in the treatment of epilepsy, especially in the developed countries. However, there is no evidence that any new AED has better efficacy compared with carbamezapine, phenytoin, or valproic acid in well-controlled trials of recent-onset epilepsy.

B. **Proper selection of AED.** Table 43.2 lists AEDs effective for managing various forms of epilepsy and epileptic syndromes.

1. **Symptomatic partial (localization-related) epilepsy.** Of the traditional AEDs, carbamazepine, phenytoin, primidone, and phenobarbital are effective in the treatment of partial epilepsy but carbamazepine and phenytoin are usually better tolerated than primidone and phenobarbital. **Carbamazepine** and **phenytoin** have been the first-line "traditional" AEDs for several decades before the introduction of the newer AEDs. They are used progressively less except in the developing countries. **Phenytoin** is relatively inexpensive, can be titrated rapidly in 2 to 3 days, is better tolerated in the initial period of therapy, and can be given in one to two divided daily doses. However, it has a high incidence of chronic dysmorphic side effects, such as hirsutism, coarsening of facial features, and acneiform eruptions, which makes its use rather unacceptable in women. Its nonlinear kinetics makes the dose adjustment difficult during maintenance therapy. **Carbamazepine** has no dysmorphic effects; hence, it is better accepted by adolescent

TABLE 43.3 Pharmacokinetics and Adult Dosages of AEDs

AEDs	Bioavailability (%)	Protein Binding (%)	Elimination Half-life (hr)	Elimination Route	Starting Adult Dose (mg/d)	Escalation Dose (mg)	Usual Adult Maintenance Dose (mg/d)	Dosing Regimen (times/d)	[a]Therapeutic Level (μg/mL)	Enzyme Induction and OCP Failure
Traditional AEDs										
Phenytoin	>90	90	10–50[b]	H	300	30–100/4 wk	300–400	1–3	10–20	↑
Carbamazepine	75–85	75	10–50[c]	H	200	200/wk	600–2,000	3	4–12	↑
Ethosuximide	>90	0	30–60	H 75, R 25	500	250/wk	500–1,500	2	40–100	—
Valproic acid	>90	70–95[d]	5–20	H	500	250/wk	750–3,000	2, 3	40–120	—
Phenobarbital	>90	40–50	50–120	H 75, R 25	60	30/4 wk	60–180	1	15–40	↑
Primidone[e]	>90	0	6–12	H	125	125/3–7 d	750–1,500	3	5–12	↑
Clonazepam	>90	85	20–40	H	1.0	0.5/3–7 d	1.5–10	1–3	0.02–0.08	—
Second-generation AEDs										
Felbamate	>90	25	15–25[f], 11–15[g]	H 50, R 50	1,200	600/wk	1,200–3,600	2, 3	40–100	↑/—
Gabapentin	30–60	0	5–9	R	300	300/2–7 d	900–3,600	3, 4	4–20	—
Lamotrigine	>90	55	24[f], 15[g], 60[h]	H 90, R 10	50[c, d], 12.5[e]	50/2 wk, 12.5/2 wk	200–600[c, d], 100–200[e]	1, 2	2–20	—
Topiramate	>80	15	20–30[f], 12–15[g]	H 40, R 60	25–50	25–50/wk	200–600	2	2–20	↑/—
Tiagabine	>90	96	6–9[f], 4–6[g]	H	4	4/wk	32–56	2–4	0.1–0.3	—
Levetiracetam	100	<10	6–8	R 66	1,000	500/wk	1,000–3,000	2	5–40	—
Zonisamide	>50	40	50–70[f], 25–40[g]	H 65, R 35	100	100/2 wk	200–600	1, 2	10–40	—
Oxcarbazepine[i]	>95	40	7–11	H	600	300/3–7 d	1,200–2,400	2	15–35	↑

(continued)

TABLE 43.3 Pharmacokinetics and Adult Dosages of AEDs (continued)

AEDs	Bioavailability (%)	Protein Binding (%)	Elimination Half-life (hr)	Elimination Route	Starting Adult Dose (mg/d)	Escalation Dose (mg)	Usual Adult Maintenance Dose (mg/d)	Dosing Regimen (times/d)	[a]Therapeutic Level (μg/mL)	Enzyme Induction and OCP Failure
Third-generation AEDs										
Pregabalin	>90	0	6–7	R	150	50–75/1–2 wk	300–600	2, 3	0.06–12.5	—
Lacosamide	100	<15	13	H 60, R 40	100	50/wk	400	2	—	—
Rufinamide	>85, ↑ by food	<34	6–10	H	400–800	400–800/2 d	3,200	2	5–55	↑/—
Vigabatrin	80–90	0	5–13	R	1,000	500/wk	3,000	2	—	—
Ezogabine	60	60	8	H.Glu	300	150/wk	1,200	3	—	↑
Clobazam	90	83	19	H	10	10/wk	20–40	2	—	↑
Perampanel	>90	95	105	H	2	2/wk	4–8	1	—	↑
Eslicarbazepine	>90	<40	13–20	H	400	400/wk	800–1,200	1	—	↑

[a]Many of these are not therapeutic ranges, but levels commonly encountered in treated patients.

[b]Elimination half-life is concentration dependent; at higher levels the half-life is long.

[c]Elimination half-life is longer in the initial 2 to 4 week of therapy before self-induction becomes significant.

[d]Concentration dependent, higher binding at low total levels.

[e]Primidone therapy produces three active metabolites: primidone, phenobarbital, and phenylethylmalonamide.

[f]When administered alone.

[g]When administered with enzyme-inducer AEDs (e.g., phenobarbital, phenytoin, carbamazepine, and primidone).

[h]When administered with valproic acid.

[i]Kinetic parameters refer to monohydroxy derivative, for which oxcarbazepine is a prodrug.

Abbreviations: AED, antiepileptic drug; H, hepatic; OCP, oral contraceptive pill; R, renal; H. glu, hepatic glucuronidation; numbers are approximate percentages for each route.

and young adult female patients. Its short half-life usually necessitates using it in three or four divided doses, but sustained-release preparations are now available and given in two daily doses. It needs to be slowly titrated over 3- to 4-week period because of autoinduction. **Valproate** is the only broad-spectrum AED of first generation, effective both in partial or generalized epilepsies. It is probably less effective than phenytoin or carbamazepine for partial epilepsy. All the three require periodic blood monitoring for bone marrow and liver functions. Most of the newer AEDs are approved by the FDA for adjunctive therapy in the treatment of partial epilepsy refractory to traditional AEDs with the exception are oxcarbazepine. **Oxcarbazepine,** which has lesser side effects, rapid titration, and no requirement for blood monitoring, has emerged a more favored newer AED alternative to carbamazepine since its approval by the FDA for monotherapy in adults with focal epilepsy. If monotherapy with oxcarbazepine fails to achieve satisfactory control, an adjunctive therapy with another second-generation AED should be strongly considered by adding levetiracetam, lamotrigine, topiramate, or zonisamide to oxcarbazepine. These four AEDs are also broad spectrum in efficacy. **Levetiracetam** is gaining more extensive use not only as adjunctive therapy but also as monotherapy (off label in the United States) because of rapid titration, no need for blood monitoring, absent hepatic metabolism, and lack of interaction with other drugs. One-fourth may develop anxiety and other behavioral side effects necessitating its discontinuation. **Lamotrigine** is another widely used newer AED in partial epilepsy, especially in women of childbearing age because of its very low teratogenic potential. However, it requires slow titration because of skin hypersensitivity. It is approved by FDA for monotherapy conversion in addition to adjunctive therapy. Although it does not affect metabolism of oral contraceptive drugs, the latter significantly decrease lamotrigine levels. Adjunctive therapy with **topiramate** (multiple mechanisms of action against epileptic process) is particularly helpful in those patients who have comorbidity of migraine and/or obesity because of its efficacy in migraine and its weight-loss effect. However, it does have significant cognitive side effects, risk for kidney stones, and relatively higher incidence of teratogenesis. Of the third-generation AEDs, **lacosamide** is being used more frequently as adjunct therapy in partial-onset seizures if lamotrigine, levetiracetam, or oxcarbazepine has not succeeded in satisfactory seizure control. Combination therapy with lacosamide is more likely to produce neurotoxic side effects. **Esclicarbazepine**, with a similar molecule as oxcarbazepine, is recently approved as monotherapy for the treatment of focal-onset epilepsy. There is yet very little clinical experience with this AED but it is reported to have a better side-effect profile than oxcarbazepine. **Felbamate**, a broad-spectrum AED, is very effective in partial epilepsy and has little or no sedative side effect. It is, however, recommended as a last resort because of its hepatic and bone marrow toxicity. One would need a signed consent form and periodic blood testing.

Even with adequate AED therapy, only 40% to 60% of patients with symptomatic partial epilepsy (the most common type of epilepsy among adults) attain full control of seizures. In one study of new-onset epileptic seizures, initial monotherapy was effective in 47% of patients. Changing to a second drug controlled another 13% of patients. Use of a third AED or combined therapy with two or more AEDs controlled just 4% of additional patients. Most experts believe that, if an adequate trial with two AEDs either as monotherapy or combined therapy fails, the patient has **medically refractory epilepsy.** Such a patient is better managed at a comprehensive epilepsy center.

2. **PGE.** Patients with PGE have either absence, myoclonic, or tonic–clonic seizures. Most, however, have more than one type of seizure, although one type may dominate. Depending on seizure type, several epileptic syndromes are identified under the heading PGE. The best example is JME, which is characterized by myoclonic seizures in the early hours after waking, but most patients also have occasional tonic–clonic seizures. Less often, even absence seizures may occur. Other syndromes include primary tonic–clonic seizures (contrasted to secondarily generalized tonic–clonic seizures, which are part of focal epilepsy), which commonly occur in the morning hours and hence are called "awakening" grand mal seizures. Absence seizures as the dominant manifestation of PGE commonly occur in childhood (childhood absence epilepsy), but in rare cases start in adolescence or early adulthood (juvenile absence epilepsy).

Patients with PGE who have absence seizures only can be treated with either ethosuximide or valproic acid because both are equally effective in controlling absences. **Ethosuximide** has narrow spectrum of efficacy being specific for absences only and not effective against myoclonic and/or tonic–clonic seizures. **Valproic acid** is the drug of choice for PGE in patients with multiple seizure types, including the syndrome of JME, primary grand mal seizures, or combined absence–grand mal epilepsy. The advantage of valproic acid is that it is effective against all seizure types comprising PGE. Because of the high incidence of fetal malformations, polycystic ovarian syndrome (PCOS), and weight gain, the use of valproic acid in women with PGE needs to be restricted because recent well-designed studies have demonstrated effectiveness of the **newer AEDs,** several of which are broad spectrum in their efficacy. **Lamotrigine** is effective against absences, has low teratogenicity, and is a weight-neutral AED. It is a good alternative for treating absences associated with childhood and juvenile absence epilepsy. Slow titration and dermatological hypersensitivity are some of the undesirable features. It is also found to be effective in JME, although it can occasionally exacerbate myoclonic seizures. **Levetiracetam** is effective in all seizure types accompanying PGE and particularly tonic–clonic and myoclonic seizures. **Topiramate** is effective in PGE manifesting with generalized tonic–clonic seizures and approved by the FDA for this indication. However, its side-effect profile (cognitive impairment, renal stones, glaucoma, and teratogenesis) limits its utility. **Perampanel** is also found to be effective and approved for tonic–clonic seizures of PGE. It may be an alternative in primary generalized tonic–clonic seizures, which have failed to respond to conventional AEDs. **Zonisamide** is probably effective, also, against all seizure types of PGE, but has more sedative side effects than lamotrigine and levetiracetam. **Clonazepam** is an effective AED for myoclonic and absence seizures but has certain disadvantages. It has a high incidence of sedative and cognitive side effects, and patients develop a tolerance to its antiepileptic potency after several months of therapy. It may be used as a bedtime medication in those who have myoclonic or generalized tonic–clonic seizures consistently during sleep or in the morning on awakening.

Although most patients with PGE can be well controlled with appropriate AEDs, some 15% are medically refractory. Some are **pseudorefractory** because they are on wrong AEDs. Sodium-channel blocking and gamma-aminobutric acid (GABA)-enhancing AEDs have been recognized to exacerbate certain seizure types in patients with PGE. Carbamazepine, oxcarbazepine, phenytoin, vigabatrin, tiagabine, gabapentin, and pregabalin commonly exacerbate absence seizures, myoclonic jerks, or both, and should not be used in the treatment of PGE. It is, therefore, critical that the patient needs to have the syndromic diagnosis of PGE established even though the precise subtype of PGE may not be identified. This will prevent iatrogenic exacerbation of seizures. In those patients where the syndromic diagnosis is yet not established, one should consider using broad-spectrum AEDs such as lamotrigine, levetiracetam, topiramate, or valproate.

In refractory cases of PGE, **combination therapy** using Depakote with either levetiracetam, lamotrigine (be aware of markedly decreased elimination of lamotrigine by valproic acid), topiramate, or zonisamide may be more effective. Combination of valproic acid and ethosuximide may control absences more effectively than either drug alone. Use of valproic acid in a woman of childbearing age should be considered as a last resort because of its high potential for teratogenesis. VNS is used, albeit rarely, in medically refractory PGE.

3. **Secondary (symptomatic) generalized epilepsy,** which is secondary to multifocal or diffuse cerebral disorders (static or progressive), occurs mostly among children and less often among adults. Patients have multiple seizure types, including atypical absence seizures, myoclonic seizures, tonic seizures, tonic–clonic seizures, and drop attacks.

In general, response to any AED is poor, with only 20% to 40% of patients attaining acceptable seizure control. Such patients commonly end up being treated with polypharmacy, which not only fails to provide better seizure control than do one or two AEDs but may even exacerbate certain types of seizures (absence seizures, myoclonic seizures, and drop attacks).

Valproic acid, being a broad-spectrum AED, is of first choice for secondarily generalized epilepsy and may be started as monotherapy. However, most patients need an addition of newer AEDs. Of these, **lamotrigine, levetiracetam, topiramate, and zonisamide** have been found useful in clinical trials. **Felbamate, rufinamide, and clobazam** have been approved by FDA for the control of seizures associated with secondary generalized epilepsy of the Lennox–Gastaut type but felbamate has potentially serious hepatic and bone marrow toxicity requiring periodic blood testing. **Clobazam** is being used progressively more since the approval by FDA in combination with valproic acid, lamotrigine, or levetiracetam to obtain a better seizure control. When drug combinations are prescribed, appropriate dosages should be used to avoid sedation, which tends to exacerbate minor seizures as well as precipitate statuses in such patients. **VNS** is another modality of treatment commonly used in this population.

C. **Pharmacokinetics of AEDs.** These are summarized in Table 43.3.

1. **Traditional (first-generation) AEDs.**

   a. Most of the **traditional AEDs** are eliminated primarily by hepatic metabolism, through microsomal cytochrome P-450 enzymes, an undesirable pharmacokinetic characteristic.

   Because of several potential drug interactions, these enzyme-inducing AEDs lower hormonal levels including oral contraceptives, warfarin, steroids, tricyclics, cyclosporine, digitalis, and antipsychotics.

   b. Carbamazepine is notorious in causing **autoinduction,** so that a smaller dose at the start is associated with blood levels, which are achievable only by two to three times that dose after a month or so. On the other hand, competitive enzymatic inhibition increases the levels of these AEDs causing clinical toxicity. Erythromycin markedly inhibits metabolism of carbamazepine. Cimetidine and propoxyphene have similar but lesser effects. These drugs, as well as grapefruit juice, may result in rise of carbamazepine to toxic levels.

   c. Valproic acid is a strong **competitive inhibitor** of certain hepatic enzymes, increasing the levels of many drugs including phenobarbital, lorazepam, lamotrigine, gonadal, and adrenal androgens.

   d. Phenytoin and valproic acid have extensive **plasma protein binding** (80% to 95%), another undesirable pharmacokinetic property. Valproic acid, in addition, has nonlinear binding; at higher levels, the proportion of protein-bound drug is less, and there is a disproportionately high level of free or unbound drug. It is the free fraction that relates to drug efficacy and clinical toxicity.

   e. Another troubling pharmacokinetic characteristic of phenytoin is its **nonlinear elimination** resulting from saturation of hepatic microsomal P-450 enzymes. Small increments (by 30 mg capsules) need to be made within the therapeutic window of 10 to 20 μg/ mL. Giving a 100 mg capsule to a patient with a blood level of 15 μg/mL on a dose of 300 mg/day may lead to levels close to 30 μg/mL with the risk of clinical toxicity. Similarly, higher serum levels require a relatively small decrease in the dose to optimize the level.

2. **Newer AEDs.**

   They have much better pharmacokinetic properties compared to those of traditional AEDs.

   a. Except zonisamide, gabapentin (dose-related absorption), and ezogabine, all the newer AEDs have 90% or more bioavailability with oral intake.

   b. Hepatic metabolism is significant only with zonisamide and tiagabine, but they do not cause significant enzymatic induction.

   c. Lamotrigine, oxcarbazepine, eslicarbazepine, and ezogabine although metabolized in the liver do not involve cytochrome P-450 enzyme system (phase I reaction). They undergo extensive metabolism by glucuronidation (phase II reaction).

   d. Topiramate, levetirecetam, gabapentin, pregabalin, and vigabatrin are eliminated either completely or largely by renal route without undergoing significant hepatic metabolism.

   e. Oxcarbazepine, eslicarbazepine, clobazam, and topiramate do induce the metabolism of oral contraceptives, but the effect of topiramate is significant only with doses over 400 mg/day.

   f. Most of the newer AEDs, with the exception of tiagabine, clobazam, and perampanel have either no or clinically insignificant binding to the plasma proteins.

g. All of the newer AEDs have linear kinetics and no autoinduction.

h. Significant drug-to-drug interactions are absent with the use of gabapentin, pregabalin, levetiracetam, zonisamide, and lacosamide.

i. Most relevant interaction is between valproic acid and lamotrigine; valproic acid decreases the metabolic elimination of lamotrigine, increasing its half-life three to four times. In patients on valproic acid, lamotrigine needs to be started at a very low dose, titrated up very slowly, and the maintenance dose needs to be much smaller (100 to 200 mg) than when lamotrigine is used either alone or with enzyme-inducing AEDs, such as carbamazepine.

j. Use of lamotrigine, topiramate, or zonisamide with cytochrome oxidase enzyme inducers such as phenytoin or carbamazepine would increase the clearance of the formal group of AEDs needing higher doses compared to when used as monotherapy.

D. **Side effects of AEDs.** These are summarized in Table 43.4.

1. **Traditional AEDs.**

a. All traditional AEDs are associated with **neurotoxic side effects** such as tiredness, somnolence, dizziness, ataxia, blurred or double vision, nystagmus, and difficulty with concentration, behavioral disturbances, and cognitive dysfunction.

b. Phenobarbital, primidone, and clonazepam have higher incidence of sedative/hypnotic side effects.

c. Phenytoin has several **cosmetic side effects** such as facial coarsening, facial/body hirsutism in women, and gum hyperplasia. These are concerning particularly to women.

d. Valproic acid, when used in larger doses, is associated with **tremor**.

e. Valproic acid and carbamazepine are commonly associated with **weight gain**.

f. **Serious reactions** to traditional AEDs are reported but are uncommon. These include **hepatotoxicity, bone marrow suppression** (aplastic anemia and agranulocytosis), **exfoliative dermatitis, and Stevens–Johnson syndrome.** HLA-B*1502 is associated with the risk of rash from carbamazepine. Valproic acid is also reported to produce **pancreatitis.** If not detected in time, these reactions may be fatal. Hence, periodic monitoring of hepatic and hematopoietic parameters is recommended, although there is no evidence that routine testing detects these serious conditions much prior to a time when the effects can still be prevented. Usually **benign leukopenia** occurs in 10% to 20% patients, especially on carbamazepine. A total white cell count of 2,000 per mm^3 and an absolute granulocyte count of 1,000 per mm^3 are well tolerated.

Valproic acid is reported to produce **thrombocytopenia**, interference in the platelet aggregation, and an increased tendency toward bleeding. However, platelet counts above 60,000 per mm^3 are acceptable.

g. Because of its inhibition of cytochrome P-450 system, valproic acid in women is associated with abnormal metabolism of gonadal and adrenal sex hormones, often resulting in **PCOS**. PCOS is characterized by infertility, hirsutism, obesity, increased serum androgen levels, frequent anovulatory cycles, and other menstrual abnormalities. The incidence of PCOS is 10% to 20% in women with epilepsy compared with 5% to 6% of women in the general population. The incidence of this syndrome is highest in women with PGE treated with valproic acid.

h. **Teratogenic effects** occur in 5% to 10% pregnancies with the use of many traditional AEDs, highest incidence with valproic acid.

i. Almost all of the traditional AEDs are associated with **bone loss,** even in young adults, and affect both genders following their use of 1 to 2 years.

2. **Newer AEDs.**

a. Many of the newer AEDs (e.g., oxcarbazepine, gabapentin, zonisamide, and tiagabine) are associated with **neurotoxic side effects** similar to those with traditional AEDs. Lamotrigine, levetiracetam, topiramate, and lacosamide have relatively less neurotoxicity in the commonly used daily doses.

b. Serious reactions are rare with newer AEDs with the exception of a high incidence of felbamate-associated **aplastic anemia and toxic hepatitis** detected after its release. This has led to a marked drop in its use and presently it is used only in medically refractory epilepsy, which has failed to respond to conventional AEDs.

TABLE 43.4 Adverse Effects Associated with Antiepileptic Drugs

AEDs	Nonserious Side-Effects	Serious but Rare Side-Effects and Black-Box Warning
Traditional AEDs		
Phenobarbital	Sedation, hyperactivity, nausea/vomiting	Hypersensitivity reaction
Primidone	Same as with phenobarbital but more side effects initially	Hypersensitivity reaction
Phenytoin	Ataxia, coarse facies, hirsutism, gum hyperplasia, skin rash	SJS/TEN, lupus, blood dyscrasia, pseudo-lymphoma, hepatitis
Carbamazepine	Sedation, dizziness, blurred/double vision, leukopenia, neutropenia, hyponatremia, skin rash, weight gain	Hepatitis, lupus, increased P-R interval, SJS/TEN especially in Asian descend with leukocyte antigen-B 1502 allele, aplastic anemia, agranulocytosis
Valproate	Hair loss, tremor, nausea/vomiting, hyperammonemia, thrombocytopenia, weight gain	SJS/TEN, PCOS, pancreatitis, hepatic toxicity, increased teratogenic effects
Clonazepam	Drowsiness, dizziness, confusion, ataxia	—
Ethosuximide	Nausea/vomiting, drowsiness	Blood dyscrasia, skin rash
Second-generation AEDs		
Felbamate	Nausea/vomiting, insomnia, dizziness, ataxia, weight loss	Aplastic anemia, hepatitis
Gabapentin	Somnolence, dizziness, ataxia, blurred vision, skin rash, weight gain	—
Lamotrigine	Dizziness, ataxia, skin rash, visual disturbance, insomnia	Severe dermatologic reactions, including SJS/TEN, aseptic meningitis
Topiramate	Concentration difficulty, slowed thought process, language dysfunction, metabolic acidosis, paresthesia, weight loss	Kidney stones, hypohydrosis (mainly children), open angle glaucoma
Tiagabine	Dizziness, drowsiness, concentration difficulty	Stupor, or spike-wave stupor
Levetiracetam	Behavior disturbance, anxiety, irritability, aggression, somnolence, dizziness	—
Oxcarbazepine	Drowsiness, dizziness, ataxia, visual disturbance, hyponatremia, skin rash	Severe dermatologic hypersensitivity, blood dyscrasia
Zonisamide	Drowsiness, irritability, skin rash, weight loss	Kidney stones, hypohydrosis (mainly children)
Third-generation AEDs		
Pregabalin	Dizziness, somnolence, ataxia, dry mouth, paresthesia, euphoria, weight gain	Angioedema, hypersensitivity reactions
Lacosamide	Dizziness, drowsiness, headache, fatigue	Prolonged P-R interval, hypersensitivity reactions
Rufinamide	Dizziness, nausea/vomiting, drowsiness	Shortened Q-T interval
Vigabatrin	Drowsiness, dizziness, weight gain	Irreversible visual field changes, permanent vision loss
Ezogabine	Drowsiness, dizziness, abnormal coordination, attention and memory impairment, visual disturbance	Urinary retention, prolonged Q-T interval
Clobazam	Drowsiness, emotional disturbance	—
Perampanel	Dizziness, gait difficulty, falls, mood changes, weight gain	Serious psychiatric/behavior reactions
Eslicarbazepine	Dizziness, gait disturbance, somnolence, visual changes, cognitive disturbance	Hyponatremia, multiorgan hypersensitivity

Abbreviations: AED, antiepileptic drug; PCOS, polycystic ovarian syndrome; SJS, Stevens–Johnson syndrome; TEN, toxic epidermal necrolysis.

c. Lamotrigine causes a **skin rash** in 5% to 10% of patients, and even **Stevens–Johnson syndrome** may occur, although rarely. These complications are more common with rapid titration of the dose and comedication with valproic acid.

d. Topiramate produces **cognitive dysfunction,** for example, slower mentation, and word-finding difficulty, problems in concentration, thinking abnormalities, impaired memory, and encephalopathy. These are less common with daily doses below 400 mg. Rarely, acute myopia associated with the secondary angle closure **glaucoma** has been reported.

e. Levetiracetam is associated with anxiety and **behavioral changes.** Similarly, parampanel is reported to produce severe **psychiatric and behavioral reaction** in significant proportion of patients.

f. Zonisamide and topiramate may produce **renal calculi** in approximately 1% patients, **paresthesiae** in the limbs and **hypohyderosis**.

g. Like carbamazepine, oxcarbazepine and eslicarbazepine are associated with **significant hyponatremia** in 1% to 3% of patients, more often in elderly patients or those who are on other medications. It becomes evident in the first few months of therapy but rarely necessitates discontinuation of the drug.

h. Lacosamide may cause **prolonged P–R interval**; hence, it should be used with caution in patients with known cardiac conditions.

i. Like several other drugs, lamotrigine is found to be associated with **aseptic meningitis,** which can manifest with headaches, meningismus, and low-grade fever.

j. Multiple AEDs are more likely to cause cognitive side effects such as sedation, dizziness, diplopia, and blurred vision. Common examples of such combinations include the use of carbamazepine or oxcarbazepine with lamotrigine or lacosamide. Reducing the dose of any one of the combination AED may eliminate or reduce the side effects.

k. There has been little available data regarding the effect of newer AEDs on bone density or teratogenicity. Most recent data of the North American Pregnancy Registry strongly suggests that lamotrigine, levetiracetam, and oxcarbazepine when used as monotherapy have lower teratogenic potential than that with many traditional AEDs (valproate, phenobarbital, phenytoin, and carbamazepine).

3. Extended-release formulations. It is well known that adherence to an AED increases from less than 50% for four-daily dosing to more than 80% with one-daily dosing. While adherence is best with one-daily dose, the risk of a breakthrough seizure may also be more after missing a dose. Extended-release products slow the absorption of drugs that showed elimination half-life, allowing only one or two daily dosing and more stable blood levels and more adherence. These formulations are now available for many AEDs including phenytoin, carbamazepine, valproate, oxcarbazepine, topiramate, lamotrigine, and levetiracetam. Extended-release products of carbamazepine and valproate are perhaps most useful because these AEDs given in a single or two daily doses have high tolerability than with multiple daily dosing of the parent drugs essentially in elderly population.

FIRST SEIZURE

AED therapy is usually not initiated after the first tonic–clonic seizure and postponed until a second seizure occurs when the diagnosis of recurrent seizures or epilepsy is made. The incidence of recurrence is 25% to 65% after the first and over 75% after the second seizure. Hence, the first seizure may be an isolated episode and not necessarily herald the onset of epilepsy. This is particularly true if a single tonic–clonic seizure was related to sleep deprivation, physical or mental stress, drug or alcohol withdrawal, or use of prescribed (e.g., Wellbutrin) or recreational drugs (e.g., cocaine). Overall, 50% of patients have recurrence over a 3-year follow-up period after the first tonic–clonic seizure. The incidence is <25% among subjects with low-risk factors to 65% or more for those with two or more of the following risk factors: strong family history of seizures in siblings, history of febrile convulsions, focal-onset seizure, postictal paralysis, abnormal cognitive and neurologic examinations, evidence of a structural cerebral lesion at neuroimaging, and the presence of epileptiform abnormalities at EEG. Patients with two or more of these risk factors therefore may need prompt initiation of AED therapy even after the first tonic–clonic seizure. American Academy of Neurology (AAN) practice parameter (2015) recommends EEG and imaging studies (MRI preferred) in the evaluation of adults presenting with the first unprovoked epileptic seizure. Management of newly diagnosed epilepsy by AED regime requires special consideration. The choice is certainly based on seizure type, epilepsy syndrome, comorbidity, concomitant medications, possible interactions, safety during pregnancy, and side-effect profile. A proper choice may improve compliance, minimizing the time before resuming driving and baseline activities. Also, once an AED is started, the clinician may be reluctant to change the AED and more likely to add another AED if the patient responds poorly, risking more side effects. **Levetiracetam** is a new-generation AED, whose use has increased tremendously owing to its ease of use, linear pharmacokinetics, lack of interaction with other drugs and broad spectrum of efficacy. In addition, there is accumulating evidence of the safety of levetiracetam in pregnancy. Several studies comparing levetiracetam with other AEDs have confirmed that it has similar but not any better efficacy compared to carbamazepine, valproate, oxcarbazepine, and others as the first-line therapy in a patient with newly diagnosed epilepsy.

STATUS EPILEPTICUS

A. **Definitions.** Status epilepticus (SE) is usually considered to be present if continuous seizure activity persists for at least 30 minutes or two or more sequential seizures repeat within 30 minutes without full recovery of consciousness between seizures. Because the neuronal injury increases with duration, experts in recent literature define SE if seizure activity persists beyond 5 minutes, or, if at least two seizures have occurred over this period without full recovery. The term **established SE** is applied to when it remains unresponsive to first line of medication (benzodiazepines), **refractory SE** refers to the one which fails to get under control by "first" and "second" line of medications (benzodiazepines and AEDs), and the term **super-refractory SE** is often applied to that which persists beyond 24 hours after the start of "third" line of drugs (general anesthesia).

B. **Types.** Overall incidence is 2 to 4 per 10,000 per year. Any type of seizure can manifest as SE, but the common forms include the following:
   1. **Generalized convulsive status epilepticus (GCSE)** manifests as repeated major motor convulsions without full recovery of consciousness between seizures. In the past, the term SE implied essentially to this form of status.
   2. **Nonconvulsive SE** produces a continuous or fluctuating "epileptic twilight" state. This includes absence status and complex partial status. Only an EEG can establish the diagnosis.
   3. **Simple partial SE** is characterized by repeated focal motor seizures, epilepsia partialis continua, and focal impairment of function (e.g., aphasia) without accompanying alteration of consciousness.

C. **Cause of GCSE.** GCSE is the most common and most serious type of SE. It occurs mainly in the following settings:
   1. **Acute cerebral insult** or **acute encephalopathy** accounts for one-half of cases of GCSE. These disorders include meningitis, encephalitis, head trauma, hypoxia, hypoglycemia, drug intoxication (e.g., cocaine), drug withdrawal, and strokes or metabolic encephalopathy.
   2. GCSE can occur in patients with a **history of chronic epilepsy**, the common precipitants being changes in AEDs, sudden discontinuation or reduction in AEDs, systemic infection, physical and emotional stress, and sleep deprivation.
   3. It can occur as an **initial unprovoked epileptic event** in an otherwise healthy person. Such "idiopathic" cases may account for one-third of all cases of GCSE.

D. **Prognosis.** GCSE is an emergency associated with substantial morbidity and mortality. The overall mortality may be as high as 30% among adults. GCSE associated with acute neurologic insults has the poorest prognosis, which essentially depends on the underlying cerebral etiologic factor. When GCSE is the first epileptic event for an otherwise neurologically intact patient, or when it occurs in a patient with chronic epilepsy, or because of drug or alcohol withdrawal, the prognosis is good if therapy is instituted promptly. Without adequate and prompt treatment, GCSE can progress to a state of electromechanical dissociation in which the patient becomes increasingly unconscious or encephalopathic from the ongoing status, but the convulsive activity becomes increasingly subtle although EEG continues to show an ictal pattern. Patients with this condition, which

TABLE 43.5 Treatment Protocol for Status Epilepticus (Generalized Tonic–Clonic) in Adults

Time (min)	Treatment
0–5	Diagnose status by observing either continued seizure activity or one additional seizure Assess vital functions, insert oral airway, and give oxygen
6–10	Establish IV infusion line with normal saline solution. Monitor temperature and BP Draw blood for electrolytes, glucose, Ca, Mg, AED levels, CBC, BUN, and AST Administer 100 mg of thiamine followed by 50 mL of 50% glucose IV push
11–20	Give lorazepam 0.1 mg/kg IV push at a rate of <2 mg/min
21–60	(a) If lorazepam stops the seizures, continue or institute appropriate AED to maintain seizure control over a long term (b) If status continues administer phenytoin 20 mg/kg IV no faster than 50 mg/min. Preferably, use fosphenytoin IV in PE doses, or (c) IV Valproic acid 20–40 mg/kg and IV levetiracetam 40–60 mg/kg are alternatives to phenytoin or fosphenytoin Monitor BP and ECG during phenytoin (or fosphenytoin) infusion, and if hypotension or ECG changes occur, slow the infusion or temporarily withhold the drug. Consider intubation at this stage, if there is evidence of respiratory depression
>60	If seizures continue, intubate the patient, transfer to ICU, and start continuous video-EEG Start pentobarbital (or propofol or midazolam or ketamine) coma. Use an IV loading dose to produce at least a suppression-burst pattern on EEG. Continue a maintenance dose by IV drip to maintain seizure-free state or at least suppression-burst pattern on EEG Slow the rate of infusion after 24–96 hr periodically to determine whether seizures have stopped clinically and on EEG Monitor continuous video-EEG, BP, ECG, and respiratory function

Abbreviations: AST, aspartate aminotransferase; Ca, calcium; CBC, complete blood count; BUN, blood urea nitrogen; BP, blood pressure; ECG, electrocardiogram; EEG, electroencephalography; ICU, intensive care unit Mg, magnesium.

is often called **subtle SE,** are considered to be candidates for an aggressive therapy, as are those with overt GCSE.

E. Management of GCSE. The treatment protocol outlined in Table 43.5 is useful in the management of GCSE.

1. Diagnose SE by observing either continued seizure activity beyond 5 minutes or two generalized convulsions without full recovery of consciousness.

2. **Assess vital functions** and systemic abnormalities and stabilize the vital functions as much as possible.

   a. *Maintain an adequate airway and oxygenation.* This can usually be accomplished with an oral airway. The airway should be suctioned periodically to maintain patency. Oxygen should be administered through a nasal cannula or with a mask and a bag-valve-mask ventilator. If, after bagging, respiratory assistance is still needed, endotracheal intubation should be considered.

   b. **Assess blood pressure (BP)** and maintain it at a normal or high-normal level during prolonged GCSE. Use vasopressors if necessary.

   c. **Establish an IV infusion line** using normal saline solution. Blood should be drawn initially for CBC, blood sugar, blood urea nitrogen (BUN), serum electrolytes (including calcium and magnesium), and AED levels, and both urine and blood should be obtained for toxicology screening.

   d. **Assess oxygenation** by means of oximetry or periodic arterial blood gas determination.

   e. *Monitor rectal temperature.* Body temperature can increase to a high level during prolonged SE as a result of increased motor activity.

   f. If hypoglycemia is documented or if it is impossible to obtain prompt blood sugar determination, **administer 50 mL of 50% glucose** by means of IV push. In adults,

thiamine (100 mg) is always given before glucose to protect a thiamine-deficient patient from exacerbation of Wernicke's encephalopathy.

g. Administer bicarbonate therapy only if serum pH is so low as to be immediately life-threatening. Acidosis commonly develops during GCSE, but acidosis usually responds promptly once the seizure activity is controlled.

h. For rare patients with GCSE resulting from hyponatremia (serum sodium concentration <120 mEq/L), hypocalcemia, or hypomagnesemia, administer appropriate electrolytes by means of IV drip.

3. **Drug therapy for the control of GCSE.** The goals of therapy are rapid termination of the clinical and EEG evidence of seizure activity and subsequent maintenance of a seizure-free state. At present, the drug treatment of GCSE is subdivided into three lines: the **first line** of treatment consisting of short-acting benzodiazepines, the **second line** comprising various AEDs, and the **third line** consisting of general anesthesia. The use of IV lorazepam (2 mg), diazepam (5 mg), or midazolam by the emergency medical personnel prior to arrival in the emergency room is increasingly recommended for out-of-the-hospital status. In the emergency room, most physicians in the United States prefer IV lorazepam as the first line of treatment.

a. **Lorazepam** is administered at 0.1 mg/kg IV at a rate of 1 to 2 mg/minute. Lorazepam has relatively rapid effectiveness and yet has a prolonged duration of action against SE; hence, it has replaced diazepam almost completely for the treatment of SE. Lorazepam like diazepam can produce serious respiratory depression or hypotension, particularly when given in combination with barbiturates.

GCSE responds to first-line treatment in approximately two-thirds of the patients. They will need to be treated further with **appropriate AEDs** to maintain seizure control. In the benzodiazepine refractory SE (established SE), one of the many IV antiepileptic medications can be used as the second line of treatment, including phenytoin, fosphenytoin, valproate, phenobarbital, levetiracetam, and lacosamide. A multicenter, randomized trial comparing the efficacy of fosphenytoin, valproate, and levetiracetam has been recently initiated but the preliminary studies suggest that these three AEDs may be equally effective. At present, fosphenytoin remains the most commonly used second-line treatment.

b. *Phenytoin or fosphenytoin.* The usual loading dose of **phenytoin** is 20 mg/kg, given through a syringe into the IV port close to the patient at a rate <50 mg/minute. Injection is preferably performed by a physician. BP and electrocardiogram (ECG) are continuously monitored throughout the infusion. The rate of infusion should be slowed or temporarily stopped if hypotension, widening of the QT interval, or arrhythmias develops.

There is a significant risk of **skin complications** when IV phenytoin is given. These include phlebitis, tissue sloughing after extravasation, and most serious, **purple glove syndrome** after infusion into a dorsal hand vein. The latter is a delayed soft tissue injury that can result in severe edema, arterial occlusion, and tissue necrosis that can necessitate amputation. These complications occur because parenteral phenytoin has 40% propylene glycol (antifreeze). Its pH is adjusted to 12.2 with sodium hydroxide (drain cleaner). Use of IV phenytoin is now virtually replaced by fosphenytoin, a much safer preparation for IV administration.

Fosphenytoin, a phosphate ester of phenytoin, is enzymatically converted to phenytoin by serum phosphatases. It is available only for parenteral use (IV or IM). Because it is dissolved in TRIS buffer at a pH of 8 to 9, fosphenytoin does not cause tissue injury as phenytoin does. Three parts of phenytoin are bioequivalent to two parts of phenytoin, but the fosphenytoin dose is labeled in phenytoin equivalents (PE), so that 150 mg of fosphenytoin is labeled 100 mg PE. Although somewhat confusing, it apparently allows easy conversion of phenytoin to fosphenytoin dosing. Fosphenytoin can be administered more rapidly, up to 150 mg PE/minute compared with <50 mg/minute for phenytoin. The shorter infusion time compensates for the time needed for its conversion to active phenytoin. The result is that peak levels of phenytoin are attainable with IV fosphenytoin as rapidly as with phenytoin infusion itself. BP and ECG monitoring are recommended during fosphenytoin infusion, as they are with IV phenytoin. **Valproate** is given intravenously in doses of 20 to 40 mg/kg over 10 minutes, whereas **levetiracetam** in doses of 40 to 60 mg/kg over 5 to 10 minutes. Because of its relative ease of administration and no required monitoring, levetiracetam may be an attractive alternative to fosphenytoin.

c. *General anesthesia.* GCSE is successfully terminated in approximately 75% of patients by lorazepam and phenytoin (or fosphenytoin) combination. Remaining 25% constitute refractory GCSE. There is a high probability that the patient has an acute cerebral insult responsible for SE and prognosis is more guarded, with mortality being around 50%. The third line of treatment is general anesthesia.

   (1) The patient must be **intubated** (if not already) and placed in intensive care unit **(ICU)** for managing refractory GCSE.

   (2) **Continuous video-EEG monitoring** must be initiated to detect subtle or electrographic status and to evaluate the effectiveness of general anesthesia.

   (3) The goal of **general anesthesia** is to eliminate not only clinical seizures but also electrical discharges indicative of continuing seizure activity. Continuous IV infusion of pentobarbital, propofol, or midazolam has been reported to be almost equally effective. The choice of a drug is largely based on the clinical experience of the physician. If one agent in optimal dosages is unsuccessful in controlling status, another should be tried. The rate of administration of the drug is adjusted to ensure cessation of all epileptiform activities, or at least suppression-burst pattern in the EEG. However, maximal EEG suppression is associated with an increased frequency of hypotension requiring the use of pressor agents. The anesthesia is continued for 1 to 2 days before an attempt is made to lighten it. If clinical seizures or ictal EEG patterns return, the infusion is appropriately increased.

   (4) **Anesthetic agents. Pentobarbital** has been used for a long period for refractory GCSE. It is started intravenously with a loading dose of 5 to 15 mg/kg, followed by a maintenance dosage of 0.5 to 1.0 mg/kg/hour.

   Propofol, a short-acting agent, is becoming the drug of choice. It is started IV with a loading dose of 1 to 2 mg/kg, given over 5 minutes, followed by a maintenance dosage of 1 to 5 mg/kg/hour.

   Midazolam is administered at a loading dose of 0.2 mg/kg by slow IV bolus followed by a maintenance dose of 0.1 to 0.5 mg/kg/hour.

   There are no prospective randomized trials comparing these three anesthetic agents for the treatment of refractory status. One systematic review demonstrated no difference between the three, at least for mortality rate. **Ketamine** may be another anesthetic agent effective in refractory SE; hypotension and cardiopulmonary depression may be less common, so that larger doses may be used to control status.

4. **Long-term antiepileptic therapy.** After the episode of GCSE has been brought under control, most patients need continuation of some form of AED therapy. Long-term AED therapy is indicated when GCSE is caused by a structural brain lesion or when the patient has a history of epileptic seizures. When GCSE constitutes the patient's first seizure and no cause is found, the decision to initiate long-term AED therapy should be individualized, but most physicians initiate long-term treatment under such circumstances. If the GCSE was caused by acute CNS involvement, such as metabolic encephalopathy, meningoencephalitis, or cerebrovascular compromise, antiepileptic therapy is continued for a short period of 3 to 6 months.

F. **Management of other types of SE.** Other forms of SE do not pose the same emergency situation that GCSE poses. **Complex partial SE** has been reported to result in long-term neurologic deficits (e.g., permanent memory impairment) and should be controlled promptly with a benzodiazepine (e.g., lorazepam) followed by IV phenytoin (or fosphenytoin) or IV levitaracetam. IV anesthesia is rarely indicated. **Absence status** is best managed with an IV benzodiazepine (diazepam or lorazepam), which is effective in most cases. If a benzodiazepine is not effective, valproic acid can be given intravenously, in a dose of 25 mg/kg to promptly achieve therapeutic blood levels. After the absence status is controlled, valproic acid therapy is continued orally. **Simple partial status, focal motor status or epilepsia partialis continua** without loss of consciousness responds to phenytoin (or fosphenytoin) usually in large doses to maintain blood levels as high as 30 μg/mL. IV levitracetam, valproic acid, and lacosamide are other alternatives. Benzodiazepines are not desirable because of their sedative side effects, except using one or two doses of IV lorazepam or diazepam initially.

MANAGEMENT OF ACUTE SEIZURE CLUSTER

Some patients have repetitive series or clusters of epileptic seizures that occur within a short period, not meeting the definition criteria of SE. Such seizure clusters can be intermittently managed with either of the following approaches:

A. Most physicians use benzodiazepine (lorazepam or diazepam) to manage a cluster. **Lorazepam** is given in doses of 2 to 4 mg orally (sublingually) or parenterally (IM or IV), usually becoming effective in approximately 30 minutes. Administration may be repeated in doses of 1 to 2 mg with a maximum dose of 6 to 8 mg in 24 hours.

B. **Rectal diazepam** (Diastat) is approved for rectal administration in the management of repetitive seizures. It is as effective, if not better, than lorazepam. Diazepam gel is administered in doses of 0.2 to 0.5 mg/kg rectally (usual adult dose is 10 to 20 mg); it is effective in 15 minutes and the effect lasts as long as 8 hours. If social or logistic reasons make the use of rectal administration difficult, sublingual, intranasal, or oral lorazepam is a better alternative.

C. **Intranasal diazepam** (0.2 mg/kg) may be more easy to deliver and acceptable than rectal diazepam. Caregiver can give the drug more easily and administer during or immediately after a seizure. Preliminary studies have shown that the intranasally delivered drug appears to achieve a peak concentration high enough to be therapeutically effective.

Home treatment with diazepam reduces the risk for subsequent status and the need for frequent visits to the emergency room in patients at risk for seizure clusters or SE.

EPILEPSY, PREGNANCY, AND OTHER WOMEN'S ISSUES

A. Major problems. Pregnancy in a woman with epilepsy (WWE) is considered to constitute a high risk and needs to be followed by a high-risk obstetrician. Recently, AAN has issued guidelines regarding the management of WWE, updated in 2009, which are incorporated in the following discussion:

1. Obstetrical complications. In short, there is no conclusive evidence of increased obstetrical complications in WWE on AEDs.

   a. There is a weak evidence that WWE on AEDs has a slightly higher (up to 1.5 times expected) risk for cesarean section but a good evidence that this risk is not >2 times expected.

   b. There is a good evidence that there is no greater risk for late pregnancy bleeding, early contractions, or early labor and delivery in WWE on AEDs. However, these complications are substantially increased in WWE who smoke.

   c. There is insufficient evidence to support or refute an increased risk for preeclampsia, hypertension, or miscarriage.

2. Effect of pregnancy on epilepsy. It is usually believed that seizures become more frequent during pregnancy in one-third WWE, especially in second and third trimesters. According to the AAN guidelines, there is insufficient evidence to support or refute an increased risk in seizure frequency or occurrence of SE. Furthermore, if a WWE has been seizure free for at least 9 months before becoming pregnant, there is a high likelihood of her remaining seizure free during pregnancy. Nonadherence to AEDs is common during pregnancy because of inadequate knowledge of the AED-induced teratogenesis. Also, the ill effects of tonic–clonic seizures do occur on the fetus and these points need to be fully discussed.

3. **Alteration of the pharmacokinetics of AEDs** (increased clearance) results in decreased serum concentrations of almost all AEDs. AAN guidelines (2009) concluded that there is a probable chance of decrease in the serum concentration of lamotrigine, phenytoin, and to a lesser degree carbamazepine, whereas a possible chance for decrease of levetiracetam and the monohydroxy derivative of oxcarbazepine. Since lamotrigine is metabolized by glucuronidation (most activated during pregnancy), its clearance is most enhanced needing an upward dosing. The clearance normalizes during the last week of pregnancy

necessitating dose reduction immediately after delivery to avoid drug toxicity. Serum concentration of most other AEDs increased gradually over 4 to 8 weeks postdelivery. Changes in AED levels and in the hormonal status, poor compliance, psychological stresses, and sleep deprivation during pregnancy are some of the factors for exacerbation of seizures in some WWE.

4. The incidence of both minor and major **fetal malformations** is two to three times higher among WWE than among women without epilepsy. **Minor malformations** are deviations from normal morphology not requiring treatment, whereas **major malformations,** which are most relevant, require medical and/or surgical treatment. The overall incidence of major malformations (oropalatal clefts, urogenital and congenital heart anomalies, and neural tube defects) among infants of epileptic mothers is approximately 3% to 10%, compared with 1.5% to 3% in women not receiving AEDs. Most of these teratogenic effects are due to intrauterine exposure to AEDs, especially during the first trimester when neural tube (4 weeks), cardiac (6 weeks), and orofacial (6 to 10 weeks) developments are happening. All major AEDs have potential teratogenic effects, but the incidence varies. The most recent prevalence data from the North American Pregnancy registry are shown in Table 43.6. There are other pregnancy registries providing similar conclusions. The findings are summarized below and are in line with the AAN practice parameter (2009):

   a. Incidence of malformation increases with polytherapy compared with monotherapy. Avoid polytherapy during pregnancy.

   b. Valproic acid is associated with the highest incidence (10%) of major malformations, which include neural tube defects, facial clefts, and hypospadias. Hence, avoid the use of valproic acid in women during childbearing years.

   c. In general, increased dose of AED correlates with higher incidence of major malformation, this being particularly the case with valproic acid, but also for carbamazepine, lamotrigine, and phenobarbital. Therefore, use lowest effective dose of AED during pregnancy.

TABLE 43.6 Prevalence of Major Fetal Malformation with AED Monotherapy in North American AED Pregnancy Registry, Fall 2014 (First Four Columns) and in Other Pregnancy Registries (Last Column)

AED/Control	Number of Pregnant Women	Mean Incidence (%) of Major Malformations	95% Confidence Interval	Incidence (%) of Major Malformations in Other Registries
Lamotrigine	1,812	2.0	1.4–2.8	AUS, 0; ILR, 2.7; UK, 3.2; NEAD, 1.0
Carbamazepine	1,078	3.1	2.1–4.3	AUS, 3.8; UK, 2.2
Levetiracetam	648	2.2	1.2–3.6	UK 2.7
Topiramate	425	4.5	2.7–6.9	UK 4.8
Phenytoin	420	2.9	1.5–5.0	AUS, 5.9; NEAD 10.7
Valproate	333	9.0	6.2–12.6	AUS, 16.8; UK, 6.2; NEAD, 20.3
Oxcarbazepine	211	1.9	0.5–4.8	–
Phenobarbital	201	6.0	3.1–10.2	–
Gabapentin	163	1.2	0.02–4.4	–
Zonisamide	119	0.0	0.0–3.3	–
Clonazepam	80	2.5	0.3–8.7	–
Internal control [a]	495	1.2	0.46–2.7	–
External control [b]	69,277	1.6	1.5–1.7	–

[a]Friends and family members were participants in the AED Pregnancy Registry.
[b]Women from the active malformations surveillance program at Brigham and Women's Hospital in Boston.
Abbreviations: AED, antiepileptic drug; AUS, Australian Registry (monotherapy); ILR, International Lamotrigine registry; NEAD, Neuro Developmental Effects of Antiepileptic Drugs (monotherapy; major malformations, and fetal deaths); UK, UK Registry (monotherapy).

d. Phenytoin, carbamazepine, and phenobarbital also increase the risk of fetal malformation: cleft palate with phenytoin use, posterior cleft palate with carbamezapine use, and cardiac malformation with phenobarbital use. Hence, avoiding these AEDs during pregnancy would reduce major malformations.

e. Lamotrigine, which is the most extensively studied new AED, appears to have the least teratogenicity (2% to 3%), probably no different from the general population. The UK registry has also shown dose–response effect of lamotrigine-associated malformations, 2% incidence with doses up to 200 mg/day compared with 5.4% for above 200 mg/day. Polytherapy use of lamotrigine with valproic acid markedly increases the incidence of malformation (12%).

f. UK and North American registries have shown higher incidence (4% to 5%) of major malformations (oral clefts, hypospadias) with topiramate, whereas a lower incidence with levetiracetam and zonisamide. Topiramate should, therefore, be avoided during pregnancy.

5. **Adverse perinatal outcomes.** There is good evidence that WWE taking AEDs have an increased risk of small-for-gestation offspring, a weak evidence for low Apgar scores at 1 minute, and a good evidence of no increase in the risk of perinatal death. **Hemorrhagic disease** is reported in newborns delivered by women who have received hepatic enzyme-inducing AEDs (phenobarbital, primidone, phenytoin, and carbamazepine) because of their effect in decreasing the vitamin K-dependent clotting factors. According to the AAN guidelines, there is insufficient evidence to support or refute an increased risk of hemorrhagic complications in the newborn of WWE taking AEDs.

6. **Cognitive outcomes.** An AAN practice parameter update (2009) concluded that children born to women, who received valproate (good evidence), phenytoin, or phenobarbital (weak evidence), have higher incidence of poor cognitive outcome compared with the offspring of WWE not taking AEDs. Carbamazepine does not have adverse effect. AED polytherapy is more likely associated with cognitive impairment compared to monotherapy. A recent study comparing monotherapy with carbamazepine, valproate, phenytoin, or lamotrigine demonstrated increased developmental delays and lower IQ at age 6 years in valproate-exposed children as well as reduced verbal IQ and increased need for special education in these children at age 6 years or above. The adverse cognitive development appears dose-dependent. The cognitive teratogenesis associated with valproate is another reason to avoid valproate in women who want to or may become pregnant.

B. **Management guidelines.** The therapeutic challenge is to keep the patient free of seizures while minimizing the adverse effects of seizures and AEDs on the course of pregnancy and the fetus. The major guidelines, which are preferably initiated before the patient becomes pregnant, are as follows:

1. Counsel the family about the higher incidence of fetal malformation, but assure the patient that >90% exposed to AEDs still bear healthy offspring.

2. May consider withdrawing AEDs before pregnancy if the patient has remained free of seizures for >2 years unless the woman has a high probability of recurrence.

3. Before conception, determine the best AED for seizure control. If the patient is on polytherapy, reduce AEDs to appropriate monotherapy. Because of the relatively high incidence of neural tube defects with valproic acid, avoid these AEDs and replace with other AEDs. For women with PGE, lamotrigine alone or with levetirecetam or zonisamide are alternative AEDs.

4. Prescribe folic acid in any sexually active woman during childbearing age to reduce the overall incidence of neural defects in the offspring.

5. Address and eliminate other risk factors, for example, drugs, alcohol, and smoking.

6. Do not stop or change AED therapy after the pregnancy has been diagnosed. The risk of fetal malformation is highest during the first 4 to 8 weeks of pregnancy. It is usually too late to protect the fetus by the time pregnancy is confirmed. Stopping or changing the drug can induce more frequent and more violent seizures with adverse consequences on both the mother and the fetus.

7. Supplemental multivitamins and folic acid are prescribed during the entire pregnancy. The precise dose for WWE has not been defined, but 1.0 mg/day is commonly used. Women at risk of having a child with neural tube defect (previous child or family history) are advised to supplement with 4.0 mg/day.

8. Monitor the AED serum level (preferably free level) before conception, at each trimester, in the last month of pregnancy, and through 8 weeks postpartum, especially if the patient is on lamotrigine, carbamazepine, or phenytoin. Adjust the dosage accordingly. Maintain lowest effective blood levels.

9. Measure serum *α*-fetoprotein and acetylcholinesterase levels at 15 to 18 weeks of gestation to be followed by high-definition **ultrasound imaging** to detect neural tube defects and other major malfunctions. Together, these detect over 99% of the major fetal abnormalities. **Amniocentesis** is indicated only if these tests do not provide positive exclusion of a neural tube defect.

10. According to AAN practice guidelines (2009), there is insufficient evidence to support or refute a benefit of vitamin K supplement for reducing the risk of hemorrhagic disease of the newborn of WWE. To the newborns exposed to enzyme-inducing AEDS in utero, administer vitamin K_1 (1.0 mg IM) to the neonate immediately after birth as is the routine practice for all neonates.

11. After delivery, check AED levels and adjust the doses of AED, usually at a lower level. Some AEDs, such as lamotrigine and oxcarbazepine, start reversing their elimination rate to the prepregnancy level even prior to the delivery. Their dose needs to be brought down within a week or so of the delivery.

12. **Breastfeeding** is allowed. Nearly all AEDs appear in breast milk at a concentration closely related to the AED's free plasma level. Hence, highly protein-bound AEDs attain only a very small concentration in the milk to produce significant clinical effects on the breast-fed baby. AAN practice parameters (2009) conclude that valproate, phenobarbital, phenytoin, and carbamazepine do not transfer into breast milk to as great an extent as gabapentin, lamotrigine, and topiramate. Levetiracetam and ethosuximide also appear in sufficient concentration in breast milk. The AAN practice parameter states that the clinical consequences for the newborns exposed to AEDs in the breast milk remains unknown. A recent Norwegian study found long breastfeeding as safe to infants exposed to carbamazepine, lamotrigine, or valproate in the breast milk. Data are still lacking for newer AEDs, which are now increasingly used such as levetiracetam, oxcarbazepine, topiramate, and zonisamide. It may take several years and extensive studies to establish the safety of these recently introduced AEDs regarding breastfeeding.

C. Prevention of pregnancy with oral contraceptives.

1. Women with epilepsy may use oral hormonal contraceptives if they wish. These do not exacerbate epilepsy despite the warnings on package inserts.

2. The major concern in using oral contraceptives is the higher failure rate (>6% per year) among women taking hepatic cytochrome-450 isoenzyme-inducing AEDs (Table 43.3 last column). This is due to increased elimination of both estrogens and progestogens by these AEDs. The effect is on many contraceptive preparations including combined contraceptive pill, combined patch, progestogen-only pill, and progestogen implants.

The most commonly used is a **combined "mini-pill"** containing 35 *μ*g or less of estrogen combined with progestogen. It may be less effective. Breakthrough bleeding can be a warning of decreased contraceptive efficiency. AAN guidelines recommend that patients taking these enzyme-inducing AEDs be placed on a medium-dose combined contraceptive pill containing at least 50 *μ*g of ethinyl estradiol. Additional use of condom is strongly recommended to assure maximum contraception efficacy. The **progestogen-only** pill is usually ineffective.

Long-acting reversible contraceptives are other desirable alternatives in patients on enzyme-inducing AEDs. **Progestogen-only implants** are not effective. Intramuscular medroxyprogesterone injections (**Depo-Provera**) appear to be very effective (>99%) but patients are advised to take injections every 10 weeks rather than 12 weeks if they are on enzyme-inducing AEDs. However, it is associated with side effects of weight gain, decreased bone mineral density (BMD), and delayed return of fertility. Contraception using **levonorgestrel-releasing intrauterine device (Mirena coils)** is effective for a period up to 5 years and is not affected by enzyme-inducing AEDs because progestogen acts by being released locally in the uterus. It is a highly effective (>99%) contraceptive option in women with poor compliance history.

Because both estrogens and progestogens are eliminated faster by enzyme-inducing AEDs, the higher dose of estrogen needs to accompany a similarly higher dose of progestogen in the combined contraceptive pill.

3. Nonenzyme inducers are unlikely to cause failure of oral contraception. Refer to Table 43.3.

4. Hormonal contraceptives have little effect on AEDs except on lamotrigine blood levels, which drop to half the precontraceptive levels because of enzyme induction. During the 7-day-off period, the levels could double back to prehormone levels. This effect may result in a breakthrough seizure during the 3 weeks of hormonal ingestion and toxicity during the off-week.

D. Catamenial epilepsy. Many women have increased frequency of seizures related to their menstrual cycle probably because of changing hormonal concentration during menstrual cycle. The term catamenial epilepsy is usually applied if seizure frequency increases by two times or more in relation to specific times of menstrual cycle. It happens in about one-third of women with partial epilepsy and increased seizures occur at three different times. Commonly, they occur either just before or during the first few days of menstruation (perimenstrual). Some have increased seizures at ovulation (midcycle), whereas others who have anovulation cycles have increased seizure activity in the second half of the menstrual cycle. **Acetazolamide** (250 to 500 mg/day) or **clobazam** (5 to 15 mg/day) may be used during the periods of increased seizure activity. An alternative is to give additional doses of the AED or use a **benzodiazepine** such as lorazepam for a few days. **Hormone therapy** is another alternative approach. Medroxyprogesterone acetate can be effective, but has undesirable side effects of weight gain and bone density loss. Progestogen supplements may be given perimenstrually or during the latter half (10 to 26 days) of the menstrual cycle. A combined oral contraceptive pill or depot progestogen may also be used.

BONE MINERAL DENSITY

Almost all of the traditional AEDs are associated with **bone mineral density (BMD) loss**, even in young adults, and affect both genders following their use of more than 1 year. The bone loss is more severe in elderly patients, with polytherapy and with prolonged use. Possible mechanisms include hepatic induction of cytochrome P-450 enzymes (phenobarbital, primidone, phenytoin, and carbamazepine) leading to increased catabolism of vitamin D, secondary hyperparathyroidism, and increased bone turnover. Valproic acid, a noninducer, does produce bone loss by increased ostoclastic activity. There is no reliable data regarding BMD loss with newer AEDs, and oxcarbazepine may not be better in this respect compared with carbamazepine.

Reduced BMD and epilepsy increase the risk, two to six times, for fractures, particularly of the hip and spine. Bone loss is best detected by dual-energy X-ray absorptiometry (DXA) and expressed as a T-score. Osteopenia is defined by a T-score of –1 to –2.5 and osteoporosis by a score –2.5 or over.

All adults with epilepsy, especially on enzyme-inducing AEDs, should receive 1,000 to 1,500 mg/day of calcium in addition to 800 to 1,600 IU of vitamin D. DXA should be performed, probably every 4 to 5 years to assess BMD loss especially in epileptic patients at greater risk (elderly, postmenopausal women on enzyme-inducing AEDs). If found to have low BMD, treatment with bisphosphonates (alendronate and risedronate), raloxifene, teriparatide, or hormonal replacement in postmenopausal women may be considered.

ANTIEPILEPTIC DRUG TREATMENT OF THE ELDERLY

The prevalence of epilepsy increases sharply in the elderly. Common causes of seizures are cerebrovascular disease, degenerative dementia, and neoplasms in that order of frequency. Seizures are nearly exclusively partial onset, being simple partial, complex partial, or secondarily generalized in type. The postictal period is often longer in the elderly and may last several days after a generalized tonic–clonic seizure. EEG shows epileptiform abnormalities in 40% patients.

A. Major problems. Elderly patients with epilepsy constitute a special patient population because of age-related changes in the pharmacokinetics of AEDs, comorbidity, and multiple drug therapy. There is a decrease in plasma albumin with resultant overall decrease in protein binding of AEDs; hence, total concentration of highly bound AEDs (valproic acid, phenytoin, and so on) becomes misleading. Hepatic drug metabolism is decreased, and there is a steady decline in glomerular filtration rate, decreased tubular secretory function, and decreased renal blood flow with normal aging. These changes lead to longer elimination half-life and reduced clearance of many AEDs, with either primarily hepatic or renal elimination. In addition, concomitant medical problems and, consequently, multiple comedications further affect the absorption, disposition, and metabolism of AEDs. Elderly patients also tend to experience more side effects of AEDs, especially somnolence, confusion, gait disturbances, and postural and other tremors.

B. **Management guidelines for using AEDs to treat the elderly.**

1. AEDs should be prescribed only when the diagnosis of epileptic seizures is firmly established and there is a high probability of recurrence.

2. AED therapy should be initiated at lower doses and titrated more slowly to a daily dose that is on average lower by 30% to 40% than used to treat younger adults.

3. For high-protein-bound AEDs, measurement of free rather than total concentration may be more useful in evaluating seizure control or drug-related toxicity.

4. "Therapeutic ranges" of the traditional AEDs do not apply to the elderly mainly because of an overall decrease tolerability for drugs in this age group. Aim for a "low therapeutic" serum level, increasing the dose only if clinically necessary.

5. Carbamazepine, phenytoin, and valproic acid have been commonly used in the past (and still used in the developing countries) because the seizures are usually focal-onset, but their pharmacokinetics makes them less ideal for the elderly. The newer AEDs should be considered early in the treatment of the elderly patient because of their fewer drug interactions, minimal or no protein binding, and predominant renal elimination. However, the dose has to be adjusted downward in the presence of renal impairment. Most of the new AEDs are approved as adjunct therapy except **oxcarbazepine** and **eslicabazepine**, which may not be well tolerated in elderly because of neurotoxicity. **Lamotrigine** (presently approved for monotherapy conversion) has only minor interactions and good tolerability; hence, it is another alternative among newer AEDs. In several studies, **levetiracetam** has been noted to have few adverse effects and many experts use it (off label) as monotherapy in elderly. It is approved as monotherapy in European Union. It appears that levetiracetam, lamotrigine, and also gabapentin may emerge as common monotherapy AEDs for elderly patients with epilepsy.

DISCONTINUATION OF ANTIEPILEPTIC DRUGS

The decision to discontinue AEDs in a patient who has been seizure-free for several years depends on many prognostic factors. The overall relapse rate after AED withdrawal is approximately 30% to 40% among adults with chronic epilepsy.

A. **Prognostic factors.**

1. **Types of epilepsy.**
   a. Some childhood forms of epilepsy (e.g., benign Rolandic epilepsy and childhood absence epilepsy) usually remit during adolescence.
   b. Patients with **PGE** with onset in adolescence or adulthood have a good prognosis. Many remit, but some (especially JME) need lifelong therapy.
   c. Adult patients with **focal epilepsy,** especially with complex partial seizures due to mesial temporal sclerosis, have a high recurrence rate (40% to 50%) after discontinuing AEDs.
   d. Patients in whom seizures occur in the setting of an acute cerebral insult (e.g., trauma, infection, or stroke) may not have chronic epilepsy. Such patients should be considered for withdrawal of AED after a seizure-free period of 6 months.

2. **EEG findings** obtained just before discontinuation of AED therapy are useful predictors of the outcome. The relapse rate is four to five times higher if EEG shows persistent epileptiform abnormalities. In the presence of these abnormalities, most physicians consider continuing AEDs.

3. **Other predictors of outcome.** A high frequency of seizures, a long duration before seizures are controlled with AEDs, and multiple seizure types in a patient carry a less favorable prognosis. Similarly, patients who have structural abnormalities responsible for seizures or who have mental retardation or neurologic deficits are more likely to have recurrence of seizures after discontinuation of AEDs.

B. **General guide lines for withdrawing AEDs.**

1. The decision to wean AED in a patient who has been seizure free has to be individualized and undertaken with the patient's full understanding of risks and benefits. There is no consensus as to how long should a patient be seizure free before AEDs could be withdrawn. In general, discontinuation of AEDs may be considered by the physician if the patient has been seizure-free for 2 to 5 years while taking AEDs, has normal neurologic examination, and normalized EEG with treatment.

2. Adult patients with PGE who have remained seizure-free for 2 to 5 years and whose EEGs show no paroxysmal abnormalities or photoparoxysmal response are good candidates for withdrawal of therapy unless they have JME.

3. Women who want to bear children and who have been seizure-free for several years should be considered for withdrawal of medication before conception to avoid possible ill-effects on the fetus.

4. However, most adults with focal epilepsy, secondary generalized epilepsy, or PGE manifesting as multiple seizure types probably need long-term AED therapy.

C. **AED withdrawal mode and precautions.**

1. AEDs must be withdrawn slowly, typically over 3 months or longer, especially in the case of barbiturates and benzodiazepines.

2. Patients taking more than one AED should have the less or least effective drug withdrawn before the first-line drug. Only after the patient has remained seizure-free for several months only on one AED, is the final drug withdrawn.

3. During the withdrawal period, the patient is advised to follow a restricted lifestyle (no driving or hazardous occupational or recreational activities) to minimize the consequences should the seizures recur.

4. If the seizures recur, the patient is promptly placed on an adequate dosage of an appropriate AED, which then probably has to be continued on a lifelong basis.

5. After the withdrawal period, attention has to be paid to such lifestyle issues as getting adequate sleep, avoiding alcohol, and avoiding stresses that can cause recurrence.

6. Epilepsy is considered to be resolved for individuals who had age-dependent epilepsy syndrome, but are now past the applicable age or those who have remained seizure free for the last 10 years with no seizure medication for last 5 years (ILAE, 2014).

SUDDEN UNEXPECTED DEATH IN EPILEPSY

The risk of dying is 3 to 4 times in patients with epilepsy and having a sudden death is about 24 times more likely compared to the general population. Increased mortality is because of multiple causes, for example, suicide, SE related to nonadherence to AEDs, and seizure-related physical injuries. In recent years, sudden unexpected death in epilepsy (SUDEP) has been recognized as an important concern in patients with epilepsy. SUDEP is defined as sudden and unexpected death in a patient with epilepsy without an obvious cause found at autopsy. At least one-sixth of all deaths in epilepsy patients represent SUDEP, risk being 5 to 7 times higher with medically refractory epilepsy.

Incidence of SUDEP is about 1 death per 1,000 epilepsy patients per year, perhaps an underestimation. The incidence rises to 1 death per 100 to 150 epilepsy patients per year in uncontrolled epilepsy.

Risk factors for SUDEP include uncontrolled and frequent seizures, especially of generalized tonic–clonic type, low AED levels, polytherapy, early onset and long duration of epilepsy, a seizure prior to the death, young adult age group (20 to 40 years), and death at night or during sleep in a prone position. The most important risk factor is the noncompliance with AEDs. SUDEP may be because of seizure-related cardiac and/or pulmonary causes. Epilepsy-related higher mortality and SUDEP are issues, which are generally ignored during patients' office visit. These issues need to be discussed at least in those patients with longstanding and poorly controlled epilepsy not only to educate the patient and the family members of the potential for this fatal complication but also to strongly emphasize the need for AED compliance.

REFERRAL FOR COMPREHENSIVE TREATMENT

A. Psychosocial problems. Patients with epilepsy face many personal and psychosocial difficulties that require **psychiatric referral** and counseling. There is a high incidence of mood disorder; **depression** occurs in 20% to 50% patients. **Citalopram** and **sertraline** are preferred antidepressants to treat coexisting depression. These have no drug–drug interaction. **Bupropion** should be avoided because of its high potential in lowering threshold for seizures. Patients who need comprehensive care should be referred to a **comprehensive epilepsy center** equipped with multidisciplinary teams capable of providing psychosocial and vocational counseling in addition to the appropriate medical therapy.

B. Experimental AEDs. Approximately 20% to 30% of patients with epilepsy who have medically intractable seizures may be helped by referral to a center, conducting ongoing clinical trials of new AEDs. Such patients often need combination therapy with two or more AEDs, or some type of surgical treatment that are best handled in a comprehensive epilepsy center.

C. Surgical treatment.
   1. Resective surgery. Epilepsy is considered medically refractory when seizure control is unsatisfactory despite trials of two or three AEDs, in monotherapy or in combination. After multimodality presurgical evaluation, if found to have a single epileptogenic focus that does not involve eloquent cortex, these patients may be candidates for resective surgery.
      a. **Anterior temporal lobectomy** is the most frequently performed resective surgery when the seizures arise from anteromedial area or the lateral cortical area of the temporal lobe on one side. Epileptic patients with mesial temporal sclerosis on the MRI are excellent candidates because they are usually medically refractory but respond very well to surgery, over two-thirds rendered seizure-free.
      b. **Extratemporal resection** for epileptogenic foci outside the temporal lobe is increasingly performed, although the success rate is 50% or less. Localizing an extratemporal seizure focus, for example, in the frontal lobe, is more challenging (may require invasive monitoring with subdural electrodes) unless a structural lesion is present on the MRI scan.
      c. **Corpus callosotomy** is performed in a few epilepsy centers for patients with secondarily generalized epilepsy who suffer from frequent drop attacks. The procedure is followed by a number of complications such as disconnection syndrome, difficulty with motor and language function, and maintenance. Although drop attacks and generalized seizures respond favorably, rarely do seizures totally remit.
      d. **Hemispherectomy** is reserved for a selected few patients (mainly children) who have unilateral hemispheric insult (Rasmussen's encephalitis, Sturge–Weber syndrome, extensive cerebral dysgenesis, hemimegalencephaly, and so on), resulting in medically refractory focal epilepsy and hemiparesis.
      e. **Subpial transection** is a surgical technique to treat focal epilepsy when the seizures arise from eloquent cortex such as the language or motor area. The procedure cuts horizontally connecting fibers so as to decrease propagation of seizure activity without resulting neurologic defects. The procedure is often combined with **corticectomy**.
   2. VNS. The FDA has approved VNS as adjunctive therapy for medically refractory seizures in adults and children. VNS is considered for patients with focal or generalized epilepsy who have undergone unsuccessful polytherapy trials of several AEDs, including newer AEDs, who are not candidates for resective surgery or have undergone unsuccessful resective surgery.

   VNS requires implantation of a programmable signal generator subcutaneously in the upper chest on the left side. This device is capable of delivering intermittent stimulation to the left vagus nerve in the neck by means of bipolar electrodes at the desired settings. In addition, the patient or a companion can activate the generator by placing the accompanying magnet over the generator for several seconds to interrupt a seizure or reduce its severity if administered at seizure onset.

   The mechanism of action of VNS is unknown, but several large trials showed that approximately 30% to 40% of patients with refractory partial-onset seizures had a 50%

or greater reduction in seizure frequency. Only a few had complete control of seizures. Overall, VNS has the same efficacy as many of the newer AEDs but without drug-related side effects. Patients with aurae are particularly helped because they can activate the device to abort an impending seizure. The common side effects include hoarseness, throat pain, coughing, dyspnea, and muscle pain. Possible surgical complications of hematoma, wound infection, left vocal cord paralysis, and injury to the vagus nerve or carotid sheath are rare when the procedure is performed by an experienced surgeon.

3. **Neuropace**, a responsive neurostimulator (RNS), has been recently (2014) approved by the FDA. It consists of placing depth or subdural electrodes in close proximity to the epileptogenic focus identified by prior presurgical evaluation. The RNS system works by detecting a seizure and then delivering an electric stimulation to abort the electrographic seizure. It is indicated in those medically refractory patients who are not candidates for resective surgery because they have either bilateral epileptogenic foci or a focus in or close to the eloquent cortex. The identification of the appropriate candidates requires surface and/or invasive monitoring by an expert team of epileptologist and surgeons in the level 4 comprehensive epilepsy center. Approximately 40% reduction in the seizures is achieved by 3 months.

4. **Future trends.** Bilateral stimulation of the anterior thalamic nucleus (**deep brain stimulation**) by placing multicontact depth electrodes stereotactically has been used in medically refractory epilepsy. Protocol-driven studies have shown a 39% median reduction of seizures in the treatment group compared to 23% in the controlled group.

Key Points

- Evaluation of a patient suspect with epilepsy should include a detailed history of episodes, MRI of the brain, and EEG studies with the goal of not only confirming that the episodes are epileptic seizures, but also defining the epilepsy syndrome.
- Patients with epilepsy, who fail to respond to two or more appropriate AEDs in monotherapy or combined therapy, are considered medically refractory. They need to be referred to comprehensive epilepsy center for further evaluation and management, which may include resective surgery, neurostimulation, or experimental medication.
- Patients with symptomatic localization-related epilepsy because of mesial temporal sclerosis are very likely to remain medically refractory and best treated by surgical resection.
- Young women with epilepsy need to be treated with AEDs with least incidence of major fetal malformation and using monotherapy in least effective dose. Appropriate AED selection needs to be planned before pregnancy and the women need to be followed closely during pregnancy to adjust doses of the medication according to the blood levels, which commonly decrease during pregnancy.
- Medically refractory patients with epilepsy, who have frequent seizures, particularly of generalized tonic–clonic type, are at increased risk for SUDEP. The incidence of this tragedy can be reduced by a rigid compliance to AEDs and reducing the frequency of seizures by more aggressive control of seizures by all options including surgical treatment.

Recommended Readings

Berg AT, Berkovic SF, Brodie MJ, et al. Revised terminology and concepts for organization of seizures and epilepsies. *Epilepsia*. 2010;51:676–685.

Bleck T, Hannah C, Chamberlain J. The established status epilepticus trial 2013. *Epilepsia*. 2013;54(suppl 6):89–92.

Cloassen J, Hirsch LJ, Emerson RG, et al. Treatment of refractory status epilepticus with pentobarbital, propofol or midazolam: a systematic study. *Epilepsia*. 2002;43:146–153.

Commission on Classification and Terminology of the International League against Epilepsy. Proposal for revised clinical and electroencephalographic classification of epileptic seizures. *Epilepsia*. 1981;22:489–501.

Commission on Classification and Terminology of the International League against Epilepsy. Proposal for revised classification of epilepsies and epileptic syndromes. *Epilepsia*. 1989;30:389–399.

Donner EJ. Explaining the unexplained; expecting the unexpected; where are we with sudden unexpected death in epilepsy? *Epilepsy Curr*. 2011;11:45–49.

Engle J Jr, Wiebe S, French J, et al. Special report, practice parameter: temporal lobe and localized neo-cortical resection for epilepsy. *Epilepsia*. 2003;44:741–751.

French JA, Chadwick WD. Antiepileptic drugs for the elderly. *Neurology*. 2005;64:1834–1835.

French JA, Kanner AM, Bautista J, et al. Efficacy and tolerability of the new antiepileptic drugs I: treatment of new onset epilepsy. *Neurology*. 2004;62:1252–1260.

French JA, Kanner AM, Bautista J, et al. Efficacy and tolerability of the new antiepileptic drugs II: treatment of refractory epilepsy. *Neurology*. 2004;62:1261–1273.

French J, Smith M, Faught E, et al. Practice advisory: the use of felbamate in the treatment of patients that intractable epilepsy. *Neurology*. 1999;52;1540–1545.

Harden CL, Hopp J, Ting TY, et al. Practice parameter update: management issues for women with epilepsy. *Neurology*. 2009;73:126–132.

Harden CL, Meador KJ, Pennell PB, et al. Practice parameter update: management issues for women with epilepsy. *Neurology*. 2009;73:133–141.

Harden CL, Pennell PB, Koppel BS, et al. Practice parameter update: management issues for women with epilepsy. *Neurology*. 2009;73:142–149.

Hernandez-Diaz S, Smith CR, Shen A, et al. Comparative safety of antiepileptic drugs during pregnancy. *Neurology*. 2012;78:1692–1699.

Hughes JR. A review of sudden unexpected death in epilepsy: prediction of patients at risk. *Epilepsy Behav*. 2009;14:280–287.

Krumholz A, Wiebe G, Gronseth S, et al. Evidence based guideline: management of an unprovoked first seizure in adult. *Neurology*. 2015;84:1705–1713.

Lamberts RJ, Blom MT, Wassenaar M, et al. Sudden cardiac arrest in people with epilepsy in the community and risk factors. *Neurology*. 2015;85:212–218.

Leppik IE. Epilepsy in elderly. *Epilepsia*. 2006;47(suppl 1):65–70.

Meador KJ, Baker GA, Browning N, et al. Fetal antiepileptic drug exposure and cognitive outcome at age 6 years (NEAD study). *Lancet Neurol*. 2013;12:244–252.

O'Brien MD, Guillebaud J. Critical review, contraception for women with epilepsy. *Epilepsia*. 2006;47:1419–1422.

Quality Standards Subcommittee of the American Academy of Neurology. Practice parameter: a guideline for discontinuing antiepileptic drugs in seizure-free patients [summary statement]. *Neurology*. 1996;47:600–602.

Sabers A, Ohman I, Christensen J, et al. Oral contraceptives reduce lamotrigine plasma levels *Neurology*. 2003;51:570–571.

Simms KM, Kortepeter C, Avigan M. Lamotrigine and aseptic meningitis. *Neurology*. 2012;78:921–927.

So NK, Sperling MR. Ictal asystole and SUDEP. *Neurology*. 2007;69:423–424.

Therapeutic and Technology Assessment Subcommittee of the American Academy of Neurology. Reassessment: vagus nerve stimulation for epilepsy. *Neurology*. 1999;53:666–669.

Treiman DM, Meyers PD, Walton NY, et al. A comparison of four treatments for generalized convulsive status epilepticus. *N Engl J Med*. 1998;339:792–798.

Trevathan E. Epilepsy associated bone mineral density loss should be prevented. *Neurology*. 2008;70:166–167.

Van Ness PC. Breast feeding in women with epilepsy. *JAMA*. 2013;70(11):1357–1358.

Zahn CA, Morrell MJ, Collins SD, et al. Management issues for women with epilepsy: a review of the literature. *Neurology*. 1998;51:949–956.

44 Multiple Sclerosis

Matthew A. McCoyd

Multiple sclerosis (MS) is a presumed autoimmune demyelinating disorder of the central nervous system (CNS). MS can cause intermittent focal neurologic symptoms (**relapses**) that typically improve over time (**remission**), but may ultimately morph into a progressively relentless neurodegenerative condition due to ongoing axonal loss. MS has likely been part of the human condition for all time—the trials and tribulations of Saint Lidwina of Holland in the 1300s are well documented and read, by today's standards, as a textbook example of relapsing–remitting MS (RR-MS). The disease was well described clinically and pathologically in the 1800s by Charcot and others. The current outlook on MS is markedly different with the steady emergence of increasingly effective therapies.

EPIDEMIOLOGY

MS is often considered a disease of young White females of Northern European descent; while this is a common face of MS, it is certainly not the only face of MS. The prevalence of MS is approximately four times higher among women than among men, the disease is more common among White people than among people of other races, and many individuals with MS have the first clinical symptoms from the ages of 20 to 40 years. However, MS is not exclusive to any age, race, or region. Symptoms can occur early in life (at least as early as age 5 years) and may present much later in life (well past the age of 50 years). The diagnosis should be considered in any patient presenting with relapsing–remitting neurologic symptoms affecting the CNS.

There appears to be a genetic susceptibility to MS, though it is not a "pure" genetic disease. First-degree relatives of the index person have a 10- to 20-fold increased risk of the disorder. This genetic risk has been borne out in twin studies, demonstrating a monozygotic concordance rate of approximately 30%, compared with 5% for dizygotic twins. Human leukocyte antigen (HLA) studies have shown a subtle but significant correlation between MS and different HLA antigens within various ethnic groups. Two different alleles have been linked to MS, but their actual influence is small. These are *HLA-DRB1* and *HLA-DQB1*. The *HLA-DRB1* has the larger effect of these genes, increasing the risk of developing MS 3-fold when present. There are also non-Major Histocompatibility Complex (MHC) genes that induce a smaller effect. However, it is also worth noting that while there is an increased risk, this rises from a lifetime risk of 0.1% to 0.2% to an absolute risk of 2% to 4% in a child or full sibling of someone with MS, meaning the vast majority of "high risk" family members will not develop MS.

Several other factors may influence risk. A geographic association has long been noted, with higher rates of MS classically being reported in latitudes farther from the equator. However, some recent data have called into question the true validity of a "latitudinal gradient" in Europe and North America. More extreme latitudes are associated with reduced sun exposure **and lower levels of Vitamin D**, which may be a contributing factor. Birth month and maternal Vitamin D levels during pregnancy may influence the risk of MS, with possibly an excess number of MS births in the spring and a decreased number of cases in the autumn in the Northern hemisphere (with inverse data noted in the Southern hemisphere). Recent findings suggest a vitamin D response element to the promoter region of *HLA-DRB1*. It is suspected that vitamin D specifically interacts with *HLA-DRB1* to alter its expression and thereby probably decrease one's susceptibility to develop MS.

No specific infectious pathogen has ever been identified as having a clear causative role in MS although several viruses have been implicated, including retroviruses such as Epstein–Barr virus (EBV). In contrast, exposure to some pathogens, such as parasites, may be associated with a *lower* risk of MS. Physical trauma and vaccinations do not increase the risk for the development of MS.

PATHOGENESIS

Substantial clinical, laboratory data, and response to immune-modulating therapy suggest an autoimmune process. There is blood–brain barrier (BBB) breakdown allowing CD4 TH1 type lymphocytes into the CNS where they secrete inflammatory cytokines resulting in damage of myelin and amplification of the immune response. This damaged myelin is then stripped by a cell such as a macrophage and conduction anomalies develop. Less frequently, the offending cell in a CD8 cytotoxic cell directly damages the oligodendroglia. There can be antibody-mediated destruction of the myelin, either directly or through activation of complement. Oligodendrocytes death may occur, with or without apoptosis, and support of development or repair of myelin ceases.

Myelin is important for saltatory axonal conduction. Demyelination frequently occurs in localized areas resulting in a pathologic lesion called a plaque. These plaques are usually located deep in the cerebral white matter, near the ventricles, but they can occur anywhere, including gray matter, cerebellum, brainstem, spinal cord, and proximal nerve roots. This almost limitless variation of plaque distribution is responsible for the variety of clinical presentations. The pathologic appearance of the plaque changes with repeated episodes of demyelination and chronicity. In an early active plaque, there is breakdown of the BBB with demyelination but typically relative sparing of the axons. Perivascular infiltrates of lymphocytes, macrophages, and occasionally plasma cells are present in small veins and venules. Demyelination may spread outward from the plaque, especially along these vessels. Perivascular and interstitial edema may be prominent. At the edge of the plaque, there is hyperplasia of oligodendrocytes and activated astrocytes. These hyperplastic oligodendrocytes are probably involved in remyelination, but thin myelin sheaths found at electron microscopic examination suggest that this remyelination often is suboptimal and incomplete. In older plaques, oligodendroglia disappear, astrocytes show hypertrophy and hyperplasia (sclerosis), and axonal loss occurs. Evidence is present, by such techniques as magnetic resonance spectroscopy (MRS) and histology studies, that there is substantial axonal dropout, in some patients, even in early disease.

The contribution of B cells, plasma cells, and antibody waxes and wanes in popularity. The recent increase in the importance of B cells partially stems from the highly beneficial effects of rituximab and ocrelizumab on the disease course. In MS patients, B cells sometimes appear in clusters or "germinal centers" in the CNS, and these areas appear to correlate with disease progression. At least a portion of these B cells may have been "immortalized" by EBV. B cells release inflammatory cytokines that upregulate T cells and antigen-presenting cells and B cells sometimes become antigen-presenting cells. Antibodies can cause demyelination directly or through complement fixation.

The more recent advances in understanding the pathogenesis of MS involves T regulatory (T REG) cells and dendritic cells (DC). T REG cells are essential for the maintenance of immuno-tolerance, and their dysfunction is associated with the development of organ autoimmunity, as shown in both animals and humans. Data suggest that the dysfunction (temporary or permanent) of suppressor function of certain T REG cells is associated with MS. "Tolerogenic" DCs can modulate the expansion and function of T REG cells during CNS inflammation, or "immunogenic" DCs can induce effector T cell that result in demyelination. This interplay results in homeostasis or disease activity. MS seems to be associated with the dysfunction or impaired maturation of certain T REG-cell and DC populations. In the future, transient or even continuous augmentation of T REG-cell function could develop as an integral component of the therapeutic management of CNS autoimmunity and the course of MS.

CLINICAL FEATURES

MS should be suspected in any individual who presents with focal neurologic symptoms localized to the CNS, particularly those with a prior history suggestive of focal symptoms that developed rapidly and resolved over days or weeks. A **relapse** (exacerbation, attack) is a patient-reported symptom or objective sign typical of an inflammatory CNS demyelinating event that lasts at least 24 hours (most lasting longer) in the absence of a fever or infection.

A. Classical presenting signs and symptoms (see Table 44.1).

1. **Optic neuritis.** Optic neuritis is the presenting feature in 15% to 20% of patients eventually diagnosed with MS, and may occur in upwards of 50% of patients at some time. Characteristic clinical features include subacute visual loss, usually progressing over hours or days; difficulty perceiving colors (**dyschromatopsia**), particularly red, which may appear less red, orange, less intense, or "washed out"; and pain with eye movements. Vision loss usually presents as a central scotoma, though many descriptions of the characteristics of the vision loss exist. Patients may report difficulty with depth perception, especially with moving objects (**Pulfrich phenomenon**) There may be recurrence of symptoms due to factors such as fever, exercise, exposure to high temperatures, or hot showers (**Uhthoff phenomenon**). Altitudinal defects, however, should raise concern for an alternate diagnosis such as anterior ischemic optic neuropathy particularly if there is no associated pain. Patients with isolated optic neuritis without classical appearing brain lesions have a low risk of eventual MS. Optic neuritis, though common in MS, is not pathognomonic (see Chapter 10).

2. **Internuclear ophthalmoplegia.** An internuclear ophthalmoplegia (INO) occurs when a lesion forms that interrupts the **medial longitudinal fasciculus (MLF)** between the abducens nuclei and the contralateral oculomotor nuclei. As this is a pathway that runs along the dorsal aspect of the brainstem close to the 4th ventricle, it is more commonly affected by demyelinating disease than vascular disease. Patients will report double vision with horizontal gaze. The affected eye will not adduct while the contralateral eye will fully abduct and may exhibit nystagmus. Bilateral INO in a young person is virtually pathognomonic for MS (Video 44.1). While INO is presented here, any isolated brain stem syndrome, including diplopia, facial weakness, and trigeminal neuralgia, particularly in a young person with no other risk factors, MS should be highly considered (see Chapter 10).

3. **Partial myelitis.** MS commonly affects the spinal cord but rarely affects the entire cross-section of the cord, creating a partial myelitis clinical picture rather than a complete myelitis (which is more common in neuromyelitis optica [NMO]). Patients often will report numbness involving both feet (due to the layering of dorsal columns fibers with the feet being closest to the midline and the upper extremities more laterally located). Any patient who reports numbness that extends above the level of the pelvis (a sensory level) should be assumed to have a spinal cord process until proven otherwise. Patients should be queried regarding "Lhermitte's sign" (which is really a symptom: an electric shock-like sensation traveling down the back induced by neck flexion). Patients should also be asked about bladder and sexual dysfunction (particularly erectile dysfunction in young men) which can indicate spinal cord pathology.

4. **Cognitive dysfunction and fatigue.** While the differential diagnosis of cognitive dysfunction and fatigue is broad, in a young person MS should be considered. Many patients with MS report fatigue that is out-of-proportion to the level of activity, and may note mild difficulty with cognition, particularly multitasking. While fatigue may be multifactorial, it may also be related to the reduced efficiency of demyelinated pathways resulting in a higher energy demand.

TABLE 44.1 Clinical Features of Multiple Sclerosis

Optic neuritis	Unilateral vision loss associated with pain and color desaturation
Internuclear ophthalmoplegia	Double vision with horizontal gaze associated with gaze palsy and monocular (dissociated) nystagmus
Partial myelitis	Numbness/sensory changes with an associated sensory level should be assumed to be spinal cord in localization until proven otherwise
Cognitive dysfunction	Usually mild subcortical cognitive impairment in a young person with no apparent risk factors

B. Chronic symptoms.

1. Fatigue. Patients with MS often report fatigue that is out-of-proportion to level of activity. It may be related to increased energy demands due to demyelination. Patients often report increased fatigue in the latter part of the day, concordant with a natural rise in body temperature. There is no single highly effective treatment. Patients should be counseled to plan their day accordingly. Temperature modification can be helpful. Patients may notice worsening of fatigue with higher temperatures (heat intolerance). Use of cooling devices (cooling scarves, cooling vests) that lower body temperature by as little as 1 degree can improve neural function. Patient should be screened for sleep disturbances. Medications that may have a modest effect on fatigue include amantadine, modafinil, and methylphenidate.

2. Spasticity. Muscle stiffness is particularly common due to involvement of the corticospinal tract. Patients often report muscle tightness especially later in the day when they are increasingly fatigued. Symptoms usually respond best to medications, with stretching providing only temporary relief. Muscle relaxants such as baclofen are used as first-line therapies. Patients need to be counseled as to the potential for withdrawal with sudden cessation of baclofen. Alternative oral therapy options include tizanidine, dantrolene sodium, and benzodiazepines. Patients with focal spasticity may benefit from botulinum toxin (Botox). More severe spasticity may be alleviated with an intrathecal baclofen pump, which seem to work better for lower extremity spasticity. Medical marijuana, while illegal at the federal level in the United States but legalized by many individual states, may theoretically be helpful for spasticity.

3. Gait impairment. Dalfampradine (4-aminopyradine or Ampyra) specifically approved for walking speed in MS, was shown to improve the average 25-foot timed walk. The medication is contraindicated in those with a history of seizures or significant renal impairment.

DIAGNOSIS

Despite many technological advances to aid in the diagnosis of neurologic disease, the core clinical diagnostic features for the diagnosis of MS, **a CNS demyelinating disorder with attacks separate in space and time,** laid out in the 1965 "Schumaker Criteria," still hold true today. MS is a **clinical** diagnosis with **paraclinical** support, which should be considered in a patient with objective abnormalities on the neurologic examination, or highly suggestive symptoms by history, attributable to dysfunction of two or more parts of the CNS involving white matter tracts that occur at separate points in time with no better explanation. It is notable that the Schumaker Criteria did not require any specific testing other than a history and neurologic examination. While this may seem "antiquated" to a current reader, it is worth highlighting that a patient presenting with objective evidence of >2 attacks, or objective evidence of 1 attack with a reasonable historical evidence of a prior attack, requires no additional testing for the diagnosis of MS in the 2010 McDonald Criteria. MS is, after all, a clinical diagnosis, and paraclinical measures are used to support the diagnosis.

However, it is also evident that paraclinical studies can be helpful in reasonably confirming the diagnosis in a patient presenting with suspicious clinical features. Brain and spinal cord magnetic resonance imaging (MRI) has been the most helpful ancillary study in the diagnosis of MS in appropriately selected patients, and can be used in the setting of a single clinical event to demonstrate prior demyelinating events involving different parts of the CNS (radiographic dissemination in space and time) that suggest a risk for future clinical relapses. Radiographic lesions due to MS usually have a typical size, appearance, and location (Figs. 44.1 to 44.5). Most lesions are >3 mm (though occasionally being as large as 2 cm or more in tumefactive MS), and have an ovoid appearance. To fulfill the 2010 McDonald Criteria for dissemination in space, lesions should be present in at least two out of four areas: periventricular, juxtacortical, infratentorial, or spinal cord (only asymptomatic spinal cord lesions are counted; Table 44.2). MS lesions tend to accumulate close to the pial surface near the ventricular system. Periventricular lesions are often best seen on sagittal fluid attenuation inversion recovery (FLAIR) imaging that demonstrates a perpendicular orientation of the lesions to the ventricle in close proximity or involving the corpus callosum ("Dawson's fingers", first described by J. W.

Dawson in 1916). Infratentorial lesions, unlike vascular lesions that appear deep in brainstem structures, tend to accumulate near the 4th ventricle, along the pontine surface or in the cerebellar peduncles, and are usually best seen on T2-weighted imaging. Spinal cord lesions are often seen in the periphery of the spinal cord, particularly in the dorsal columns, are typically <1 vertebral segment in length, and seldom involve the entire cross-section of the cord. It is unusual for any disease other than MS to affect the brain and spinal cord. Dissemination in time is demonstrated by the appearance of a new T2 lesion at any point in time compared to a reference scan, irrespective of the timing of the first scan (older criteria required a 30-day gap), or the presence of an asymptomatic gadolinium-enhancing lesion on even the baseline

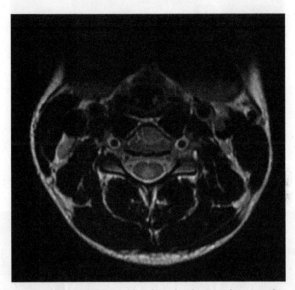

FIGURE 44.1 Spinal cord lesion involving the dorsal columns abutting the pial surface.

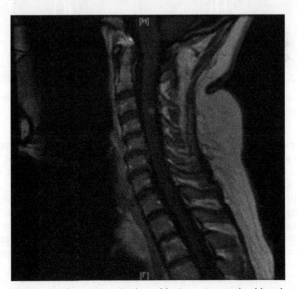

FIGURE 44.2 Gadolinium-enhancing spinal cord lesion <1 vertebral level, typical of MS. MS, multiple sclerosis.

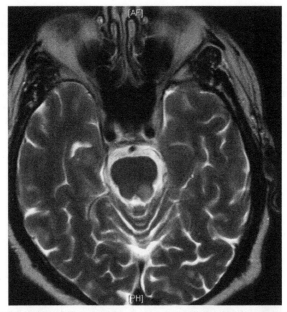

FIGURE 44.3 Infratentorial brainstem lesion close to the pial surface of the brainstem.

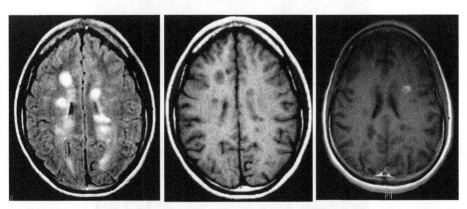

FIGURE 44.4 Periventricular lesions (FLAIR, T1 hypointense "black hole," and characteristic gadolinium-enhancing lesion). FLAIR, fluid attenuation inversion recovery.

scan. Gadolinium-enhancing lesions are often incompletely enhancing, and indicate recent (several days to several weeks) or active demyelination. The presence of T1 hypointense lesions, though suggestive of chronic lesion formation that would support dissemination in time, is not included in the criteria.

The concept of "**radiographically isolated MS**" (RIS) has been introduced in the literature, referencing a situation in which a patient is imaged for presumably alternative reasons (such as headaches) that are not felt to be demyelinating in nature, and the imaging reveals lesions characteristic in appearance for MS. RIS is not currently included as an MS phenotype, though patients may require close clinical and radiographic follow-up to assess for signs and symptoms suggestive of MS.

MRI has become clearly the leading paraclinical study, and most other "classic" paraclinical studies now having diminishing clinical relevance. For example, though a historic biomarker for the disease, spinal fluid analysis is no longer considered mandatory for the diagnosis of MS and is not included in the 2010 McDonald Criteria for relapsing forms of MS. While this may

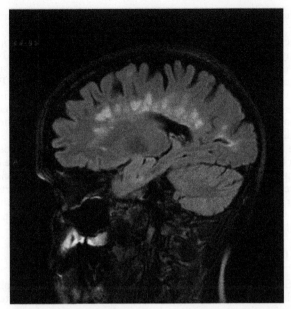

FIGURE 44.5 Perpendicularly oriented periventricular lesions (Dawson's fingers).

TABLE 44.2 2010 MRI Criteria for Dissemination in Space and Time

Dissemination in space	Juxtacortical	Periventricular	Infratentorial	Spinal cord
Dissemination in time	Asymptomatic Gd-enhancing lesion (at any time)	New T2 lesion irrespective of baseline scan		

Abbreviation: MRI, magnetic resonance imaging.

induce chest pain and rage in older neurologists, its inclusion was not felt to be necessary. In the past, "positive" cerebrospinal fluid (CSF) could be used to reduce MRI requirements for the diagnosis of MS. As the 2010 McDonald criteria simplified imaging requirements, further "liberalizing" MRI requirements with CSF was felt to be unnecessary.

Though CSF is **not required,** it can still provide important information and should be used in appropriate situations where the information may influence clinical decisions. The basic CSF profile (white blood cell count [WBC], protein, glucose) in MS is usually normal, though mild elevations in the WBC count and protein content can be seen. A higher than normal ($>5 \times 10^6$/L) WBC count is seen in upwards of one-third of MS patients and a mildly elevated protein count (>54 mg/dL) in as many as one-fourth. However, extreme elevations such as a very elevated WBC count ($>50 \times 10^6$/L) or protein count (>100 mg/dL) are unusual and should prompt consideration of an alternate diagnosis. Oligoclonal bands (OCBs) represent IgG unique to the CSF, and suggest immunologic activity of clonally expanding lymphocytes within the CNS. Qualitative assessment of CSF for IgG is likely the most informative analysis, and is considered superior to quantitative IgG analysis (IgG index). While commonly assumed to be "diagnostic" of MS, OCBs are not unique to MS and may alternatively be absent in patients with MS. OCBs may have some prognostic role, with the presence of OCBs possibly being associated with an increased risk of converting from clinically isolated syndrome (CIS) to MS. Other historic markers, such as myelin basic protein (MBP) which may be a marker of acute demyelination, are nonspecific. There has been great interest in other CSF biomarkers for diagnostic and prognostic purposes in MS but, to date, have shown minimal real-world clinical promise.

Evoked potentials have also been classically used as a paraclinical support for clinically silent CNS demyelination. The American Academy of Neurology (AAN) has published recommendations that **visual evoked potentials (VEPs)** are "probably" useful to identify patients at risk to develop MS, **somatosensory evoked potentials (SSEPs)** are "possibly" useful, and **brainstem auditory evoked potentials (BAEPs)** have insufficient evidence be recommended as useful. With advances in MRI technology, and the emergence of **ocular coherence tomography (OCT)**, VEPs will likely take a placed next to "hot bath tests" as a footnote to the diagnostic history of MS.

Perhaps the key questions for the neurologist facing a patient with possible MS are: (1) Does the patient have concerning signs or symptoms for MS? (2) Does the MRI of the brain and spinal cord appear characteristic for MS? and (3) Is there any more reasonable explanation? If the answers are satisfactory for each, the patient has MS. It is also important to remember that diagnostic criteria exist to aid the diagnosis, and the clinician is not completely beholden to criteria in the face of a clear clinical presentation. As Admiral John Kurtzke noted, "MS is what a good clinician would call MS."

Defining the Course of Multiple Sclerosis

Patients with MS have MS independent of the relatively arbitrary labels placed on them by clinicians. It is clear, however, that some patients with MS have intermittent inflammatory relapses that recover in time, some patients have steady progression of symptoms without clear recovery, and some patients have both inflammatory relapses and concomitant progression.

In 1996, several subtypes of MS were defined by the United States National Multiple Sclerosis Society (NMSS). Four clinical courses were defined at that time: (1) relapsing–remitting (RR) (2) secondary progressive (SP) (3) primary progressive (PP), and (4) progressive relapsing (PR). At that time of publication, it was noted that the subtypes lacked objective biomarkers such as MRI (which was still in its relative infancy, and not even included in the existing diagnostic criteria for MS).

The subtypes of MS were updated in 2013. Key updates include the following:

1. **Clinically isolated syndrome.** The first clinical presentation of an inflammatory CNS demyelinating condition suggestive of MS, but not meeting full criteria. Perhaps ironically, though now "officially" recognized, the changes in the diagnostic criteria for MS have made the use of the term "clinically isolated syndrome" somewhat academic as patients with a single clinical event meeting current MRI criteria can simply be defined as having MS based on a single scan.

2. **Assessment of disease activity by clinical or radiographic features as "active" or "not active."** Evidence of disease activity and clinical progression, either clinically or radiographically, reflects ongoing risk of inflammatory disease or neurodegenerative progression. Disease activity can be assessed by annual clinical assessment and *annual cranial imaging* for patients deemed to be at risk of inflammatory attacks. The role of annual imaging for patients with progressive disease is less clear.

3. A patient with RR-MS with a clinical relapse or evidence of a gadolinium-enhancing lesion would be considered "RR-active"; a patient with RR-MS without clinical or radiographic activity would be considered "RR-not active."

4. The use of disease activity as a modifier allows for the elimination of the PR-MS subtype. A patient previously considered PR-MS would not be classified as PP-active or PP-not active.

5. Assessment of disease progression, independent of relapses. Progression can be determined by history or objective measure of change. Though labeled "progressive," not all progressive forms of MS progress over a specified period of time, and no two cases necessarily progress at the same rate.

6. A patient with SP-MS without progression would be considered SP-MS-not progressing.

7. A patient with SP-MS with new lesions and gradual clinical worsening would be considered SP-MS-active and progressing.

What remains to be seen is how quickly, if at all, the 2013 revisions to the clinical course of MS are incorporated into regular clinical practice. The four subtypes of MS (RR-MS, SP-MS, PP-MS, PR-MS) seem to have become relatively ingrained in the MS vernacular, despite their existence for barely two decades. However, the 2013 revisions do emphasize a key point—is the patient at risk for future clinical or radiographic relapses, which is a pivotal decision point in the treatment algorithm. The revisions are also seemingly one of the first "authoritative" recommendations for annual imaging in patients with relapsing forms of MS as a means of surveillance.

TREATMENT OF ACUTE RELAPSES

An MS relapse has classically been defined as a new or worsening neurologic deficit lasting >24 hours in the absence of a fever or infection. The goal of treating acute inflammatory MS attacks is to restore neurologic function as quickly as possible. Treatment is not absolutely necessary—many patients will regain function within several months independent of treatment. Before treatment, concurrent infection should be excluded. Infections or other active medical issues can cause recurrence of prior MS symptoms, often termed a "**pseudo-relapse**."

The mainstay of acute treatment has been high-dose corticosteroids, administered in one of several fashions. The first medication proven to be effective at treating an MS relapse in a well-designed, multicenter randomized clinical trial was corticotropin gel (ACTH). ACTH is still available for use, but is often used only in patients who have had an inadequate response to high-dose steroids or cannot tolerate steroids for some reason.

Intravenous (IV) methylprednisolone (MP) has become the "standard" treatment for MS relapses based on clinical trial experience in the 1980s. IV MP was found to be comparable to ACTH (and at a lower cost) in several head-to-head trials. The Optic Neuritis Treatment Trial in 1992 seemed to suggest that IV MP was superior to oral prednisone. The IV MP had faster recovery of visual function and the oral prednisone group had a higher relapse recurrence rate than IV steroids. However, it is entirely possible the response was *dose-dependent* and not *route-dependent*. In the study, patients received 1,000 mg of IV MP (divided 250 mg every 6 hours for 3 days) followed by an oral course of prednisone for 11 days, or 1 mg/kg/day of oral prednisone for 14 days—a substantially lower dose. IV MP has close to a 1:1 conversion rate to oral steroids. Interestingly, low-dose IV MP (40 mg/day for 7 days, 20 mg/day for 4 days, and 10 mg/day for 3 days) was not shown to be as effective in the treatment of relapses in 1989. Several studies have shown that equally dosed oral and IV steroids have a similar impact on recovery and rate of recurrence. For patients who can tolerate high-dose oral prednisone, oral treatment may be an option.

For patients who do not respond to high-dose oral steroids, plasma exchange (PLEX) may be an option. The American Academy of Neurology published guidelines in 2011 in support of PLEX for steroid-refractory MS relapses, recommending that PLEX be considered for the adjunctive treatment of exacerbations in relapsing forms of MS, and that it may be considered in the treatment of fulminant CNS demyelinating diseases that fail to respond to high-dose corticosteroid treatment. Intravenous immunoglobulin (IVIG) has also been used, though the efficacy data are less clear with conflicting data in the literature.

DISEASE-MODIFYING THERAPIES

A cure for MS has long been sought for, and has long been equally elusive. Charcot once remarked regarding treatment for MS that "I can only tell you of some experiments, the results of which have, unfortunately, not been very encouraging." This was largely true in MS until the early 1990s when interferon beta-1b was shown to reduce the risk of MS relapses and radiographic lesion formation. As Dr. Barry Arnason editorialized, though not "the long-awaited cure. . . . half a loaf is better than no bread." Since the early 1990s, there has been a significant change in the landscape for the treatment of MS. Whereas in the past physicians had little to offer patients in the way of treatment, the current challenge is in trying to navigate all of the treatment options.

There is no "perfect" treatment for MS, and the variability of the disease makes an algorithmic approach problematic. There are few head-to-head studies comparing treatment options to guide decision making. Cross-study analysis is fraught with statistical peril, as MS clinical trials have changed substantially in the last 30 years in regards to patient demographics, in part reflective of changes in the diagnostic requirements for MS (the placebo annualized relapse rate [ARR] for the original interferon trial was >1.0; in many modern studies, the ARR is closer to 0.5).

Many factors should be taken into account when selecting a therapy. Reasonable therapeutic questions include:

1. **Is the medication effective at treating MS?** Most clinical trials have measured the effectiveness of MS therapies on the relative reduction in the relapse rate compared to placebo, the reduction in the formation of new radiographic lesions (new or unequivocally enlarging T2 lesions or new gadolinium-enhancing lesions), and the reduction in risk of disability progression. While data on the long-term impact of treatment on disease impact are somewhat lacking (in part because therapies have only been available just over 20 years), extension data from the original Interferon (IFN) clinical trial clearly show a mortality and quality-of-life benefit from treatment.

2. **Is the medication reasonably safe?** Many patients who start therapy are young, often in child-bearing years, and can reasonably expect to be on treatment for many years, possibly many decades. A reasonable risk–benefit analysis must be favorable in the treatment of a disease that can cause significant disability but a less clear impact mortality.

3. **Is the medication reasonably tolerated?** A patient with a "high" relapse rate may have new symptoms due to MS as infrequently as once a year, and many patients having relapses "only" once every 2 to 3 years. Medications must be taken with regularity to be effective. If the day-to-day experience of a medication is worse than the disease, few patients will take it.

4. **Will the patient be compliant with the medication?** Few medications work less well than the one not taken. Physicians should discuss at length with patients lifestyle factors including family life, work, personal preferences, in selecting a therapy for a patient.

APPROVED THERAPIES FOR RELAPSING MS (TABLE 44.3)

A. **Injectable therapies.**
   1. **Interferons (IFN).** Though the exact mechanism of action is unknown, IFNs are believed to prevent the migration of self-reactive immune cells across the blood brain barrier. All IFNs have similar side-effect profiles, most notably including the potential for liver function abnormalities, flu-like reactions following injections, and depression. Monitoring requirements include baseline liver function tests (LFTs) and routine blood counts, which should be periodically repeated (usually at 3 months, then 6 months, then 12 months, and every 6 to 12 months thereafter). IFNs are most notably differentiated by the dosing regimen. There are very limited head-to-head studies comparing the individual therapies.
      a. **IFN beta**-1b (Betaseron, Extavia) is given subcutaneously (SC) every other day
      b. **IFN beta**-1a (Avonex) is given intramuscularly (IM) once weekly
      c. **IFN beta**-1a (Plegridy) is given IM once every 2 weeks
      d. **IFN beta**-1a (Rebif) is given SC 3 days weekly
   2. **Glatiramer acetate (GA).** The exact mechanism of action is unknown, but is believed to induce a shift from a proinflammatory state to an anti-inflammatory state within the CNS. Notable side effects include the potential for a chest-tightening reaction (usually within a few minutes of injection and lasting several minutes), and focal lipoatrophy at injection sites. No routine laboratory monitoring is required. There are currently three formulations of GA available.
      a. **GA** (Copaxone) 20 mg given SC on a daily basis
      b. **GA** (Copaxone) 40 mg given SC three times weekly
      c. **GA** (Glatopa) 20 mg given SC on a daily basis
B. **Oral therapies.**
   1. **Dimethyl fumarate (Tecfidera).** Fumarates have been used for many years for the treatment of psoriasis. In part due to reports of patients with MS and psoriasis responding well, dimethyl fumarate (DMF) was studied in relapsing forms of MS. The mechanism of

TABLE 44.3 Therapies Approved for Relapsing Forms of Multiple Sclerosis

Disease-Modifying Therapy	Administration	Common Side Effects	Black Box Warning
Interferon beta 1B (Betaseron/Extavia)	SC qod	Flu-like reactions Liver function abnormalities Depression Injection site reactions	None
Interferon beta 1A (Avonex)	IM qwk	Flu-like reactions Liver function abnormalities Depression Injection site reactions	None
Interferon beta 1A (Plegridy)	SC q2wk	Flu-like reactions Liver function abnormalities Depression Injection site reactions	None
Interferon beta 1A (Rebif)	SC 3×wk	Flu-like reactions Liver function abnormalities Depression Injection site reactions	None
Glatiramer acetate (Copaxone/Glatopa)	SC qd (20 mg)	Injection reaction Lipoatrophy	None
Glatiramer acetate (Copaxone)	SC 3×wk (40 mg)	Injection reaction Lipoatrophy	None
Natalizumab (Tysabri)	IV q28d	Infusion reaction Liver function abnormalities	Progressive multifocal leukoencephalopathy
Fingolimod (Gilenya)	PO qd	Transient bradycardia Macular edema Liver function abnormalities	None (PML cases reported)
Teriflunomide (Aubagio)	PO qd	Transient hair thinning	Hepatotoxicity Teratogenicity
Dimethyl fumarate (Tecfidera)	PO bid	GI intolerance Flushing	None (PML cases reported)
Alemtuzumab (Lemtrada)	Annual infusion	Infection Thyroid dysfunction	Autoimmunity Infusion reaction Risk of malignancies

Abbreviations: bid, twice a day; GI, gastrointestinal; IM, intramuscularly; PML, progressive multifocal leukoencephalopathy; PO, by mouth; qd, every day; qod, every other day; SC, subcutaneously.

action of DMF is unknown, but it has been theorized that it may interfere with the NrF2 pathway, a proinflammatory pathway. Notable side effects include gastrointestinal upset that typically occurs for the first few days to a week after initiation, and may possibly be ameliorated by taking the medication with foods high in fat content, and a flushing reaction variably described as a reddening of the skin and/or itching that often randomly occurs and usually lasts for several minutes following ingestion. There have been, to date, a very limited number of case reports of progressive multifocal leukoencephalopathy (PML) in patients taking DMF, none of whom had known prior exposure to or concomitant use of medications associated with PML. Monitoring includes a baseline complete blood count (CBC) and follow-up studies every 6 months. A small percentage of patients may show a significant and sustained drop in lymphocyte count that may be a risk factor for opportunistic infection.

    a. Dimethyl fumarate (Tecfidera) 240 mg by mouth (PO) twice daily

2. **Fingolimod (Gilenya).** Fingolimod was the first oral therapy approved for the treatment of relapsing MS. It is believed to affect sphingosine-1-phosphate (S1P) receptors. S1P is involved in the egress of lymphocytes from lymph nodes. The presumed mechanism of action is the reversible sequestration of autoreactive lymphocytes from lymph nodes. S1P receptors are also found on cardiac tissue, and may be cause for the transient drop in heart rate following first dose. Notable side effects include the potential for macular edema (particularly in those with diabetes mellitus), which typically occurs within the first few months of starting the medication, transient cardiac changes, and the potential for some infections. Monitoring requirements include baseline LFTs and CBC, examination of the fundus (either formal funduscopic examination or OCT), reasonable confirmation of prior varicella-zoster virus (VZV) exposure (either by history or, more commonly, testing for serum VZV antibodies to confirm immunologic surveillance), and first dose observation (FDO). FDO includes a baseline electrocardiogram (ECG) to evaluate for a prolonged QT interval and second-degree, type 2, or third-degree heart block (both of which are contraindications to fingolimod and should prompt immediate cardiology consultation). After taking the medication, the patient is monitored for 6 hours with periodic evaluation of the heart rate and blood pressure. Following FDO, patients should undergo a repeat fundus examination after 3-to-4 months to evaluate for macular edema. Follow-up blood studies include periodic surveillance of LFTs. CBC surveillance often reveals a drop in the total WBC count and lymphocyte count, sometimes to dramatically low levels (<500). However, the clinical significance of the lymphopenia is unclear; based on the available clinical trial data, there was not an association between lymphopenia and infection, and is not a reason to reflexively discontinue treatment. There have been, to date, a small number of case reports of individuals taking fingolimod developing PML. The majority of cases have occurred in those who switched from natalizumab to fingolimod, often with a short interval between the last dose of natalizumab and first dose of fingolimod, and virtually all having a known John Cunningham virus (JCV) positive antibody status. There are also a smaller number of cases of cases in which individuals with no prior exposure to natalizumab who were on fingolimod who developed PML.

3. **Teriflunomide (Aubagio).** Teriflunomide is a derivative of leflunomide, which has been used for the treatment of rheumatoid arthritis (an autoimmune inflammatory condition directed against joints). Teriflunomide is given as a once-daily pill. Its presumed mechanism of action is inhibition of the enzyme dihydro-oratate dehydrogenase (DHOD), an enzyme critical in the de novo cell synthesis pathway. Notable side effects include the potential for LFT abnormalities, transient hair thinning (occurring around 3 months after treatment initiation and usually resolving around 6 months after treatment initiation), and a possible increased risk for peripheral neuropathy (especially mononeuropathies such as median neuropathy at the wrist). Effective forms of birth control are recommended as the medication has been classified as pregnancy Category X by the Food and Drug Administration (FDA). Though the medication has a considerably long half-life, and can theoretically linger as long as 2 years, it can be eliminated with cholestyramine, usually over the course of 11 days. Activated charcoal would also theoretically eliminate the medication and is included in the package insert, but its availability and tolerability make it a moot point. Monitoring requirements include baseline and monthly LFTs for the first 6 months of therapy, baseline and periodic CBC, screening for tuberculosis (either tuberculin skin testing or quantiferon gold testing), and exclusion of pregnancy.

C. **Intravenous therapies.**

1. **Natalizumab (Tysabri).** Natalizumab is a once-every-28-day monoclonal antibody that is believed to bind to integrin, which prevents the adherence of WBCs to the blood vessel wall, a necessary step for access to the CNS across the BBB. While considered a highly effective therapy for MS, it was briefly pulled from the market after its approval in 2004 due to the occurrence of treatment-related PML. Natalizumab has been definitively associated with the risk of PML. Patients considered at the highest risk include those

with history of prior immunosuppressant exposure, on therapy for greater than 2 years, and who have a positive JCV Ab status.

2. **Alemtuzumab (Lemtrada).** Alemtuzumab is a CD52 monoclonal antibody that causes the rapid depletion of T- and B-cell lines, with a slow return to baseline over many months. It is uniquely dosed in annual courses, with five consecutive daily infusions given in year 1 and three consecutive daily infusions in year 2. The need for a third course or beyond is case dependent, but many patients do not require re-treatment in year 3 or 4. Notable side effects include the potential for an infusion reaction that may be reduced with concomitant IV MP for at least the first three infusions. Interestingly, patients can develop delayed secondary autoimmunity. Rare but significant side effects include immune thrombocytopenic purpura (ITP) and rapidly progressive glomerulonephritis. Autoimmune thyroid dysfunction, either hypo- or hyperthyroidism, occurs more commonly (30% to 40%), usually between 1 and 4 years from the last infusion. As a result, a comprehensive risk mitigation program is required that includes monthly blood and urine studies for 48 months after the last infusion.

D. **Emerging therapies.**

Rapid evolution of MS treatment options often relegate virtually all literature outdated almost as soon as it is published. At the present time, at least two therapies are close to approval for use, including ocrelizumab and daclizumab. Several others are under investigation including laquinimod and ofatunamab. A number of treatments are showing promise for remyelination including anti-LINGO, RhMIg22, and high-dose biotin. Some of these therapies will eventually be available for use, while others may never bear out the promise of initial studies. But for patients, it is clear that more and more options are readily emerging.

MULTIPLE SCLEROSIS AND PREGNANCY

As MS commonly affects women of child-bearing potential, it is fairly common for the neurologist to offer an opinion in regard to obstetric management. MS appears to have little impact on pregnancy and pregnancy little impact on MS. While there is an increase in relapses in the 3 months after delivery, the relapse rate declines during pregnancy and during the "pregnancy year" (pregnancy plus 3-month postpregnancy period) the relapse rate is unaffected. Factors that may influence the intra- and postpregnancy relapse rate include the prepregnancy relapse rate and higher expanded disability status scale (EDSS). Pregnancy does not appear to impact the long-term course of the disease. There is no evidence that MS increases the risk of miscarriages, ectopic pregnancies, premature delivery, or fetal malformations. There is no medical reason to discourage women with MS from considering pregnancy.

If a woman does experience a relapse during pregnancy, a decision can be made as to whether it is significant enough to require treatment. Prednisone is classified a Category C medication. It may cross the placenta and could possibly contribute to miscarriage, preterm labor and cleft palate if used in the first trimester. It is probably safe to use in the 2nd or 3rd trimester. IVIG does not appear to affect the fetus though it does cross the placenta and could be used if deemed clinically appropriate (see Chapter 62).

Most patients with MS do well during their pregnancy and do not require disease-modifying therapies (DMTs). The majority of DMTs are pregnancy Category C medications, with glatiramer acetate classified a B, leflunomide an X, and mitoxantrone a D. While there are no clear data, patients are generally advised to stop DMTs before becoming pregnant. Medications can be found in the breastmilk. As there are no adequate studies, resumption of a DMT is usually held until after the mother has stopped breastfeeding.

MS should have **no impact** on most obstetric decisions, including pain management. There are outdated, flawed reports that epidural anesthesia may increase the risk of a postpartum relapse. Consistent studies have shown this to not be true. Epidural analgesia does not increase the risk of relapse of the level of disability following pregnancy. There is no contraindication to vaginal or caesarean delivery. Most patients with MS will have routine deliveries. Patients with significant pelvic floor weakness (due to spinal cord lesions) may have prolonged labor, and may experience increased muscle fatigue due to a rise in body temperature.

Key Points

- MS is an inflammatory demyelinating condition of the CNS
- The hallmark of MS is the occurrence of acute, focal neurologic symptoms (relapses) with gradual, though sometimes incomplete, recovery of function (remission)
- In time, after repeated inflammatory attacks, progressive neurologic deterioration may occur (progressive multiple sclerosis)
- The diagnosis is made based on the presence of characteristic clinic events corroborated by paraclinical evidence (specifically MRI) demonstrating a disease that is disseminated in space and time
- There is an ever-expanding arsenal of treatment options to slow, or halt, the disease

Recommended Readings

Arnason BG. Interferon beta in multiple sclerosis. *Neurology.* 1993;43:641–643.

Barkhof F, Filippi M, Miller DH, et al. Comparison of MRI criteria at first presentation to predict conversion to clinically definite multiple sclerosis. *Brain.* 1997;120:2059–2069.

Bar-Or A. The immunology of multiple sclerosis. *Semin Neurol.* 2008;28:29–45.

Berkovich R. Treatment of acute relapses in multiple sclerosis. *Neurotherapeutics.* 2013;10:97–105.

Bove R, Alwan S, Friedman JM, et al. Management of multiple sclerosis during pregnancy and the reproductive years: a systematic review. *Obstet Gynecol.* 2014;124:1157–1168.

Cortese I, Chaudhry V, So YT, et al. Evidence-based guideline update: plasmapheresis in neurologic disorders. *Neurology.* 2011;76:294–300.

D'hooghe MB, Nagels G, Bissay V, et al. Modifiable factors influencing relapses and disability in multiple sclerosis. *Mult Scler.* 2010;16:773–785.

Freedman MS, Hughes B, Mikol DD, et al. Efficacy of disease-modifying therapies in relapsing remitting multiple sclerosis: a systematic comparison. *Eur Neurol.* 2008;60:1–11.

Freedman MS, Thompson EJ, Deisenhammer F, et al. Recommended standard of cerebrospinal fluid analysis in the diagnosis of multiple sclerosis: a consensus statement. *Arch Neurol.* 2005;62:865–870.

Frohman TC, Davis SL, Beh S, et al. Uhthoff's phenomena in MS—clinical features and pathophysiology. *Nat Rev.* 2013;9:535–540.

Giesser BS. Diagnosis of multiple sclerosis. *Neurol Clin.* 2011;29:381–388.

Hauser SL. The Charcot lecture | beatin MS: a story of B cells, with twists and turns. *Mult Scler J.* 2015;21:8–21.

Koch-Henriksen N, Sorensen PS. The changing demographic pattern of multiple sclerosis epidemiology. *Lancet.* 2010;9:520–532.

Langer-Gould A, Qian L, Tartof SY, et al. Vaccines and the risk of multiple sclerosis and other central nervous system demyelinating disease. *JAMA Neurol.* 2014;71:1506–1513.

Lublin FD, Reingold SC, Cohen JA, et al. Defining the clinical course of multiple sclerosis: the 2013 revisions. *Neurology.* 2014;83:278–286.

Miller DH, Weinshenker BG, Filippi M, et al. Differential diagnosis of suspected multiple sclerosis: a consensus approach. *Mult Scler.* 2008;14:1157–1174.

Montalban X. Review of methodological issues of clinical trials in multiple sclerosis. *J Neurol Sci.* 2011;311(S1):S35–S42.

Polman CH, Reingold SC, Banwell B, et al. Diagnostic criteria for multiple sclerosis: 2010 revisions of the McDonald critera. *Ann Neurol.* 2011;69:292–302.

Poser CM, Paty DW, Scheinberg L, et al. New diagnostic criteria for multiple sclerosis: guidelines for research protocols. *Ann Neurol.* 1983;13:227–231.

Schumacher GA, Beebe G, Kibler RF. Problems of experimental trials of therapy in multiple sclerosis: report by the panel on the evaluation of experimental trials of therapy in multiple sclerosis. *Ann N Y Acad Sci.* 1965;122:552–568.

Scolding N. The differential diagnosis of multiple sclerosis. *J Neurol Neurosurg Psychiatry.* 2001;71(suppl II):ii9–ii15.

Swanton JK, Fernando K, Dalton CM, et al. Modification of MRI criteria for multiple sclerosis in patients with clinically isolated syndrome. *J Neurol Neurosurg Psychiatry.* 2006;77:830–833.

Tintore M, Rovira A, Rio J, et al. Do oligoclonal bands add information to MRI in first attacks of multiple sclerosis? *Neurology.* 2008;70:1079–1083.

Wallin MT, Wilken JA, Kane R. Cognitive dysfunction in multiple sclerosis: assessment, imaging, and risk factors. *J Rehabil Res Dev.* 2006;43:63–72.

45 Movement Disorders

Andrew P. Duker and Alberto J. Espay

Movement disorders can be divided into **hypokinetic** and **hyperkinetic.** Hypokinetic movement disorders refer primarily to disorders with decreased amplitude and/or speed of movement (parkinsonism), whereas hyperkinetic movement disorders are those displaying excess of movement (chorea, dystonia, myoclonus, tics, and tremor).

HYPOKINETIC MOVEMENT DISORDERS

A. **Parkinson's disease (PD)** is the most common cause of degenerative parkinsonism. PD's response to dopaminergic medications is robust, compared with the atypical parkinsonisms (previously referred to as Parkinson-plus syndromes) in which the response, if any, is partial and transient.

1. **Nonpharmacologic management** of PD includes education about the disease, support of patient and family, appropriate nutrition, and exercise. Exercise can improve symptoms and their response to treatment, in addition to reducing fatigue, enhancing sleep, and potentially yielding a disease-modifying effect in the long run. A well-balanced diet is essential for PD patients because of the increased risk of malnutrition and weight loss. Redistribution of dietary protein can be beneficial in the care of patients with advanced PD as protein interferes with absorption of levodopa in the gastrointestinal tract.

2. **Pharmacologic therapy for PD.**

   a. **Neuroprotection.** None of the currently available therapies is firmly acknowledged as disease modifying. The selective monoamine oxidase B (MAO-B) inhibitors selegiline (Eldepryl) and rasagiline (Azilect) have been tested in designs suggestive of such an effect, but their symptomatic benefit may be masking any putative neuroprotective effects. Levodopa's introduction in the 1970s dramatically reduced the mortality from this disease, but this is believed to result from purely symptomatic effects.

   b. **Symptomatic management of PD.** Many drugs are useful for improving parkinsonian symptoms. Initiation of PD treatment can be tailored to patients' age, employment status, predominant PD symptoms, severity of illness, intercurrent medical problems, side-effect profile of previous medications, and cost.

      (1) **Selegiline** (Eldepryl) and **rasagiline** (Azilect) are irreversible, selective inhibitors of MAO-B at the recommended doses of up to 5 mg twice a day and 1 mg every day, respectively. MAO-B inhibition blocks one of the degradation pathways for dopamine, thus increasing its availability. **Zydis selegiline** (Zelapar) is an orally disintegrating formulation of selegiline, taken at 2.5 mg/day. MAO-B inhibitors can be used alone in the management of the mild symptoms of early PD, or as adjunctive therapy to extend the duration of benefit from levodopa.

      Adverse effects of selegiline are relatively infrequent when the drug is used early in the disease. Occasional patients report insomnia related to its amphetamine-like metabolite. To minimize insomnia, selegiline should not be used late in the afternoon or evening. Rasagiline, on the other hand, does not produce amphetamine-like metabolites. Although a restricted low-tyramine diet has been recommended by the American Food and Drug Administration to minimize the "cheese effect," such effect is not expected at the recommended doses, designed to maintain selectivity of MAO-B receptors.

      Patients taking MAO-B inhibitors should not be given meperidine (Demerol; Sanofi) for pain control or **dextromethorphan.** Although serotonin syndrome has been reported in patients taking selegiline with selective serotonin reuptake inhibitors (SSRIs), many patients are on this combination without adverse effects, and the incidence of this serious complication has been estimated to be 0.04%.

(2) Amantadine (Symmetrel) is used in the management of mild-to-moderate PD and is most helpful in addressing tremor and levodopa-induced dyskinesias. The various mechanisms of action include N-methyl-D-aspartate receptor antagonism, blockade of dopamine reuptake, stimulation of dopamine receptors, and promotion of dopamine release.

Amantadine is excreted unchanged in the urine. The usual dosage range is 100 mg two or three times a day (Table 45.1). Elderly patients and those sensitive to the effects of medications should probably start with 25 mg/day for a few days, using a syrup formulation.

Adverse effects of amantadine may be mild, but some are intolerable. The most common are leg edema and **livedo reticularis**, a mottling discoloration of the lower limbs, as well as effects associated with its anticholinergic properties which occur principally in older patients, such as disorientation, hallucinations, dry mouth, and blurry vision.

(3) Anticholinergic drugs are some of the oldest pharmacologic therapies for the management of PD. Dopamine depletion in the striatum causes a relative "hypercholinergic" state that responds to the use of anticholinergic drugs. Many centrally acting anticholinergic drugs are available, but the two most commonly used in the United States are **trihexyphenidyl** (Artane) and **benztropine** (Cogentin).

Anticholinergics may be used early in the course of PD. Tremor remains the only practical indication for their use given the poor side-effect profile (see below). Typically, **trihexyphenidyl** is started at doses of 1 mg/day and increased weekly up to 2 mg four times per day until symptomatic control is obtained or side effects develop. **Benztropine** usually is started at 0.5 mg/day and titrated up to 4 mg/day. If anticholinergics are to be discontinued, this should be done gradually to avoid withdrawal effects.

TABLE 45.1 Antiparkinsonian Medications

Drug	Total Daily Dose (mg)	Frequency
Selegiline	5–10	b.i.d. (morning and noon)
Zydis selegiline	1.25–2.5	q.d.
Rasagiline	1	q.d.
Amantadine	200–300	b.i.d.–t.i.d.
Trihexyphenidyl	4–8	b.i.d.–q.i.d.
Benztropine	2–4	b.i.d.–q.i.d.
Pramipexole	1–4.5	t.i.d.
Ropinirole	3–24	t.i.d.
Rotigotine	2–8	q.d.
Apomorphine	2–6 mg (0.2–0.6 mL) per dose	q.d.–6/d p.r.n.
Levodopa	300–3,000	q.i.d.–q 2 h
Levodopa CR[a]	200–400	q.h.s.
Levodopa extended-release capsules[b]	285–3,900	t.i.d.–5×/d
Levodopa enteral suspension[b]	300–2,000	Continuous 16 hr/d
Entacapone (with levodopa)	300–500	t.i.d.–5/d

[a] Levodopa CR is no longer recommended for daily use given its unpredictable pharmacokinetic profile. Its use is restricted to bedtime to address nocturnal or early-morning PD symptoms.
[b] Levodopa extended-release capsules (Rytary) and Levodopa enteral suspension (Duopa) were approved by the FDA in 2015.
Abbreviations: ACR, controlled-release; b.i.d., twice a day; FDA, Food and Drug Administration; PD, Parkinson's disease; p.r.n., as needed; q.d., every day; q.i.d., four times a day; q.h., every hour; t.i.d., three times a day.

Adverse effects of anticholinergic medications include both **peripheral antimuscarinic side effects** (e.g., dry mouth, impaired visual accommodation, urinary retention, constipation, tachycardia, and impaired sweating) and **central effects** (e.g., sedation, dysphoria, memory difficulties, confusion, and hallucinations).

(4) **Dopamine receptor agonists** directly stimulate dopamine receptors. The current commercially available oral dopamine agonists used for the treatment of PD in the United States are **pramipexole** (Mirapex) and **ropinirole** (Requip). Once-daily extended-release formulations are available for both pramipexole and ropinirole. **Rotigotine** (Neupro) is a transdermally delivered dopamine agonist, and **apomorphine** (Apokyn) is administered subcutaneously with a rapid onset of action but very short duration of benefit (60 to 90 minutes). The long-acting ergot derivatives **bromocriptine** and **cabergoline** are rarely used for the treatment of PD. Their use in North America has been largely restricted to the treatment of hyperprolactinemia.

Dopamine receptor agonists may relieve all of the cardinal manifestations of PD. Despite the theoretical advantages over levodopa by acting directly on striatal dopamine receptors while circumventing the degenerating dopaminergic neurons, dopamine agonists are less effective than levodopa, yielding a lower risk of **dyskinesia** and **motor fluctuation** compared with it, and have an extensive list of potential side effects. Agonists can be used both as monotherapy and as adjuncts to levodopa. To minimize side effects, the dosage of a dopamine agonist should be increased gradually until the desired effect is obtained. Table 45.1 shows common dosages for different antiparkinsonian drugs. Currently, apomorphine can only be administered subcutaneously as a rescue treatment for intractable and disabling wearing off, although it is available as a subcutaneous infusion therapy in Europe. Apomorphine titration in the clinic or under the supervision of a nurse at home to monitor for emesis and orthostatic hypotension is required to determine the correct dose of the drug while the patient is pretreated with an antiemetic, such as **domperidone** or **trimethobenzamide**.

Dopaminergic adverse effects of dopamine agonists include **nausea, vomiting, orthostatic hypotension, excessive daytime sleepiness**, and **psychiatric manifestations** including visual hallucinations and impulse-control disorders. Elderly and cognitively impaired patients are more prone to psychiatric side effects. **Impulse-control disorders** (excessive shopping, compulsive gambling, and hypersexuality, among others) may develop even after 20 months have elapsed after the onset of therapy, which demands regular monitoring. Also in the long term, dopamine agonists can cause **leg edema** and livedo reticularis. Older **ergot-derived dopamine agonists** such as bromocriptine and cabergoline in rare instances cause **pulmonary** and **retroperitoneal fibrosis, cardiac valvulopathy, vasospasm,** and **erythromelalgia** and can exacerbate **angina** and **peptic ulcer disease**.

(5) **Levodopa** is the most effective antiparkinsonian medication (Video 45.1). It is mainly absorbed in the proximal small intestine by a carrier-mediated process for neutral amino acids and is similarly transported across the blood–brain barrier. Once in the brain, it is converted to dopamine by the enzyme aromatic L-amino acid decarboxylase. Levodopa is administered in combination with a peripheral dopa decarboxylase inhibitor (carbidopa in North America or benserazide in Europe) which markedly reduces the required total daily dose of levodopa and minimizes the gastrointestinal side effects and hypotension caused by peripheral conversion of levodopa to dopamine.

Currently available preparations of carbidopa–levodopa include **immediate-release carbidopa–levodopa** (Sinemet), an orally disintegrating tablet (Parcopa), a **controlled-release** preparation (Sinemet CR), an **extended-release capsule** formulation (Rytary), and an **enteral suspension** (Duopa) for continuous administration through a portable infusion pump. A minimum of 75 mg/day of carbidopa is required for appropriate peripheral decarboxylation. While both controlled- and extended-release preparations are less bioavailable than immediate-release carbidopa–levodopa, the erratic pharmacokinetics of the CR form generally limits its use to nighttime administration for the treatment of nocturnal or early-morning reemergence of parkinsonian symptoms. The ER capsule formulation comprises different types of beads including immediate-release and extended-release beads combined in a specific ratio, designed to allow for an onset as rapid that of IR, but allowing for a longer duration of benefit.

Levodopa generally relieves all of the cardinal signs of PD—bradykinesia, tremor, and rigidity. It should be the first-line treatment in any patient older than 70 years of age or in younger individuals with moderate-to-severe disability. Unlike the core deficits of tremor, bradykinesia, and rigidity, axial deficits, such as impaired postural reflexes, hypophonia, and dysphagia, are less reliably improved. A lack of response to levodopa may suggest a diagnosis of one of the atypical parkinsonisms, but an adequate trial with doses up to 1,500 mg of levodopa should be tried before considering anyone a nonresponder. Treatment with carbidopa–levodopa usually is initiated using 25 per 100 immediate-release tablets titrating slowly upward to minimize any acute side effects.

As the disease progresses, patients may develop motor complications in the form of motor fluctuations with **wearing off** toward the end of a dose cycle (reemergence of parkinsonian deficits or appearance of end-of-dose or early-morning dystonia) or choreic or choreathetoid movements (**dyskinesia**). **Wearing off** can be improved by decreasing the interdose interval of levodopa, increasing the individual levodopa doses, changing to the ER capsule formulation, adding a catechol-o-methyl-transferase (COMT) or MAO-B inhibitor, or considering apomorphine subcutaneous injections. Choreic movements of the upper body, predominantly head and neck, are often indicative of **peak-dose dyskinesia** and require lowering the levodopa dose, increasing the interdose interval, or adding amantadine. Choreic movements predominantly of the lower body, especially legs, feet, and pelvis, may occur at the beginning of or at the end of a dose cycle of levodopa and are referred to as **diphasic dyskinesia**. Unlike peak-dose dyskinesias, diphasic dyskinesias are treated by increasing the dose of levodopa or decreasing the interdose interval. In general, motor complications, particularly dyskinesia, begin after 2 to 10 years of levodopa therapy. Younger patients are more prone to dyskinesia and motor fluctuations earlier in the course of the disease. When medication adjustments do not improve these motor complications, deep brain stimulation (DBS) of the subthalamic nucleus (STN) or internal segment of the globus pallidus (GPi) may be considered (see section **A.3** under Hypokinetic Movement Disorders, below). Alternatively, prominent motor fluctuations can also be improved by implanting a percutaneous gastrojejunostomy tube and administering a continuous infusion of carbidopa–levodopa enteral suspension via a portable infusion pump.

Adverse effects of levodopa can be classified into acute and chronic. In the short term, **nausea, vomiting,** and hypotension-related lightheadedness can be addressed by adding extra carbidopa (Lodosyn), 25 to 75 mg three times per day, to enhance the peripheral decarboxylation and minimize bioavailability of dopamine outside the brain, where this is typically toxic. Another option is to use a peripheral dopamine receptor blocker such as **domperidone**. Due to the possibility of ventricular arrhythmia and QT prolongation, doses of domperidone should be kept ideally at 10 mg three times a day, and raised only if needed to 20 mg three times per day. Domperidone is not currently available in the United States but can be readily obtained from Canadian online pharmacies.

In the long term, patients may develop behavioral complications in the form of psychosis, paranoia, sexual preoccupation, impulse-control disorder, mania, or agitation. **Visual hallucinations** can be quite vivid in the form of people or animals. The psychosis is usually dose-dependent and typically lessens with medication reduction, although at the expense of deterioration of motor function. **Quetiapine** (Seroquel) or **clozapine** (Clozaril) may be considered in these cases, as the only antipsychotics safe to use in PD. **Pimavanserin** (Nuplazid), a selective serotonin 5-HT2A inverse agonist, is the first FDA-approved medication for psychosis associated with PD. Reports of accelerated melanoma growth in PD patients taking levodopa have been published. However, melanoma seems to be more prevalent among PD patients regardless of their exposure to levodopa or other PD drugs.

(6) **COMT inhibitors** are used as adjuncts to levodopa. By blocking the peripheral conversion of levodopa to 3-o-methyldopa, COMT inhibitors increase the bioavailability of levodopa. Two COMT inhibitors are available—**tolcapone** (Tasmar) and **entacapone** (Comtan). A combination carbidopa–levodopa–entacapone preparation (Stalevo) is also available. Tolcapone is used in doses of 100 to 200 mg three times a day, and entacapone 200 mg is given with each dose of levodopa up to 2,000 mg/day. If tolcapone is used, liver function tests should be monitored periodically at least for the first 6 months because of earlier reports of rare cases of tolcapone-induced **liver failure**, some fatal. Side effects of COMT inhibitors are related to increased bioavailability of levodopa. In addition, **diarrhea** and a **brownish-orange discoloration of the urine** may occur.

(7) **Visual hallucinations** and **psychosis** are adverse effects that can occur in association with any antiparkinsonian medication. Any potential triggering event, such as infections or metabolic derangements, should be actively sought and treated, if present. Otherwise, decreasing or discontinuing the dose of dopaminergic medications is warranted, in the following order if hallucinations persist: anticholinergics, amantadine, selegiline/rasagiline, and dopamine agonists. If worsening of motor symptoms make such a reduction impossible, the judicious use of one of the safe atypical antipsychotics quetiapine or clozapine, or an acetylcholinesterase inhibitor, such as rivastigmine, may be necessary. **Clozapine** (Clozaril) is typically started at a dose of 12.5 mg at bedtime, and increased slowly to benefit. Because 1% to 2% of patients taking clozapine may experience **agranulocytosis,** patients should be monitored with weekly blood counts. **Quetiapine** (Seroquel) is effective in the management of dopaminergic-induced psychosis at doses of 12.5 mg to 300 at night without worsening parkinsonism. Pimavanserin (Nuplazid) can also be used at a dose of 34 mg daily.

(8) **Constipation** is a common problem among PD patients. Management should include dietary modifications, increasing fluid and fiber intake, exercise, and minimizing or eliminating the use of anticholinergic medications. **Psyllium** (Metamucil), **polyethylene glycol** (Miralax), **sorbitol** and **lactulose** can be helpful, as well as agents that stimulate intestinal motility such as **bisacodyl** (Dulcolax). Some patients may need enemas.

(9) Other potential problems of patients with PD include **nocturia, urinary urgency and frequency, erectile dysfunction, dysphagia, orthostatic hypotension,** and **sleep problems** (see Chapters 7, 9, 18, and 32). **Depression** requires special mention as it affects about 50% of patients with PD and may respond to antidepressant medications such as SSRIs and SNRIs, given the involvement of serotonin but importantly of norepinephrine in PD.

3. **Surgical treatment of PD.** The neurosurgical treatment of PD has progressed from destructive and lesional procedures to focused and targeted brain stimulation. The success of surgical treatment depends on a careful selection of the appropriate candidates. First, only patients with idiopathic PD should be considered. Patients with advanced disease, poor response to levodopa, dementia, uncontrolled depression, uncontrolled hallucinations, and unstable medical problems are unlikely to benefit from these procedures. Surgical candidates should undergo a presurgical neuropsychological evaluation to rule out substantial cognitive dysfunction. The effects of DBS typically mirror the benefits of levodopa, however, with the benefit of reducing motor fluctuations and off time, as well as decreasing dyskinesia. The two main targets for DBS in PD, the subthalamic nucleus (STN) and internal segment of the globus pallidus (GPi), appear to give similar outcomes, although individual patient factors and surgeon expertise may be important.

   a. **Thalamic DBS** is effective at reducing tremor in PD, and although the benefit is sustained, Vim DBS does not address bradykinesia or other PD symptoms, which invariably progress over time.

   b. **STN DBS** yields excellent antiparkinsonian benefit and allows for greater medication reduction than GPi stimulation.

c. **Pallidal DBS,** targeting the posteroventral GPi, is more effective at reducing dyskinesia and secondary dystonia. Although there is some suggestion that GPi DBS is "safer" from a neurocognitive standpoint, leading some to suggest this target for cognitively impaired patients who are otherwise good candidates, controlled clinical trials have not demonstrated significant cognitive differences in outcomes between the two targets.

B. **Atypical parkinsonism** are a group of rare degenerative conditions within the akinetic-rigid syndrome to which PD belongs.

1. **Multiple system atrophy (MSA)** is a progressive neurodegenerative disease characterized by a combination of **parkinsonism, cerebellar dysfunction,** and **autonomic failure.** The nomenclature MSA-P and MSA-C are used when parkinsonian or cerebellar features predominate, respectively. The parkinsonism tends to be tremorless. Clinical features that suggest the diagnosis are hyperreflexia or other corticospinal signs, severe early orthostatic hypotension and/or urinary incontinence, atypical levodopa-induced dyskinesias (affecting face [sardonic grin] and feet), Pisa syndrome (lateral truncal deviation), and inspiratory stridor.

a. Levodopa may provide transient improvement of parkinsonian sympoms albeit rarely sustained beyond 1 year. Other dopaminergic drugs are not indicated.

b. Orthostatic hypotension may be the greatest source of disability and can be worsened by levodopa. Nonpharmacologic measures include liberalizing salt and water intake, using waist or thigh-high compressive leg stockings during the day, and raising the head of the bed 8 inches (20 cm) at night to minimize supine hypertension and excessive nocturnal diuresis. Patients should be careful rising from the sitting or supine positions and should avoid heavy meals. When pharmacotherapy is required, the peripheral α-1-adrenergic receptor agonist **midodrine** (ProAmatine) may be used, starting at 2.5 mg three times a day, increasing by 2.5-mg weekly increments up to a maximum of 10 mg three times a day. When midodrine is insufficient, treatment with the mineralocorticoid **fludrocortisone** (Florinef) may be added at doses of 0.1 to 0.3 mg/day, as needed. The norepinephrine precursor **droxidopa** (Northera), starting at 100 mg and increasing up to 600 mg three times a day, as tolerated, has also been shown to improve postural lightheadedness in patients with orthostatic hypotension. Other potentially useful drugs are methylphenidate, pyridostigmine, erythropoietin, ergots, and desmopressin.

c. **Urinary frequency** or **incontinence** should be evaluated with the assistance of an urologist. Treatments such as **oxybutynin** (Ditropan), **solifenacin** (Vesicare), **tolterodine** (Detrol), **darifenacin** (Enablex), or **trospium chloride** (Sanctura) for a spastic bladder or **bethanechol** (Urecholine) for a hypotonic bladder may provide relief. Some patients need intermittent or continuous catheterization. **Sildefanil** (Viagra), **tadalafil** (Cialis), and **vardenafil** (Levitra) may be useful for management of erectile dysfunction.

d. Dysarthria and dysphagia may benefit from evaluation by a speech therapist. Some patients with severe dysphagia need percutaneous gastrostomy. Gait difficulties and instability may necessitate use of supportive devices and physical therapy. Patients with MSA and inspiratory stridor should undergo a sleep study to determine whether concurrent obstructive sleep apnea requires treatment.

2. **Progressive supranuclear palsy (PSP)** is an atypical parkinsonism characterized by early postural instability and falls, disproportionate neck rigidity (sometimes with retrocollis), facial dystonia, supranuclear vertical gaze abnormalities, pseudobulbar affect, subcortical frontal dementia, and apathy.

a. **Management** of PSP is extremely limited. Antiparkinsonian medications are rarely helpful, although a trial of levodopa is prudent.

b. Symptomatic palliative therapies for PSP include management of dysarthria and dysphagia with the assistance of a speech therapist and may include the use of a gastrostomy tube among other measures. Because of the significantly decreased blinking rate, patients with PSP are at increased risk of keratitis and should use artificial tears. Blepharospasm and neck dystonia can be managed with botulinum toxin injections. Depression can be managed with serotonergic and/or noradrenergic antidepressants and emotional incontinence **(pseudobulbar affect)** with **dextromethorphan/quinidine** (Nuedexta). Dystonia may benefit from amantadine. Gait instability can be managed with physical therapy and supportive devices.

HYPERKINETIC MOVEMENT DISORDERS

A. **Chorea** is an involuntary movement disorder characterized by irregular, dance-like jerky movements occurring within or between body parts in a random sequence. It can result from a variety of disorders of the basal ganglia.

1. **Huntington's disease (HD)** is an autosomal-dominant degenerative brain disorder characterized by the insidious development of motor, cognitive, and psychiatric symptoms progressing toward death on average of about 20 years after onset of symptoms. The underlying genetic defect is the expansion of a CAG trinucleotide repeat of the *htt* gene, the product of which is a protein called **huntingtin.** Symptomatic treatment is directed at the major clinical features of the disease.

   a. Choreiform movements can be reliably controlled with **neuroleptics** that have potent postsynaptic dopamine blocking effects such as haloperidol. Benzodiazepines such as lorazepam and clonazepam may also decrease chorea. **Tetrabenazine** (Xenazine), a reversible dopamine depleter and mild postsynaptic dopamine blocker, is effective in reducing chorea. Effective doses range from 12.5 to 50 mg three times a day.

   b. **Depression** affects at least 30% to 50% of patients with HD. In HD patients, the suicide rate is four to eight times greater than in the general population. Depression can be managed with all standard agents used for the management of major depression. **SSRIs** typically are the drugs of choice for HD. **Mirtazapine** (Remeron) can be helpful in the care of HD patients with cachexia, anxiety, and insomnia because it can increase body weight and assist in sleep induction.

   c. **Irritability and aggressive behavior** are common psychiatric manifestations in HD. First-line therapy for these symptoms is typically an SSRI or neuroleptic. Propranolol (Inderal), valproic acid (Depakote), and carbamazepine (Tegretol) are also potentially useful to treat aggressive behavior related to frustration and impatience.

   d. **Mania** and **hypomania** can occur, although they may be difficult to distinguish from impulsivity and disinhibition associated with the dysexecutive syndrome common in HD. Approximately 10% of HD patients may exhibit hypomanic behavior. Therapeutic alternatives include valproic acid, **lamotrigine** (Lamictal), and carbamazepine, whereas lithium is less effective.

   e. **Psychosis** has an estimated frequency of 3% to 25% among patients with HD and is more common among patients with early-onset disease. Antipsychotic medications such as **risperidone** (Risperdal) or **olanzapine** (Zyprexa) can be effective at reducing these symptoms, and can also help with chorea.

2. Other causes of chorea include neurodegenerative disorders (e.g., chorea-acanthocytosis, Wilson's disease [WD], and dentatorubropallidoluysian atrophy), Sydenham's chorea, systemic lupus erythematosus, hyperthyroidism, and drug-induced chorea (e.g., phenytoin, oral contraceptives, stimulants, or antiparkinsonian drugs). Regardless of the underlying cause, the movements can be improved with the use of neuroleptics. However, disease-specific treatments should be pursued as appropriate (e.g., warfarin in antiphospholipid antibody syndrome, penicillin in Sydenham's chorea). The risk of tardive dyskinesia (TD) is uncertain when neuroleptics are used in the treatment of chorea.

3. **NMDA-receptor antibody encephalitis** is an autoimmune disorder associated with ovarian teratoma due to antibodies against the NMDA receptor. It is most common in young African-American women with choreoathetotic (dyskinetic) movements of the craniofacial region in the setting of "wakeful unresponsiveness," particularly if preceded by psychotic features and seizures. Treatment includes **first-line immunotherapy (steroids, intravenous immunoglobulin, plasmapheresis),** second-line immunotherapy (rituximab, cyclophosphamide), and teratoma removal.

4. **Hemiballismus** is a severe form of chorea, with violent, flailing movements of the proximal aspect of the limbs on one side of the body. It is classically caused by lesions in the **contralateral** STN, but lesions outside the STN are more common. Non-ketotic hyperglycemia is the most common metabolic cause. Treatment includes supportive care, prevention of self-injury, and pharmacologic agents such as benzodiazepines, neuroleptics, and catecholamine-depleting agents (reserpine or tetrabenazine). Valproic acid and other gamma-aminobutyric acid (GABA)-ergic drugs may be alternative therapeutic options. Surgical alternatives exist for patients who do not appropriately respond to medical therapy.

B. Tics are common movement disorders, affecting as many as 20% of children. They are brief, rapid, purposeless, repetitive movements involving one or more muscular groups. They are differentiated from other paroxysmal movement disorders by their partial voluntary control with suppressability when performing complex tasks, premonitory "urge," and stereotypic appearance.

1. **Tourette's syndrome (TS)** is a childhood-onset neuropsychiatric disorder characterized by motor and phonic tics. Tics wax and wane and tend to improve considerably during adulthood. **Obsessive–compulsive behavior** and **attention deficit disorder (ADD)** are comorbid conditions frequently associated with TS and may be more disabling than tics themselves.

   a. **Tics** do not require treatment unless they are troublesome to the patient. The first step in treatment is education and reassurance. Cognitive behavioral therapy has emerged as an effective nonpharmacologic intervention. If further symptomatic improvement is needed, **clonidine** (Catapres) starting at 0.05 mg at bedtime and increased 0.05 mg every few days can be considered. The efficacy of clonidine for tic control is modest, however. **Guanfacine** (Tenex) starting at 0.5 to 1 mg at bedtime is another option that may be less sedating than clonidine.

   Neuroleptics are the most efficacious agents for tic suppression. **Haloperidol** is probably the most commonly used neuroleptic for tics. **Pimozide** (Orap) was developed specifically for use in TS and may cause less sedation than haloperidol does. Other typical neuroleptics such as fluphenazine, **trifluoperazine**, and **thiothixene** can also be helpful. Atypical antipsychotics such as **risperidone** (Risperdal), **ziprasidone** (Geodon), **aripripazole** (Abilify), and **olanzapine** (Zyprexa) may be used. The necessary dosage can vary widely among patients and at different times for a given patient, given the fluctuating severity of the natural history of tics. Sedation and depression may be troublesome side effects, and the risk of QT interval prolongation should be noted. Although the risk of TD appears to be low among patients with TS, this potential long-term adverse effect must be discussed with patients and documented in the medical record. Tetrabenazine (Xenazine) is effective for tic suppression and is not linked with TD. **Clonazepam** (Klonopin) and baclofen may be helpful to some patients. Botulinum toxin injections may be helpful for some tics.

   b. Management of **obsessive–compulsive behavior** associated with TS is identical to that of the purely psychiatric condition. SSRIs and **clomipramine** (Anafranil), may be used in this regard. The major adverse effects of clomipramine are sedation and anticholinergic effects.

   c. **ADD** and other behavioral disorders of children may be difficult to control. Clonidine, tricyclic antidepressants, or selegiline may be effective. Use of central nervous system (CNS) stimulants such as **methylphenidate** (Ritalin) may ease ADD. **Modafinil** (Provigil) may be useful as well. The diverse behavioral abnormalities sometimes exhibited by children with TS not infrequently necessitate family counseling and other nonpharmacologic approaches.

C. Myoclonus is a shock-like, brief, involuntary movement caused by muscular contraction (positive myoclonus) or muscular inhibition (negative myoclonus). Myoclonus can originate from the cortex, subcortical areas, brainstem, or spinal cord. Common causes of myoclonus include metabolic derangements, such as renal and hepatic failure, epileptiform disorders, and neurodegenerative disorders.

1. **Diagnosis** should include a thorough history and physical examination plus blood glucose and electrolytes, drug and toxin screen, renal and hepatic function tests, brain imaging, and EEG. A search for inborn errors of metabolism and paraneoplastic antibodies may be indicated in some cases.

2. The ideal therapy for myoclonus is to manage the underlying condition. However, symptomatic treatment should be used if treatment is likely to make a significant functional impact (Table 45.2). **Clonazepam** at 2 to 6 mg/day, **valproic acid** (Depakote) 250 to 1,500 mg/day, **levetiracetam** (Keppra) 500 to 4,000 mg/day, and **piracetam** up to 24 g/day (not available in the United States) are first-line drugs for the management of myoclonus. Many patients need polytherapy to control myoclonus.

D. Tardive Dyskinesia is a generic term used to describe persistent involuntary movements that occur as a consequence of long-term treatment with dopamine receptor antagonists.

TABLE 45.2 Medications Used in the Management of Myoclonus

Drugs	Total Daily Dose (mg)	Frequency
Usually Helpful Drugs		
Clonazepam	0.5–20	b.i.d.–t.i.d.
Valproic acid	250–2,500	b.i.d.–q.i.d.
Piracetam	1,000–24,000	t.i.d.
Levetiracetam	500–3,000	b.i.d.–t.i.d.
Occasionally Helpful Drugs		
Zonisamide	100–600	q.d.–b.i.d.
Primidone	125–1,500	b.i.d.–t.i.d.
5-hydroxytryptophan (with carbidopa)	100–3,000	q.i.d.
Tetrabenazine	50–200	b.i.d.–t.i.d.
Trihexyphenidyl	1–60	t.i.d.
Propranolol	40–240	b.i.d.–t.i.d.

Abbreviations: b.i.d., twice a day; q.i.d., four times a day; q.d., every day; t.i.d., three times a day.

Antipsychotics are the main causative group of medications, but antiemetics such as metoclopramide, prochlorperazine, and promethazine may also induce TD. The risk factors for development of classic TD include old age, female gender, mood disorder, and "organic" brain dysfunction. Classic TD usually consists of oral–buccal–lingual dyskinesia that may be associated with a variety of repetitive limb or trunk stereotyped movements.

1. The pathophysiologic mechanism of TD is not completely understood, but it is thought to be related to an increased number and affinity of postsynaptic D2 dopamine receptors in the striatum. The patient's condition may initially improve after the offending agent is restarted or after the dosage is increased. Unfortunately, this is likely to perpetuate the problem.

2. The ideal management of TD would be prevention of this condition by avoiding unnecessary use of dopamine receptor antagonists and using the minimally effective dose. Anticholinergic medications can worsen classic TD.

   a. **Dopamine depleters** such as **reserpine** or **tetrabenazine** have been among the most useful medications to treat TD. Dosages of reserpine usually are started at 0.10 to 0.25 mg three times a day and may be gradually increased to 3 to 5 mg/day. Reserpine may cause parkinsonism, depression, orthostatic hypotension, and peptic ulcer disease. Tetrabenazine can be started at 25 mg/day and gradually increased up to 150 mg/day in divided doses. The most common limiting side effects are sedation, depression, and parkinsonism.

   b. **Benzodiazepines** may prove useful for patients with mild symptoms. Long-acting agents such as clonazepam (usually 1.5 to 3 mg/day) provide the most consistent relief of symptoms.

   c. **Branched-chain amino acids** (Tarvil) have been shown to significantly decrease TD symptoms in males. It is used at a dose of 222 mg/kg three times a day.

   d. **Neuroleptics,** used in the lowest possible dosages, may be necessary if symptoms markedly interfere with activities of daily living.

   e. **Tardive dystonia** is a subtype of TD that typically affects younger people. It usually involves the neck and trunk muscles. Management of tardive dystonia differs from that of classic TD in that anticholinergics are potentially beneficial, and botulinum toxin can be used in focal or segmental forms. Dopamine depleters are also useful. GPi DBS may also be considered.

   f. For many patients, combination therapy is most effective. The use of a benzodiazepine with either a dopamine depleter or a low dosage of an atypical neuroleptic may be necessary. Vitamin E might prevent further deterioration of TD, but it is not really clear if it can improve TD symptoms. The eventual rate of remission is approximately 60% and improvement is slow, taking as long as 2 years.

E. **Dystonia** is a syndrome of sustained muscle contraction causing abnormal repetitive movements, twisting, or abnormal postures. Numerous genetic forms of dystonia exist, and are typically designated as DYTn. Idiopathic dystonia can be generalized or restricted to a particular muscle group. With the exception of DYT3 (X-linked Lubag disease), patients with primary idiopathic dystonia have no gross or microscopic abnormalities. Secondary dystonia includes several inherited inborn errors of metabolism such as dopa-responsive dystonia (DRD or DYT5) and WD. Trauma, vascular disease, space-occupying lesions, drugs, and toxins are other causes of secondary dystonia.

1. **DRD** or **DYT5** is an autosomal-dominant disorder caused by a mutation in the *GTP cyclohydrolase I gene*. It usually becomes apparent during childhood with a gait disorder, foot cramping, or toe walking. It can involve the trunk and arms and can be misdiagnosed as cerebral palsy. Patients with this form of dystonia have few symptoms after first awakening but the symptoms progress throughout the day. This disorder is exquisitely sensitive to small doses of levodopa (50 to 200 mg). A brief trial of levodopa for childhood-onset dystonia is frequently recommended to exclude DRD.

2. Medical management of dystonia of any cause can be attempted with the medications listed in Table 45.3. None of these medications provides complete relief of symptoms. Combinations of medications can be beneficial. Extremely high doses of anticholinergic drugs such as trihexyphenidyl have been reported to benefit more than 50% of patients in some trials (sometimes at doses greater than 100 mg/day). Therapy usually is started with 1 mg/day and increased 1 to 2 mg/week divided on a three times a day schedule until control of symptoms is achieved or intolerable adverse effects appear. The combination of a dopamine depleter such as reserpine, an anticholinergic, and a postsynaptic dopamine blocker may be beneficial to patients with severe dystonia. GPi DBS can be offered to patients to with pharmacologically intractable and disabling dystonia.

3. Injection of **botulinum toxin** is the first line of treatment of many patients with focal and segmental dystonia. There are seven botulinum toxin serotypes, but only types A and B are available in the United States—**botulinum toxin type A** -(onabotulinumtoxinA [Botox], abobotulinumtoxinA [Dysport], and incobotulinumtoxinA [Xeomin]) and **botulinum toxin type B** (rimabotulinumtoxinB [MyoBloc]). The toxin is injected directly into the affected muscle, producing reversible pharmacologic denervation. Injections usually are repeated at an average interval of 12 to 16 weeks. Potential side effects include excessive transient weakness of the injected and adjacent muscles, dry mouth, and local hematoma.

F. **Tremor** is probably the most common movement disorder. It is defined as a rhythmic oscillation around an axis of a given body part.

1. **Essential tremor (ET)** is a default diagnosis for a range of tremor disorders that predominantly include postural and kinetic tremor of the hands and, variably, head and

TABLE 45.3 Medications Used in the Management of Dystonia

Class	Example	Dosage
Anticholinergics	Trihexyphenidyl	6–100 mg/d
Dopaminergics	Levodopa	50–300 mg/d
Antidopaminergics	Haloperidol	2–20 mg/d
Benzodiazepines	Diazepam	5–20 mg/d
	Clonazepam	1–10 mg/d
GABA agonists	Baclofen	15–240 mg/d
Antidepressants	Amitriptyline	25–150 mg/d
Anticonvulsants	Carbamazepine	300–1,200 mg/d
	Valproic acid	500–1,500 mg/d
Dopamine depleters	Reserpine	0.5–5 mg/d
	Tetrabenazine	50–300 mg/d
Toxins	Botulinum toxin type A or B	Varies

Abbreviation: MU, mouse units.

TABLE 45.4 Medications Used in the Management of Tremor

Drug	Dose (mg)	Frequency
Propranolol	60–800	b.i.d.–q.i.d.
Propranolol LA	80–320	q.d.
Atenolol	50–150	q.d.
Nadolol	120–240	q.d.
Sotalol	75–200	b.i.d.
Primidone	50–750	q.d.–t.i.d.
Alprazolam	0.125–3	b.i.d.–q.i.d.
Clonazepam	0.5–6	t.i.d.
Topiramate	100–400	q.d.–b.i.d.
Gabapentin	1,200–1,800	t.i.d
Nimodipine	120	q. 4 hr

Abbreviations: b.i.d., twice a day; q., every; q.i.d., four times a day; q.d., every day; t.i.d., three times a day.

vocal cords. A positive family history of tremor is common among ET patients. Tremor typically may improve with small amounts of alcohol. Generally, it is not possible to completely eliminate the tremor, and the goal of therapy should be to normalize activities of daily living. One-half to two-thirds of patients with ET benefit from pharmacologic therapy (Table 45.4). In some cases, the tremor may be quite refractory, and surgical treatment should be considered.

a. **β-Adrenergic receptor antagonists** are used most extensively to manage ET. The clinical response to β-blockers is variable and usually incomplete. These drugs reduce tremor amplitude but not tremor frequency and appear to be less effective in managing voice and head tremor. Nonselective β-blockers such as **propranolol** (Inderal) are preferred. Propranolol should be started at small doses (e.g., 10 mg three times a day) and titrated upward as needed. Doses larger than 320 mg/day usually do not confer additional benefit. Potential side effects of β-blockers include congestive heart failure, second- or third-degree atrioventricular block, worsening of obstructive lung disease, and masking of signs of hypoglycemia. The β-blockers can also cause fatigue, nausea, diarrhea, rash, erectile dysfunction, and depression. **Nadolol** (Corgard) is an option if propranolol causes CNS side effects, as this drug does not readily cross the blood–brain barrier. **Atenolol** (Tenormin), **sotalol** (Betapace), **metoprolol** (Lopressor), and **timolol** are potentially useful in the treatment of ET.

b. **Primidone** (Mysoline) may improve ET. The mechanism of action of primidone for management of tremor is unknown. Primidone decreases the amplitude of tremor but does not alter its frequency. Treatment usually is started at 25 mg at bedtime, and a response may begin at doses between 50 and 350 mg/day. Doses up to 750 mg/day divided three times a day may be required for benefits to appear. Side effects include vertigo, nausea, unsteadiness, and drowsiness.

c. **Benzodiazepines** may be used if the above drugs do not provide sufficient control of symptoms. Long-acting agents such as **clonazepam** can be used, but some patients may respond better to the use of a shorter-acting agent such as **alprazolam** (Xanax). Clonazepam at 1 to 3 mg/day can be very effective in orthostatic tremor. Potential adverse effects include sedation, ataxia, tolerance, and potential for abuse.

d. **Botulinum toxin injections** of limb tremor in ET may offer modest improvement of tremor that might be more cosmetic than functional as no improvement has been seen in functional scales. Transient weakness is the most common side effect.

e. **Other drugs** that may be considered for the management of ET are **gabapentin** (Neurontin), **topiramate** (Topamax), and **zonisamide** (Zonegran).

f. **Surgery** should be considered when activities of daily living are severely affected despite medical management. Stereotactic thalamotomy or Vim DBS improves contralateral tremor.

2. **Fragile X tremor-ataxia syndrome (FXTAS)** is an ET-like X-linked disorder due to premutation expansions in the *FMR1* gene (CGG repeats, 55–200), typically among grandfathers of children with fragile X syndrome. The tremor has a cerebellar component (worsening with action) and patients also exhibit progressive truncal ataxia and cognitive impairment. Family history of mental retardation in children and early menopause or infertility in women are important historical clues. While treatments for ET may work, ataxia and dementia become intractable sources of disability with disease progression. Response to Vim DBS may be short lived.

G. **Wilson's disease** is a rare but treatable autosomal recessive disorder of copper accumulation caused by a defect in copper excretion into the bile. Low-plasma levels of **ceruloplasmin** characterize WD. Copper deposits typically occur in the liver, iris, and basal ganglia. Other organs may be affected as well. A variety of movement disorders can accompany WD, including tremor, dystonia, chorea, dysphagia, dysarthria, and parkinsonism. Symptomatic management of the movement disorder is as discussed in other sections of this chapter.

1. **Recommended screening** methods for patients with neurologic signs and symptoms of WD are as follows:

   a. **Serum ceruloplasmin and slit-lamp examination for Kayser–Fleischer (KF) rings.** Approximately 90% of WD patients who have neurologic symptoms have a low-ceruloplasmin level. KF rings are present in 99.9% of WD patients who have neurologic symptoms.

   b. **24-hour urine copper.** In patients with neurologic WD, the 24-hour urine copper level is always more than 100 μg before chelation treatment. This value may be falsely elevated in patients with long-standing liver disease.

2. Copper-rich foods such as shellfish, chocolate, liver, nuts, and soy products should be avoided. However, this is not sufficient to avoid further accumulation, and **zinc acetate** is used to block mucosal absorption of copper. Zinc acetate is taken at a dose of 50 mg three times a day between meals. The toxicity of zinc is negligible, although it can cause abdominal discomfort. Zinc is the drug of choice for maintenance therapy after chelation and in presymptomatic or pregnant patients.

3. **Penicillamine** (Cuprimine) acts by means of reductive chelation of copper. It mobilizes large amounts of copper, mainly from the liver. The standard dose after a titration phase is 250 mg four times a day, each dose separated from food. Doses up to 1,500 mg/day can be used. Several potentially serious adverse effects are associated with penicillamine. Approximately 50% of patients treated with penicillamine have **marked neurologic deterioration,** and half of these patients do not recover to the pre-penicillamine level of function. Approximately one-third of patients who start taking penicillamine have an **acute hypersensitivity reaction.** Other subacute potential toxicities include **bone marrow suppression,** membranous glomerulopathy, myasthenia gravis, reduced immune response, hepatitis, pemphigus, and a lupus erythematosus-like syndrome with a positive antinuclear antibody. A CBC with platelets and urinalysis are recommended every 2 weeks for the first 6 months of therapy and monthly thereafter.

4. **Trientine** (Syprine) is a chelating agent that induces urinary excretion of copper and has a more favorable side-effect profile than penicillamine, with a lower risk of neurologic deterioration (25%), which makes it more favorable for consideration as initial WD treatment. Dosage and administration are identical to those of penicillamine. Although trientine promotes less copper excretion than does penicillamine, it does not cause a hypersensitivity reaction. The other toxicities are somewhat similar to those of penicillamine but less frequent.

5. **Tetrathiomolybdate** is an experimental drug that prevents absorption of copper from the intestine and is absorbed into the blood, where it binds to copper to form nontoxic complexes. It has been used successfully at a dose of 120 mg/day to manage acute WD with neurologic manifestations.

6. **Liver transplantation** is curative of WD.

Key Points

- Exercise should be considered an essential initial and adjunctive treatment for Parkinson's disease (PD).
- Levodopa is the most effective medical therapy for PD, and therapeutic doses of this medication will bring the most improvement in a patient's function.
- Treatment of the nonmotor symptoms in PD can improve quality of life as they become a disproportionately greater source of disability with disease progression.
- Treatment of the motor and psychiatric symptoms of Huntington's disease can benefit from a multidisciplinary approach.
- Tics do not require treatment unless they are troublesome to the patient; cognitive behavioral therapy may be an effective nonpharmacologic intervention.
- Common causes of myoclonus are metabolic, epileptic, and neurodegenerative; treatment should be targeted to the underlying etiology if possible.
- A trial of levodopa is indicated in childhood-onset (predominantly leg) dystonia, in order to assess for the possibility of dopa-responsive dystonia.
- It is generally difficult to completely abate essential tremor, but medical and surgical therapies can diminish its disability.

Recommended Readings

Albanese A, Bhatia K, Bressman SB, et al. Phenomenology and classification of dystonia: a consensus update. *Mov Disord.* 2013;28(7):863–873.

Connolly BS, Lang AE. Pharmacological treatment of Parkinson disease: a review. *JAMA.* 2014;311(16):1670–1683.

Duker AP, Espay AJ. Surgical treatment of Parkinson disease: past, present, and future. *Neurol Clin.* 2013;31(3):799–808.

McNaught KSP, Mink JW. Advances in understanding and treatment of Tourette syndrome. *Nat Rev Neurol.* 2011;7(12):667–676.

Nance M, Paulsen JS, Rosenblatt A, et al. A Physician's Guide to the Management of Huntington's Disease. 3rd ed. New York, NY: Huntington's Disease Society of America; 2011. http://hdsa .org/wp-content/uploads/2015/03/PhysiciansGuide_3rd-Edition.pdf

Postuma R, Lang A. Hemiballism: revisiting a classic disorder. *Lancet Neurol.* 2003;2(11):661–668.

Stamelou M, Bhatia KP. Atypical parkinsonism: diagnosis and treatment. *Neurol Clin.* 2015;33(1):39–56.

Titulaer MJ, McCracken L, Gabilondo I, et al. Treatment and prognostic factors for long-term outcome in patients with anti-NMDA receptor encephalitis: an observational cohort study. *Lancet Neurol.* 2013;12(2):157–165.

Zesiewicz TA, Elble RJ, Louis ED, et al. Evidence-based guideline update: treatment of essential tremor: report of the Quality Standards subcommittee of the American Academy of Neurology. *Neurology.* 2011;77(19):1752–1755.

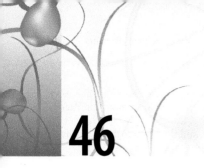

46

Dementia

Annya D. Tisher and Arash Salardini

Dementia is a syndrome of chronic progressive decline in cognition that results in loss of independence and functioning. In 2010, the prevalence of dementia among Americans over the age of 70 years was 14.7% affecting 4.2 million adults. The yearly estimated monetary cost, including estimates for unpaid care provided by families, was between $41,689 and $56,293 per person, contributing to an overall cost of $157 to $215 billion. The prevalence of dementia increases with age. As the global median age increases, the economic costs of dementias become more burdensome. The prevalence of dementia is projected to increase 3-fold by 2050.

Medical management of dementia represents an opportunity to maximize function, reduce harm, improve quality of life, and provide support. We discuss management of dementias and their symptoms.

The goals of treatment are:
- Disease modification
- Cognitive remediation
- Treatment of neuropsychiatric comorbidities
- Harm minimization

TREATMENT MODALITIES

A. **Disease modification.** Where possible, disease modification is the holy grail of dementia treatment. As of yet, there are no specific disease-modifying treatments for neurodegenerative conditions. This is likely to change in the next few years. Presently, disease modification takes the following forms:
1. **Vascular risk factor modification.** The relationship between vascular risk factors and dementias, especially Alzheimer's disease (AD) and vascular dementia, is well established. One possible explanation for increased risk of AD is that the "glymphatic" system, which removes large molecules from the brain, relies on the pulsatility of cerebral vessels. The modifiable vascular risk factors established as contributing to AD include: diabetes mellitus, arterial hypertension, obesity, cigarette smoking, alcohol abuse, high serum cholesterol levels, coronary heart disease, renal dysfunction, high unsaturated fat intake, and inflammation.

   Prediabetes (metabolic syndrome) and diabetes increase the risk of progression from mild cognitive impairment (MCI) to AD. People with treated diabetes are less likely to progress from MCI to AD. Diabetes and metabolic syndrome are associated with atherosclerosis, brain infarcts, and microvascular abnormalities leading to vascular lesions that accumulate to cause vascular dementia. Insulin has also been found to inhibit beta amyloid degradation and has been specifically associated with cognitive decline and AD. Hyperinsulinemia is seen in type 2 diabetes.
2. **Prevention of delirium.** Patients with dementia are at increased risk for delirium (See Chapter 1). Delirium itself is associated with an elevated risk of long-term cognitive impairment. While onset of delirium is usually acute, patients with dementia can take months to recover fully from an episode of delirium and may not return to their previous level of functioning. There is data suggesting that delirium is a neurotoxic condition. Delirium risk can be minimized by simple nonpharmacologic interventions such as reorienting a patient frequently, having a consistent daily schedule with daily rituals,

maintaining a normal sleep wake cycle, and encouraging time with family, loved ones, and familiar care givers.

Medications should be reviewed and patients should be taken off medications that can affect cognition. Below is a list of medications known to be delirogenic (Table 46.1).

a. Anticholinergic medications are of particular concern as they can cause acute cognitive impairment even after a single dose. There is also evidence that higher cumulative use of anticholinergic medications increases the risk of dementia.

b. Benzodiazepines are also of significant concern and are heavily prescribed to elderly patients. Benzodiazepine use is known to be amnestic even at single low doses. It is also a frequently documented contributor to delirium. An association exists between long-term use of benzodiazepines and AD, although this remains controversial.

3. Lifestyle changes which may help with disease progression.

a. Supplements. The golden rule of over-the-counter supplementation is the following: there is no strong evidence for any of them, but if they are benign in terms of side effects and are cheap, then they may be tried by the patient. Potential candidates for this include resveratrol (found in wine but not at biologically active concentrations), curcumin (found in turmeric with questionable penetration across the blood–brain barrier), coconut oil and medium chain fatty acids (released under the brand name of Axona and approved by the Food and Drug Administration (FDA) as a medical food supplement), and omega 3 polyunsaturated fats as they have a proven cardiovascular benefit.

b. Mediterranean diet. A diet rich in complex carbohydrates and mono-unsaturated oils may be protective against disease progression. It has been shown in several prospective studies to be protective against AD as well as cardiovascular disease, hypertension, and obesity.

c. Exercise. Aerobic exercise, even 20 minutes three times per week, may have positive effects on the brain independent of its vascular benefits. Exercise has been shown to improve cardiovascular function, bone health, mood, and sleep. It has also been shown to have a protective effect against cognitive decline even in institutionalized individuals with dementia. The mechanisms by which exercise may be protective include improvement in insulin resistance and central adiposity, decrement of oxidative stress and inflammation, improvement in vascular function, increased cerebral blood flow (CBF), and direct increases in the production of neurotrophic factors in the brain.

d. Mental engagement. An intellectually enriched life, which includes taking up new hobbies and knowledge, may increase brain connectivity and partially counteract the effects of synaptic loss. Studies have shown benefits of cognitive stimulation in cognitive function and quality of life but not in functional status, behavior, or mood. Activities should, however, be appropriate for the patient's mental abilities; otherwise, excessive frustration can worsen behavior and mood.

e. Social engagement similarly is thought to increase brain connectivity and mood. Positive relationships have been shown to have healing effects on mood and emotional regulation. Social engagement is key to a high quality of life. Social withdrawal is a common reaction to receiving the diagnosis of dementia or MCI as patients feel a decreased sense of self-worth. This often leads to depression and patients should be counseled about this and encouraged to keep up with social activities as much as they feel able.

4. Clinical trials. The neurologist is often the source of information for trial participation by patients with new diagnoses of dementia. Many trials are presently being conducted on potentially disease-modifying agents. A list of these trials is available from http://www.trials.gov.

AD is by far the most common type of dementia and comprises 50% to 75% of all cases. The vast majority of dementia-related research is currently directed at efforts to create disease-modifying drugs for the treatment of AD. AD is defined by the presence of β-amyloid plaques and neurofibrillary tangles made up of hyperphosphorylated tau protein. A number of promising drugs are in trials targeting β-amyloid.

a. One approach has been the development of monoclonal antibodies targeted at various forms of the β-amyloid peptide in an effort to remove these from the brain. This has been shown to cause cognitive improvement in mouse models of AD. Solanezumab

TABLE 46.1 2012 Beers Criteria for Potentially Inappropriate Medication Use in Older Adults

Medication Class	Medications	Recommendation	Rationale
Anticholinergic	Brompheniramine, carbinoxamine, clemastine, cyproheptadine, dexbrompheniramine, diphenhydramine (oral), doxylamine, hydroxyzine, promethazine, triprolidine	Avoid, except diphenhydramine in the case of acute allergic reaction	Highly anticholinergic, clearance reduced with age.
Antiparkinson agents	Benztropine, trihexyphenidyl	Avoid	Better tolerated Parkinson's treatments exist
Antispasmodics	Belladonna alkaloids, clidinium-chlordiazepoxide, dicyclomine, hyoscyamine, propantheline, scopolamine	Avoid except in short-term palliative care to decrease oral secretions	Highly anticholinergic, uncertain effectiveness
Antithrombotic	Dipyridamole (oral short acting), ticlopidine	Avoid, IV form of dipyridamole acceptable for use in cardiac stress testing	Orthostatic hypotension, safer alternatives available
Anti-infective	Nitrofurantoin	Avoid for long-term suppression	Potential pulmonary toxicity, lack of efficacy if CrCl <60 mL/min due to inadequate drug concentration in urine
Alpha₁ blockers	Doxazosin, prazosin, terazosin	Avoid	High risk of orthostatic hypotension
Alpha blockers, central	Clonidine, guanabenz, guanfacine, methyldopa, reserpine (>0.1 mg/d)	Avoid	High risk of adverse CNS effects, bradycardia, orthostatic hypotension
Antiarrhythmic drugs (Class Ia, Ic, III)	Amiodarone, dofetilide, dronedarone, flecainide, ibutilide, procainamide, propafenone, quinidine, sotalol	Avoid as first line treatment of atrial fibrillation	Rate control has less potential for harm in older adults, amiodarone is associated with toxicities
Miscellaneous cardiovascular medications	Disopyramide	Avoid	Potential negative inotrope, may induce heart failure
	Dronedarone	Avoid in atrial fibrillation and heart failure	Worse outcomes have been reported
	Digoxin >0.125 mg/d	Avoid	Higher doses show no additional benefit and increase risk of toxicity.
	Nifedipine, immediate release	Avoid	Potential for hypotension, risk of precipitating myocardial ischemia
Tertiary TCAs	Amitriptyline, chlordiazepoxide-amitriptyline, clomipramine, doxepin >6 mg/d, imipramine, perphenazine-amitriptyline, trimipramine	Avoid	Highly anticholinergic, sedating, may cause orthostatic hypotension

Antipsychotics	Typical: Chlorpromazine, fluphenazine, haloperidol, loxapine, molindone, perphenazine, pimozide, promazine, thioridazine, thiothixene, trifluoperazine, triflupromazine Atypical: Aripiprazole, asenapine, clozapine, iloperidone, lurasidone, olanzapine, paliperidone, quetiapine, risperidone, ziprasidone	Avoid unless other treatments have failed	Increased risk of stroke and mortality
Barbiturates	Thioridazine, mesoridazine	Avoid	Greater risk of QTc prolongation
	Amobarbital, butabarbital, butalbital, mephobarbital, pentobarbital, phenobarbital, secobarbital	Avoid	High rates of dependence, tolerance, risk of overdose
Benzodiazepines	Alprazolam, estazolam, lorazepam, oxazepam, temazepam, triazolam, chlorazepate, chlordiazepoxide, clonazepam, diazepam, flurazepam, quazepam	Avoid except in the management of seizures, rapid eye movement disorders, withdrawal from alcohol or benzodiazepines	Decreased metabolism makes older adults more sensitive. Causes amnesia, increased risk of cognitive impairment, delirium, falls, fractures, and motor vehicle accidents.
Non-benzodiazepines	Eszopiclone, zolpidem, zaleplon	Avoid chronic use	Have adverse reactions similar to benzodiazepines as they both act on GABA.
Androgens	Methyltestosterone, testosterone	Avoid unless for moderate to severe hypogonadism	Potential for cardiac problems in men with prostate cancer
Estrogens with or without progestins		Avoid oral and topical patch. Topical vaginal cream acceptable	Evidence of carcinogenic potential, lack of cardiac or cognitive protection.
	Growth hormone	Avoid except has hormone replacement following pituitary gland removal	Associated with edema, arthralgias, carpal tunnel, gynecomastia and impaired fasting glucose.
	Insulin sliding scale	Avoid	Higher risk or hypoglycemia without improvement in hyperglycemia.
	Megestrol	Avoid	Minimal effect on weight, increased risk of thrombotic events and early death.
Sulfonylureas, long-duration	Chlorpropamide, glyburide	Avoid	Longer half-life in older adults can cause prolonged hypoglycemia.

(continued)

TABLE 46.1 2012 Beers Criteria for Potentially Inappropriate Medication Use in Older Adults (*continued*)

Medication Class	Medications	Recommendation	Rationale
Gastrointestinal	Metoclopramide	Avoid unless for gastroparesis	Can cause extrapyramidal effects, parkinsonism and tardive dyskinesia
	Mineral oil, given orally	Avoid	Potential for aspiration
	Trimethobenzamide	Avoid	Poor antiemetic effects, Causes extrapyramidal side effects.
Pain medications	Meperidine	Avoid	Poor efficacy and can cause neurotoxicity.
NSAIDS	Aspirin >325 mg/d, diclofenac, diflunisal, etodolac, fenoprofen, ibuprofen, ketoprofen, meclofenamate, mefenamic acid, meloxicam, nabumetone, naproxen, oxaprozin, piroxicam, sulindac, tolmetin, indomethacin, ketorolac	Avoid chronic use. Use with a proton pump inhibitor or other gastroprotective agent.	Increases risk of GI bleed.
Opiates	Pentazocine	Avoid	CNS adverse effects, confusion, hallucinations.
Skeletal muscle relaxants	Carisoprodol, chlorzoxazone, cyclobenzaprine, metaxalone, methocarbamol, orphenadrine	Avoid	Poorly tolerated. Anticholinergic side effects, sedation, increased fracture risk.

Abbreviations: CNS, central nervous system; GI, gastrointestinal; GABA, gamma–aminobutyric acid; NSAIDS, nonsteroidal anti-inflammatory drugs.

is one such antibody targeted at a monomeric (not plaque) form of the β-amyloid peptide with the assumption that the monomeric form is the toxic species. Phase III trials showed that it reduced cognitive decline in mild AD though this trend was not statistically significant. It is, however, thought to be disease modifying. Crenezumab is a monoclonal antibody that binds all forms of β-amyloid. Higher doses showed some slowing of cognitive decline though this did not reach statistical significance. This effect was especially pronounced in those with mild disease. Gantenerumab is a monoclonal antibody designed to bind fibrillar β-amyloid acting to disassemble and degrade amyloid plaques by recruiting microglia and activating phagocytosis. The investigation progressed to phase III but was halted due to a lack of efficacy.

b. MK-8931 is an inhibitor of the β-secretase cleaving enzyme (BACE) 1 and 2. This enzyme acts to prevent the production of β-amyloid which is done through the cleavage of the amyloid precursor protein (APP). This has advanced to phase II/III trials after promising phase I trials showed significantly reduced β-amyloid levels in CSF.

c. Another approach is the development of vaccines in an effort to induce antibody formation against β-amyloid proteins. ACC-001 is a vaccine intended to induce antibodies to beta-sheet conformation regions of β-amyloid. It is currently in phase II trials. CAD106 is another vaccine made up of multiple β-amyloid proteins in an effort to produce a strong antibody response without producing inflammatory T-cell activation. This did well in phase I trials.

d. β-amyloid oligomers are the most toxic forms of amyloid-β and they bind to the cellular prion receptor. This receptor activates an intracellular Fyn kinase which leads to synaptotoxicity. AZD0530 (saracatinib) is an inhibitor of Fyn kinase that has done well in Phase Ib trials.

B. **Cognitive remediation.** This can be either by pharmacotherapy or with behavioral interventions.

1. **Cholinesterase inhibitors.** Cholinesterase inhibitors are the mainstay of dementia treatment. The most commonly used and studied is donepezil, but rivastigmine and galantamine are also US FDA approved. These medications work by blocking the metabolism of the neurotransmitter acetylcholine in the synaptic cleft. Acetylcholine is important for attention, memory and neuronal plasticity and there is a decrease in this neurotransmitter in AD. Data have shown that these medications provide small but statistically significant improvements in cognition, behavior, and function. As a class, data support their use in Parkinson's disease dementia, Lewy body disease (LBD) and vascular dementia. They may worsen symptoms in frontotemporal lobar degeneration (FTLD). Side effects include nausea, vomiting, and diarrhea and these are the primary reasons cited for stopping these medications. Additional side effects include syncope, bradycardia, and falls.

2. **Memantine.** The NMDA receptor antagonist memantine is approved for moderate-to-severe dementia. It is thought to be neuroprotective by preventing the pathologic over-activation of the NMDA receptor. It has not been shown to be of benefit in mild AD. There is some evidence that it may be effective in vascular dementia, but there is inconsistent evidence in Parkinson's, LBD, and FTLD. Our practice is to combine memantine and a cholinesterase inhibitor in moderate-to-severe AD, although there is no good evidence to demonstrate an added benefit.

3. **Cognitive intervention.** The advantage of cognitive intervention is that it has little side effect compared to pharmacotherapy. However, presently, cognitive interventions are not reimbursed by most insurance companies. Traditionally, cognitive interventions have been divided into:

a. **Cognitive enrichment.** Which is creating an intellectually stimulating environment for the cognitively at-risk patient. Its main benefits may be related to improved mood and sense of self-worth.

b. **Cognitive neurorehabilitation.** This involves the use of compensatory mechanism to overcome deficits. The exercises are geared to particular tasks with which the patient may have problems. Both internal and external aids such as diaries and alarm clocks may be used. There is no expectation of improvement in cognition but rather use of compensatory strategies to use the limited cognitive resources available optimally. For these strategies to be useful executive function needs to be relatively intact. As such, cognitive neurorehabilitation appears to work better in AD patients than frontotemporal dementia in which the executive dysfunction is an earlier sign. Various guidelines are available including from American Congress of Rehabilitation Medicine.

   c. Brain training uses high repetition of a skilled purposeful task to improve cognition via neuroplasticity. Brain training is likely to be useful only at high intensities and with high numbers of repetitions, for this reason batteries of entertaining games used casually at home is unlikely to create the desired effect. The dual n-back training exercise has the greatest weight of evidence behind its efficacy especially for executive function and attention. It is particularly useful in patients with impairment in complex and simple attention, as is the case in traumatic brain injury for example. The exercise should be given daily for a period of weeks for the effects to be useful. No data exist regarding "refreshers" after this initial training period.

C. **Treatment of neuropsychiatric comorbidities.** These include

1. **Depression.** The importance of depression and treatment in dementia are several folds:

   a. Lifelong depression is a risk factor for the development of dementia. Treatment of depression may reduce the rate of decline in patients with neurodegenerative pathologies. There is some evidence, for example, that the presence of depression predicts conversion from MCI to dementia.

   b. Rates of depression are higher in patients with dementia. Approximately 50% of patients with AD have co-occurring depression.

   c. Depression in dementia is caused by a combination of physiologic changes in the brain as a result of neurodegeneration but also due to reaction to cognitive decline and loss of independence.

   d. Depression can affect attention, memory, motivation, processing speed, and organization. These manifest as real cognitive and executive deficits on neuropsychiatric testing.

   e. Pseudo-dementia is a term used to describe a depression that presents with primarily cognitive deficits. It is now thought to be associated with an underlying dementia, and though treatable, it is likely a prodromal phenomenon.

   f. **Treatment options.**

      (1) **Medications.** The choice of treatment will depend on the comorbidities present in the patient. Table 46.2 shows medication options, important side effects, and dosing guidelines.

      For patient with comorbid anxiety, the use of nonactivating selective-serotonin reuptake inhibitors (SSRIs) may be the initial treatment. Citalopram has a good side-effect profile and is often not activating. Citalopram can increase QT interval. Sertraline is a similarly low-activating antidepressant that is well tolerated. Both Sertraline and Citalopram have been studied in this population to good effect.

      Patients with comorbid apathy or loss of motivation may benefit from bupropion, which increases dopamine transmission in the brain. This medication can reduce seizures threshold and is contraindicated in patients with comorbid seizures. This medication has not been specifically studied in this population.

      Patient with fatigue or chronic pain and depression may prefer serotonin–norepinephrine reuptake inhibitors (SNRIs) such as duloxetine. Again, there are no studies specifically in patients with dementia or MCI.

      Trazadone can be used as a sleep aid and antidepressant. Its sedating effects last through the night so it is helpful for people that wake frequently. Conversely, patients complain of residual grogginess upon waking. Mirtazepine at a dose of 15 mg PO nightly improves sleep but may increase appetite. This latter side effect may be useful in end stage dementia when anorexia is a major problem. The drawback of both of these medications is that they are weaker antidepressants and have not been studied in patients with dementia.

      Avoid tricyclic antidepressants because of potential anticholinergic effects that adversely influence memory.

      (2) **Meditation.** There is some evidence that meditation reduces the activation in the brain and helps with depression.

(3) **Talking therapy.** Ultimately this is one of the most useful tools in the arsenal of the physician, whether this is done formally (psychiatrist) or informally in the neurologist's office. There are many therapeutic approaches that have been shown to have efficacy in the treatment of depression including psychodynamic therapy, cognitive behavioral therapy, and mindfulness-based therapy. Finding the appropriate therapeutic treatment for a particular patient is best done via a referral to a psychiatrist who can assess the psychological, social, and biological factors influencing a patient's depressive illness along with their goals and preferences to connect them to an appropriate therapist. At a minimum psychoeducation and supportive therapy should be a part of the clinical approach to these patients as they grapple with their limitations and diagnosis.

(4) **Transcranial magnetic stimulation.** Although data for the use of this modality in dementias is as yet lacking, there are good theoretical reasons to think that the method may hold promise for resistant cases of depression in dementia populations.

2. Anxiety.

a. Anxiety is more common amongst patients with neurodegenerative dementias.

b. Anxiety is caused by both physiologic changes in the brain especially with systems involved in emotional regulation; as well as in reaction to circumstances. The risk of social embarrassment appears to be a strong provoker of anxiety in patients with cognitive problems. Anxiety in neurodegenerative dementias may be physiological, for example due to the loss inhibition of ventromedial frontal lobe or in response to perceived social stigma and feeling of reduced self-efficacy.

c. High levels of anxiety interfere with prefrontal function: Prefrontal function has an "inverted U curve" relationship with anxiety. In other words at very low and very high levels of anxiety, executive function suffers. Different patients have different needs in terms of how best to maximize their cognition along this curve (Fig. 46.1).

d. Taking a careful history is important in the assessment of anxiety as patients mean different things when they use this term. Often patients will not endorse anxiety if they feel their symptoms are in proportion to, or appropriate for, their situation.

e. Treatment options include.

(1) **Medication.**

Use of nonactivating SSRIs, primarily Citalopram and Sertraline.

Avoid use of benzodiazepines except for short period of time. Benzodiazepines have immediate amnestic affects, increase risk of delirium, and long-term use increases risk of dementia and MCI converting to dementia.

We have tried Buspirone in the clinic and anecdotally we have not had as much success with this as with SSRIs.

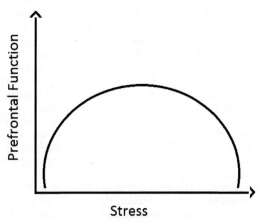

FIGURE 46.1 The inverted U curve relationship between stress/arousal and prefrontal function. At low levels of arousal such as fatigue or ADHD the prefrontal function is poor. In very high levels of stress/anxiety the prefrontal function also suffers. ADHD, attention deficit hyperactivity disorder.

    (2) Psychotherapy. Cognitive behavioral therapy may be particularly useful for anxiety in early dementias. The patient's thought patterns related to reduced self-worth due to reduced cognitive abilities needs to be addressed. It is helpful for patients suffering from social withdrawal and isolation to be encouraged to speak about their predicament and be taught strategies to mitigate social embarrassment.

    (3) Other. Adjunctive therapies may include massages, meditation (both directive and mindfulness), and exercise. Exercise has the added benefit that it may slow dementia progression as previously mentioned.

3. Sleep disturbance.
   a. Sleep deprivation is a risk factor for dementia especially AD.
   b. Sleep deprivation is a risk factor for delirium in neurodegenerative dementias.
   c. Loss of sleep architecture may be caused by neurodegenerative changes in the brain.
   d. Sleep deprivation worsens cognition.
   e. Sleep disorders including nocturnal parasomnias, rapid eye movement (REM) behavior disorder, and daytime hypersomnolence are prodromal features of Lewy body dementia and Parkinson's disease dementia.
   f. Treatment options. Treatments are generally similar to treatments for elderly patients without dementia.

    (1) Sleep hygiene. Strict day–night precautions should be observed: during the day, the patient should be exposed to natural light and encouraged to sit out of bed or to be active. Naps should be discouraged. During the night, the room should be darkened, television and other source of artificial light should be turned off, and patient be encouraged to sleep. Avoid caffeine in the afternoon and avoid strenuous exercise or meals right before bed. A bedtime routine and set times may help with better sleep.

    (2) Addressing sleep disorders. Untreated obstructive sleep apnea should be addressed. A sleep study may be indicated if the patient appears to dose off during the day, to rule out and treat periodic leg movement or hypnic jerks. REM behavior disorder, often more of a nuisance to the spouse than the patient, is common in Parkinson's dementia and LBD and may be treated with clonazepam.

    (3) Addressing comorbidities. Pain and discomfort can be reasons for lack of sleep and in late dementia may be unexpressed by the patient. Especially in patients with advanced dementia, regular use of acetaminophen for pain should be encouraged if there are no contraindications. When in doubt, the trial of a small dose of an opiate may be indicated.

    (4) Medications. Trazadone or mirtazapine are both antidepressants that are frequently and effectively used off label for sleep.

    Melatonin: Regular use of melatonin has been shown to reduce delirium risk in patients with dementia. It is not effective as a one-time or as needed sleep aid but rather it has a beneficial effect on circadian rhythm if used nightly for at least 2 weeks. Its potential as a disease modifying agent in AD is under investigation.

    Non-benzodiazepines such as zolpidem or eszopiclone can be tried at low doses. Both these medications act on the GABA receptor in a similar fashion to benzodiazepines (BZD). In contrast to BZD these drugs have less anxiolytic properties and are less likely to cause dependence or be abused. They are however associated with amnestic and cognitive side effects.

    Avoid benzodiazepines for all the reasons previously discussed. TCA such as doxepin are often used off label for sleep but this should be avoided in patients with dementia due to anticholinergic effects. Diphenhydramine should be avoided for the same reason and patients should be cautioned about its presence in most over-the-counter sleep aids.

4. Fatigue. Fatigue may be related to sleep disturbance or be independent of it. If sleep related then the treatment is often addressing the underlying cause. The use of amantadine is anecdotally helpful but there is no evidence behind its use for this indication. The use of stimulants both amphetamines and modafinil (Table 46.2) is usually not indicated.

5. Apathy. The term apathy refers to a lack of interest or concern as well as a lack of emotional feeling. Apathetic patients initiate very few activities and often ignore personal hygiene and show decreased social engagement. An apathy syndrome occurs when

TABLE 46.2 List of Psycho-Pharmaceuticals used in the Management of Patients with Dementia

Medication	Indication	Mode of Action	Important Side Effects	Dosing Recommendations
Citalopram	Depression, anxiety, agitation	Selective serotonin reuptake inhibitor (SSRI)	Gastrointestinal (GI) upset, QT prolongation, sexual dysfunction, headache, increased bleeding risk, SIADH	Start at 10 mg daily and titrate up to a maximum of 40 mg daily.
Sertraline	Depression, anxiety, agitation	SSRI	GI upset, sexual dysfunction, headache, increased bleeding risk, SIADH	Start at 25–50 mg depending on patient's prior sensitivity to medications. Can be titrated up to doses as high as 150–200 mg.
Bupropion	Depression, apathy, inattention	Inhibits dopamine and norepinephrine reuptake	Anxiety or agitation, GI upset, decreased seizure threshold, insomnia, weight loss, tremor, headache	Start at 75 mg daily and increase up to 450 mg daily. BID dosing for IR formulation or once daily for XR formulation.
Duloxetine (Cymbalta)	Depression, anxiety, pain	Serotonin–norepinephrine reuptake inhibitors (SNRIs)	GI upset, orthostatic hypotension, SIADH	Start at 20 mg daily and increase to 60 mg daily.
Trazodone	Depression, sleep	Inhibits serotonin reuptake and antagonizes serotonin 5-$HT_{2A/C}$ and α_1- adrenergic receptors	Sleep/sedation, orthostatic hypotension, headache, priapism	Start at 25 mg qhs and increase to doses up to 200 mg.
Mirtazapine	Depression, sleep	Increases serotonin and norepinephrine release and antagonizes 5_$HT_{2A/C}$	At doses of 15 mg and below it stimulates appetite and causes sedation, weight gain, dizziness, constipation, orthostatic hypotension	7.5 mg or 15 mg qhs for sleep, higher doses for depression.
Melatonin	Sleep	Hormone regulating circadian rhythm	Daytime sleepiness, decreased libido at high doses,	0.25–0.3 mg/d to start, increasing up to 5 mg daily.
Zolpidem	Sleep	Acts at GABA receptor	Sleep walking and eating, confusion, amnesia	Start at 2.5 mg qhs. Max dose of 10 mg daily.
Eszopiclone	Sleep	Acts at GABA receptor	Sleep walking and eating, confusion, amnesia	Start at 1 mg qhs, maximum dose of 3 mg qhs.
Methylphenidate	Apathy, inattention	Blocks reuptake and increases release of norepinephrine and dopamine	Insomnia, tremor, decreased appetite, palpitations, constipation, dizziness	Start at 5 mg BID and increase to 80 mg daily with BID or TID dosing.

(continued)

Medication	Indication	Mode of Action	Important Side Effects	Dosing Recommendations
Risperidone	Agitation	Blocks D_2 dopamine receptors	Extrapyramidal symptoms (EPS) including akathesia, parkinsonism and tardive dyskinesia; weight gain; metabolic syndrome; risk of early death; Neuroleptic malignant syndrome; hyperprolactinemia; QT prolongation; sexual dysfunction	Start at 0.5 mg. Can be dosed up to 8 mg. Suggest not going above 4 mg daily for agitation. Dosing can be targeted to times or situations when agitation is worse.
Olanzapine	Agitation	Blocks D_2 dopamine receptors	Same as risperidone. Olanzapine is most likely to have metabolic side effects but less likely to have QT prolongation.	Start at 2.5 mg and increase to a maximum dose of 10 mg. Dosing can be targeted to times or situations when agitation is worse.
Aripiprazole	Agitation	Partial agonist of D_2 receptors	Same as risperidone. Aripiprazole is the least likely to have metabolic side effects of all the antipsychotics. It is also less likely to cause EPS.	Start at 5 mg and increase up to a maximum dose of 15 mg. Dosing can be targeted to times or situations when agitation is worse.
Quetiapine	Agitation in PDD	Blocks D_2 dopamine receptors	Same as risperidone. Quetiapine is more likely to be sedating than other antipsychotics and has a significant risk of metabolic side effects.	Start at 25 mg daily. Can be tolerated up to 750 mg but in this population would suggest a maximum dose of 200 mg. Dosing can be targeted to times or situations when agitation is worse.
Clozapine	Agitation in PDD	Blocks D_2 dopamine receptors	Same as risperidone. Clozapine is associated with significant metabolic side effects.	Starting dose 12.5 mg, tolerated to doses as high as 900 mg. Suggest not going above 300 mg for agitation. Dosing can be targeted to times or situations when agitation is worse.
Haloperidol	Agitation	Blocks D_2 dopamine receptors	Same as risperidone. As a potent "typical antipsychotic" it is more likely to cause EPS.	Start at 0.5 mg daily and increase to a maximum of 5 mg. Dosing can be targeted to times or situations when agitation is worse.

Abbreviations: BID, twice a day; GABA, gamma–aminobutyric acid; IR, immediate release; PDD, pervasive developmental disorder; SIADH, syndrome of inappropriate antidiuretic hormone secretion; TID, three times a day; XR, extended release.

there is damage to the medial prefrontal cortex including the anterior cingulate cortex which is necessary for motor and emotional motivation. This leads to less goal-directed behavior and psychomotor slowing.

This area of the brain is often damaged early in behavioral variant frontotemporal dementia (bvFTD). AD and other dementia will often affect these brain regions later in the course of the disease as damage progresses to affect more cortical regions.

It is important to note that this is a distinct condition from depression which is also quite commonly co-occurring in dementias. Apathetic patients do not endorse sadness, do not cry, and are not easily upset by people or things in their environment. Clinically differentiating between these two conditions can be challenging.

Estimates of prevalence in AD range from 25% to 90% of individuals. In Parkinson's disease, dementia estimates are from 20% to 70%. The presence of apathy is associated with poorer cognitive and executive function.

Apathy has been shown to respond to treatment with acetylcholinesterase inhibitors and dopaminergic medications such as methylphenidate. However, a 2009 systematic review found insufficient evidence that dementia-related apathy improves with pharmacologic treatment and no subsequent studies have shown otherwise. Nevertheless, we use dopaminergic medications such as bupropion and methylphenidate in our patients and have had some success with these medications. Buproprion has the added benefit of an antidepressant effect if the clinician is also treating depression or is unsure which of these they are treating.

6. **Inattention.** During delirium, cognitive impersistence may improve with a neuroleptic/antipsychotic. Although the better option in that case is to remove the underlying cause of the delirium. If there are reasons to treat delirium, we prefer to use risperidone due to its relatively high affinity for dopamine receptors and its low affinity for histaminergic or cholinergic receptors which can cause the opposite of the intended treatment effect. It is usually effective at low doses when there is less risk for extrapyramidal or parkinsonian side effects. If delirium has been ruled out as the cause of inattention then dopaminergic medications such as bupropion or stimulants such as methylphenidate can be effective. Often inattention is associated with anxiety and depression and will improve with treatment of these conditions so these should be screened for first.

7. **Agitation and aggression.** These are the two most problematic and intractable problems in late stage dementias. There is no FDA approved medications for agitation and aggression so all medications discussed below are used off label and a number of them are controversial. There are a number of steps which may be used to improve these symptoms:

   a. The first step is to make sure that the aggression is not due to an unmet need. Pain in particular can cause agitation. Scheduled acetaminophen can be tried and when uncertain, a small dose of an opiate may be tried.

   b. The triggers for agitation should be addressed. A lack of understanding is often frightening for these patients and can lead to symptoms of paranoia. A common trigger for agitation is suspicion by the patient that something sinister might be going on. To minimize this, the patient should be included in conversation even if they do not understand. Kind prosody should be used when talking to them, and eye contact is important. Minimizing discussions about patients in front of them and working with consistent caregivers as much as possible can also help.

   c. Agitation and aggression with a sudden onset or exacerbation can often be the first symptom of a hyperactive delirium. Rule out a urinary tract infection or other metabolic disturbances.

   d. If the patient is not on a cholinesterase inhibitor and memantine, then these may be started. The exception is for frontotemporal dementia which may worsen with the introduction of these medications.

   e. If the patient is not on an SSRI, then this should also be tried. Note that the effect is going to take weeks to reach an optimum level. Non-activating SSRIs such as citalopram or sertraline might be the medication of choice in this setting. Our clinical experience suggests that often these medications are under dosed in elderly patients perhaps due to tolerability concerns. Starting at a low dose always makes sense but they should be titrated upwards before they are considered to have failed.

    f. Mood stabilizers, especially Depakote, may be tried in some cases but often the results are disappointing and there is no evidence that these medications are effective for behavioral symptoms of dementia.

    g. Benzodiazepines should only be used as "rescue" medication if the patient's agitation is severe enough that they are at acute risk of harming themselves or others. Benzodiazepines increase the risk of confusion, falls, and delirium. Benzodiazepine gel formulations are poorly absorbed and are essentially placebos.

    h. Antipsychotics are used off label in as many as 20% to 30% of patients with dementia though their use is controversial. There is no evidence supporting the use of typical antipsychotics in this group with the exception of haloperidol used at low doses for aggression (1.2 to 3.5 mg/day). Meta-analyses of 15 randomized controlled trials of atypical antipsychotics showed efficacy of risperidone, aripiprazole, and olanzapine (in that order). There is insufficient evidence regarding the use of quetiapine though it is often used due to a more favorable side-effect profile. Side effects of antipsychotics are of significant concern and include anticholinergic effects, hyperprolactinemia, prolonged QT interval, orthostatic hypotension, extrapyramidal symptoms (EPS), weight gain, metabolic syndrome, diabetes, somnolence, sexual dysfunction, seizures, cognitive decline, and increased risk of stroke. Risperidone is the most likely atypical antipsychotic to cause EPS and hyperprolactinemia. Olanzapine is the most likely to cause weight gain, metabolic syndrome, diabetes, orthostatic hypotension, and somnolence. Aripiprazole has a more tolerable side-effect profile. Additionally, both typical and atypical antipsychotics are associated with an increased risk of death which has led the USFDA to give both classes black box warnings regarding their use in patients with dementia. Recent data show that this risk is worse with haloperidol followed by risperidone, then olanzapine, and finally quetiapine. Patients with Lewy body dementia are especially likely to have adverse effects with antipsychotics.

        Therefore, antipsychotics should be used sparingly in dementias and a careful risk–benefit analysis should be made and discussed with the patient's medical decision maker. When patients are severely agitated, we believe the humane thing to do is to treat that agitation, trying more conservative approaches first. Ultimately, despite the risks, there are instances when antipsychotic use is important and can prevent hospitalization and dramatically improve quality of life. When used in Parkinson's disease dementia and in LBD, only quetiapine and clozapine should be trialed. Quetiapine is preferred as it has the least potential to exacerbate the symptoms of Parkinson's. If there is evidence of EPS with the start of neuroleptics then they need to be stopped. We recommend only using antipsychotics for which there is evidence of efficacy: risperidone, olanzepine, haloperidol, and aripiprazole.

      (1) Electroconvulsive therapy (ECT) is an additional option with significant literature supporting its safety and effectiveness for the treatment of the most agitated and aggressive patients as well as patients with pathologic yelling. It has several obvious benefits: it can be effective quickly and can permit minimal use of potentially harmful medications. Clinicians are often reluctant to consider ECT in this population as it is known to have cognitive side effects. Usually this manifests as amnesia surrounding the procedure. More lasting effects on short- and long-term memory are rare. Studies have failed to show that ECT worsens cognition in patients with dementia. Often, any amnestic effects are far outweighed by an improvement in a patient's ability to attend to, focus on, and interact with their environment leading to a net positive cognitive effect.

D. Harm minimization.

    1. Caregiver training. Caregiver training is an approach that involves problem solving with a family to identify precipitating and modifiable causes of symptoms and working with them to create a specific tailored approach. Several models for this have been studied to good effect for both the patient's symptoms and for caregiver well-being.

        Training may include setting realistic expectation and goals. Also equally as important is to avoid attributing all symptoms to dementia. Intervention is taught to caregivers including reduction of triggers for wandering and aggression. Prompted bladder evacuation can reduce risk of incontinence.

2. **Environmental modification.** Home safety checks should be done where available to address hazards such as carpets, stairs, and bathrooms. Modifications should be made to reduce fall risk. Adequate lighting may help with orientation and navigation. In facilities clear signs, clocks, and calendars can help to orient a person to the new environment. A consistent daily routine can reduce anxiety.

3. **Caregiver support.** Over 75% of people with dementia are cared for by family or friends at home. Support includes caregiver respite, day programs, financial and legal advice, and home help. These supportive services may increase the ability of the patient to stay independent for longer.

4. **Dementia groups.** These provide participants with practical advice, ability to network and mutual support. They are highly recommended.

COUNSELING AND EDUCATION

A. **Prognostication.** This is one of the most important tasks for the neurologist, as it allows the patient and her family to plan for the future and allows the patient to complete "unfinished business." By the same token the ability to prognosticate is severely impeded by a lack of reliable data. Most of the data which does exist pertains to AD and VD. There are higher rates of mortality amongst patients with dementia, at least in part due to concomitantly higher vascular risk factors. Aspiration pneumonia is one of the most common causes of death in late stage disease. Life expectancy is often reported to be of the order of 5 years or less from the time of diagnosis. But given the average age of diagnosis in AD is around 75 years, it is likely that the major cause of death in this population is cerebrovascular and cardiovascular disease. Improved survival reported in more recent literature is likely related to earlier diagnosis and better cardiovascular risk factor management. The best guide to prognosis is the patient's progression in the last few years: if decline has been rapid then it is likely to remain so and vice versa. Symptoms begin with impairment in just a couple domains and broaden overtime as the disease progresses.

B. **Hereditary risk.** The family often likes to know whether they are at increased risk of developing dementias. Family history of late onset dementias in particular late onset AD (>65 years) only confers slightly increased risk of developing the disease. Early-onset dementias however are much more likely to be due to autosomal dominant genetic mutations. In such cases the patient may require genetic testing and counseling. Although no disease modifying medication exists as yet, it is likely that regardless of the mechanism of future treatments, disease modification will be effective only in the earliest stage of the disease. Knowing the genetic status of pre-symptomatic patient might allow them to position themselves better with regards to future clinical trials.

SPECIAL GROUPS

A. **Early-onset dementia.** Early-onset dementia is dementia that presents before the age of 65. AD is the most common cause of dementia and it is similarly the most common cause of dementia in younger patients followed by vascular disease and FTLD. In patients younger than 35 years of age, most dementias are caused by metabolic disturbances. A large proportion of early-onset AD are caused by autosomal dominant mutations in either the amyloid precursor protein, presenilin-1 or presenilin-2 genes. The presentation is usually similar to later-onset sporadic disease, i.e., patients present with amnesia plus visuospatial problems. However, the incidence of less common neuropsychological types of AD, such as posterior cortical atrophy and executive variant of AD, is relatively higher in the young-onset group compared to the late onset presentation. These rarer neuropsychological presentations are likely to be more rapidly progressive compared to the more common amnesia plus visuospatial subtype (Videos 46.1 and 46.2).

Frontotemporal lobar degeneration refers to a group of degenerative dementias where the neuronal damage is preferentially in the frontal and temporal lobes. The presenting syndromes reflect the functions of the cortical regions within these lobes that are affected first. Two main categories include primary progressive aphasias where damage is primarily in the left hemisphere's language regions and behavioral variant where damage is primarily in the non-language of the frontal lobes. These illnesses are all likely to have an earlier onset and therefore comprise a larger proportion of early-onset dementias. They are also more highly heritable, about 20% to 40%.

People with Down's syndrome have a special vulnerability to early-onset AD. This is due to the fact that the gene for amyloid precursor protein is found on chromosome 21 leading to over production of this protein in these individuals and a corresponding increase in accumulation of β-amyloid.

The diagnosis of AD is always difficult but it is especially devastating in younger patients. Because of the increased incidence of hereditary disease it is important to make the correct diagnosis and to refer patient's to genetic counseling to know if other family members are at risk. Additionally it is often important to refer patients and their families to counselors and psychiatry to process their grief surrounding the diagnosis. Community support groups can also be very helpful for patients and families.

B. **Asymptomatic patients with strong genetic risk.** This special group of patients have unique needs. They should be referred to genetic counseling and to psychiatry. Many will ask about prevention and ways to delay presentation of the disease. While it is not clear to what extent this can be done the psychological benefits to patients of feeling like they can be proactive is significant so education about risk factor minimization should be offered. But they should also be cautioned about the limited benefits of many of the products marketed with high promise. These patients are also often highly motivated to participate in clinical trials if they are available in your region.

C. **Anosognosia.** Anosognosia is an unawareness of a neurological deficit. It is a problem in dementia patients because their compliance with safety measures and treatments will be affected. There are three reasons why a dementia patient may not accept her diagnosis:

1. **Denial.** The main reason people deny having cognitive problems is that their self-worth is in some ways tied in with their mental capacity. Counseling that addresses feeling of self-worth will help with denial.

2. **Loss of self-monitoring mechanism.** Self-monitoring is a cortical function. Often this skill can become impaired or lost. The patient may be helped by education about the high prevalence of anosognosia in dementia populations. It is also useful to go through the cognitive test results to convince the patient of the fact of their cognitive decline. Working with care givers to understand and accommodate for this is also important.

3. The patient does not have the intellectual capacity to understand the disease. This is usually in end stage disease and the patient should be approached with kindness and understanding.

D. **Difficult diagnosis.** Some people may not be diagnosed even after genetic testing, lumbar puncture (LP) and positron emission tomography (PET) scanning. The strategy may be to **repeat** neuropsychological testing in 6 months or a year. If rapidly progressive and no diagnosis then brain biopsy may be considered.

Key Points

- Management of vascular risk factors, especially hypertension currently shows the most promise for disease modification in AD and vascular cognitive impairment (VCI).
- The main treatments are currently cholinesterase inhibitors, which have been shown to be of modest benefit in most dementia's with the exception of FTLD, and memantine, which has been shown to be beneficial in moderate-to-severe AD or VCI.
- Screen for and treat comorbid depression and anxiety. Depression often presents similar to dementia and both conditions worsen cognitive function.
- Harm reduction is key: treat and take measures to avoid delirium, address polypharmacy and minimize use of medications such as benzodiazepines medications with anticholinergic effects as they worsen cognition.
- In advanced dementia behavioral symptoms can be a challenge for clinicians and we recommend an approach focused on quality of life and risk benefit analysis.
- Early-onset dementias, presenting prior to age 65, are more likely to be heritable so correct diagnosis and genetic testing and counseling are important for these patients and their families.

Recommended Readings

Aguero-Torres H, von Strauss E, Viitanen M, et al. Institutionalization in the elderly: the role of chronic diseases and dementia. Cross-sectional and longitudinal data from a population-based study. *J Clin Epidemiol*. 2001;54(8):795–801.

American Geriatrics Society 2012 Beers Criteria Update Expert Panel. American geriatrics society updated beers criteria for potentially inappropriate medication use in older adults. *J Am Geriatr Soc*. 2012;60(4):616–631.

Arrighi HM, Neumann PJ, Lieberburg IM, et al. Lethality of Alzheimer disease and its impact on nursing home placement. *Alzheimer Dis Assoc Disord*. 2010;24(1):90–95.

Azermai M. Dealing with behavioral and psychological symptoms of dementia: a general overview. *Psychol Res Behav Manag*. 2015;8:181–185.

Baker LD, Frank LL, Foster-Schubert K, et al. Aerobic exercise improves cognition for older adults with glucose intolerance, a risk factor for Alzheimer's disease. *J Alzheimers Dis*. 2010;22(2):569–579.

Bang J, Price D, Prentice G, et al. ECT treatment for two cases of dementia-related pathological yelling. *J Neuropsychiatry Clin Neurosci*. 2008;20(3):379–380.

Billioti de Gage S, Moride Y, Ducruet T, et al. Benzodiazepine use and risk of Alzheimer's disease: case-Control study. *BMJ*. 2014;349:g5205.

Bolduc V, Thorin-Trescases N, Thorin E. Endothelium-dependent control of cerebrovascular functions through age: exercise for healthy cerebrovascular aging. *Am J Physiol Heart Circ Physiol*. 2013;305(5):H620–H633.

Cancela JM, Ayan C, Varela S, et al. Effects of a long-term aerobic exercise intervention on institutionalized patients with dementia. *J Sci Med Sport*. 2015;19(4):293–298. http://dx.doi/10/1016/j.jsams.2015.05.007

Carlyle W, Killick L, Ancill R. ECT: an effective treatment in the screaming demented patient. *J Am Geriatr Soc*. 1991;39:637–639.

Coley N, Gallini A, Andrieu S. Prevention studies in Alzheimer's disease: progress towards the development of new therapeutics. *CNS drugs*. 2015;29(7):519–528. doi: 10.1007/s40263-015-0256-9.

Cooper C, Sommerlad A, Lyketsos CG, et al. Modifiable predictors of dementia in mild cognitive impairment: a systematic review and meta-analysis. *Mech Psychiatr Illn*. 2015;172(4):323–334.

Cummings J, Friedman JH, Garibaldi G, et al. Apathy in neurodegenerative diseases: recommendations on the design of clinical trials. *J Geriatr Psychiatry Neurol*. 2015;28(3):159–173. doi: 10.1177/0891988715573534.

Cunningham EL, MCGuiness B, Herron B, et al. Dementia. *Ulster Med J*. 2015;84(2):79–87.

Deckers K, van Boxtel MP, Schiepers OJ, et al. Target risk factors for dementia prevention: a systemic review and Delphi consensus study on the evidence from observational studies. *Int J Geriatr Psychiatry*. 2015;30(3):234–246.

Dishman RK, Berthoud HR, Booth FW, et al. Neurobiology of exercise. *Obesity*. 2006;14(3):345–356.

Drijgers RL, Aalten P, Winogrodzka A, et al. Pharmacological treatment of apathy in neurodegenerative diseases: a systematic review. *Dement Geriatr Cogn Disord*. 2009;28(1):13–22.

Fong TG, Davis D, Growdon ME, et al. The interface between delirium and dementia in elderly adults. *Lancet Neurol*. 2015;14(8):823–832.

Fujita S, Rasmussen BB, Cadenas JG, et al. Aerobic exercise overcomes the age-related insulin resistance of muscle protein metabolism by improving endothelial function and Akt/mammalian target of rapamycin signaling. *Diabetes*. 2007;56(6):1615–1622.

Goodpaster BH, Kelley DE, Wing RR, et al. Effects of weight loss on regional fat distribution and insulin sensitivity in obesity. *Diabetes*. 1999;48(4):839–847.

Gorelick PB, Scuteri A, Black SE, et al. Vascular contributions to cognitive impairment and dementia: a statement for healthcare professionals from the American Heart Association/American stroke association. *Stroke*. 2011;42(9):2672–2713.

Grant JE, Mohan SN. Treatment of agitation and aggression in four demented patients using ECT. *J ECT*. 2001;18(3):205–209.

Gray SL, Anderson ML, Dublin S, et al. Cumulative use of strong anticholinergic and incident dementia: a prospective cohort study. *JAMA Int Med*. 2015;175(3):401–407.

Haskins EC. *Cognitive Rehabilitation Manual: Translating Evidence-Based Recommendations into Practice*. Reston, VA: American Congress of Rehabilitation Medicine; 2012.

Hildreth KL, Church S. Evaluation and management of the elderly patient presenting with cognitive complaints. *Med Clin North Am*. 2015;99(2):311–335.

Hurd MD, Martorell P, Delavande A, et al. Monetary costs of dementia in the United States. *N Engl J Med*. 2013;368(14):1326–1334.

Hurd MD, Martorell P, Langa K. Future monetary costs of dementia in the United States under alternative dementia prevalence scenarios. *J Popul Ageing*. 2015;8(1–2):101–112.

Kales HC, Gitlin LN, Lyketsos CG. Assessment and management of behavioral and psychological symptoms of dementia. *BMJ*. 2015;350:h369.

Lanata SC, Miller BL. The behavioral variant frontotemporal dementia (bvFTD) syndrome in psychiatry. *J Neurol Neurosurg Psychiatry*. 2015;0:1–11.

Li J, Wang YJ, Zhang M, et al. Vascular risk factors promote conversion from mild cognitive impairment to Alzheimer's disease. *Neurology*. 2011;76(17):1485–1491.

Li KZ, Roudaia E, Lussier M, et al. Benefits of cognitive dual-task training on balance and mobility in healthy older adults. *J Gerontol A Biol Sci Med Sci*. 2010;65(12):1344–1352.

Lin L, Huang Q-X, Yang S-S, et al. Melatonin in Alzheimer's disease. *Int J Mol Sci*. 2013;14: 12575–14593.

MacLullich AM, Beaglehole A, Hall RJ, et al. Delirium and long-term cognitive impairment. *Int Rev Psychiatry*. 2009;21(1):30–42.

McKhann GM, Knopman DS, Chertkow H, et al. The diagnosis of dementia due to Alzheimer's disease: recommendations from the national institute on aging-Alzheimer's association workgroups on diagnostic guidelines for Alzheimer's disease. *Alzheimers Demen*. 2011;7(3):263–269.

Nestel P, Clifton P, Colquhoun D, et al. Indications for Omega-3 long chain polyunsaturated fatty acid in the prevention and treatment of cardiovascular disease. *Heart Lung Circ*. 2015;24(8):769–779.

Nygaard HB, Wagner AF, Bowen GS, et al. A phase Ib multiple ascending dose study of safety, tolerability and central nervous system availability of AZD0530 (saracatinib) in Alzheimer's disease. *Alzheimers Res Ther*. 2015;7(1):35.

Philibert RA, Richards L, Lynch CF, et al. Effect of ECT on mortality and clinical outcome in geriatric unipolar depression. *J Clin Psychiatry*. 1995;56(9):390–394.

Prince M, Guerchet M, Prina M. *Policy Brief for Heads of Government: The Global Impact of Dementia 2013-2050*. London, England: Alzheimer's Disease International; 2013.

Rafii MS, Aisen PS. Advances in Alzheimer's disease drug development. *BMC Med*. 2015;13:62.

Roccaforte WH, Wengel SP, Burke WJ. ECT for screaming in dementia. *Am J Geriatr Psychiatry*. 2000;8(2):177–179.

Rodakowski J, Safhafi E, Butters MA, et al. Non-pharmacological interventions for adults with mild cognitive impairment and early stage dementia: an updated scoping review. *Mol Aspects Med*. 2015;43–44:38–53. doi: 10.1016/j.mam.2015.06.003.

Rossor MN, Fox NC, Mummery CJ, et al. The diagnosis of young-onset dementia. *Lancet Neurol*. 2010;9(8):793–806.

Ryan AS. Insulin resistance with aging: effects of diet and exercise. *Sports Med*. 2000;30(5):327–346.

Saava GM, Wharton SB, Ince PG, et al. Age, neuropathology, and dementia. *N Engl J Med*. 2009;360(22):2302–2309.

Salminen TT, Frensch P, Strobach T, et al. Age specific differences of dual n-back training. *Aging Neurophychol Cogn*. 2016;23(1)2:18–39.

Schenk D, Barbour R, Dunn W, et al. Immunization with amyloid-beta attenuates Alzheimer-disease-like pathology in the PDAPP mouse. *Nature*. 1999;400:173–177.

Sofi F, Valecchi D, Bacci D, et al. Physical activity and risk of cognitive decline: a meta-analysis of prospective studies. *J Int Med*. 2011;169:107–117.

Teixeira-Lemos E, Nunes S, Teizeira F, et al. Regular physical exercise training assists in preventing type 2 diabetes development: focus on its antioxidant and anti-inflammatory properties. *Cardiovasc Diabetol*. 2011;10:12.

Tschanz JT, Welsh-Bohmer KA, Lyketsos CG, et al. Conversion to dementia from mild cognitive disorder: the Cache County Study. *Neurology*. 2006;67(2):229–234.

Ujkaj M, Davidoff DA, Seiner SJ, et al. Safety and efficacy of electroconvulsive therapy for the treatment of agitation and aggression in patients with dementia. *Am J Geriatr Psychiatry*. 2012;20(1):61–72." above the reference "Visioli".

Visioli F, Burgos-Ramos E. Selected micronutrients in cognitive decline prevention and therapy. *Mol Neurobiol*. 2015;53(6):4083–4093. doi 10.1007/s12035-015-9349-1.

Wu Q, Prentice G, Campbell JJ. ECT Treatment for two cases of dementia-related aggressive behavior. *J Neuropsychiatry Clin Neurosci*. 2012;22(2):E10–E11.

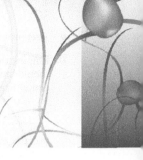

47 Central Nervous System Infections

Karen L. Roos

BACTERIAL MENINGITIS

The initial signs and symptoms of bacterial meningitis are fever, stiff neck, headache, lethargy, confusion or coma, nausea and vomiting, and photophobia (see Video 47.1). Examination of the cerebrospinal fluid (CSF) shows an elevated opening pressure (>180 mm H_2O), a decreased glucose concentration (<40 mg/dL), polymorphonuclear pleocytosis, and an elevated protein concentration. The diagnosis is made by demonstrating the organism with Gram's stain or in culture. Polymerase chain reaction (PCR) to detect bacterial nucleic acid in CSF is available at some centers. *Bacterial meningitis is a neurologic emergency*, and initial treatment is empiric until a specific organism is identified.

A. **Therapeutic approach.**

1. Dexamethasone therapy. The American Academy of Pediatrics recommends consideration of dexamethasone in the treatment of infants and children 2 months of age and older with proven or suspected bacterial meningitis on the basis of findings on CSF examination. The Infectious Diseases Society of America (IDSA) Practice Guidelines for the Management of Bacterial Meningitis and the European Federation of Neurological Societies Guideline on the Management of Community-Acquired Bacterial Meningitis recommend the use of dexamethasone in adults with suspected or proven pneumococcal meningitis (based on CSF gram-positive diplococci or blood or CSF cultures that are positive for *Streptococcus pneumoniae*). The IDSA Practice Guidelines also acknowledge that some authorities would initiate dexamethasone in all adults with suspected bacterial meningitis because the etiologic organism is not known at initial evaluation. Recent studies have demonstrated a favorable trend toward reduced rates of death and hearing loss and no evidence that dexamethasone was harmful in meningococcal meningitis. In clinical trials, dexamethasone improves the outcome of meningitis. In experimental models of bacterial meningitis, dexamethasone inhibits synthesis of the inflammatory cytokines, decreases leakage of serum proteins into the CSF, minimizes damage to the blood–brain barrier (BBB), and decreases CSF outflow resistance. Dexamethasone also decreases brain edema and intracranial pressure (ICP).

   The recommended dosage of dexamethasone is 0.15 mg/kg intravenous (IV) every 6 hours for the first 4 days of therapy. The initial dose of dexamethasone should be given before or at least with the initial dose of antimicrobial therapy for maximum benefit. Dexamethasone is not likely to be of much benefit if started >24 hours or more after antimicrobial therapy has been initiated. The concomitant use of a histamine-2 receptor antagonist is recommended with dexamethasone to avoid gastrointestinal bleeding.

2. Antimicrobial therapy. If bacterial meningitis is suspected, antimicrobial therapy must be initiated immediately. This should be done before the performance of computed tomography (CT) or lumbar puncture. Initial antimicrobial therapy is empiric and is determined by the most likely meningeal pathogen according to the patient's age and underlying condition or predisposing factors.

   a. The most likely etiologic organisms of bacterial meningitis in **neonates** are group B streptococci, enteric gram-negative bacilli (*Escherichia coli*), and *Listeria monocytogenes*. Empiric therapy for bacterial meningitis in a neonate should include a combination of ampicillin and either a third- or fourth-generation cephalosporin (cefotaxime or cefepime).

b. Empiric therapy for community-acquired bacterial meningitis in **infants and children** should include coverage for *S.pneumoniae* and *Neisseria meningitidis.* A third- or fourth-generation cephalosporin (ceftriaxone, cefotaxime, or cefepime) and vancomycin are recommended as initial therapy for bacterial meningitis in children in whom the etiologic agent has not been identified. Cefuroxime, also a third-generation cephalosporin, is not recommended for therapy for bacterial meningitis in children because of reports of delayed sterilization of CSF cultures associated with hearing loss in children treated with cefuroxime.

c. Empiric therapy for community-acquired bacterial meningitis in **adults** (15 to 50 years of age) should include coverage for *S. pneumoniae* and *N. meningitidis.* A third-generation cephalosporin (ceftriaxone or cefotaxime) or a fourth-generation cephalosporin (cefepime) plus vancomycin is recommended for empiric therapy. All CSF isolates of pneumococci and meningococci should be tested for antimicrobial susceptibility. Cefotaxime, ceftriaxone, or cefepime is recommended for relatively resistant strains of pneumococci (penicillin minimal inhibitory concentrations [MIC], 0.1 to 1.0 μg/mL and MICs of cefotaxime or cefepime $\leq$0.5 μg/mL). For highly penicillin-resistant pneumococcal meningitis (MIC >1.0 μg/mL), a combination of vancomycin and a third-generation or fourth-generation cephalosporin is recommended. Penicillin G or ampicillin can be used for meningococcal meningitis.

d. Initial therapy for meningitis in **postneurosurgical patients** should be directed against gram-negative bacilli, *Pseudomonas aeruginosa,* and *Staphylococcus aureus.* Ceftazidime or meropenem is recommended for management of gram-negative bacillary meningitis in neurosurgical patients. Ceftazidime is the only cephalosporin with sufficient activity against *P. aeruginosa* in the central nervous system (CNS). Vancomycin should be added until infection with staphylococci is excluded.

e. In infants, children, and adults with **CSF ventriculoperitoneal shunt infections,** initial therapy for meningitis should include coverage for coagulase-negative staphylococci and *S. aureus.* The assumption can be made that the organism will be resistant to methicillin; therefore, initial therapy for a shunt infection should include IV vancomycin. Intrashunt or intraventricular vancomycin may also be needed to eradicate the infection.

f. In **immunocompromised patients,** the infecting organism can be predicted on the basis of the type of immune abnormality. In patients with neutropenia, initial therapy for bacterial meningitis should include coverage for *L. monocytogenes,* staphylococci, and enteric gram-negative bacilli. Patients with defective humoral immunity and those who have undergone splenectomy are unable to mount an antibody response to a bacterial infection or to control an infection caused by encapsulated bacteria. These patients are at particular risk of meningitis caused by *S. pneumoniae, Haemophilus influenzae* type b (Hib), and *N. meningitidis.*

g. The most common organisms causing meningitis in the **older adult** (50 years or older) are *S. pneumoniae* and enteric gram-negative bacilli; however, meningitis caused by *Listeria* organisms and Hib are increasingly recognized. The recommended initial therapy for meningitis in the older adult is either ceftriaxone, cefotaxime, or cefepime in combination with vancomycin and ampicillin. Table 47.1 lists empiric antimicrobial therapy for bacterial meningitis by age group. Tables 47.2 and 47.3 list the recommended antimicrobial therapy for bacterial meningitis in neonates, infants and children, and adults by meningeal pathogen.

3. Management of increased ICP. Increased ICP is an expected complication of bacterial meningitis and should be anticipated.

a. **Elevation of the head of the bed** 30 degrees.

b. **Hyperventilation** to maintain Paco$_2$ between 30 and 35 mm Hg.

c. Mannitol.

   (1) **Children.** 0.5 to 2.0 g/kg infused over 30 minutes and repeated as necessary.

   (2) **Adults.** 1.0 g/kg bolus injection and then 0.25 g/kg every 2 to 3 hours. A dose of 0.25 g/kg appears as effective as a dose of 1.0 g/kg in lowering ICP. The main exception is that the higher dose has a longer duration of action. Serum osmolarity should not be allowed to rise above 320 mOsm/kg.

TABLE 47.1 Empiric Antimicrobial Therapy for Bacterial Meningitis

Age Group	Antimicrobial Agent
Neonates	Ampicillin plus cefotaxime or cefepime
Infants and children	Ceftriaxone, cefotaxime, or cefepime plus vancomycin
Adults (15–50 yr)	
Community acquired	Ceftriaxone, cefotaxime, or cefepime plus vancomycin
Otitis, mastoiditis, sinusitis	Ceftriaxone plus vancomycin plus metronidazole
Postneurosurgical	Ceftazidime or meropenem plus vancomycin
Immunocompromised	Ceftazidime or meropenem plus ampicillin
Older adults	Ceftriaxone, cefotaxime, or cefepime plus vancomycin plus ampicillin

TABLE 47.2 Recommended Antimicrobial Therapy for Bacterial Meningitis in Neonates, Infants, and Children by Organism

	Total Daily Dose		
Organism	Neonates (<1 wk)	Neonates (1–4 wk)	Infants and Children (>4 wk)
Hib	Cefotaxime 100 mg/kg/d q12h or Cefepime 100 mg/kg/d q12h	Cefotaxime 150–200 mg/kg/d q8h or cefepime 100 mg/kg/d q12h	Ceftriaxone 100 mg/kg/d IV in a once or twice daily dosing regimen, or cefotaxime 225 mg/kg/d IV in divided doses q6h or cefepime 150 mg/kg/d in divided doses q8h
S. pneumoniae[a]	Cefotaxime	Cefotaxime	Ceftriaxone or cefotaxime or cefepime
Group B streptococci	Ampicillin 100–150 mg/kg/d q8h	Ampicillin 200 mg/kg/d q8h	Ampicillin 200–300 mg/kg/d q4–6h
L. monocytogenes[b]	Ampicillin with or without gentamicin 5 mg/kg/d q8h	Ampicillin with or without gentamicin 7.5 mg/kg/d q8h	Ampicillin with or without gentamicin 5 mg/kg/d q8h
N. meningitidis	Penicillin G 50,000–150,000 U/kg/d q8h, or ampicillin 100–150 mg/kg/d q12h	Penicillin G 150,000–200,000 U/kg/d q6h, or ampicillin 200 mg/kg/d q8h	Penicillin G 250,000–400,000 U/kg/d q4h, or ampicillin IV in divided doses q4–6h
Enteric gram-negative bacilli[a]	Cefotaxime or cefepime	Cefotaxime or cefepime	Ceftriaxone or cefotaxime or cefepime
S. aureus	Oxacillin 50–100 mg/kg/d q6h	Oxacillin 100–200 mg/kg/d q6h	Oxacillin 200–300 mg/kg/d q4h
Methicillin-resistant staphylococci	Vancomycin 20–30 mg/kg/d q12h	Vancomycin 40 mg/kg/d q6h	Vancomycin 40–60 mg/kg/d q6h, may also add intrashunt or intraventricular vancomycin 10 mg once a day

[a]Dosages are the same as for Hib.
[b]Dosages are the same as for group B streptococci.

TABLE 47.3 Recommended Antimicrobial Therapy for Bacterial Meningitis in Adults by Organism

Organism	Antimicrobial Agent
S. pneumoniae	Ceftriaxone 4 g/d (q12h) or cefotaxime 12 g/d (q4h) or cefepime 6 g/d (q8h) plus vancomycin 45–60 mg/kg/d (q6–12h)
N. meningitidis	Penicillin G 20–24 miU/kg/d (q4h) or ampicillin 12 g/d (q4h)
Gram-negative bacilli (except P. aeruginosa)	Ceftriaxone 4 g/d (q12h) or cefotaxime 12 g/d (q4h) or cefepime 6 g/d (q8h)
P. aeruginosa	Ceftazidime 8 g/d (q8h) or meropenem 6 g/d (q8h)
H. influenzae type b	Ceftriaxone or cefotaxime or cefepime
S. aureus (methicillin-sensitive)	Oxacillin 9–12 g/d (q4h) or nafcillin 12 g/d (q4h)
S. aureus (methicillin-resistant)	Vancomycin 45–60 mg/kg/d (q6–12h)
L. monocytogenes	Ampicillin 12 g/d (q4h) with or without gentamicin
Enterobacteriaceae	Ceftriaxone or cefotaxime or cefepime

    d. Pentobarbital.
      (1) Loading dose. 10 mg/kg over 30 minutes.
      (2) 5 mg/kg/hour for 3 hours, supplemented with 200-mg IV boluses until a burst-suppression pattern is obtained on an EEG.
      (3) Maintenance dosage. 1 mg/kg/hour by constant IV infusion.
  4. Seizure activity is such a common complication of bacterial meningitis in adults, especially pneumococcal meningitis, for which prophylactic anticonvulsant therapy is not unreasonable.
    a. Prophylactic therapy. Phenytoin is administered at a dosage of 18 to 20 mg/kg at a rate no faster than 50 mg/minute. Propylene glycol, the diluent of IV phenytoin, can cause bradycardia, hypotension, and cardiac dysrhythmias. IV phenytoin should be administered via central access while the ECG and BP are monitored. If these side effects are observed, the rate of administration should be decreased. It is recommended that phenytoin be administered no faster than 25 mg/minute in the elderly.

        Fosphenytoin, the prodrug to phenytoin, is administered at a dosage of 18 to 20 mg (phenytoin equivalents) PE per kg at a rate no faster than 150 mg/minute. IV fosphenytoin does not contain propylene glycol and thus can be administered at a faster rate than phenytoin. A standard maintenance dosage is 100 mg of phenytoin or 100 mg PE of fosphenytoin every 8 hours. A serum concentration of 10 to 20 μg/mL should be maintained.

        Levetiracetam is an alternative option for parenteral seizure prophylaxis therapy. The loading dose is 1,000 to 1,500 mg intravenously, followed by a maintenance dose of 500 mg every 12 hours. Levetiracetam dosing should be adjusted for creatinine clearance.
    b. Status epilepticus.
      (1) Lorazepam (0.1 mg/kg for adults; 0.05 mg/kg/dose for children) or diazepam (5 to 10 mg for adults; 0.2 to 0.3 mg/kg/dose for children) is administered IV.
      (2) Phenytoin is administered in a dose of 18 to 20 mg/kg as described in Section **A.4.a** under Bacterial Meningitis. Fosphenytoin is administered in a dose of 20 mg PE/kg as described in Section **A.4.a** under Bacterial Meningitis. If seizures are not controlled, a repeat bolus of 10 mg PE/kg fosphenytoin or 500 mg phenytoin can be given.
      (3) If phenytoin fails to control seizure activity, phenobarbital is administered intravenously at a rate of 100 mg/minute to a loading dose of 20 mg/kg. The loading dose of phenobarbital for children is also 20 mg/kg. The most common adverse effects of phenobarbital loading are hypotension and respiratory depression. Before phenobarbital loading, ensure that an endotracheal tube has been placed

and mechanical ventilation begun. The primary reason for failure to control seizure activity is either that anticonvulsants are administered in subtherapeutic dosages or, as is the case for phenobarbital, the rate of administration is too slow.

(4) For more information on the management of refractory status epilepticus, see Chapters 42, 43, and 63.

5. **Fluid management.** Most children with bacterial meningitis have hyponatremia (serum sodium concentration <135 mEq/L) at the time of admission. For this reason, fluid restriction to correct the serum sodium level is important, but this must be done taking into consideration the adverse effects of hypovolemia on cerebral perfusion pressure. The recommended initial rate of IV fluid administration is approximately three-fourths normal maintenance requirements, or approximately 1,000 to 2,000 mL/m²/day. A 5% dextrose solution with one-fourth to one-half normal saline solution and 20 to 40 mEq/L potassium is recommended. The volume of fluids administered can be gradually increased when serum sodium concentration increases to >135 mEq/L.

B. **Expected outcome.** Despite appropriate antimicrobial therapy, patients with bacterial meningitis are very sick. Prognosis depends on age, underlying or associated conditions, time from onset of illness to institution of appropriate antimicrobial therapy, the infecting organism, and the development of brain edema, coma, arterial and venous cerebrovascular complications, hydrocephalus, or seizures. Pneumococcal meningitis has the worst prognosis, and a poor prognosis is associated with the extremes of age.

C. **Prevention.**

1. Rifampin is recommended for all close contacts with a patient who has **meningococcal meningitis.** Rifampin is given in divided doses at 12-hour intervals for 2 days as follows: adults, 600 mg; children, 10 mg/kg; neonates (younger than 1 month), 5 mg/kg. It should not be given during pregnancy. Pregnant and lactating women may be given intravenous or IV ceftriaxone (a single injection of 250 mg).

   The Advisory Committee on Immunization Practices recommends that adolescents and college freshmen be vaccinated against meningococcal meningitis with the tetravalent (Men A, C, W135, Y) meningococcal polysaccharide vaccine. This vaccine does not include serotype B.

2. The vaccination of infants with the Hib conjugate vaccine has greatly decreased the incidence of **Hib.** Rifampin prophylaxis should be given to children younger than 4 years of age who have not been fully vaccinated against Hib disease and who come in contact with a patient with Hib meningitis. It is recommended for all adults who have close contact with the patient and for the patient, because the organism usually is not eradicated from the nasopharynx with systemic antimicrobial therapy. Rifampin in the following dosages is recommended: adults, 20 mg/kg/day orally for 4 days; children, 20 mg/kg/day orally (maximum 600 mg/day) for 4 days; and neonates (younger than 1 month), 10 mg/kg/day for 4 days. Rifampin is not recommended for pregnant women.

HERPES ENCEPHALITIS

Encephalitis is inflammation of the brain parenchyma. Herpes simplex virus (HSV-1) is the principal cause of herpes encephalitis. Initial infection occurs either after exposure to infected saliva or respiratory secretions, the virus gaining access to the CNS along the olfactory nerve and tract into the limbic lobe, or as a result of reactivation of latent virus from the trigeminal ganglion. Virus is transmitted from infected persons to other persons only through close personal contact. The typical clinical presentation is a several-day history of fever and headache followed by memory loss, confusion, olfactory hallucinations, and seizures. The hallmark sign is a focal neurologic deficit suggestive of a structural lesion in the frontotemporal area. On CT scans, there is a low-density lesion within the temporal lobe with mass effect. On magnetic resonance imaging (MRI), the infection appears as an area of high signal intensity on T2-weighted (Fig. 47.1), diffusion-weighted, and fluid-attenuated inversion recovery images. Examination of the CSF shows a lymphocytic pleocytosis (with an average WBC count of 50 to 500 cells per mm³), elevation in protein concentration, and normal or mildly decreased glucose concentration. CSF should be sent for the PCR assay to detect nucleic acid of HSV-1 and it should be examined for HSV-1 antibodies. Antibodies to HSV-1 do not appear in the

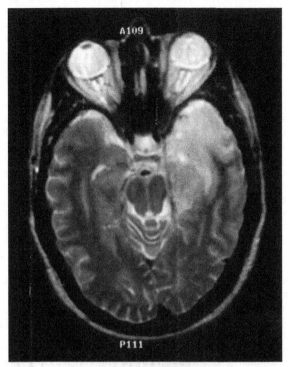

FIGURE 47.1 T2-weighted MRI shows classical high signal intensity lesion in left temporal lobe in herpes encephalitis. MRI, magnetic resonance imaging.

CSF until approximately 8 to 12 days after symptom onset, and increase significantly during the first 2 to 4 weeks of infection. In order to determine if there is an intrathecal synthesis of antibodies against HSV-1, send CSF and serum samples. A serum:CSF ratio of <20:1 is considered diagnostic of HSV-1 infection. Because this infection produces areas of hemorrhagic necrosis, the CSF may contain RBC or xanthochromia. RBC in the CSF may inhibit the PCR, giving a false-negative result.

The EEG often is abnormal, demonstrating periodic sharp-wave complexes from one or both temporal regions. The abnormalities on the EEG arise from one temporal lobe initially but typically spread to the contralateral temporal lobe over a period of 6 to 10 days.

A. **Therapeutic approach.**

1. **Antiviral activity.** Acyclovir is the antiviral drug of choice for HSV-1 encephalitis. It is given at a dosage of 10 mg/kg every 8 hours (30 mg/kg/day) IV, each infusion lasting >1 hour, for a period of 3 weeks. IV acyclovir can cause transient renal insufficiency secondary to crystallization of the drug in renal epithelial cells. For this reason, it is recommended that acyclovir be infused slowly over a period of 1 hour and that attention be paid to adequate IV hydration of the patient.

2. **Anticonvulsant therapy.** Seizure activity, either focal or focal with secondary generalization, occurs in two-thirds of patients with HSV-1 encephalitis. Anticonvulsant therapy is indicated if seizure activity develops, and the following drugs are recommended.

   a. **Lorazepam** at dosages of 0.1 mg/kg for adults and 0.05 mg/kg for children, or diazepam at 5 to 10 mg for adults and 0.2 to 0.3 mg/kg/dose for children.

   b. **Fosphenytoin** at a dose of 18 to 20 mg PE/kg no faster than 150 mg/minute. The daily maintenance dosage of fosphenytoin should be determined by serum levels.

   c. **Levetiracetam** or **valproic acid** or **lacosamide** can also be used. All three can be given intravenously.

Therapy for increased ICP. Increased ICP is a common complication of herpes encephalitis and is associated with a poor outcome. Increased ICP should be aggressively managed as outlined in Section **A.3** under Bacterial Meningitis.
B. Expected outcome. Among untreated patients with HSV-1 encephalitis, the mortality is higher than 70%, and only 2.5% of patients return to normal function after recovery. Patients treated with acyclovir have a significantly lower mortality of 19%, and 38% of these patients return to normal function.
C. Referrals. Because the clinical diagnosis of herpes encephalitis typically requires interpretation of the neurologic presentation, the EEG, neuroimaging studies, and CSF, the diagnosis of this severe and devastating neurologic illness should be made in consultation with a neurologist.

HERPES ZOSTER (SHINGLES)

A. Therapeutic approach. Oral valacyclovir 1,000 mg three times a day has been found superior to acyclovir in reducing zoster-associated pain. Oral acyclovir 800 mg five times a day and valacyclovir accelerate the rate of cutaneous healing and reduce the severity of acute neuritis and are most beneficial if treatment is initiated within 48 hours. Neither valacyclovir nor acyclovir reduces the incidence or severity of postherpetic neuralgia. For immunosuppressed patients, and for those with zoster ophthalmicus, many experts recommend the use of IV acyclovir. Ganciclovir can be considered an alternative agent for treatment. Corticosteroids have been proposed as adjunctive therapy in immunocompetent patients with varicella-zoster virus encephalitis.
B. Side effects. Oral acyclovir therapy has not been associated with renal dysfunction, but IV acyclovir can cause renal insufficiency. The risk of this complication is decreased by a slow rate of infusion.
C. Prevention. A varicella-zoster vaccine is available to decrease the risk of herpes zoster. Individuals with primary or acquired immunosuppression should not receive the vaccine.

LYME DISEASE

Lyme disease is caused by the spirochete *Borrelia burgdorferi*, which is transmitted by the bite of an infected tick. It is endemic in the coastal northeast from Massachusetts to Maryland (particularly in New York), in the upper Midwest in Minnesota and Wisconsin, and on the Pacific coast in California and southern Oregon.

In the majority of patients, initial infection is manifested by the appearance of an annular erythematous cutaneous lesion with central clearing of at least 5 cm in diameter, called erythema migrans. This lesion appears within 3 days to 1 month after a tick bite. Early disseminated Lyme disease is characterized by cardiac conduction abnormalities, arthritis, myalgia, fatigue, fever, meningitis, and cranial and peripheral neuropathy and radiculopathy. The most common neurologic abnormality during early disseminated Lyme disease is meningitis. The clinical features are typical of viral meningitis with symptoms of headache, mild neck stiffness, nausea, vomiting, low-grade fever, and photophobia. These symptoms may be associated with unilateral or bilateral facial nerve palsy or with symptoms of radiculitis (paresthesia and hyperesthesia) with or without focal weakness, transverse myelitis, or mononeuritis multiplex.

The majority of patients with Lyme disease have or have had an erythema migrans lesion. The diagnosis of Lyme disease begins with a serologic test for antibodies against *B. burgdorferi*. Most laboratories use an enzyme-linked immunosorbent assay technique. False-positive serologic results are a problem with this test for two reasons:

1. Tests can be performed on identical sera in different laboratories with different results. Because these tests are not well standardized, it is important to use a laboratory that is reliable in performing this test. A positive test result may indicate only exposure to *B. burgdorferi* rather than active infection. Persons who live in high-risk areas may have measurable antibodies without having Lyme disease.

2. False-positive serologic results can occur with rheumatoid arthritis, Rocky Mountain spotted fever, infectious mononucleosis, syphilis, tuberculous meningitis, and leptospirosis. When the ELISA is positive, then a Western blot should be obtained. The CSF is generally abnormal in neurologic Lyme disease. The typical spinal fluid abnormalities include lymphocytic pleocytosis (100 to 200 cells per mm^3), an elevated protein concentration, and a normal glucose concentration. The CSF should be examined for intrathecal production of anti-*B. burgdorferi* antibodies, and an antibody index should be calculated. The antibody index is determined as the ratio of (anti-*Borrelia* IgG in CSF/ anti-*Borrelia* IgG in serum) to (total IgG in CSF/total IgG in serum) and is defined as positive when the result is >1.3 to 1.5. The use of the antibody index to determine that there is an intrathecal production of antibodies is important as antibodies can be passively transferred from serum to CSF giving a false-positive result, and Lyme antibodies may persist in CSF for years.

A. **Therapeutic approach.**
   1. Patients with facial nerve palsy without other neurologic manifestations can be treated with doxycycline 100 mg by mouth twice a day for 14 days. *Doxycycline should not be given to pregnant women.*
   2. Parenteral ceftriaxone is recommended for patients with neurologic complications of Lyme disease, although oral doxycycline may be equally effective in the absence of brain or spinal cord involvement. The adult dosage of ceftriaxone is 2 g/day, which may be given in a single daily dose, and the dosage for children is 75 to 100 mg/kg/day (up to 2 g/day). Treatment is given for at least 2 weeks and should be continued for an additional 2 weeks if the response to treatment is slow or there is severe infection.
   3. Alternatives to ceftriaxone are penicillin G and cefotaxime. Penicillin G is administered at an adult dosage of 3 to 4 million units (miU) every 4 hours for 10 to 14 days or at a child dosage of 250,000 U/kg/day in divided doses. The major side effect of penicillin G is hypersensitivity reaction. Cefotaxime is given at dosages of 2 g three times a day for adults and 150 to 200 mg/kg/day (every 6 hours) for children.

B. **Expected outcome.** The condition of patients with neurologic complications of early disseminated Lyme disease (meningitis, cranial neuropathy, and peripheral neuropathy) should improve clinically within days, although improvement of facial weakness and radicular symptoms can take weeks. Prolonged antimicrobial therapy does not improve symptoms of post-Lyme syndrome and is not recommended.

C. **Prevention.** The deer tick is the usual vector of Lyme disease in the northeastern and the midwestern United States. Wearing protective clothing can help decrease the risk of infection. Transmission of infection is unlikely if the tick has been attached for <24 hours.

CRYPTOCOCCAL MENINGITIS

The diagnosis of cryptococcal meningitis is made when examination of the CSF shows lymphocytic pleocytosis, a decreased glucose concentration, and a positive result of a CSF cryptococcal antigen assay, fungal smear, or culture.

A. **Therapeutic approach.** The management of cryptococcal meningitis is divided into induction, consolidation, and maintenance (suppressive therapy). Induction therapy includes amphotericin B 0.7 to 1 mg/kg/day in combination with flucytosine 100 mg/kg/day divided into four daily doses for at least 4 weeks. Treatment then is switched to consolidation therapy with fluconazole 400 mg/day for a minimum of 8 weeks. Present guidelines recommend slight modifications for induction and consolidation therapy in HIV-infected patients and in organ transplant recipients. In the treatment of patients with HIV infection, fluconazole 200 mg/day is continued for lifelong suppressive therapy.

B. **Side effects.** The most important adverse effect of amphotericin B is renal dysfunction, which occurs in 80% of patients. Renal function, hemoglobin concentration, and electrolytes should be monitored closely. Renal toxicity appears to be reduced or prevented by means of careful attention to serum sodium concentration at the time of administration of amphotericin B. If renal insufficiency develops, AmBisome (Fujisawa, Deerfield, IL, USA) 5 mg/kg/day or amphotericin B lipid complex 5 mg/kg/day can be substituted for amphotericin B.

Flucytosine is generally well-tolerated; however, bone marrow suppression with anemia, leukopenia, or thrombocytopenia can develop. These hematologic abnormalities occur more often when serum concentrations of the drug exceed 100 mgmL; therefore, serum concentrations of flucytosine should be monitored and the peak serum concentration kept well below 100 mg/mL.

NEUROSYPHILIS IN IMMUNOCOMPETENT PATIENTS

In immunocompetent patients, the clinical presentation of neurosyphilis falls into one or more of the following categories: (1) asymptomatic neurosyphilis, (2) meningitis, (3) meningovascular syphilis, (4) dementia paralytica, and (5) tabes dorsalis. The diagnosis of neurosyphilis is based on a reactive serum treponemal test and CSF abnormalities. In neurosyphilis, there is often a mild CSF mononuclear pleocytosis with a mild elevation in the CSF protein concentration or a reactive CSF venereal disease research laboratory (VDRL) test. A positive CSF VDRL test establishes the diagnosis of neurosyphilis. A nonreactive CSF VDRL result does not exclude neurosyphilis. The CSF VDRL test is nonreactive in 30% to 57% of patients with neurosyphilis. A nonreactive CSF fluorescent treponemal antibody absorption test (FTA-ABS) excludes the diagnosis of neurosyphilis in all cases except early syphilis. A reactive CSF FTA-ABS is nonspecific and cannot be used to make a diagnosis of neurosyphilis.

A. **Therapeutic approach.** The regimen recommended by the CDC for management of neurosyphilis is IV aqueous penicillin G at 18 to 24 miU/day (3 to 4 miU every 4 hours) for 10 to 14 days. An alternative regimen is intramuscular procaine penicillin at 2.4 miU/day and oral probenecid at 500 mg four times a day, both for 10 to 14 days.

B. **Expected outcome.** The serum VDRL titer should decrease after successful therapy for neurosyphilis. The serum fluorescent treponemal antibody absorption test and the microhemagglutination—*Treponema pallidum* test remains reactive for life. The CSF WBC count should be normal 6 months after therapy is completed. If on reexamination of the CSF, the WBC count remains elevated, repetition of treatment is indicated.

TUBERCULOUS MENINGITIS

A. **Clinical presentation.** Tuberculous meningitis manifests as either subacute or chronic meningitis, as a slowly progressive dementing illness, or as fulminant meningoencephalitis. The intradermal tuberculin skin test is helpful when the result is positive. Radiographic evidence of pulmonary tuberculosis is found more often in children with tuberculous meningitis than in adults with tuberculous meningitis. The classical abnormalities at CSF examination are decreased glucose concentration, elevated protein concentration, and polymorphonuclear or lymphocytic pleocytosis. The CSF pleocytosis is typically neutrophilic initially, but then becomes mononuclear or lymphocytic within several weeks. Acid-fast bacilli are difficult to find in smears of CSF. Culture of CSF is the standard for diagnosis but is insensitive. Cultures are reported to be positive in 25% to 75% of cases of tuberculous meningitis, requiring 3 to 6 weeks for growth to be detectable. PCR assays that detect *Mycobacterium tuberculosis* rRNA in CSF have shown good results in clinical trials.

B. **Therapeutic approach.** Current recommendations for the management of tuberculous meningitis in children and adults include a combination of isoniazid (5 to 10 mg/kg/day up to 300 mg/day), rifampin (10 to 20 mg/kg/day up to 600 mg/day), and pyrazinamide (25 to 35 mg/kg/day up to 2 g/day). If the clinical response is good, pyrazinamide is discontinued after 8 weeks, and isoniazid and rifampin are continued for an additional 10 months. Ethambutol is added, and the course of treatment is extended to 1 to 2 years for immunocompromised patients. The American Academy of Pediatrics recommends addition of streptomycin at 20 to 40 mg/kg/day to the foregoing regimen for the first 2 months. Pyridoxine may be administered at a dosage of 25 to 50 mg/day to prevent the peripheral neuropathy that can result from use of isoniazid. Corticosteroid therapy is recommended when clinical deterioration occurs after treatment has begun. Dexamethasone can be administered at a dosage of 0.3 to 0.5 mg/kg/day for the 1st week of treatment and followed by oral prednisone.

NEUROCYSTICERCOSIS

A diagnosis of neurocysticercosis should be considered when a patient has seizures and neuroimaging evidence of cystic brain lesions. Cysticercosis is acquired by ingesting the eggs of the *Taenia solium* tapeworm shed in human feces.

A. Principal forms. The lesions of neurocysticercosis can be found in the brain parenchyma, the ventricles, the subarachnoid space, or in the basilar cisterns (racemose forms). In the parenchymal form, single or multiple cysts are found in the gray matter in the cerebrum and cerebellum. Cysticercal intraparenchymal cysts evolve through four stages with different appearances on neuroimaging. In the vesicular stage, the cyst contains a living larva. The scolex is often seen on CT and MRI. In the colloidal stage, the larva degenerates and on neuroimaging, the lesion is surrounded by edema. In the granulo-nodular stage, the membrane of the cyst thickens. In the final stage, the lesion is a calcified lesion. The most common clinical manifestation of parenchymal neurocysticercosis is new-onset seizure activity. In the ventricular form, single or multiple cysts are adherent to the ventricular wall or free in the CSF. Cysts are most common in the area of the fourth ventricle. In subarachnoid neurocysticercosis, cysts are found in the subarachnoid space or fixed under the pia and burrowed into the cortex. In the racemose form, cysts grow, often in clusters, in the basilar cisterns and obstruct the flow of CSF. Hydrocephalus and cysticercotic encephalitis, a severe form of neurocysticercosis due to intense inflammation around cysticerci and cerebral edema, are the most common cause of increased ICP.

B. Diagnosis. The diagnosis of neurocysticercosis depends on clinical features and evidence of cystic lesions demonstrating the scolex at CT or MRI, or other neuroimaging abnormalities (ring enhancing cystic lesions and intraparenchymal calcifications) (Fig. 47.2) suggestive of neurocysticercosis. Serum may be sent for enzyme-linked immunoelectrotransfer blot assay. Biopsy for histologic demonstration of the parasite is rarely done.

C. Therapeutic approach.

1. **Cysticidal therapy** consists of praziquantel at a dose of 50 mg/kg/day for 15 days, or praziquantel 100 mg/kg in three divided doses at 2-hour intervals (single day course) or albendazole at a dosage of 15 mg/kg/day for 8 days.

2. Corticosteroids. Cysticidal therapy frequently causes an inflammatory response with an increase in CSF protein concentration and CSF pleocytosis. This may result in an

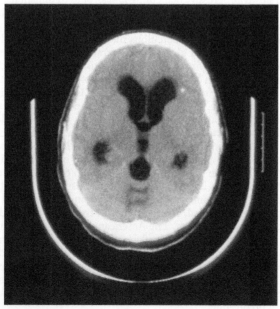

FIGURE 47.2 CT scan shows parenchymal brain calcification and hydrocephalus due to neurocysticercosis. CT, computed tomography.

exacerbation of signs and symptoms. The incidence of an inflammatory response is reduced by the concomitant use of corticosteroids, and their use is recommended both before and during treatment with anticysticidal therapy. Plasma levels of albendazole are increased by dexamethasone; plasma levels of praziquantel are decreased by dexamethasone therapy. This should be taken into consideration when corticosteroid therapy is used to decrease the headaches and vomiting induced by the destruction of parasites in cysticidal therapy. Dexamethasone 24 to 32 mg/day is recommended for patients with subarachnoid cysts, encephalitis, angiitis, or arachnoiditis.

3. **Side effects.** Phenytoin and carbamazepine decrease serum praziquantel levels due to their induction of the cytochrome P-450 liver enzyme system. If one of these anticonvulsants is used with praziquantel, it is recommended that oral cimetidine be added at a dosage of 800 mg twice a day. Cimetidine inhibits the cytochrome P-450 enzyme system, and in this way increases serum levels of praziquantel.

4. **Surgical therapy.** Intraventricular cysts necessitate surgical therapy, and when they obstruct the flow of CSF with resulting hydrocephalus, an intraventricular shunting device is indicated.

D. **Expected outcome.** The prognosis of patients with parenchymal neurocysticercosis is very good with cysticidal therapy. Cystic lesions should disappear within 3 months of treatment. The mortality is higher among patients with increased ICP, hydrocephalus, or the racemose form of the disease.

E. **Prevention.** Humans can acquire cysticercosis by eating food handled and contaminated by *T. solium* tapeworm carriers. Persons at high risk of tapeworm infestation who are employed as food handlers should be screened for intestinal parasites. Improved sanitation can decrease the incidence of cysticercosis from contaminated food or drinking water.

Key Points

- Bacterial meningitis is a neurologic emergency, and initial treatment is empiric until a specific organism is identified. Obtain blood cultures and begin antimicrobial therapy prior to neuroimaging or CSF analysis.
- Empiric therapy for community-acquired meningitis in infants, children, and adults (15 to 50 years of age) is the combination of a third- or fourth-generation cephalosporin plus vancomycin.
- Add ampicillin to empiric antimicrobial therapy (a third- or fourth-generation cephalosporin and vancomycin) in adults 50 years of age or older.
- Every patient with fever and headache, in whom herpes simplex virus-1 encephalitis is a possibility, should be treated with acyclovir 10 mg/kg/every 8 hours as soon as possible to decrease mortality and morbidity.
- The CSF HSV-1 PCR may be negative in the first 72 hours of symptoms of HSV encephalitis.
- Magnetic resonance fluid-attenuated inverse recovery (FLAIR) and diffusion-weighted sequences demonstrate an abnormal lesion of increased signal intensity in the temporal lobe in 90% of adult patients with herpes simplex virus encephalitis 48 hours after symptom onset.
- Neurologic Lyme disease may manifest as a seventh nerve or bilateral seventh nerve palsies (cranial nerves III, IV, and VI may also be involved), a radiculitis, a mononeuritis multiplex, and/or a lymphocytic meningitis.
- A positive CSF VDRL—treat for neurosyphilis.
- Negative CSF FTA-ABS, negative CSF VDRL, no CSF pleocytosis, normal protein concentration—no treatment for neurosyphilis is required.
- Negative CSF VDRL, increased white blood cell count, and/or protein concentration—treat for neurosyphilis.
- In neurocysticercosis, only cysts in the vesicular and colloidal stages contain live larva and are amendable to anticysticercal treatment. On neuroimaging, the scolex can often be seen in a cyst in the vesicular stage. As the larva degenerates, the cyst enters the colloidal stage and on neuroimaging, edema surrounds the lesion.

Recommended Readings

Baird A, Wiebe S, Zunt J, et al. Evidence-based guideline: treatment of parenchymal neurocyticercosis: report of the Guideline Development Subcommittee of the American Academy of Neurology. *Neurology.* 2013;80:1424–1429.

Brouwer MC, Heckenberg SGB, de Gans J, et al. Nationwide implementation of adjunctive dexamethasone therapy for pneumococcal meningitis. *Neurology.* 2010;75:1533–1539.

Cadavid D. Spirochetal infection. In: Roos KL, Tunkel AR, eds. *Handbook of Clinical Neurology. Bacterial Infections of the Central Nervous System.* Edinburgh, UK: Elsevier; 2010:179–219.

Corona T, Lugo M, Medina R, et al. Single day praziquantel therapy for neurocysticercosis. *N Engl J Med.* 1996;334:125.

Del Brutto OH, Wadia NH, Dumas M, et al. Proposal of diagnostic criteria for human cysticercosis and neurocysticercosis. *J Neurol Sci.* 1996;142:1–6.

Halperin JJ, Shapiro ED, Logigian E, et al. Practice parameter: treatment of nervous system Lyme disease (an evidence-based review). *Neurology.* 2007;69:91–102.

Kent SJ, Crowe SM, Yung A, et al. Tuberculous meningitis: a 30-year review. *Clin Infect Dis.* 1993;17:987–994.

Marra CM. Syphilis and human immunodeficiency virus infection. *Semin Neurol.* 1992;12:43–50.

Newton RW. Tuberculous meningitis. *Arch Dis Child.* 1994;70:364–366.

Perfect JR, Dismukes WE, Dromer F, et al. Clinical practice guidelines for the management of cryptococcal disease: 2010 update by the Infectious Diseases Society of America. *Clin Infect Dis.* 2010;50:291–322.

Roos KL, Tunkel AR, van de Beek D, et al. Acute bacterial meningitis. In: Scheld WM, Whitley RJ, Marra CM, eds. *Infections of the Central Nervous System.* Philadelphia, PA: Wolters Kluwer Health; 2014:365–419.

Roos KL, Tyler KL. Meningitis, encephalitis, brain abscess and empyema. In: Fauci AS, Braunwald E, Kasper DL, et al. eds. *Harrison's Principles of Internal Medicine.* 19th ed. New York, NY: McGraw-Hill; 2015.

Skoldenberg B. Herpes simplex encephalitis. *Scand J Infect Dis.* 1991;78:40–46.

Tunkel AR, Hartman BJ, Kaplan SL, et al. Practice guidelines for the management of bacterial meningitis. *Clin Infect Dis.* 2004;39:1267–1284.

Wood MJ, Shukla S, Fiddian AP, et al. Treatment of acute herpes zoster: effect of early (<48 h) versus late (48–72 h) therapy with acyclovir and valacyclovir on prolonged pain. *J Infect Dis.* 1998;178(suppl 1):S81–S84.

48 Neurologic Complications in Acquired Immune Deficiency Syndrome

Krutika Kuppalli and Paul O'Keefe

GENERAL CONSIDERATIONS

At the end of 2013, according to the World Health Organization (WHO), there were 35.0 million people living with human immunodeficiency virus (HIV)/acquired immune deficiency syndrome (AIDS) (PLWHA) globally and an additional 1.5 million people who died of AIDS-related complications that same year. At this time, sub-Saharan Africa continues to remain most severely affected, accounting for 71% of PLWHA. Introduction of antiretroviral therapy (ART) has aided in the decline of HIV infections globally, as new HIV infections have fallen by 38% since 2002 and AIDS-related deaths have decreased by 35% since 2005. Despite widespread availability of effective ART, central nervous system (CNS) involvement in PLWHA continues to be a serious threat worldwide with patients at risk for significant morbidity and mortality.

The CNS is involved early in the course of HIV infection and may produce the presenting clinical manifestations. Early natural history studies found neurologic signs and symptoms in 40% to 70% of patients during the course of the disease, whereas autopsy series demonstrated neuropathologic changes in 90% to 100% of PLWHA, affecting all levels of the neuraxis. These neurologic manifestations can result from effects of HIV itself or opportunistic infections (OIs). Acute meningitis, meningoencephalitis, peripheral facial nerve palsy, or polyneuritis can mark HIV seroconversion. Subsequently, neuropathy, encephalopathy, myelopathy, or myopathy may occur with OIs of the CNS occurring in conjunction with marked immune suppression.

Current therapeutic advances with combinations of antiretroviral agents known as highly active antiretroviral therapy (HAART) have had a profound effect on the frequency of HIV-induced neurologic manifestations and CNS OIs. Neurologic complications continue to occur, although more commonly as a presentation in persons not aware of their HIV status, or among those who fail ART due to medication noncompliance or development of drug-resistant HIV strains. The most common neurologic complications seen in PLWHA are listed in Table 48.1. More recently, it has become apparent that subtle neurologic manifestations of HIV infection occur in patients on ART, including those who appear to be responding to treatment and have suppression of plasma viral load. Given these subtle findings, when evaluating a PLWHA with neurologic disease, general considerations include:

A. The imaging modality of choice in HIV-related CNS disease is magnetic resonance imaging (MRI); however, particular imaging patterns may be nonspecific.

B. Multiple pathologic conditions in the CNS may occur concurrently in patients with profound immune suppression.

C. Most OIs appear with significant immune suppression (CD4 <200 cells/mm^3).

D. Neurologic manifestations of OIs in patients with AIDS can be subtle and lack classical disease features seen in immune competent hosts.

E. Specific diagnosis of an OI requires confirmation by culture, or demonstration of genetic material in cerebrospinal fluid (CSF) or biopsied tissue.

F. Empiric therapy based on a presumptive diagnosis is appropriate in some circumstances; however, the absence of a typical treatment response should prompt early further evaluation.

G. HIV-associated cognitive deficits are becoming more subtle in the era of successful ART and may occur in patients who appear to have successful control of systemic disease.

H. Not all neurologic symptoms occurring in HIV-infected patients result from HIV or OIs, particularly when the HIV infection appears to be well controlled. Such patients are subject to all of the common neurologic conditions that affect other populations.

I. Treatment strategies in AIDS are continuously evolving, particularly ART regimens.

TABLE 48.1 Entities Causing Neurologic Complications in AIDS

Encephalopathy

Diffuse

HIV
PML
CMV
VZV
Syphilis
Toxoplasmosis
Aspergillosis
Toxic (medications)
Metabolic (e.g., hypoxia and sepsis)

Focal

Toxoplasmosis
PML
Lymphoma
Cryptococcus
CMV
HSV
VZV
Syphilis
Tuberculosis
Fungal abscess
Nocardia species
Pyogenic abscess

Myelopathy

HIV
CMV
VZV
Syphilis
Lymphoma
Tuberculosis
Toxoplasmosis
Vitamin B_{12} deficiency
Nocardia species
Pyogenic abscess

Meningitis

HIV
Cryptococcus neoformans
Syphilis
Tuberculosis
Lymphoma
CMV
HSV
VZV
Fungi (*Histoplasma capsulatum*, Blastomycoses, Coccidiomycosis)

Neuropathy

HIV
Toxic (e.g., di-deoxynucleosides)
CMV

TABLE 48.1 Entities Causing Neurologic Complications in AIDS (*continued*)

Lymphoma
Syphilis
Vitamin B$_{12}$ deficiency
Myopathy
HIV
Toxic (Zidovudine)
Toxoplasmosis
Pyogenic
CMV

Abbreviations: AIDS, acquired immune deficiency syndrome; CMV, cytomegalovirus; HIV, human immunodeficiency virus; HSV, herpes simplex virus; HZV, herpes zoster virus; PML, progressive multifocal leukoencephalopathy; VZV.

CONDITIONS ATTRIBUTED TO HUMAN IMMUNE DEFICIENCY VIRUS INFECTION

A. HIV-associated neurocognitive disorder.
   1. Epidemiology. HIV-associated neurocognitive disorder (HAND) is the impaired cognition caused by HIV; and despite advances in the treatment of HIV with more effective ART, the CNS continues to be affected by this disease. Although the incidence of the most severe form of HAND, HIV-associated dementia (HAD), has declined due to effective ART, the incidence of milder forms of HAND (asymptomatic neurocognitive impairment [ANI] and mild neurocognitive disorder [MND]) remains stable. Even in its mildest form, HAND has been associated with lower medication adherence, decreased ability to perform the most complex daily tasks, difficulty finding employment, worse quality of life, and shorter survival. A recent study employing neurocognitive testing found that 69% of patients with HIV infection taking ART and without detectable plasma HIV VL or cognitive complaints had subtle cognitive impairments. With individuals surviving longer due to effective ART and the independent evolution of HIV in the relatively sequestered CNS, there could be a rise in HAND. Studies have demonstrated discordant presence of HIV VL in CSF despite undetectable plasma viral load and differing HIV viral strains in CSF compared to those found in plasma, which may have different resistance-associated mutations (RAMs) to ART.

   In addition to HIV infection itself, several factors may predispose HIV-infected individuals to cognitive impairment, such as concurrent hepatitis C virus infection, the use of psychoactive medications, substance use, mood disorders, low educations, and age-related cognitive changes. ART may alter lipid metabolism with accelerated atherosclerosis increasing the risk of cerebrovascular disease with related cognitive deficits.

   Three categories have been proposed to describe the current spectrum of HAND (Table 48.2):
   a. Asymptomatic neurocognitive impairment. Individuals with acquired subclinical impairment in at least two cognitive domains on neurocognitive testing, without delirium, symptomatic complaints, or impaired daily activities.
   b. Mild neurocognitive disorder. Individuals with clear sensorium and acquired impairments in at least two cognitive domains causing at least mild interference with daily activities.
   c. HIV-associated dementia. Individuals with clear sensorium and more severe acquired impairments in at least two cognitive domains sufficient to produce marked interference with daily activities.
   2. Pathogenesis. The pathogenesis of HAND is not well understood. Pre-ART autopsy studies demonstrated multinucleated giant cells containing HIV, myelin pallor, microglial nodules, and loss of neurons and synaptic density. ART era studies have found less significant correlations between the first three elements and clinical impairments. Neurons are not infected by HIV and die in locations remote from the perivascular macrophages and microglia that harbor the virus. Indirect neurotoxicity resulting from

TABLE 48.2 Criteria for HIV-Associated Neurocognitive Disorder (HAND)

HIV-associated asymptomatic neurocognitive impairment (ANI)
Acquired impairment in cognitive functioning involving at least two ability domains
Cognitive impairment does not interfere with daily functioning
Criteria for dementia or delirium are not present
No evidence for an alternative etiology for the ANI
HIV-associated mild neurocognitive disorder (MND)
Acquired impairment in cognitive functioning involving at least two ability domains
Cognitive impairment produces at least mild interference in function at work, home or in social activities
Criteria for dementia or delirium are not present
No evidence for an alternative etiology for the MND
HIV-associated dementia (HAD)
Acquired impairment in cognitive functioning involving at least two ability domains
Marked interference in function (e.g., inability to work, manage affairs, etc.)
Criteria for delirium not present (clear sensorium)
No evidence of another cause for the dementia

Abbreviation: HIV, human immunodeficiency virus.
Adapted from Antinori A, Arendt G, Becker JT, et al. Updated research nosology for HIV-associated neurocognitive disorders. *Neurology*. 2007;69:1789–1799.

soluble factors released by infected cells causing activation of inflammatory mechanisms and disruption of critical trophic influences which culminate in neuronal apoptosis and neuron damage are currently favored as the pathogenesis for HAND.

3. Clinical features. A clinical triad of cognitive impairment, behavioral changes, and motor impairment was described early in the AIDS pandemic. Cognitive features include slowness of thought processing, perseveration, impairments of complex attention, and impaired recall of acquired memories. Behavioral features include apathy, withdrawal from social interaction, and depression. Uncommonly, mania or atypical psychoses occur. Motor features include hyperreflexia, hypertonia, ataxia, and tremors, typically affecting the legs initially but also involving fine motor coordination of the upper extremities. Extrapyramidal features including bradykinesia, facial masking, rigidity, and postural instability may be seen.

In patients on ART, the features may be attenuated and the temporal course prolonged. Psychomotor slowing, lassitude, and mild extrapyramidal or fine motor impairments are most commonly seen. The impact can still be significant both on the more demanding aspects of daily activities and by altering adherence to ART regimens resulting in loss of viral suppression. Individuals may have mild cognitive abnormalities on testing but no apparent changes in daily functioning. Performance fluctuation on cognitive tests is seen in more mildly affected individuals with some improving and others evolving to more severe impairments.

4. Diagnosis. A clear sensorium is required for the diagnosis of HAND. Evidence of functional impairment often comes to attention from impaired work performance or reports from a companion who assumes responsibility for handling funds and documents. Withdrawal from social activities is common, and depression may be a comorbid feature. Neuropsychometric testing should be employed for both diagnosis and monitoring. OIs must be excluded with neuroradiographic imaging and CSF analysis. Other comorbid conditions also need to be evaluated such as metabolic abnormalities, use of psychotropic medications, and the presence of substance abuse.

In patients with HAND, CSF is normal or shows mild-to-moderate protein elevation. Occasionally HIV emerges in the CSF along in the presence of plasma virologic control. This phenomenon of viral escape is uncommon but should be a sign to assess the CSF if new or active neurologic symptoms are present that are not otherwise explained. In the ART era, many patients with asymptomatic or mild impairments are not severely immunosuppressed. Neurocognitive measures are sensitive but must be compared with appropriate normative populations with similar age, educational level, ethnicity, and gender.

MRI in HAND may be normal, demonstrate atrophic changes, or reveal a confluent symmetric leukoencephalopathy. More recent radiologic studies have focused on evaluating the use of newer MRI techniques such as diffusion tensor imaging (DTI) and functional MRI (fMRI). DTI has been shown to be a sensitive tool in detecting white matter changes in various CNS diseases. fMRI makes use of the blood oxygen level dependent contrast to provide dynamic information during resting state or performance of cognitive tasks. Abnormal activation and connectivity have been seen on fMRI among HIV patients with mild cognitive impairment. Studies have demonstrated that functional connections within and between particular networks may be compromised in HAND.

5. **Management.**
   a. **Antiviral agents.** There are increasing data demonstrating there is variable CSF concentration achieved by antiretrovirals (ARVs). The variable CSF penetration of different ARVs may help explain the discordance in CSF viral escape and paradoxical cognitive deterioration in patients with HAND who have plasma viral suppression. ARVs with greater CNS penetration are thought to be more effective at treating HAND. To address this issue, CNS penetration effectiveness (CPE) was developed and assigns a number to each ARV based on its chemical properties, CSF concentration, and effectiveness at achieving a reduction in CSF VL based on available data. The higher the CPE number, the better the CNS availability and chance of obtaining an undetectable CNS HIV VL. There is no established optimal ART regimen for HAND; however, antiretroviral resistance testing of recovered virus from blood and CSF can aid in the selection of a regimen, ideally one with a higher CPE score and minimal adverse effects. Zidovudine (AZT), a nucleoside reverse transcriptase inhibitor (NRTI) that penetrates into CSF reasonably well, was the first antiretroviral agent shown in a prospective randomized controlled trial (RCT) to have efficacy in HAND, as measured by serial cognitive testing. ARVs with highest CPE score of four (Zidovudine, Nevaripine, Indinavir) are followed by those with a score of three (Abacavir, Emtricitabine, Efavirenz, Darunavir, Fosamprenavir, Kaletra, Maraviroc, and Raltegravir). Other strategies for treatment of HAND include targeting mediators of neurotoxicity and a searching for reliable and timely surrogate markers of CNS disease.
   b. **Supportive therapy.**
      (1) **Apathy and withdrawal** can be managed with modafenil 200 to 400 mg daily (not an FDA-approved indication) or methylphenidate at 5 to 10 mg two or three times a day.
      (2) **Depression** is usually managed with selective serotonin reuptake inhibitors (SSRIs) such as fluoxetine or others. Tricyclic antidepressants (TCAs) such as nortriptyline at initial dosages of 25 mg at bedtime, increasing in 25-mg increments every 1 to 2 weeks (or similar agents at comparable doses) are alternatives; however, anticholinergic effects of these drugs can precipitate delirium.
      (3) **Seizures** occur with increased frequency in HIV-infected patients. Because of potential interactions with ART, non–enzyme-inducing antiepileptic drugs (AEDs), which are not metabolized by the cytochrome P-450 system, such as levetiracetam, lamotrigine, gabapentin, or pregabalin, are preferred.
      (4) **Supervision.** Progression of HIV-associated cognitive change results in loss of ability to manage personal business and financial affairs. Provisions for assistance and ultimately legal transfer of decision-making powers for both financial and healthcare decisions, and advanced healthcare directives, should be arranged. Assistance in the home may be needed for the provision of meals and facilitation of personal care. Residence in a sheltered facility can be considered when the need for assistance precludes independent living.
6. **Outcomes.** ART has reduced the severity and mortality of HAND. By prolonging survival of patients with HIV infection, ART may also lead to an increase in prevalence of cognitive impairment. The natural history of HAND in the era of successful ART continues to evolve.

B. HIV myelopathy.

1. **Epidemiology.** This condition is symptomatic in 5% to 10% of patients, although neuropathologic evidence of myelopathy has been found at the time of autopsy in up to 50% of patients with AIDS. In the era of effective ART, the frequency appears to be decreasing.

2. **Pathogenesis.** Vacuolar changes with foamy macrophages are found predominantly in the myelin of the dorsal and lateral columns of the thoracic spinal cord, resembling changes seen in subacute combined degeneration. Occasionally diffuse cord changes are seen. Signs of active HIV infection such as microglial nodules and infected macrophages are not thought to be associated. Pathologic evidence of productive HIV infection within the spinal cord is only found in about 6% of patients. The specific cause is unknown; however, a deficiency of transmethylation pathways and cytokines, such as tumor necrosis factor, may be important.

3. **Clinical features.** Progressive painless spastic paraparesis, with sensory ataxia and neurogenic bladder, is consistent with vacuolar myelopathy.

4. **Diagnosis.** HIV myelopathy is a diagnosis of exclusion and should be made based on clinical features in the setting of HIV. CSF should be obtained to exclude other conditions and etiologies, such as B_{12} deficiency, syphilitic myelitis, tuberculous myelitis, human T-cell lymphotropic virus type I (HTLV-1), cytomegalovirus (CMV) myeloradiculitis, and varicella zoster virus (VZV) myelitis. MRI of the spinal cord can be normal, reveal atrophy, or rarely have increased T2 signal.

5. **Management.** No specific therapy has been shown to prevent progression of myelopathy. Optimizing ART is recommended although it has not been demonstrated to have a favorable effect on neurologic deficits. Spasticity can be managed with baclofen or tizanidine and painful dysesthesias may be treated with lamotrigine or desipramine. Urinary frequency, urgency, and incontinence may be relieved with anticholinergic agents such as oxybutynin.

   External supports enhance safer mobility in patients with sufficient leg strength. Motorized scooters or wheelchairs can maintain mobility in weaker patients who are otherwise capable of independent activity.

6. **Outcomes.** Most individuals have a slow progressive course over time. Since patients have prolonged survival due to effective ART, the focus is now on managing chronic disability with routine neurologic evaluation to adjust supportive therapy. Abrupt neurologic changes should prompt evaluation for superimposed OIs.

C. HIV distal sensory polyneuropathy (HIV-DSP).

1. **Epidemiology.** HIV-DSP is the most common neurologic complication in HIV with an estimated incidence of 33% to 50%. Prior to the widespread use of effective ART, risk factors were thought to be low CD4 count, elevated HIV viral load, and use of neurotoxic ART (didanosine, stavudine, and zalcitabine). More recent studies have demonstrated that there appears to be an increased risk in patients with a history of substance abuse, older age, diabetes, hypertriglyceridemia, and that longer survival in HIV-infected patients may result in continued significant morbidity from this condition.

2. **Pathogenesis.** HIV-DSP is due to distal degeneration of long axons, macrophage infiltration, and a loss of neurons in the dorsal root ganglion (DRG). The process predominately affects distal small unmyelinated fibers with involvement of myelinated fibers in more severe cases. Neurotoxicity can occur by direct infection of the peripheral nerve by the virus or various indirect immunomodulatory mechanisms. HIV-DSP can also be associated with ART, most commonly the di-deoxynucleosides, which are thought to cause neurotoxicity by causing mitochondrial dysfunction.

3. **Clinical features.** The most prominent symptom of HIV-DSP is a symmetric, burning, stabbing, or shooting pain that can be disabling in severity. Initial symptoms include paresthesias and numbness starting at the feet which may gradually ascend. Balance can be affected if involvement of larger fibers occurs. Physical examination demonstrates impaired vibratory sensation, pin-prick and temperature perception, and absent/diminished ankle reflexes. Sensory ataxia and weakness of small muscles in the feet is also common.

4. **Diagnosis.** HIV-DSP is a diagnosis of exclusion of other small fiber neuropathies, particularly toxic neuropathy associated with di-deoxynucleosides which appears clinically similar. Other causes of neuropathy need to be excluded, such as vitamin B_{12} deficiency,

diabetes, uremia, alcoholism, hypothyroidism, and hepatitis C which may mimic or influence the neuropathic features.

Confirmatory diagnostic tests may include electromyography (EMG), nerve conduction studies (NCS), and skin biopsy. EMG may show active or chronic denervation patterns, NCS may show decreased amplitude or absence of sural nerve sensory potentials, and skin biopsy may show a decrease in epidermal nerve fiber density.

5. **Management.**
   a. There is no established therapy for HIV-DSP, and treatment should be directed at symptomatic relief.
   b. No agents are currently FDA approved for the treatment of HIV-DSP. Pain relief is important to optimize function and improve quality of life. Medications for treating other neuropathic pain syndromes are typically used including AEDs, antidepressants, and nonspecific analgesics including opioids.
   c. ART has not been convincingly shown to modify the course of the neuropathy; however, higher plasma viral load has been associated with pain severity in some studies.
   d. Neurotoxic agents should be discontinued whenever possible, particularly di-deoxynucleosides. Toxic neuropathy may persist for 6 to 8 weeks after discontinuation of these agents, and occasionally may temporarily worsen.
   e. Any metabolic deficiencies should be corrected.
   f. Topical lidocaine or capsaicin formulations may be effective adjuvants.
   g. Nonpharmacologic approaches such as acupuncture, transcutaneous electrical nerve stimulation, biofeedback, and relaxation therapies can be tried.

6. **Outcomes.** Symptomatic management can be helpful in alleviating discomfort; however, reversal of HIV-DSP is unlikely. Acute worsening of symptoms may arise when concurrent pathologies are present; and if this occurs, should be further investigated.

D. **Inflammatory demyelinating polyneuropathy (IDP).**
   1. **Epidemiology.** Individuals with HIV rarely develop acute inflammatory demyelinating polyneuropathy (AIDP) or chronic inflammatory demyelinating polyneuropathy (CIDP), with the incidence of these neuropathies unknown. AIDP is similar to Guillain–Barré syndrome (GBS) in non–HIV-infected persons. It usually occurs early in the course of HIV infection and may represent a response to seroconversion. CIDP results from immune-mediated demyelination and may be relapsing or progressive.
   2. **Pathogenesis.** IDP at the time of HIV seroconversion is thought to result from an immune reaction to HIV and targets peripheral myelin.
   3. **Clinical features.** Individuals with IDP present with progressive, symmetric motor weakness, variable sensory and autonomic features, and areflexia. Symptoms usually begin in the distal lower extremities and ascend over days with some individuals progressing to respiratory failure requiring mechanical ventilatory support. Patients with clinical progression after the first 4 to 6 weeks by definition have CIDP. CIDP may follow a progressive or relapsing course over months with motor weakness and areflexia but with more prominent sensory impairment.
   4. **Diagnosis.** There are typical features suggestive of IDP which help assist with the diagnosis. Electrophysiologic studies reveal prominent slowing and motor nerve conduction blocks, prolonged or absent F-wave responses, and variable degree of axonal damage and denervation. CSF may demonstrate a moderate mononuclear pleocytosis up to 50 cells/μL along with a prominent protein elevation.
   5. **Management.**
      a. Plasma exchange (PLEX) with a course of 200 to 250 mL/kg divided into five or six exchanges over a 2-week period has been shown to be effective. Intravenous immune globulin (IVIG) (400 mg/kg/day for 5 days) is an alternative therapy shown to be beneficial. Individuals with CIDP need maintenance therapy with one treatment every 2 to 4 weeks.
      b. Individuals with impending respiratory failure need elective intubation with ventilator support until adequate respiratory function returns.
      c. Adjunctive therapy is important to prevent complications of immobility and maintain function in anticipation of neuromuscular recovery. Physical therapy should be initiated at the bedside with passive range of motion to prevent contractures and advance as strength is improved. Neuralgic pain can be treated as in patients with HIV-DSP. As strength improves, mobilization may require support devices and orthotics.

6. **Outcomes.** AIDP usually resolves and most individuals have recovery. CIDP has a more variable outcome with residual impairment often persisting.

E. **HIV myopathy.**

1. **Epidemiology.** Symptomatic and primary muscle disease is uncommon in HIV-infected individuals, however rarely a polymyositis-like syndrome can occur. In the latter half of the 1980s, after the widespread use of zidovudine (AZT) was initiated, a secondary myopathy attributable to muscle toxicity began to emerge. Zidovudine myopathy usually appears after at least 6 months of treatment and is thought to be a result of mitochondrial toxicity. A study of 86 patients on AZT for more than 6 months revealed 16% had persistently elevated creatine kinase (CK) and 6% had symptomatic myopathy. Uncommonly, OIs may cause myositis (i.e., toxoplasmosis) and should also be investigated if medication cessation does not lead to resolution of symptoms.

2. **Pathogenesis.** AZT likely causes mitochondrial toxicity in muscle through inhibition of the mitochondrial enzyme DNA polymerase gamma. The cause of myopathies unassociated with AZT is unknown, but pathologic findings include rod body myopathy, necrotizing and nonnecrotizing inflammatory myopathy, and type 2 muscle fiber atrophy found in HIV-1–associated muscle wasting syndrome. Immunologic factors are also thought to play an important role.

3. **Clinical features.** Individuals typically present with symmetric proximal muscle weakness of the hip or shoulder girdle muscles. Difficulty squatting, rising from a chair, or walking up stairs are typical presenting symptoms of myopathy. Some individuals also have myalgias and muscle tenderness.

4. **Diagnosis.** In addition to having clinical features suggestive of myopathy, serum CK is typically elevated. EMG of weak muscles demonstrates small myopathic motor unit potentials with increased recruitment, fibrillation, and complex discharges. Muscle biopsy may reveal scattered muscle fiber degeneration and inflammatory infiltrates of CD8+ T lymphocytes and macrophages. Mitochondrial abnormalities and inclusions such as nemaline rod bodies may be present.

5. **Management.** In patients taking AZT, discontinuation of the medication may result in improvement of the myopathy. In patients who continue to deteriorate after AZT is stopped, biopsy to evaluate for opportunistic or inflammatory myositis should be considered. Prednisone has been used with variable success in patients with polymyositis or rod body myopathy, although the natural history of these myopathies is uncertain and the relation of improvement to treatment is unclear.

6. **Outcomes.** Most patients respond to discontinuation of toxic medications (i.e., AZT) or treatment with corticosteroids. Lack of response to empiric therapy should prompt a muscle biopsy.

F. **Aseptic meningitis.**

1. **Epidemiology.** HIV is often overlooked as a cause of aseptic meningitis, meningoencephalitis, or encephalitis. It can cause neurologic features in up to 17% of patients and acute aseptic meningitis in 1% to 2% of all primary HIV infections. Neurologic symptoms may occur or develop up to 3 months after the onset of symptoms of acute HIV when the other symptoms have resolved.

2. **Clinical features.** Patients may present with headache, fever, and neck stiffness. They may occasionally have a positive Kernig's or Bruzdinski's sign, cranial neuropathy, confusion, or lethargy.

3. **Diagnosis.** Patients with HIV may have a chronic, subclinical aseptic meningitis. CSF analysis may show a modest lymphocytic pleocytosis, mild elevation of protein, and elevated gamma globulin index.

4. **Management.** The importance of this condition is in its potential for causing diagnostic confusion particularly in the evaluation of neurosyphilis or other CNS OIs. Practitioners should also be cognizant of the fact that aseptic meningitis or meningoencephalitis can be a presenting symptom of acute HIV and individuals with this clinical presentation should be tested for HIV and if deemed appropriate, started on effective ART without delay.

5. **Outcomes.** Aseptic meningitis is often self-limited but can recur at any time following the initial infection. It is possible that it may be associated with a more rapid progression of HIV-related disease.

OPPORTUNISTIC INFECTIONS

Advances in ART have decreased the incidence of CNS OIs; however, they continue to occur as presenting manifestations of AIDS, particularly in patients who have poor responses to ART or have limited access to medications. Most OIs that affect the CNS are AIDS-defining conditions. They include cryptococcal meningitis, toxoplasmosis, primary CNS lymphoma (PCNSL), progressive multifocal leukoencephalopathy (PML), CNS infection by CMV, CNS varicella zoster virus (VZV), CNS tuberculosis (TB), and have a high associated mortality. The above conditions including neurosyphilis will be reviewed as they are the most common CNS infections affecting PLWHA worldwide. Only the most common OIs are reviewed here.

A. **Cryptococcal meningitis.**
1. **Epidemiology.** Cryptococcal meningitis is a fungal infection most commonly caused by *Cryptococcus neoformans* (Video 48.1). It is a ubiquitous environmental encapsulated yeast found in the soil and pigeon droppings, acquired through inhalation and spreads to the CNS hematogenously. It is more common than any other systemic fungal infection in PLWHA and is the most common opportunistic pathogen causing meningitis in PLWHA. In addition to meningitis, it can cause localized cryptococcomas in brain parenchyma and extra-neurologic cryptococcal infection in the lung, bone marrow, liver, urinary tract (prostate), and skin. It usually occurs in patients with HIV/AIDS who have a CD4 count ≤ 100 cells/mm^3. The incidence of cryptococcal meningitis has declined as patients have had increased access to effective ART; however, this infection continues to remain one of the leading causes of mortality in regions where access to effective ART is limited and diagnosis of HIV is delayed.
2. **Pathogenesis.** Cryptococcal spores enter the body via inhalation, which leads to primary pulmonary infection, latent infection, or disseminated systemic infection with a tendency to localize to the CNS. In patients with HIV, most cases of cryptococcal meningitis represent reactivation of latent infection.
3. **Clinical features.** The most common presentation of *C. neoformans* is meningitis with symptoms of headache, malaise, and fever. It can cause increased intracranial pressure (ICP); thus some patients may present with altered mental status, papilledema, personality changes, hearing loss, lethargy, or memory loss. Peripheral facial nerve involvement associated with AIDS is the most common cranial neuropathy. Seizures and focal CNS signs may be observed with parenchymal involvement and cerebral infarctions been reported.
4. **Diagnosis.** In patients with meningitis, radiographic imaging may be normal or show meningeal enhancement. Brain MRI is recommended in HIV patients to evaluate for space-occupying lesions, in patients with focal neurologic deficits, or clinical manifestations of increased ICP prior to obtaining a lumbar puncture (LP). An LP for CSF examination is essential in making the diagnosis of cryptococcal meningitis. CSF opening pressure should be measured at the time of LP. CSF usually demonstrates a lymphocytic pleocytosis, elevated protein, and low glucose. It is important to note, the CSF profile can be normal in 30% of patients. India Ink stain of the CSF can be done quickly, but requires an experienced technician and if positive can show round encapsulated yeast. It has a low sensitivity in early infection and is not diagnostic in 10% to 30% of HIV-infected patients. Detection of the CSF cryptococcal antigen (CrAg) supports the diagnosis of cryptococcal meningitis with sensitivity of 93% to 100% and specificity of 93% to 98%. CSF culture is usually positive in a patient with meningitis within 3 to 7 days; however, results may be negative when cryptococcomas are present, thus requiring biopsy of the lesion. Serum CrAg is highly sensitive and positive in 91% to 92% of cases, and should be performed in patients with suspected cryptococcal meningitis.
5. **Management.** Treatment of cryptococcal meningitis is comprised of three phases: induction, consolidation, and maintenance.
   a. **Induction therapy.** Mortality in cryptococcal meningitis often occurs in the first 2 weeks of therapy. Induction therapy with Amphotericin B plus Flucytosine for 2 weeks is recommended in patients with cryptococcal meningitis or extrapulmonary cryptococcosis. Flucytosine is recommended since it leads to rapid sterilization of the CSF and is associated with increased rates of survival. For patients unable to

tolerate Amphotericin B or those in resource-limited countries where access to the medication may be limited, high-dose fluconazole has been used. Induction is usually continued for at least 14 days, but in seriously ill patients, therapy may be extended.

b. **Consolidation therapy.** After at least 14 days of successful induction therapy. Defined as substantial clinical improvement and negative CSF culture after repeat LP. Patients are treated with fluconazole 400 mg daily for 8 weeks.

c. **Maintenance therapy.** Fluconazole 200 mg daily is continued for at least 1 year. Maintenance therapy can be terminated when the following criteria are met: completion of initial (induction and consolidation) therapy and at least 1 year of maintenance therapy; patient remains asymptomatic from cryptococcal infection; and CD4 count remains at 100 cells/mm^3 for 3 or more months with suppressed HIV RNA on effective ART. If CD4 falls below 100 cells/mm^3 maintenance therapy should be re-initiated and patients should be reevaluated for cryptococcal meningitis if deemed appropriate.

d. **Adjunctive therapy.** Elevated ICP is a common and serious complication in cryptococcal meningitis and occurs in over 50% of patients. It is vital to aggressively manage increased ICP with serial LPs, and, if necessary, lumbar drains or ventriculo-peritoneal shunts (VPS). The goal of treatment is to have ICP within normal range. Acetazolamide or mannitol therapy is not recommended as it has been associated with adverse events. ART should be initiated; however, the timing of this is still uncertain as it may be associated with immune reconstitution inflammatory syndrome (IRIS) in up to 30% of cases (Section **J** under Opportunistic Infections) and may be associated with increased morbidity and mortality.

e. **Timing of ART.** ART should be initiated, however the timing of this in acute disease is controversial as studies have shown conflicting data. Currently, the Panel on Opportunistic Infections in HIV-Infected Adults and Adolescents recommends delaying ART until induction therapy or induction/consolidation therapy has been completed in those with severe disease. It is noted that in patients with severe immune deficiency (CD4 <50 cells/mm^3), earlier initiation of ART may be needed. If ART is initiated in these individuals, they should be monitored for signs and symptoms of IRIS.

6. **Outcomes.** Acute mortality from cryptococcal meningitis in patients with HIV/AIDS ranges from 11% to 45%, with the majority of deaths occurring during the first 2 weeks. Important prognostic factors are the degree of obtundation at presentation and the presence and response to treatment of increased ICP. Other factors reported to negatively affect prognosis are CSF CrAg >1:1,024, extra-neurologic cryptococcal infection, low CSF and WBC count, and hyponatremia. CSF should be sampled after completion of induction therapy and those with persistently positive cryptococcal cultures should be managed with continued higher doses of anti-fungals. Serum CrAg cannot be used to manage disease response.

B. **CNS toxoplasmosis.**

1. **Epidemiology.** *Toxoplasma gondii* is an intracellular protozoan most commonly acquired by consumption of undercooked or contaminated meat or ingestion of oocysts in an environment contaminated with cat feces. The prevalence in the U.S. is about 11%. The parasite typically remains dormant in the absence of immune suppression and disease develops through reactivation of latent cysts, with greatest risk in those with CD4 <100 cells/mm^3. Seropositive individuals not on effective prophylaxis have a 30% risk of reactivation. The widespread use of ART and the practice of using trimethoprim-sulfamethoxazole for the prevention of *Pneumocystis Jirovecii* (PJP) Pneumonia has helped decrease the incidence of CNS toxoplasmosis.

2. **Pathogenesis.** Toxoplasma protozoa invade the intestinal epithelium and spread throughout the body leading either to primary infection, or more commonly, establishment of latent infection in various tissues. In immune compromised hosts, clinical disease results from reactivation of latent disease with the most common site being the CNS. Toxoplasmosis is considered the most common cause of HIV-associated focal CNS disease.

3. **Clinical features.** The most common presentation is a focal encephalitis with headache (55%), confusion (52%) and fever (47%). Common manifestations are seizures, impaired

mentation and focal abnormalities such as hemiparesis, hemiplegia, hemisensory loss, cerebellar ataxia, visual field defects, cranial nerve palsies, and aphasia. Involvement of the basal ganglia can result in movement disorders.

4. **Diagnosis.** Definitive diagnosis of CNS toxoplasmosis requires a compatible clinical syndrome, identification of one or more mass lesions by brain imaging, and detection of the organism in a specimen.

   Presumptive diagnosis of CNS toxoplasmosis is made if the patient has a CD4 count less than 100 cells/mm^3, compatible clinical syndrome and not been on effective prophylaxis, positive serum toxoplasma serology, and characteristic brain imaging. Based on this criteria, there is a 90% probability the diagnosis is CNS toxoplasmosis. Patients should be started on therapy with repeat brain imaging performed in 2 weeks to evaluate for response.

   Brain MRI usually shows multiple ring enhancing lesions which often involve the basal ganglia and gray-white junction in 90% of patients (Fig. 48.1A and B). The appearance of the mass lesions is nonspecific, although a signet ring sign has been suggested to be highly suggestive when present. An isolated mass lesion can occur in up to 14% of patients, and non-enhancing infarction-like patterns, meningoencephalitis, and myelitis have been reported. Radionuclide imaging with thallium single-photon emission computed tomography (SPECT) can be helpful in differentiating abscesses from primary CNS lymphoma (PCNSL), but does not distinguish toxoplasmosis from other abscesses.

   Toxoplasma IgG antibodies are present in the blood in almost all cases, although rare cases of seronegative pathologically proven toxoplasmosis have been described. Specific antibodies to *T. gondii* and Toxoplasma DNA can be detected in the CSF which can assist with the diagnosis, having a sensitivity of 68.8% and specificity of 100%. Definitive diagnosis requires pathologic demonstration of organisms or their DNA. Diagnostic brain biopsy is indicated in patients with negative serology for *T. gondii* and single lesions, worsening lesions, or those failing to respond after 2 weeks to antibiotic therapy directed at the organism.

5. **Management.**
   a. **Prophylaxis.** Patients who have a positive serum toxoplasma IgG with a CD4 count <100 cells/mm^3 should be placed on primary prophylaxis. The preferred drug of choice is trimethoprim-sulfamethoxazole since most patients are placed on it for PJP prophylaxis which is initiated when CD4 count <200 cells/mm^3. Alternative regimens for primary prophylaxis are available and should be initiated with the assistance of a specialist. Prophylaxis can be discontinued once a patient's CD4 count exceeds 200 cells/mm^3 for 3 or more months in response to effective ART.
   b. **Treatment.** Management of CNS toxoplasmosis includes an induction phase for acute symptoms followed by a maintenance phase to prevent recurrence of infection. Patients with cerebral toxoplasmosis typically have a rapid response to therapy thus empiric treatment in patients with cerebral lesions suggestive of the infection and positive serology is warranted. A clinical response is expected within 2 weeks. The treatment of choice is oral sulfadiazine + pyrimethamine + leucovorin; however, pyrimethamine + clindamycin + leucovorin is the preferred alternative regimen in those unable to tolerate sulfadiazine. Patients who are severely ill and unable to take oral medications can be treated with IV trimethoprim-sulfamethoxazole. Corticosteroids can be used in those with increased ICP; however, if possible should be avoided in those empirically treated for CNS toxoplasmosis as their use can lead to diagnostic confusion with CNS lymphoma.

   Induction therapy is continued for at least 6 weeks or until there is regression of all lesions. Once this has occurred, patients are placed on maintenance therapy with a lower dose of the same regimen to reduce risk of recurrent infection until their CD4 count remains >200 cells/mm^3 for at least 6 months in response to effective ART.

6. **Outcomes.** Therapeutic monitoring is particularly important for patients treated empirically for CNS toxoplasmosis. Imaging should be repeated approximately 2 weeks after the initiation of antibiotic therapy. Failure of lesions to respond to therapy or worsening lesions should prompt a brain biopsy to evaluate for an alternate or concurrent process.

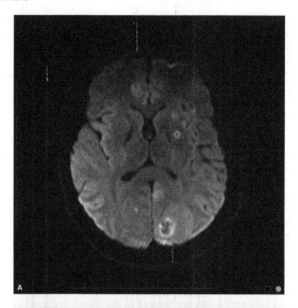

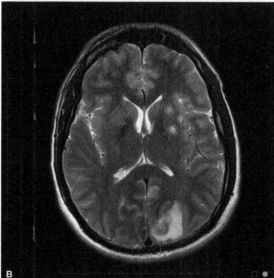

FIGURE 48.1 (A) Axial Diffusion weighted image (DWI) and **(B)** T2 weighted images in a 28-year-old man HIV+ with CNS toxoplasmosis. CNS, central nervous system; HIV, human immune deficiency virus. (Courtesy of Dr. Jordan Rosenblum)

C. **Primary CNS lymphoma.**
  1. Epidemiology. Primary CNS lymphoma (PCNSL) became an AIDS-defining malignancy in 1983 and accounts for 15% of non-Hodgkin lymphoma (NHL) in HIV-infected populations. It is a subtype of diffuse large B cell lymphoma (DLBCL) containing Epstein–Barr virus (EBV) and is 1,000 times more common in HIV-infected patients. PCNSL typically presents in patients with advanced HIV disease having a CD4 count ≤50 cells/mm³ and most have had a prior OI. The widespread use of ART in PLWHA has significantly decreased the incidence of PCNSL after 1996 from 313.2 per 100,000 person-years to 77.4 per 100,000 person-years.

2. **Pathogenesis.** PCNSL is strongly associated with the Epstein–Barr virus (EBV), a member of the herpes virus family and correlated to HIV immunodeficiency. Studies have demonstrated that EBV is incorporated into the genome of neoplastic cells and as HIV infection progresses infected B cells reach the CNS. EBV infection can lead to PCNSL in patients with advanced AIDS by transforming B cells due to its oncogenic properties, enhanced stimulation and reduced immunosurveillance against B cells, depletion of EBV-specific CD8+ T cells by HIV, and EBV induced mutations of tumor-suppressor genes and proto-oncogene activation.

3. **Clinical features.** Patients with PCNSL tend to have nonspecific clinical features and diagnosis may be delayed by empiric treatment for CNS toxoplasmosis. Common symptoms on presentation are subacute progressive headache, lethargy, cognitive impairment, seizures, and focal neurologic deficits related to tumor location, such as hemiparesis, aphasia, ataxia, or visual field deficits. Signs and symptoms of increased ICP such as headache, nausea, vomiting, and papilledema may be present. Meningitis, meningoencephalitis, or meningoradiculitis with cranial nerve abnormalities are commonly seen in patients with leptomeningeal lymphoma. Typical B systemic symptoms are not usually present.

4. **Diagnosis.** As with other CNS malignancies, diagnosis of PCNSL is made radiographically in conjunction with CSF analysis. CT or MRI can be used to characterize CNS lesions, although the latter is preferred since it is more sensitive, accurate, and can detect smaller lesions. Brain MRI tends to show solitary or multiple contrast enhancing, irregularly shaped lesions most commonly located in the periependymal area, corpus callosum, or periventricular area. Lesions may be difficult to differentiate from CNS toxoplasmosis or other cerebral abscesses by MRI. Thallium single-photon emission CT (SPECT) can show increased uptake in PCNSL and can be used to differentiate from toxoplasmosis with a sensitivity and specificity of about 90%.

   Routine CSF analysis yields a diagnosis of PCNSL in about 25% of patients. CSF examination tends to reveal normal glucose and protein with normal or increased lymphocytes. The detection of EBV DNA in the CSF by polymerase chain reaction (PCR) suggests lymphoma and is nearly 100% sensitive and about 50% specific.

   Brain biopsy is the gold standard to assist with diagnosis of focal brain lesions. Usually patients with brain lesions are empirically treated for toxoplasmosis despite their serologic status and may also receive corticosteroids which can confuse the biopsy results. This can delay diagnosis and expose patients to potentially dangerous medication side effects particularly in those with negative serology for toxoplasmosis. Thus, unless there is an absolute contraindication in a patient with AIDS sterotactic brain biopsy should be performed to make a diagnosis if lesions fail to respond to empiric therapy or if they are worsening.

5. **Management.** The cornerstone of therapy in patients with PCNSL is ART with the goal of effective immune reconstitution. In the pre-HAART era, outcomes were poor as patients with PCNSL had an overall median survival of 2.6 months. There is debate about the use of anticonvulsants and steroids since there is the potential for the latter to confound histologic diagnosis. A few days of steroid treatment may be useful particularly when there is mass effect, however prolonged course would not be recommended.

   Radiation therapy has been the mainstay of management along with ART, however it can be associated with delayed CNS toxicity. More recently, high-dose methotrexate in combination with rituximab administered for eight cycles with or without radiotherapy has been shown to be effective. A recent report also described five HIV-infected patients with PCNSL who underwent autologous stem cell transplant after induction chemotherapy, with two of them in remission 2 years post-transplant and two doing well 7 months post-transplant.

6. **Outcomes.** HIV seropositive status is typically an exclusion criteria for prospective PCNSL studies, thus therapeutic regimens have been adopted from data in immune competent patients. Large population-based studies have shown with the widespread use of ART, there are reasonable 1-year survival rates of about 54% and 5-year survival rates of about 23%.

D. **Progressive multifocal leukoencephalopathy.**

1. **Epidemiology.** PML is a demyelinating disease of the CNS caused by reactivation of the John Cunningham virus (JCV). It is a polyoma virus which causes asymptomatic primary infection in childhood and remains latent in the kidneys, bone marrow, and

lymphoid tissue. Prior to the ART era, the prevalence of PML was 0.3% to 8% with less than one-tenth surviving more than 1 year.

2. **Pathogenesis.** Primary JCV infection is typically asymptomatic and the virus remains latent in the kidneys, bone marrow, and lymphoid tissue. The events leading to PML remain uncertain. About 50% to 90% of individuals are seropositive for JCV and once cellular immunosuppression occurs, it can reactivate and spread to the brain, primarily infecting oligodendrocytes, astrocytes, and occasionally cerebellar granular cells eventually leading to demyelination in white matter. HIV may be a cofactor for JCV replication by the HIV TAT protein which may provide another mechanism of pathogenesis.

3. **Clinical features.** PML usually occurs in patients with CD4 <100 cells/mm^3 however it has been described in those with higher CD4 counts. JCV leads to demyelination of the white matter leading to cognitive impairment and focal neurologic deficits. Common signs and symptoms include subacute cognitive impairment, visual field defects, hemiparesis, ataxia, and speech or language disturbances evolving over weeks. Some patients come to medical attention with seizures or acute stroke-like presentations while others may evolve over several months with eventual progression to dementia followed by coma and death.

   In the pre-ART era, median survival was about 6 months, although those with less immune suppression survived longer. Effective ART therapy has extended survival to years although patients often have residual neurologic impairments. Higher JC virus load in the CSF may be associated with poorer prognosis while the presence of specific JC virus CD8+ immune cells has been associated with better prognosis.

4. **Diagnosis.** PML can be diagnosed based on clinical presentation in conjunction with neuroimaging and detection of JCV DNA in the CSF or brain biopsy. MRI typically demonstrates asymmetric lesions in cerebral white matter on T2-weighted sequences. A scalloped appearance reflecting involvement of the subcortical arcuate fibers is suggestive when present (Fig. 48.2). Frontal, parietal, temporal, basal ganglia, cerebellar and brainstem lesions may be seen. In contrast to other settings in which the disease occurs, PML lesions in AIDS enhance following contrast infusion in a minority of cases, usually in relatively less immunosuppressed patients. Single lesions are sometimes seen. Definitive diagnosis requires confirmation of JCV infection, by brain biopsy, or by demonstration of JCV DNA in CSF in a patient with compatible clinical and imaging features. High-sensitivity JCV PCR assays which can detect 50 copies/mL or less should be used to analyze CSF.

5. **Management.** Currently only effective ART to help restore immune function has been shown to benefit AIDS-associated PML. Reports show that survival rates have increased from 10% in the pre-ART era to 50% to 75% since. CNS IRIS is a potential complication following initiation of ART and may be difficult to distinguish from worsening PML (see discussion of IRIS in Section J under Opportunistic Infections). Controlled trials with cytosine arabinoside and cidofovir failed to show any benefit. Case reports suggest possible benefit with mirtazapine.

6. **Outcomes.** The prognosis of PML is poor with a median survival of about 6 months in HIV-infected patients. Prolonged survival is associated with the use of ART, elevated CD4 count at the time of diagnosis, increased CD4 count by 100 cells/mm^3, low HIV RNA, PML as an initial AIDS diagnosis, low JCV levels in CSF, clearance of JCV in CSF, and lack of neurologic progression after diagnosis.

E. **Cytomegalovirus.**

1. **Epidemiology.** CMV is a double-stranded DNA virus that belongs to the herpes virus family. CMV is ubiquitously acquired, and serologic evidence of exposure is present in most adults. Although some may have a transient systemic illness on acquisition, normal immune function prevents further manifestations. Clinical evidence of disease in HIV-infected patients is typically seen in individuals with a CD4 count ≤50 cells/mm^3 with retinitis being the most common end-organ presentation of disease, occurring in 30% of PLWHA in the pre-ART era. Prior to the advent of ART, neurologic complications of CMV occurred in about 2% of patients with AIDS and could be fatal.

2. **Pathogenesis and clinical features.** In PLWHA, CMV disease is due to reactivation of latent infection with end-organ disease resulting from hematogenous spread of the virus. Risk factors for CMV infection include CD4 count ≤50 cells/mm^3, HIV RNA >100,000 copies/mL, high level of CMV viremia, and history of prior OI.

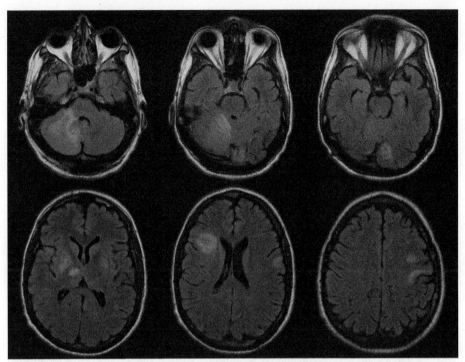

FIGURE 48.2 A 38-year-old man with cortico-subcortical type of suprabulbar palsy. MRI demonstrated patchy areas of abnormal increased T2 and FLAIR signal abnormality involving bilateral frontal lobe subcortical white matter, bilateral basal ganglion and thalami with some extension into the right cerebral peduncle, as well as right cerebellum. FLAIR, fluid-attenuated inversion recovery; MRI, magnetic resonance imaging. (Courtesy of Dr. José Biller)

Neurologic manifestations of CMV infection include encephalitis, polyradiculomyelitis, multifocal neuropathy, meningomyelitis, and myositis. CSF analysis typically demonstrates a lymphocytic pleocytosis, low to normal glucose, and normal to elevated protein content.

a. **CMV encephalitis (CMVE)** usually presents in advanced HIV/AIDS infection and is characterized by subacute confusion, delirium, impaired attention, memory, and cognitive processing with varying focal signs, including cranial neuropathy, nystagmus, weakness, spasticity, and ataxia. Focal encephalitis with mass lesions or aseptic meningitis can also occur.

b. **CMV polyradiculomyelitis (CMVRM)** presents as a subacute motor weakness with areflexia and sphincter dysfunction (usually urinary and/or bowel) that evolves over days to weeks. Painful paresthesias in the perineum and lower-extremities along with features of myelopathy such as a sensory level and Babinski's signs, may be found on examination. Symptoms in the lower extremities may ascend resembling GBS.

c. **CMV multifocal neuropathy** is characterized by motor weakness, depressed reflexes, and sensory deficits. It involves nerves of both upper and lower extremities in an asymmetric pattern evolving over weeks to months. Motor features overshadow the sensory findings.

d. CMV can less commonly cause myositis or meningomyelitis.

3. **Diagnosis.** The clinical syndromes are suggestive but not pathognomonic for CMV infection in severely immunosuppressed patients with AIDS. MRI with contrast may reveal enhancement of ventricular ependyma in CMVE, of meninges in some patients with meningoencephalitis or meningomyelitis, and of lumbar nerve roots or conus medullaris in some patients with CMVRM. Normal findings or nonspecific atrophic changes may also be seen.

CSF analysis in CMVRM characteristically reveals a polymorphonuclear pleocytosis, elevated protein, and low glucose. In CMVE, CSF pleocytosis is less common, and in CMV multifocal neuropathy CSF is usually normal or reveals a nonspecific protein elevation. Detection of CMV DNA in CSF using PCR amplification techniques is a sensitive and specific indicator of active CMV infection, exceeding 80% and 90%, respectively, thus avoiding the need for a brain biopsy. Patients with AIDS and CMV infection of the nervous system typically have systemic viremia as well; however, the level of viremia does not correlate with end-organ disease and has poor diagnostic and predictive value.

4. **Management.** No randomized controlled studies of treatment of CMV CNS OIs have been conducted. There are three available agents for the management of CMV infection. Given the poor prognosis with monotherapy, combination therapy with ganciclovir and foscarnet is now recommended by the panel on Opportunistic Infections in HIV-Infected Adults and Adolescents.

   a. **Ganciclovir (GCV)** is administered as an induction dose of 5 mg/kg IV twice daily in those with normal renal function for 21 days followed by a maintenance dose of 5 mg/kg daily. Potential adverse effects include thrombocytopenia, anemia, nausea, vomiting, and abdominal pain.

   b. **Foscarnet (FOS)** is thought to have greater CNS penetration than Ganciclovir; however, it has more adverse effects. An induction dose of 90 mg/kg IV twice daily in those with normal renal function for 21 days is followed by a maintenance dose of 90 mg/kg daily. Potential adverse effects include renal dysfunction, proteinuria, nephrogenic diabetes insipidus (hypokalemia, hypocalcemia, hypomagnesemia), headache, nausea, fatigue, and leukopenia.

   c. **Cidofovir (CDV)** is administered at 5 mg/kg in 1L of IV fluids once a week for two successive weeks and then every 2 weeks in those with normal renal function. Probenecid 2 g orally is given 2 hours prior to the infusion and 1 g orally is given 2 and 8 hours upon completion of the infusion. Patients should have ocular monitoring for hypotony and renal function for acute kidney injury. Other adverse events include dose-dependent proximal tubular injury (Fanconi-like syndrome, with proteinuria, glycosuria, bicarbonaturia, phosphaturia, polyuria), nephrogenic diabetes insipidus, acidosis, nausea, fever, and alopecia.

   d. **Viral resistance** may develop during prolonged therapy. CMV neurologic disease emerging while on maintenance therapy for another etiology of CMV disease (i.e., retinitis or enteritis) should be managed with an alternative agent while viral resistance testing is sent. The most common resistance mutations occur in the viral UL97 kinase or the UL54 DNA polymerase gene. GCV resistance mutations have been identified in both genes, while FOS and CDV mutations occur in only the DNA polymerase gene.

5. **Outcomes.** There are no RCTs to help guide therapy for AIDS-related CMV neurologic disease as responses to therapy are reported anecdotally. The optimal regimen remains unknown with each therapeutic option having pros and cons. Immunosuppressed patients should receive induction therapy and then transition to maintenance therapy. CSF evaluation may be the best marker of CNS disease activity and should be performed at the completion of induction therapy and if worsening neurologic functioning occurs.

F. **Varicella Zoster virus.**

1. **Epidemiology.** VZV commonly occurs in patients with HIV infection at multiple stages of the disease and may produce encephalitis, myelitis, and mono or polyradiculitis. Patients with radiculitis often have self-limited dermatologic eruptions, which may be accompanied by prolonged neuralgia. CNS extension may be marked by vasculitis resulting in cerebral infarction, particularly after ophthalmic zoster, and can result in necrotizing myelitis and brainstem, focal or diffuse cerebral encephalitis.

2. **Pathogenesis.** VZV, the virus which causes chicken pox, is acquired early in life and resides latently in sensory ganglia where it can intermittently produce recurrent radiculitis. Retrograde extension to the CNS along contiguous sensory roots and fiber tracts has also been demonstrated. This can lead to vasculitis, meningitis, or encephalitis.

3. **Clinical features.**

   a. **VZV radiculitis** is characterized by painful paresthesias in a restricted dermatomal distribution of a spinal or trigeminal nerve root. A vesicular rash usually follows, but VZV can occur without a rash. The skin eruption typically heals over weeks; however, pain may persist.

b. **VZV myelitis** may be limited or progressive resulting in spastic weakness, sensory impairment, and sphincter dysfunction. It is sometimes associated with myoclonus or meningitis. Dermatomal VZV may or may not be present.

c. **VZV meningitis** presents with headache, fever, altered mental status. CSF examination demonstrates a lymphocytic pleocytosis, increased protein, and normal to decreased glucose.

d. **Polyradiculitis** is clinically indistinguishable from CMVRM. It can also be caused by VZV.

e. **VZV encephalitis** can be focal or diffuse in PLWHA. It can manifest as seizures, confusion, progressive language and cognitive impairment, and sensory or motor abnormalities. Progression can be gradual and meningitis may be associated.

f. **VZV vasculitis** can cause focal features resulting from cerebral or spinal cord infarction or diffuse leukoencephalitis due to small vessel involvement.

4. **Diagnosis.** When the characteristic dermatologic eruption occurs, diagnosis of radiculitis is not difficult. In patients with CNS disease, MRI may demonstrate focal or diffuse areas of high-signal intensity on T2-weighted images of the brain or spinal cord. Enhancing focal lesions and meningeal enhancement may also be seen. Diagnosis is confirmed by demonstration of VZV DNA in CSF or tissue or an elevated VZV antibody index in CSF.

5. **Management.** Patients with HIV and VZV radiculitis should be treated with valacyclovir or famciclovir for 7 to 10 days. Neuralgia can be managed with pregabalin 75 to 150 mg twice a day, or gabapentin 300 to 600 mg three to four times daily. Amitriptyline 25 mg at bedtime may be added and titrated to 100 mg at bedtime.

Patients with VZV encephalitis, meningitis, or myelitis should be treated with IV Acyclovir at 10 mg/kg every 8 hours for 14 to 21 days, adjusted for renal function. Resistance of VZV to acyclovir has been reported and refractory disease should be managed with foscarnet.

6. **Outcomes.** Most patients with VZV radiculitis achieve resolution of the acute symptoms, although recurrences are common in immunosuppressed individuals and may involve different dermatomes. The prognosis for progressive myelitis and encephalitis varies; however, limited anecdotal data suggest some patients respond to antiviral therapy.

G. **CNS tuberculosis.**

1. **Epidemiology.** *Mycobacterium tuberculosis* (MTB) is the second most common infectious diseases cause of death worldwide after HIV/AIDS and the most common cause of death in HIV-infected patients in resource-limited countries. MTB is transmitted via droplet nuclei, and thus the lungs are the most common organ involved. The organism causes extrapulmonary and disseminated infection more commonly in HIV-infected individuals, especially those with advanced disease (CD4 count <200 cells/mm^3). Of all sites of infection, tuberculosis involvement of the CNS is the most severe and has the highest mortality with a poor prognosis despite therapy. TB meningitis (TBM) occurs in about 7% to 12% of individuals with TB, having a subacute or chronic presentation usually preceded by a systemic illness. Individuals may also have mass lesions such as tuberculomas or cerebral abscesses which may evolve more acutely. Up to 20% to 30% of survivors manifest various neurologic sequelae. In the United States, increased risk is associated with intravenous drug use, history of incarceration, homelessness, migration from countries with high MTB prevalence, and close contact with those who have MTB infection.

2. **Pathogenesis.** MTB belongs to the family of *Mycobacteriaceae* and is the most common causative agent of TB. MTB enters the body when a person inhales droplet nuclei containing the organism. An individual with intact T-cell–mediated immunity will have limited growth of MTB which helps prevent its spread. Viable bacilli can persist for years as walled-off foci leading to latent TB infection (LTBI). TB can occur in two forms: primary infection or reactivation of latent infection. From either form, the organism can reach the CNS hematogenously and form granulomas or Rich foci in the subependymal layers and later form tuberculomas. In many of these cases, the granulomas rupture and cause meningitis. HIV patients have a 10% per year risk of reactivation of LTBI and progression to active TB disease.

3. **Clinical features.** Staging of TBM has been established by the Medical Research Council based on mental status at the time of diagnosis. *Stage I:* Patients are alert with no focal neurologic signs; *Stage II:* Patients are confused with or without focal neurologic deficits; *Stage III:* Patients are stuporous or comatose. The most common presentation is meningitis or meningoencephalitis marked by headaches, fevers, anorexia, meningismus, emesis, myalgia, confusion, lethargy, cranial neuropathy, ataxia, seizure or hemiparesis. Patients may also have meningoradiculitis, myelitis, anterior spinal artery infarction, and epidural or intramedullary abscess formation. The mortality and neurologic sequelae of TBM is related to the stage of disease on admission, and the duration of symptoms before presentation.

4. **Diagnosis.** Early diagnosis and initiation of TB therapy is vital to the management of TBM. Diagnosis is based on clinical presentation, radiographic findings, CSF examination, and response to therapy.

   With imaging, MRI is superior to CT at defining lesions in the basal ganglia, midbrain, and brainstem. Neuroimaging with either CT or MRI can demonstrate hydrocephalus (45% to 87%), basilar meningeal enhancement (23% to 38%), infarct (20% to 38%), and tuberculomas (12% to 16%). Neuroimaging may show brain abscesses that may be difficult to distinguish from toxoplasmosis or CNS lymphoma. MRI of the spine may demonstrate abscesses and vertebral body collapse in patients with meningitis or myelitis.

   CSF typically reveals a mixed or predominantly lymphocytic pleocytosis, elevated protein, and low glucose. Detection of MTB in the CSF is the gold standard for diagnosis of TBM. However smears for acid-fast bacteria (AFB) are rarely positive, and the growth of the organism is slow in culture. CSF culture may be negative in up to one-third of cases, although in some reports, diagnostic yield of AFB staining can increase up to 87% when four serial CSF examinations were performed. Detection of MTB DNA by PCR and MTB antigen assays provide more rapid detection in CSF. Diagnosis of tuberculomas and abscesses may require biopsy with demonstration of granulomas and AFB on pathology along with positive culture for MTB.

5. **Management.**
   a. **TB therapy.** If there is a strong clinical suspicion of TBM, then therapy should not be delayed until a microbiologic diagnosis can be confirmed, as outcomes are dependent on the stage of disease at which therapy is initiated. Patients should be started on "Intensive Phase" therapy, which consists of a four-medication regimen of isoniazid (INH), rifampin (RIF), pyrazinamide (PZA) and a fourth agent, either ethambutol (ETB) or streptomycin (SM), for at least 2 months. Pyridoxine is added for patients taking INH. Drug susceptibility testing to first-line TB medications (INH, RIF, PZA, ETB) should be performed on all patients with MTB disease as these results impact therapeutic regimens. Upon completion of the "Intensive Phase" the "Continuation Phase" of therapy includes INH/RIF for pan-sensitive TB for 9 to 12 months.

      Multidrug-resistant TB (MDR-TB) is increasingly more common and refers to an isolate resistant to INH and RIF. Extensively drug-resistant TB (XDR-TB) refers to an isolate resistant to INH, RIF, Fluoroquinolones (FQ), and Aminoglycosides (AG). Patients with either MDR or XDR TB require more complex and prolonged therapy and should be referred to a specialist for care.

   b. **Corticosteroids.** Adjunctive use of corticosteroids in TBM has been shown to improve survival. The Panel on Opportunistic Infections in HIV-Infected Adults and Adolescents recommends using tapering doses of dexamethasone in the treatment of TBM. In patients with TBM, dexamethasone 0.3 to 0.4 mg/kg/day or prednisone 1 mg/kg/day should be added for the first 3 weeks and then tapered over the next 3 to 5 weeks. IRIS is not uncommonly seen with reversal of immune suppression following cART (see Section J under Opportunistic Infections.).

   c. **ART.** Treatment of TB and HIV can be challenging due to problems of noncompliance from high pill burden, medication side effects from both therapies, drug–drug interactions among agents, and the development of IRIS. Due to the numerous considerations which must be taken into account the Panel on Opportunistic Infections in HIV-Infected Adults and Adolescents currently recommends that in ART-naive patients with a CD4 count <50 cells/mm^3, ART should be initiated within 2 weeks of diagnosis, and by 8 to 12 weeks for all others. There are no clear guidelines for when to initiate ART in HIV-infected individuals with TBM. Thus, caution must be taken when initiating ART in patients with TBM, particularly those with low CD4 counts as they must be monitored closely.

6. **Outcomes.** The mortality of HIV-associated TBM often exceeds 50% and is related to the degree of immune suppression. Patients with TBM need follow-up CSF studies to ensure there is not persistent infection. Tuberculomas can be followed with serial imaging in the absence of life-threatening mass effect. Lesions that enlarge despite therapy should be reevaluated and considered for biopsy to detect resistant organisms or concurrent opportunistic processes.

H. **Neurosyphilis.**

1. **Epidemiology.** Syphilis is a sexually transmitted infection caused by *Treponema pallidum*. The disease is divided into stages based on clinical findings, which guides treatment and follow-up. It is associated with increased risk of sexual acquisition and transmission of HIV. Although not strictly an opportunistic pathogen, overlapping risk factors and a potentially more aggressive course make it an infection of particular concern in patients with HIV infection. Increased frequency of CNS involvement and occasional failure of conventional therapy with emergence or recurrence of neurosyphilis despite standard courses of penicillin have been reported.

2. **Pathogenesis.** Neurosyphilis occurs when *T. pallidum* invades the CSF. This can occur during any stage of disease as CSF abnormalities are common in individuals with early syphilis even in the absence of neurologic findings. Invasion of the CSF with *T. pallidum* does not always cause persistent infection and in some cases spontaneous resolution may occur without an inflammatory response.

3. **Clinical features.** All persons with HIV infection and syphilis should undergo a careful neurologic exam and those with abnormal neurologic signs or symptoms should undergo CSF examination. In the absence of neurologic symptoms, CSF examination has not been associated with improved clinical outcomes and is not recommended. The exception to this is patients with tertiary syphilis who should also receive a CSF exam prior to initiation of therapy to see if they have neurosyphilis.

   Neurosyphilis can be categorized into early and late forms. Early forms of the disease include asymptomatic neurosyphilis, symptomatic meningitis, ocular syphilis, otosyphilis, and meningovascular syphilis. Late forms of disease include general paresis and tabes dorsalis.

   Clinical evidence of neurologic involvement can be meningitis, encephalitis, cognitive dysfunction, motor or sensory dysfunction, cranial nerve palsies, signs or symptoms of stroke, motor or sensory deficits, and visual or auditory symptoms. Syphilitic uveitis or other ocular manifestations (neuroretinitis and optic neuritis) can also be associated with neurosyphilis, thus a CSF examination should be performed in all cases of ocular syphilis even if there are no neurologic findings.

4. **Diagnosis.** Early syphilis is best diagnosed by using darkfield exam and tests to detect *T. pallidum* directly from the lesion exudate or tissue. A diagnosis of syphilis requires two tests: a non-treponemal test (i.e., Venereal Disease Research Laboratory [VDRL] or Rapid Plasma Reagin [RPR]) and a treponemal test (i.e., fluorescent treponemal antibody absorbed [FTA-ABS] tests, the *T. pallidum* passive particle agglutination [TP-PA] assay, various enzyme immunoassays [EIAs], chemiluminescence immunoassays, immunoblots, or rapid treponemal assays). Use of only one type of serologic test can lead to false-negative or positive results.

   The diagnosis of neurosyphilis is complex and depends on the combination of CSF tests (cell count, protein, and reactive VDRL), in the presence of reactive serologic tests and neurologic abnormalities. CSF leukocyte count is usually elevated in patients with HIV, so a cutoff of >20 WBC/mm^3 is recommended to improve the specificity of neurosyphilis diagnosis. The CSF-VDRL is specific but insensitive. If it is negative, and there is a high clinical suspicion for neurosyphilis additional evaluation using the FTA-ABS testing on the CSF should be considered.

5. **Management.** Neurosyphilis should be treated with intravenous aqueous crystalline penicillin G 18 to 24 million units per day, administered as 3 to 4 million units every 4

hours (or as a continuous infusion) for 14 days. An alternative regimen, is 2.4 million units of intramuscular procaine penicillin G once daily plus probenecid 500 mg orally four times a day for 14 days. This regimen can be used in patients who are thought to be compliant and not allergic to sulfa medications. Benzathine penicillin, 2.4 million units IM once a week for three doses can be considered after completion of treatment for neurosyphilis.

6. **Outcomes.** Although initial response to treatment is good, the risk of recurrent neurosyphilis is increased in the setting of HIV infection. If initial CSF examination demonstrates pleocytosis, a repeat CSF examination should be performed every 6 months until the cell count is normal. Follow-up CSF examination should also be used to evaluate changes in CSF-VDRL or protein; however, changes to these parameters occur more slowly than the cell count. If the cell count has not decreased after 6 months or if the CSF cell count or protein is not normal after 2 years, retreatment should be considered. Additionally new onset of neurologic symptoms should prompt evaluation for neurosyphilis.

I. **Other OIs.** Numerous other OIs have been described in HIV-infected patients. A more complete compilation is beyond the scope of this chapter. More extensive reviews are contained in the references below.

J. **Immune reconstitution inflammatory syndrome.**

1. **Epidemiology.** IRIS is a potentially life-threatening condition that occurs in approximately 35% of patients following initiation of ART. It is a potential consequence of rapid restoration of the patient's immune system in the setting of improving HIV disease markers (i.e., HIV VL and CD4 count). IRIS is characterized by a paradoxical worsening in the patient's clinical condition. Some cases occur in the absence of OIs and are presumed to be an inflammatory response to HIV-related antigens. In other cases, a resident OI may be unmasked by initiation of ART and the vigorous immune response which follows, whereas in other instances, an initial improvement in an OI may be followed by clinical worsening. In this scenario it may be difficult to distinguish between treatment failure of the OI versus IRIS.

   CNS IRIS is rare and has an incidence of 0.9% to 1.5%. It can be seen in the setting of AIDS-related OIs, such as PML, CMV, cryptococcal disease, CNS tuberculosis, or toxoplasmosis. Individuals who are ART naive, have a low CD4 T-cell count, high HIV VL, and show rapid improvement in immunologic and virologic markers in response to ART appear to be at greatest risk for IRIS. A majority of cases occur within the first 8 weeks of initiation of ART and likelihood of IRIS may be increased when ART is initiated in close proximity to treatment for an OI. This can become difficult when initiating ART in a patient with a CNS OI and such patients should be monitored closely for IRIS.

2. **Pathogenesis.** The pathogenesis of IRIS remains unclear. Following initiation of ART there is a rapid recovery of memory T cells. These lymphocytes penetrate peripheral nonlymphoid sites, recognize previously encountered antigens and mount an inflammatory response. Most paradoxical inflammatory responses are against opportunistic pathogens already present when ART is initiated. Pathologic reports of CNS IRIS most commonly have identified CD8+ lymphocytic infiltration from the perivascular space along with activated macrophages.

3. **Clinical features.** Patients with CNS IRIS may present with signs and symptoms consistent with an infectious or inflammatory condition temporally related to initiation of ART. Patients may develop recurrence of the initial symptoms associated with their infection or may develop new inflammatory symptoms such as fever, enlarged lymph nodes, headache, AMS, meningitis, encephalitis, or cranial nerve palsies after initiation of ART.

4. **Diagnosis.** A diagnosis of IRIS requires exclusion of recurrent or new concurrent infection or neoplasm to explain the clinical syndrome. In cases where biopsy is pursued, a vigorous CD8+ inflammatory response in the absence of active infections suggests the diagnosis. MRI may show enlarged space enhancing lesions with edema and mass effect suggestive of an inflammatory response in patients with CNS parenchymal disease. Individuals should be suspected of having CNS IRIS when they present with the following:

   a. Rapid deterioration of clinical and neurologic status following initiation of ART
   b. Decrease of HIV RNA greater than 1 log
   c. Clinical, laboratory, and radiologic signs and symptoms concerning for inflammation

d. Lack of correlation between symptoms and a newly acquired infection, a previously present OI, or drug toxicity.
5. **Management.** There are no RCTs addressing management of IRIS. Stopping ART is not recommended as resumption of HIV viral replication will allow for disease progression. Both spontaneous resolution and resolution associated with corticosteroid therapy have been reported. Current practice favors high-dose steroids for patients with severe neurologic symptoms and IRIS. Steroids may be required for several weeks or months and should be gradually tapered to prevent rebound inflammation on withdrawal.
6. **Outcomes.** IRIS can affect any organ system in the body, however when it affects the CNS it can cause significant morbidity and mortality. Mortality rates range from 5% to 15% as it can be difficult to manage the inflammatory response in the setting of an OI. Ultimately, if the inflammatory response can be contained as the patient's immune system recovers, the patient's long-term outcome will be improved.

Key Points

- HIV may involve the CNS directly or through causing opportunistic diseases
- Even on effective ART, subtle findings of HAND may be present in over half of patients
- In cryptococcal meningitis, elevated ICP must be aggressively managed
- A 2-week trial of therapy in a toxoplasma seropositive patient with encephalitis and compatible imaging may obviate the need for brain biopsy
- Detection of Epstein–Barr virus DNA by PCR in CSF strongly supports the diagnosis of primary CNS lymphoma
- Progressive multifocal leukoencephalopathy (PML) can be diagnosed with compatible clinical presentation, neuroimaging and detection of JC Virus DNA in CSF or tissue
- Nervous system involvement by CMV is uncommon and can present as encephalitis, radiculitis, myelitis, or multifocal neuropathy
- If TB is highly suspected as a cause of meningitis, therapy should commence **before** diagnosis can be confirmed
- Invasion of the nervous system by *T. pallidum* (syphilis) occurs in early stages of the disease but may resolve spontaneously
- The immune reconstitution inflammatory syndrome (IRIS) follows initiation of ART and is characterized by paradoxical worsening either of HIV itself or an OI.

Recommended Readings

Antinori A, Arendt G, Becker JT, et al. Updated research nosology for HIV-associated neurocognitive disorders. *Neurology*. 2007;69:1789–1799.
Boulware D, Meya D, Moozura C, et al. Timing of antiretroviral therapy after diagnosis of cryptococcal meningitis. *N Engl J Med*. 2014;370:2487–2498.
Canestri A, Lescure FX, Jaureguiberry S, et al. Discordance between cerebral spinal fluid and plasma HIV replication in patients with neurological symptoms who are receiving suppressive antiretroviral therapy. *Clin Infect Dis*. 2010;50:773–778.
Chan P, Brew B. HIV-associated neurocognitive disorders in the modern antiviral treatment era: prevalence, characteristics, biomarkers, and effects of treatment. *Curr HIV/AIDS Rep*. 2014;11:317–324.
Clifford D, Ances B. HIV-associated neurocognitive disorder. *Lancet Infect Dis*. 2013;13:976–986.
Cysique LA, Vaida F, Letendre S, et al. Dynamics of cognitive change in impaired HIV-positive patients initiating antiretroviral therapy. *Neurology*. 2009;73:342–348.
Garvey L, Winston A, Walsh J, et al. Antiretroviral therapy CNS penetration and HIV-1-associated CNS disease. *Neurology*. 2011;76:693–700.
Gendelman H, Grant I, Everall IP, et al. eds. *The Neurology of AIDS*, 3rd Edn. Oxford University Press, New York, NY; 2012.
Johnson T, Nath A. Neurological complications of immune reconstitution in HIV-infected populations. *Ann N Y Acad Sci*. 2010;1184:106–120.
Kaplan JE, Benson C, Holmes KK, et al. Guidelines for prevention and treatment of opportunistic infections in HIV-infected adults and adolescents. *Clin Infect Dis*. 2014;58(9):1308–1311.

Panel on Opportunistic Infections in HIV-Infected Adults and Adolescents. Guidelines for the prevention and treatment of opportunistic infections in HIV-infected adults and adolescents: recommendations from the Centers for Disease Control and Prevention, the National Institutes of Health, and the HIV Medicine Association of the Infectious Diseases Society of America. Available at http://aidsinfo.nih. gov/contentfiles/lvguidelines/adult_oi.pdf.

Letendre S, Marquie-Beck J, Capparelli E, et al. Validation of the CNS penetration-effectiveness rank for quantifying antiretroviral penetration into the central nervous system. *Arch Neurol*. 2008;65:65–70.

Nightingale S, Winston A, Letendre S, et al. Controversies in HIV-associated neurocognitive disorders. *Lancet Neurol*. 2014;13:1139–1151.

Portegies P, Berger JR, eds. HIV/AIDS and the nervous system. In: Aminoff MJ, Boller F, Swaab DF, eds. *Handbook of Clinical Neurology*. Vol 85, 3rd series. Amsterdam, Netherlands: Elsevier; 2007.

Tan IL, Smith BR, Von Gelden G, et al. HIV-associated opportunistic infections of the CNS. *Lancet Neurol*. 2013;11:605–617.

The Mind Exchange Working Group. Assessment, diagnosis, and treatment of HIV-associated neurocognitive disorder: a consensus report of the mind exchange program. *Clin Inf Dis*. 2013;56(7): 1004–1017.

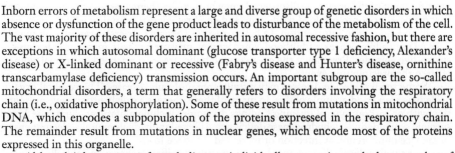

49 Inherited Metabolic Neurologic Disorders

Marc C. Patterson

Inborn errors of metabolism represent a large and diverse group of genetic disorders in which absence or dysfunction of the gene product leads to disturbance of the metabolism of the cell. The vast majority of these disorders are inherited in autosomal recessive fashion, but there are exceptions in which autosomal dominant (glucose transporter type 1 deficiency, Alexander's disease) or X-linked dominant or recessive (Fabry's disease and Hunter's disease, ornithine transcarbamylase deficiency) transmission occurs. An important subgroup are the so-called mitochondrial disorders, a term that generally refers to disorders involving the respiratory chain (i.e., oxidative phosphorylation). Some of these result from mutations in mitochondrial DNA, which encodes a subpopulation of the proteins expressed in the respiratory chain. The remainder result from mutations in nuclear genes, which encode most of the proteins expressed in this organelle.

Although inborn errors of metabolism are individually rare, owing to the large number of these disorders, they are collectively rather common, and constitute a significant public health problem. Since most of these disorders in their more severe forms impinge on the nervous system, it is essential that neurologists be aware of their manifestations and the means with which to diagnose and manage them (Video 49.1).

INCIDENCE AND PREVALENCE

Inborn errors of metabolism are individually rare. Most data in the past have relied on studies of prevalence, which are highly dependent on ascertainment of cases. This has tended to bias such numbers in favor of more severe cases, particularly those first presenting in children. In more recent years, the availability of disease-modifying therapies for many of these disorders has led to pressure for newborn screening to be performed. In the Unites States, many states now screen for 50 or more diseases, most of which qualify as inborn errors of metabolism. The institution of newborn screening has given greater insight into the birth incidence of these diseases. In some cases, it has become apparent that preexisting estimates were far too low. For example, it was thought that the birth incidence of Fabry's disease was approximately 1 in 50,000. A study that screened more than 30,000 consecutive newborn males in the Piedmont region of Italy found that the birth incidence was closer to 1 in 3,000. Of note, the majority of these cases were predicted to be late onset, as opposed to the classical childhood onset form of the disease. More widespread application of such screening has confirmed that previous figures were too low and that it is likely that the majority of cases of inborn errors of metabolism are actually those with milder phenotypes, which may go unrecognized or misdiagnosed. Thus, it is incumbent on all neurologists, including adult neurologists, to be familiar with these disorders, which can present at any age and in many guises.

CLASSIFICATION

The complexity of metabolic pathways in the cell is such that mutations in any one gene may lead to a large variety of downstream consequences. Any classification is thus an oversimplification. Nevertheless, for practical purposes, a division of inborn errors of metabolism into small and large molecule diseases is clinically useful.

The small molecule diseases are those involving amino acids, organic acids, the urea cycle, the respiratory chain and the synthesis of neurotransmitters, among others. In their most severe form, these disorders present in neonates or young children, in whom the deficiency of the enzyme or other gene product is so profound that these children are unable to metabolize even normal substrate loads. They will often present with catastrophic deterioration in the newborn period when they are first exposed to a normal substrate load, typically when they begin to feed.

Alternatively, those with less severe loss of activity of the gene product may present only when they are confronted with an increased substrate load, such as that which occurs in a hypercatabolic state associated with fever, or in association with a change in diet. Common presenting features may include coma, seizures, acidosis or movement disorders. There may be evidence of multiorgan failure in many of these phenotypes.

A prime example is the X-linked disorder, ornithine transcarbamylase deficiency, the most frequent of the urea cycle disorders. In newborn males (hemizygotes), this presents after first exposure to a protein load with coma and cerebral edema; mortality is high, even with timely and aggressive intervention. In heterozygotes (female carriers), presentation may be delayed until adolescence or adulthood, when women may present with migrainous features or stroke-like episodes. Pregnancy, the greatest metabolic stress experienced by normal women, is often the precipitating event.

Some small molecule diseases may mimic large molecule diseases. The cerebral organic acidemias are a good example of this. In many of these, there is a slowly progressive presentation with or without typical imaging findings. Examples include glutaric aciduria type 1, and succinic semialdehyde dehydrogenase deficiency. Affected individuals may also decompensate in the face of intercurrent infection or increased substrate loads.

The small molecule diseases may be conveniently classified as shown on Table 49.1. Typical presentations and abnormal substrates for analytic purposes are also shown here.

TABLE 49.1 Small Molecule Disorders

Disorder	Clinical Features	Key Laboratory Findings	Management
Amino acidopathies	ND, ED, DD	Specific amino acid patterns in blood and urine	Dietary restriction; cofactor supplementation; dialysis or hemoperfusion (acute decompensation)
Organic acidopathies	ND, ED, DD	Specific organic acid pattern in urine; neutropenia, thrombocytopenia	Dietary restriction; cofactor supplementation; dialysis or hemoperfusion (acute decompensation)
Urea cycle disorders	ND, ED, DD	Marked hyperammonemia; specific amino acid patterns; orotic aciduria; respiratory alkalosis	Protein restriction; cofactor therapy; dialysis or hemoperfusion (acute decompensation)
Fatty acid oxidation disorders	MY, DD, ED	Hypoketotic hypoglycemia; low total carnitine, elevated acylcarnitine	Dietary restriction; cofactor supplementation
Oxidative phosphorylation disorders	MY, DD, ED, MD, SZ	Elevated lactate; (mild) hyperammonemia; low total carnitine, elevated acylcarnitine	Ketogenic diet (selected disorders); cofactor supplementation ("mitochondrial cocktail")
Neurotransmitter disorders	Dopa-responsive dystonia; DD; SZ	Low CSF neurotransmitter metabolites; low CSF pterins; low 5MTHF	Product replacement therapy (L-dopa); cofactor therapy (folinic acid, pyridoxine)

Abbreviations: CSF, cerebrospinal fluid; DD, developmental delay; ED, episodic decompensation; MD, movement disorders; MY, myopathy; ND, neonatal depression and coma; SZ, seizures; 5MTHF, 5-methyltetrathydrofolate.

LARGE MOLECULE DISORDERS

These are the disorders typically described as "storage diseases." They usually have an insidious, slowly progressive presentation in which what is initially thought to be intellectual disability may eventually declare itself as dementia. Organomegaly and changes in the eyes, skin, hair, and nails are commonly seen, but need not be present to diagnose one of these disorders. They are usually classified based on the biochemistry of the accumulating substrate. In addition, the organelle to which they are localized is used as part of an overarching classification. Thus, lysosomal storage diseases, first characterized in the 1950s, when the ultrastructural anatomy of the cell first began to be appreciated, are subclassified as sphingolipidoses (disorders in which there is excessive storage of lipids), mucopolysaccharidoses (complex polymers of sugars accumulate), neuronal ceroid lipofuscinoses (proteins accumulate in excess), mucolipidoses (overlapping features of sphingolipodoses and mucopolysaccharidoses) and glycoprotein storage diseases (glycans [glycosylated proteins] accumulate in excess). Peroxisomal disorders are classified according to the nature of the deficiency of the gene product; elevated very long-chain fatty acids are characteristic. In the classic archetype, the Zellweger's syndrome, unusual facial features, organomegaly, bone abnormalities (chondrodysplasia punctata) and neurodegeneration are characteristic. The Zellweger phenotype is in fact a family of diseases in which mutations involving different transport proteins (peroxins) lead to deficiency of multiple enzymes within the peroxisomal matrix. In other disorders, a single gene product may be defective. Thus, X-linked adrenoleukodystrophy, commonly presenting in boys in middle childhood with various agnosias, spasticity and rapid neurologic deterioration, result from deficiency of a single enzyme transported into the peroxisome by the ALD protein.

Table 49.2 summarizes the findings in these disorders.

Some disorders defy easy categorization into small and large molecule disorders. The rapidly expanding family of congenital disorders of glycosylation (CDG; more than 90 types at the time of writing) comprise such a group. The most prevalent type, comprising about 80% of all CDG cases, is phosphomannosmutase 2 (PMM2) deficiency, which features episodic metabolic decompensation, stroke-like episodes and seizures in infancy and early childhood, but a more slowly progressive, large molecule disorder-like course in those who survive to the second and later decades. Similar diversity is encountered among the other N- and O-linked disorders of glycosylation, ranging from nonsyndromic intellectual disability in TUSC3-CDG, to congenital muscular dystrophy phenotypes (Walker-Warburg syndrome, Fukuyama congenital muscular dystrophy) to severe neurologic phenotypes with essentially no development and intractable seizures (ALG8-CDG).

DIAGNOSIS

The most important element in making a diagnosis of an inborn error of metabolism affecting the nervous system is a high index of suspicion. Any individual presenting with characteristic features of these phenotypes should be investigated. However, we increasingly recognize that late-onset diseases may have fragmentary or atypical phenotypes. Inborn errors of metabolism should be included in the differential diagnosis of any neurologic disorder. When the phenotype is typical, diagnostic testing may be focused to a specific enzyme, substrate, or gene. However, in cases presenting in more nondescript fashion, such as children with developmental delay with or without hypotonia and other suggestive features, or adults with early-onset dementias or treatment-resistant psychiatric illness, more broad screening may be appropriate. It is important to remember that screening tests have false negatives and false positives and, particularly in the case of small molecule diseases, that the ideal time to obtain a sample is when the patient is most symptomatic. Unfortunately, this commonly seems to occur after hours when regular services may not be available. Thus, it is important to obtain, collect and transport such samples in such a fashion that they will be in suitable condition for analysis. If there is any suspicion of an inborn error of metabolism in an adult or child who has decompensated, it is prudent to discuss the case with the biochemical genetics laboratory to ensure that appropriate samples are obtained.

Typical screening profiles will include quantitative plasma amino acids, urine organic acids, plasma lactate, pyruvate and ammonia, serum carnitine profile, complete blood count and biochemical profile plus blood gas analysis. Such investigations will enable diagnosis of

TABLE 49.2 Large Molecule Disorders

Disorder	Clinical Features	Key Laboratory Findings	Management
Lysosomal	PD, HS (±); FA (mucopolysaccharidoses, glycoprotein storage disorders, mucolipidoses); retinal and other ocular findings; peripheral neuropathy (metachromatic leukodystrophy, Krabbe's disease)	Enzyme deficiencies; oxysterols for Niemann-Pick diseases; characteristic storage (light microscopy) and inclusions (electron microscopy) on tissue biopsy (rarely required now)	Enzyme replacement (non-neurologic manifestations); hematopoietic stem cell transplantation; substrate reduction therapy; chaperone (enzyme enhancement) therapy
Peroxisomal	PD; peripheral neuropathy (X-ALD, AMN)	Very long-chain fatty acids; enzyme deficiencies	Hematopoietic stem cell transplantation; gene therapy (experimental); dietary therapy (erucic acid; Lorenzo's oil)
Glycogen storage	PW, HS; muscle enlargement	Glycogen storage on muscle biopsy + enzyme deficiency; hypoglycemia, hyperuricemia in some forms	Dietary therapy (cornstarch, sucrose)

Abbreviations: AMN, adrenomyeloneuropathy; FA, characteristic facial features (previously referred to as coarsening); HS, hepatosplenomegaly; PD, progressive neurodegeneration; PW, progressive weakness; X-ALD, X-linked adrenoleukodystrophy.

most of the amino acid, organic acid, and urea cycle disorders and may provide clues to the diagnosis of a respiratory chain or fatty acid oxidation disorder. Confirmation of the diagnosis is by sequencing of the relevant gene (individually or in a panel) in most cases; this information is important for prognosis and allows for antenatal diagnosis for couples who wish to avail themselves of this option.

More specialized testing is required in the case of neurotransmitter disorders in which cerebrospinal fluid must be obtained and rapidly cooled on dry ice, then promptly shipped to a reference laboratory. When obtaining cerebrospinal fluid (CSF), it is important to measure CSF glucose with simultaneous serum glucose to permit appropriate interpretation. In addition, any time that the cerebrospinal fluid glucose is measured, the lactate and pyruvate should also be measured. Disorders with hypoglycorrhachia and increased CSF lactate may result from bacterial infection or respiratory chain disorders. On the other hand, a low (less than 40% of serum glucose) CSF glucose and low CSF lactate point strongly to glucose transporter type 1 deficiency, a disorder readily treatable with the ketogenic diet in children.

A child with weakness attributed to muscle disease who presents with decompensation and hypoglycemia without ketonuria may have a disorder of fatty acid oxidation. Assay of serum fatty acids, a carnitine profile, acyl carnitines and acyl glycines can help round out the evaluation of such a child and are likely to detect disorders of fatty acid oxidation and many respiratory chain disorders. Urine screening is helpful for disorders of creatine synthesis, complemented by magnetic resonance spectroscopy of the brain.

Urine screens for purine and pyrimidine disorders may be helpful in patients presenting with delay or autistic features, particularly if they are associated with megaloblastic anemia or hyperuricemia.

In patients with slowly progressive loss of neurologic function (cognitive decline, progressive spasticity, weakness, movement disorders) particularly with evidence of systemic storage, the urine may be screened for mucopolysaccharides and oligosaccharides; false negatives may occur with some of these disorders. More sophisticated mass spectrometry techniques have improved the sensitivity and detection ability of urinalyses for these conditions. Direct assay of one or more lysosomal enzymes in white cells, serum, or fibroblasts is often employed when these disorders are suspected, although in certain cases (e.g., in at-risk populations with a high frequency of specific mutations), direct molecular analysis may be appropriate.

As next-generation DNA-sequencing technology continues to fall in cost, and as software algorithms for analysis of the massive data produced by these techniques are refined, whole-exome, and eventually, whole-genome sequencing will eventually become first-line screening and diagnostic techniques for inborn errors of metabolism. Because these methods find many DNA sequence variants whose pathogenicity is unclear, sophisticated biochemical analytical techniques will not be supplanted, since these will be critical in establishing the functional significance of DNA variants.

TREATMENT

In general, the small molecule disorders have a wider range of treatment options than the large molecule disorders. The prototype of these disorders is phenylketonuria, in which a phenylalanine-restricted diet applied early, and maintained rigorously, clearly improves the outcome. Since newborn screening for this disorder was instituted a half century ago in the United States, the prevalence of individuals impaired by phenylketonuria has dropped dramatically. It has been learned, however, that dietary restriction must be maintained at least through the adult years and perhaps lifelong, since failure to adhere to the diet can lead to recurrence or the development of new neurologic symptoms. Many of the amino acid and organic acid disorders can be managed with specific diets that qualify as medical foods. In some cases, the administration of specific cofactors may be highly beneficial. Thus, some forms of homocystinuria may respond to cobalamine and others to pyridoxine, depending on the precise enzymatic deficiency. Biotinidase deficiency, which can present with developmental delay, dermatitis and myoclonic seizures, with or without abnormal organic acids in the urine, responds well to the administration of pharmacologic doses of biotinidase. Disorders for which disease-modifying therapy is of proven value, and is readily available, should take priority in diagnostic workup.

In some cases, definitive therapy may take the form of organ transplantation and gene therapy is beginning to be investigated for these disorders.

Progress in large molecule diseases has been slower, but hematopoietic stem cell transplantation, enzyme replacement therapy, and small molecule therapy all have now established places in the treatment of these disorders, particularly the so-called lysosomal storage diseases.

It is clear, even if definitive therapy is not available, that early diagnosis is beneficial to affected individuals. Not only does this mean that clinical problems may be anticipated and managed expectantly, but it also allows the diagnostic odyssey to be ended and to provide the family with useful information for family planning, should the diagnosis be made sufficiently early. The impact of newborn screening on these diseases has yet to be assessed. However, preliminary data suggest that many patients will be detected as newborns, who would not be expected to present until much later in life. How to manage these individuals both medically and from the psychosocial point of view is proving to be a challenge, which has not yet been fully met.

PREVENTION

Given difficulties in diagnosis and continuing limitations in disease-modifying therapies, the ideal approach to inborn errors of metabolism is to prevent their occurrence. The greatest success story in this regard is the carrier screening program for Tay–Sachs disease. Tay–Sachs disease is a form of GM2 gangliosidosis, inherited in autosomal recessive fashion, which classically presents in infants with developmental stagnation and regression associated with hypotonia, macrocephaly, seizures and an exaggerated startle response. Children typically have cherry-red spots at the macula. This disease has a carrier frequency in the Ashkenazi Jewish population of approximately 1 in 30. After the enzymatic deficiency was discovered in 1969, it was found that carriers could be identified by screening blood tests and a prevention program was established. This has proven to be an enormous success, whose widespread implementation led to a dramatic reduction in the incidence of Tay–Sachs disease in the Ashkenazi Jewish population. Indeed, most cases of Tay–Sachs disease are now seen in non-Ashkenazi subjects.

The availability of a simple screening test, and a high carrier frequency in the at-risk population were key factors in the success of this approach. These factors are not present in many other inborn errors of metabolism. However, progress in DNA-sequencing technologies, particularly the widespread application of next-generation sequencing techniques, has raised the possibility of broad screening for rare diseases on a population basis. There are still many practical, ethical and social issues to be addressed before this can be implemented, but this new technology does hold the promise of eventually dramatically reducing the incidence and prevalence of these diseases, which are individually devastating and collectively costly.

Key Points

- Inherited metabolic neurologic disorders are individually rare, but collectively common, owing to the large (and growing) number of such disorders.
- Neurologists must be familiar with these disorders because they may present at any time during the life span, because many have disease-modifying therapy available, and because accurate and timely diagnosis ends what is often a prolonged diagnostic odyssey, allows the neurologist to intervene appropriately, and provides data for prognostication and counseling.
- Although no classification is entirely satisfactory, grouping these disorders into small and large molecule disorders is of practical value.
- Small molecule disorders typically result from enzyme deficiencies. Complete deficiency results in presentation in the newborn, when first exposed to a substrate load, often the first feeding. Less profound deficiencies result in episodic presentations in older children, or even adults, where the residual enzyme activity is sufficient for everyday demands, but decompensates in the face of intercurrent infection, pregnancy, or other hypercatabolic states.
- Samples of blood, urine, or CSF for metabolic testing should be obtained when the patient is acutely ill; normal assays when the patient is well do not rule out small molecule diseases.
- Large molecule disorders are the classic "storage" disorders, in which macromolecules accumulate in specific tissues, leading to distinct phenotypes.
- Patients with large molecule diseases may present with
  - Developmental delay
  - "Cerebral palsy"—with progressive physical findings
  - Epilepsy, particularly if intractable
  - Psychiatric symptoms, often refractory to therapy
  - Early-onset dementia
  - All of the above with varying combinations of somatic findings—organomegaly need not be present to diagnose "storage" disorders.
- All patients with inherited disorders benefit from accurate and timely diagnosis, and all are helped by treatment, even if specific disease-modifying therapy is not yet available.

Recommended Readings

Ahrens-Nicklas RC, Slap G, Ficicioglu C. Adolescent presentations of inborn errors of metabolism. *J Adolesc Health.* 2015;56:477–482.

Campistol J, Plecko B. Treatable newborn and infant seizures due to inborn errors of metabolism. *Epileptic Disord.* 2015;17:229–242.

Dulac O, Plecko B, Gataullina S, et al. Occasional seizures, epilepsy, and inborn errors of metabolism. *Lancet Neurol.* 2014;13:727–739.

Freeze HH, Eklund EA, Ng BG, et al. Neurology of inherited glycosylation disorders. *Lancet Neurol.* 2012;11:453–466.

Ginocchio VM, Brunetti-Pierri N. Progress toward improved therapies for inborn errors of metabolism. *Hum Mol Genet.* 2016;25(R1):R27–R35.

McLauchlan D, Robertson NP. Refining the phenotype of inborn errors of metabolism. *J Neurol.* 2015;262:2396–2398.

Rahman S, Footitt EJ, Varadkar S, et al. Inborn errors of metabolism causing epilepsy. *Dev Med Child Neurol.* 2013;55:23–36.

Sedel F, Barnerias C, Dubourg O, et al. Peripheral neuropathy and inborn errors of metabolism in adults. *J Inherit Metab Dis.* 2007;30:642–653.

Sedel F, Baumann N, Turpin JC, et al. Psychiatric manifestations revealing inborn errors of metabolism in adolescents and adults. *J Inherit Metab Dis.* 2007;30:631–641.

Sedel F, Fontaine B, Saudubray JM, et al. Hereditary spastic paraparesis in adults associated with inborn errors of metabolism: a diagnostic approach. *J Inherit Metab Dis.* 2007;30:855–864.

Sedel F, Gourfinkel-An I, Lyon-Caen O, et al. Epilepsy and inborn errors of metabolism in adults: a diagnostic approach. *J Inherit Metab Dis.* 2007;30:846–854.

Sedel F, Saudubray JM, Roze E, et al. Movement disorders and inborn errors of metabolism in adults: a diagnostic approach. *J Inherit Metab Dis.* 2008;31:308–318.

Sedel F, Tourbah A, Fontaine B, et al. Leukoencephalopathies associated with inborn errors of metabolism in adults. *J Inherit Metab Dis.* 2008;31:295–307.

Therrell BL Jr, Lloyd-Puryear MA, Camp KM, et al. Inborn errors of metabolism identified via newborn screening: ten-year incidence data and costs of nutritional interventions for research agenda planning. *Mol Genet Metab.* 2014;113:14–26.

van Karnebeek CD, Stockler-Ipsiroglu S. Early identification of treatable inborn errors of metabolism in children with intellectual disability: the Treatable Intellectual Disability Endeavor protocol in British Columbia. *Pediatr Child Health.* 2014;19:469–471.

Vernon HJ. Inborn errors of metabolism: advances in diagnosis and therapy. *JAMA Pediatr.* 2015;169:778–782.

Walterfang M, Bonnot O, Mocellin R, et al. The neuropsychiatry of inborn errors of metabolism. *J Inherit Metab Dis.* 2013;36:687–702.

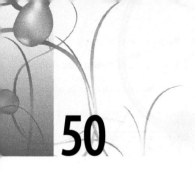

50   Spinal Cord Disorders

Athena Kostidis

DEVELOPMENTAL DISORDERS

Developmental disorders occasionally cause pain or progressive neurologic dysfunction in adults. Others are found incidentally.

A. **Chiari malformations** are characterized by descent of the cerebellar tonsils by 5 mm beyond the foramen magnum, with downward displacement of the medulla and kinking of the cervical spinal cord. Hydrocephalus, bony abnormalities of the skull base, and syringomyelia in the cervical cord are frequently found. Chiari I malformations (not associated with meningomyelocele) frequently do not manifest themselves until adulthood. Approximately 80% of patients will have syringomyelia.

   1. No treatment is warranted if the patient has no symptoms. Cranial nerve signs, a history of sleep apnea, and radiologic evidence of syringomyelia should be sought. Neurologic and radiologic follow-up evaluation is warranted, especially for children and young adults.

   2. If the patient has symptoms, decompressive suboccipital craniectomy and upper cervical laminectomy with or without ventricular shunting are required. However, patients may be stratified to a more or less aggressive surgical approach, based on structural features of the cisterna magna, extent of tonsillar descent, presence of a syrinx, and intraoperative ultrasound findings.

      a. Respiratory depression is the most common postoperative complication necessitating close monitoring.

      b. Approximately 75% of patients benefit, 17% have no change, and 9% deteriorate.

      c. Syringomyelia improved or resolved in 78% of patients.

B. **Spina bifida occulta** is the anomalous development of the posterior neural arch without an extraspinal cyst. The condition is found in 5% of the population. Cutaneous anomalies often overlie the bony defect. Evidence of other lumbosacral anomalies may be found by means of ultrasonography in infants younger than 3 months or by means of magnetic resonance imaging (MRI) in older patients. Dermal sinus tracts can cause recurrent meningitis. Lipomas and dermoids can impinge on the cord or the cauda equina.

   1. Dermal sinus tracts are closed to prevent meningitis.

   2. Biopsy is indicated for tissue diagnosis of mass lesions.

   3. Surgery is indicated for progressive deficits.

C. **Tethering of the cord** by adhesions, lipomas, or a tight filum terminale is the most common finding associated with spina bifida occulta. The syndrome often manifests itself after growth spurts or minor trauma. Pain can be the predominant presentation in adults, whereas scoliosis is more common in children. Bladder and bowel symptoms are common in both.

   1. Surgery is controversial in the care of children who have no symptoms. Arguments for early prophylactic surgery are strong because symptoms stabilize but are often not relieved after surgery. Intraoperative electromyography (EMG) monitoring can reduce the risk of surgical complications such as incomplete detethering. Patients should undergo EMG and urodynamic evaluations before a final decision is made.

   2. In follow-up care, the possibility of retethering of the spinal cord has to be monitored.

D. **Diastematomyelia** is splitting of the spinal cord by a bony or fibrous septum. The anomaly can become evident during growth spurts or minor trauma. Spina bifida occulta often is present. Pain is prominent in adults but not in children. Treatment should depend on the intensity of local pain and the degree of neurologic deficit.

   1. The septum is removed in children in response to expected progression.

E. **Platybasia** (upward displacement of the floor of the posterior fossa) and **basilar invagination** (protrusion of the odontoid through the foramen magnum) decrease the diameter of the foramen magnum. In adults, these conditions manifest as spastic tetraparesis or lower cranial nerve dysfunction.

   1. Surgical options include decompressive suboccipital craniectomy with upper cervical laminectomy.
   2. Counseling is indicated for the apparent genetic basis of skull-base disorders.

F. **Syringomyelia** is a congenital pericentral cavity of the cervical spinal cord that may extend into the thoracic cord or upward into the medulla (syringobulbia). Most lesions are between C2 and T9. It most frequently occurs in the setting of Chiari I malformation, but other etiologies include Klippel–Feil syndrome, tethered spinal cord, postinfectious, postinflammatory, posttraumatic, and spinal neoplasms.

   1. Syringomyelia usually manifests itself in adolescence or adulthood. The classic syndrome of upper-extremity weakness and atrophy (often asymmetric) with dissociated sensation in a "cape distribution" is found in 75% of cases. Enlargement of the syrinx can result in Horner's syndrome and myelopathy. Sleep-related respiratory disturbances are not uncommon, especially in syringobulbia.
   2. Although this disorder often is slowly progressive, long periods of stabilization, as well as of acute deterioration, can occur. Neck or arm pain often is a prominent problem among older patients. Scoliosis may be prominent in younger patients.
      a. Surgery may not be indicated if symptoms are minimal or very severe, if symptoms have been present longer than 5 years, or if the cord is of normal size on MRI.
      b. Surgery may be indicated in the presence of mild deficits of short duration, enlargement of the cord on MRI, and predominant symptoms of pain or spasticity.

      Surgery is indicated in progressive cases. Pain and paraparesis show the best response postoperatively. Sensory loss, lower motor neuron signs and brainstem findings are the symptoms least likely to be relieved.

VITAMIN DEFICIENCIES

A. **Vitamin B$_{12}$ (cobalamin) deficiency** is the most common disorder of the spinal cord for which specific medical therapy exists.

   1. **Pernicious anemia** is the most common cause of vitamin B$_{12}$ deficiency and is thought to be an autoimmune disorder affecting all races and both sexes. Antibodies to parietal cells are found in almost 90% of patients, and antibodies to intrinsic factor are found in somewhat more than 60%. Increased clinical suspicion, automated red blood cell (RBC) indices, and insidious onset (it takes 5 to 10 years to deplete normal body stores of cobalamin) make the fully developed classic hematologic and neurologic manifestations clinical rarities today.
   2. **Other causes** of vitamin B$_{12}$ deficiency include **gastrectomy, diseases of the terminal ileum** (Crohn's disease and diverticulosis), and less severe **gastric atrophy** (causing food-bound malabsorption). Dietary causes, once thought to be uncommon except in vegans and their breast-fed infants, may be an increasing problem among the elderly. **Nitrous oxide exposure** during anesthesia can result in precipitous neurologic manifestations in patients with "silent" deficiencies or marginal body stores. Nitrous oxide can also be the cause of an insidious myelopathy if abused. Certain medications such as colchicine can impair B$_{12}$ absorption.
   3. Clinical features.
      a. Hematologic features. The classic severe megaloblastic anemia of insidious onset is relatively rare. Approximately 25% of patients have normal hemoglobin values, 25% have normal RBC indices, and 10% to 20% have completely normal complete blood counts (CBCs).
      b. Neurologic features. Approximately 25% to 50% of patients with vitamin B$_{12}$ deficiency have neurologic symptoms or signs at diagnosis. One study showed that 27% of patients were without neurologic problems but had abnormal signs. Most patients experience leg dysesthesia as the first symptom. Neurologic presentations include the following:
         (1) **Polyneuropathy,** autonomic disturbances, and decreased visual acuity.

(2) **Subacute combined degeneration of the spinal cord** affecting the posterior and lateral columns. T2 hyperintensity in the posterior columns may be apparent on spinal MR.

(3) **Personality changes, dementia,** and psychiatric illness, including psychosis.

4. Diagnosis. In large-scale screening of elderly persons without symptoms, between 10% and 20% may have cobalamin deficiency.

   a. **Serum vitamin B$_{12}$** (cobalamin). The sensitivity, specificity, and accuracy of this commonly used assay are controversial. Patients can have normal levels and cobalamin-responsive neurologic disorders; low levels and nonresponsive deficits; or low levels but no other evidence of deficiency. Despite these severe shortcomings, measurement of cobalamin in the serum is the screening test that is the most widely available. For most patients, serum folate should be measured at the same time. Cobalamin levels in blood are light and temperature sensitive.

   b. The **peripheral blood smear** should be examined for macro-ovalocytes and hypersegmentation of neutrophils. It may be abnormal in the absence of clinically significant anemia, although the sensitivity is low in mild vitamin B$_{12}$ deficiency.

   c. **Methylmalonic acid (MMA)** (urine and serum) and serum **homocysteine** (HCYS) accumulate in vitamin B$_{12}$ deficiency. HCYS level is also elevated in folate deficiency. Assays for these metabolites can be helpful in selected cases. In comparison with serum cobalamin measurement, these assays are characterized by the following:

      (1) **Advantages** include possibly better sensitivity and specificity.

      (2) **Disadvantages** are expense and limited availability.

         (a) Elevated MMA and HCYS levels are found in hypovolemia, renal failure, and inherited disorders.

         (b) HCYS level is elevated in hypothyroidism, pyridoxine deficiency, and psoriasis.

         (c) **Intrinsic factor antibody testing** is specific but suffers from low sensitivity (<60%). However, its low cost and simplicity make this test useful as an alternative confirmation of pernicious anemia.

         (d) **Parietal cell antibody testing** is sensitive (>90%) but suffers from low specificity. A negative result makes pernicious anemia unlikely.

5. Treatment.

   a. For patients with pernicious anemia, severe deficits, or poor compliance, the usual treatment is cyanocobalamin in the following dosages: 1 mg/day intramuscularly (IM) for 7 to 12 days, then 1 mg/week IM for 3 weeks, and then 1 mg every 1 to 3 months IM for life. Less severe deficiencies can be initially treated with every other day injections for the first week, then weekly injections for the first month. Monthly injection is the standard maintenance regimen and provides the greatest ease of compliance. If longer intervals are used, MMA levels should document adequate treatment and compliance.

   b. The unusual patient with pernicious anemia and a strong aversion to injections may be offered **oral therapy** after initial cobalamin repletion. Large doses are needed, because only 1% to 3% of cobalamin is absorbed independently of intrinsic factor. Monitoring of cobalamin levels is needed until compliance is assured. The usual dosage is 1 to 2 mg/day by mouth for life. Recent evidence suggests oral therapy is at least as efficacious as parenteral therapy in reversing the clinical and biochemical indicators of vitamin B$_{12}$ deficiency.

   c. For patients who are compliant, absorb oral vitamin B$_{12}$ (the results of a standard Schilling test is normal and serum cobalamin level normalizes), have mild deficits, and want to avoid monthly injections, cyanocobalamin can be given at 50 to 1,000 µg/day by mouth for life. Cobalamin or MMA levels or both should document adequacy of the dosing schedule.

6. Prognosis. Degree of recovery depends on the severity and duration of deficits at diagnosis. Severe deficits or symptoms that have existed for more than 1 year often respond incompletely. Most improvement occurs within 6 to 12 months. If a patient has not shown some improvement after 3 months, a response is unlikely. Either the diagnosis was in error or a vitamin B$_{12}$ deficiency was coexistent but not causal (commonly observed in dementia).

7. **Therapeutic strategy.** Predicting which neurologic deficits will respond to vitamin B_{12} is imprecise. Patients with symptoms or signs consistent with vitamin B_{12} deficiency and laboratory evidence of a possible vitamin B_{12} deficiency should be given a 6-to 12-month trial of vitamin B_{12} if other treatable disorders (including folic acid deficiency) have been eliminated.

B. **Folic acid deficiency** is not generally appreciated as a cause of neurologic dysfunction similar to that found in vitamin B_{12} deficiency. As in vitamin B_{12} deficiency, the neurologic deficits can develop with normal or mildly abnormal hematologic values. The incidence of severe neurologic deficits is lower in folate deficiency than in cobalamin deficiency.

1. **Dietary inadequacy** is the most common cause of folate deficiency, especially among the elderly. Pregnancy, alcoholism, generalized malabsorption, antiepileptic medication, chemotherapy, and congenital defects in absorption or one-carbon enzymes are other potential causes.

2. Clinical features.

   a. Instances of dementia, depression, psychosis, polyneuropathy, and subacute combined degeneration of the spinal cord all have been shown to be responsive to folate supplementation. Changes in mental status and higher cortical functions may be the most common presentations in adults.

   b. An association between maternal folate supplementation and prevention of neural tube defects in the offspring has been found. Folate appears to correct a subtle block in one-carbon metabolism rather than replenish a deficiency.

3. Diagnosis.

   a. A low-**serum folate** level indicates a negative balance and predicts the likelihood of folate deficiency if uncorrected. The serum level is a poor predictor of total body stores. Because RBC folate level is much greater than serum folate level, hemolyzed specimens should be rejected.

   b. **RBC folate** level indicates body stores during the lifetime of the RBC. The specificity, sensitivity, and usefulness of the value obtained by means of radioassay (the most common technique) are controversial. If both the serum and RBC folate levels are low, ongoing folate deficiency is suggested.

   c. Elevated **serum HCYS** level with a normal serum MMA level is also a marker of folate deficiency and can be helpful in equivocal cases. Because cobalamin deficiency also elevates HCYS level, MMA has to be measured at the same time to differentiate the two deficiencies.

   d. A search for a gastrointestinal disorder should be undertaken when signs of malabsorption exist or if a dietary cause is not clear. Gastroenterologic referral and jejunal biopsy should be considered. Concurrent vitamin B_{12} deficiency can cause folate malabsorption and result in low serum and RBC folate levels. (Vitamin B_{12} deficiency is more likely to elevate serum folate levels consistent with the methylfolate trap hypothesis.)

4. **Treatment** with folic acid at a dosage of 3 mg to 10 mg/day by mouth is sufficient in dietary deficiency. Parenteral (IM) doses are given in malabsorption syndromes. Treatment is for life or until body stores are replete and etiologic factors corrected. A multivitamin should also be taken. Compliance and adequacy of treatment can be monitored with HCYS levels.

5. There is uncertainty concerning the possible **epileptogenic properties** of folic acid. Folate deficiency should be confirmed with serum HCYS measurement in the care of patients with seizures. Unless severe hematologic or neurologic deficits are present, less aggressive dosing (1 to 2 mg/day) may be best. Normalization of serum HCYS level is necessary to document compliance and to verify adequate treatment.

6. **Prognosis** is generally good if treatment is started early. Poor responses in cases of dementia or depression with folate deficiency probably represent the concurrence of two common disorders in the elderly.

C. **Vitamin E deficiency** can cause polyneuropathy, myopathy, scotomata, and demyelination within the posterior columns and spinocerebellar tracts of the spinal cord. The ataxia and posterior column manifestations of abetalipoproteinemia, a rare autosomal recessive disorder of lipoprotein metabolism are responsive to vitamin E supplementation. Rare cases of vitamin E deficiency usually manifest as long-standing malabsorption and steatorrhea. An isolated autosomal recessive defect in transport also exists. Reversal of neurologic deficits with vitamin E supplementation is variable but can be dramatic. Because prognosis appears related to duration of symptoms, a high index of symptoms is warranted. Large oral dosages of vitamin E (800 to 3,600 U/day) or semiweekly injections of α-tocopherol have been used.

D. **Copper deficiency** can cause a myelopathy marked by a spastic gait and sensory ataxia. An axonal, sensorimotor polyneuropathy frequently coexists. The myelopathy is most pronounced in the cervical cord compared with the thoracic and lumbar segments. It most frequently presents in the fifth and sixth decades and is more common in women. The clinical and radiographic features are often similar to those seen in subacute combined degeneration from B_{12} deficiency. In fact, the two conditions may coexist. Causes of copper deficiency include prior gastric surgery, malabsorption (e.g., in celiac disease), parenteral feeding deficiency, and excessive zinc intake (as can be seen with use of certain denture creams). However, in many cases, the cause remains unclear. Hematologic manifestations of copper deficiency include anemia or neutropenia. Treatment with copper supplementation may prevent further neurologic deterioration, and variably can improve symptoms. Supplementation is typically oral, at 8 mg/day for 1 week, then 6 mg/day for 1 week, then 4 mg/day for 1 week and 2 mg/day thereafter.

VASCULAR MALFORMATIONS OF THE SPINAL CORD

A. **Classification.** Spinal cord vascular malformations can be classified into intramedullary arteriovenous malformations (AVMs), perimedullary AVMs, spinal-dural arteriovenous fistulas, epidural AVMs, paravertebral vascular malformations, vertebral hemangiomas, and complex angiomatosis. Of these, spinal-dural arteriovenous fistulas (DAVFs) are the most common, making up about 70% of all lesions, and thus the rest of this section will focus on this entity.

B. **Clinical features.** Patients present with a variety of symptoms distal to the malformation, including progressive paraparesis or radiculopathy, sensory impairment, sphincter disturbances, and pain. Usually the deficits are slowly progressive. When hemorrhage occurs within the lesion, it may result in an acute medullary syndrome.

C. **Diagnosis.** Most DAVFs are located in the mid to lower dorsal spinal cord (T6–T12). Enhanced MRI is the screening modality of choice, but a spinal-dural fistula may escape detection even on high quality MRI. MR angiography (MRA) is a useful noninvasive tool that can aid in diagnosis by localizing the level of the fistula and course of drainage. Nonetheless, selective spinal arteriography is the gold standard for diagnosis and classification of these fistulas.

D. **Treatment.** Endovascular embolization can often cure these lesions. Open surgery is indicated if embolization fails. In some patients, a combination of both embolization and open surgery is the best therapeutic option.

E. **Prognosis.** DAVFs in the mid to lower thoracic cord respond best to treatment. Motor symptoms tend to improve most (up to two-thirds of patients), followed by pain and sensory disturbances (up to one-third of patients), and finally sphincteric dysfunction, which is less likely to be reversible.

SPINAL CORD INFARCTION

Although spinal cord infarctions account for only about 1% of all strokes, they are a cause of significant morbidity. Some common etiologies include prolonged episodes of arterial hypotension, surgical procedures, and pathologies affecting the aorta, disk prolapse or herniation, and arteriopathy; however, in some cases, no cause can be identified. Rarely, spinal cord infarction may be a complication of transforaminal cervical epidural steroid injection. In terms of prevention, motor evoked potentials are commonly been used during aortic surgeries (e.g., during thracoabdominal aortic aneurysm repair) to alert the surgeon to impending spinal cord ischemia, thus reducing the incidence of paraplegia. Other forms of prevention which have shown clinical benefit during aortic surgeries include spinal fluid drainage, hypothermia and increased mean arterial pressure. The neurologic symptoms of spinal cord ischemia are referable to the involved artery or segment of the spinal cord. Pain at the level of infarction is also a common finding. Diagnosis is aided by contrast-enhanced MRI. This should include diffusion-weighted imaging as well, as it may take up to 24 hours for ischemic lesions to appear on conventional sequences (Fig. 50.1). Therapeutic interventions include

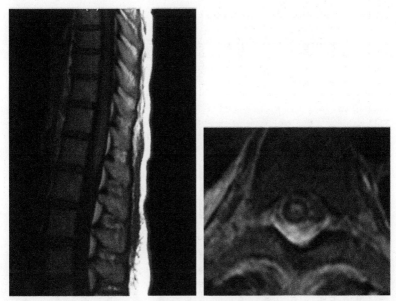

FIGURE 50.1 A 33-year-old woman with systemic lupus erythematosus, antiphospholipid antibody syndrome, status postquintuple coronary artery bypass graft, who developed acute cardiac tamponade and hepato-renal syndrome. She was found to have flaccid paraplegia of the lower extremities. Pre- and postcontrast MRI (sagittal and axial) of the lower thoracic spinal cord and conus medullaris demonstrates abnormal high signal intensity most prominent at the levels of T11 and T12, as seen on the T2-weighted images. These findings are consistent with spinal cord ischemia. (Courtesy of Dr. José Biller.). MRI, magnetic resonance imaging.

lumbar cerebrospinal fluid (CSF) drainage with or without vasopressor therapy. Treatment is also supportive and focused on the underlying pathology and secondary stroke prevention (patients generally receive an antiplatelet unless there is a contraindication). Unilateral infarcts have a more favorable prognosis; however, prognosis is largely dependent on the severity of the initial deficit. There is some evidence to suggest that intact proprioception at the onset of the deficit also carries a more favorable prognosis.

ACUTE SPINAL CORD INJURY

A. **Etiology.** The major causes of acute spinal cord injury are motor vehicle accidents, falls, recreational injuries, and acts of violence. Fracture and compromise of the spinal cord (or cauda equina) occur most often at cervical and thoracolumbar levels. Although thoracic fractures are less common, neurologic injury is more common because of the narrowness of the spinal canal.

B. **Prevention.** Proper use of passive and active restraints in automobiles and use of helmets by motorcyclists and bicyclists prevent head and spinal injuries. For example, the Think First program, which addresses educational issues for youth in kindergarten through 12th grade and is actively supported by the neurosurgical community, should be embraced by health care providers.

C. **Prognosis.** Improvement of even one level can have a dramatic effect on function, especially in cervical cord injuries (Table 50.1). Final neurologic function depends on severity of initial injury, prevention of secondary damage, and successful management of the complications and sequelae of the acute injury and intensive rehabilitation. Neurologic assessment 72 hours after injury according to American Spinal Injury Association guidelines is useful in estimating outcome.

1. Features suggesting a possibility of neurologic improvement are as follows:
    a. Motor or sensory function below neurologic level (incomplete lesion).
    b. Degree to which motor strength is preserved below neurologic level.

TABLE 50.1 Expected Functional Outcomes in Spinal Cord Injury

Function	C1–C4	C5	C6	C7–C8	T1–T9	T10–S5
Respiratory	Ventilator dependent[a]	Assisted cough	Assisted cough	Assisted cough	Decreased endurance	Intact
Bowel	Total assist	Total assist	Moderate assist	Moderate assist	Independent	Independent
Bladder	Total assist	Total assist	Moderate assist	Variable assist	Independent	Independent
Bed mobility	Total assist	Some assist	Some assist	Variable assist	Independent	Independent
Transfers	Total assist	Total assist	Variable assist	Variable assist	Independent	Independent
Pressure relief, positioning	Total assist	Independent with equipment	Independent with equipment	Independent	Independent	Independent
Eating	Total assist	Independent with equipment and setup	Variable assist	Independent	Independent	Independent
Dressing	Total assist	Near total assist	Moderate assist	Variable assist	Independent	Independent
Grooming	Total assist	Moderate assist	Independent with equipment	Independent	Independent	Independent
Bathing	Total assist	Total assist	Moderate assist	Variable assist	Independent	Independent
Wheelchair	Power with special controls	Near total assist or power	Moderate assist or power	Minimal assist	Independent	Independent
Ambulation	Not indicated	Not indicated	Not indicated	Not indicated	Typically not functional	Functional with variable assist
Communication	Moderate assist with equipment	Independent with equipment	Independent with equipment	Independent	Independent	Independent
Transportation	Total assist	Highly custom van with lift	Modified van with lift	Modified vehicle	Hand controls	Hand controls
Homemaking	Total assist	Total assist	Moderate assist	Variable assist	Independent, moderate assist	Independent, minimal assist
Assist required	24 hr/d	16 hr/d	10 hr/d	8 hr/d	3 hr/d	0–2 hr/d

[a]C4 level may be ventilator independent needing assisted cough.

Data from Consortium for Spinal Cord Medicine. Outcomes following traumatic spinal cord injury: clinical practice guidelines for health care professionals. Paralyzed Veterans of America, 1999.

c. Preservation of pinprick response in addition to light touch below neurologic level.
d. Age <30 years.
e. Residual anal sphincter tone.
f. Relatively well-preserved vertebral alignment.
2. Features suggesting a poor prognosis are as follows:
a. Absence of residual function (complete lesion).
b. Hemorrhage or multilevel edema on MRI.
D. Principles of treatment.
1. **Immobilization of the spine** at the scene, in transport, and in the emergency department is critical in preventing further damage.
2. **ABCs of trauma care;** supplemental oxygen should be provided.
3. **Primary survey** of associated damage.
a. Alteration of sensorium necessitates investigation for accompanying head injury.
b. Neurologic level may mask the usual symptoms and signs of thoracic, abdominal, pelvic, or extremity injury. More reliance is placed on objective tests.
4. **Radiologic evaluation** of level of skeletal injury.
5. **Skeletal traction** for stabilization and closed reduction if indicated.
6. Assessment of **neurologic level of injury.**
a. The neurologic level of injury is the most caudal segment at which both motor function and sensory function are intact bilaterally (Table 50.2).

TABLE 50.2 Key Muscles and Sensory Areas for Determination of Neurologic Level of Injury

Level	Muscle Action	Key Muscle	Key Sensory Area
C2	–	–	Occipital protuberance
C3	–	–	Supraclavicular fossa
C4	–	–	Top anterior shoulder
C5	Elbow flexion	Biceps brachialis	Lateral antecubital fossa
C6	Wrist extension	Extensor carpi radialis	Thumb
C7	Elbow extension	Triceps	Dorsal middle finger
C8	Finger flexion (third)	Extensor digitorum profundus	Dorsal little finger
T1	Finger abduction (fifth)	Abductor digiti minimi	Medial antecubital fossa
T2	–	–	Apex of axilla
T3	–	–	Third intercostal space
T4	–	–	Nipple line
T5	–	–	Midway between T4 and T6
T6	–	–	Xiphisternum
T7	–	–	Midway between T6 and T8
T8	–	–	Midway between T6 and T10
T9	–	–	Midway between T8 and T10
T10	–	–	Umbilicus
T11	–	–	Midway between T10 and T12
T12	–	–	Midpoint of inguinal ligament
L1	–	–	Midway between T12 and L2
L2	Hip flexion	Iliopsoas	Mid-anterior thigh
L3	Knee extension	Quadriceps	Medial femoral condyle
L4	Ankle dorsiflexion	Tibialis anterior	Medial malleolus
L5	Toe extension (first)	Extensor hallucis longus	Dorsum of foot at third metatarsophalangeal joint
S1	Ankle plantar fexion	Gastrocnemius, soleus	Lateral heel
S2	–	–	Mid-popliteal fossa
S3	–	–	Ischial tuberosity
S4–S5	–	–	Perianal sensation

Data from Maynard FM, Bracken MB, Creasey G, et al. International standards for neurological and functional classification of spinal cord injury. *Spinal Cord.* 1997;35:266–274.

    b. The completeness of the injury is defined by American Spinal Injury Association classes grades A through E, which describe function at least three levels below the neurologic level of injury. Grade A indicates a complete level, grade E indicates recovery, and grades B through D describe incomplete levels.

7. **Secondary survey** and stabilization of patient's condition.
8. **Transport** to spinal cord injury center.
9. **Surgical decompression** preferably done within 24 hours in select cases.
10. **Medications** to prevent secondary (oxidative) damage.
    a. The National Acute Spinal Cord Injury Study 2 (NASCIS 2) showed a modest but significant benefit compared with placebo for high-dose methylprednisolone if started within 8 hours of injury. The initial dose of 30 mg/kg intravenous bolus is followed by 5.4 mg/kg/hour infusion for 23 hours. Complications include pneumonia, sepsis, and gastrointestinal hemorrhage.
    b. NASCIS 3 showed an additional 24 hours of steroid infusion to be beneficial to patients who received the initial bolus between 3 and 8 hours after injury. Treatment started at later than 8 hours after injury resulted in poorer outcomes than did placebo treatment.
    c. However in 2013, based on further data, the American Association of Neurological Surgeons (AANS)/Congress of Neurological Surgeons (CNS) Guidelines for the Management of Acute Cervical Spine and Spinal Cord Injury issued a level 1 recommendation that administration of MP for the treatment of acute spinal cord injury is not recommended.
    d. There is some controversy around this change of guideline, and some physicians advocate treating on a patient to patient basis, balancing the potential risks and benefits for each patient. Specifically, patients with cervical spinal cord injury have been found to be less prone to the complications of methylprednisolone.
11. **Restoration and maintenance** of spinal alignment.

SEQUELAE OF SPINAL CORD INJURIES

A. **Pressure sores** are the most preventable complication of spinal cord injury.
1. **Prevention.** Patient and family education are important. Pressure is relieved by turning in bed every 2 hours and "wheelchair" lifts for 5 to 10 seconds every 15 to 30 minutes. Special mattresses and wheelchair cushions do not obviate proper positioning and frequent repositioning. The skin is kept clean, dry, and inspected daily. Attention is paid to nutritional requirements.
2. **Pressure relief.** A repositioning schedule ensuring that the sore is always pressure free needs to be rigidly followed because the reduced number of possible weight-bearing position makes another sore more likely. Simultaneous management of more than one pressure sore requires special frames or flotation beds.
3. **Debridement.** Saline wet-to-dry gauze and whirlpool therapy are standard, but commercial enzyme preparations are less labor intensive. If the eschar is hard and blackened, necrotic tissue is removed surgically.
4. **Dressings.** Shallow ulcers are covered with sterile gauze. Occlusive dressings may promote more rapid healing and have to be changed less often but are much more expensive. Deeper, pear-shaped ulcers are loosely packed with saline-soaked gauze to prevent abscess formation and to promote "bottom-up" healing. The goal is to keep the wound moist, whereas the surrounding tissue is kept dry.
5. **Electrical stimulation** may accelerate wound healing.
6. **Surgical excision** with a myocutaneous flap to fill the cavity is usually required for deeper ulcers. Reduction of bony prominences may be necessary.
B. **Deep venous thrombosis** is a serious concern after spinal cord injury. Pain may not be felt below a sensory level, and swelling may be masked by edema and vasomotor changes.
1. **Prophylaxis** is needed for up to 3 months or until discharge from the rehabilitation unit. Intermittent pneumatic compression devices or compression stockings are used for the

2 weeks after injury. Anticoagulation with low-molecular-weight heparin or adjusted-dose unfractionated heparin should be started 48 to 72 hours after injury and continued 8 to 12 weeks depending on associated risk factors. Vena caval filters are placed in patients with contraindications to or who have undergone unsuccessful anticoagulation therapy. Filters should also be considered in addition to anticoagulation in the care of patients with complete C2 or C3 neurologic levels of injury.

2. **Treatment** is the same as that of patients without spinal cord injury. Mobilization and exercise of the lower extremities should be withheld 48 to 72 hours until anticoagulation is adequate. Pain relief should be provided to lessen the possibility of autonomic dysreflexia.

C. Autonomic dysreflexia. From 30% to 85% of patients with quadriplegia or high paraplegia have paroxysmal episodes of severe hypertension, sweating, flushing, and piloerection accompanied by headache, chest pain, and bradycardia or tachycardia in response to relatively benign stimuli below the level of injury. Pulmonary edema, intracranial hemorrhage, cerebral infarction, seizures, or death can result. Bladder and bowel distention, instrumentation, or irritation are the most common precipitating stimuli.

1. Etiology. In the setting of a spinal lesion above the major splanchnic outflow tract (T6–L2), reflex activation of sympathetic discharge occurs below the lesion unchecked by descending inhibitory pathways from supraspinal centers.

2. Management. Initial treatment entails removal of the precipitating stimulus and medication for the hypertensive crisis.

   a. Removal of precipitating stimulus.

      (1) Stop procedure.

      (2) Check for urinary catheter blockage.

      (3) Remove tight clothing, shoes, straps, and other restrictive items.

      (4) Catheterize carefully with 2% lidocaine jelly.

      (5) Perform kidney, ureter, and bladder and rectal examination with lidocaine jelly to check for impaction.

      (6) Check for sores, infection, trauma, and fractures.

      (7) Consider acute abdomen and deep venous thrombosis.

   b. Management of hypertension.

      (1) Elevate head of bed or place patient in sitting position to induce postural changes in blood pressure.

      (2) Drug therapy.

         (a) Nifedipine 10 mg by mouth (immediate release form—bite through capsule and swallow); monitor response *or*

         (b) Nitroglycerin 2% ointment—1 inch (2.5 cm) applied above neurologic site of injury; monitor response.

      (3) If blood pressure remains critical, intravenous protocols (e.g., hydralazine, diazoxide, and sodium nitroprusside) for hypertensive crisis must be initiated.

   c. Management of profuse sweating without hypertension. Give propantheline at 15 mg by mouth (may be repeated after 10 minutes) or oxybutynin at 5 mg by mouth (may be repeated after 10 minutes).

3. Prophylactic medications.

   a. Nifedipine 10 mg by mouth 30 minutes before procedure.

   b. Phenoxybenzamine 10 to 20 mg by mouth three times a day.

   c. Scopolamine patch may help with reflex sweating.

D. **Depression** must be continually assessed and managed.

E. Central pain syndrome. Development of chronic dysesthesia or central (neuropathic) pain above, at, or distal to the level of injury poses therapeutic challenges. Central pain is in addition to the musculoskeletal and visceral pain experienced by patients with spinal cord injuries.

1. Etiology.

   a. Above level of injury. Compressive mononeuropathy (e.g., ulnar and median) and posttraumatic syringomyelia formation.

   b. At level of injury. Central pain from cord damage, radicular pain from root damage, and complex regional pain syndrome.

   c. Below level of injury. Central pain.

2. **Pharmacologic approach** is trial and error.
   a. **Tricyclic antidepressants** for nonlancinating pain.
      (1) Amitriptyline (Elavil) or nortriptyline (Pamelor) 10 to 25 mg by mouth at bedtime; increase by 10 to 25 mg every 5 to 7 days as tolerated to 75 to 150 mg at bedtime.
      (2) Side effects include sedation, anticholinergic effects, orthostatic hypotension, weight gain, and cardiac arrhythmia.
      (3) If side effects are not tolerable, a chemically unrelated compound, such as duloxetine (Cymbalta) at 30 to 60 mg/day by mouth, may be tried.
   b. **Anticonvulsants** (frequently in combination with tricyclic antidepressants) for lancinating central pain.
      (1) Carbamazepine (Tegretol) 100 mg twice a day increased 100 mg every 3 days as tolerated to a serum level of 8 to 10 mg/mL in three or four doses per day.
         (a) Side effects include sedation, diplopia, gastrointestinal upset, ataxia, weakness, rash, and bone marrow suppression.
         (b) Monitor CBC with platelets every 2 weeks for 3 months, then CBC, platelets, and liver function every 3 to 6 months.
      (2) Gabapentin (Neurontin) 100 mg three times a day increased 100 to 300 mg every 3 days as tolerated up to 600 to 900 three or four times a day.
         (a) Side effects include drowsiness and dizziness.
         (b) Blood levels are not used clinically, and no monitoring is needed.
      (3) Pregabalin (Lyrica) 50 mg three times a day increased to 100 mg three times a day after 1 week as tolerated.
         (a) Side effects include peripheral edema, weight gain, constipation, dizziness, and somnolence.
         (b) Blood levels are not used clinically and no monitoring is needed.
3. **Physical methods** may provide some temporary relief for central pain at the level of the injury.
   a. Transcutaneous electrical nerve stimulation.
   b. Warm or cool packs, ultrasound and massage.
4. Surgical treatment should be considered only after conservative therapy has failed.
   a. Dorsal root entry zone (DREZ) surgery.
      (1) Laminectomy and radiofrequency ablation of DREZ is performed two levels above and one level below the site of injury.
      (2) Improvement is realized in 60% to 90% of patients. Best results are achieved in patients with pain at or just below the level of injury.
      (3) Complications include loss of one or two sensory levels, CSF leakage, hematoma, and bowel, bladder, and sexual dysfunction.
   b. Avoid sympathectomy, rhizotomy, and cordotomy.
5. **Narcotic therapy** is indicated only after both conservative and surgical therapies have failed.
   a. Combination with tricyclic antidepressants may be synergistic.
   b. The patient must be carefully selected and carefully supervised.
   c. Methadone (Dolophine) sustained release oxycodone (Oxycontin), and an intrathecal morphine pump (if possible) are options for selected patients.
      (1) A formal contract detailing expectations and criteria for termination of treatment are made with the patient.
      (2) Periodic attempts should be made to wean the medication.
      (3) Side effects include sedation and cognitive slowing, respiratory depression, constipation, and reduced sexual function.

SPINAL EPIDURAL ABSCESS

A. Etiology. Epidural abscesses occur in patients with predisposing conditions, such as a chronic disease (alcoholism and immunodeficiency states), a spinal abnormality or intervention, or a source for local or systemic infection. Bacteria seed the epidural space by either contiguous spread or hematogenous dissemination (about half of cases). Methicillin-sensitive *Staphylococcus aureus* accounts for 40% of cases, Methicillin-resistant *S. aureus* account for 30% of cases, other gram-positive cocci account for 13% and gram-negative bacteria occur in about 15% of cases.

B. Clinical features. Back pain, fever, and neurologic deficits are the most common symptoms; however, this triad is not often found in all patients. The clinical features are divided into four stages:
   1. Back pain at the level of the abscess.
   2. Radicular pain from the involved level of the spinal column.
   3. Motor weakness, sensory deficit, and bowel and bladder dysfunction.
   4. Paralysis.
      The rate of progression between stages can vary between a few hours to days.
C. Diagnosis. Two-thirds of patients will have a leukocytosis. The vast majority of patients will also have an elevated erythrocyte sedimentation rate upon presentation. CRP levels are also useful, but processing can take hours to days, which may unnecessarily delay the diagnosis. The initial CRP value is useful for comparison to repeat values as a measure of treatment response. Bacteremia can be detected in up to 60% of cases. However, definitive diagnosis is best established by contrast-enhanced MRI of the affected area.
D. Treatment. Emergent surgical decompression and debridement combined with systemic antibiotics for at least 6 weeks is the treatment of choice. Empiric antibiotic therapy should provide coverage against staphylococci and gram-negative bacilli.
E. Prognosis. Prompt diagnosis and the patient's neurologic status prior to surgical drainage are the most important predictors of outcome.

DEMYELINATING LESIONS OF THE SPINAL CORD

The most common cause of demyelination in the spinal cord is multiple sclerosis (MS). Up to 50% of cases will involve the spinal cord. The lesions are typically dorsolateral, longitudinal, and flame-shaped (Video 50.1). Another less common cause of demyelination in the spinal cord is neuromyelitis optica (NMO) or Devic's disease. It is currently recognized as its own distinct disorder, separate from MS. Diagnostic criteria for NMO include optic neuritis, acute myelitis, and at least two of the three following supportive criteria: (1) contiguous spinal cord MRI lesion extending three or more vertebral segments (Fig. 50.2), (2) brain MRI not meeting diagnostic criteria for MS, and (3) NMO-IgG seropositivity. The NMO-IgG antibody has a sensitivity of 74% and a specificity of >90%. Treatment of acute attacks of optic neuritis or myelitis often only partially respond, or do not respond at all to high-dose glucocorticoids. In this setting, plasmapheresis is often used. Maintenance of remission in NMO requires long-term immunosuppressive therapy. There has been evidence for the use of azathioprine, methotrexate, mitoxantrone, mycophenolate mofetil, and rituximab.

CENTRAL CORD SYNDROME

A. Etiology. Hyperextension injuries may produce a spinal cord contusion primarily affecting the central gray matter. Lamination of tracks in the cervical cord (sacral fibers, lateral; cervical fibers, and medial) explains the clinical signs and symptoms.
B. Clinical features. Patients have "inverted quadriparesis," in which upper-extremity weakness exceeds lower extremity weakness. Transient burning dysesthesia in the hands with little weakness, or urinary dysfunction can also occur. With recovery, the leg, bladder, and upper-extremity weaknesses improve. The fingers are last to recover.
C. Treatment.
   1. **Medical management** consists of intensive care unit (ICU) care, rigid immobilization of the neck, and physical therapy.
   2. Surgical therapy. Surgery is recommended for patients with focal cord compression or instability of the spine. Surgical management for patients without bony injury is a subject of debate in recent literature, and should be decided on a patient to patient basis.
D. Prognosis. Almost all patients have improvement, but often to an incomplete degree among the elderly. Delayed progressive myelopathy can develop in approximately 25% of cases.

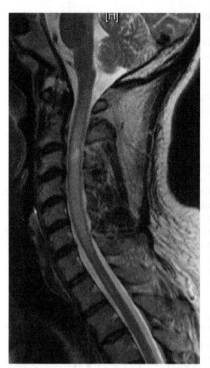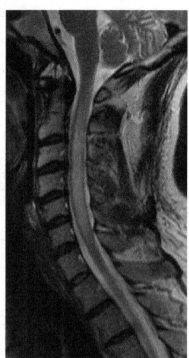

FIGURE 50.2 A 44-year-old African American man with neuromyelitis optica (Devic's disease). MRI of the cervical spine without and with contrast shows contiguous cord signal abnormality identified involving the cervical spinal cord from the craniocervical junction to the C6–C7 level. The spinal cord signal abnormality involves nearly the entire central spinal cord symmetrically with relative sparing of the lateral portions bilaterally. The cervical spinal cord signal abnormality is associated with tapered cord expansion resulting in circumferential, partial to complete effacement of the thecal sac at the involved levels. (Courtesy of José Biller, MD). MRI, magnetic resonance imaging.

HYPEREXTENSION–FLEXION INJURY (WHIPLASH INJURY)

A. **Etiology.** Automobile accidents account for approximately 85% of whiplash injuries. The cardinal symptoms of neck pain and headache are musculoskeletal. Concomitant symptoms may include dizziness, visual impairments, nausea, tinnitus, deafness, paresthesias, lower back pain, arm or shoulder pain, posttraumatic stress disorder, and cognitive dysfunction. The roles of mild CNS injury and psychosocial factors are controversial and have led to biopsychosocial models of outcome in the disorder.

B. **Prevention.** Automobile head restraints reduce flexion–hyperextension motion of the head in automobile accidents, especially during rear-end collisions. However, surveys have shown that the restraints frequently are adjusted incorrectly.

C. **Natural history.** Rear-end collisions are involved in most whiplash injuries. Cynicism and controversy exist over the cause of chronic whiplash syndrome. Although figures vary widely, approximately 15% to 30% of patients continue to have symptoms 6 months after the injury. By 12 months, 80% of patients have no symptoms, whereas 5% of patients remain severely affected. Results of fluoroscopically guided nerve block studies suggest that zygapophyseal joint pain (usually C2–C3) accounts for 50% of chronic neck pain after whiplash.

D. **Treatment.** Compensation concerns hinder controlled clinical trials of treatment.

1. Positive attitude and encouragement.
2. Ice for first 24 hours.

3. Muscle relaxants, nonsteroidal anti-inflammatory drugs, and adequate pain relief in the first 7 to 14 days.
4. Resumption of most normal activities together with active therapy or home exercises results in better outcome than with conventional regimens of restricted activity, rest, and soft cervical collar.
5. Heat, ultrasound, massage, and trigger-point injections often make patients more comfortable but remain unproven.
6. Percutaneous radiofrequency neurotomy for cervical zygapophysial joint pain has been showed to be effective in several studies, but the pain frequently returns and necessitates repeated procedures.

SPASTICITY

Spasticity is one of the cardinal manifestations of chronic spinal cord disease. In acute spinal lesions, spasticity develops after a variable period of spinal shock, whereas in disorders with insidious onset, it may be the first symptom noticed.

A. The decision to treat a patient must be made on an individual basis. Treatment is indicated when the advantages of spasticity outweigh the disadvantages. Specific treatment goals need to be formulated.
   1. Advantages.
      a. Bowel training maintains sphincter tone.
      b. "Internal crutches" are available for ambulation.
      c. Weight-bearing is possible in transfers.
      d. Osteopenia is reduced.
      e. Muscle bulk is increased.
      f. Venous tone is increased, and deep venous thrombosis may be decreased.
   2. Disadvantages.
      a. Pain and falls result from paroxysmal spasms.
      b. Hygiene is impaired owing to hip adductor spasticity.
      c. Joint contractures occur.
      d. Pressure sores form.
      e. Renal damage occurs because of external sphincter spasticity.
      f. Movements required for activities of daily living are impaired or interrupted.
B. **Assessment** of severity can be made with the modified Ashworth scale (Table 50.3).
C. A **changing pattern in a previously stable degree of spasticity** should alert the clinician to varying etiologic factors.
   1. Medication: fluoxetine, sertraline, or trazodone.
   2. Anxiety.
   3. Tight clothing or shoes.
   4. Inadequate or prolonged postures.
   5. Formation of pressure sores.
   6. Development of deep venous thrombosis.
   7. Ingrown toenails.

TABLE 50.3 Modified Ashworth Scale for Measuring Spasticity

Grade 0: Normal muscle tone
Grade 1: Slight increase in muscle tone; "catch" or minimal resistance at end of ROM
Grade 2: Slight increase; "catch" followed by minimal resistance for remainder of ROM
Grade 3: More marked increase in tone through most of ROM; parts moved easily
Grade 4: Considerable increase in tone; passive movement difficult
Grade 5: Affected part or parts rigid in flexion or extension
Total score is the average of bilateral hip flexion and abduction, knee flexion, and ankle dorsiflexion.

Abbreviation: ROM, range of motion.
Adapted from McLean BN. Intrathecal baclofen in severe spasticity. *Br J Hosp Med.* 1993;49:262–267.

8. Spinal instability.
9. Fractures.
10. Posttraumatic syringomyelia.
11. Gastrointestinal dysfunction: impaction, hemorrhoids, and acute abdomen.
12. Genitourinary dysfunction: infection, stones, blocked catheters, and disorders of testicle, prostate, vagina, uterus, or ovary.
D. **Management** is based on a multidisciplinary approach with a rigorous program of both passive and active stretching.
   1. Physical modalities.
      a. Range of motion and stretching exercises.
      b. Heat or cold.
      c. Vibration (increases presynaptic spinal inhibition).
      d. Splints, casts, and orthotics to prevent contractures and increase mobility.
   2. **Useful medications** are summarized in Table 50.4. Muscle relaxants (antispasmodics) are not used in the long-term management of spasticity.
   3. Nerve blocks.
      Botulinum toxin type A (Botox; Allergan, Irvine, CA, USA) injection has been found effective for focal spasticity at a variety of sites.
      a. The discomfort and expense of numerous injections in large lower extremity muscles limit this technique to relatively small muscles.
      b. Transient postinjection discomfort and side effects are generally well-tolerated. Excessive weakness and flu-like syndromes may be experienced at initiation of treatment.

TABLE 50.4 Drug Management of Spasticity

Drug	Daily Dosage[a] (Starting Dosage)	Side Effects and Comments
Baclofen (Lioresal; Novartis, Hanover, NJ, USA)	10–160 mg (5 mg b.i.d.)	Drowsiness, weakness, tremor, ataxia, abrupt withdrawal with seizures, confusion, hallucinations
Tizanidine (Zanaflex; Athena Neurosciences, Inc., San Francisco, CA, USA)	8–32 mg (2 mg at bedtime)	Use with caution in liver disease
		Dry mouth, sedation, dizziness, risk of hypotension, insomnia, hallucinations, hepatotoxicity Liver monitoring at 1, 3, and 6 mo Somewhat less weakness than with baclofen
Gabapentin (Neurontin; Parke-Davis, Morris Plains, NJ, USA)	300–3,600 mg (100 mg t.i.d.)	Nausea, sedation, ataxia, dizziness
Diazepam (Valium; Roche Products, Nutley, NJ, USA)	4–60 mg (2 mg at bedtime)	Sedation, cognitive changes, depression, weakness, dependence, abuse, withdrawal syndrome
Dantrolene[b] (Dantrium; Procter and Gamble Pharmaceuticals, Inc., Cincinnati, OH, USA)	25–400 mg (25 mg once a day)	Weakness, hepatotoxicity, confusion, sedation, nausea, diarrhea Monitor liver function closely

[a]It is important to start with a low dosage and gradually build to a target dosage as tolerance of the sedation and most other side effects of the medication develops.
[b]The potentially fatal hepatotoxicity of dantrolene is more common among adults and those taking estrogens. This drug probably should be avoided by those with preexisting liver disease.
Abbreviations: b.i.d., twice a day; t.i.d., three times a day.

Botulinum injections should be avoided by patients receiving aminoglycosides. Neutralizing antibodies are more common with larger, more frequent doses.

c. Advantages are reversible block (2 to 6 months) and selectivity toward motor fibers.

d. Disadvantages are expense and need for repeated injections.

4. Neurosurgical procedures.

a. An **intrathecal baclofen pump** is a safe alternative to ablative surgery for intractable spasticity at experienced centers.

(1) Referral to an experienced center should be considered for patients with stable neurologic disorders accompanied by spasticity seriously interfering with quality of life. Oral agents should have been found ineffective or limited owing to intolerable side effects.

(2) Patients are selected after a test dose of 50 to 75 mg baclofen administered by lumbar puncture. Spasticity is assessed 1, 2, 4, and 8 hours after injection with the modified Ashworth scale (Table 50.3). If two-point improvement is not documented and side effects are tolerable, a second larger test dose (75 to 100 mg) is given the next day.

(3) During the first year after implantation, daily doses generally increase before stabilizing in the range of 300 to 800 mg/day.

(4) Improvement is observed in muscle tone, mobility, and bladder function, and spasms and musculoskeletal pain are relieved. There is little or no relief of central pain.

(5) Systemic side effects are less than with oral therapy. Drowsiness, nausea, hypotension, headache, and weakness may be experienced during the dose titration phase. Infections and catheter or pump complications are rare but potentially serious side effects.

(6) Depletion of the pump battery in 5 to 7 years necessitates replacing the entire pump unit.

(7) Although life-threatening, all instances of drug overdose have been completely reversible. Experience and better pump design have decreased the complication rate to <5%. In early series of patients, surgical revision was needed in 20% of cases for catheter-related problems.

b. **Selective posterior rhizotomy** with intraoperative EMG selection of lumbosacral rootlets for sectioning is useful in the management of cerebral palsy. Two-thirds of patients' conditions are improved with minimal sensory loss and few side effects. DREZ operations are functionally similar microsurgical procedures.

c. Percutaneous posterior rhizotomy is technically more difficult, and recurrence may be more of a problem.

d. Efficacy of spinal cord stimulators is controversial.

e. Peripheral neurectomy is occasionally used to relieve specific joint contractures.

f. Longitudinal myelotomy, nonselective posterior rhizotomy, and anterior rhizotomy are rarely performed.

5. **Orthopedic procedures** are used most often performed in a supportive role to relieve pain, increase mobility, and decrease deformity in cerebral palsy.

a. Tendon release, lengthening, and transfer.

b. Osteotomy and arthrodesis.

Key Points

- Spinal cord disorders can be due to various etiologies: developmental, nutritional, vascular, infectious, demyelinating and traumatic.
- MRI is the preferred method of initial diagnosis in any disorder of the spinal cord. Other testing is then needed on an individual basis, based on clinical judgment.
- Specific treatment should be instituted as soon as the diagnosis has been made.
- In any traumatic spinal cord disorder, it is important to stabilize the spine first.
- In chronic spinal cord disorders, one must manage sequelae appropriately for best patient outcome.

Recommended Readings

Aarabi B, Hadley M, Dhall S. Management of acute traumatic central cord syndrome. *Neurosurgery.* 2013;72(3):195–204.

Arnautovic, A, Splavski, B, Boop F, et al. Pediatric and Adult Chiari Malformation Type I surgical series 1965-2013: a review of demographics, operative treatment and outcomes. *J Neurosurg Pediatr.* 2015;15(2):161–177.

Belanger E, Levi AD. The acute and chronic management of spinal cord injury. *J Am Coll Surg.* 2000;190:603–618.

Bryce TN, Ragnarsson KT. Pain after spinal cord injury. *Phys Med Rehabil Clin N Am.* 2000;11:157–168.

Darouiche RO. Spinal epidural abscess. *N Engl J Med.* 2006;355:2012–2020.

Davis EC, Barnes MP. Botulinum toxin and spasticity. *J Neurol Neurosurg Psychiatry.* 2000;69:143–147.

Fehlings M, Wilson J, Cho N. Methylprednisolone for the treatment of acute spinal cord injury: counterpoint. *Neurosurgery.* 2014;61(suppl 1):36–42.

Goodman, B. Metabolic and toxic causes of myelopathy. *Continuum (Minneap Minn).* 2015;21(1):84–99.

Green R, Kinsella LJ. Current concepts in the diagnosis of cobalamin deficiency. *Neurology.* 1995;45:1435–1440.

Jaiser S, Winston G. Copper deficiency myelopathy. *J Neurol.* 2010;27:869–881.

Kita M, Goodkin DE. Drugs used to treat spasticity. *Drugs.* 2000;59:487–495.

Marcus J, Schwarz J, Singh P, et al. Spinal dural arteriovenous fistula: a review. *Curr Atheroscler Rep.* 2013;15:335.

Maynard FM Jr, Bracken MB, Creasey G, et al. International standards for neurological and functional classification of spinal cord injury. American Spinal Injury Association. *Spinal Cord.* 1997;35:266–274.

McIntyre A, Mays R, Mehta S, et al. Examining the effectiveness of intrathecal baclofen in spasticity in individuals with chronic spinal cord injury: a systematic review. *J Spinal Cord Med.* 2014;37(1):11–18.

Newey ML, Sen PK, Fraser RD. The long-term outcome after central cord syndrome: a study of the natural history. *J Bone Joint Surg Br.* 2000;82:851–855.

Shamji MF, Ventureyra EC, Baronia B, et al. Classification of symptomatic Chiari I malformation guide to surgical strategy. *Can J Neurol Sci.* 2010;37:482–487.

Teasell RW, Mehta S, Aubut JA, et al. A systematic review of pharmacologic treatments of pain after spinal cord injury. *Arch Phys Med Rehabil.* 2010;91:816–831.

Tompkins M, Panuncialman I, Lucas P, et al. Spinal epidural abscess. *J Emerg Med.* 2010;39(3):384–390.

Van Suijlekom H, et al. Whiplash-associated disorders. *Pain Pract.* 2010;10(2):131–136.

Wynn M, Acher CW. A modern theory of spinal cord ischemia/injury in thoracoabdominal aortic surgery and its implications for prevention of paralysis. *J Cardiothorac Vasc Anesth.* 2014;28(4):1088–1099.

51 Peripheral Neuropathy

John C. Kincaid

Peripheral neuropathy is the general term for diseases that affect the peripheral nervous system (PNS). The primary sites of pathology are the cell bodies, the axons, and the myelin sheath. Terms used to describe peripheral lesions in a proximal to distal sequence are:

Neuronopathy: Abnormality of the nerve cell body, usually producing motor, sensory, or autonomic dysfunction independently.

Radiculopathy: Abnormality of the spinal nerve, most often at a single spinal level and due to compression by a herniated disc or osteophyte.

Polyradiculopathy: Abnormality involving the nerve roots or spinal nerves at many spinal levels and most often caused by inflammation, infection, or infiltration by neoplastic cells.

Plexopathy and plexitis: Abnormality affecting the brachial or lumbosacral plexus. Plexopathy is the more general term while plexitis implies an inflammatory etiology.

Polyradiculoneuropathy: Abnormality affecting both the nerve roots and the peripheral nerve trunks.

Polyneuropathy: Abnormality affecting multiple peripheral nerve trunks, usually in a length-dependent symmetrical pattern.

Axonal neuropathy: Neuropathy in which the primary site of pathology is the axons.

Demyelinating neuropathy: Neuropathy in which the primary site of pathology is the myelin sheaths.

Mononeuropathy: Abnormality of an individual peripheral nerve trunk most often due to entrapment or local trauma.

Mononeuritis multiplex: Abnormality of multiple, individual nerve trunks occurring in a serial fashion most often due to vasculitis involving the vasa nervorum.

SYMPTOM-BASED MANAGEMENT

Whether or not the specific cause of a neuropathy is known and a specific treatment is available, the patient often reports a group of symptoms which are relatively similar. Following a standard approach to management of these symptoms is useful. Neuropathic symptoms may include the following:

Pain
Paresthesias
Sensory loss
Weakness
Cramping
Unstable balance

A. **Pain** is often the most bothersome symptom and may have several different characters. The paradigm described below is based on symptomatic treatment of painful diabetic neuropathy but should be applicable to other neuropathies. **(See Chapter 55)**

1. **Fiery, burning pain** is most often experienced in the toes, bottoms of the feet, and fingertips. If the symptom is bothersome enough for the patient to request treatment, mild analgesics such as aspirin or acetaminophen can help relieve low-level pain. Nonsteroidal anti-inflammatory drugs usually do not help this type of pain but can be tried. An antiepileptic drug (AED) such as gabapentin is more likely to help these types of symptoms. An initial dose of 300 mg once or twice daily is reasonable. If a benefit

is going to occur, some improvement often begins within a day or two of starting the medication. The dosage may need to be increased to three times daily if symptoms exacerbate before the next dose. The dose can be increased at weekly intervals to optimize the response, but doses above 2,400 mg/day often provide no further benefit. Improvement rather than full relief of the symptoms is the realistic treatment goal. Pregabalin may also provide symptomatic relief. This drug is only approved for use in symptomatic diabetic neuropathy and postherpetic neuralgia but may help symptoms in other neuropathies. Approval for payment by insurance often limits the use of this medication in other neuropathies.

Burning pain can often be improved by tricyclic antidepressants. Medications such as amitriptyline, nortriptyline, and doxepin are the preferred agents. Antidepressants of the selective serotonin reuptake inhibitor class do not seem to provide much pain-modulating benefit. Medications which have both serotonergic and adrenergic effects like duloxetine may help this type of pain and may have fewer side effects than the tricyclic drugs. When starting one of the tricyclic medications, inform the patient that side effects such as morning sedation, dry mouth, and blurred vision may occur. These effects usually lessen within a few days. Start these medications at a low dosage, such as 25 mg/hour before bedtime. Benefit may begin within a few days but may take several weeks to become evident. Increase the dosage by 10 to 25 mg every 1 to 2 weeks if there has been no benefit at the initial dosage. A dose of 35 to 75 mg is usually sufficient, but higher doses can be used within the bounds of the particular drug if the pain worsens after initial benefit at a particular dose. If a medication is beneficial, it should be continued for at least 6 months. At that point, a taper of 10 to 25 mg should be tried to determine whether the drug is still providing benefit. If symptoms worsen, the drug should be returned to the previous level. Long-term use will likely be needed.

Pain not sufficiently responsive to the agents above may require analgesics such as tramadol, codeine, hydrocodone, or oxycodone in combination with acetaminophen. Longer-acting opioids such as sustained-release oxycodone, morphine, or methadone may provide smoother pain control for patients with severe symptoms. Methadone is the least expensive of these. It is important for the patient and physician to understand that even major analgesics will usually not provide complete relief. Achieving mild to moderate improvement is a reasonable goal. Neuropathic pain is often worse when the patient retires for sleep, and, if possible, the stronger analgesics should be reserved for that time.

Topical capsaicin creams also may be helpful for this type of pain. Depletion of neurotransmitters in pain-sensing neurons is the proposed mechanism of action. These preparations are applied to the painful areas three or four times a day. Several weeks are required for benefit to appear, and a short-term increase in the pain may occur before the benefit begins. This medication is cumbersome to use. Topical lidocaine patches may be helpful if the pain is localized. Topical agents which contain multiple medications like amitriptyline, baclofen, clonidine, gabapentin, and ketoprofen are available from compounding pharmacies. The role of these preparations in treating neuropathic pain needs to be investigated further.

2. **Short electric-like jabs of pain** are another form of neuropathic pain. These are often felt in the toes, feet, lower legs, or fingers. Each lasts a second or two, and tends to migrate from one site to another. The patient may gasp due to the intensity of the pain. This type of pain often responds to gabapentin or pregabalin. Other AEDs such as phenytoin at 100 mg two or three times a day or carbamazepine at 100 mg twice a day up to 200 mg three times a day may help. Benefit from any of the medications often begins within a few days. The dosage may need to be increased if the initial benefit lessens. Monitoring of drug levels is probably not helpful in maximizing benefit. Complete blood count (CBC) should be monitored for patients undergoing maintenance therapy with carbamazepine.

3. **Tight or band-like pressure pain** in the feet or lower parts of the legs is resistant to symptomatic treatment. Encourage your patients or referring physicians to not expect relief from this type of pain.

4. **Allodynia,** pain to nonnoxious stimuli, often is an accompaniment to spontaneous pain. The patient perceives light touch in the involved area as exquisitely uncomfortable during and a few seconds after the touch. Wearing light cotton socks or gloves can lessen these

sensations, as can tents in the foot end of the bed linens to keep the toes from being touched. The antidepressants discussed above may improve these sensations.

B. **Paresthesia** is another form of sensory abnormality. This phenomenon takes the form of feelings of repetitive prickling, or "pins and needles" sensations. These sensations are felt in larger areas than the discrete sharp jabs of pain discussed in Section **A.2** under Symptom-Based Management, and may be felt in the toes, the feet, or the hands. They occur spontaneously or may be provoked by touching of the body part. These sensations tend to improve with antiepileptic medications discussed above. Lessening of the intensity and frequency should be the goal of treatment rather than complete relief. Analgesics tend to not help these symptoms.

C. **Sensory loss** can cause the affected areas to be perceived as "dead, woody or leathery." Sensations such as these do not respond to symptomatic treatment. Because of the loss of sensation underlying these symptoms, it is important for the patient to visually inspect the bottoms of the feet at least twice daily for local trauma such as blisters or cuts. Unrecognized lesions may lead to more serious problems such as ulcers and infections. Properly fitting shoes are important.

D. **Weakness** can occur focally in radiculopathy, plexopathy, mononeuropathy, or polyneuropathy. Bracing with an orthotic may partially compensate the deficit. Mobilization of the weak body part through a complete range of motion should be done at least daily to prevent contracture formation.

1. Patients with polyneuropathy tend to have **distal, symmetric weakness.** Weakness limited to the intrinsic foot muscles manifesting as difficulty abducting the toes is not clinically significant. Spread of the deficits to the toe extensors or flexors, and particularly the ankle musculature can impair balance. Ankle–foot orthotics may greatly improve standing and walking stability. Use of large-handled utensils may help compensate for finger and hand weakness. Physical and occupational therapy can help the patient maximize function when these type deficits are present.

2. **Proximal, symmetric weakness** in the legs causing difficulty in getting up from chairs or with stairs or of arm weakness causing lifting difficulty is relatively distinct and most often suggests inflammatory demyelinating neuropathy (**Guillain–Barré syndrome [GBS] or its chronic variants**).

3. **Unilateral proximal leg weakness** can occur in lumbar plexopathy, such as diabetes. Knee weakness can predispose patients to falling. Patients compensate by keeping the knee locked in extension. Minor dislodgment from that position, caused by a shift in body position or a slight bump from a passerby, exposes the weakness. Successful bracing of this joint is more difficult than at the ankle. A lift chair may help with getting up from a sitting position.

4. Evaluation by a physical therapist and a physical medicine rehabilitation physician can be very helpful in optimally managing all of these situations.

E. **Cramping** can be a bothersome component of peripheral neuropathy. Intrinsic foot and leg muscles like the gastrocnemius and hamstrings are the more common sites. Cramps may be provoked by movement or occur spontaneously. Successful treatment can be a challenge. Maintenance of proper hydration and serum potassium levels are important first steps. Use of quinine sulfate before bedtime had been the traditional mainstay of symptomatic treatment for prevention of nocturnal leg cramps. The 260-mg over-the-counter preparation was withdrawn by the U.S. Food and Drug Administration (FDA) over concern for rare but potentially serious hematological reactions. Despite its long-time use and anecdotal support, no clinical study done to modern levels of design rigor is available to support quinine's use in treating muscle cramps. No other medication is currently approved for the treatment of this bothersome symptom. Traditional muscle relaxers do not help. Low doses of benzodiazepines like diazepam or clonazepam or the directly acting muscle relaxer dantrolene can be tried.

F. **Unstable balance** can arise from sensory loss, cerebellar dysfunction, or leg weakness. Mild imbalance may require no active management other than caution on the patient's part. More pronounced deficits that put the patient at risk of falling require intervention. The intervention can be informal such as another person's arm to hold, strategically placed furniture, or use of a shopping cart at the store. More formal aids include a cane, walker, wheelchair, or motorized scooter. Patients may have increased difficulty in darkness or in situations in which their eyes are temporarily closed, such as showering. A patient who has had several falls should be encouraged to use a wheelchair to avoid further injury. Physical therapy and physical medicine rehabilitation evaluations can help determine the best management.

DIAGNOSIS AND MANAGEMENT OF SPECIFIC CONDITIONS

A. Autoimmune inflammatory neuropathies/acute inflammatory demyelinating neuropathy (GBS).

1. Clinical features. GBS manifests as weakness and sensory loss, usually beginning in the feet and then spreading into the legs and arms. The onset may follow a viral or other infectious-type illness by a week or 2, but can also develop spontaneously. The condition evolves and usually reaches maximum severity by 4 but not more than 8 weeks. The maximum impairment can vary between mild up to the need of ventilation support. Weakness is usually the cause for the patient seeking medical attention. Generalized loss of muscle stretch reflexes (MSRs) is an expected finding. Sensory deficits tend to be mild.

2. **Laboratory findings** of increased cerebrospinal fluid (CSF) protein concentration along with a normal to minimally elevated white blood cell (WBC) count support the diagnosis. Nerve conduction studies (NCS) that show slowing of velocity to <70% of normal or prolongation of distal latencies >125% of normal support the diagnosis but this "demyelinating" pattern may not always be found. Screening for arsenic intoxication and acute intermittent porphyria should be performed because these disorders can produce a similar clinical picture. Tick bite paralysis also can mimic this condition.

3. Treatment. Patients with this working diagnosis should be admitted to a hospital. Mild cases may not need active intervention but should be observed closely for at least several days to ensure the deficits have stabilized. Weakness of a degree that impairs walking or use of the upper limbs justifies active treatment. Two treatments—plasma exchange (PLEX) and intravenous gamma globulin (IVIG) infusion—have produced shortening of the duration of the weakness. Better benefits tend to result if treatment is begun within the first week or two of onset.

   a. **PLEX** is done by removing a portion of the plasma to eliminate components that are the mediators of the attack. The treatment usually consists of five exchanges done on every other day schedule. Vascular access through peripheral veins may be possible, but a central line is usually required. Treatment is generally well tolerated. Transient hypotension can occur, and therefore this mode may not be optimal for patients with labile cardiovascular systems.

   b. **IVIG infusion** is most commonly done on a 0.4 g/kg/day 5 days schedule. The total target dose of 2 g/kg can also be given on a shorter schedule. This treatment has been shown to be equally effective to PLEX and is often logistically easier. Headache and pruritus are the more common side effects of the infusions. Major complications are infrequent but thrombotic events and aseptic meningitis can occur.

   c. **Improvement may begin as early as a few days with either of these treatments** but may not appear for weeks and only manifest as a shortened duration of the major motor deficits. Lack of improvement over the first week or so of treatment is not a valid reason to switch from the initial treatment method to another. About 10% of the patients whose condition improves with treatment may have a partial relapse within a few weeks. In such instances, another one or two sessions of plasma exchanges or gamma globulin infusions will usually reestablish the improvement. Major improvement eventually occurs in a high percentage of patients, but even with these immune-modulating treatments, some still have a prolonged course necessitating weeks if not months of hospitalization. Some patients are left with distal weakness and sensory disturbances. Corticosteroids do not benefit patients with the acute form of inflammatory demyelinating neuropathy.

B. Chronic inflammatory demyelinating neuropathy.

1. Clinical features. The neuropathy is similar to the acute form described above but has a slower evolution which extends over at least 8 weeks and more commonly over many months. Generalized arreflexia is an expected feature which distinguishes this neuropathy from other slowly evolving conditions which are not autoimmune/inflammatory in origin.

This condition usually does not improve without active treatment. The laboratory and NCS results are similar to those of the acute form. Monoclonal gammopathy of the IgM type can produce a very similar neuropathy, and initial evaluation should include a serum protein electrophoresis. If an IgM protein is found, a myelin-associated glycoprotein antibody test (MAG) should also be performed because the presence of this antibody strongly supports the gammopathy being the cause of the neuropathy.

2. Treatment. The options are the same as for GBS with the exception that corticosteroids are an effective option. IVIG infusion or PLEX are the more commonly chosen options. The schedules given for GBS should be followed. If steroid treatment is chosen, prednisone at 1 mg/kg/day can be used. If the initially chosen treatment is going to help, some signs of improvement should become evident within 1 month of initiation. Further improvement is then likely over the next few months. If steroids are chosen, a tapering schedule of 10 mg/month can be followed after the initial 4- to 6-week period of 1 mg/kg dosing. If worsening occurs after a dose decrease, an increase back to the previous effective dose should be made. After a dose decrease, some steroid-treated patients report symptoms of general aching, stiffness, and listlessness. These types of symptoms are not usually due to true exacerbation of the neuropathy but rather are nonspecific effects of the steroid dose decrease. These types of symptoms improve a week after the dose decrease. If no true improvement has occurred within 8 weeks of starting either of these treatments, benefit is unlikely, and an alternative treatment be started. Treatment with steroids is much less expensive than PLEX or IVIG infusion but long-term steroid side effects are factors in the decision about treatment type. Patients who show a good initial response to IVIG infusion or PLEX may need recurring treatment. Reexacerbation within 4 to 8 weeks of the initial treatment dictates retreatment. One to two days of PLEX or IVIG should be repeated and the patient observed for the next month. The need for further treatment is then dictated by reexacerbation versus sustained improvement. In some patients recurring treatment every 3 to 6 weeks over many months or years may be required to maintain the improvement. If the patient has shown sustained improvement after several cycles of treatment lengthening the interval between treatments, or not retreating unless definite worsening occurs, should be considered because remission is possible. The roles of other immune suppressants like azathioprine, mycophenolate, and rituximab have not been established in the longer term management of this condition.

C. Vasculitic neuropathy.

Vasculitic neuropathy occurs due to inflammation of the vasa nervorum. The vasculitis is usually a component of a more generalized systemic disease but in rare cases may be limited to the peripheral nerves alone.

1. Clinical features. The presentation and evolution of this type of neuropathy are distinct. Progression occurs in a patchy manner in that a single nerve in a limb malfunctions and then another nerve in that limb or another limb does the same. Individual deficits often appear over hours to a few days, and then accumulate at other sites over days to weeks. This stepwise, cumulative pattern is termed mononeuritis multiplex. If left unchecked, the condition often evolves into what appears to be a generalized, symmetric polyneuropathy. Careful history taking identifies the stepwise pattern of progression.

Vasculitic neuropathy can be serious and usually continues to progress unless treated. The neuropathy may occur in association with polyarteritis nodosa, rheumatoid arthritis (RA), systemic lupus erythematosus (SLE), or granulomatosis with polyangiitis and may be a presenting feature of these conditions. It may also occur in the absence of other organ involvement and is then termed nonsystemic vasculitic neuropathy.

2. The **diagnosis** is supported by results of laboratory studies that identify any of the aforementioned systemic illnesses. Electromyogram (EMG) can help by showing a patchy "axonal" type pattern of involvement. Biopsy of a peripheral nerve in an area of clinical involvement, such as the sural or a superficial radial nerve, establishes the diagnosis if the results are positive.

3. **Treatment** requires **immunosuppressive therapy.** Prednisone or solumedrol at 1 mg/kg/day is the initial treatment, but an additional agent like **cyclophosphamide** will likely be required for sustained benefit. Cyclophosphamide should be given by physicians familiar with its use. It can be administered by means of daily oral dosage or monthly intravenous pulses. The initial response to treatment declares itself as a

cessation of further spread. Improvement requires axonal regeneration and occurs over months to several years. Severely affected areas may show persistent deficits despite overall improvement.

D. **Brachial plexitis,** also known as **Parsonage–Turner syndrome** or **neuralgic amyotrophy,** is easily diagnosable once it is fully manifest but can be difficult to differentiate from cervical nerve-root compression or intrinsic shoulder disease in its early stages. Brachial plexitis can be idiopathic or may appear a few weeks after an infection or immunization. Surgery, which can be on structures remote from the shoulder, can also provoke an attack. A dominantly inherited familial form is also known. Brachial plexopathy can develop years to decades after therapeutic radiation therapy given to treat neoplastic disease. The upper trunk of the brachial plexus tends to be most often involved despite the etiology.

1. Clinical features. Pain is usually the initial symptom in brachial plexitis and begins in the neck, shoulder, or upper arm. It has a "deep in the bone" character and is usually unilateral. The pain intensifies over days to weeks and can become excruciating. Neck movement tends not to worsen the pain, but arm or shoulder motion may. Several weeks after the onset of pain, symptoms of sensory loss and weakness appear. The sensory deficits tend to occur in the lateral arm and forearm and first two digits. Weakness most often occurs in the deltoid, biceps, supraspinatus, infraspinatus, and serratus anterior muscles (Video 51.1). Significant atrophy can occur in the affected muscles. The pain usually lessens within 3 to 6 weeks. Sensory loss and weakness improve over months, but long-term deficits may persist. The acquired form tends not to recur but the familial form can.

Differentiation from cervical radiculopathy requires cervical spine imaging. Imaging of the plexus may show signal enhancement or enlargement in the affected portions. In a plexus lesion electro diagnostic studies show acute denervation on needle EMG in limb muscles but sparing of the parapinals. The postradiation type lesion often shows myokymic discharges in the needle exam. Conduction studies show low amplitude sensory nerve action potentials in affected nerves, a finding that also helps distinguish plexopathy from radiculopathy. Sensory action potentials should be normal in radiculopathy.

2. Treatment. The lesion is presumably inflammatory in nature but treatment with oral or intravenous corticosteroids have shown no consistent benefit in small trials. The pain is often poorly responsive to even major analgesics but should be managed symptomatically as best as possible. The pain improves over several months. Pain is usually not a prominent feature of the postradiation plexopathy. The motor and sensory deficits in this specific condition slowly worsen over many years. No specific treatment is available.

Toxic or Metabolic Polyneuropathies

A. **Alcoholic neuropathy** is a sensorimotor polyneuropathy that primarily affects the distal legs but can also produce mononeuropathies.

1. Clinical features and diagnosis. The onset of the polyneuropathy is insidious, and progression takes place over months or longer. Sensory symptoms include numbness, paresthesia, and fiery pain. Motor abnormalities in the form of deficits of toe abduction or extension are present in many patients. Foot drop can occur in more advanced cases. Electro diagnostic studies show a pattern of axonal disease. Supporting laboratory findings include liver enzyme abnormalities and red cell macrocytosis.

2. **Treatment** consists of discontinuance of alcohol and establishment of an adequate diet plus supplementation of the diet with thiamine at 100 mg/day. Improvement takes place over months. Unstable walking resulting from concomitant alcoholic cerebellar disease recovers less well than the neuropathy and can limit overall improvement.

B. **Critical illness polyneuropathy** occurs in patients who experience severe episodes of sepsis and multiorgan failure that require days to weeks of treatment in the intensive care unit.

1. Clinical features. The neuropathy typically becomes evident when respiratory support is withdrawn and the patient remains severely weak. Sensory loss may be found in patients with sensorium clear enough for a detailed neurologic examination. GBS is often considered in this setting. The CSF protein content tends to be normal in critical illness polyneuropathy in contrast to the latter. NCS show axonal rather than demyelinating patterns. Critical illness myopathy can also occur in this same setting.

This condition is distinguished from the neuropathy by the finding of normal sensory examination and normal sensory NCS. The myopathy patients have often received high-dose corticosteroids and nondepolarizing neuromuscular blocking agents as part of the ventilator support during the critical illness.

2. **Treatment.** Management is supportive. Recovery occurs over months. Aggressive management of hyperglycemia, which can occur in the acute phase of the critical illness, appears to lessen the occurrence of this neuropathy.

C. **Diabetic neuropathy** can appear in several different forms, which are not mutually exclusive. Other than optimal control of blood glucose levels there is still no specific therapy for biochemical abnormalities underlying the neuropathy. **The principles of general symptom management outlined in Section Symptom-Based Management should be followed.**

1. **Sensorimotor polyneuropathy** causing bilateral foot numbness with or without a painful component is the most common type of diabetic neuropathy. Good control of blood glucose is the foundation of management, but neuropathic symptoms may still develop.

2. **Lumbosacral plexopathy,** also termed diabetic amyotrophy or radiculoplexus neuropathy, is a distinctive syndrome (**see Chapter 25**). The condition usually begins with spontaneous unilateral pain in the low back, hip, or proximal leg. The pain can become severe over the next week or two. A few weeks after onset of the pain, paresthesia and sensory loss appear in the thigh and at times in the medial lower leg. Weakness most often affects the quadriceps and appears about the same time as the sensory loss. Notable muscle atrophy can occur in the affected muscles. The pain is often only partially responsive to even major analgesics but tends to begin improving within a month or two after onset. Considerable weight loss may occur with this condition. Occasionally, as the initially involved side is improving, the opposite side becomes involved. The long-term prognosis tends to be good, but recovery can extend over a year or more. Some patients have persisting motor deficits. Several small series in the literature suggest that a course of IVIG or corticosteroids by the oral or intravenous route may shorten the course of this syndrome.

3. **Thoracic radiculopathy** is somewhat similar to lumbosacral plexopathy in terms of onset and time course. Unilateral band-like pain in the chest or upper lumbar region is the main symptom. The pain can be severe. Cutaneous hypersensitivity that makes the touch of clothing uncomfortable in the involved area also may be reported. Localized weakness of the lateral or anterior abdominal muscles may produce localized bulging of the abdominal wall. Analgesics can provide at best partial relief. Gabapentin and tricyclic antidepressants may partially improve the pain. Local anesthetic nerve blocks or topical lidocaine patches in the involved dermatome may help to some degree, as can use of a transcutaneous electrical nerve stimulation unit. The pain persists for some months but eventually resolves or greatly improves.

MEDICATION-INDUCED POLYNEUROPATHIES

A. **Medication-**induced polyneuropathy can occur during treatment for neoplasms, autoimmune disorders, chronic infections, and cardiac arrhythmia. Vincristine, paclitaxel and docetaxel, cis and carboplatinum, and bortezemab are the antineoplastic drugs most often associated with neuropathy. Colchicine, hydroxychloroquine, leflunomide, and thalidomide used for treatment of inflammatory and autoimmune disorders can cause neuropathy. The antibiotics dapsone, isoniazid, metronidazole, and nitrofurantoin have been reported to cause neuropathy. The antiarrythmic amiodarone can cause neuropathy.

1. **Clinical features.** All of these except the platinum-based medications produce a sensorimotor neuropathy and the sensory deficits are usually the prominent features. The platinum compounds tend to affect only sensory neurons and can produce both sensory loss and ataxia. A significant painful component may develop with vincristine and bortezemab. If sensory deficits progress proximally to the mid-shin and fingertip levels, foot drop and weakness of the intrinsic hand muscles can occur. The occurrence and severity of chemotherapy-related neuropathy tend to be dose related and usually begin after several cycles of administration. Neuropathy may develop or worsen after completion of the chemotherapy. This pattern is termed

"coasting." Neuropathies related to antibiotics and the rheumatologic modulating agents tend to occur after prolonged exposure except for nitrofurantoin, which can produce an acute syndrome similar to GBS. Amiodarone-related neuropathies occur after prolonged exposure.

2. **Treatment.** When repeated or prolonged use of the medication is required for treatment of the primary illness, lengthening of the interval between chemotherapy treatment or reduction of the dose at each treatment may allow the neuropathy to stabilize. When neuropathy is related to antibiotic, rheumatologic agent or amiodarone use the medication has to be stopped. Improvement is the expected course but the time interval may extend over many months. Symptoms should be managed as described above in Section under Symptom-Based Management.

POLYNEUROPATHIES DUE TO INFECTIONS

A. **Lyme disease** can produce several different types of peripheral neuropathy. The bites of certain ticks of the *Ixodes* genus (e.g., *Ixodes dammini*, most often) transmit the infectious agent *Borrelia burgdorferi*. Endemic areas include southern New England and the Mid-Atlantic states, the central regions of Wisconsin and neighboring states, and north coastal California plus Oregon.

1. **Clinical features.** The characteristic skin lesion erythema chronic migraines develops 3 to 20 days after the bite, as does a general flu-like syndrome of fever, malaise, and myalgia. The skin lesion occurs in approximately 80% of cases. Frank neurologic involvement occurs in approximately 15% of cases and tends to appear 1 to 3 months after the initial infection in the time frame termed the *early disseminated phase* of the illness. Less specific symptoms of headache occur in more than half of patients. A positive serologic result for antibodies against the infectious agent is helpful for establishing the cause, but test results may be negative for a month or so after the initial infection. An ELISA or immunofluorescence assay should be done first and if positive be followed up by an immunoblot test for IgM or IgG antibodies. The latter test helps to identify false-positive results.

2. **Treatment.** Antibiotic treatment appears to relieve all of the manifestations, either by shortening the duration of episodes or by alleviating more persistent symptoms such as polyneuropathy. Oral antibiotics can be used to manage the rash and flu-like phase of the initial stage of the infection. For adults, doxycycline 100 mg twice a day, amoxicillin 500 mg three times a day, or cefuroxime 500 mg twice a day for 2 to 3 weeks are recommended. PNS and central nervous system (CNS) manifestations are best managed with intravenous penicillin G, 20 million U/day, or ceftriaxone, 2 g daily for the same 2 to 3 weeks.

3. **Types of neuropathy of the early disseminated phase.**
   a. **Facial nerve involvement** produces typical peripheral facial nerve palsy (often resembling Bell's palsy), including pain in the ear region. Bilateral facial nerve involvement occurs more frequently with Lyme disease than in the idiopathic form.
   b. **Radiculitis** producing a syndrome similar to that described for diabetic thoracic radiculopathy (see Section **C.3** under Toxic or Metabolic Polyneuropathies) and consisting of dermatomal pain, which can reach a high level of intensity, sensory loss, and focal weakness. Limb as well as truncal spinal segments can be involved.

B. **Human immunodeficiency virus (HIV)** infection can be associated with several types of peripheral neuropathy.

1. Typical **acute inflammatory demyelinating neuropathy (GBS)** can occur early in the course of the infection. CSF pleocytosis with white cell counts of 10 or more is the only feature that distinguishes this form from the idiopathic variety. Therapy should be the same as for the idiopathic form of the disorder (**see** Section **A.3** under Diagnosis and Management of Specific Conditions).

2. **Distal symmetrical polyneuropathy** with predominant painful symptoms can also occur in up to a third of patients and is more likely when viral load becomes greater than 10,000 copies per mL. Patients report painful paresthesia consisting of pressure- or burning-type sensations in the feet and distal legs. The hands can be involved to a lesser

extent. Weakness is minimal. CSF tends to be normal to minimally abnormal. NCS show a pattern of axonal damage. Management of this type of neuropathy is symptomatic only, and the general guidelines for painful neuropathy presented in Section **A** under Symptom-Based Management. should be followed. A similar type of neuropathy can occur in patients being actively treated with high-activity antiretroviral therapy (HAART). This type neuropathy has symptoms and signs very similar to those produced by the HIV infection. A potential clue that the neuropathy is treatment-related is its appearance after HAART has been begun. Dosage reduction or substitution of potentially less neurotoxic medications should be considered if the status of the infection permits.

3. **Polyradiculitis** resulting from infection by **cytomegalovirus (CMV)** is another distinctive form of neuropathy that affects patients with AIDS in the advanced stage of the illness. Patients report pain and weakness in the lower extremities and the back. The onset may be asymmetrical but becomes bilateral within days to weeks. Sensory loss develops in the limbs and perineal area. Bladder and bowel incontinence are also regular features. Progression to arm involvement is infrequent. CSF shows pleocytosis and elevated protein level. Pathologic specimens show inflammation of the nerve roots of the lumbar and sacral areas. Treatment with ganciclovir and foscarnet may stabilize the condition, but this lesion tends to be a poor prognostic indicator.

C. Inherited polyneuropathies.

A genetic etiology should always be considered in patients with neuropathies which evolve over many years and for which another etiology is not obvious.

1. **Clinical features** of a length-dependent motor greater than sensory neuropathy is typical but multifocal pattern occurring over many years is seen in the hereditary liability to pressure palsy variant. Bothersome paresthesia and neuropathic pain tend to not be present. Anatomical features like abnormally high foot arches and hammer toes further support a genetic etiology. A dominant pattern of inheritance is most common but X-linked and recessive patterns also occur.

NCS tend to show demyelinating features that are often more uniform in degree from one nerve to the next in contrast to acquired demyelinating conditions in which action potential dispersion is the more common finding. Genetic studies available through commercial testing labs can help make a specific diagnosis.

2. **Treatment.** Ankle bracing may be required for foot drop. Significant hand weakness may be partly compensated for by input from occupational therapy.

NEW DEVELOPMENTS IN PERIPHERAL NEUROPATHY

A. Small fiber neuropathy. This diagnosis is being more commonly considered in the differential diagnosis for patients who have widespread pain. Fibromyalgia is often the alternate clinical diagnosis.

1. Clinical features. A formal definition of small fiber neuropathy has not been established. The following parameters have been suggested: spontaneous and stimulus evoked pain, deficits in pain and temperature sensation on clinical examination, preservation of light touch, position and vibration sensory functions, normal limb strength and reflexes, abnormalities in the autonomic domains of cardiovagal, adrenergic and sweat gland function, abnormalities in cold and warm sensory functions in quantitative sensory testing and decrease in the number of epidermal nerve fibers in skin biopsies. Potential etiologies include glucose intolerance, autoimmune conditions like Sjögren's syndrome, and hepatitis C. Many cases remain idiopathic.

2. Treatment. Managing symptoms is the mainstay of treatment. Identifiable etiologies like impaired glucose tolerance and autoimmune disorders should be managed as best as possible. At this point in our knowledge of this disorder, I consider treatment of idiopathic cases by immune-modulating treatments such as IVIG to be inappropriate.

B. Amyloid neuropathy.

Although amyloidosis is a very rare cause of polyneuropathy the advancements in the treatment of familial amyloid neuropathy (FAP) which result from mutations in the transthyretin protein provide an exciting example the potential for direct treatment of a neuropathy. FAP results from deposition of protein fibrils composed of normal and mutant transthyretin. The peripheral nerve and cardiac tissue are the most common sites of pathological accumulation. The typical neuropathy involves small and then large fiber modalities. The accompanying cardiomyopathy can be fatal. Liver transplantation has been the mainstay of therapy for reducing production of the abnormal protein but over the last 5 years several compounds have been discovered which can either alter the potential for deposition of or synthesis of the abnormal protein. The use of oligonucleotide mechanisms to suppress production of the abnormal protein by the liver is the focus of the most recent research.

Key Points

- Peripheral neuropathies are classified based on the sites of pathology and the etiology
- Symptoms and signs of the neuropathies correlate with the structures affected by the disease process
- Symptom management is a key component of treatment regardless of the etiology of the neuropathy
- Polyneuropathies due to inflammatory processes are directly treatable
- Knowledge of the course of neuropathies due to systemic causes allow improved patient and referring provider education

Recommended Readings

Amato AA, Russell JA. *Neuromuscular Disorders*. New York, NY: McGraw Hill Medical; 2008.

Berk J, Suhr O, Obici L, et al. Repurposing difunisal for familial amyloidotic polyneuropathy. *JAMA*. 2013;310:2658–2667.

Bromberg MB, Smith AG, eds. *Handbook of Peripheral Neuropathy*. Boca Raton, FL: Informa Healthcare; 2005.

Dyck PJ, Thomas PK, eds. *Peripheral Neuropathy*. 4th ed. Philadelphia, PA: WB Saunders; 2005.

McKahnn GM. Guillain–Barré syndrome: clinical and therapeutic observations. *Ann Neurol*. 1990;27(suppl):S13–S16.

Oaklander A, Herzog Z, Downs H, et al. Objective evidence that small-fiber polyneuropathy underlies some illness currently labeled a fibromyalgia. *Pain*. 2013;154:2310–2316.

Van Doorn PA, Vermeulen M, Brand A, et al. Intravenous gamma globulin in treatment of patients with chronic inflammatory demyelinating polyneuropathy. *Arch Neurol*. 1991;48:217–220.

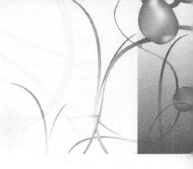

52 Myopathy

Holli A. Horak and Raul N. Mandler

Myopathy is an abnormality of the skeletal muscle in which striated muscle cells are damaged. Myopathy can result from abnormalities of skeletal muscle proteins (Duchenne muscular dystrophy), alterations of the sarcolemmal ion channels (hyperkalemic periodic paralysis), mitochondrial alterations (mitochondrial myopathy), or cell-mediated autoimmune mechanisms (polymyositis), to name a few examples. Because of the myriad abnormal mechanisms, treatments vary from one condition to the next. Progress in molecular biology, genetics, and immunology has considerably expanded our understanding of these diseases. This chapter emphasizes current therapeutic approaches to the care of patients with relatively common forms of myopathy.

IDIOPATHIC INFLAMMATORY MYOPATHY

Idiopathic inflammatory myopathies are autoimmune diseases characterized by muscle weakness, pain, and fatigue. Inflammatory damage of muscle fibers is the underlying pathology. **Polymyositis** can occur in isolation or accompany other connective tissue disorders or associated systemic autoimmune disorders. **Dermatomyositis, inclusion body myositis (IBM),** and **polymyalgia rheumatica (PMR)** are the other major categories of idiopathic inflammatory myopathies. The incidence of these diseases is approximately 1 case among 100,000 persons.

A. Natural history and prognosis.

1. **Polymyositis** is more common in adults and usually affects upper and lower girdle muscles in a symmetric pattern. Patients with no family history of muscle abnormalities have subacute (weeks to months) progressive weakness of the shoulder and hip girdles, bulbar muscles and neck flexor and extensors.

   Patients characteristically have problems arising from a sitting position, using stairs or lifting their arms (such as washing their hair). Muscle pain may accompany the weakness. Pharyngeal muscle compromise can lead to dysphagia and choking. The tongue, extraocular muscles, and facial muscles are usually spared. Sensation is not affected. Cardiac involvement can occur in as many as 40% of cases. Pulmonary involvement can result from primary weakness of respiratory muscles or from pulmonary interstitial fibrosis.

   Polymyositis can occur in association with connective tissue and systemic autoimmune disorders. Polymyositis is not associated with an increased incidence of malignant disease. T-cell-mediated immunity plays a prominent role in the pathogenesis of polymyositis.

2. A rash that accompanies or precedes muscle weakness characterizes dermatomyositis. The characteristic skin abnormality is a heliotrope rash around the orbits and zygomatic arch with erythema on the rest of the face, upper trunk, and knuckles (Gottren's papules). Subcutaneous nodular calcifications and dilated capillaries in the nail beds may occur.

   In children, extramuscular manifestations are more frequent than they are in adults. Dermatomyositis usually occurs alone but may be associated with systemic sclerosis, mixed connective tissue disease, or malignant lesions. Ten percent of patients with dermatomyositis will be found to have an underlying malignancy. It is a humorally mediated microangiopathic disorder with vascular deposition of immunoglobulin G (IgG), C3, and membrane attack complex. This suggests that the primary immunologic event is generation of antibodies against antigens within the walls of intramuscular blood vessels.

3. **IBM** involves distal and proximal muscles. Weakness and atrophy can be slightly asymmetric; quadriceps and finger flexors are commonly affected. It is a late-onset myopathy (sixth or seventh decade). It is treatment resistant. Occasionally, the diagnosis of IBM is made retrospectively when a patient fails to respond to treatment for polymyositis. Hereditary forms of IBM have been described: an autosomal dominant variant, which has a younger age of onset and an autosomal recessive variant, caused by a mutation in the *GNE* gene, on chromosome 9. Most cases are thought to be autoimmune but again, are treatment resistant.

4. **PMR** is technically a rheumatologic myopathy and not myositis. The muscle cells do not show direct damage or inflammation. PMR affects older patients with a peak incidence at 74 years of age. Patients describe diffuse muscle aching with neck and shoulder stiffness. Pain predominates over weakness and atrophy. Approximately 15% of the patients also have temporal arteritis. The erythrocyte sedimentation rate (ESR) is elevated to >40 mm/hour.

5. Noninfectious inflammatory myositis can also occur in the context of systemic lupus erythematosus, progressive systemic sclerosis, Sjögren's syndrome, rheumatoid arthritis, mixed connective tissue disease, sarcoidosis, hypereosinophilic syndromes, and other disorders.

B. **Diagnosis.** In addition to the clinical features, the diagnosis of inflammatory myopathy is supported by measurement of muscle enzymes, electromyography (EMG), and muscle biopsy.

1. **Muscle enzymes.** Creatine kinase (CK) is released from the sarcoplasm into the serum after muscle destruction, and the level may be elevated as much as 50-fold in polymyositis/dermatomyositis. Other muscle enzymes such as lactate dehydrogenase, aldolase, and aminotransferases are commonly elevated. In IBM, CK level may be elevated as much as 10-fold or remain normal. In childhood dermatomyositis and in patients with myopathy associated with connective tissue diseases, CK levels may be normal. ESR should be determined, especially for suspected PMR.

2. The main value of **EMG** resides in its ability to show that peripheral neuromuscular weakness originates from the muscle itself and not from denervation or from a defect in neuromuscular transmission. It can also help ascertain the presence of disease activity. The classic EMG findings include short-duration, small-amplitude motor unit potentials, and increased insertional activity. These findings should not be considered specific for inflammatory myopathy because they can also be found in acute toxic or metabolic myopathy and in dystrophy.

3. **Muscle biopsy** helps establish the diagnosis.

   a. In **polymyositis,** light microscopic examination displays intrafascicular inflammatory infiltrates, necrosis, atrophy and regeneration of muscle fibers, and increased amounts of connective tissue.

   b. In **dermatomyositis,** the inflammatory infiltrates are present around the vessels or in the interfascicular septa, and perifascicular atrophy is characteristic. Small blood vessels may be occluded.

   c. **IBM** is characterized by basophilic granular inclusions around the edges of vacuoles (rimmed vacuoles). However, these findings can be missed due to sampling error. One should alert the pathologist that IBM is suspected, and so extra sections can be evaluated.

   d. Muscle biopsy has **limitations.** A biopsy sometimes fails to disclose abnormalities expected from the clinical presentation. Also, biopsy changes are a result of muscle injury and are not specific: an end-stage dystrophy and myopathy will have similar findings on biopsy.

C. **Therapy.**

1. **Prednisone.**

   a. **Administration.** High-dose prednisone is the initial line of therapy for polymyositis and dermatomyositis. For prednisone, the recommended dosage is 1.0 mg/kg/day in a single daily dose for 60 days or more. The total dose should not exceed 100 mg. Daily administration should be used until there is unquestionable improvement muscle strength with recovery of ambulation. Then the dosage can be slowly reduced over 10 weeks to 1 mg/kg every other day. If no clinical deterioration occurs, the dose is further reduced by 5 to 10 mg every 3 to 4 weeks until the lowest dose that controls the disease is reached. The dose should not be reduced if strength decreases. If treatment is effective, strength should improve within 3 months. If after 3 months of therapy no improvement has been achieved, prednisone should be tapered off and another immunosuppressant medication begun.

   b. **Side effects.** Patients need to be alerted to the numerous side effects of long-term prednisone treatment. Infections, fluid retention, potassium depletion, hypertension, diabetes, osteoporosis, premature cataracts, peptic ulcer disease, and skin bruising are some of the side effects that can occur.

      Prevention of osteoporosis requires supplemental calcium gluconate or carbonate (500 to 1,000 mg/day) and calcitriol (0.2 to 0.5 mg/day) as well as axial exercise and adequate passive range of motion maneuvers. Bisphosphonates (alendronate and risedronate, among others) can be used. A baseline dual-energy X-ray absorption densitometry (DEXA) scan to measure bone density should be obtained for every patient before steroid treatment is started. The scan should be repeated every 6 months.

      Proton-pump inhibitors should be used to prevent peptic ulcers. Periodic eye examinations are needed for diagnosis of incipient cataracts or glaucoma. Periodic laboratory tests for serum glucose and electrolytes are recommended. Steroid myopathy, a side effect of long-term steroid use, will be addressed later in this chapter.

2. Sometimes patients with dermatomyositis need separate therapy for the rash.

3. Steroid-sparing agents are often used. These are most often immunosuppressants. They all carry the risk of bone marrow suppression, hepatotoxicity, risk of reactivation of latent infections and increasing risk of future hematologic malignancy. One should aim for the lowest possible dose needed to control symptoms with the goal of tapering the dose if possible.

4. **Azathioprine** is considered when complications preclude use of steroids, or when the disease is not responding to adequate dosages of prednisone. A therapeutic response may take 3 to 6 months.

   a. **Administration.** Azathioprine can be administered at 2 to 3 mg/kg/day. The initial dose should be approximately 50 mg/day, gradually increasing to BID dosing.

   b. **Side effects.** The most common side effects of azathioprine are nausea or rash. However, bone marrow suppression and liver toxicity can occur. Complete blood count (CBC) with differential and platelets and liver function tests should be performed weekly for the first month and monthly thereafter. Patients with absent thiopurine S-methyltransferase (TPMT) enzyme activity are at high risk for azathioprine toxicity. TPMT testing is commercially available and may be considered before beginning treatment with azathioprine. Allopurinol will potentiate bone marrow toxicity: avoid concurrent use with azathioprine if possible.

5. **Mycophenylate mofetil** inhibits proliferation of T and B lymphocytes and can be used as an alternative to azathioprine. Doses typically start at 500 mg/day and are increased to 1,000 mg twice a day. Side effects include immunosuppression, gastrointestinal side effects, hepatotoxicity, and bone marrow inhibition. CBC and metabolic profile (CMP) monitoring are recommended.

6. **Methotrexate** (15 to 25 mg/week by mouth) is used as another method to spare use of prednisone or if prednisone has not been effective. Hepatotoxicity, leukopenia, alopecia, stomatitis, and risk of neoplasia can occur. Methotrexate should not be used in patients with anti-Jo-1 antibodies and polymyositis because they are at increased risk for pulmonary fibrosis.

7. **Intravenous gamma globulin (IVIG)** is effective in the management of acute polymyositis and in dermatomyositis. A typical dosage is 0.5 g/kg IV for 4 days, repeated monthly if needed. Side effects include headaches, hypertension, acute renal failure, and hyperviscosity. Aseptic meningitis can occur, it typically responds to prednisone. IgA-depleted preparations reduce the risk of reactions related to anti-IgA antibodies. Treatments are expensive. Despite these reservations, high-dosage IV gamma globulin might benefit patients who have been unresponsive to other medications.

8. In refractory cases, or if interstitial lung disease occurs, **cyclophosphamide** (1 to 2 g/m^2 a month IV) may be considered. Side effects include nausea, vomiting, alopecia, hemorrhagic cystitis, teratogenicity, bone marrow suppression, carcinogenesis, and pulmonary fibrosis. Cyclophosphamide can also be used orally at doses of 1 to 2 mg/kg/day.

9. **Rituximab,** a CD20 monoclonal antibody that depletes B cells, is being investigated for use in resistant disease. It is administered at a dose of 375 mg/m² every week for a month, with possible repeat courses in 6 months or 1 year. Opportunistic infections have occurred with this medication.

10. In **PMR,** prednisone rapidly provides benefits. Duration of treatment and dosage have to be individualized. In general, a starting dosage of 1 mg/kg/day should be appropriate. In patients suffering from temporal arteritis, corticosteroid treatment needs to be initiated immediately.

D. **Prognosis.** Dermatomyositis and, to a lesser degree, polymyositis are responsive to treatment, whereas IBM is usually resistant. Patients with interstitial lung disease have a higher mortality rate. When management of polymyositis is unsuccessful, the patient should be reevaluated and the muscle biopsy specimen reexamined to exclude IBM or muscular dystrophy of the limb-girdle type. Finally, it is important to emphasize the need to evaluate the patient's strength and activities of daily living as measures of improvement, rather than simply adjusting treatment on the basis of CK levels alone.

VIRAL INFLAMMATORY MYOPATHY

Viruses and retroviruses can cause acute or subacute inflammatory myopathy.

A. **Reye's syndrome** is acute encephalopathy with fatty degeneration of the liver that develops after varicella or influenza infections. This rare condition that affects children and adolescents begins with repeated vomiting and continues with confusion, lethargy, and coma. The mortality is high. There is acute liver dysfunction. The level of CK MM isoenzyme may be increased 300-fold. The level of CK correlates with prognosis. Salicylates may precipitate the syndrome. Treatment is supportive. The incidence of this syndrome has decreased over the years because aspirin is no longer being used in children.

B. **HIV** may cause subacute or chronic myopathy early or late in relation to the infection. Proximal, symmetric involvement of lower or upper limbs manifests as weakness with or without atrophy. Serum CK levels may be elevated 10 to 15 times. The syndrome is almost identical to polymyositis. Thus, in the evaluation of patients with polymyositis, evaluation for HIV is recommended.

PARASITIC INFLAMMATORY MYOPATHY

In North America, **trichinosis, cysticercosis,** and **toxoplasmosis** are rarely the cause of a myopathy. These causes may need to be considered in an acute–subacute onset myopathy in an immunocompromised patient or one who has been in an endemic area or has had possible exposure to the parasite.

PERIODIC PARALYSES

Periodic paralyses are disorders characterized by episodes of flaccid muscle weakness that can evolve into paralysis. Attacks usually last hours. Periodic paralysis is either a primary autosomal dominant disorder or a secondary disorder. The inherited forms of these diseases are caused by **channelopathies,** or defects in genes coding for muscle membrane ion channels (Table 52.1).

A. **Natural history and prognosis.**

1. **Primary hypokalemic periodic paralysis** affects young and middle-aged persons. Attacks usually occur at night or after strenuous exercise. On awakening, patients may be paralyzed and unable to get out of bed. The flaccid paralysis usually spares the respiratory and cranial muscles. During attacks, serum potassium level decreases. An electrocardiogram (ECG) may reveal hypokalemic changes, including progressive flattening of T waves, depression of the ST segment, and appearance of U waves. Some patients eventually develop a progressive myopathy.

   Seventy percent of patients with this disorder have a defect in the calcium channel gene: *CACNA1S,* which is located on chromosome 1q31. A small percentage of patients, however, have a sodium channel defect (*SCN4A*). For approximately 20% of patients the gene defect is yet to be identified.

TABLE 52.1 Channelopathies

Channel	hypoK+ PP	hyperK+ PP	Andersen–Tawil	Paramyotonia Congenita	Myotonia Congenita
SCN4A	+	+		+	
CLCNI					+
CACNAIS	+				
KCNJ2			+		
Myotonia on EMG	+/−			+	+
Acetazolamide responsive	+	+	+/−		

Abbreviations: EMG, electromyography; hypoK+ PP, hypokalemic periodic paralysis; hyperK+ PP, hyperkalemic periodic paralysis.

2. Secondary hypokalemic periodic paralysis.
   a. **Thyrotoxic periodic paralysis** occurs 70 times more often in men than in women, despite the increased prevalence of hyperthyroidism among women. In nearly all cases, the condition is sporadic and the attacks cease when thyroid function is normalized. Every patient with hypokalemic periodic paralysis needs screening for thyrotoxicosis. This condition is more common in patients of Asian, Hispanic American, and Amerind origin.
   b. **Periodic paralysis secondary** to urinary or gastrointestinal potassium loss can result from primary hyperaldosteronism, excessive thiazide therapy, excessive mineralocorticoid therapy for Addison's disease, renal tubular acidosis, the recovery phase of diabetic coma, sprue, laxative abuse, villous adenoma of the rectum, or prolonged gastrointestinal intubation or vomiting.
3. **Hyperkalemic periodic paralysis** produces episodic attacks of weakness accompanied by elevations in serum potassium level (up to 5 to 6 mmol/L). It can be associated with myotonia (inability to relax the muscle) or paramyotonia (muscle stiffness worsened by exercise or cold). It is inherited in an autosomal dominant manner. Attacks start in the first decade of life. Patients usually have brief periods of generalized weakness. Static weakness is rare. Sustained mild exercise may prevent attacks. Cardiac arrhythmias can occur.
   a. The **genetic abnormality** is a mutation in the *SCN4A* (sodium channel) gene.
   b. **Needle EMG** may detect myotonia, which supports the diagnosis.
4. **Andersen's syndrome (or Andersen–Tawil syndrome)** is a triad of facial dysmorphism, long QT syndrome, and periodic paralysis. Short stature is often also present. Andersen syndrome is an autosomal dominantly inherited disease with a young age of onset and phenotypic variability. Fatal cardiac dysrhythmias may occur, making early recognition of this condition important. Mutations in the *KCNJ2* gene, which codes for an inward-rectifying potassium channel, have been found in some patients.
5. **Chloride channel mutations** produce **myotonia congenital** with dominant and recessive forms (Thomsen and Becker, respectively), and with more myotonia than weakness. The dominant form manifests as painless muscle stiffness. Muscle stiffness is relieved after repeated exercise (warm-up), but it returns after rest. Cooling does not produce a significant change. These disorders result from missense mutations in the chloride channel gene *CLCN1*.

B. Prevention and therapeutic approach.
   1. Primary hypokalemic periodic paralysis. Mild attacks may not require treatment. For attacks of general paralysis, oral potassium chloride can be used (0.25 mEq/kg), repeated every 30 minutes until the weakness is relieved. Muscle strength usually recovers within approximately 1 hour. IV potassium is not recommended because of the danger of cardiac arrhythmias and should be avoided.

   For **prevention** of attacks, acetazolamide is the drug of choice, starting at 125 mg every other day, which can be increased to 250 mg three times a day. Side effects include increased incidence of nephrolithiasis, paresthesia, anorexia, and metallic taste. In severe cases, patients should eat a low-salt diet and be given the aldosterone antagonist spironolactone (100 mg twice a day) or triamterene (150 mg/day). Both drugs promote renal potassium retention.

2. **Thyrotoxic periodic paralysis.** Return to euthyroid status is curative. Propranolol (40 mg four times a day) and other β-adrenergic blocking agents may prevent attacks, possibly by suppressing the adrenergic overactivity induced by hyperthyroidism.

3. **Hyperkalemic periodic paralysis.**

   a. **Preventive measures** consist of low-potassium diet, avoidance of fasting, and avoiding strenuous exercise. Slight exercise or ingestion of carbohydrates at the onset of weakness may prevent or abort attacks.

   b. A thiazide diuretic, acetazolamide, or inhalation of a β-adrenergic agent (metaproterenol or salbutamol) may **abort an attack.** Dilantin (300 mg/day) can also be useful. For **long-term preventive therapy,** a thiazide diuretic or acetazolamide is recommended at the lowest possible dosage (hydrochlorothiazide, 25 mg every other day).

4. In **myotonia congenita,** mexiletine has been used. The starting dose is 150 mg by mouth twice a day, up to 1,200 mg/day. Mexiletine is contraindicated in the case of patients with second- and third-degree heart block; other cardiac arrhythmias can occur.

MUSCULAR DYSTROPHY

Muscular dystrophy is the term for inherited defects of cellular muscle structure, producing intrinsic muscle weakness. Some forms present at childbirth, others as late as the seventh decade. Family history, clinical examination, and temporal profile are necessary when considering a muscular dystrophy. The number of inherited dystrophies and the enormous variety of phenotypes prevent complete coverage in this forum. The following dystrophies will be discussed: **X-linked dystrophinopathy (Duchenne and Becker muscular dystrophy), facioscapulohumeral dystrophy, myotonic, limb-girdle,** and **oculopharyngeal.**

A. **Natural history and prognosis.**

   1. **Dystrophinopathy** is an X-linked disorder caused by a mutation in the short arm, locus 21, of the X chromosome in the enormous gene that codes for the protein dystrophin. Dystrophin is a filamentous protein present in striated and cardiac muscle and other tissues. Although the role of dystrophin is not precisely known, anchoring and structural functions have been proposed for this protein.

      In the most severe form of dystrophinopathy—Duchenne muscular dystrophy— almost no dystrophin is detected in skeletal muscle. In milder forms—phenotypically denominated as Becker muscular dystrophy—some muscle fibers express dystrophin, which may be structurally abnormal. Almost all patients with dystrophinopathy are male. The disease can be caused by spontaneous mutations, which are more common than in other genetic disorders, probably because of the large size of the gene. Approximately 70% of patients with Duchenne and Becker muscular dystrophy have detectable mutations on routine DNA testing of peripheral blood. Deletions of varying sizes can be found in approximately 65% of cases; 5% of patients have gene duplications. The remaining patients have a point mutation. The diagnosis in some cases of previously unreported point mutations is confirmed with dystrophin analysis at muscle biopsy.

      a. **Duchenne muscular dystrophy** affects children early in life. Motor developmental delay is noticeable after the first year, but muscle necrosis and serum enzyme elevation can be found in neonates. Onset of walking may be delayed past 15 months of age. Signs are present before the age of 5 years. They include difficulties in running and climbing stairs.

         Children have hyperlordosis with a prominent abdomen and calf pseudohypertrophy. Toe walking is common. To stand up from the floor, patients use their hands (**Gower's sign**). Joint contractures of the iliotibial bands, hip flexors, and heel cords develop in most patients by 6 to 9 years of age. By the age of 10 years, many of these patients lose the ability to walk or stand and must use a wheelchair. By the midteens they lose upper-extremity function. Cognitive dysfunction occurs in 10% of cases. Although patients are living longer due to improved medical interventions, these patients have a shortened life span. Death is due to pulmonary infection, respiratory failure, or cardiomyopathy. Approximately 8% of female carriers have myopathy of the limb-girdle type. Female carriers may also have isolated cardiomyopathy.

Muscle biopsy specimens from patients with Duchenne muscular dystrophy have abnormal variations in fiber size, fiber splitting, central nuclei, and replacement by fat and fibrous tissues. The diagnosis of Duchenne's muscular dystrophy on biopsy can be confirmed by an **absence of dystrophin immunostaining.**

An EMG obtained early in the course of the disease shows findings compatible with those of myopathy. In end stage, there are decreased numbers of muscle fibers and the tissue can even become inexcitable.

   b. **Becker's muscular dystrophy** is a milder variety of dystrophinopathy in terms of severity and molecular abnormality. The diagnosis has been typically defined as a patient who remains ambulatory after age 12. There is a wide range of phenotypic variability; some patients may live decades with mild symptoms, indistinguishable from those of limb-girdle dystrophy. All Becker-type patients are at risk for cardiomyopathy.

2. **Facioscapulohumeral muscular dystrophy** is an autosomal dominant disease that has high penetrance. It affects both men and women, most often presenting before 30 years of age. Ninety-five percent of patients have a deletion in a sequence of a 3.3-kb repetitive unit (known at D4Z4) in chromosome 4q35.

   Clinically, facial muscles are affected early. Bell's phenomenon (failure of eyelids to close completely when the patient is sleeping or blinking) and drooping of the lower lip are noticeable. Patients may be unable to whistle. Facioscapulohumeral muscular dystrophy also involves the trapezius, rhomboid, and serratus anterior scapular muscles. Scapular winging is noticed with forward arm movement because of serratus anterior weakness. Deltoid function and rotator cuff muscles are better preserved. Lower-extremity weakness is found later in the disease.

   This disorder has wide phenotypic variability, even within the same family. Some patients remain ambulatory all their lives, whereas others progress to using a wheelchair. The heart is usually spared but cardiac monitoring is recommended.

3. **Oculopharyngeal muscular dystrophy** is an autosomal dominant disease of later onset. It is a GCG repeat disorder (8 to 13 repeats) involving the polyadenylate binding protein nuclear gene (PABPN) on chromosome 14. This dystrophy manifests as ptosis and progressive dysphagia. Muscle biopsy shows rimmed vacuoles in muscle biopsy specimens, and tubulofilamentous inclusions within the striated muscle cell nucleus. The differential diagnosis includes myasthenia gravis and mitochondrial myopathies (Kearns–Sayre syndrome).

4. **Limb-girdle muscular dystrophy** is a heterogeneous collection of both autosomal recessive and autosomal dominant disorders that affect pelvic and upper girdle muscles and spare the face. Some disorders present in childhood, others into late adulthood. There is CK, clinical phenotype and biopsy variability. In 2015, this remains a clinical diagnosis, but genetic testing with gene panels is improving.

5. **Myotonic dystrophy** is the most common muscular dystrophy among adults. Rather than being restricted to the skeletal muscle, it is a multisystemic, autosomal dominant disorder. It also involves the pancreas, gonads, thyroid, myocardium, and brain. Myotonic dystrophy is produced by a CTG trinucleotide repeat expansion in chromosome 19 (19q13.2–13.3) that codes for myotonin protein kinase, a ubiquitous enzyme related to protein phosphorylation. Patients are symptomatic when the CTG expansion is >80 repeats and the length of the repeat roughly correlates with severity of the disease. Clinical diagnosis is supported by the presence of myotonic discharges on EMG.

   a. **Muscle features.** Weakness of facial muscles is typical. The face is hatched and thin with early frontal balding. Ptosis is present but is not as severe as in myasthenia gravis or Kearns–Sayre syndrome. Temporalis and masseter atrophy is a characteristic feature. Limb involvement is predominantly distal. Proximal limb muscles are usually preserved until the late stages. Myotonia, which is the delay of muscle relaxation after contraction, is present. Percussion of the thenar eminence or tongue can elicit myotonia. Patients may be unable to release their grip after a handshake.

   b. **Generalized features.** Many patients have prominent systemic symptoms. Common abnormalities include cataracts, testicular atrophy, adult-onset diabetes mellitus, thyroid dysfunction, heart block, and arrhythmias. Hypersomnia and excessive daytime somnolence are reported and patients are often found to have mixed obstructive and central apneas. Because of the cardiorespiratory compromise, patients are susceptible to complications during surgery and anesthesia. Cognitive dysfunction, apathy, and lethargy are seen in more severely affected patients.

6. **Myotonic dystrophy type 2 or proximal myotonic myopathy** is an autosomal dominant disorder characterized by progressive weakness, myotonia, and cataracts. This is caused by a tetranucleotide repeat (CCTG) in the zinc finger protein 9 gene (*ZNF9*). These patients are a phenotypically milder form of myotonic dystrophy, with a later onset of symptoms.

7. **Mitochondrial myopathies** are a category of inherited diseases in which the genetic defect is either in the mitochondrial DNA or in a nuclear DNA gene that encodes for a protein involved in the mitochondrial respiratory chain. Because these defects all produce mitochondrial dysfunction, leading to decreased cellular energy production, patients manifest with symptoms related to oxidative stress. Seizures, encephalopathy, strokes, cardiomyopathy, muscle weakness (especially extraocular muscles), short stature, and hearing loss are common symptoms. The genetics underlying mitochondrial myopathies are complex. Mitochondrial DNA defects are maternally inherited and heteroplasmy (unequal distribution of affected mitochondria) may occur. Nuclear DNA genetic abnormalities follow Mendelian genetics.

Measurement of function of the components of the respiratory chain, muscle biopsy, MRI of affected organs, pedigree analysis, and genetic analysis of the mitochondrial genome can assist in making the diagnosis. Some of the more common phenotypes are mitochondrial encephalopathy with ragged red fibers, mitochondrial encephalopathy with lactic acidosis and stroke-like syndrome, chronic progressive external ophthalmoplegia, Kearns–Sayre syndrome, and Leigh's disease.

B. Therapeutic approach.

1. Duchenne muscular dystrophy.

   a. **Family and patient education** is important. A multidisciplinary clinic, which specializes in muscular dystrophy, can provide specialists and support to the patient and families.

   Genetic counseling is recommended. Mothers and female siblings can be assessed for carrier status by assessment of serum CK or, if the patient has a documented genetic defect, through peripheral blood genetic analysis. However, negative results of mutation analysis in the mother do not rule out the risk of Duchenne muscular dystrophy affecting future pregnancies. Even with normal results of peripheral blood gene analysis, a mutation can be present in a percentage of oocytes (germline mosaicism).

   b. **Physical therapy** is used to preserve mobility and to prevent early contractures. Passive range of motion exercises and adequate orthotics may prolong ambulation but do not stop disease progression.

   Orthotics and splints can assist with managing contractures. All patients progress to wheelchair dependency: proper wheelchair assessments and fittings can lessen the development of scoliosis.

   Patients with Duchenne muscular dystrophy are at high risk of side effects of general anesthesia. Succinylcholine or halothane should not be used because of the risk of episodes that resemble malignant hyperthermia. Adverse effects can be reduced with the use of nondepolarizing muscle relaxants.

   c. Respiratory therapy. In later stages, noninvasive intermittent positive-pressure ventilation is useful, especially when patients retain carbon dioxide. Pulmonary exercises, use of a cough assist device and use of a respiratory vest may prevent pulmonary infections.

   d. Medications. Prednisone (0.75 mg/kg/day) is recommended when children are still ambulatory to prolong this phase of life. Prednisone can improve neuromuscular strength after 1 month of treatment. The maximum effect is reached by 3 months. Side effects need to be addressed and close monitoring is needed.

   e. Therapy for **Becker muscular dystrophy** follows principles similar to those of therapy for Duchenne disease, tailored to each patient's level of strength.

2. In **facioscapulohumeral muscular dystrophy and limb-girdle muscular dystrophy,** treatment varies with individual patients. In patients with minimal symptoms, screening for cardiomyopathy and genetic counseling may be all that is needed. For patients with a foot-drop, ankle-foot orthoses may be prescribed. Physical therapy will be useful for range of motion, stretching, and gait assessment. When ambulation is impaired, a mobility evaluation can assess for wheelchair or motorized scooter needs.

3. In **oculopharyngeal muscular dystrophy,** blepharoplasty with resection of the levator palpebrae muscles may be needed. Dysphagia may be relieved with cricopharyngeal myotomy.

4. In **myotonic dystrophy,** only when myotonia is disabling, phenytoin (100 mg by mouth three times a day) can alleviate myotonia. In general, patients with myotonic dystrophy are not greatly concerned about the myotonia. The main goals are prevention and management of the systemic disease, especially cardiac arrhythmias.

5. Treatment of **mitochondrial myopathies** depends upon which organ systems are involved. Avoiding oxidative stress (hypoxia, ischemia, hypoglycemia, and infection) may help prevent exacerbations or worsening. A "mitochondrial cocktail" of antioxidants and vitamins has been developed to promote respiratory chain function and includes co-enzyme Q10, riboflavin, creatine, carnitine, B complex vitamins, and vitamins E and C.

METABOLIC MYOPATHY

Metabolic myopathies comprise a group of inherited disorders in which the defect is an alteration in the processing of carbohydrates or fats. **Acid maltase deficiency, McArdle's disease,** and **carnitine-O-palmitoyltransferase (CPT II) deficiency** are reviewed (Table 52.2).

A. Natural history, prognosis, and treatment.

1. **Acid maltase deficiency (Pompe's disease)** is an autosomal recessive glycogen storage disease caused by a deficiency in lysosomal α-glucosidase, which participates in the metabolism of glycogen into glucose. The infantile form is often fatal; there is also a less severe juvenile and adult-onset form. Infants with Pompe's disease have hypotonia, macroglossia, cardiomegaly, and hepatomegaly. Adults suffer from slowly progressive myopathy with respiratory failure. Diaphragm and thigh adductor muscles are preferentially affected.

   The cause of this disorder is a mutation in the acid alpha-glucosidase gene (GAA), located on chromosome 17q25. GAA enzyme activity evaluation is used for screening, but in borderline cases, molecular genetic testing is available.

TABLE 52.2 Metabolic Myopathies

Clinical Finding	Acid Maltase Deficiency	Myophosphorylase Deficiency	CPT II Deficiency
Gene defect	GAA	PYGM	CPT II
Age of onset	Infant–adult	Late childhood–adult	Adult
Muscle weakness	Progressive	Intermittent	Intermittent
Respiratory involvement	Yes	–	–
CK	Elevated	Elevated	Normal between attacks
Myoglobinuria	–	Yes	Yes
Electrical myotonia	Yes	–	–
Abnormal ischemic forearm exercise test	–	Yes: no rise in lactate	–
Muscle pathology	Vacuolar myopathy with elevated glycogen storage	Subsarcolemmal deposits of glycogen; absence of myophosphorylase staining	Normal or slight increase in lipid droplets in muscle fibers

Abbreviations: CK, creatine kinase; GAA, acid alpha-glucosidase; PYGM, glycogen phosphorylase; (−), negative or absent.

Treatment is now available for acid maltase deficiency, in the form of recombinant human α-glucosidase (Myozyme; Genzyme, Cambridge, MA, USA), given as repeated infusions. Enzyme replacement therapy has been clinically shown to lengthen the time before ventilator dependence in the infantile form. Adults have been documented to show increased strength and increased respiratory function.

2. **McArdle's disease,** or myophosphorylase deficiency, affects children and adults and manifests with myalgia, fatigue, and muscle stiffness. Myoglobinuria and renal failure can develop. CK level is increased. EMG shows myopathic changes. The forearm ischemic exercise in affected patients shows no increase in venous lactate (unlike in normal controls). Muscle biopsy discloses subsarcolemmal deposits of glycogen. Immunohistochemistry staining of muscle biopsy tissue will show absence of myophosphorylase.

   The disease is autosomal recessive, caused by homozygous or compound heterozygous mutations in the glycogen phosphorylase (PYGM) gene.

   Prognosis is rather benign. Some patients can tolerate the deficits and learn to avoid brief, strong exercises that precipitate attacks. No definite treatment is available.

3. **Carnitine-O-palmitoyltransferase II (CPT II) deficiency** manifests in the adult patient with intermittent cramps, myalgia, and myoglobinuria. Renal failure, resulting from myoglobinuria, or respiratory failure may ensue. CK and EMG are normal between attacks. The symptoms are precipitated by intense exertion. The capacity to perform short exercise is not impaired. Fasting, exposure to cold, high fat intake, viral infections, and general anesthesia can precipitate rhabdomyolysis. Increased lipid content may be seen on histochemical staining on muscle biopsy, but is not always present. The disease is autosomal recessive. The diagnosis is made by sequencing and mutation analysis of the carnitine palmitoyltransferase II (CPT2) gene. Therapy includes avoidance of triggers (general anesthesia, prolonged exercise, cold exposure and prolonged fasting) and a diet high in carbohydrates and low in fats.

TOXIC MYOPATHY

Toxic myopathy is myopathy associated with either systemic disease or medication effect. Some medications produce direct muscle fiber necrosis, while others produce electrolyte imbalances with rhabdomyolysis. The most important types of toxic myopathy are **necrotizing, autophagic, antimicrotubular,** and **steroid** (Video 52.1).

A. Natural history, prognosis, and treatment.
   1. Endocrine myopathy.
      a. **Thyrotoxic myopathy** manifests as weakness and muscle wasting. Fatigue and heat intolerance are also present. Hypokalemic periodic paralysis (see Section A.2.a under Periodic Paralyses) and myasthenia gravis are associated with hyperthyroidism and should be included in the differential diagnosis. Treatment relies on correcting the hyperthyroid state; β-adrenergic blocking agents may be of help. Glucocorticoids should be used in thyroid storm to block the peripheral conversion of thyroxine to triiodothyronine.
      b. **Hypothyroid myopathy** manifests as enlargement of muscles, weakness, painful cramps, myoedema, and slow-recovery reflexes. This disease is more common among women. Rhabdomyolysis or respiratory muscle involvement may be present. Serum level of CK may be elevated. The diagnosis is supported by abnormal results of thyroid function tests. Treatment is to restore the euthyroid state.
   2. Toxic necrotizing myopathy. HMG-CoA reductase inhibitors (statins), used for cholesterol management, can cause a myopathy. Onset can be acute or insidious, often with myalgia, occasionally with myoglobinuria, and more often involving the proximal lower-extremity muscles. Patients with renal failure are especially predisposed. Elevated serum CK levels are common, and the EMG findings are abnormal. Muscle fiber necrosis with phagocytosis and small regenerating fibers are found on biopsy. When the medication is stopped, symptoms should resolve when the medication is stopped.
      a. Asymptomatic elevations of CK level occur in about 1% of patients taking statins. These patients will need monitoring for muscle weakness.
      b. **Cyclosporine** and **tacrolimus** have also been associated with toxic myopathy.

3. **Autophagic myopathy** can occur with **chloroquine** (and its derivatives) or **amiodarone**; it can be seen with systemic lupus erythematosus, scleroderma, and rheumatoid arthritis. The myopathy of chloroquine affects the proximal lower-extremity muscles and is usually not painful. The course is subacute or chronic. The heart can be affected. Elevation in CK level and myotonic potentials on the EMG can be found. Muscle biopsy shows vacuoles (lysosomes), which stain for acid phosphatase and contain debris and curvilinear structures (autophagic vacuoles). With amiodarone, severe proximal and distal weakness may occur in combination with distal sensory loss, tremor, and ataxia. The treatment is to discontinue the medication.

4. **Antimicrotubular myopathy** is produced by **colchicine** and **vincristine**. These drugs bind to nerve and muscle tubulin. The toxic etiology of this myopathy is often not recognized because of the insidious onset in patients who may have been taking colchicine for years. Concomitant axonal sensorimotor neuropathy occurs. Weakness resolves slowly. Because of the neuromyopathy, a mixed pattern of denervation and myopathy is seen on electrophysiologic studies. Muscle biopsy shows acid-phosphatase-positive autophagic vacuoles.

5. The effects of **zidovudine** can be indistinguishable from the myopathy of HIV infection. It is due to mitochondrial toxicity associated with this agent. CK levels are normal or mildly elevated. Differentiation from HIV myopathy can be difficult solely on a clinical basis. The muscle biopsy may show "ragged red fibers," a sign of mitochondrial disease. Treatment consists of stopping the medication. Whereas myalgia (muscle pain) is usually relieved within weeks of discontinuing zidovudine, muscle weakness can persist for months.

6. **Steroid myopathy** is a type-2 fiber atrophy of muscles associated with long-term corticosteroid exposure. Doses of prednisone >30 mg/day carry the risk of myopathy. Fluorinated compounds (triamcinolone, betamethasone, and dexamethasone) have a greater risk. Patients have predominantly proximal muscle weakness and atrophy. Serum level of CK is usually normal. EMG findings are normal. Muscle biopsy shows type-2 fiber atrophy, especially type 2B (fast twitch glycolytic). Tapering to an alternate-day regimen, use of "steroid-sparing" drugs (e.g., azathioprine), use of nonfluorinated steroids, and exercise may reduce the incidence of this myopathy.

In polymyositis or dermatomyositis, clinical worsening in a patient being treated with steroids may represent either a progression of the primary disease or the onset of steroid myopathy. The decision to raise or lower the prednisone dose has to be made after evaluation of the patient's muscle strength, mobility, CK levels, and medication changes in the preceding months.

Key Points

- Early and precise diagnosis of inflammatory myopathies is mandatory to initiate a correct treatment course, for the patient to get a good quality of life and a better prognosis.
- Care providers need to be aware of the myopathic consequences of statins, colchicine and chloroquine.
- Neurogenetics of muscle disorders has enormously expanded; new findings are leading to rational therapies.
- Care providers need to recognize the muscle complications of endocrine disorders, particularly those of thyroid, parathyroid, and adrenal glands.
- Specific treatments are now available for patients with acid maltase deficiency; therefore, this disease should be screened in all myopathic patients with diaphragmatic or thigh adductor weakness.

Recommended Readings

Amato AA, Darras BT, Greenberg SA, et al. Muscle diseases. *AAN Continuum*. 2006;12(3):140–168.

Dalakas, MC. Inflammatory muscle diseases. *N Engl J Med*. 2015;372:1734–1747.

King WM, Kissel JT. Multidisciplinary approach to the management of myopathies. *Continuum*. 2013;19(6):1650–1673.

Narayanaswami P, Weiss M, Selcen D, et al. Evidence-based guideline summary: diagnosis and treatment of limb-girdle and distal dystrophies: report of the guideline development subcommittee of the American Academy of Neurology and the practice issues review panel of the American Association of Neuromuscular & Electrodiagnostic Medicine. *Neurology*. 2014;83:1453–1463.

Statland J, Phillips L, Trivedi JR. Muscle channelopathies. *Neurol Clinics*. 2014;32:801–815.

Turner C, Hilton-Jones D. Myotonic dystrophy: diagnosis, management and new therapies. *Curr Opin Neurol*. 2014;27(5):599–606.

53 Disorders of the Neuromuscular Junction

Robert M. Pascuzzi and Cynthia L. Bodkin

MYASTHENIA GRAVIS

Myasthenia gravis (MG) is an autoimmune disorder of neuromuscular transmission involving the production of autoantibodies directed against the neuromuscular junction (most commonly the nicotinic acetylcholine (ACh) receptor). ACh receptor antibodies are detectable in the serum of 80% to 90% of patients with MG. The prevalence of MG is about 1 in 10,000 to 20,000 persons. Women are affected about twice as often as men. Symptoms may begin at virtually any age with a peak in women in the second and third decades, whereas the peak in men occurs in the fifth and sixth decades. Associated autoimmune diseases such as rheumatoid arthritis, systemic lupus erythematous (SLE), and pernicious anemia are present in about 5% of patients. Thyroid disease occurs in about 10%, often in association with antithyroid antibodies. About 10% to 15% of MG patients have a thymoma, whereas thymic lymphoid hyperplasia with proliferation of germinal centers occurs in 50% to 70% of cases. In most patients, the cause of autoimmune MG is unknown. However, there are three iatrogenic causes for autoimmune MG. D-penicillamine (used in the treatment of Wilson's disease and rheumatoid arthritis) and α-interferon therapy are both capable of inducing MG. In addition, bone marrow transplantation is associated with the development of MG as part of the chronic graft-versus-host disease.

A. **Clinical features.** The hallmark of MG is fluctuating or fatigable weakness. The presenting symptoms are ocular in half of all patients (25% of patients initially present with diplopia, 25% with eyelid ptosis), and by 1 month into the course of illness, 80% of patients have some degree of ocular involvement. Presenting symptoms are bulbar (dysarthria or dysphagia) in 10%, leg weakness (impaired walking) in 10%, and generalized weakness in 10%. Respiratory failure is the presenting symptom in 1% of cases. Patients usually complain of symptoms from focal muscle dysfunction such as diplopia, ptosis, dysarthria, dysphagia, inability to work with arms raised over the head, or disturbance of gait (Video 53.1). In contrast, patients with MG tend not to complain of "generalized weakness," "generalized fatigue," "sleepiness," or muscle pain. In the classic case, fluctuating weakness is worse with exercise and improved with rest. Symptoms tend to progress later in the day. Many different factors can precipitate or aggravate weakness, such as physical stress, emotional stress, infection, or exposure to medications that impair neuromuscular transmission (perioperative succinylcholine, aminoglycoside antibiotics, quinine, quinidine, and botulinum toxin).

B. **Diagnosis.** The diagnosis is based on a history of fluctuating weakness with corroborating findings on examination (Video 53.2). There are several different ways to validate or confirm the clinical diagnosis.

1. **Edrophonium test.** The most immediate and readily accessible confirmatory study is the edrophonium test. To perform the test, choose one or two weak muscles to judge. Eyelid ptosis, dysconjugate gaze, and other cranial deficits provide the most reliable endpoints. Use a setting where hypotension, syncope, or respiratory failure can be managed as patients occasionally decompensate during the test. If the patient has severe dyspnea, defer the test until the airway is secure. Start an intravenous (IV). Have IV atropine 0.4 mg readily available in the event of bradycardia or extreme gastrointestinal (GI) side effects. Edrophonium 10 mg (1 mL) is drawn up in a syringe, and 1 mg (0.1 mL) should be given as a test dose while checking the patient's heart rate (to assure the patient is not supersensitive to the drug). If no untoward side effects occur after 1 minute, another 3 mg is given. Many MG patients will show improved power within 30 to 60 seconds of

giving the initial 4 mg at which point the test can be stopped. If after 1 minute there is no improvement, give additional 3 mg, and if there is still no response, 1 minute later give the final 3 mg. If the patient develops muscarinic symptoms or signs at any time during the test (sweating, salivation, and GI symptoms), or should fasciculations be detected then one can assume that enough edrophonium has been given to see improvement in strength and the test can be stopped. When a placebo effect or examiner bias is of concern, the test is performed in a double-blind placebo control fashion. The 1 mL control syringe contains either saline, 0.4 mg atropine, or nicotinic acid 10 mg. Improved strength from edrophonium lasts for just a few minutes. When improvement is clear-cut, the test is positive. If the improvement is borderline, it is best to consider the test negative. The test can be repeated several times. Sensitivity of the edrophonium test is about 90%. The specificity is difficult to determine because improvement following IV edrophonium has been reported in other neuromuscular diseases including Lambert–Eaton myasthenic syndrome (LEMS), botulism, Guillain–Barré syndrome (GBS), motor neuron disease, and with lesions of the brainstem, pituitary, and cavernous sinus. Neostigmine has a longer duration of effect and in selected patients may be an alternative cholinesterase inhibitor (CEI) for diagnostic testing, especially in children. For performance of a "neostigmine test," 0.04 mg/kg is given intramuscularly or 0.02 mg/kg intravenously (one time only).

2. **ACh receptor antibodies.** The primary serologic test is the immunoprecipitation assay for ACh receptor binding antibodies. In addition, assays for receptor modulating and blocking antibodies are available. Binding antibodies are present in about 80% of all MG patients (40% to 50% of patients with pure ocular MG, 80% of those with mild generalized MG, and 90% of patients with moderate to severe generalized MG, and 70% of those in clinical remission). By also testing for modulating and blocking antibodies, the sensitivity improves to 90% overall. Specificity is superb with false positives exceedingly rare in reliable labs.

3. **MuSK antibodies.** Approximately 25% of patients seronegative for ACh receptor antibodies have antibodies to muscle-specific kinase (MuSK). The clinical features of MuSK positive patients may differ from non-MuSK MG patients. Such patients tend to be younger women (under age 40) with disproportionate bulbar, neck extensor, shoulder, and respiratory symptoms with increased likelihood of "fixed weakness" and have a lower likelihood of abnormal repetitive stimulation and edrophonium test results. MuSK patients have no associated thymus abnormalities and are more likely to be refractory to conventional medical management.

4. **LRP4** (low-density lipoprotein receptor-related protein 4) and agrin antibodies present in a small number of patients.

5. **EMG (electrophysiological testing).** Repetitive stimulation testing is widely available and has variable sensitivity depending on the number and selection of muscles studied and various provocative maneuvers. However, in most laboratories, this technique has a sensitivity of about 50% in all patients with MG (lower in patients with mild or pure ocular disease). In general, the yield from repetitive stimulation is higher when testing muscle groups having clinically significant weakness. Single-fiber EMG (SFEMG) is a highly specialized technique, usually available in major academic centers, with a sensitivity of about 90%. Abnormal single-fiber results are common in other neuromuscular diseases; therefore, the test must be used in the correct clinical context. The specificity of SFEMG is an important issue in that mild abnormalities can clearly be present with a variety of other diseases of the motor unit including motor neuron disease, peripheral neuropathy, and myopathy. Disorders of neuromuscular transmission other than MG can have abnormalities on SFEMG. In contrast, ACh receptor antibodies (and MuSK antibodies) are not found in non-MG patients. In summary, the two highly sensitive laboratory studies are SFEMG and ACh receptor antibodies; nonetheless, neither test is 100% sensitive.

C. **Prognosis.** Natural course: Appropriate management of the patient with autoimmune MG requires understanding of the natural course of the disease. The long-term natural course of MG is highly variable but generalizations are as follows. About half of MG patients present with ocular symptoms (ptosis or diplopia) and by 1 month 80% have eye findings. The presenting weakness is bulbar in 10%, limb in 10%, generalized in 10%, and respiratory in 1%. By 1 month, symptoms remain purely ocular in 40%, generalized in 40%, limited to the limbs in 10%, and limited to bulbar muscles in 10%. Weakness remains restricted to the ocular muscles on a long-term basis in about 15% to 20% (pure ocular MG). Most patients with initial ocular involvement tend to develop generalized weakness within the first year of the disease (90% of those who generalize do so within the initial 12 months). Maximal weakness occurs within the initial 3 years in 70% of patients. In the modem era, death from MG is rare. Spontaneous long-lasting remission occurs in about 10% to 15%, usually in the first or second year of the disease. Most MG patients develop progression of clinical symptoms during the initial 2 to 3 years. However, progression is not uniform, as illustrated by 15% to 20% of patients whose symptoms remain purely ocular and those who have spontaneous remission.

D. **Treatment.**

1. **First-line therapy.** CEIs are safe, effective, and first-line therapy in all patients. Inhibition of acetylcholinesterase (AChE) reduces the hydrolysis of ACh, increasing the accumulation of ACh at the nicotinic postsynaptic membrane. The CEIs used in MG bind reversibly (as opposed to organophosphate CEIs, which bind irreversibly) to AChE. These drugs cross the blood–brain barrier poorly and tend not to cause central nervous system (CNS) side effects. Absorption from the GI tract tends to be inefficient and variable, with oral bioavailability of about 10%. Muscarinic autonomic side effects of GI cramping, diarrhea, salivation, lacrimation, and diaphoresis are common and dose-related, and occasional patients may have bradycardia. A feared potential complication of excessive CEI use is skeletal muscle weakness (cholinergic weakness). Patients receiving parenteral CEI are at the greatest risk to have cholinergic weakness. It is uncommon for patients receiving oral CEI to develop significant cholinergic weakness even while experiencing muscarinic cholinergic side effects. Generally available CEIs are summarized in Table 53.1.

   a. **Pyridostigmine (Mestinon)** is the most widely used CEI for long-term oral therapy. Onset of effect is within 30 minutes of an oral dose, with peak effect within 1 to 2 hours, and wearing off gradually at 3 to 4 hours postdose. The starting dose is 30 to 60 mg three to four times per day depending on symptoms. Optimal benefit usually occurs with a dose of 60 mg every 4 hours. Muscarinic cholinergic side effects are common with larger doses. Patients with significant bulbar weakness will often time their dose about 1 hour before meals in order to maximize chewing and swallowing.

TABLE 53.1 Cholinesterase Inhibitors

	Unit Dose	Average Dose (Adult)
Pyridostigmine bromide tablet (Mestinon)	60 mg tablet	30–60 mg every 4–6 hr
Pyridostigmine bromide syrup	12 mg/mL	30–60 mg every 4–6 hr
Pyridostigmine bromide timespan (Mestinon Timespan)	180 mg tablet	1 tablet twice daily
Pyridostigmine bromide (Parenteral)	5 mg/mL ampoules	1–2 mg every 3–4 hr (1/30 of oral dose)
Neostigmine bromide (Prostigmin)	15 mg tablet	7.5–15 mg every 3–4 hr
Neostigmine methylsulfate (Parenteral)	0.25–1.0 mg/mL	0.5 mg IM, IV, or SC ampoules every 2–3 hr
Children's dosing		

Edrophonium (Tensilon)
   Diagnosis: 0.1 mg/kg IV (or 0.15 mg/kg IM or SC, which prolongs the effect), preceded by a test dose of 0.01 mg/kg
Pyridostigmine bromide (Mestinon)
   Treatment: oral dose is about 1.0 mg/kg every 4–6 hr, as tablets or syrup (60 mg/5 mL)
Neostigmine methylsulfate (Parenteral)
   Diagnosis: 0.1 mg/kg IM or SC X1 or 0.05 mg/kg IV X1
   Treatment: 0.01–0.04 mg/kg/dose IM, IV, or SC q 2–3 hr p.r.n.

Abbreviations: IM, intramuscular; p.r.n., as needed; q, every; SC, subcutaneous.

Of all the CEI preparations, pyridostigmine has the least muscarinic side effects. Pyridostigmine may be used in a number of alternative forms to the 60 mg tablet. The syrup may be necessary for children or for patients with difficulty swallowing pills. Sustained-release pyridostigmine 180 mg (Mestinon Timespan) is sometimes preferred for night time use. Unpredictable release and absorption limit its use. Patients with severe dysphagia or those undergoing surgical procedures may need parenteral CEI. IV pyridostigmine should be given at about 1/30 of the oral dose. Neostigmine (prostigmine) has a slightly shorter duration of action and somewhat greater muscarinic side effects.

b. For patients with intolerable muscarinic side effects at CEI doses required for optimal power, a concomitant anticholinergic drug such as atropine sulfate (0.4 to 0.5 mg orally) or glycopyrrolate (Robinul) (1 to 2 mg orally) on a p.r.n. basis or with each dose of CEI may prevent the side effects. Patients with mild disease can often be managed adequately with CEIs. However, patients with moderate, severe, or progressive disease will usually require more effective therapy.

2. **Thymectomy.** Association of the thymus gland with MG was first noted around 1900 and thymectomy has become standard therapy for over 50 years. A large randomized international multicenter controlled trial demonstrated that thymectomy improved clinical outcomes over a 3 year period in patients with nonthymomatous MG. The general consensus is that thymectomy should be considered for patients with moderate to severe MG, especially those inadequately controlled on CEI, and those under age 55 years. All patients with suspected thymoma undergo surgery. About 75% of MG patients appear to benefit from thymectomy. Patients may improve or simply stabilize. For unclear reasons, the onset of improvement tends to be delayed by a year or two in most patients (some patients may improve 5 to 10 years after surgery). The majority of centers use the transsternal approach for thymectomy with the goal of complete removal of the gland. The limited transcervical approach has been largely abandoned due to the likelihood of incomplete gland removal. Many centers perform a "maximal thymectomy" in order to ensure complete removal. The procedure involves a combined transsternal–transcervical exposure with en bloc removal of the thymus. Thorascopic and video-assisted thymectomy offer less invasive options. If thymectomy is to be performed, choose an experienced surgeon, anesthesiologist, and a medical center with a good track record and insist that the entire gland is removed.

a. Which patients do not undergo thymectomy? Patients with very mild or trivial symptoms do not have surgery. Most patients with pure ocular MG do not undergo thymectomy even though there has been some reported benefit in selected patients. Thymectomy is often avoided in children due to the theoretical possibility of impairing the developing immune system. However, reports of thymectomy in children as young as 2 to 3 years of age have shown favorable results without adverse effects on the immune system. Thymectomy has been largely discouraged in patients over age 55 because of expected increased morbidity, latency of clinical benefit, and frequent observation of an atrophic, involuted gland. Major complications from thymectomy are uncommon so long as the surgery is performed at an experienced center with anesthesiologists and neurologists familiar with the disease and perioperative management of MG patients. Common, though less serious, aspects of thymectomy include postoperative chest pain (which may last several weeks), a 4- to 6-week convalescence period, and cosmetically displeasing incisional scar.

3. **Corticosteroids.** There are no controlled trials documenting the benefit of corticosteroids in MG. However, nearly all authorities have personal experience attesting to the virtues (and complications) of corticosteroid use in MG patients. In general, corticosteroids are used in patients with moderate to severe disabling symptoms that are refractory to CEI. Patients are commonly hospitalized to initiate therapy due to the risk of early exacerbation. Opinions differ regarding the best method of administration. For patients with severe MG it is best to begin with high-dose daily therapy of 60 to 80 mg/day orally. Early exacerbation occurs in about half of patients, usually within the first few days of therapy and typically lasting 3 or 4 days. In 10% of cases, the exacerbation is severe, requiring mechanical ventilation or a feeding tube (thus, the need to initiate therapy in the hospital). Overall, about 80% of patients show a favorable response to steroids (with 30% attaining

remission and 50% having marked improvement). Mild to moderate improvement occurs in 15%, and 5% have no response. Improvement begins as early as 12 hours and as late as 60 days after beginning prednisone, but usually the patient begins to improve within the first or second week. Improvement is gradual, with marked improvement occurring at a mean of 3 months, and maximal improvement at a mean of 9 months. Of those patients having a favorable response, most maintain their improvement with gradual dosage reduction at a rate of 10 mg every 1 to 2 months. More rapid reduction is usually associated with a flare-up of the disease. Although many patients can eventually be weaned off steroids and maintain their response, the majority cannot. They require a minimum dose (5 to 30 mg alternate day [AD]) in order to maintain their improvement. Complications of long-term high-dose prednisone therapy are substantial, including cushingoid appearance, hypertension, osteoporosis, diabetes, cataracts, aseptic necrosis, and the other well-known complications of chronic steroid therapy. Older patients tend to respond more favorably to prednisone. An alternative prednisone regimen involves low-dose AD gradually increasing schedule in an attempt to avoid the early exacerbation. Patients receive prednisone 25 mg AD with increase by 12.5 mg every third dose (about every fifth day) to a maximum dose of 100 mg AD or until sufficient improvement occurs. Clinical improvement usually begins within 1 month of treatment. The frequency and severity of early exacerbation is less than that associated with high-dose daily regimens. High-dose IV methylprednisolone (1,000 mg IV daily for 3 to 5 days) can provide improvement within 1 to 2 weeks but the clinical improvement is temporary.

4. Alternative immunosuppressive drug therapy.

   a. **Mycophenolate mofetil** (CellCept) is a purine inhibitor widely used in recent years for the treatment of MG. Anecdotal uncontrolled experience would suggest that about 75% of MG patients benefit from the drug with the typical onset of improvement within 2 to 3 months. The drug is generally well tolerated. Typically begin with 250 to 500 mg orally twice a day, and over 2 to 4 weeks increase the dose to 1,000 mg orally twice a day. Two recently completed prospective controlled double-blind trials failed to demonstrate a benefit from mycophenolate in selected MG patients leading to a reevaluation of its role and suggesting that the anecdotal reports of benefit may be incorrect. Complications are uncommon and include GI intolerance and occasional patients with hepatic or hematologic abnormalities.

   b. **Azathioprine** (Imuran) is a cytotoxic purine analog with extensive use in MG (but largely uncontrolled and retrospective). The starting dose is 50 mg by mouth daily, with complete blood count (CBC) and liver function tests weekly in the beginning. If the drug is tolerated and if the blood work is stable, the dose is increased by 50 mg every 1 to 2 weeks aiming for a total daily dose or about 2 to 3 mg/kg/day (about 150 mg/day in the average-sized adult). When azathioprine is first started, about 15% of patients will have intolerable GI side effects (nausea, anorexia, and abdominal discomfort) and sometimes associated with fever, leading to discontinuation. Bone marrow suppression with relative leukopenia (white blood cells (WBCs) 2,500 to 4,000) occurs in 25% of patients but is usually not significant. If the WBC count drops below 2,500 or the absolute granulocyte count goes below 1,000, the drug is stopped (and the abnormalities usually resolve). Macrocytosis is common and of unclear clinical significance. Liver enzymes elevate in 5% to 10% but are usually reversible, and severe hepatic toxicity occurs in only about 1%. Infection occurs in about 5%. There is a theoretical risk of malignancy (based on observations in organ transplant patients), but this increased risk has not been clearly established in the MG patient population. About half of MG patients improve on azathioprine with onset about 4 to 8 months into treatment. Maximal improvement takes about 12 months. Relapse after discontinuation of azathioprine occurs in over half of patients, usually within 1 year.

   c. **Cyclosporine** is used in patients with severe MG who cannot be adequately managed with corticosteroids or azathioprine. The starting dose is 3 to 5 mg/kg/day given in two divided doses. Cyclosporine blood levels should be measured monthly (aiming for a level of 200 to 300) along with electrolytes, magnesium, and renal function (in general, serum creatinine should not exceed one and one-half times the pretreatment level). Blood should be sampled before the morning dose is taken. Over half of patients improve on cyclosporine. The onset of clinical improvement occurs about 1 to 2 months after beginning therapy, and maximal improvement occurs at about 3 to 4 months. Side effects include renal toxicity and hypertension. Nonsteroidal anti-inflammatory drugs (NSAIDs) and potassium-sparing diuretics are among the list of drugs that should be avoided while on cyclosporine. In patients on corticosteroids, the addition of cyclosporine can lead to a reduction in steroid dosage (although it is usually not possible to discontinue prednisone).

d. **Methotrexate** has been used in selected patients for decades with clinical response the subject of sporadic anecdotal reports.

e. **Tacrolimus** has been reported to be beneficial in several series and in some parts of the world is among the more commonly prescribed immunosuppressive options.

f. **Rituximab** has been reported to be effective in treating MG in selected patients (the anecdotal reports tend to involve relatively refractory patients who have done poorly with alternative treatment options). The anecdotal reports of rituximab benefits in MuSK patients are particularly notable given the disproportionate tendency for such patients to be refractory to many other immunosuppressive options.

g. **Eculizumab** has been reported to be effective in treating MG and is completing a large randomized trial. This monoclonal antibody blocks C5 and ostensibly reduces compliment mediated lysis of the postsynaptic membrane.

5. **Plasma exchange** (PLEX or plasmapheresis) removes ACh receptor antibodies and results in rapid clinical improvement. The standard course involves removal of 2 to 3 L of plasma every other day or 3 times per week until the patient improves (usually a total of three to five exchanges). Improvement begins after the first few exchanges and reaches the maximum within 2 to 3 weeks. The improvement is moderate to marked in nearly all patients but usually wears off after 4 to 8 weeks due to the reaccumulation of pathogenic antibodies. Vascular access may require placement of a central line. Complications include hypotension, bradycardia, electrolyte imbalance, hemolysis, infection, and access problems (such as pneumothorax from placement of a central line). Indications for PLEX include any patient in whom a rapid temporary clinical improvement is needed. Patients with MuSK antibodies who are refractory to other modalities may respond favorably to PLEX.

6. **High-dose IV and subcutaneous immunoglobulin (IVIG)** administration is associated with rapid improvement in MG symptoms in a time frame similar to plasma exchange. The mechanism is unclear but may relate to down-regulation of ACh receptor antibody production or to the effect of anti-idiotype antibodies. The usual protocol is 2 g/kg spread out over 5 consecutive days (0.4 g/kg/day). Different IVIG preparations are administered IV at different rates (contact the pharmacy for guidelines). The majority of MG patients improve, usually within 1 week of starting IVIG. The degree of response is variable and the duration of response is limited, as with plasma exchange, to about 4 to 8 weeks. Complications include fever, chills, and headache, which respond to slowing down the rate of the infusion and giving diphenhydramine. Occasional cases of aseptic meningitis, renal failure, nephrotic syndrome, and stroke have been reported. Also, patients with selective IgA deficiency can have anaphylaxis, best avoided by screening for IgA deficiency ahead of time. The treatment is relatively expensive, comparable to PLEX. In patients with problematic IV access or those using IG for long-term maintenance therapy a subcutaneous IG preparation is an alternative.

E. General guidelines for management.

1. Be certain of the diagnosis.

2. Patient education. Provide the patient with information about the natural course of the disease (including the variable and somewhat unpredictable course). Briefly review the treatment options outlined above pointing out effectiveness, time course of improvement, duration of response, and complications. Provide the patient with educational pamphlets prepared by the Myasthenia Gravis Foundation or the Muscular Dystrophy Association.

3. When to hospitalize the patient. Patients with severe MG can deteriorate rapidly over a period of hours. Therefore, those having dyspnea should be hospitalized immediately in a constant observation or intensive care setting. Patients with moderate or severe dysphagia, weight loss, as well as those with rapidly progressive or severe weakness

should be admitted urgently. This will allow close monitoring and early intervention in the case of respiratory failure and will also expedite the diagnostic workup and initiation of therapy.

4. **Myasthenic crisis (Table 53.2)** is a medical emergency characterized by respiratory failure from diaphragm weakness or severe oropharyngeal weakness leading to aspiration. Crisis can occur in the setting of surgery (post-op), acute infection, or following rapid withdrawal of corticosteroids (though some patients have no precipitating factors). Patients should be placed in an intensive care unit (ICU) setting and have forced vital capacity (FVC) checked every 2 hours. Changes in arterial blood gases occur relatively late in neuromuscular respiratory failure. There should be a low threshold for intubation and mechanical ventilation. Criteria for intubation include a drop in the FVC below 15 mL/kg (or below 1 L in an average-sized adult), severe aspiration from oropharyngeal weakness, or labored breathing regardless of the measurements. If the diagnosis is not clear-cut, it is advisable to secure the airway with intubation, stabilize ventilation, and only then address the question of the underlying diagnosis. If the patient has been taking CEI, the drug should be temporarily discontinued in order to rule out the possibility of "cholinergic crisis."

5. Screen for and correct any underlying medical problems such as systemic infection, metabolic problems (like diabetes), and thyroid disease (hypo or hyperthyroidism can exacerbate MG).

6. Drugs to avoid in MG. Avoid using D-penicillamine, α-interferon, chloroquine, quinine, quinidine, procainamide, and botulinum toxin. Aminoglycoside antibiotics should be avoided unless needed for a life-threatening infection. Fluoroquinolones (ciprofloxacin) and erythromycin have significant neuromuscular blocking effects. Telithromycin (Ketek) has been reported to cause life-threatening weakness in patients with MG and should not be used. Neuromuscular blocking drugs such as pancuronium and D-tubocurarine can produce marked and prolonged paralysis in MG patients. Depolarizing drugs such as succinylcholine can also have a prolonged effect and should be used by a skilled anesthesiologist who is well aware of the patient's MG.

F. Guidelines for specific therapies. Treatment must be individualized. Mild diplopia and eyelid ptosis may not be disabling for some patients, but for a pilot or neurosurgeon, mild intermittent diplopia may be critical. In a similar fashion, some patients may tolerate side effects better than others.

1. Mild or trivial weakness, either localized or generalized, should be managed with a CEI such as pyridostigmine.

2. Moderate to marked weakness, localized or generalized, should initially be managed with a CEI. Even if symptoms are adequately controlled, patients under age 55 should be considered for thymectomy early in the course of the disease (within the first year). In older patients, thymectomy is usually not performed unless the patient is thought to have a thymoma. Thymectomy is performed at an experienced medical center with

TABLE 53.2 The Acutely Deteriorating Myasthenic Patient

Myasthenic Crisis	Cholinergic Crisis
Respiratory distress	Abdominal cramps
Respiratory arrest	Diarrhea
Cyanosis	Nausea and vomiting
Increased pulse and blood pressure	Excessive secretions
Diaphoresis	Miosis
Poor cough	Fasciculations
Inability to handle oral secretions	Diaphoresis
Dysphagia	Weakness
Weakness	Worse with edrophonium
Improves with edrophonium	

the clear intent of complete removal of the gland. All patients with suspected thymoma (by chest scan) should have thymectomy, even if their myasthenic symptoms are mild. Unless a thymoma is suspected, patients with pure ocular disease are usually not treated with thymectomy.

3. If symptoms are inadequately controlled on CEI, immunosuppression is used. High-dose corticosteroid therapy is the most predictable and effective long-term option. If patients have severe, rapidly progressive, or life-threatening symptoms, the decision to start corticosteroids is clear-cut. Patients with disabling but stable symptoms may instead receive a nonsteroidal immunosuppressive drug such as azathioprine.

4. PLEX or IVIG are indicated in:
   a. Rapidly progressive, life-threatening, impending myasthenic crisis or actual crisis, particularly if prolonged intubation with mechanical ventilation is judged hazardous.
   b. Preoperative stabilization of MG (such as prior to thymectomy or other elective surgery) in poorly controlled patients.
   c. Disabling MG refractory to other therapies (maintenance therapy).

5. If these options fail, then use mycophenolate, cyclosporine, tacrolimus, or rituximab.

6. If the patient remains poorly controlled despite appropriate treatment, then perform a repeat chest computed tomography (CT) scan looking for residual thymus. Some patients improve after "repeat thymectomy." Check for other medical problems (diabetes, thyroid disease, infection, and coexisting autoimmune diseases).

7. Referral to a neurologist or center specializing in neuromuscular disease is advised for all patients with suspected MG and can be particularly important for complicated or refractory patients.

G. **Transient neonatal myasthenia** occurs in 10% to 15% of babies born to mothers with autoimmune MG. Within the first few days after delivery the baby has a weak cry or suck, appears floppy, and on occasion, requires mechanical ventilation. The condition is caused by maternal antibodies that cross the placenta late in pregnancy. As these maternal antibodies are replaced by the baby's own antibodies, the symptoms gradually disappear, usually within a few weeks, and the baby is normal thereafter. Infants with severe weakness are treated with oral pyridostigmine 1 to 2 mg/kg every 4 hours.

H. **Congenital myasthenia** represents a group of rare hereditary disorders of the neuromuscular junction. The patients tend to have lifelong relatively stable symptoms of generalized fatigable weakness. These disorders are nonimmunologic, without ACh receptor antibodies, and therefore patients do not respond to immune therapy (steroids, thymectomy, and plasma exchange). Most of these patients improve on CEI. Even though there are many established subtypes of congenital MG, several are worth noting due in part to specific therapeutic implications. The **fast channel congenital myasthenic syndrome** tends to be static or slowly progressive, but usually very responsive to combination therapy with 3,4-diaminopyridine (enhances release of ACh) and pyridostigmine (reduces metabolism of ACh). **Slow channel congenital myasthenic syndrome** typically worsens over years as the endplate myopathy progresses. Although CEIs typically worsen symptoms, quinidine and fluoxetine, which reduce the duration of ACh receptor channel openings, are both effective treatments for slow channel syndrome. **The congenital myasthenic syndrome associated with ACh receptor deficiency** tends to be relatively nonprogressive and may even improve slightly as the patient ages. The disorder typically responds to symptomatic therapy with pyridostigmine and/or 3,4-diaminopyridine. Ephedrine produces benefit in some cases. **Patients with endplate AChE deficiency** usually present in infancy or early childhood with generalized weakness, underdevelopment of muscles, slowed pupillary responses to light, and either no response or worsening with CEIs. No effective long-term treatment has been described for congenital endplate AChE deficiency. A homozygous mutation of **Dok-7** is responsible for a form of congenital myasthenia characterized by weakness in limbs and trunk but largely sparing the face, eyes, and oropharyngeal muscles. The formation of neuromuscular synapses requires the muscle-specific receptor tyrosine kinase (MuSK). Dok-7 is necessary and sufficient for the activation of MuSK. Albuterol was effective in treating patients with **endplate acetylcholinesterase deficiency** and also **Dok-7** forms of congenital myasthenia.

LAMBERT–EATON MYASTHENIC SYNDROME

Lambert–Eaton myasthenic syndrome (LEMS) is a presynaptic disease characterized by chronic fluctuating weakness of proximal limb muscles. Symptoms include difficulty walking, climbing stairs, or rising from a chair. In LEMS there may be some improvement in power with sustained or repeated exercise. In contrast, eyelid ptosis, diplopia, dysphagia, and respiratory failure are far less common. In addition, LEMS patients often complain of myalgias, muscle stiffness of the back and legs, distal paresthesias, metallic taste, dry mouth, impotence, and other autonomic symptoms of muscarinic cholinergic insufficiency. LEMS is rare compared to MG, which is about 100 times more common. About half of LEMS patients have an underlying malignancy that is usually small-cell carcinoma of the lung. In patients without malignancy, LEMS is an autoimmune disease and can be associated with other autoimmune phenomena. In general, patients over age 40 are more likely to be men and have an associated malignancy whereas younger patients are more likely to be women and have no neoplasm malignancy. LEMS symptoms can precede detection of the malignancy by 1 to 2 years. Of all patients with small cell lung cancer, 4% have LEMS.

A. The examination typically shows proximal lower extremity weakness, although the objective bedside assessment may suggest relatively mild weakness relative to the patient's history. The muscle stretch reflexes are absent. On testing sustained maximal grip there is a gradual increase in power over the initial 2 to 3 seconds (Lambert's sign).

B. The **diagnosis** is confirmed with EMG studies, which typically show low amplitude of the compound muscle action potentials and a decrement to slow rates or repetitive stimulation. Following brief exercise, there is marked facilitation of the compound motor action potential (CMAP) amplitude. At high rates of repetitive stimulation, there may be an incremental response. SFEMG is markedly abnormal in virtually all patients with LEMS. The pathogenesis involves autoantibodies directed against voltage-gated calcium channels at cholinergic nerve terminals. These IgG antibodies also inhibit cholinergic synapses of the autonomic nervous system. Over 90% of LEMS patients demonstrated these antibodies to voltage-gated calcium channels in serum, providing another useful diagnostic test.

C. Treatment.

1. In patients with associated malignancy, successful treatment of the tumor can lead to improvement in the LEMS symptoms if the malignancy is successfully treated.

2. Symptomatic improvement in neuromuscular transmission may occur with the use of CEIs such as pyridostigmine.

3. 3,4-Diaminopyridine (DAP) increases ACh release by blocking voltage-dependent potassium conductance and thereby prolonging depolarization at the nerve terminal and enhancing the voltage-dependent calcium influx. 3,4-DAP has been shown to clearly improve most patients with LEMS with relatively mild toxicity and is becoming increasingly available, such that it represents first-line symptomatic therapy for LEMS. The typical beginning dose is 10 mg every 4 to 6 hours with gradual increase as needed up to a maximum of 100 mg/day. 3,4-DAP base and 3,4-DAP phosphate salt (amifampridine) two preparations.

4. Immunosuppressive therapy is used in patients with disabling symptoms. Long-term high-dose corticosteroids, plasma exchange, and IVIG have all been used with moderate success. In general, the use of these therapies should be tailored to the severity of patient's symptoms.

BOTULISM

Consumption of sausage spoiled by *Clostridium botulinum* resulted in an outbreak of this paralytic illness in the 1700s in Germany, leading to the name botulism, derived from the Latin term for sausage, *botulus*. Botulinum toxin blocks ACh release at the presynaptic motor nerve terminal (and causes dysautonomia by blocking muscarinic autonomic cholinergic function as well). The intracellular target of botulinum toxin appears to be a protein of the ACh vesicle membrane. The toxin is a zinc-dependent protease that cleaves protein components of the neuroexocytosis apparatus.

A. **Classic botulism** occurs after ingestion of food contaminated by botulinum toxin. Eight different toxins have been identified, but disease in humans is caused by types A, B, and E.

Type E is associated with contaminated seafood. All types produce a similar clinical picture, although type A may produce more severe and enduring symptoms. In all three types, the condition is potentially fatal. Most cases result from ingestion of bottled or canned foods that have not been properly sterilized during preparation, especially "home-canned foods." Today's tomatoes used in home canning may have a low acid content and therefore may be more vulnerable for contamination. Foods cooked on an outdoor grill and then wrapped in foil for a day or two, creating an anaerobic environment, can lead to toxin production. Home-bottled oils should also be considered; in the case of children, honey may be contaminated.

1. **Clinical features** begin 12 to 48 hours after ingestion of tainted food. Bulbar symptoms including diplopia, ptosis, blurred vision, dysarthria, and dysphagia occur initially, and are followed by weakness in the upper limbs and then in the lower limbs. In contrast to the typical patient with GBS, botulism is sometimes said to produce an acute "descending paralysis." Severe cases result in respiratory failure, requiring mechanical ventilation. Botulism produces autonomic dysfunction, including constipation, ileus, dry mouth, and dilated pupils. (Note: Some of these signs are seen in most but not all patients; normal pupils do not rule out the diagnosis of botulism.)

2. Diagnosis. The CMAP amplitudes are typically low on the motor nerve conduction studies. Repetitive stimulation studies before and following exercise may show a decrement to low rates of repetitive stimulation and postexercise facilitation of the CMAP amplitude. It is wise to send both stool and serum specimens to the lab for detection of the toxin. The specimen is injected into the peritoneum of a mouse, while neutralized or inactivated specimen is injected as the control. If the mouse becomes paralyzed and dies, the diagnosis is secure. Toxin is found in blood samples 30% to 40% of the time, while stool samples have a somewhat higher yield (thus the need to send both). Newer polymerase chain reaction tests for the clostridial genes and ELISA identification of the toxin have been used to screen for the bacteria in food but are not widely available for clinical usage.

3. **Management** involves placement of the patient in the ICU and assiduous monitoring of pulmonary function every few hours. When the FVC falls below 15 mL/kg or below 1 L or if the patient appears to be having respiratory difficulty, intubation and mechanical ventilation are necessary.

   a. There is a **trivalent botulinum antitoxin,** but its use is inconsistent, in part because of adverse side effects that occur in about 10% to 20% of patients. There is evidence that antitoxin shortens the course of the illness, especially the one associated with type E. If a diagnosis can be made early, it may be worth using the antitoxin. Serious complications from antitoxin therapy include serum sickness (4%), urticaria (3%), and anaphylaxis (2% to 3%).

   b. The Center for Disease Control and Prevention (CDC) recommends administration of one vial of antitoxin for adult patients with botulism as soon as diagnosis is made, without waiting for laboratory confirmation; before administration of antitoxin, consider skin testing for sensitivity to serum or antitoxin. One vial of trivalent botulism antitoxin administered IV results in serum levels of type A, B, and E antibodies capable of neutralizing serum toxin concentrations in excess of those reported for botulism patients.

   c. Antitoxin packages, including instructions for skin or conjunctival testing for hypersensitivity, are available through the CDC and state health departments. Antitoxin neutralizes toxin not yet bound to nerve terminals and has circulating half-life of 5 to 8 days. Patients who do not receive antitoxin treatment show free toxin in serum for up to 28 days.

4. Clinical course. With aggressive support, the overall mortality remains about 5% to 10%, usually the result of respiratory or septic complications. The other patients improve over a period of several weeks to several months. In those who survive, the eventual level of recovery usually is nearly complete. Several years after the illness, some patients have subjective fatigue and autonomic symptoms including constipation, impotence, and dry mouth. Clinical recovery results from brisk sprouting of new motor axons from the nerve terminal with reinnervation of denervated muscle fibers.

B. **Infant botulism** is probably the most frequent form of botulism. The infant ingests the spores of *C. botulinum*, which lodge in the intestinal tract, germinate there, and produce botulinum toxin in the gut. Honey has often been implicated as the contaminated food in the infant disease (25% of honey samples may contain spores). In adults, the small amount of *C. botulinum* in honey appears inadequate to colonize the GI tract. The typical presentation is an infant between the ages of 6 weeks and 6 months of age who exhibits generalized weakness and constipation. The weakness may start in the cranial muscles and then descend, causing a weak suck, a poor cry, and reduced spontaneous movement. The cranial muscles are weak, with poor extraocular movements, reduced gag reflex, and drooling. Finding *C. botulinum* in feces validates the diagnosis. The toxin is usually not detectable in the serum. EMG studies can point to the diagnosis in 80% to 90% of cases. Infantile botulism can range from mild to severe. Management centers on observation and general support (including respiratory stability). The recovery is usually excellent and runs a course of several weeks to several months. For infant botulism, IV botulinum immune globulin (BIG) trials in California were completed in early 1997 demonstrating safety and efficacy of human-derived BIG (BabyBIG) and a reduced mean hospital stay from 5.5 to 2.5 weeks. BIG is Food and Drug Administration (FDA) approved and is available from the California Department of Health Services. Antibiotic use is not recommended for infant botulism because cell death and lysis may result in the release of more toxin.

C. **Wound botulism** occurs when toxin is produced from *C. botulinum* infection of a wound. The symptoms are similar to those of classic botulism except that the onset may be delayed for up to 2 weeks after contamination of the wound. The diagnosis is supported by EMG studies, demonstration of toxin in the patient's blood, or finding the organism in the patient's wound. Wounds that lead to botulism include direct trauma, surgical wounds, and wounds associated with drug use (such as IV and intranasal cocaine). The use of local antibiotics such as penicillin G or metronidazole may be helpful in eradicating *C. botulinum* in wound botulism.

Key Points

- Half of all MG patients present with either diplopia or ptosis or both and within several months 80% of patients have ocular involvement.
- 20% of MG patients have pure ocular disease, 20% have a spontaneous long-lasting remission, and 10% have thymoma.
- A recent prospective controlled trial has demonstrated clear benefit of thymectomy in the treatment of MG.
- Patients with MuSK myasthenia who are refractory to conventional first-line treatment respond disproportionately well to plasma exchange and rituximab.
- Patients with Lambert–Eaton syndrome present with fluctuating proximal lower extremity weakness, dry mouth, and absent muscle stretch reflexes and half of them have small cell lung cancer.
- The most effective first-line treatment for Lambert–Eaton syndrome is 3,4 diaminopyridine.

Recommended Readings

Aban IB, Wolfe GI, Cutter GR, et al. The MGTX experience: challenges in planning and executing an international, multicenter clinical trial. *J Neuroimmunol.* 2008;201–202:80–84.

Benatar M, Rowland LP. The muddle of mycophenolate mofetil in myasthenia. *Neurology.* 2008;71:390–391.

Gozzard P, Woodhall M, Chapman C, et al. Paraneoplastic neurologic disorders in small cell lung carcinoma. A prospective study. *Neurology.* 2015;85(3):235–239.

Ibrahim H, Dimachkie MM, Shaibani A. A review: the use of rituximab in neuromuscular diseases. *J Clin Neuromuscul Dis.* 2010;12:91–102.

Keogh M, Sedehizadeh S, Maddison P. Treatment for Lambert-Eaton myasthenic syndrome. *Cochrane Database Syst Rev.* 2011. doi:10.1002/14651858.CD003279.pub3.

Mehrizi M, Fontem RF, Gearhart TR, et al. Medications and Myasthenia Gravis (A Reference for Health Care Professionals) prepared for the Myasthenia Gravis Foundation of America. http://www.myasthenia.org. Accessed August, 2012.

Pasnoor M, Wolfe GI, Nations S, et al. Clinical findings in MuSK-antibody positive myasthenia gravis: a U.S. experience. *Muscle Nerve.* 2010;41:370–374.

Rosow LK, Strober JB. Infant botulism: review and clinical update. *Pediatr Neurol.* 2015;52:487–492.

Sanders DB, Hart IK, Mantegazza R, et al. An international, phase III, randomized trial of mycophenolate mofetil in myasthenia gravis. *Neurology.* 2008;71:400–406.

Sieb JP. Myasthenia gravis: an update for the clinician. *Clin Exp Immunol.* 2014;175:408–418.

Spillane J, Beeson DJ, Kullmann DM. Myasthenia and related disorders of the neuromuscular junction. *J Neurol Neurosurg Psychiatry.* 2010;81:850–857.

Spillane J, Ermolyuk Y, Cano-Jaimez M, et al. Lambert-Eaton syndrome IgG inhibits transmitter release via P/Q Ca2+ channels. *Neurology.* 2015;84:575–579.

Wolfe GI, Kaminski HJ, Aban IB, et al. Randomized trial of thymectomy in myasthenia gravis. *N. Engl. J. Med.* 2016;375,511–522.

Yuan J, Inami G, Mohle-Boetani J, et al. Recurrent wound botulism among injection drug users in California. *Clin Infect Dis.* 2011;52:862–866.

Zinman L, Ng E, Bril V. IV immunoglobulin in patients with myasthenia gravis: a randomized controlled trial. *Neurology.* 2007;68:837–841.

54

Therapy of Migraine, Tension-Type, and Cluster Headache

Amy R. Tso and Peter J. Goadsby

MIGRAINE THERAPY

Worldwide, migraine is the most disabling of all neurologic disorders and the sixth most common cause of disability overall. In addition to headache, migraine attacks may be accompanied by sensitivity to sensory stimuli, nausea, vomiting, and cognitive or emotional dysfunction. A range of theories have been advanced for migraine, including as a primarily vascular, inflammatory, or peripheral disorder, although migraine is now best understood as a brain disorder, with functional imaging studies consistently showing subcortical structures active in all stages of the attacks. Although many treatments exist, migraine-related disability remains an enormous burden on societies and increasingly diverse approaches targeting neuronal mechanisms have been investigated in recent years. Perhaps the most exciting development is the first class of migraine mechanism specific treatments that target calcitonin gene-related peptide (CGRP), which are now in phase III development.

Clinically, migraine has a wide spectrum of severity that is dichotomized by the number of days affected by the disorder per month into episodic migraine (<14) or chronic migraine (≥15). Accordingly treatment options range widely, and some patients may be successfully managed with nonpharmacologic approaches while others will fail outpatient treatments and require inpatient therapy.

NONPHARMACOLOGIC

A. **Avoidance of migraine triggers.** Migraine attacks are said to be commonly triggered by changes in physiologic state, for instance variations in stress, amount of sleep, frequency of meals, or in women with onset of menses. Lifestyle modifications to maintain a regular sleep, meal, and exercise schedule and avoidance of known triggers for a specific patient, such as alcohol or heat, can be beneficial. Some currently accepted triggers, such as light or sound, may indeed be features of premonitory phase photophobia or phonophobia, respectively, and with time may be less emphasized. Indeed there is a school of thought that has suggested trigger confrontation, an analogy with desensitization; much is yet to be done to establish the science of triggers.
B. **Acupuncture.** Multiple studies have examined whether acupuncture is effective for migraine prevention when compared to either no preventive treatment, sham acupuncture, where needles are placed but not in accordance with acupuncture principles, or proven pharmacologic treatments. Taken together, the evidence suggests there is no difference between true and sham acupuncture methods. Advocates would contend acupuncture is no less effective than pharmaceuticals; more data are required to settle this issue.
C. **Behavioral treatments.** Methods such as relaxation, biofeedback, and cognitive behavioral therapy, often used as an adjunctive treatment, have been shown to be useful for reducing migraine frequency in both adult and pediatric populations although the quality of studies varies widely.

PHARMACOTHERAPY

Migraine pharmacotherapy falls broadly into two categories: acute treatment of attacks as they occur and preventive therapy, which has the primary goal of reducing attack frequency. For patients in whom attacks can be effectively aborted without medication overuse, preventive therapy may not be necessary.

A. **Acute attack treatments (Table 54.1).** Acute treatments are taken at the onset of an attack to abort the headache, or at least reduce the severity. However, regular, frequent use of acute attack medications ("medication overuse") in a patient with underlying migraine may increase the frequency of attacks. The biologic basis for this is not fully understood but may be related to alterations in receptor physiology, including agonist-induced tachyphylaxis, particularly in the endogenous nociceptive and descending pain control pathways. Functional neuroimaging studies of migraineurs with medication overuse have demonstrated hypometabolism in areas involved in pain processing and the orbitofrontal cortex that normalize after withdrawal of the overused substances. Medication-overuse headache (MOH) is defined in the *International Classification of Headache Disorders-III beta (ICHD-3β)* as headache occurring on 15 or more days per month for more than 3 months as a consequence of medication overuse, which is defined as 10 or 15 days per month or more, depending on the agent. Thus, appropriate selection and restricted use of acute treatments is an important principle in migraine therapy.

1. **Simple analgesics.** This category includes medications with nonspecific pain efficacy, that is, may be used to treat pain other than headache. These medications are the first line of acute migraine treatment and many are available without a prescription. *ICHD-3β* defines overuse of these medications as 15 or more days per month. Acetaminophen 1,000 mg may be used for acute treatment without the gastrointestinal adverse effects of nonsteroidal anti-inflammatory drugs (NSAIDs). Acetaminophen is safe to use in anticoagulated patients or those with peptic ulcer or renal disease, and is the safest option for acute migraine treatment during pregnancy. The main contraindication for use is liver disease or active alcoholism. Aspirin 900 mg can be an effective acute attack treatment, if tolerated, and is often used with an antiemetic, such as metoclopramide or ondansetron. Aspirin has similar gastrointestinal problems to those of the NSAIDs below.

2. **Nonsteroidal anti-inflammatories (NSAIDs).** NSAIDs exert their analgesic effect via inhibition of the cyclooxygenase pathways and include naproxen, ibuprofen, tolfenamic acid, and diclofenac. Naproxen has the longest half-life allowing it to be taken twice daily. Relatively higher doses (e.g., naproxen 500 to 1,000 mg, ibuprofen 800 mg) may be needed. The NSAIDs share a similar side effect profile, with gastrointestinal symptoms,

TABLE 54.1 Acute Treatments for Migraine. Mode of Administration Is Oral unless Otherwise Specified

Medication	Overuse[a]
Simple analgesics	
Naproxen 500–1,000 mg Ibuprofen 400–800 mg Aspirin 650–975 mg Acetaminophen 650–1,000 mg	15 d or more per month
Combination analgesics	
Acetaminophen/aspirin/caffeine Acetaminophen/dichloralphenazone/isometheptene	10 d or more per month
Headache-specific treatments	
Dihydroergotamine 0.5–1 mg (intramuscular, intravenous, nasal) Triptans (see Table 54.2)	10 d or more per month
Avoid if possible	
Opioids or opioid-containing compounds Butalbital-containing compounds	10 d or more per month

[a]As defined in the *International Classification of Headache Disorders-III beta (ICHD-3β)*.

such as dyspepsia and nausea, being the most common. NSAIDs are contraindicated in patients who are anticoagulated or have peptic ulcer disease, and may be contraindicated for patients with severe renal impairment, ongoing alcohol abuse, severe gastroesophageal reflux disease, or a history of gastric bypass or Nissen fundoplication. There is increasing evidence that long-term use of NSAIDs may increase the risk of heart attack or stroke.

3. **Combination analgesics.** Various combinations of NSAIDs, acetaminophen, caffeine, and aspirin are available and should be restricted to less than 10 days per month.

4. **Headache-specific treatments.** These medications are commonly referred to as "migraine-specific" therapy even though they can be effective for cluster headache. They are employed if simple analgesics and NSAIDs are not sufficiently effective at aborting attacks. In addition, various combinations of nonspecific and headache-specific analgesics are available both with and without a prescription. *ICHD-3β* defines overuse of these medications as 10 or more days per month.

   a. **Ergot alkaloids.** In the 19th century, ergotamine, and later in the 20th century, dihydroergotamine, were the first medications to be used specifically for acute migraine treatment. Both have a wide spectrum of pharmacologic activity at serotonergic, adrenergic, and dopaminergic receptors. Although effective, these medications are burdened by side effects, the most significant of which are nausea, vomiting, and vasoconstriction with a subsequent labeled contraindication for patients with coronary or cerebrovascular disease. Of historical note, the efficacy of ergotamine derivatives was attributed to their vasoconstrictor effects and the triptans were developed to retain this property with fewer side effects. Nowadays, ergotamine derivatives are not as commonly used as the better-tolerated triptan class. Ergotamine is available in oral, sublingual, and rectal formulations. Dihydroergotamine has intramuscular, intravenous, and intranasal formulations; in addition, an orally inhaled formulation is in late-stage development.

   b. **Triptans.** Triptans are serotonin $5\text{-HT}_{1B/1D}$ receptor agonists. Sumatriptan first became available in 1991; six additional triptans are now available that differ in their pharmacokinetic and side-effect profiles, which can be used to clinical benefit (Table 54.2). In addition, sumatriptan and zolmitriptan are available as a nasal spray

---

TABLE 54.2 Selection of Triptan Based on Clinical Scenario. Mode of Administration Is Oral unless Otherwise Specified

Insufficient response to other acute treatments
Sumatriptan 50 or 100 mg
Zolmitriptan 2.5 or 5 mg
Eletriptan 40 mg
Rizatriptan 10 mg
Problematic adverse effects
Almotriptan 12.5 mg
Naratriptan 2.5 mg
Frovatriptan 2.5 mg
Early nausea/vomiting or other absorption concern
Zolmitriptan 5 mg nasal spray
Sumatriptan 20 mg nasal spray
Sumatriptan 4 or 6 mg subcutaneous injection
Rizatriptan 10 mg orally disintegrating tablet
Rapidly intensifying attacks
Zolmitriptan 5 mg nasal spray
Sumatriptan 6 mg subcutaneous injection
Headache recurrence
Naratriptan 2.5 mg
Eletriptan 40 mg

and sumatriptan as an injection, which can benefit patients with significant nausea, vomiting, or attacks that intensify rapidly. In terms of efficacy, most triptans achieve a 2-hour pain freedom rate in the range of 25% to 40%. Common side effects include tingling paresthesias and warm sensations in the head, neck, chest, and limbs. Less common but perhaps more concerning to patients are chest-related symptoms-chest pressure, which can radiate into the arm, shortness of breath, palpitations, anxiety, or drowsiness. Triptans have vasoconstrictor actions mediated by their effects on the 5-HT_{1B} receptor, and thus also have a labeled contraindication for patients with coronary or cerebrovascular disease and for use within 24 hours of other vasoconstrictors such as dihydroergotamine. However, triptans are currently considered to exert their antimigraine effect via neuronal mechanisms, and in line with this, agents selectively active at the 5-HT_{1F} receptors (the "ditans") are being developed and have efficacy against migraine without vascular effects.

5. **Other abortive approaches.** A range of other approaches are used in Emergency Departments, or indeed in outpatients, for the treatment of acute migraine. Chlorpromazine has been used and there is some evidence for this treatment. Corticosteroids offer no better pain relief than placebo when they have been studied systematically. Nerve block procedures are used, including greater occipital nerve (GON) injection and other cranial nerve injections, although there is no systematic well-controlled evidence supporting the practice.

6. **In development: CGRP mechanism antagonists.** This is the first class of agents (the "gepants") to target a migraine-specific mechanism. CGRP is a peptide formed from alternative splicing of the calcitonin gene. CGRP is released into the jugular venous system after activation of the trigeminovascular system during migraine attacks. Serum CGRP levels are also elevated interictally in chronic migraine and to a lesser extent in episodic migraine. Finally, infusion of CGRP can trigger migraine-like attacks in migraineurs. Six CGRP receptor antagonists have been through at least phase II studies and each is reported to be more effective than placebo. Telcagepant and MK-3207 have had their programs terminated due to hepatic toxicity, while olcegepant has not been progressed as it is not orally bioavailable. Rimagepant and BI44370TA are not currently being developed, while ubrogepant (MK-1604) was effective in a phase II study and has moved to phase III studies. No data exist regarding the effects of overuse of this class of agents, although since telcagepant has been shown to be effective also as a preventive, it is entirely possible that medication overuse will not be a class issue. Supporting this conclusion, biologics targeting the same mechanism with long-lasting antagonism reduce attack frequency (see Section **B** under Pharmacotherapy). Importantly, CGRP receptor antagonists do not have vasoconstrictor effects and will not be contraindicated for patients with cerebral or coronary vascular disease.

7. **Opioids and barbiturates.** Barbiturates have no useful place in modern migraine therapy. Opioids may have limited uses in particular settings over the short term. These medications present several issues: first, they are the most prone to causing medication-overuse headache, particularly barbiturates. Second, they may render both acute and preventive therapy less effective. Third, frequent use often engenders tolerance or dependence, requiring escalating doses over time. Last, withdrawal of the offending substance in a patient taking high doses may not be possible as an outpatient, and access to an inpatient withdrawal program may be limited. In the case of opioids, clonidine may be useful for mitigating withdrawal symptoms. Barbiturates carry the additional risk of withdrawal seizures and may require a supervised taper to be safely discontinued.

8. **Antiemetics.** Nausea is often overlooked and is an important symptom to treat if present. Phenothiazine antiemetics (D2 dopamine receptor antagonists), such as prochlorperazine and chlorpromazine, have been shown in placebo-controlled trials to also be effective for headache. Possible adverse effects shared by most anti-dopaminergic medications include drowsiness, akathisia, dystonia, and prolongation of the QT interval at higher doses. Serotonin (5-HT_3 receptor) antagonists, such as ondansetron or granisetron, may be better tolerated. For patients with significant vomiting, sublingual dissolving tablets or suppositories may be useful.

B. **Preventive treatments (Table 54.3).** Preventive therapies are meant to reduce headache frequency and must be taken daily, except for onabotulinumtoxinA, which is injected every 3 months. The decision to initiate preventive therapy is individualized and may depend on

TABLE 54.3 Preventive Treatments for Migraine

Medication	Dose	Adverse Effects
Beta-blockers		
Propranolol	40–120 mg twice daily	Fatigue, exercise intolerance, orthostatic symptoms, can exacerbate asthma
Metoprolol	25–100 mg twice daily	
Antidepressants		
Amitriptyline	25–100 mg nightly	Drowsiness, dry mouth, weight gain, urinary retention, arrhythmias
Venlafaxine	75–150 mg daily	Nausea, drowsiness, dry mouth, arrhythmias
Antiepileptics		
Valproate	250–750 mg twice daily	Weight gain, nausea, hair loss, drowsiness, tremor; teratogenic
Topiramate	50–100 mg twice daily	Cognitive difficulties, tingling paresthesias, weight loss, metallic taste
Calcium channel blockers[a]		
Flunarizine[b]	5–15 mg daily	Drowsiness, weight gain, depression, and extrapyramidal symptoms
Candesartan	16 mg daily	Fatigue, dizziness; teratogenic
OnabotulinumtoxinA	155 units by PREEMPT protocol	Ptosis, neck pain; contraindicated during pregnancy
Nutraceuticals		
Riboflavin	400 mg daily	Brightly colored urine
Magnesium	600 mg daily	Diarrhea
Feverfew	6.25 mg three times daily	Rash
Coenzyme Q10	100 mg three times daily	Gastrointestinal upset

[a]Verapamil is commonly used in clinical practice but has insufficient supporting evidence.
[b]Not FDA-approved in the United States; widely used elsewhere in the world.

several factors in addition to attack frequency, such as the severity and disability associated with attacks, their duration and responsiveness to acute therapies, and the patient's willingness and ability to comply with the preventive medication regimen. Preventive treatment should certainly be considered if abortive use is increasing and especially if bordering on medication overuse. An important principle in migraine prevention is that an adequate dose is reached and maintained for at least 6 to 8 weeks before judging the efficacy. Currently, migraine preventives comprise a diverse group of medicines developed for other diseases; the arrival of the previously discussed antagonists targeting the migraine-specific CGRP receptor mechanism will be a welcome addition.

1. *β*-Adrenoceptor antagonists. Multiple agents in this class have randomized, double-blinded, controlled clinical trial data to support their use for migraine prevention. Propranolol and metoprolol are perhaps the most commonly used, although timolol, atenolol, and nadolol may be used as well. One small trial suggests that nebivolol may be effective. Beta-blockers should be avoided in patients with asthma, and used with good discussion in athletes.
2. Antidepressants.
   a. Tricyclic antidepressants. Amitriptyline is a serotonin and norepinephrine reuptake inhibitor and was first shown to be effective for migraine prevention in the 1970s. The tricyclic antidepressants also antagonize histamine and muscarinic receptors; side effects include drowsiness, dry mouth, and weight gain. Nortriptyline is a metabolite

of amitriptyline with different receptor binding affinities and is often better tolerated. Caution should be used in the presence of other serotonin-promoting medications (e.g., selective serotonin reuptake inhibitors) to minimize the risk of serotonin syndrome.

b. **Venlafaxine.** Venlafaxine is a selective serotonin and norephinephrine reuptake inhibitor (SNRI). Two clinical trials, one placebo-controlled and one crossover comparator study with amitriptyline, support its use for migraine prevention. The most common side effect in both trials was nausea.

c. **Other antidepressants.** Other antidepressants are sometimes used to treat migraine, but this clinical practice is not evidence-based as most have not been formally studied in blinded, randomized, controlled trials. Multiple trials of fluoxetine for migraine prevention have yielded mixed results and many are of poor quality; the overarching outcome is a lack of effect. Fluvoxamine has no placebo-controlled data but one study comparing it to amitriptyline found comparable efficacy. One placebo-controlled, crossover study supports the use of trazodone for prevention of pediatric migraine but no controlled data exist for adults. Other antidepressants including citalopram, escitalopram, and duloxetine only have uncontrolled, open-label data.

3. **Antiepileptic drugs.**

   a. **Valproate.** Both divalproex and sodium valproate have been shown to be effective for migraine prevention. Studies suggest that efficacy is comparable to propranolol or amitriptyline. Side effects can be troublesome and include weight gain, nausea, hair loss, drowsiness, and less commonly tremor. Valproate is teratogenic (neural tube defects in particular) and should only be used in women of reproductive age if a reliable form of contraception is used. Caution should be used in pediatric populations with underlying metabolic or mitochondrial disorders as hepatoxicity has been reported.

   b. **Topiramate.** Multiple large randomized, controlled, double-blinded trials have shown topiramate to be effective for prevention of both episodic and chronic migraine. Topiramate's mechanism of action against migraine is not fully understood, but it inhibits excitatory glutamatergic activity, enhances GABA receptor type A-mediated inhibition, and inhibits cortical spreading depression in animal models. Side effects include cognitive difficulties, tingling paresthesias, metallic taste, and in contrast to other migraine preventives, may suppress appetite and cause weight loss. Caution should be used in patients with a history of nephrolithiasis or glaucoma.

   c. **Gabapentin.** In the past, gabapentin was recommended for migraine prevention based on two placebo-controlled trials. However, full disclosure of the studies demonstrated they were both negative. In addition, a large, randomized, controlled trial of gabapentin enacarbil, a prodrug that is rapidly converted to gabapentin after absorption, was reported in 2013 and was negative. The case of gabapentin emphasizes the need for transparency of data from industry-sponsored trials and careful diligence by investigators to see the data from a study that is being reported.

4. **Calcium channel blockers.**

   a. **Flunarizine.** Flunarizine is a selective calcium channel antagonist with a long half-life of approximately 18 days. Although numerous randomized, placebo-controlled clinical trials have shown flunarizine to be effective for migraine prevention and at least as effective as propranolol, metoprolol, and pizotifen ($5\text{-}HT_2$ serotonin antagonist), it is not FDA-approved for use in the United States. It is widely used for migraine prevention elsewhere in the world. Side effects include drowsiness, weight gain, depression, and extrapyramidal symptoms with long-term use, likely owing to its antidopaminergic properties. It is particularly useful in hemiplegic migraine.

   b. **Verapamil.** Although verapamil is commonly used in clinical practice for migraine prevention, only two randomized, controlled trials exist and each included less than 15 patients. More data are needed to support or refute its use in migraine. Side effects include constipation and ankle edema.

5. **Candesartan.** Two randomized, double-blinded, controlled clinical trials have shown candesartan to be effective for migraine prevention, with efficacy comparable to propranolol. Side effects include fatigue and dizziness.

6. **OnabotulinumtoxinA.** Multiple clinical trials have shown onabotulinumtoxinA injections are not effective for episodic migraine. Two clinical trials (PREEMPT 1 and 2) demonstrated efficacy for chronic migraine, and only this group should be treated

with onabotulinumtoxinA using the protocol employed in these trials. The PREEMPT protocol consists of 31 injection sites in the head and neck totaling 155 units and is generally very well tolerated. Side effects include forehead weakness and possible ptosis or neck pain. Use is contraindicated during pregnancy.

7. **Nutraceuticals.** A number of naturally occurring supplements such as vitamins, minerals, and herbal extracts have been studied for migraine prevention. Two double-blinded, randomized, controlled trials have shown efficacy for butterbur, an extract from *Petasites hybridus*. However, this plant also contains hepatotoxic elements (pyrrolizidine alkaloids) that pose serious safety concerns. Riboflavin 400 mg daily, magnesium 600 mg daily, feverfew 6.25 mg three times daily, and coenzyme Q10 100 mg three times daily may be used for migraine prevention; although much of the clinical trial data have significant methodologic limitations, each of these has at least one positive double-blind, randomized, controlled trial. Nutraceuticals may be useful for patients who are hesitant to take prescription medications or are particularly prone to side effects.

8. **GON block.** The GON carries sensory information for most of the posterior aspect of the head and is derived primarily from the C2 dorsal root. GON blocks have been employed in the treatment of various headache types although its mechanism is unknown. Upper cervical and trigeminal afferents converge onto second-order neurons in the trigeminocervical complex which then project rostrally from the brainstem, and the effect of GON blocks may be mediated by modulation of this activity. The existing literature on GON blockade for migraine is difficult to interpret. Most studies are open-label and uncontrolled, and patient blinding is problematic since nerve blocks typically result in hypoesthesia in the affected distribution. Many studies have significant methodologic flaws, and in addition heterogeneous outcome measures are used, with some studies examining acute pain relief at 20 minutes and others examining reduction of frequency or severity at weeks to months. Likewise, methods vary considerably including the use of repetitive blocks versus single injections, the addition of corticosteroids to anesthetic or not, and unilateral versus bilateral injections. Despite the lack of definitive evidence supporting the use of GON blocks for migraine, many clinicians and patients feel they are useful and they are commonly utilized in clinical practice.

9. **In development: CGRP mechanism antagonists.** Inhibition of this mechanism (see Section **A** under Pharmacotherapy for more detail) is being targeted for migraine prevention in addition to acute treatment. Currently there are four biologics, monoclonal antibodies, in development, three aimed at CGRP itself and one at the CGRP (CLR/RAMP1) receptor and one small molecule CGRP receptor antagonist (atogepant). Initial results have been promising, and the success of these agents in phase III trials would mark the beginning of a new era in migraine therapy with the first migraine-specific target. Long-term safety data are needed, as CGRP may have important nonmigraine functions that are not yet known or understood.

C. **Inpatient therapies.** For the most refractory patients who do not respond satisfactorily to outpatient treatments, admission for a course of intravenous therapy may be useful. The literature on inpatient treatments is uncontrolled and observational; the most evidence exists for dihydroergotamine and lidocaine.

1. **Dihydroergotamine (DHE).** Repetitive dosing of intravenous DHE every 8 hours for 3 days for intractable migraine was first described by Raskin in 1986. Headache-freedom was achieved within 48 hours for 89% of 55 patients who had continuous headache for at least 2 months, with most reporting lasting benefit at follow-up. Two large, retrospective studies have since supported the efficacy and safety of DHE used in this manner, although one study was confounded by concurrent use of corticosteroids and nonsteroidal anti-inflammatories. The other study extended DHE administration to 5 days finding that higher total DHE dose produced a better outcome. Two studies show that good nausea control improves the outcome from DHE. Nausea is the most common side effect of DHE, requiring premedication with antiemetics.

2. **Lidocaine.** Two retrospective reviews have reported improvement in chronic daily headache, mostly migraine, with intravenous lidocaine infusion for 7 to 10 days. In one study, the majority of patients reported benefit lasting at least 6 months. The other study was confounded by concurrent use of intravenous DHE or corticosteroids as needed. Side effects include nausea, hypotension, psychiatric side effects, hallucinations, and arrhythmia.

3. **Valproate.** One uncontrolled study of ten chronic migraine patients found that repetitive dosing of intravenous valproate every 8 hours for 2 to 7 days led to improvement in eight patients.
4. **Lysine acetylsalicylate (aspirin).** For patients using high doses of acute medications such as opioids or barbiturates, admission may be necessary to provide a supervised environment in which to discontinue the overused agents with aggressive management of withdrawal symptoms. Cessation of the overused acute medications often results in worsened headache that is in itself intolerable to the patient, and for this intravenous aspirin may be useful. One gram of intravenous aspirin, given primarily for medication withdrawal headache in an inpatient setting, was moderately effective or better in 89% of 91 migraine patients and was well tolerated, even in patients with a history of upper gastrointestinal problems or NSAID intolerance.

NEUROMODULATION

For many patients, current pharmacologic therapies offer insufficient efficacy and a high rate of adverse effects. Neuromodulation is increasingly being explored for both acute and preventive treatment of migraine. Peripheral nerve stimulation has long been used to treat other types of chronic pain and was the first approach applied to migraine. Evaluation of such devices is plagued by blinding difficulties because nerve stimulation is perceptible and may produce paresthesias or pain. Transcranial magnetic stimulation (TMS) offers another approach to neuromodulation by using a fluctuating magnetic field to induce an electrical current in the underlying cortex which can either inhibit or potentiate cortical excitability depending on the frequency and pattern of stimulation used.

A. **Peripheral nerve or ganglion stimulation.** The mechanism by which peripheral neurostimulation impacts migraine is not known but may be related to the convergence of upper cervical and trigeminal afferents onto second-order neurons in the medullary trigeminocervical complex. These neurons then project rostrally in the brainstem and to the diencephalon, and are anatomic pathways by which peripheral afferent input might modulate central processes. The occipital nerves (upper cervical roots) and supraorbital nerves (ophthalmic division of trigeminal nerve) have been targeted for neuromodulation with modest results. The sphenopalatine ganglion (SPG) and vagus nerve are under investigation as new potential targets.

1. **Occipital nerve stimulation.** The multicenter ONSTIM trial examined occipital nerve stimulation using implanted leads as a preventive treatment for chronic migraine. The primary outcome was 50% reduction of pain severity, and there was no significant difference between the 105 patients randomized to active stimulation and the 52 sham stimulation patients. In addition, there was a high rate of device-related adverse events, with lead migration in 19% of patients and persistent pain or numbness at the lead site in 22%. The PRISM trial, available only in abstract form, and a third trial also did not show a statistically significant difference in primary outcome between groups.
2. **Supraorbital neurostimulation.** In the PREMICE trial, noninvasive supraorbital transcutaneous stimulation for 20 minutes daily with the Cefaly device reduced the number of monthly migraine days after 3 months of treatment when compared to a sham stimulation group. The treatment is remarkably well tolerated, with only 4.3% of over 2,300 users reporting minor adverse events and 2% discontinuing use.
3. **SPG stimulation.** The sphenopalatine gangnalion (SPG) is an extracranial ganglion located in the pterygopalatine fossa. Its postganglionic parasympathetic fibers innervate the lacrimal and salivary glands and blood vessels of the nasal mucosa, playing a central role in the cranial autonomic symptoms seen in both migraine and the trigeminal autonomic cephalalgias (TACs). Reversible blockade of this ganglion via electrical stimulation was first studied for cluster headache and appeared to have both acute and preventive effects, leading to exploration of its use in migraine. In a small pilot study, stimulation of the SPG with a temporary lead aborted or relieved migraine headache in 5 of 11 patients. An exploratory study in three patients with episodic migraine has gathered preliminary safety and efficacy data on an implanted SPG stimulator for both acute and preventive treatment of migraine (ClinicalTrials.gov NCT01294046), and a

trial for prevention in chronic migraine is underway (NCT01540799). A slightly different approach to SPG blockade with twice weekly, trans-nasal pharmacologic blocks did not find statistically significant differences between bupivacaine and saline groups within 2 hours of treatments or after 6 weeks.

4. **Vagal nerve stimulation.** Anecdotal reports of migraine improvement in epileptic patients treated with implanted vagal nerve stimulators led to two open-label, pilot studies for acute treatment of migraine using a noninvasive device held against the neck (GammaCore). Both have shown some efficacy for acute migraine treatment, and a preliminary trial investigating this device for chronic migraine prevention has been completed and was reported as negative in an abstract (NCT01667250). Adverse effects include paresthesias or redness at the site of device application, neck twitching, or raspy voice.

B. **Transcranial magnetic stimulation.** Two single-magnetic pulses delivered 30 seconds apart to the back of the head with the Cerena Transcranial Magnetic Stimulator at aura onset resulted in a higher rate of pain freedom at 2 hours (39% vs. 22% in the sham group) and sustained pain freedom at 48 hours (27% vs. 13% in the sham group). The Food and Drug Administration (FDA) approved this device for acute treatment of migraine with aura in December 2013 on the basis of this study. A similar but smaller product, the Spring TMS, is available for clinical use in the United Kingdom. The device is very well tolerated, with transient lightheadedness being the most common adverse effect reported in a postmarketing survey. Repetitive TMS is under investigation for prevention of chronic migraine (NCT02122744).

SURGICAL TREATMENT

Surgical procedures targeting extracranial nerves of the head and face, for example, branches of the trigeminal nerve or greater or lesser occipital nerves, are sometimes advertised to migraine patients for prevention. Options include nerve "decompression" via removal of overlying muscle or the nerve sheath, or even radiofrequency ablation or resection. Although reports of benefit have been published, no true randomized, double-blind, placebo-controlled trials of such procedures exist. Given the irreversible nature of many treatments and potential risks of anesthesia, such an approach does not seem warranted.

TENSION-TYPE HEADACHE THERAPY

The *ICHD-3β* defines tension-type headache as the absence of the features used to define migraine headache, requiring two of the following four: bilateral (vs. unilateral for migraine), nonthrobbing (vs. throbbing), mild or moderate intensity (vs. moderate or severe), and absence of movement sensitivity (vs. presence for migraine). Photophobia or phonophobia but not both may be present, and mild nausea is permitted only if photophobia and phonophobia are absent; the presence of either photophobia with phonophobia or nausea defines migraine. Appendix criteria define tension-type headache as having none of nausea, photophobia, or phonophobia; this definition sharpens the distinction and is recommended for clinical practice. Like migraine, tension-type headache is categorized as episodic (14 or fewer days per month) or chronic (15 or more days per month), with episodic tension-type headache further subdivided into infrequent (less than 1 day per month) or frequent forms.

In clinical practice, migraineurs often report also having headaches that phenotypically meet criteria for tension-type headache, and this is reflected in clinical trials for migraine which frequently include both migraine days and total headache days as separate outcomes. Ascribing two distinct biologic entities to explain the observed range of headaches, rather than viewing migraine and tension-type headaches as lying on a continuum in terms of severity and associated features, seems unnecessarily complicated. Notably, many migraine treatments are also effective for tension-type headache.

Patients with infrequent or low-frequency episodic tension-type headache often do not come to medical attention, as their symptoms can typically be managed with nonprescription analgesics. For patients with chronic tension-type headache, treatments that have randomized, double-blinded, controlled trials to support their use include amitriptyline, sodium valproate, stress management, and acupuncture (for prevention). If these are not effective, use of proven migraine treatments is a logical approach.

CLUSTER HEADACHE THERAPY

Cluster headache is one of the trigeminal autonomic cephalalgias (TACs), a group of primary headache disorders characterized by lateralized attacks of varying duration that may be associated with particularly prominent, ipsilateral cranial autonomic symptoms, such as conjunctival injection, lacrimation, nasal congestion or rhinorrhea, or ptosis. The TACs also share imaging properties featuring activation of the posterior hypothalamic region. Cluster headache is characterized by attacks of excruciating, unilateral pain typically lasting from 45 to 90 minutes but with a wider range of 15 to 180 minutes allowed, with attacks occurring from every other day up to several times per day. For most cluster headache patients, attacks are not always present; the periods during which attacks occur are referred to as cluster periods or bouts, with bouts typically lasting for weeks to months. The *ICHD-3β* defines episodic cluster headache as having at least 1 month annually without attacks; if attacks are present continuously or remissions are shorter than 1 month, the condition is chronic cluster headache. Periodicity is a hallmark feature of the disorder, with attacks frequently displaying a circadian pattern and, in episodic cluster headache, bouts often exhibiting a circannual pattern (Video 54.1).

PHARMACOTHERAPY

Similar to migraine pharmacotherapy, cluster headache treatments fall into two categories: acute treatment of attacks as they occur and preventive therapy which has the primary goal of ending the bout by suppressing attacks.

A. Acute/abortive treatments (Table 54.4). In general, the severity of cluster headache attacks intensifies too rapidly for oral formulations to be useful or practical. Inhaled or injectable treatments form the mainstay of acute cluster headache therapy, with high-flow oxygen and triptans being the primary treatments. In contrast to migraine, it is not clear whether frequent abortive use increases the frequency of cluster headache attacks. Conflicting reports describe chronic subcutaneous sumatriptan use both with and without a subsequent increase in attack frequency; some were confounded by the withdrawal of prophylactic agents immediately prior. In a retrospective review of 430 cluster headache patients, 4% described chronic daily headache associated with medication overuse, nearly all of whom had a personal or family history of migraine. In addition, tachyphylaxis does not appear to be of significant concern for acute cluster headache treatment.

1. High-flow oxygen inhalation. Although reports of oxygen inhalation to treat cluster headache attacks had existed for decades, it was not systematically studied until 1981, albeit in an unblinded fashion. Delivery of 100% oxygen at 7 L/minute by face mask for 15 minutes aborted attacks in 75% of patients. A crossover comparison with sublingual ergotamine showed comparable efficacy and faster onset of relief with oxygen. A small,

---

TABLE 54.4 Acute Treatments for Cluster Headache

100% oxygen inhalation (minimum 12 L/min, non-rebreather face mask)
Triptans
  Sumatriptan 6 mg subcutaneous injection
  Sumatriptan 20 mg nasal spray
  Zolmitriptan 5 or 10 mg nasal spray
Intranasal Lidocaine 10% solution (applied by swab near sphenopalatine ganglion)
Octreotide 100 μg subcutaneous injection
Sphenopalatine ganglion electrical stimulation for 15 min

double-blinded, crossover study of pure oxygen versus compressed room air corroborated oxygen's abortive effect, which was later confirmed by a large randomized, double-blinded, crossover study of 100% oxygen at 12 L/minute by non-rebreather face mask for 15 minutes. A small double-blinded, crossover study showed no difference between pure oxygen and normoxic air given under hyperbaric conditions. High-flow oxygen can be used repetitively without adverse effects and is relatively free of medical contraindications given the short duration of use, which is of particular benefit to patients with several attacks per day.

2. Triptans. Sumatriptan and zolmitriptan have randomized, double-blinded, placebo-controlled data showing efficacy for acute treatment in both episodic and chronic cluster headache. The efficacy of subcutaneous injection of sumatriptan 6 mg was reported in 1991, which offered considerable convenience and portability advantages over oxygen tanks. Subsequently, both sumatriptan 20 mg nasal spray and zolmitriptan 5 and 10 mg nasal spray were shown to be effective, offering cluster headache patients additional options with cost and tolerability advantages. Zolmitriptan 10 mg tablet was also shown to be effective for aborting cluster attacks but only met the primary endpoint in patients with episodic cluster headache. Patients are generally advised to limit triptan use to no more than twice daily given their vasoconstrictor effects.

3. Ergot derivatives. Only one placebo-controlled, crossover trial has examined intranasal dihydroergotamine (DHE) 1 mg for acute treatment of cluster headache. It found that DHE reduced the intensity but not duration of attacks. Of note, this trial used a smaller dose than is typically used for migraine (4 mg). Other outpatient delivery methods of DHE have not been formally studied for cluster headache. Historically, oral, sublingual, inhaled, or intravenous formulations of ergotamine were used to treat cluster headache, but reports of their efficacy were open label and uncontrolled. Given the medical contraindications and side effects, ergotamine has generally been abandoned in favor of treatments with better evidence and tolerability.

4. Intranasal lidocaine. Two open-label series in the 1980s reported that lidocaine 4% solution applied as drops intranasally, targeting the pterygopalatine fossa, was effective at aborting nitroglycerin-induced and spontaneous cluster attacks. A larger series using sprays of lidocaine solution had more modest results. A small double-blinded study comparing lidocaine 10% solution to saline, applied by nasal swab targeting the pterygopalatine fossa, found lidocaine to be significantly more effective but required a mean of 37 minutes to fully abort an attack.

5. Subcutaneous octreotide. During a cluster attack, calcitonin gene-related peptide and vasoactive intestinal polypeptide are released; somatostatin is an endogenous peptide that inhibits their release. Subcutaneous injection of octreotide, a somatostatin analog with a longer half-life, was shown in a double-blinded, two-attack crossover study to be more effective than placebo for acute treatment of cluster headache.

B. Preventive/prophylactic treatments (Table 54.5). Preventive treatment for cluster headache has the goal of suppressing attacks and either terminating the bout or reducing the frequency of attacks. Verapamil, the first-line cluster headache preventive therapy, requires a slow titration and thus other short-term preventive treatments may be used in combination.

1. Short-term prevention.
   a. GON block. The preventive effect of GON block in cluster headache was first reported by Anthony in 1985. Subsequent open-label studies of GON block with steroids, some with the addition of local anesthetic, have had variable outcomes. Two randomized, double-blinded, controlled studies including both episodic and chronic cluster headache patients have examined suboccipital steroid injections for cluster headache prophylaxis. The first study compared betamethasone with a small amount (0.5 mL) of lidocaine to saline with lidocaine and found that attacks ceased within 5 days for 12 of 13 patients in the steroid group; 9 of 13 remained attack-free 4 weeks after injection. In contrast, 0 of 10 patients injected with saline and anesthetic were attack-free 1 week and 4 weeks after treatment. The second study compared a total of three injections of cortivazol, a potent and long-acting steroid, versus saline when given every 2 to 3 days as add-on preventive therapy, most commonly in conjunction with verapamil. The baseline attack frequency was higher in this study, and it showed

TABLE 54.5 **Preventive Treatments for Cluster Headache**

Medication	Adverse Effects
Short-term	
Suboccipital steroid injections, with or without local anesthetic	Alopecia at injection site
Corticosteroids[a]—best used as a short taper in conjunction with a long-term preventive	Dyspepsia, nausea, hyperglycemia, euphoria, insomnia, avascular bone necrosis
Long-term	
Verapamil 240–960 mg daily, split into three times daily dosing	Arrhythmias (particularly heart block) with frequent ECG monitoring required, constipation, edema
Lithium 600–1,200 mg daily, split into three times daily dosing (monitor serum level)	nausea, thirst, tremor, dysarthria, confusion, ataxia; nephrogenic diabetes insipidus and hypothyroidism with long-term use
Melatonin 10 mg nightly (episodic only)	Daytime drowsiness
Topiramate[a] 50–200 mg daily	Cognitive difficulties, tingling paresthesias, weight loss
Methysergide[b] 1–4 mg three times daily	Rare but serious fibrosis (retroperitoneal, pulmonary, cardiac), nausea, vasoconstriction
Neuromodulation[a]	
Hypothalamic deep brain stimulation	Intracerebral hemorrhage, death, diplopia
Occipital nerve stimulation	Side-switch of attacks with unilateral stimulation, infection, lead migration, recurrent surgery for battery replacement
Spenopalatine ganglion stimulation	Facial dysesthesia or hypoesthesia, infection, lead revision

[a]No randomized, double-blinded, controlled trials.
[b]No longer available in the United States, but sometimes used in other countries.

a significantly greater reduction in mean attack frequency and sumatriptan usage for 15 days after treatment in the steroid group.

b. Corticosteroids. High-quality evidence supporting the use of corticosteroids in cluster headache is lacking. Several open-label and uncontrolled studies suggested an effect but had wide variability in the dose, formulation, and duration of corticosteroid use. Some studies have demonstrated a recurrence of attacks upon discontinuation of steroids in as little as 2 days, and corticosteroids are necessarily for short-term use only given their multiple adverse effects with prolonged use. Thus, steroids are best used in conjunction with a long-term preventive therapy to provide initial relief. A randomized, double-blinded, placebo-controlled trial of prednisone as add-on therapy to verapamil for episodic cluster headache is underway in Germany (PredCH).

2. Long-term prevention.

a. Verapamil. Open-label reports on the efficacy of verapamil for cluster headache prophylaxis led to two randomized, double-blinded trials. A crossover study in chronic cluster headache patients comparing 8 weeks of treatment with verapamil 120 mg three times daily or lithium 300 mg three times daily, the standard of care at the time, with 2-week washout (placebo) periods, found both to be efficacious in reducing attack frequency and analgesic use. Verapamil had a shorter latency period and fewer side effects. A parallel-group study in episodic cluster headache showed verapamil 120 mg three times daily for 2 weeks to be more effective than placebo in reducing attack frequency. Verapamil is the first-line preventive therapy for cluster headache, and the dose may need to be increased to a maximum of 960 mg daily to achieve full effect. Electrocardiographic (ECG) abnormalities are the primary safety concern, and in a retrospective review of 108 cluster headache patients who had taken verapamil, arrhythmias were present in 19%. First-degree heart block was the most common finding (62% of the abnormalities), but second-degree heart block, junctional rhythm, and right bundle branch block were also seen. Patients with arrhythmias were not taking higher doses of verapamil than those without. In another retrospective study of 29 patients taking verapamil 720 mg daily or higher, 14% presented with first-, second-, or third-degree heart block. Both series reported cases of heart block appearing years after reaching a stable verapamil dose. Thus, patients on verapamil therapy must be closely monitored with ECGs throughout the duration of therapy. Other common side effects include fatigue, constipation, and ankle edema.

b. **Lithium.** Lithium's use in cluster headache was inspired by its efficacy in other diseases with a marked cyclical nature such as bipolar disorder, and it was first reported to be effective for three cluster headache patients by Ekbom in 1974. Numerous open-label case series subsequently corroborated its effect, suggesting in sum that lithium is more effective for chronic cluster headache than episodic, that its therapeutic effect can begin within days and likewise withdrawal of the medication can result in rapid worsening, and that its effect may wane with long-term use although tolerance was an inconsistent finding. Lithium has been studied in two randomized, double-blinded studies including the aforementioned crossover study with verapamil in chronic cluster headache patients showing comparable efficacy. The other study attempted to compare 1 week of slow-release lithium 800 mg daily to placebo in episodic cluster headache patients, but assumed zero placebo response which proved to be untrue, rendering the study underpowered for drawing any conclusions. Lithium 600 to 1,200 mg daily can be used for cluster headache prevention and is typically titrated to a serum concentration between 0.4 and 0.8 mEq/L or to cessation of attacks. Lithium has a narrow therapeutic window and possible side effects include nausea, thirst, tremor, dysarthria, confusion, and ataxia. Renal and thyroid function tests prior to treatment are necessary as long-term use may cause nephrogenic diabetes insipidus and hypothyroidism.

c. **Melatonin.** One small, randomized, double-blinded, placebo-controlled trial of melatonin 10 mg nightly suggested that melatonin may reduce attack frequency in patients with episodic cluster headache.

d. **Topiramate.** All studies examining topiramate for cluster headache prevention have been open-label and uncontrolled. While initial reports suggested a response, the largest series of 36 patients found no difference in attack frequency after 20 days of treatment.

e. **Methysergide.** Methysergide is a serotonin antagonist that is no longer available in the United States due to its risk of fibrosis with long-term use, primarily retroperitoneal although pulmonary and cardiac effects have also been seen. In other countries, it is still sometimes used for cluster headache not responsive to other preventives; to minimize risk of fibrosis, a 1-month drug holiday should be taken every 6 months.

f. **Intranasal capsaicin and civamide.** Two studies have reported on intranasal capsaicin for prevention of cluster headache. One reported a decrease in severity but not frequency of attacks in the week following 1 week of treatment, and the other reported a decrease in attack frequency for 2 months following intranasal capsaicin ipsilateral but not contralateral to the side of pain. Intranasal civamide, a synthetic isomer of capsaicin, was found to reduce attack frequency compared to vehicle placebo, but only in the first week after treatment. These treatments are not recommended for routine use.

C. **Inpatient treatment.** Two series have reported improvement in cluster headache attack frequency after repetitive dosing of intravenous dihydroergotamine (DHE) every 8 hours for 2 to 6 days, with headache-freedom achieved during treatment in nearly all patients. In both series, improvement in attack frequency lasted for months in a subset of patients.

NEUROMODULATION

A. **Deep brain stimulation (DBS).** Hypothalamic DBS was first reported to be effective at reducing attack frequency in a case of chronic cluster headache in 2001. The posterior hypothalamus was chosen as a target based on functional and structural imaging studies showing alterations in this region and the clinical features of circadian and circannual periodicity, functions attributed to the hypothalamus. A number of open-label series subsequently supported the long-term preventive efficacy of hypothalamic DBS in refractory chronic cluster headache patients. However, a randomized, double-blinded, crossover study did not find a difference in attack frequency between active and sham stimulation periods; this may have been due to a short treatment period. Nonetheless, when also considering that one patient in Belgium died from intracerebral hemorrhage along the electrode track, DBS has largely been abandoned in favor of less invasive approaches.

B. **Occipital nerve stimulation.** Occipital nerve stimulation has been explored as a safer neuromodulation option for prevention of cluster headache. Several series have reported improvement in medically refractory chronic cluster headache patients, with two-thirds of patients in the worldwide literature experiencing at least 50% reduction in attack frequency. All have been open-label and uncontrolled, and blinding presents considerable methodologic difficulty since effective occipital nerve stimulation produces paresthesias. The therapeutic effect takes weeks or months to appear and can be long-lasting, although attacks recur within days if the stimulation is discontinued. Bilateral lead implantation is recommended as side-shift of attacks can occur with unilateral treatment. The main adverse effects are related to hardware, including immediate or delayed infection requiring lead or battery explantation, lead migration, or additional surgery for battery replacement.

C. **SPG stimulation.** The SPG sits extracranially in the pterygopalatine fossa and its postganglionic, parasympathetic fibers serve as the major outflow pathway for the cranial autonomic symptoms that are a clinical hallmark of the TACs. It has been targeted with pharmacologic blocks with transient results. Radiofrequency ablation of the SPG in chronic cluster headache patients resulted in sustained improvement in frequency and intensity of attacks. Nondestructive functional inhibition can be achieved with electrical stimulation. A small series examining SPG stimulation with a temporary lead for acute treatment of both spontaneous and triggered cluster headache attacks resulted in complete relief within 3 minutes for 11 of 18 attacks, with at least 50% relief in another three attacks. A multicenter, randomized, sham-controlled, multiple-attack study (Pathway CH-1) examined an implanted, remote control-activated SPG microstimulator as an acute treatment in chronic cluster headache patients. Pain relief after 15 minutes of treatment was achieved in 67% of attacks, with pain freedom achieved in 34% of attacks, compared with 7% and 2% of attacks, respectively, after sham stimulation. In addition, an unexpected preventive effect was seen, with 12 of 28 patients experiencing at least 50% reduction in attack frequency. A similar study is underway in a larger population of chronic cluster headache patients (Pathway CH-2, ClinicalTrials.gov NCT02168764). SPG stimulation is minimally invasive, relatively safe, and its potential as an acute treatment without daily usage limits that has concurrent preventive effects is an exciting development for a population in dire need of additional treatment options.

D. **Vagus nerve stimulation.** A preliminary, open-label, observational study of a noninvasive vagus nerve stimulator has suggested benefit for both acute and preventive treatment of cluster headache, warranting further study with randomized, controlled trials.

SURGICAL TREATMENT

Surgical treatments for chronic cluster headache patients comprise a range of approaches to disrupt or destroy either trigeminal sensory or cranial parasympathetic fibers. These include glycerol application, radiofrequency ablation, or gamma knife surgery to the trigeminal ganglion or nerve or SPG. With trigeminal procedures affecting the V1 distribution, corneal anesthesia is a major issue that can lead to abrasions, ulcerations, and visual loss. Facial dysesthesias, sometimes painful, can also occur.

In contrast to neuromodulatory approaches, bilateral destructive procedures are not recommended given the significant ophthalmologic risks. Studies supporting these procedures are often small, uncontrolled, and without long-term follow-up. Given the many new therapies and approaches, destructive procedures cannot be recommended.

Key Points

- Migraine is highly prevalent and the most disabling of neurologic disorders.
- Migraine therapy is divided into acute treatment of attacks as they occur and preventive therapy which has the goal of reducing attack frequency.
- Regular, frequent use of acute medications ("medication overuse") can increase migraine frequency; appropriate selection and limitation of abortive use is of utmost importance.
- Finding an effective migraine preventive may take time, as each medication should be trialed at an adequate dose for at least 2 months.
- Tension-type headache can often be managed with over-the-counter analgesics as needed. Tension-type headaches that are frequent enough to require preventive therapy can be treated with migraine preventives.
- Cluster headache is characterized by excruciating, unilateral attacks often associated with prominent, ipsilateral cranial autonomic symptoms. High-flow oxygen and injectable or inhaled triptans are the mainstay of acute therapy. Preventive therapy to suppress attacks may require a combination of short- and long-term strategies.
- Neuromodulation is an area of increasing interest and development for treatment of primary headache disorders.

Recommended Reading

Akerman S, Holland PR, Lasalandra MP, et al. Oxygen inhibits neuronal activation in the trigeminocervical complex after stimulation of trigeminal autonomic reflex, but not during direct dural activation of trigeminal afferents. *Headache*. 2009;49:1131–1143.

Ambrosini A, Vandenheede M, Rossi P, et al. Suboccipital injection with a mixture of rapid- and long-acting steroids in cluster headache: a double-blind placebo-controlled study. *Pain*. 2005;118:92–96.

Bigal ME, Serrano D, Buse D, et al. Acute migraine medications and evolution from episodic to chronic migraine: a longitudinal population-based study. *Headache*. 2008;48:1157–1168.

Bigal ME, Walter S. Monoclonal antibodies for migraine: preventing calcitonin gene-related peptide activity. *CNS Drugs*. 2014;28:389–399.

Cittadini E, May A, Straube A, et al. Effectiveness of intranasal zolmitriptan in acute cluster headache: a randomized, placebo-controlled, double-blind crossover study. *Arch Neurol*. 2006;63:1537–1542.

Cohen AS, Burns B, Goadsby PJ. High-flow oxygen for treatment of cluster headache: a randomized trial. *JAMA*. 2009;302:2451–2457.

Cohen AS, Matharu MS, Goadsby PJ. Electrocardiographic abnormalities in patients with cluster headache on verapamil therapy. *Neurology*. 2007;69:668–675.

Ferrari MD, Goadsby PJ, Roon KI, et al. Triptans (serotonin, 5-HT1B/1D agonists) in migraine: detailed results and methods of a meta-analysis of 53 trials. *Cephalalgia*. 2002;22:633–658.

Fumal A, Laureys S, Di Clemente L, et al. Orbitofrontal cortex involvement in chronic analgesic-overuse headache evolving from episodic migraine. *Brain*. 2006;129:543–550.

Goadsby PJ. Decade in review – migraine: incredible progress for an era of better migraine care. *Nat Rev Neurol*. 2015; 11:621–622.

Goadsby PJ, Sprenger T. Current practice and future directions in the prevention and acute management of migraine. *Lancet Neurol*. 2010;9:285–298.

Headache Classification Committee of the International Headache Society. The International Classification of Headache Disorders, 3rd edition (beta version). *Cephalalgia*. 2013;33:629–808.

Ho TW, Rodgers A, Bigal ME. Impact of recent prior opioid use on rizatriptan efficacy. A post hoc pooled analysis. *Headache*. 2009;49:395–403.

Holland S, Silberstein SD, Freitag F, et al. Evidence-based guideline update: NSAIDs and other complementary treatments for episodic migraine prevention in adults: report of the Quality Standards Subcommittee of the American Academy of Neurology and the American Headache Society. *Neurology*. 2012;78:1346–1353.

Magis D, Schoenen J. Advances and challenges in neurostimulation for headaches. *Lancet Neurol*. 2012;11:708–719.

Mather PJ, Silberstein SD, Schulman EA, et al. The treatment of cluster headache with repetitive intravenous dihydroergotamine. *Headache*. 1991;31:525–532.

Nagy AJ, Gandhi S, Bhola R, et al. Intravenous dihydroergotamine for inpatient management of refractory primary headaches. *Neurology*. 2011;77:1827–1832.

Orr SL, Venkateswaran S. Nutraceuticals in the prophylaxis of pediatric migraine: evidence-based review and recommendations. *Cephalalgia*. 2014;34:568–583.

Paemeleire K, Bahra A, Evers S, et al. Medication-overuse headache in patients with cluster headache. *Neurology*. 2006;67:109–113.

Schoenen J, Jensen RH, Lanteri-Minet M, et al. Stimulation of the sphenopalatine ganglion (SPG) for cluster headache treatment. Pathway CH-1: a randomized, sham-controlled study. *Cephalalgia*. 2013;33:816–830.

Silberstein SD, Holland S, Freitag F, et al. Evidence-based guideline update: pharmacologic treatment for episodic migraine prevention in adults: report of the Quality Standards Subcommittee of the American Academy of Neurology and the American Headache Society. *Neurology*. 2012;78:1337–1345.

Tfelt-Hansen P, Saxena PR, Dahlof C, et al. Ergotamine in the acute treatment of migraine: a review and European consensus. *Brain*. 2000;123(pt 1):9–18.

Treatment of acute cluster headache with sumatriptan. The Sumatriptan Cluster Headache Study Group. *N Engl J Med*. 1991;325:322–326.

Vos T, Flaxman AD, Naghavi M, et al. Years lived with disability (YLDs) for 1160 sequelae of 289 diseases and injuries 1990-2010: a systematic analysis for the Global Burden of Disease Study 2010. *Lancet*. 2012;380:2163–2196.

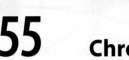

55   Chronic Pain

Troy Buck and Walter S. Jellish

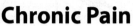

Chronic pain is often defined as any pain lasting more than 12 weeks. Chronic pain can persist for months or even longer. It may arise from an initial injury such as spine injury or any traumatic injury. However, there may be no clear underlying cause. Persistent pain is a serious health problem because it dramatically impacts the **economic, physical**, and **bio-psychosocial** well-being of society. Chronic pain is characterized by relatively ambiguous neuroanatomic pathways, mediating somatic effects. Transmission of information may perpetuate protective responses of limited adaptive value, especially to the extent that there is a lack of underlying tissue damage and/or decrease in avoidance of activity, inhibiting rehabilitation. Often, there is a protracted course of medication use and minimally effective medical services with marked behavioral and emotional changes including restriction in daily activities. In addition, there is an association between psychological distress and cognitive impairment in patients with chronic pain. The anterior cingulate cortex (ACC) appears to play a role in the cognitive induction of negative affect in depression. This area modulates emotional reactivity and contributes to an executive attention system and appears to be an integral component of the neural system that mediates the impact of pain-related emotional distress on cognitive function. Physiologic responses to repeated stress have also been related to changes in brain structure and function. An intriguing possibility is that anticipation of pain symptoms that are difficult to predict is a significant stressor that repeatedly activates the ACC area resulting in cognitive impairment. This chapter presents an overview of the classification and treatment of chronic pain states.

TYPES OF CHRONIC PAIN

The sensation of pain can be broadly classified into somatic, visceral, and neuropathic.

Somatic pain. This is the pain typically thought of when pain comes to mind. If you cut your finger or burn yourself on a hot stove, this is the type of pain you would experience. The pain is typically sharp and well localized, and in the acute setting, often associated with a reflex withdrawal of the affected area.

Visceral pain. Often associated with pain from an organ, the pain is often poorly localized and frequently described as dull and aching. Not uncommonly this type of pain refers into an area distant to the affected area (i.e., an irritated diaphragm resulting in shoulder pain).

Neuropathic pain. This type of pain is often the most unpredictable and difficult to treat. Neuropathic pain is often described as sharp, stabbing, and shooting, though the descriptors icy, achy, throbbing, squeezing, itching, or crawling are often used.

MANAGEMENT OF CHRONIC PAIN

Treatment may involve pharmacologic therapy, interventional options, and biofeedback.

A. **Medications.**

1. **Nonsteroidal anti-inflammatory drugs (NSAIDs).** These agents lead to analgesia via central and peripheral mechanisms. NSAIDs inhibit the arachidonic acid cascade, leading to decreased prostaglandins production. Patients may have varying responses to different NSAIDs. These drugs can be classified on the basis of their action against **cyclooxygenase I/II activity (COX)**. COX I/II nonselective agents include ibuprofen, naproxen, and piroxicam. Celecoxib is currently the only COX II selective agent available in the United States. Parecoxib, an intravenous COX II selective agent, is not currently available in the United States. Common side effects of NSAIDs include renal dysfunction,

gastrointestinal (GI) bleeding, and ulcer formation. The antiplatelet effects are not seen with celecoxib and other COX II selective agents.

2. Opioids. These drugs are either naturally occurring alkaloids or are synthetically produced. They function, to varying degrees, at opioid receptors in the central nervous system (CNS) and periphery. Opioids are classified on the basis of chemical structure. Opium plant derivatives (**phenanthrenes**) include morphine and codeine. Agents synthetically derived from the phenanthrenes (**semisynthetic**) are hydrocodone, oxymorphone, and oxycodone. Synthetic agents not derived from the phenanthrenes include the **aniliodopiperidines**, fentanyl, sufentanil, and remifentanil. The **phenylpiperidines** include meperidine and tramadol. The **phenylpropylamines** include propoxyphene, methadone, and loperamide. Pentazocine is a **benzomorphane**, **oripavane** (buprenorphine), and **morphinan** drugs include butorphanol and nalbuphine. Buprenorphine is an opioid receptor agonist/antagonist also used in pain management (Table 55.1).

TABLE 55.1 Opioids

Drug	Starting Dose	Goal Dose	Side Effects
Morphine (available in immediate release, continuous extended release, and elixir)	15–30 mg q4–6h immediate release	Use preparation with least abuse potential	Respiratory distress
Codeine (available in various combinations with acetaminophen)	15–60 mg P.O. q4–6h, not to exceed 360 mg/24 hr	Use combination agents that contain an anti-inflammatory to decrease opioid dose	Sedative, cognitive impairment
Oxycodone (also available with acetaminophen—percocet)	10–30 mg q4h	May utilize narcotic contract to control abuse	Liver dysfunction with long-term use
Oxymorphone	1 mg IV q4–6h		Testosterone deficiency
Hydrocodone (available with acetaminophen—norco, vicodin, lorbab, available with ibuprofen–vicoprofen)	1 tablet q4–6h, not to exceed 3–4 g of acet-aminophen q.d.		Tolerance
Fentanyl	Patch: start with 12 mcg q72h		Addiction potential
Meperidine	15–35 mg/hr IV		Withdrawal with cessation
Tramadol (also available in combination with acetaminophen)	50–100 mg P.O. q.i.d., max 400 q.d. if >75 yr, hepatic or renal dysfunction, max daily dose 200 mg q.d.		
Methadone and loperamide	2.5–10 mg q8–12h		
Pentazocin in formulation with aspirin and/or naloxone	1 tablet q4h p.r.n.		
Buprenorphine (also available in formulation with naloxone)	Variable with formulation		
Butorphanol	1–4 mg q3–4h by MDI		
Nalbuphine	10 mg/70 kg body wt 3–4 hr p.r.n. Total daily dose ≤160 mg q.d.		

Abbreviations: P.O., orally; p.r.n., as needed; q.d., every day; MDI, multi dose injection.

Preparations with the least abuse potential and side effects should be utilized. Agents containing an anti-inflammatory/acetaminophen, to decrease the dose of opioid required for analgesia, should be considered first-line drugs. Careful consideration must be given to the total daily dosage of acetaminophen/NSAIDS when using a combination drug. Common side effects of opioids include respiratory depression, sedation, cognitive impairment, liver dysfunction, and testosterone deficiency in men with long-term use. Tolerance, addiction potential, and withdrawal from sudden cessation are also common.

3. Antidepressants. Antidepressants are also utilized in chronic pain management. Mechanisms of action include a direct antidepressant effect, a decrease in synaptic transmission, and enhancement of the action of endogenous opioids (Table 55.2). Antidepressants are classified on the basis of their mechanism of action. **Tricyclic antidepressants** include amitriptyline and nortriptyline. Common side effects include dry mouth, sedation, sexual dysfunction, hyponatremia, and risk of withdrawal if discontinued. **Serotonin norepinephrine reuptake inhibitors (SSNRI)**, another class of antidepressants, include fluoxetine and duloxetine. Duloxetine is a **dopamine, serotonin, and norepinephrine reuptake inhibitor**. These drugs can be used for diabetic neuropathy and are contraindicated in patients with concomitant monoamine oxidase inhibitor (MAOI) therapy, hypersensitivity, and narrow angle glaucoma. Common side effects of SSNRI include dry mouth, constipation, orthostatic hypotension, weight gain, dizziness, unmasking of mania in bipolar patients, and risk of seizures in patients receiving tramadol. Other agents in this class include milnacipran, levomilnacipran, and desvenlafaxine. Lower doses of antidepressants are usually used for analgesia.

4. Antiepileptic drugs (AEDs). AEDs are also used in the treatment of chronic pain. AEDs **increase inhibitory neurotransmission, decrease excitatory transmission**, and **block ion channels**. AEDs are most effective for managing neuropathic pain (Table 55.2).

Phenytoin is used to treat diabetic neuropathy; treatment is initiated at 300 mg/day, with increased dosage as needed. Side effects include gingival hyperplasia, hirsutism, acne, and coarsening of facial features. Phenytoin activates the P-450 enzyme system in the liver, resulting in a decreased efficacy of mexiletine, haloperidol, and carbamazepine. Coadministration with antidepressants may lead to increased blood levels of phenytoin.

Carbamazepine is used for trigeminal neuralgia (tic douloureux), poststroke pain, postherpetic neuralgia, and diabetic neuropathy. Carbamazepine is believed to act via central and peripheral mechanisms, selectively targeting actively firing C and A delta fibers. Treatment is started at 100 mg twice a day and titrated to effect; typical dose range is 300 to 1,000 mg/day in divided doses. Side effects include gait imbalance, hyponatremia, leukopenia, aplastic anemia, and agranulocytosis. Because of these serious, though rare, side effects, carbamazepine is seldom used as a first-line agent for chronic pain. As a result of these potential hematologic alterations, blood tests are recommended every 2 to 4 months. Oxcarbazepine, an analog of carbamazepine, is less likely to cause CNS/hematologic alterations. Side effects include hyponatremia, sedation, and dizziness.

Lamotrigine prevents the release of glutamate in addition to blocking active sodium channels. Lamotrigine is used for cold-induced discomfort, trigeminal neuralgia, and diabetic and HIV neuropathy. Starting dose is 20 to 50 mg at bedtime, slowly increased to 300 to 500 mg/day in twice daily divided doses (over 2 weeks). A rash, the most common side effect, is commonly seen in pediatric patients, those receiving valproic acid, or patients receiving rapid titration of lamotrigine. The rash may also lead to Stevens–Johnson syndrome. Concomitant administration of carbamazepine and phenytoin leads to a decreased efficacy of lamotrigine.

Topiramate acts at both sodium and calcium channels, enhancing the action of gamma-aminobutyric acid (GABA) and inhibiting AMPA receptors. Topiramate is used in diabetic neuropathy, postherpetic and intercostal neuralgia, and complex regional pain syndrome (CRPS) (see Chapter 56). Initial dosing is begun at 50 mg at bedtime, increasing to 200 mg twice daily. Side effects include sedation, kidney stones, and acute-angle closure glaucoma. Another channel-blocking agent, levetiracetam, is started at 500 mg P.O. twice daily and adjusted to a target of 1,500 mg twice a day. Side effects include rash, hives, itching, and dizziness.

TABLE 55.2 Non-Narcotics

Drug	Use	Starting Dose	Goal Dose	Side Effects
Amitriptyline	Neuropathic pain	50 mg q.h.s.	150 mg q.h.s.	Sedation, dry mouth, impotence, hyponatremia, withdrawal, and possible dementia with long-term use
Nortriptyline	Diabetic neuropathic pain	25 mg P.O. q.h.s.	150 mg q.h.s.	Sedation, dry mouth, impotence, hyponatremia, withdrawal, and possible dementia with long-term use
Duloxetine	Diabetic neuropathic pain	60 mg q.d.	120 mg q.d.	Dry mouth constipation, orthostatic hypotension, weight gain, dizziness, unmasking of mania in bipolar patients, and seizure risk in patients on tramadol
Phenytoin	Diabetic neuropathy	300 mg/d	300–400 mg/d	Gingival hyperplasia, hirsutism, coarsening of features
Carbamazepine	Trigeminal neuralgia, poststroke pain, postherpetic neuralgia, neuropathy	100 mg b.i.d.	300–1,000 mg/d in divided doses	Gait disturbances, hyponatremia, leucopenia, aplastic anemia, agranulocytosis
Lamotrigine	Cold-induced pain, trigeminal neuralgia, neuropathy	20–50 mg P.O. q.h.s.	300–500 mg/d in divided b.i.d. doses over 2 wk	Rash, Stevens–Johnson syndrome, decreased efficacy with coadministration of carbamazepine, phenytoin
Topiramate	Diabetic neuropathy, postherpetic neuralgia, intercostal neuralgia, CRPS	50 mg q.h.s.	200 mg P.O. b.i.d.	Sedation, kidney stones, acute-angle closure glaucoma
Levetiracetam	Neuropathic pain	500 mg P.O. b.i.d.	1,500 mg b.i.d.	Rash, hives, itching, dizziness
Gabapentin	Diabetic neuropathy, postherpetic neuralgia, CRPS	100–300 mg q.h.s.	4,800 mg P.O. divided in t.i.d. dosing	Fatigue, somnolence, dizziness
Pregabalin	Neuropathic pains, fibromyalgia	50–150 mg/d	Max of 300 mg/d	Dizziness, blurred vision, weight gain, memory disturbance
Zonisamide	Neuropathic pain	100 mg/d	600 mg/d	Ataxia, rash, kidney stones, oligohydramnios, pediatric hyperthermia

Drug	Indication	Starting dose	Maximum dose	Side effects
ω-conopeptide	Cancer pain, HIV neuropathy	0–3–1 ng/hr		Sedation, tremor, hypotension, histaminergic reaction, psychosis
Baclofen	Spinal cord injury, spasticity	5 mg t.i.d.	80–100 mg/d in divided doses	Confusion, ataxia, hallucinations, life-threatening withdrawal
Tiagabine	Neuropathic pain, spasticity	4 mg q.d.	12–22 mg q.d. for patients not on epileptic drugs; 32–53 mg q.d. for patients one AEDs	Seizures, aphasia, sedation
Diazepam	Muscle spasms, spasticity	2 mg b.i.d.	20–30 mg q.d.	Sedation, dependence, risk of seizure, and death with withdrawal
Tizanidine	Muscle spasms, spasticity, spinal cord injury, poststroke pain	4 mg q.d.	Increase by 4–6 mg/wk to 36 mg q.d.	Headache, digestive changes, dry mouth
Cyclobenzaprine	Muscle spasms	30–40 mg q.d.	30–40 mg q.d.	Sedation, dry mouth
Chlorzoxasone	Muscle spasms	250 mg t.i.d./q.i.d.	1,000–2,000 mg q.d.	GI disturbances, liver dysfunction, sedation
Carisoprodol	Muscle spasms, spasticity	350 mg t.i.d./q.i.d.	350 mg PO. t.i.d./q.i.d.	Sedation, tremor, altered cognition, addiction potential
Methocarbamol	Muscle spasms	1,000 mg/t.i.d.	3,000–4,000 mg q.d.	Sedation, altered cognition
Metaxolone	Muscle spasms	800 mg t.i.d./q.i.d.	800 mg t.i.d./q.i.d.	Hemolytic anemia, elevated liver function tests
Orphenadrine	Neuropathic pain, muscle spasms	60–80 mg q8h	60–80 mg q8h	Orthostatic hypotension, urinary retention, dizziness, euphoria
Botulinum toxin	Dystonia, spasticity, migraine, torticollis, myofascial pain, GI, GU spasms	Varies based on site of injection		Myalgias, dysphagia, discomfort

Abbreviations: AEDs, antiepileptic drugs; b.i.d., twice a day; CRPS, complex regional pain syndrome; GI, gastrointestinal; GU, genitourinary; P.O., orally; q.d., every day; q.i.d., four times a day; q.h.s., every night at bedtime; t.i.d., three times a day.

5. **Local anesthetics.** Lidocaine, available in salve and patch (5%) forms, is used for postherpetic neuralgia, postthoracotomy pain, intercostal neuralgia, and fibromyalgia. The patch is used 12 hours/day and may be cut to size and shape. Lidocaine side effects include bradycardia, dizziness (at plasma level of 10 mg/mL), cardiac depression (at 20 to 25 mg/mL plasma level), blurred vision, and seizures. Mexiletine, an oral analog of lidocaine, is used for poststroke pain, myotonia, spasticity, and diabetic neuropathy. Treatment is initiated at 150 mg/day up to a goal of 300 to 450 mg/day. The side-effect profile is similar to lidocaine.

6. **Calcium channel blockers.** Gabapentin is a membrane stabilizer that binds at the alpha-2-delta subunit of the L-calcium channel (Table 55.2). Gabapentin is used for many neuropathic pain states including diabetic neuropathy, postherpetic neuralgia, and CRPS. Treatment is started at 100 to 300 mg at bedtime, increasing to 3,600 mg/day divided in three doses. Common side effects include fatigue, somnolence, and dizziness.

   Pregabalin also binds to the alpha-2-delta subunit at voltage-dependent calcium channels. Pregabalin is used for neuropathic pain states and for fibromyalgia. The starting dose is 50 to 150 mg/day titrated to 300 mg/day for neuropathic pain states; for fibromyalgia, the maximum daily dose is 300 mg/day. Side effects include dizziness, blurred vision, weight gain, and diminished cognition.

   Zonisamide acts at T calcium and sodium channels. This drug increases GABA release. Zonisamide is started at 100 mg daily and increased after 2 weeks by 200 mg/week for a goal of 600 mg/day. Common side effects include ataxia, rash, kidney stones, oligohydramnios, and pediatric hyperthermia.

   ω-Conopeptides (ziconotide) acts on N-type calcium channels. Used intrathecally at 0.3 to 1 ng/kg/hour, the drug has been studied in patients with cancer and HIV/AIDS. Side effects include sedation, tremor, hypotension, a histaminergic reaction, and psychosis. Nimodipine, diltiazem, verapamil, and nifedipine are calcium channel blockers that may have a role in association with other agents in pain management.

7. **Gabaergic agents.** Baclofen, a derivative of GABA with activity at GABA-b channels, has both spinal and supraspinal activity (Table 55.2). Baclofen is used for spinal cord injury and spasticity. Initial therapy begins at 5 mg three times a day with titration to a daily dose of 100 mg if necessary. Baclofen may also be given intrathecally. Common side effects include confusion, somnolence, ataxia, and hallucinations. Sudden cessation of therapy may lead to a potentially life-threatening withdrawal syndrome, particularly in the setting of chronic intrathecal administration.

   Tiagabine, a GABA reuptake inhibitor, is started at 4 mg daily and increased by 4 to 8 mg/day to a final goal of 12 to 22 mg/day for patients not on AEDs, or 32 to 52 mg/day for patients on AEDs. Common side effects include risk of seizures in patients without history of seizure disorder, aphasia, and sedation.

   Diazepam is a benzodiazepine and muscle relaxant that enhances the inhibitory action of GABA-A receptors especially in patients with spinal cord disease and muscle spasms. Diazepam is usually started at 2 mg twice daily to a total dose of 20 to 30 mg/day. Side effects include sedation and dependence; a withdrawal or sudden cessation may lead to seizures and death.

8. **Muscle relaxants.** Tizanidine is a centrally active alpha-2 adrenergic agonist used for spasticity, spinal cord injury, and poststroke pain (Table 55.2). Dosing starts at 4 mg/day and is increased by 4 to 6 mg/week to a total of 36 mg/day. Side effects include headache, indigestion, and dry mouth. Concomitant use of other alpha-2 agonists increases the risk of arterial hypotension. Cyclobenzaprine is a muscle relaxant that primarily acts at the brainstem, although it is not effective for centrally mediated spastic states. The dose is 30 to 40 mg/day and side effects include sedation and dry mouth. Liver function tests are recommended with long-term use.

   Chlorzoxazone is centrally acting with a target dose of 1,000 to 2,000 mg/day. Side effects include GI disturbances, sedation, and liver dysfunction. Carisoprodol is a muscle relaxant that acts centrally at the reticular activating system and the spinal cord. The treatment goal is 350 mg three to four times a day. Side effects include sedation, tremor, altered cognition, and possible addiction potential. Methocarbamol is used at

3,000 to 4,000 mg/day. Metaxolone is dosed at 800 mg three to four times a day; this drug may lead to hemolytic anemia and abnormal liver function tests.

Orphenadrine, an NMDA receptor antagonist with anticholinergic effects, acts via central and peripheral mechanisms. This drug is used for neuropathic pain and muscle spasms. It potentiates the analgesic effects of opioids. Orphenadrine is started at 60 to 80 mg every 8 hours. Side effects include orthostatic hypotension, urinary retention, dizziness, and euphoria.

Botulinum toxin acts at the neuromuscular junction and inhibits the release of acetylcholine presynaptically. Its effect lasts for approximately 3 months. This agent is used for dystonias, spasticity, chronic migraine, hyperhidrosis, myofascial pain, and GI and genitourinary (GU) spasm. Botulinum toxin should not be used in patients with neuromuscular junction or motor neuron disorders such as myasthenia gravis (MG), Lambert–Eaton myasthenic syndrome (LEMS), and amyotrophic lateral sclerosis (ALS). Side effects include myalgia, dysphagia, and local discomfort. The amount injected is tailored to the site of injection, degree of spasm and musculature being injected.

9. **Other agents.** Clonidine, an alpha-2 agonist that potentiates the analgesic action of opioids, is useful for managing neuropathic pain. A transdermal patch is started at a dose of 0.1 mg/day and changed every 7 days. Side effects include sedation, dry mouth, and orthostatic hypotension. Capsaicin, an extract of chili pepper, is thought to cause analgesia by depletion of substance P. Recent approval by the US FDA for an 8% topical patch has shown some success in the treatment of postherpetic neuralgia. Its application may lead to discomfort and irritation before analgesia.

Chronic pain states often differentially engage different types of glutamate receptors as the source, time course, and quantities of released glutamate and co-transmitters are different. Glutamate is released from central terminals in the spinal cord upon noxious stimulation activating amino-3-hydroxy-5-methyl-4-isoxazole propionic acid (AMPA). Prolonged activation of nociceptors from tissue damage evokes continuous release of glutamate that, in combination with co-released neuropeptides like substance P, causes long-lasting membrane depolarization. Presynaptic GLuR's localized on central terminals of primary afferents also play a role in segmental nociceptive transmission. These include kainate, NMDA, and some metabotropic GLuR. There are a great variety of GLuR's that can be used as targets for pharmacological intervention for the treatment of pain. The NMDA receptor has been considered an important target for the treatment of chronic pain. However, the use of clinically available NMDA antagonists is limited because of unacceptable side effects like psychotomimesis, ataxia, and sedation. These side effects appear to be related to the mechanism of action as they are observed with both channel blockers and competitive agonists. With channel blockers, the neurotoxicity is lower with low-affinity compounds (memantidine) compared to high-affinity drugs (MK 801). One of the most promising strategies to dissociate the analgesia from side effects is the development of the subtype NMDA antagonists ifemprodil and eliprodil that are highly selective for the NMDA receptor containing NR2B sub units. The reason for the low side-effect profile of NR2B selective NMDA antagonists is unclear. However, they have a restricted CNS localization pattern and are present in structures specifically involved in nociceptive transmission implying a stronger inhibition of the transmission involving greater receptor activation for chronic pain versus normal physiologic transmission.

Ketamine has also been used to treat various chronic pain syndromes, especially those with a neuropathic component presumably by inhibition of NMDA receptors, though other mechanisms could be involved including enhancement of descending inhibition and anti-inflammatory effects at central sites. Short-term infusions of ketamine produces potent analgesia during administration only, while prolonged infusions (4 to 14 days) showed long-term effects for up to 3 months. Side effects of ketamine include psychedelic symptoms, memory deficits, nausea, vomiting, somnolence, and cardiovascular stimulation. The recreational use of ketamine is increasing and additional risks including bowel and bladder and renal complications. In clinical settings, ketamine is well tolerated, especially when used with benzodiazepines. Close monitoring of patients receiving ketamine is mandatory, particularly aimed at CNS, hemodynamics, renal, and hepatic symptoms. Further research is needed to determine if benefits outweigh risks and costs. Until definite proof is obtained, ketamine use should be restricted to patients with resistant severe neuropathic pain.

AMPA receptor antagonists are a new class of drugs seemingly devoid of the typical neurotoxic effects of NMDA antagonists. A recent finding notes that antinociceptive doses of gabapentin, known to be useful for the treatment of neuropathic pain, selectively inhibit AMPA responses of dorsal spinal horn neurons. The use of selective glutamate receptor antagonists and NMDA blockers has been demonstrated to have high analgesic efficacy. The major problem with previous generations of these drugs has been side effects. The new classes of glutamate modulation have positive side-effect profiles, and continued research into these therapies is promising.

B. Nonpharmacologic treatments.

Physical therapy and occupational therapy. The use of heat, ultrasound, electrical stimulation, and deep tissue massage may reduce the discomfort associated with chronic pain states. Goals of physical therapy include: decreasing pain, improving range of motion, improving strength, and improving functional status. Patients should focus therapy in the plane of comfort: meaning if it is painful to flex the lumbar spine then extension-based exercises should be utilized, and vice versa. Therapy should also improve the pain rather than worsen it.

1. **Electrical stimulation** involves the use of either **transcutaneous electrical nerve stimulation (TENS), spinal cord (dorsal column)**, or **thalamic stimulators**. Patients with neuropathic pain states, muscular pain, central pain, and axial low back pain may benefit from these therapies. The classical "gate control" theory postulates that stimulation of large fiber (a beta) neurons closes the gate that has been opened or initiated by the smaller diameter nociceptors.

2. **Spinal cord stimulation** has become more refined and more widely used and is particularly useful in the setting of chronic neuropathic pain not responsive to more conservative options.

3. A trial initially performed before permanent implantation affords the patient the experience of the stimulation sensation and also to determine the level of pain relief before the more invasive permanent implantation. Most of the time, the trial is performed percutaneously during an outpatient procedure and left in for a period varying from 3 to 7 days.

4. **Transmagnetic stimulation** is a form of neuromodulation that potentiates or inhibits the transmission of nerve signals, but it is not the actual means of transmission itself. Transcranial magnetic stimulation is a noninvasive method enabling the stimulation of specific cortical areas by an electric current induced by a coil placed on the scalp. A rapidly varying electric current (1 ms) flows through a wiring system and creates an electromagnetic field that produces a current a few centimeters inside the brain parenchyma. This focused electrical current may depolarize neurons and creates evoked responses or changes neuronal plasticity. This repetitive transcranial magnetic stimulation (rTMS), especially when applied to the dorsolateral prefrontal cortex, has been found to be effective in treating major depression. Other studies have shown it to be effective in reducing pain especially if rTMS is performed at a high frequency of 10 Hz over the M1 and the current is delivered in a posterior/anterior direction. rTMS has been shown to be effective in reducing neuropathic pain in some individuals; the greatest effect has been noted with a figure 8 coil over the hand or face area of M1. There has also been a therapeutic effect of rTMS for fibromyalgia pain with treatment to the right M1 for 10 consecutive days, producing a long-term analgesic effect. rTMS has also been noted to be effective in reducing pain associated with CRPS. Patients are treated with pharmacologic and rehabilitation treatment as per standard practice with rTMS applied as additional treatment.

Mounting evidence suggests that stimulation of M1 and prefontal cortex activates distant brain areas. Electrophysiologic studies have shown that motor cortex stimulation has inhibitory effects on thalamic and spinal nociceptive neurons. M1 stimulation decreases the availability of opioid receptors in the periaqueductal gray area and the magnitude of pain reduction correlates with the availability of μ-opioid receptors. High frequency of >10 Hz stimulations seem to be the most effective in reducing pain. New rTMS paradigms have been proposed to increase the size and duration of long-term potentiation. One such treatment is theta-burst stimulation (TBS). This is based on studies suggesting that this pattern of stimulation is able to induce long-term synaptic changes. Various protocols of TBS are used consisting of a short burst of 3 TMS pulses with inner high frequency (50 Hz within the gamma range) that are delivered at 5 Hz (in the theta range). These different stimulation protocols have been noted to decrease overall pain at a higher percentage than standard rTMS techniques. The total number of pulses per session seems to be related to the net analgesic effects, but it is not clear whether a minimum number of pulses is required to obtain this effect and if there is a ceiling effect to this therapy. The major limitation of rTMS is the short duration of analgesia achieved with transcranial stimulation, and therefore the efficacy of this modality is not totally established in patients with chronic pain. Multiple sessions of rTMS and increased number of pulses per session have cumulative analgesic effects with long-lasting pain control in patients with chronic pain syndrome.

5. Interventional modalities can occasionally be useful in the setting of chronic pain. The modalities chosen need to be tailored to the individual patient and treatment goals. Constant evaluation/monitoring of the responses to these interventional modalities also needs to be undertaken, as repeated procedures can expose the patient to increasing risk.

6. Several types of steroid injections can be performed, depending on the suspected diagnosis. In general, whatever the injection being considered, it should be clear to patients that steroid injections do not cure the underlying pathology. Reasons to consider injections is to potentially help ameliorate the pain and to get the patient back to a reasonable level of function.

    While there is conflicting evidence on the efficacy of epidural injections in treating low back pain alone, the evidence does point to short-term benefits for relief in the setting of radicular leg pain associated with lumbar disc herniations. Advanced imaging is recommended before epidural injections, MRI being the preferred modality, though computed tomography (CT) scans of the lumbar spine can also be appropriate.

    Several other types of injections can be performed, depending on the diagnosis and the underlying pathology (see Video 55.1). Injections for low back pain include epidural injections (see Video 55.2), sacroiliac joint injections, lumbar facet injections, piriformis injections, quadratos lumborum injections, trigger point injections, and intaarticular hip joint injections (see Video 55.3). Again, similar to epidural injections, these injections do not cure or heal the underlying pathology.

    Sympathetic blocks have the potential to offer pain relief in specific subsets of patients. They also have the added benefit of being a diagnostic procedure in that they help differentiate sympathetically maintained pain from sympathetically independent pain (see Video 55.4). In general, sympathetic blocks are more effective in the long run if they are combined with a course of physical therapy or a home exercise program.

7. Peripheral nerve blocks can have some benefit in certain patients, particularly when combined with physical therapy or a home exercise regimen.

8. It should be noted that while most of the above-mentioned procedures are performed with the use in fluoroscopy as the imaging modality of choice, there is a gradual movement toward ultrasound as a modality used in conjunction with or independently from fluoroscopy. Ultrasound technology does show promise in the arena of interventional pain as it has the ability to show superior soft tissue structures including blood vessels, nerves and nerve roots. It also has the added advantage of not exposing the patient and practitioner to radiation during the procedure.

9. Psychological treatment is also an important component of the patient's overall pain treatment plan. A support network for patients, involving family and friends, may be conducive to the healing process. Additionally, the use of biofeedback along with adjunctive physical therapy may help a patient with their discomfort.

    Finally, the ultimate goal in the management of patients with chronic pain is the precise diagnosis with appropriate treatment for the painful condition. Referral to an interventional pain physician may benefit patients after conservative therapy has failed.

Disease processes difficult to treat, such as CRPS, diabetic neuropathy, and peripheral neuropathies, may be addressed with a specialist versed in providing interventional modalities along with pharmacotherapy. Physical therapy is also vital to the patient's treatment in decreasing discomfort. It is crucial to have honest communication with the patient about treatment goals, expectations, and the possibility of achieving those expectations.

10. **Hypnosis.** Training patients in self-hypnosis is an attractive component in pain therapy. Hypnosis incorporates relaxation, focused attention, imaging, interpersonal processing, and suggestion. Response to hypnosis treatment is highly variable. Recent studies use a 30% reduction in average daily pain intensity to represent clinically meaningful improvement in chronic pain states. Certain pain types respond to hypnosis better than others. In most instances, neuropathic pain seems to respond to hypnosis better than non-neuropathic pain. There is also a hypnotizability factor, which reflects a person's tendency or trait to respond positively to a variety of different suggestions following a hypnotic induction. One of the most important findings from recent neurophysiologic studies of pain is that there is no single "pain center" in the brain responsible for processing pain. Cortical areas most often activated during pain are the thalamus, ACC, insular cortex (IC), primary and secondary sensory cortices and prefrontal cortex. Hypnotic suggestion to reduce pain and unpleasantness influences activity in the ACC but not in other brain areas including the sensory cortex. It is also noted that cortical neurons fire at different frequencies and the speed at which they fire is associated with different brain states. Pain is associated with more neuron firing at relatively fast beta (13 to 30 Hz) frequencies and fewer neurons firing at slow alpha (8 to 13 Hz) frequencies. Hypnotic suggestion result in changes in brain activity consistent with those observed in individuals who experience pain relief (decrease in beta activity and an increase in alpha activity). Therefore, hypnotic analgesia may influence pain both by altering activity in specific areas and by facilitating shifts in general brain states. There are two current theories as to how hypnosis affects chronic pain. One is neodissociation where a state of effortlessness is thought to be associated with a shift in the control of responses from higher executive function to cognitive subsystems that have a direct influence on the behavioral responses with the usual layer of judgment or critical screening. Dissociation theories hypothesize that hypnosis involve a qualitative shift in the nature of cognitive processes. Hypnosis creates a shift from an active to a passive form of attention. These attentional shifts are associated with a reduction in the monitoring of control and the censoring experience. The sociocognitive model of hypnosis argues that the concept of an altered state is not required to understand hypnosis but that it is best explained by the same sociopsychological factors that explain all behaviors. Several mechanisms have been offered as important elements of hypnosis. These include relaxation, use of distracting imagery, focused attention, and expectancy. Patients who manage their chronic pain through mindfulness meditation training and therapies incorporating mindfulness are becoming very popular. In these approaches, efforts to directly resist or reduce chronic pain are thought to contribute to suffering, and having a direct goal of a reduction in chronic pain might decrease the quality of life in some patients. Hypnosis can be used to reduce pain; however, in many instances it serves as a tool to help patients better cope and accept their pain rather than seek to change their experience.

Hypnosis for chronic pain states has few negative side effects. In fact, with hypnosis most patients report positive side effects such as improved sense of well-being, greater sense of control, improved sleep, and increased satisfaction with life, all independent of whether they report reductions in pain. Hypnotic suggestion can target specific pain domains and outcomes as well as activities in specific brain regions.

Key Points

- Chronic pain is any pain lasting 12 weeks or more which may be secondary to traumatic injury, but in many instances there may be no clear cause.
- Pain may be somatic, visceral, and/or neuropathic. Somatic pain is typical pain that occurs after an injury. It is sharp and well localized. Visceral pain is often associated with organ pain. It is poorly localized, dull, and achy. Neuropathic pain is the most difficult to treat, could be sharp, stabbing but also described as achy, throbbing, squeezing, itching, or crawling.
- Chronic pain can be managed by medications. The most common of which are opioids which have side effects with possible tolerance, addiction, or withdrawal with discontinuation.
- Other medications such as NSAIDs, AEDs, SNRIs, GABAergic agents, and muscle relaxants can be used in combination with opioids or other medications to produce analgesia.
- Nonpharmacologic therapies to treat chronic pain include electric stimulation either by transcutaneous methods (TENS), spinal cord (dorsal column stimulator), or thalamic stimulation. TMS of cortical areas can also help control pain. All of these effect pain by neuromodulation.
- Hypnosis may also benefit patients with chronic pain by incorporating a number of components including relaxation techniques, focused attention, imaging, and suggestions to help modulate pain.
- Interventional modalities can be useful in the setting of chronic pain. The use of epidural steroid injection to treat chronic back pain can be coupled with local anesthetic injections of sacroiliac joints, lumbar facet, and trigger points to reduce pain.
- Sympathetic blocks have the ability to reduce certain types of pain, especially neuropathic. These blocks can be used for diagnosis and treatment of both upper and lower extremity pain.

Recommended Readings

Benzon H, Raja S, Molloy R, et al, eds. *Essentials of Pain Medicine and Regional Anesthesia.* 2nd ed. Philadelphia, PA: Elsevier; 2005.

Chizh BA. Novel approaches to targeting glutamate receptors for the treatment of chronic pain: review article. *Amino Acids.* 2002;23:169–176.

Dickenson AH, Ghandehari J. Anticonvulsants and antidepressants. *Handb Exp Pharmacol.* 2007;177:145–177.

Ettinger AB, Argoff CE. Use of antiepileptic drugs for nonepileptic conditions: psychiatric disorders and chronic pain. *Neurotherapeutics.* 2007;4:75–83.

Hart RP, Martelli MF, Zasler ND. Chronic pain and neuropsychological functioning. *Neuropsychol Rev.* 2000;10:131–149.

Jensen MP, Patterson DR. Hypnotic approaches for chronic pain management: clinical implications of recent research findings. *Am Psychol.* 2014;69:167–177.

Lachkar Y, Bouassida W. Drug induced angle closure glaucoma. *Curr Opin Ophthalmol.* 2007;18(2):129–133.

Loeser JD, Chapman CR, Fordyce WE, eds. *The Management of Pain.* 2nd ed. Philadelphia, PA: Lea & Feibiger; 1990.

Nikolaus T, Zeyfang A. Pharmacological treatments for persistent non-malignant pain in older persons. *Drugs Aging.* 2004;21:19–41.

Ross JC, Cook AM, Stewart GL, et al. Acute intrathecal baclofen withdrawal: a brief review of treatment options. *Neurocrit Care.* 2011;14:103–108.

Sullivan MD, Robinson JP. Antidepressant and anticonvulsant medications in chronic pain. *Phys Med Rehabil Clin N Am.* 2006;17:381–400.

Wall P, Melzack R, eds. *Textbook of Pain.* 4th ed. Edinburgh, UK: Churchill Livingstone; 1999.

Wallace JM. Update on the pharmacotherapy guidelines for treatment of neuropathic pain. *Curr Pain Headache Rep.* 2007;11:208–214.

Young NA, Sharma M, Deogaonkar M. Transcranial magnetic stimulation for chronic pain. *Neurosurg Clin N Am.* 2014;25:819–832.

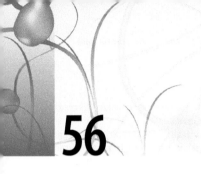

56

Complex Regional Pain Syndrome

Joseph R. Holtman, Jr. and Michael J. Frett, Jr.

Complex regional pain syndrome (CRPS) is a term used by the International Association for the Study of Pain (IASP) to describe a chronic pain disorder that is localized regionally, typically in a distal extremity, with spontaneous and evoked pain out of proportion in degree or duration to the expected course after an injury or trauma. The clinical picture of CRPS involves pain accompanied by sensory, autonomic, and motor dysfunction as well as characteristic trophic changes. Specifically, patients present with a limb that features to varying degrees: (1) spontaneous pain, allodynia, and hyperalgesia; (2) edema, changes in skin color and temperature along with sweating; (3) weakness, tremors, and dystonia and (4) abnormal skin, hair, and nail growth (Fig. 56.1). Although resolution of CRPS has been described, without treatment, atrophy and contracture of the limb may occur. CRPS is divided into two types—CRPS I and CRPS II. The distinguishing feature between CRPS I (previously known as reflex sympathetic dystrophy) and CRPS II (previously known as causalgia) is the presence of an identifiable nerve injury, typically a peripheral nerve, in CRPS II. CRPS I typically presents after trauma such as fracture or sprain. Nonetheless, the subsequent clinical presentation in both types is similar. Treatment approaches are also in general similar for both types of CRPS.

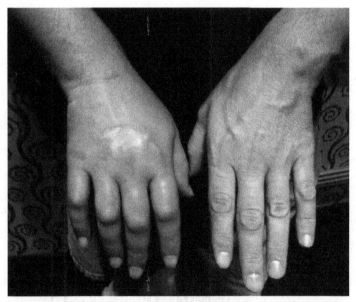

FIGURE 56.1 CRPS I of Upper Extremity. Patient had minor injury to right hand following a fall. Edema and erythema are evident along with allodynia, hyperalgesia, and decreased range of motion of hand. Patient failed to get significant relief from medication and stellate ganglion block. A spinal cord stimulator was placed for patient. The results of stimulation are presented in <u>Video 56.1</u>. (See color plates.)

TABLE 56.1 Budapest Criteria for CRPS

- Continuing pain, which is disproportionate to any inciting event.
- Must report at least one symptom in three of the four following categories:
  - Sensory: Reports of hyperalgesia and/or allodynia
  - Vasomotor: Reports of temperature asymmetry and/or skin color changes and/or color asymmetry
  - Sudomotor/Edema: Reports of edema and/or sweating changes and/or sweating asymmetry
  - Motor/Trophic: Reports of decreased range of motion and/or motor dysfunction (weakness, tremor, dystonia) and/or trophic changes (hair, nails, skin)
- Must display at least one sign at time of evaluation in two or more of the following categories:
  - Sensory: Evidence of hyperalgesia and/or allodynia
  - Vasomotor: Evidence of temperature asymmetry and/or skin color changes and/or asymmetry
  - Sudomotor/Edema: Evidence of edema and/or sweating changes and/or sweating asymmetry
  - Motor/Trophic: Evidence of decreased range of motion and/or motor dysfunction (weakness, tremor, dystonia) and or trophic changes (hair, nails, skin)
- There is no other diagnosis that better explains the symptoms and signs

Abbreviation: CRPS, complex regional pain syndrome.

DIAGNOSIS OF COMPLEX REGIONAL PAIN SYNDROME

A. IASP diagnostic criteria.

The diagnosis of CRPS as adopted by the IASP in 2012 is based upon a set of criteria known as the Budapest Criteria. They are presented in Table 56.1. The criteria list symptoms and signs in the following categories: sensory, vasomotor, sudomotor, and motor. At least one symptom in three of four of these categories and one sign in two categories must be present for the CRPS diagnosis. Pain must be chronic and disproportionate to any inciting event. No other diagnosis should better explain the symptoms and signs. In research settings, in order to maximize specificity, all four of the symptom categories and two of the sign categories must be present for a positive diagnosis.

B. Differential diagnosis.

At least some of the symptoms and signs of CRPS can present in a variety of other conditions. Therefore, the differential diagnosis can be somewhat extensive. Conditions with features of CRPS can include neuropathies, vascular disorders, inflammatory disorders, infection, and trauma. A differential diagnosis list is presented in Table 56.2.

C. Diagnostic tests.

A standardized test for CRPS does not exist. The diagnosis of CRPS is based on history and clinical findings. The use of tests is often done to exclude other diagnoses. Both imaging tests and tests of sympathetic nervous system activity are employed typically comparing the affected to the unaffected limb.

1. Imaging techniques.

a. Plain film radiography.

Plain film radiographs are performed on the affected distal extremity. Some of the features on plain radiograph suspicious for a diagnosis of CRPS include soft tissue swelling, osteopenia, cortical bone resorption, and articular erosion. Plain radiography is also useful in identifying or ruling out other bone diseases (e.g., Paget's disease).

b. Triple-phase bone scan.

Bone scintigraphy is a nuclear imaging test that helps diagnose and follow several types of bone disease. It typically uses a technetium 99 m tracer and gamma counter. It can be used to detect a number of bone-related conditions including malignant lesions, infection (osteomyelitis), arthritis, fractures not evident on plain film, and potentially metabolic bone diseases (e.g., Paget's disease, osteomalacia).

The triple-phase bone scan is more useful in CRPS diagnosis than plain film radiography. The scan has three phases: (1) Phase 1 (Blood flow)—images are obtained immediately after imaging and demonstrate the perfusion to a region; (2) Phase 2 (Blood pool)—images are obtained 1 to 5 minutes after injection and demonstrate

TABLE 56.2 **CRPS Differential Diagnosis**

Neurologic

Nerve entrapment
Diabetes
Erythromelalgia
Chronic inflammatory demyelinating polyneuropathy
Thoracic outlet syndrome
Peripheral neuropathy
Carpal tunnel syndrome

Vascular

Compartment syndrome
Thrombophlebitis
Vascular insufficiency
Deep vein thrombosis
Raynaud's disease
Lymphedema

Inflammatory

Septic arthritis
Rheumatoid arthritis

Trauma

Fracture
Ligament damage
Surgery

Infections

Osteomyelitis
Viral, fungal, or bacterial infections skin or soft tissue

Abbreviation: CRPS, complex regional pain syndrome.

relative vascularity of the region; (3) Phase 3 (Bone scan)—images are obtained 1.5 to 4 hours after injection and reflect tracer uptake within bone demonstrating relative bone turnover. The third phase has been shown to be the most reliable phase for supporting a diagnosis of CRPS. The images consistent with a diagnosis of CRPS are characterized by diffusely increased periarticular uptake to joints of the affected extremity.

2. Sympathetic function tests.

Clinical features of CRPS I can include sympathetic nervous system dysfunction. Changes in both vasomotor and sudomotor activity can occur in the affected extremity.

a. Sympathetic block.

A diagnostic/therapeutic block of the stellate ganglion (upper extremity CRPS) or lumbar sympathetic nerve block (lower extremity CRPS) can be performed with local anesthetic to assess the involvement of the sympathetic nervous system. An increase of skin temperature of 1 to 1.5°C is generally considered to be evidence of a successful block when associated with relief of pain.

b. Thermal testing.

Temperature in the affected and nonaffected extremity in CRPS can be assessed by placing temperature sensors on the surface of both extremities. More detailed assessment of temperature can be done with infrared thermography. Early acute CRPS I often presents as a warm, red, edematous extremity, whereas chronic CRPS more often presents as a cold, mottled, and sweaty extremity.

    c. Quantitative sudomotor axon testing.

QSART is a test to assess postganglionic sympathetic cholinergic function by evaluating resting and stimulated sweat production. Increased sweat production in the affected extremity is consistent with a CRPS I diagnosis.

3. Nerve function.

Electromyography and nerve conduction velocity studies can also be considered in order to rule out some neuropathies (see Table 56.2) from CRPS I. However, these studies may be difficult to obtain given the degree of pain some CRPS I patients have in the affected extremity.

EPIDEMIOLOGY

A. Occurrence.

The incidence and prevalence of CRPS are not well established. A large population-based study in the United States showed an incidence of 5.5/100,000 and a prevalence of 21/100,000 for CRPS I. In the same study CRPS II had an incidence of 0.8/100,000 and a prevalence of 4/100,000.

B. Gender, age, race.

The incidence of CRPS I is three to four times more common in women compared to men. CRPS can occur at any age. However, it is less likely to occur in the pediatric population. It is more likely to occur in adolescence than in younger patients. Again, there is a female predominance. The highest incidence of CRPS I occurs between 40 and 70 years of age with a peak in the 40- to 50-year age group. It has been suggested that CRPS in adults and children is more common in Caucasian populations. However, there is insufficient data on which to make a definitive conclusion. CRPS appears to affect all races.

C. Location.

In adults with CRPS I the upper extremity (60%) is typically more often affected than the lower extremity (40%) with equal involvement of left and right sides of the body. In pediatric CRPS I a lower extremity (80%) is more commonly involved again with typically equal left and right sides of the body.

D. Common causes.

In the general population the most common precipitating events for CRPS I include fractures (45%), sprains (18%), and surgery (12%).

PATHOPHYSIOLOGY

Several mechanisms involving both the peripheral and central nervous systems (CNS) have been proposed in the development of CRPS. The syndrome is likely caused by the interaction of several mechanisms rather than a single one. However, it is not clear how and in what proportion these various mechanisms interact to produce CRPS.

A. Inflammation.

Several of the classic inflammatory signs occur in CRPS including pain, edema, erythema, and warmth. These findings are especially evident in early acute CRPS. This acute phase of CRPS has sometimes been identified as "warm CRPS." Chronic CRPS is more often associated with a cold, mottled, and sweaty extremity. This has been sometimes identified as "cold CRPS." Both classic inflammatory mechanisms as well as neurogenic inflammation likely contribute to the clinical features in an extremity affected by CRPS. Inflammatory mediators (e.g., cytokines, tumor necrosis factor) as well as proinflammatory neuropeptides (e.g., substance P, calcitonin gene-related peptide) have been found to be present at elevated levels in the affected extremity of patients with CRPS. These substances are involved in the processes leading to vasodilation and protein extravasation resulting in a warm, red, edematous extremity.

B. Immune mechanisms.

Immune mechanisms have also been proposed as being involved in CRPS. An elevation of proinflammatory monocytes as well as mast cells has been seen in patients with CRPS I. It has been suggested that an autoimmune process may contribute to CRPS.

C. Peripheral and central sensitization.

Peripheral and central sensitization are likely both involved in the pathology of CRPS. This is evidenced by the presence of spontaneous pain, allodynia, and hyperalgesia in the CRPS-affected extremity.

Changes in the sensitivity of peripheral nociceptors occur as a result of the effects of proinflammatory mediators. The actions of these mediators result in an increase in firing of the nociceptors at lower thresholds—a process known as peripheral sensitization. This results in primary hyperalgesia.

Changes in the CNS are also evident in CRPS. Central sensitization occurs in the dorsal horn of the spinal cord. N-methyl-D-aspartate receptor mechanisms appear to be involved in this process. Microglia in the spinal cord may also be involved in central sensitization. The net effect is an increased throughput of nociceptive signals likely involved in the chronicity of the CRPS pain state. Central sensitization is directly involved in secondary hyperalgesia.

D. Sympathetic nervous system.

Alterations in sympathetic nervous system function can also be seen after injury in CRPS. This is evident by occurrence of changes in skin temperature, skin color, and sweating in the extremity affected by CRPS.

The type of autonomic dysfunction likely depends on the time frame of the disease. Acute "warm CRPS" more likely involves sympathetic nervous system inhibition with resultant erythema and warmth (vasodilation) in the affected limb. As the syndrome becomes more chronic ("cold CRPS"), sympathetic nervous system hyperactivity may become more evident, manifesting in vasoconstriction and a cold, mottled appearance and sweaty extremity. It has been demonstrated in CRPS that there are newly expressed catecholamine receptors on nociceptive nerve fibers. Therefore, an increase in sympathetic nervous system activity or in circulating catecholamines can result in an increased firing of nociceptive neurons. This phenomenon is known as sympatho-afferent coupling. Activation of these receptors would be expected to increase pain.

E. CNS changes.

CNS changes also play an important role in CRPS. Both alterations in CNS function and structure appear to be present in CRPS. Imaging and functional studies (e.g., functional magnetic resonance imaging) have identified changes in brain regions including primary and secondary somatosensory cortex, motor cortex, and the insula and cingulate cortex. Thus, alterations in cortical function and structure likely contribute to the CRPS presentation, in particular, the motor and sensory deficits seen in the CRPS patient.

F. Psychological changes.

As has been done with other chronic pain disorders it has been questioned that patients with CRPS have certain psychological issues. This has not been demonstrated to be the case. Depression as in the chronic pain population is common in CRPS (25% to 50%). A greater degree of anxiety in response to injury or surgery has been identified as a factor contributing to patients more likely to develop and have a poorer outcome with CRPS.

CLINICAL PRESENTATION AND COURSE

A. Precipitating events.

CRPS presents with a triad of sensory, autonomic, and motor disturbances. CRPS I typically presents after tissue injury. Most commonly it presents after fracture (e.g., wrist, ankle) or sprain. However, there are other potential precipitating events (Table 56.3). About 10% of patients do not recall a specific event. CRPS II is associated with an identifiable nerve injury. This could be from trauma (e.g., brachial plexus avulsion) or surgery (e.g., carpal tunnel).

B. Sensory changes.

CRPS is characterized by pain disproportionate in intensity and/or duration to what would be expected with the initial injury. The pain is not in an area typically associated with a single dermatome. Spontaneous pain accompanied by allodynia and hyperalgesia is present. The pain is typically characterized as burning and tingling but has also been described as a deep, dull aching pain.

TABLE 56.3 Precipitating Events CRPS I

Fracture
Sprain
Surgery
Immobilization of limb
Spinal cord injury
Stroke
Infection skin or joint
Injections
Venipuncture
Burn
Frostbite

Abbreviation: CRPS, complex regional pain syndrome.

C. Autonomic/trophic changes.

Initially, patients with CRPS present with a warm, erythematous and edematous extremity. This acute presentation often develops into a chronic presentation characterized by a cold, mottled extremity. Sudomotor changes can also occur evidenced typically by hyperhidrosis and accompanied by trophic changes. The trophic changes can include thin, shiny skin as well as changes in hair distribution, loss more common than gain. Atrophy of muscle and bone loss (osteopenia) can also be present.

D. Motor changes.

A majority of patients with CRPS will develop motor changes. Most commonly this will manifest as extremity weakness. Tremor, myoclonus, and dystonia have also been described.

E. Spread of CRPS.

CRPS may spread from the originally affected limb. Proximal spread in the affected limb is not uncommon. It can also spread to other extremities. Spread from one upper extremity to the contralateral extremity is more common than spread to an ipsilateral lower extremity. All four limbs may be affected.

F. Stages in Presentation of CRPS.

It is generally accepted that there are at least two identifiable presentations of CRPS—acute, so called "warm CRPS" and chronic so called "cold CRPS." There can be considerable overlap in these presentations. The acute phase of CRPS is evidenced by a warm, erythematous, edematous extremity with spontaneous pain as well as allodynia and hyperalgesia. Chronic CRPS manifests as an extremity that is cold, mottled, and sweaty. Spontaneous pain, allodynia, and hyperalgesia can be present but often to a lesser degree than acute CRPS. Trophic changes and motor dysfunction are also present in CRPS. These features may be more prominent in chronic CRPS. There is no clear time course for either stage. However, the inflammatory changes characteristic of acute CRPS have been shown to be significantly diminished in treated patients with CRPS at 1 year.

Classically, CRPS I has been divided into three sequential stages or phases—stage 1 (acute), stage 2 (dystrophic), and stage 3 (atrophic). Stage 1 has been characterized by pain, sensory abnormalities, edema, and sudomotor changes with less motor change. Stage 2 has been characterized by more significant pain and sensory changes as well as trophic and motor changes. Finally, stage 3 has been characterized by a decrease in pain and sensory abnormalities with persisting vasomotor changes (vasoconstriction) and advanced trophic and motor disturbances. It has been proposed that these classic stages are more likely to represent distinct subtypes of CRPS rather than sequential stages of the syndrome.

TREATMENT OPTIONS

CRPS can be a very challenging syndrome to effectively treat. While some data suggest that acute CRPS may resolve with conservative medical treatment, chronic CRPS is a challenging condition that likely requires a multidisciplinary approach that includes medical, interventional, psychological, physical therapy (PT) and occupational therapy (OT) components. Review of the most recent literature regarding treatment modalities for CRPS demonstrates that there is little support from high-quality randomized controlled trials (RCTs) for many of the most accepted treatment strategies. Therefore, until more high-quality studies can be done to support specific treatments, clinicians must rely on collective clinical experience by experts in the field and standards of care. The currently accepted treatment modalities for CRPS are discussed in this section.

A. Pharmacologic therapy.
  1. Anti-inflammatory treatments.

     Systemic anti-inflammatory medications [nonsteroidal anti-inflammatory drugs (NSAIDs)] are often started as a primary treatment modality in patients with symptoms of CRPS. Many times, anti-inflammatories have been initiated prior to referral to a pain specialist. To date, it has not been possible to gather good data from trials regarding efficacy of NSAIDs because of a wide range of intervention strategies and outcomes. Symptomatic relief reported by patients taking NSAIDs is also variable.

  2. Systemic glucocorticoids.

     An early trial of oral corticosteroids is often used in the acute phase of CRPS. The rationale is to inhibit the expression of proinflammatory cytokines (e.g., tumor necrosis factor, interleukin 1), production of inflammatory mediators (e.g., prostaglandins), and reduce the expression of neuropeptides in afferent neurons. The goals are to decrease the inflammatory component believed to be part of acute CRPS and to decrease the likelihood of developing peripheral and central sensitization.

     There is very low-quality evidence that oral corticosteroids improve CRPS symptoms when compared to placebo. Oral prednisolone has been used for CRPS. Currently accepted dosages are 30 to 40 mg/day of oral prednisolone for 2 weeks followed by a scheduled taper.

  3. Anticonvulsants.

     Gabapentin, a medication originally designed to treat epilepsy, currently has a wide range of applications in chronic pain conditions. Gabapentin binds with high affinity to the alpha-2-delta subunit of voltage-gated calcium channels in both peripheral and central neurons. It is believed to exert its effect by stabilizing abnormal hyperexcitability in these neurons. One RCT suggests that gabapentin may have a small effect on pain in CRPS, with a somewhat larger effect on sensory deficits.

     There is evidence that participants taking gabapentin experience a variety of adverse events more frequently than those taking placebo. It is typically dosed three times daily up to a maximum of 3,600 mg/day. Dosing should be reduced in patients with impaired renal function.

  4. Antidepressants.

     Antidepressants are another class of medication, which are commonly utilized in chronic pain conditions including CRPS. They have been shown to exert direct effects on neuropathic pain as well as treat frequently encountered comorbid psychiatric conditions including depression and anxiety. There are a wide range of agents within this class of drugs and selection is often empiric.

     Amitriptyline, a tricyclic antidepressant, is the prototypical antidepressant agent used to treat chronic pain. Low doses of the medication (10 to 25 mg) are started orally at bedtime as it can cause sedation and may help with concurrent sleep disturbance. Amitriptyline can be slowly titrated to clinical effect. Side effects include sedation, orthostatic hypotension, dry mouth, blurred vision, and urinary retention.

     Duloxetine, a serotonin and norepinephrine reuptake inhibitor, is a newer class of antidepressant medication used to treat major depression as well as chronic pain. Duloxetine has also been effective in treating pain and fatigue associated with other pain conditions such as fibromyalgia.

     While there are no RCTs to provide data on the efficacy of antidepressants in CRPS specifically, they are frequently used in conjunction with other medications to treat CRPS-related symptoms. Patient response is variable.

5. **Opioids.**

Opioids are rarely effective in pain conditions with a large neuropathic component such as CRPS. Opioids are occasionally added short-term if additional pain control is needed to facilitate fuller participation in functional therapies.

6. **Sympathetics.**

Calcium-channel blockers are occasionally used as part of a medication regimen in patients with CRPS. In particular, they are utilized in cases of CRPS that appear to have more of a component of sympathetic dysregulation. The rationale is that they produce vasodilatory effects, improving blood flow to the affected area. Side effects may include increase in pain symptoms, arterial hypotension, myocardial depression, and cold intolerance.

Clonidine, a centrally acting α2-agonist, can also be used in cases with suspected inappropriate sympathetic activity. It acts by decreasing sympathetic outflow resulting in vasodilation. Clonidine may be administered transdermally over the affected area. It works by inhibiting norepinephrine release from peripheral presynaptic adrenergic terminals, leading to decreases in hyperalgesia in the areas directly below the patch. Less data are available to support the use of systemic clonidine. Side effects more prominently associated with systemic clonidine include sedation, arterial hypotension, and bradycardia.

7. **Inhibition of osteoclastic activity.**

The efficacy of bisphosphonates in CRPS has been demonstrated in RCTs. Effects on pain, swelling, and mobility are apparent. One agent that is used is alendronate.

B. **Interventional therapy.**

1. **Sympathetic ganglion blocks.**

Based on the understanding that CRPS can have a significant component of sympathetic dysregulation as part of its pathophysiology, directed injections targeting sympathetic ganglia are commonly used as an adjunct to medication and PT and OT. Stellate ganglion sympathetic blockade is utilized for patients with CRPS of the upper extremity, and lumbar sympathetic blockade is utilized for CRPS of the lower extremity. If the sympathetic block is helpful, meaning the patient experiences a subjective improvement in pain relief extending longer than the duration of the local anesthetic or has an objective improvement in function of the affected limb, the injections can be repeated at 1- to 2-week intervals. There is no evidence that sympathetic blocks are curative for CRPS. However, they can be effective if they produce a decrease in pain symptoms allowing the patient to participate more fully in PT and OT.

A stellate ganglion block is performed by injecting local anesthetic at the anterior tubercle of C6, also known as Chassaignac's tubercle. A successful stellate ganglion block is evidenced by an increase in temperature in the affected extremity ($\geq$1 to 1.5°C) along with pain relief. In addition, an ipsilateral Horner's syndrome and hoarseness due to a transient, recurrent laryngeal nerve palsy may also occur. Other potential complications include respiratory distress secondary to phrenic nerve block, inadvertent vertebral artery injection with seizures, inadvertent epidural or intrathecal injection of local anesthetic resulting in high spinal, osteitis of transverse process or soft tissue infection, pneumothorax, and brachial plexus dysfunction.

A lumbar sympathetic block is performed by targeting the sympathetic ganglia supplying the legs. The target ganglia are located at anterolateral portions of the L2–L4 vertebral bodies. Potential complications include pain or infection at the injection site, epidural or intrathecal injection of local anesthetic, intravascular injection, and trauma to adjacent structures including the kidney and bowel. Again, a successful block is evidenced by an increase in temperature ($\geq$1 to 1.5°C) in the affected extremity with pain relief.

2. **Spinal cord stimulation.**

If the above-mentioned modalities are ineffective, or if sympathetic blocks are effective for only short amounts of time, it is reasonable to proceed to a trial of spinal cord stimulation (SCS). The principles of SCS are based upon a theory proposed by

Patrick Wall, a neurophysiologist and Ronald Melzack, a psychologist, known as the gate-control theory. This theory proposes that second-order neurons at the level of the dorsal horn act as a "gate" through which noxious stimuli from the periphery must pass in order to reach the higher centers of pain perception in the brain. However, if these same nerve fibers simultaneously receive a non-noxious stimulus, this can serve to "close the gate." Noxious pain signals from the periphery will thus be inhibited from ascending to the brain. SCS functions by creating this non-noxious stimulus that closes the gate. The spinal cord stimulator lead is placed directly into the epidural space during a trial. During the trial, the stimulator is activated in order to achieve coverage over the painful body region. The trial typically lasts 5 to 7 days. If it is successful, the patient can then proceed to implantation of a permanent spinal cord stimulator.

There is evidence to suggest that SCS + physiotherapy is more effective than physiotherapy alone. Additionally, there is evidence that SCS is effective at improving patients' own perception of overall improvement for up to 2 years.

3. Sympathectomy.

Surgical sympathectomy is a procedure that has been used to treat multiple conditions with sympathetically mediated pain for many years. Some of these syndromes include hyperhydrosis, Raynaud's, and CRPS. The procedure involves extensive ablation of the thoracic sympathetic ganglia (T1–T6/7) for conditions affecting the upper extremities and the lumbar sympathetic chain (L2–L4) for lower extremity symptoms. Initially, these were done as open surgical procedures. With medical advancements, these procedures can be done endoscopically or via percutaneous neurolysis with radiofrequency or chemical destruction (alcohol or phenol).

Review of available literature revealed a high failure rate (up to 35%), which was attributed to poor patient selection. Other suggested causes of procedure failure include incorrect diagnosis, inadequate resection, reinnervation, and contralateral innervations. In addition to initial failure, there is also concern for post-sympathectomy neuralgia, which can occur 6 months to 2 years after the initial ablation procedure. One study reports a 44% rate of occurrence of this syndrome.

C. Physical and behavioral therapy.

1. PT and OT.

Many of the pharmacologic and procedural interventions described above are used as a means to allow the patient with CRPS to participate more fully in PT and OT. PT and OT continue to be the mainstay of therapy of CRPS in order to restore function and avoid atrophy and contractures in the affected limb. Patient education regarding the extent to which they should participate in PT and OT and the amount of pain control they should have is important. There should be an understanding that with any physical exercise there may be some increase in pain symptoms. However, it is imperative not to undergo inappropriately aggressive PT, which can result in extreme pain, edema, distress, fatigue, and exacerbation of inflammatory and sympathetic symptoms. The therapy should be directed at gradual increases in strength and flexibility of the affected limb. Some experts have also advocated the use of massage to facilitate lymphatic drainage and improve edema. At this time, this is not a strong evidence to suggest that there is an advantage to lymphatic drainage techniques.

Desensitization therapy is a graded approach to helping a patient overcome associated allodynia and hyperesthesia. In this therapy, the affected limb is incrementally exposed to a wide range of sensations including light touch with soft and coarse fabrics and temperature changes achieved by submerging the limb in cool and warm water baths. The goal of the therapy is to retrain the hyperactive nerves in the affected area to begin interpreting and transmitting sensory input in a normalized fashion.

Transcutaneous electrical nerve stimulation (TENS) is a portable device composed of an electrical generator and conducting pads, which can be applied directly to the skin over the area of pain. The unit provides a buzzing sensation of varying intensities and is again based upon the gate theory described in section on SCS. A trial with a TENS unit can be performed during PT sessions. If it is successful in alleviating pain symptoms, the patient may benefit from having a TENS unit at home to use as needed.

2. **Behavioral therapy.**

In the setting of chronic pain, comorbid conditions such as depression, anxiety, suicidal ideation, and opioid dependence are commonly present. This is certainly true for CRPS, and the help of a trained behavioral specialist is often a helpful adjunct to medications and interventions.

Psychotherapeutic management of CRPS typically involves counseling, whereby a patient is instructed on pain coping strategies. Attempts are made to identify past or current stressors that may be contributing to the patient's pain perception. Cognitive-behavioral therapy (CBT), including biofeedback, relaxation, and hypnosis, may also be explored. Finally, additional psychiatric diagnoses that may be present should be identified and treated accordingly.

COMPLEX REGIONAL PAIN SYNDROME IN CHILDREN

Currently, the diagnosis of CRPS in patients under the age of 18 is made using the same criteria used to diagnose adults. Regarding demographics in pediatric patients, there appears to be higher incidence of CRPS in girls, and it seems to be more common in Caucasians. There also appears to be a higher incidence of CRPS affecting the lower extremities compared to the upper extremities.

Although there is a commonly held belief among clinicians that CRPS in children is in some way intrinsically different from CRPS in adults, there is not sufficient empiric evidence to support this claim. Initially, this was based on a series of case reports from the 1970s giving the perception that children may have a milder course of the disease or that they respond more favorably to conservative therapy. Consequently, there were suggestions that CRPS was a self-limited disease in children and risks of side effects from various therapies were not warranted. However, a more recent longitudinal study of adult patients diagnosed with CRPS as children found that on long-term follow-up 52% of these patients still experienced pain and 36% had documented recurrence of CRPS.

A commonly accepted viewpoint is that intensive PT may offer complete resolution of CRPS symptoms in children. Therefore, all other treatment modalities should be utilized for the main goal of facilitating a PT regimen. Numerous studies in the past have supported this claim, some of which reported cure rates of greater than 90% with regimens of intensive PT and no injections or medications. Some experts have suggested that children may have a greater willingness to actively participate in PT, which may lead to the perceived higher resolution of symptoms with PT compared to adults. Many pediatric centers also advocate a trial of TENS as part of a multimodality approach to CRPS. There are no prospective RCTs validating any medication regimens in the treatment of pediatric CRPS. Therefore, there is a wide range of clinical practice utilizing various combinations of tricyclic and other antidepressants, anticonvulsants, steroids, NSAIDs, and opioids to facilitate more meaningful participation in PT. Additionally, there are no prospective RCTs directly comparing outcomes in pediatric CRPS with or without sympathetic blocks. Advocacy of their use is variable among clinicians.

Multiple authors have written about psychological aspects of children with CRPS. Some have even suggested that pediatric CRPS is entirely a psychological or psychosomatic disease process. This misconception likely came from the presentation of CRPS, namely, pain, which is out of proportion to the inciting event and pain patterns, which cross multiple dermatomes and areas of innervations by single nerves. Based on multiple studies, the current consensus is that children who are considered "overachievers" or have significant enmeshment with their parents may have a higher incidence of CRPS. However, aside from this, there is no compelling evidence that children with CRPS are psychologically unique compared with other children with chronic pain or adults with CRPS. A pediatric psychologist, who is trained specifically in chronic pain, is an invaluable addition to the multidisciplinary approach to treating CRPS. They are especially helpful in identifying other psychiatric diagnoses or external stressors (i.e., school or academic stressors, bullying, or psychological/physical abuse) that may be creating obstacles for improvement in symptoms. In addition to meeting with the patient as part of a multidisciplinary team approach, a pediatric psychologist also can meet individually with the child to help cultivate pain management techniques such as relaxation, meditation, and CBT.

ADDITIONAL TREATMENT OPTIONS

At this time, there are emerging therapies for CRPS that go beyond the current standard of care. Some of these therapies have already been studied and advocated by other countries around the world.

Free radical scavengers have been proposed for use in the treatment of CRPS. Both intravenous (IV) (mannitol) and topical [50% dimethyl sulfoxide (DMSO)] preparations have been studied. One RCT has shown some improvement in pain and inflammatory signs with application four times daily of 50% DMSO to the affected area. The rationale for this therapy is based on the understanding that there may be episodes of ischemia followed by reperfusion and increased free radical damage to tissues and nerves. Others have also advocated the use of oral Vitamin C and *N*-acetyl-cysteine for the same purpose.

NMDA receptor antagonists have also been studied and utilized. The prototypical NMDA receptor antagonist, ketamine, has been administered both topically and via a series of daily subanesthetic infusions in patients with refractory CRPS symptoms. Some placebo-controlled studies have demonstrated that this may be useful. Care should be taken with the administration of ketamine. Potential side effects include sympathetic stimulation, increased secretion production, and psychiatric manifestations including disturbing dreams and hallucinations.

When common treatment modalities are not effective, several studies have investigated the initiation of a 5-day IV lidocaine administration with an escalating dose schedule. The rationale for this therapy is based on studies demonstrating upregulation of tetrodotoxin-resistant sodium channels on primary nociceptive afferent fibers and small dorsal root ganglia pain transmission neurons following peripheral nerve injury. IV lidocaine selectively inhibits these channels and, therefore, decreases neural transmission in a use-dependent manner. One study of 49 patients with refractory CRPS demonstrated a significant decrease in pain parameters and other symptoms and signs of CRPS following a 5-day continuous lidocaine infusion. The pain reduction lasted an average of 3 months and was particularly effective for thermal and mechanical allodynia. Careful monitoring for local anesthetic toxicity is necessary, as faster infusion rates and a duration of treatment longer than 5 days have resulted in dizziness, dysphoria, and hypotension.

Other new and emerging modalities include IV immunoglobulin, oral tadalafil, and low-dose naltrexone. Given the wide range of treatments with different mechanisms of action, it is again apparent that CPRS is a very complex condition and often requires a varied multimodality approach to effectively treat it.

CONCLUSION

CRPS is a challenging condition that often requires a multidisciplinary approach that includes medical, interventional, psychological, and PT and OT components. A wide range of pharmacologic approaches is used in practice. Interventional procedures are also often added to these medication regimens. There is little RCT-supported data for any of these pharmacologic and interventional modalities and current standard of care is based upon expert opinion. PT/OT and pain psychology are important adjuncts to this multidisciplinary approach as well.

Key Points

- CRPS is a chronic pain condition characterized by pain out of proportion to the inciting event. Diagnosis based on the Budapest Criteria relies upon clinical findings including sensory (allodynia, hyperalgesia), vasomotor, sudomotor, and trophic changes.
- CRPS is divided into type I and type II. The distinguishing feature is the presence of an identifiable nerve injury in CRPS II.

- CRPS is a diagnosis of exclusion. The differential diagnosis may include vascular disorders, inflammatory disorders, infection, trauma, and surgery.
- Standard diagnostic testing does not exist for CRPS. Imaging such as X-rays and triple-phase bone scan as well as sympathetic testing, nerve testing, and thermal testing can be used to support the diagnosis.
- CRPS I in adults is more common in women and has the highest incidence between ages 40 and 70. CRPS is more common in the upper extremity in adults.
- Common inciting events for CRPS I include fractures, sprains, and surgery.
- The pathophysiology of CRPS is complex and likely multimodal including components of inflammation, immune mechanisms, peripheral and central sensitization, CNS changes, sympathetic dysregulation, and psychological changes.
- Early CRPS presents with a warm, erythematous, and edematous extremity. Chronic CRPS is characterized by a cold, mottled, and sweaty extremity with trophic changes.
- CRPS can spread from one limb to another.
- There is little RCT data to support most pharmacologic treatments for CRPS. Current standards of care are based on expert opinion and on current understanding of CRPS pathophysiology and on medication use in other chronic pain disorders.
- Sympathetic blocks including stellate ganglion block and lumbar sympathetic block can be useful in the diagnosis and treatment of CRPS.
- SCS is a potentially useful treatment modality in patients with CRPS not controlled with medications and sympathetic blocks.
- PT and OT remain cornerstones of therapy for CRPS treatment focusing on range of motion, muscle strength, and desensitization.
- CRPS in children is diagnosed using same criteria as adults. It is more common in females as in adults. Unlike adults, CRPS more commonly affects the lower extremity in children.
- Treatment of CRPS in children utilizes a multidisciplinary approach including pain physician, child psychologist, social worker, and physical therapist. Intensive PT is considered paramount in the treatment of CRPS in children.
- New therapeutic options are being investigated for the treatment of CRPS. These include free radical scavengers, IV immunoglobulin, tadalafil, and low-dose naltrexone.

Recommended Readings

Bernstein BH, Singsen BH, Kent JT, et al. Reflex neurovascular dystrophy in childhood. *J Pediatr.* 1978;93:211–215.

Borchers AT, Gershwin ME. Complex regional pain syndrome: a comprehensive and critical review. *Autoimmun Rev.* 2014;13:242–265.

Bruehl S. Complex regional pain syndrome. *BJM.* 2015;350:h2730.

Cappello ZJ, Kasdan ML, Louis DS. Meta-analysis of imaging techniques for the diagnosis of complex regional pain syndrome, type I. *J Hand Surg Am.* 2012;37A:288–296.

Finsh PM, Knudson L, Drummond PD. Reduction of allodynia in patients with complex regional pain syndrome: a double-blind placebo-controlled trial of topical ketamine. *Pain.* 2009;145:18–25.

Goebel A, Blaes F. Complex regional pain syndrome, a prototype of a novel kind of autoimmune disease. *Autoimmun Rev.* 2013;12:682–686.

Kalita J, Vajpayee A, Misra UK. Comparison of prednisolone with piroxicam in complex regional pain syndrome following stroke: a randomized controlled trial. *QJM.* 2006;99:89–95.

Kim K, DeSalles A, Johnson J, et al. Sympathectomy: open and thoracoscopic. In: Burchiel K, ed. *Surgical Management of Pain.* New York, NY: Thieme Publishers; 2002:688–700.

Kozin F, Soin JS, Ryan LM, et al. Bone scintigraphy in the reflex sympathetic dystrophy syndrome. *Radiology.* 1981;138:437–443.

Lee GW, Weeks PM. The role of bone scintigraphy in diagnosing reflex sympathetic dystrophy. *J Hand Surg.* 1995;20A(3):458–463.

Maihöfner C, Seifert F, Markovic K. Complex regional pain syndromes: new pathophysiological concepts and therapies. *Eur J Neurol.* 2010;17:649–660.

Marnus J, Moseley GL, Birklein F, et al. Clinical features and pathophysiology of complex regional pain syndrome. *Lancet Neurol.* 2011;10:637–648.

Matles AI. Reflex sympathetic dystrophy in a child: a case report. *Bull Hosp Jt Dis.* 1971;32:193–197.

Mockus MB, Rutherford RB, Rosales C, et al. Sympathectomy for causalgia: patient selection and long-term results. *Arch Surg.* 1987;122:668–672.

O'Connell NE, Wand BM, McAuley J, et al. Interventions for treating pain and disability in adults with complex regional pain syndrome- an overview of systemic reviews (Review). *The Cochrane Collaboration.* 2013;(4):1–68. http://www.the cochranelibrary.com

Schürmann M, Gradl G, Wizgal I, et al. Clinical and physiologic evaluation of stellate ganglion blockade for complex regional pain syndrome type I. *Clin J Pain.* 2001;17:94–100.

Schürmann M, Zaspel J, Löhr P, et al. Imaging in early posttraumatic complex regional pain syndrome: a comparison of diagnostic methods. *Clin J Pain.* 2007;23(5):449–457.

Schwartzman RJ, Alexander GM, Grothusen JR, et al. Outpatient intravenous ketamine for the treatment of complex regional pain syndrome: a double-blind placebo-controlled study. *Pain.* 2009;147:107–115.

Schwartzman RJ, Patel M, Grothusen JR, et al. Efficacy of 5-day continuous lidocaine infusion for the treatment of refractory complex regional pain syndrome. *Pain Med.* 2009;10(2):401–412.

Sherry DD, Wallace CA, Kelley C, et al. Short- and long-term outcomes of children with complex regional pain syndrome type I treated with exercise therapy. *Clin J Pain.* 1999;15:218–223.

Tan EC, van de Sandt-Renkema N, Krabbe PF, et al. Quality of life in adults with childhood-onset of complex regional pain syndrome type I. *Injury* 2009;40:901–904.

Wilder RT. Management of pediatric patients with complex regional pain syndrome. *Clin J Pain.* 2006;22:443–448.

Wüppenhorst N, Maier C, Frettlöh J, et al. Sensitivity and specificity of 3-phase bone scintigraphy in the diagnosis of complex regional pain syndrome of the upper extremity. *Clin J Pain.* 2010;26(3):182–189.

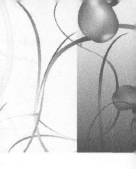

57 Primary Central Nervous System Tumors

Edward J. Dropcho

More than 40,000 new cases of primary central nervous system (CNS) tumors are diagnosed each year in the United States (Video 57.1). Brain tumors are the second most frequent cause of cancer-related death among children. Brain tumors may affect adults at any age, and often have a devastating effect on patients and their families. This review will summarize the current clinical approaches to the most common primary brain tumors. For most if not all brain tumors the therapeutic strategies are in a state of evolution, and there are more than a few uncertainties and controversies. The past several years have seen an explosion of new knowledge of the molecular genetics and basic biology of brain tumors. Although the clinical progress seems painfully slow, these new discoveries are gradually being translated into more precise disease stratification, into targets for new therapies, and into "personalized" tumor therapy.

HIGH-GRADE GLIOMAS IN ADULTS

A. **Course of disease.**

The World Health Organization (WHO) stratifies "malignant" or "high-grade" gliomas (HGGs) into histologic grade 3 tumors (anaplastic astrocytoma, anaplastic oligodendroglioma, and anaplastic oligoastrocytoma) and grade 4 glioblastoma (GBM) based on the degree of hypercellularity, nuclear pleomorphism, mitoses, microvascular proliferation, and necrosis. GBM is the most common glioma in adults, accounting for at least 50% of all cases. Unfortunately, this tumor is also the most deadly. Grade 3 tumors together account for approximately 20% of adult gliomas. There is a slight male predominance. Median age at diagnosis for GBM is 55 to 60 years and for grade 3 tumors 40 to 45 years. Recent epidemiologic evidence suggests an increasing incidence of GBM, especially among elderly persons. Approximately 5% to 8% of patients with GBM had a prior histologically proven diagnosis of astrocytoma or other lower-grade glioma. These patients with "secondary" GBM are on average younger than the great majority of patients with de novo or "primary" GBM.

Patients with HGG generally present with a fairly short history of some combination of headache, seizures, and focal neurologic symptoms determined by the tumor location. HGG appears on magnetic resonance imaging (MRI) scans as an irregular mass lesion with heterogeneous or ring enhancement (Fig. 57.1). Central necrosis with peripheral ring enhancement is more likely GBM than a grade 3 tumor. There is a predilection for infiltrating tumor to extend across the corpus callosum or to spread along other major white matter pathways. T2-weighted and fluid-attenuated inversion recovery (FLAIR) images typically show hyperintense signal extending in an irregular shape for considerable distance beyond the margins of contrast enhancement. In most if not all patients there are infiltrating tumor cells within and beyond the area of abnormal T2/FLAIR signal. The variable topography and distance of tumor cell infiltration are serious obstacles to attempts at surgical resection or other "focal" therapies for these tumors.

B. **Therapy.**

Standard treatment for patients with newly diagnosed GBM is maximal tumor resection consistent with preservation of neurologic function, followed by limited-field radiation therapy (RT), and for most patients chemotherapy begun during or after RT. Several modern techniques facilitate the aggressive resection of gliomas and reduce the risk of neurologic morbidity for selected patients. Preoperative functional MRI, diffusion-tensor MRI, and intraoperative cortical and subcortical mapping can determine the tumor's

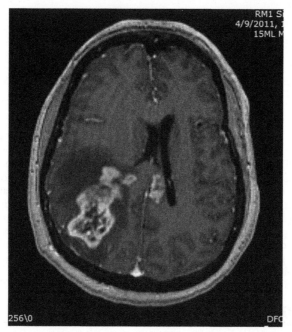

FIGURE 57.1 Axial T1-weighted MRI scan of a patient with a right parietal GBM, showing heterogeneous tumor enhancement, moderate surrounding cerebral edema and associated mass effect, and extension of tumor enhancement across the corpus callosum into the deep left hemisphere. GBM, grade 4 glioblastoma; MRI, magnetic resonance imaging.

proximity to and involvement of motor and speech structures. Intraoperative MRI allows the surgeon to assess the degree of resection and possibly continue the resection to remove more residual tumor.

For patients with symptomatic tumor mass effect, aggressive surgery usually improves neurologic function. All published data regarding the impact of extent of initial resection of GBM on overall survival are retrospective and nonrandomized. Most (not all) retrospective studies show a survival advantage for patients who undergo an "aggressive" resection. The cutoff value of how much of the enhancing tumor needs to be resected to impact survival ranges from 75% to almost 100% in various studies. In studies where multivariate analysis showed the extent of resection to be an independent prognostic factor, the impact on survival was nearly always less than that for patient age, tumor histology, and pretreatment performance status.

Standard postoperative RT for GBM is 60 Gy "focal" or "limited-field" RT delivered to a target encompassing a 2 to 3 cm margin around the radiographically visible tumor area.

GBM occasionally spreads through the leptomeninges or recurs far from the initial tumor site, but for the vast majority of patients the ultimate cause of death is tumor recurrence within the initial RT target area. There is no evidence that higher doses of fractionated RT or a "boost" of stereotactic radiosurgery or brachytherapy in addition to conventional RT provide any survival advantage.

Based on a randomized prospective study, the current standard chemotherapy regimen for patients with newly diagnosed GBM is daily oral temozolomide taken concurrently during RT, followed by six or more monthly cycles of temozolomide after completion of RT. Temozolomide is an alkylating agent, which has excellent oral bioavailability and shows good penetration across the blood–brain barrier. Noncumulative myelosuppression is the dose-limiting toxicity. For selected GBM patients another chemotherapy option is surgical implantation of carmustine-containing wafers at the time of initial resection.

Nearly all GBMs recur despite aggressive multimodality treatment. The median time to tumor progression after initial diagnosis of GBM is 6 to 9 months. For selected patients with relatively young age, good performance status, and accessible lesions, a second surgical resection may improve neurologic function, and modestly prolongs survival. Depending on tumor size and location, some patients may benefit from stereotactic radiosurgery or a second course of fractionated RT. For many if not most patients with recurrent or progressive GBM, further surgery or RT is judged not to be feasible or advisable. Systemic chemotherapy options for recurrent GBM include a retrial of temozolomide, carboplatin, or lomustine.

In the United States the most commonly used drug treatment for recurrent GBM is bevacizumab, a humanized monoclonal antibody against vascular endothelial growth factor. In addition to its antiangiogenic and antitumor effect, bevacizumab is a potent inhibitor of vascular permeability and cerebral edema. Two large phase 3 randomized studies of patients with newly diagnosed GBM did not show an overall survival advantage among those who received upfront bevacizumab in addition to RT and temozolomide, though bevacizumab did prolong median time to tumor progression. At this time bevacizumab is not considered standard care for newly diagnosed GBM patients.

NovoTTF treatment is a portable device that applies an electrical field to the tumor area through the scalp. There is no systemic or neurologic toxicity. This device is approved in the United States for treatment of patients with recurrent GBM, and has recently been approved for patients with newly diagnosed GBM following initial RT and temozolomide.

Current clinical trials for treatment of GBM include agents that inhibit growth factor receptors, intracellular or extracellular signaling pathways, angiogenesis, or tumor cell migration. Immunotherapy trials include autologous dendritic cell vaccination, immunologic "checkpoint inhibitors," and active immunization with mutant epidermal growth factor receptor protein. Several viruses including poliovirus have been genetically modified to selectively attack tumor cells rather than normal neurons.

The treatment of patients with newly diagnosed grade 3 glioma is similar to that for patients with GBM, that is, maximal safe surgical resection followed by fractionated RT and chemotherapy. For patients with newly diagnosed anaplastic astrocytoma, the efficacy of concurrent RT + temozolomide, followed by monthly temozolomide has not been definitively proven, but it is common practice to administer the same regimen as for patients with GBM.

Two prospective randomized studies of patients with newly diagnosed anaplastic oligodendroglioma showed that adding procarbazine/CCNU/vincristine chemotherapy (the PCV regimen) to surgery and RT significantly prolonged time to tumor progression and overall survival. The benefit of PCV was strongly linked to the presence of chromosome 1p/19q codeletion and to isocitrate dehydrogenase (IDH) mutation, though the genetic markers are not an absolute predictor of response or outcome. It is common practice to administer temozolomide rather than PCV for these patients, because of temozolomide's greater simplicity and better toxicity profile, though the relative efficacy of temozolomide versus PCV is not clearly known. It is also not clear whether chemotherapy (PCV or temozolomide) without RT could be an equally effective option for patients with anaplastic oligodendroglioma and a favorable genetic profile.

Supportive care for patients with HGG includes varying doses of dexamethasone to reduce peritumoral edema and increase neurologic function, and aggressive treatment of pain and/or depression if they occur. The concepts and strategies for treating glioma-associated seizures are the same as those for treating localization-related epilepsy in general. There is no definite evidence that any particular antiepileptic drug is differentially effective for glioma-related seizures versus epilepsy caused by other structural brain lesions. For patients taking dexamethasone or receiving chemotherapy agents metabolized by the liver, the non-enzyme-inducing antiepileptic drugs (e.g., levetiracetam or valproate) may offer fewer drug interactions than enzyme-inducing drugs (e.g., phenytoin or carbamazepine). For patients who do not have seizures at initial presentation, there is no definite evidence to support long-term prophylactic antiepileptic medication.

C. Prognosis.

Patient age, tumor histology, and performance status are independent prognostic factors for survival of patients with HGG. These are useful as predictors of individual patient outcome and are critically important in designing and interpreting clinical trials. With standard multimodality treatment, patients with GBM have a median survival of about 18 months and only about 25% survive 24 months. Patients with anaplastic astrocytoma have a median survival of 3 to 4 years, and for those with anaplastic oligodendroglioma 4 to 6 years. Median survival is inversely proportional to age throughout all decades of adult life; older patients have a worse prognosis. Patients with a better performance status at the time of diagnosis have a better survival outlook than patients who present with severe neurologic impairment.

Gene expression profiling studies have identified four major molecular subclasses of GBM based on their transcriptional patterns: classical, proneural, mesenchymal, and neural. Patients with proneural GBM have a somewhat better survival outcome than those in the other classes. The proneural group contains an over-representation of patients with secondary GBM. At the present time the molecular subclass of GBM does not influence treatment choices for individual patients.

The molecular genetic profile of grade 3 (and grade 2) gliomas has a major impact on patient outcome and is becoming an integral part of tumor classification. Approximately 75% of grade 2 or grade 3 gliomas of any histologic type (astrocytoma, oligodendroglioma, or oligoastrocytoma) show mutation of the gene encoding *IDH*. This mutation is believed to be a very early event in tumorigenesis. Tumors with *IDH* mutation and mutation of the *p53* tumor suppressor gene tend to show astrocytic differentiation, whereas tumors with *IDH* mutation and codeletion of chromosome 1p and 19q tend to have an oligodendroglial phenotype. *P53* mutation and chromosome 1p/19q codeletion are almost always mutually exclusive. Grade 2 or grade 3 gliomas can roughly be divided into three subgroups based on their *IDH* and 1p/19q status: (1) tumors with *IDH* mutation and 1p/19q codeletion have the most favorable survival outcome; (2) tumors with *IDH* mutation but not 1p/19q codeletion (nearly all with *p53* mutation) have an intermediate survival outlook; and (3) tumors with wild-type *IDH* and not 1p/19q codeletion are most often classified as anaplastic astrocytoma, and have other molecular genetic features resembling GBM; these tumors have the least favorable outcome. Recent studies show that stratification of clinical outcome on the basis of *IDH*/chromosome 1p/19q status is more accurate than prediction based on histologic phenotype.

LOW-GRADE GLIOMAS IN ADULTS

A. Course of disease.

Low-grade gliomas (LGGs) in adults include WHO grade 2 astrocytoma, oligodendroglioma, and mixed oligoastrocytoma. Together these comprise about 30% of all gliomas in adults. LGGs should not be considered "benign" tumors, as they generally lead to a fatal outcome. Low-grade astrocytomas are poorly circumscribed and are characterized by diffuse infiltration of atypical astrocytes with hyperchromatic nuclei. Gross and microscopic boundaries are difficult to define. Immunocytochemical staining for the intermediate filament glial fibrillary acidic protein is a marker for astroglial derivation. The classic histologic features of oligodendrogliomas are tumor cells with uniform round nuclei and clear perinuclear halos ("fried-egg appearance"), with a "chicken wire" network of branching capillaries. Microcalcifications and microcystic spaces are common. Mixed oligoastrocytomas contain some tumor cells with astrocytic morphology and other cells with oligodendrocytic morphology. The two elements are either spatially separate, or more often intermingled.

The median age at diagnosis of supratentorial LGG in adults is 35 to 40 years. There is a slight male predominance. In the era of MRI scanning at least 70% of patients with LGG present only with seizures, and no headache or other neurologic symptoms. LGG usually appears as a poorly demarcated mass lesion hypointense on T1-weighted MR images and hyperintense on T2-weighted and FLAIR images (Fig. 57.2). Gadolinium enhancement is present in 10% to 30% of cases, and if present is usually faint and patchy. Imaging alone does not clearly distinguish the histologic subtypes of LGG, though calcification is more common among oligodendrogliomas or oligoastrocytomas than among astrocytomas. Infiltration of tumor cells nearly always extends beyond the margins of radiographically visible tumor. Serial MRI scans show variable growth rates of LGG over time; some tumors, especially oligodendrogliomas, grow very slowly.

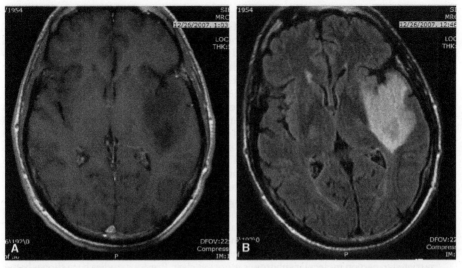

FIGURE 57.2 Axial MRI scan from a patient with a left temporal low-grade oligodendroglioma, showing no contrast enhancement on T1-weighted images **(A)** and diffuse hyperintensity on FLAIR images **(B)**. FLAIR, fluid-attenuated inversion recovery; MRI, magnetic resonance imaging.

B. Therapy.

Few of the key issues regarding treatment of patients with LGG have been studied in well-designed prospective or randomized clinical trials. It is therefore difficult to dogmatically state the "conventional" treatment for these tumors. The proper treatment for patients needs to be individualized and based on several factors, including patient age, clinical presentation, tumor size and location, tumor histology, and molecular genetic profile.

The fact that MRI identifies most patients with LGG early in their natural course raises the question of whether all patients require immediate treatment when the lesion is discovered. Currently the unequivocal indications for early intervention for patients with a presumed or proven LGG include neurologic signs and symptoms other than seizures; presence of significant mass effect on neuroimaging; growth of the lesion on serial scans; and patient age ≥50 years. It is unclear whether the presence of MRI contrast enhancement should be an indication of early treatment, assuming the area of enhancement is biopsied and shown to be histologically low-grade. For younger patients with presumed LGG who have no neurologic symptoms other than seizures, the recent trend has been to offer early surgery if aggressive resection can be done safely (see next paragraph). A reasonable alternative approach is to follow these patients closely with serial MRI scans, and defer treatment until clinical or radiographic tumor progression occurs.

Surgical resection of LGG is rarely curative. The potential goals of surgery are to relieve neurologic symptoms caused by mass effect, to improve seizure control, and to improve long-term survival. The impact of the extent of surgical resection on patients' ultimate survival has never been studied prospectively in which "ideal candidates" with LGG were randomly assigned to undergo varying degrees of surgical resection. Patients who have extensive resection are more likely to be younger, have better performance status, and have small, unilateral, relatively well-circumscribed tumors in noncritical locations than patients who have more conservative surgery. These features are probably in themselves favorable prognostic factors. Several retrospective series indicate a survival advantage for LGG patients who underwent extensive surgical resection as compared with those who had only biopsy or "partial" tumor excision. Some studies suggest a lower risk of subsequent "malignant transformation" (see Section C) for patients with LGG who undergo a more extensive initial resection.

RT is generally recommended for patients with LGG who require treatment and who do not undergo aggressive surgical resection. There is uncertainty whether all patients with LGG should receive RT early in their course. In a large prospective multicenter study, patients with newly diagnosed LGG were randomized to either receive 54 Gy RT immediately after initial biopsy or resection, or to receive no RT until tumor progression. There was no difference in overall survival of patients who received early RT compared to patients in whom RT was deferred, though there was suggestion of delayed time to tumor progression in patients receiving early RT.

A major reason for not treating all patients with newly diagnosed LGG with early RT is concern over long-term neurocognitive toxicity of RT. This is a significant concern for patients with LGG, because at the time of initial diagnosis most patients are young, have mild or no neurologic deficits, and have an anticipated survival of at least several years. Recent evidence suggests worsening neurocognitive function as LGG patients are followed for many years after RT. The question of whether early RT is more likely to have a positive or a negative effect on patients' long-term neurologic function and quality of life is still unanswered.

The role of chemotherapy for patients with LGG is in a state of evolution. A recent randomized study of patients with newly diagnosed "high-risk" LGG (i.e., patients over age 40 years, or undergoing less than a "complete" surgical resection) showed significantly prolonged progression-free survival and overall survival among patients who received postoperative RT plus PCV chemotherapy, versus patients randomized to surgery + RT and no chemotherapy. Whether the benefit of RT + chemotherapy applies to all patients with "high-risk" LGG or is restricted to certain molecular subgroups is not yet clear. Previous studies have shown better response to PCV or to temozolomide among low-grade oligodendrogliomas with chromosome 1p/19 codeletion. It is not known whether RT + PCV should be offered to all LGG patients, including those under age 40 or who undergo extensive initial resection. The relative efficacy of PCV versus temozolomide for LGG is unclear. Finally, it is not known whether a subset of patients could derive survival benefit from upfront chemotherapy only, rather than RT + chemotherapy, thus avoiding or at least deferring the risk of neurotoxicity of RT.

C. Prognosis.

In recent series the median survival of adults with supratentorial grade 2 astrocytoma is 5 to 9 years, and with grade 2 oligodendroglioma 8 to 12 years. Patient age at diagnosis is a strong independent predictor of outcome: time to tumor progression and overall survival are significantly shorter for older patients, particularly those over 50 years of age. Significant neurologic impairment at diagnosis has a negative impact on survival. Patients who present with a long history of seizures and no other neurologic deficits have a relatively favorable prognosis. In some series, the presence of contrast enhancement on initial computed tomography (CT) or MRI scans was predictive of shorter survival. Larger pretreatment tumor size (>4 to 5 cm) is predictive of shorter survival. This at least partly reflects the greater difficulty in resecting larger tumors. It is also possible that larger tumors are inherently more aggressive.

At the time of tumor recurrence or progression, about 75% of initially grade 2 astrocytomas and about 50% of initially grade 2 oligodendrogliomas will have undergone "malignant transformation" to a grade 3 or grade 4 tumor. Malignant transformation of LGG tends to occur sooner and more frequently among older patients than in younger patients. This histologic and phenotypic transformation reflects the acquisition of several genetic abnormalities. Unfortunately, it is not rare for LGG that has remained stable for several years to eventually show progression leading to a fatal outcome. There does not seem to be a time point beyond which patients with LGG can be confidently declared to be "cured" of their tumor.

As discussed above, the *IDH* and chromosome 1p/19q status of LGGs has prognostic significance independent of histologic subtype. Unfortunately, several large recent studies of LGG were carried out and published before this information was recognized. Future advances in management of patients with LGG will certainly incorporate molecular profiling of patients' tumors.

MENINGIOMA

A. Course of disease.

Meningioma is the most common primary CNS tumor in adults. The majority of meningiomas are asymptomatic and discovered incidentally by neuroimaging studies or at autopsy (see Section B). Symptomatic meningiomas are twice as common among women than men and account for approximately 20% of primary brain tumors in adults. There is a steadily increasing incidence above 20 years of age, with peak incidence during the seventh decade.

The WHO classification uses hypercellularity, nuclear pleomorphism, mitotic rate, focal necrosis, and infiltration of brain parenchyma to divide meningiomas into "benign" (grade 1, accounting for 85% of cases), "atypical" (grade 2, 5% to 15% of cases), and "malignant" or "anaplastic" (grade 3, 1% to 5% of cases). There is a variety of histologic subtypes of meningiomas, including meningothelial, transitional, and fibrous; these subtypes generally do not have prognostic significance, except for more aggressive clinical behavior among the clear-cell, chordoid, rhabdoid, and papillary subtypes. Brain invasion is associated with a higher rate of tumor recurrence after therapy.

The clinical presentation of meningiomas is determined by their anatomic site. The most common sites of origin are along the cerebral convexity, parasagittal area and falx, and along the sphenoid ridge; together these sites account for at least two-thirds of cases. The slow growth of these tumors is reflected in the slow progression of signs and symptoms.

Meningiomas arise adjacent to dural surfaces and have a characteristic diffuse, homogeneous contrast enhancement on CT or MRI scans (Fig. 57.3). Calcification is present in at least one-third of cases. Peritumoral cerebral edema is variable and in some cases dramatic. Approximately 20% of patients have hyperostosis in the skull adjacent to the tumor; this bone is usually invaded by tumor cells. Approximately 5% of patients have two or more meningiomas at separate sites. The neuroimaging features of atypical or malignant meningiomas do not differ reliably from those of benign tumors. Arteriography or MR angiography/venography is frequently required to delineate the tumor's blood supply in consideration of surgery or preoperative embolization.

B. **Therapy.**

Modern neuroimaging techniques have led to increased detection of incidentally discovered, asymptomatic meningiomas. Serial MRI scans in these patients usually show

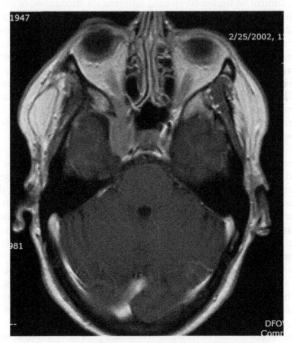

FIGURE 57.3 Axial T1-weighted MRI scan from a patient with a right parasellar meningioma, showing homogeneous contrast enhancement extending into the adjacent cavernous sinus and orbit. MRI, magnetic resonance imaging.

slow or no growth over several years. It is reasonable to defer surgery or other interventions, especially in elderly patients, unless symptoms develop or the tumor clearly enlarges.

The optimum treatment for symptomatic meningiomas is total surgical resection, if it can be done safely. The success (and morbidity) of aggressive surgery depends mainly on tumor location. Overall, gross total resection can be achieved in approximately 75% of patients. Tumors along the hemispheric convexity, anterior falx, or olfactory groove are most amenable to complete excision. For meningiomas arising in some anatomic locations such as petroclival, parasellar, cavernous sinus, or orbital tumors, gross total resection is often not possible without causing unacceptable neurologic morbidity. Some patients with recurrent meningioma are candidates for a second surgical resection, depending on tumor size and location.

RT is not given following gross total resection of benign meningioma, but is generally recommended for patients with (1) symptomatic benign meningioma not amenable to aggressive surgical resection; (2) significant residual benign meningioma following attempted resection; (3) recurrent tumor following surgery; and (4) newly diagnosed atypical or anaplastic meningioma, regardless of the extent of initial surgical resection. Of these indications for RT, perhaps the most controversial is the group of patients with subtotally resected benign meningioma. The weight of retrospective data suggests a significantly lower long-term recurrence rate for these patients if they receive RT shortly after surgery, but it is common practice to defer RT and monitor serial MRI scans.

RT options for meningioma include "standard" fractionated conformal RT, intensity-modulated RT, single-dose or fractionated stereotactic radiosurgery, interstitial brachytherapy, and proton beam therapy. Intensity-modulated RT, stereotactic radiosurgery, and proton beam therapy offer the theoretical advantage of being able to deliver a therapeutic dose to an irregularly shaped target, with reduced risk to nearby normal structures such as the optic pathways or brainstem. Published series report partial tumor shrinkage in 30% to 50% of patients and "tumor control" (stable or improved MRI scans) in up to 90% of patients, at least over a 5-year follow-up period. There are only a few studies that have determined control rates over 10 years or longer. Despite the common occurrence of meningiomas, there are virtually no prospective or controlled studies comparing different RT modalities, or establishing optimal patient selection, RT doses, tumor target volumes, or fractionation schemes.

A significant proportion of patients with recurrent meningioma have tumors, which are not surgically resectable, have exhausted options for RT, and would therefore benefit from effective systemic treatment. Unfortunately, meningiomas are generally not sensitive to currently available chemotherapy agents. There are a few reports of partial response or prolonged tumor stabilization in patients with recurrent or anaplastic meningiomas treated with hydroxyurea, temozolomide, other chemotherapy regimens, tamoxifen, antiprogesterone agents, interferon-alpha, somatostatin, bevacizumab, or sunitinib. To date, molecularly targeted agents such as the tyrosine kinase inhibitors imatinib or erlotinib have not shown significant efficacy.

C. Prognosis.

The most important prognostic factors for meningioma are the extent of initial resection and the histologic tumor grade. Following gross total resection of benign meningioma, recurrence-free survival rates are close to 90% at 5 years, declining to 75% at 10 years and 65% at 15 years. A high percentage of these patients never have tumor recurrence during their lifetime. Following subtotal resection alone, tumor recurrence rates at various time points are at least twice as high as for patients with gross total resection. Retrospective studies suggest improved outcome for patients who receive postoperative RT after incomplete resection.

Patients with atypical and malignant meningiomas clearly have a higher tumor recurrence rate and a shorter survival outlook than benign tumors. Approximately 50% of patients with atypical or malignant meningioma have tumor recurrence within 5 years of initial treatment. Reported median overall survival times vary between 2 and 10 years.

There are recent studies correlating molecular genetic changes in meningiomas with patient outcomes. For example, tumors with complex karyotypic abnormalities at diagnosis tend to behave more aggressively. Molecular profiling of meningiomas is not yet part of standard clinical practice.

PRIMARY CENTRAL NERVOUS SYSTEM LYMPHOMA

A. Course of disease.

The great majority of primary CNS lymphomas (PCNSLs) occur sporadically in persons with no apparent immune deficiency. The peak incidence among immunocompetent persons occurs between age 60 and 65 years. Recent epidemiologic studies suggest an increasing incidence among older adults. PCNSL accounts for about 3% of all primary brain tumors in adults. PCNSL is disproportionately common among patients with HIV infection, though the incidence has dropped dramatically with the advent of modern antiretroviral therapy. PCNSL may also occur in recipients of organ transplants or in persons with other iatrogenic immunodeficiency states.

More than 90% of PCNSLs are classified as diffuse large-cell B-lymphocyte tumors. The Epstein–Barr virus is detected in 90% of PCNSLs associated with HIV infection or organ transplants, but only rarely in sporadically occurring tumors. The origin and pathophysiology of PCNSL in immunocompetent persons are poorly understood.

Patients generally present with a combination of altered mental status and focal neurologic symptoms. Neurologic deficits often progress rapidly and the diagnosis is usually made within 2 to 3 months. Seizures are less common than among patients with gliomas. PCNSL has a predilection for arising in deep or midline brain structures. On MRI scans PCNSL characteristically appears as a bright fairly homogeneously enhancing mass lesion (Fig. 57.4). About one-half of patients have multifocal lesions. Lymphomatous infiltration of the posterior vitreous and/or retina (often asymptomatic) occurs in 10% to 20% of patients. Leptomeningeal dissemination occurs at some time in 10% to 40% of patients and is usually asymptomatic when present at the time of initial diagnosis.

B. Therapy.

PCNSL is unique among primary brain tumors in that corticosteroids not only reduce peritumoral cerebral edema, but also have a direct oncolytic effect and can produce

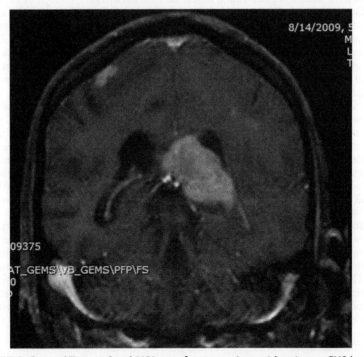

FIGURE 57.4 Coronal T1-weighted MRI scan from a patient with primary CNS lymphoma, showing a large area of bright homogeneously enhancing tumor centered in the left thalamus, and a smaller focus of enhancing tumor in the superficial right frontal lobe. CNS, central nervous system; MRI, magnetic resonance imaging.

significant (but temporary) clinical and radiographic improvement. Whenever clinically possible, steroids should be withheld prior to biopsy of patients with suspected PCNSL because their oncolytic effect may render the biopsy nondiagnostic.

There is no definite evidence that attempted surgical resection provides a survival benefit for patients with PCNSL. The role of surgery for suspected PCNSL is to provide a histologic diagnosis.

Patients with newly diagnosed PCNSL should have a staging workup including MRI of the brain and total spine, cerebrospinal fluid (CSF) exam (if safe) for cytology and flow cytometry studies, slit lamp ophthalmologic exam, CT scans of the chest and abdomen, serum lactate dehydrogenase, and HIV serology. *Immunoglobulin H* gene rearrangement analysis of CSF may show evidence for leptomeningeal tumor when other studies are negative or equivocal. It is not clear whether all patients should have a bone marrow biopsy and/or total-body 18-fluoro-deoxyglucose positron emission tomography scan.

High-dose intravenous methotrexate is the mainstay of treatment for PCNSL. When given in sufficient doses methotrexate penetrates into the brain parenchyma regardless of the state of the blood–brain barrier, and also produces cytotoxic concentrations in the CSF. The optimal methotrexate dose, schedule, and number of treatment cycles are not clearly known. For patients treated with high-dose intravenous methotrexate, upfront intrathecal chemotherapy is generally not recommended in the absence of definite radiographic or CSF evidence for leptomeningeal tumor.

Rituximab is a monoclonal antibody against the CD20 B-lymphocyte cell-surface marker, and is cytolytic for B-cell lymphomas. Current regimens for newly diagnosed PCNSL generally combine rituximab with methotrexate. High-dose intravenous cytarabine also achieves good brain and CSF concentrations. Two cycles of cytarabine are commonly given as "consolidation therapy" following methotrexate and rituximab. There are numerous published studies of multiagent regimens in which other chemotherapy drugs, including temozolomide or procarbazine, are added to high-dose methotrexate, but no randomized comparative studies demonstrating a clear survival advantage.

Other chemotherapy options for newly diagnosed PCNSL include hyperosmolar disruption of the blood–brain barrier followed by a combination of intra-arterially and systemically administered drugs. In patients who achieve a complete radiographic response (no residual contrast-enhancing tumor) to initial methotrexate-based chemotherapy, subsequent high-dose chemotherapy with autologous stem-cell rescue may provide good overall survival outcomes. Most published series of this approach preselected patients for younger age and good performance status.

PCNSL is highly responsive to RT, but following RT alone the tumor recurs quickly and the median survival is only 12 to 18 months. Whole-brain RT (35 to 50 Gy) is generally given after the "induction" methotrexate-based chemotherapy. Whole-brain RT should be given to all patients who do not attain a complete radiographic remission following induction chemotherapy. It is less clear whether all patients who achieve a complete radiographic remission to initial methotrexate-based chemotherapy should then receive "consolidation" whole-brain RT. There are conflicting data whether consolidation RT necessarily extends overall survival in these patients, versus deferring RT until the time of tumor recurrence.

C. Prognosis.

Younger age and good initial performance status are the two most important prognostic factors for survival outcome in PCNSL. The median survival of patients initially treated with methotrexate-based chemotherapy is 3 to 5 years. Overall survival is better among patients who achieve a complete remission to the initial chemotherapy regimen.

There is concern over delayed neurotoxicity of PCNSL treatment: the risk of severe neurocognitive decline and leukoencephalopathy in survivors increases with patient age and among patients who receive methotrexate plus RT, versus patients who receive chemotherapy only.

MEDULLOBLASTOMA

A. Course of disease.

Medulloblastoma is the most common malignant brain tumor of childhood, comprising 20% of brain tumors occurring before age 18 years. There is a bimodal incidence peak, at

3 to 4 years and 8 to 10 years of age, with a slight male predominance. About 20% of all medulloblastomas occur in adults, usually before age 30 years.

The WHO classification divides medulloblastomas into three main histologic groups. At least two-thirds of tumors have a "classic" histology, with sheets of "small, round, blue" tumor cells with hyperchromatic nuclei. The nodular/desmoplastic histologic pattern is present in 10% to 20% of cases, and is disproportionately common in adults and in children under 3 years of age. The third histologic group shows severe anaplasia and/or large tumor cells, accounting for 5% to 20% of cases.

Medulloblastomas in children usually arise in or near the cerebellar vermis and fourth ventricle, and thus present with a combination of headache, vomiting (often occurring in the morning), lethargy, and gait ataxia. Tumors arising more laterally in the cerebellar hemisphere present with ipsilateral ataxia, with or without signs and symptoms of increased intracranial pressure. Tumor enlargement or invasion into the brainstem causes cranial nerve palsies and long-tract findings. The diagnosis is usually made within 2 to 3 months of symptom onset.

Medulloblastoma is the primary brain tumor most likely to disseminate in the subarachnoid space, and is also the brain tumor most likely to metastasize outside the CNS, usually in the setting of recurrent disease at the primary site.

On MRI scans medulloblastoma usually appears as a homogeneously or heterogeneously enhancing mass filling and distorting the fourth ventricle. The tumor may be centered more laterally in the cerebellar hemisphere (Fig. 57.5). Calcifications or hemorrhage may be present. Hydrocephalus is present in at least 75% of cases at diagnosis. At initial diagnosis all patients should have total spine MRI and CSF exam to look for leptomeningeal tumor dissemination, present in about 25% of patients.

B. Therapy.

Multimodality treatment for medulloblastoma includes aggressive surgical resection, followed by "risk-adapted" RT and chemotherapy. Gross total resection can be performed in approximately 75% of patients. One-half of patients require placement of a permanent CSF shunt. Postoperatively, children are clinically stratified into "average-risk" and "high-risk" prognostic subgroups based on the extent of initial surgical resection and the presence or absence of leptomeningeal dissemination. Average-risk patients (about two-thirds of the total) have a gross total or nearly gross total tumor resection, negative CSF cytology, and no leptomeningeal spread on brain and total spine MRI scans. Patients are designated high-risk if they have a less complete tumor resection, and/or evidence for leptomeningeal dissemination at diagnosis.

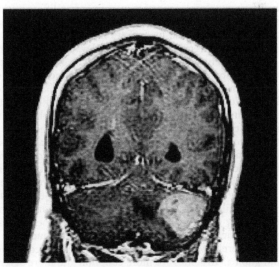

FIGURE 57.5 Coronal contrast-enhanced T1-weighted MRI scan from a young man with a desmoplastic medulloblastoma in the left cerebellar hemisphere. MRI, magnetic resonance imaging.

Average-risk children older than 3 years of age receive RT to the craniospinal axis (23 to 25 Gy), plus a higher RT dose to the tumor site (55 Gy) and posterior fossa (36 Gy). Proton beam RT reduces toxicity to nearby non-neural organs. Multiagent chemotherapy (usually including cisplatin, cyclophosphamide, and vincristine) is given for several months after RT.

Children over age 3 years with high-risk disease also receive postoperative RT, usually at a higher craniospinal axis dose than average-risk patients. There is a general strategy to give more intensified chemotherapy regimens to high-risk than to average-risk children, though there is no clear evidence establishing the best approach.

Children younger than 3 years of age have a higher incidence of leptomeningeal dissemination at diagnosis. The risk of severe neurocognitive toxicity in survivors is much higher if RT is given early in childhood, so these patients generally receive intensive chemotherapy regimens after surgery with the goal of avoiding or at least deferring RT for as long as possible.

Following tumor resection, adults with medulloblastoma are stratified into average-risk and high-risk groups as are older children, and treated with RT and chemotherapy accordingly. Adults tend to tolerate the multiagent "childhood medulloblastoma" chemotherapy regimens less well than do children.

Recent identification of key molecular signaling pathways in medulloblastoma and the recognition of different molecular subgroups (see Section C) are gradually leading to trials of molecular targeted therapies. In the future these therapies will hopefully provide more individualized approaches to increase efficacy and reduce toxicity.

C. Prognosis.

The most frequent mode of treatment failure for medulloblastoma is recurrence in the posterior fossa, with or without leptomeningeal dissemination. In modern series that include chemotherapy as part of multimodality treatment, the 5-year progression-free survival rate for older children with average-risk disease is 80% to 90%. The majority of these children are cured. The 5-year progression-free survival rate is 50% to 60% for older children with high-risk disease, and 30% to 50% for children younger than 3 years of age. Large-cell/anaplastic medulloblastomas generally carry a worse outcome. The nodular/desmoplastic variant in young children is associated with better survival outcome. Metastatic disease at diagnosis carries a worse prognosis at any age. The present clinical staging scheme is not able to identify which average-risk patients are more likely to develop tumor recurrence and therefore require more aggressive initial treatment, nor to identify which patients could be cured with less aggressive treatment (especially the dose of craniospinal RT) so as to reduce the incidence and severity of long-term treatment sequelae.

Recent gene expression profiling studies divide medulloblastomas into four major subgroups with differing molecular genetics and somewhat different (though overlapping) representation of patient age, gender, tumor histology, and clinical outcomes. These groups are designated SHH (characterized by activation of sonic hedgehog or SHH pathway signaling), Wnt (featuring upregulation of Wnt pathway signaling), Group 3, and Group 4. Patients in the Wnt subtype (about 10% of the total) have the best clinical outcome, whereas Group 3 patients have the least favorable outcome. Infants in the SHH group (usually desmoplastic or nodular tumors) actually have excellent outcomes even without RT. Most adult medulloblastomas are in the SHH subtype, though with a different gene expression profile from infants. It is hoped that molecular subtyping will further refine the current clinical patient staging and help to individualize therapy.

The relatively favorable survival outcome and potential curability of medulloblastoma are tempered by significant treatment sequelae in the majority of survivors. About 25% of children develop the "cerebellar mutism syndrome" within a few days after surgery. This consists of mutism, axial hypotonia, ataxia, and irritability. Patients eventually recover, but one-half of severely affected children have long-term speech, motor, and cognitive deficits. Survivors of childhood medulloblastoma have a high incidence of other long-term sequelae, including growth failure and other neuroendocrine dysfunction, hearing loss, neurocognitive deficits that may be progressive, requirement for special education, behavioral disorders, cerebrovascular disease, and the risk of second neoplasms including meningioma and glioma. Toxicities are more common and more severe among children treated at a younger age.

Key Points

- Brain tumors may affect adults at any age and are the second most frequent cause of cancer-related death among children.
- Brain tumors are classified on the basis of histopathology into tumors of neuroepithelial tissue (gliomas), tumors of the meninges (meningiomas), germ cell tumors, and tumors of the sellar region.
- The World Health Organization stratifies "high-grade gliomas" into histologic grade 3 tumors (anaplastic astrocytoma, anaplastic oligodendroglioma, and anaplastic oligoastrocytoma) and grade 4 glioblastoma.
- Meningiomas, approximately twice as common in women, are the most common primary central nervous system tumor in adults, and the majority are asymptomatic and discovered incidentally by neuroimaging or at autopsy.
- Most primary central nervous system lymphomas are sporadic and occur in persons with no apparent immune deficiency.
- Medulloblastomas are the most common malignant brain tumor in childhood.

Recommended Readings

Brat DJ, Verhaak RG, Aldape KD, et al. Comprehensive, integrative genomic analysis of diffuse lower-grade gliomas. *N Engl J Med*. 2015;372:2481–2498.

Buckner JC, Shaw EG, Pugh SL, et al. Radiation plus procarbazine, CCNU, and vincristine in low-grade glioma. *N Engl J Med*. 2016;374:1344–1355.

Cairncross JG, Wang M, Jenkins RB, et al. Benefit from procarbazine, lomustine, and vincristine in oligodendroglial tumors is associated with mutation of IDH. *J Clin Oncol*. 2014;332:783–790.

Duffau H, Taillandier L. New concepts in the management of diffuse low-grade glioma: proposal of a multistage and individualized therapeutic approach. *Neurooncol*. 2015;17:332–342.

Gajjar AJ, Robinson GW. Medulloblastoma – translating discoveries from the bench to the bedside. *Nat Rev Clin Oncol*. 2014;11:714–722.

Korfel A, Thiel E, Martus P, et al. Randomized phase III study of whole-brain radiotherapy for primary CNS lymphoma. *Neurology*. 2015;84:1242–1248.

Omuro A, DeAngelis LM. Glioblastoma and other malignant gliomas: a clinical review. *JAMA*. 2013;310:1842–1850.

Rogers L, Barani I, Chamberlain M, et al. Meningiomas: knowledge base, treatment outcomes, and uncertainties: a RANO review. *J Neurosurg*. 2015;122:4–23.

Stupp R, Hegi ME, Mason WP, et al. Effects of radiotherapy with concomitant and adjuvant temozolomide versus radiotherapy alone on survival in glioblastoma in a randomized phase III study: 5-year analysis of the EORTC-NCIC trial. *Lancet Oncol*. 2009;10:459–466.

Thomas AA, Brennan CW, DeAngelis LM, et al. Emerging therapies for glioblastoma. *JAMA Neurol*. 2014;1437–1444.

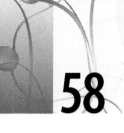

58 Nervous System Complications of Cancer

Rimas V. Lukas

We will organize our discussion of nervous system complications of cancer into those which are a direct result of cancer involving the nervous system and those which are not. Direct nervous system involvement of cancer will be evaluated anatomically. We will begin with central nervous system (CNS) involvement, which will be further subdivided into brain, spinal cord, cerebrospinal fluid (CSF), and dural, and then move into peripheral nervous system (PNS) where we will review involvement of the plexuses and the peripheral nerves. After addressing CNS and PNS metastases we will shift focus to nervous system complications not directly related to metastases. These will be divided into those that are secondary to the cancer (and will include immune-mediated complications) and those that are secondary to the treatment of cancer both within the nervous system and outside of it.

METASTASES TO THE NERVOUS SYSTEM

A. Brain metastases.
  1. Epidemiology.
    a. ~8 to 11/100,000 in the United States
    b. Incidence is likely increasing, although longitudinal epidemiologic data are lacking to confirm this. Brain metastases are likely the most common malignant tumor within the CNS.
    c. The most common solid tumors to have metastases to the brain are from lung, breast, and melanoma primaries (in descending likelihood). Although many cancers rarely metastasize to the brain, reports can be found of most cancers causing brain metastases.
  2. Pathophysiology.
    a. The majority of brain metastases reach their destination through a hematogenous route. A smaller number arrive through direct extension from extra-CNS sites of disease.
      (1) The majority are found within the vascular territory of the anterior circulation, although there appears to be some histology-specific intracerebral localization of brain metastases.
      (2) Metastatic cells or clusters of cells lodge in very small-caliber vessels. This may explain their predisposition to the gray–white interface.
      (3) Different tumor histologies appear to demonstrate different growth patterns within the CNS ranging from early angiogenesis to cooptation of existing CNS vasculature.
    b. Ongoing research supports the clonal nature of brain metastases, which diverge from the primary tumor and extra-CNS metastases with respect to mutational profiles.
    c. A growing understanding of the underlying biology of brain metastases will influence both therapeutic and preventative strategies.
  3. Clinical presentation.
    a. Signs/Symptoms.
      (1) Focal/localizable symptoms. Patients may experience symptomatology based on the location and size of the tumor as well as its associated edema. Often the edema may be the predominant contributing factor to a patient's symptoms.
      (2) Patients may develop seizures. The semiology of the seizures may allow for localization.

(3) Nonfocal symptoms. Symptoms of increased intracranial pressure (ICP) such as headache (particularly one present upon first awakening or which awakes a patient from sleep or worsens with Valsalva), diplopia (a false localizing sign due to compression of CN VI), and nausea/vomiting may be present.

b. Imaging.

(1) Magnetic resonance imaging (MRI) is more sensitive than computed tomography (CT) in detecting metastases (Figs. 58.1 and 58.2). Imaging with contrast is preferred. Brain metastases are often round, sometime ring-enhancing, lesions which may or may not have surrounding edema. As they are spread predominantly hematogenously the majority are often supratentorial with a higher likelihood at the interface between the gray and white matter in narrow-caliber blood vessels. In comparison to cerebral abscesses, brain metastases are less likely to have restricted diffusion in their centers on diffusion-weighted imaging. There are often multiple lesions present.

(2) Formal Response Assessment for Neuro-Oncology criteria for Brain Metastases (RANO-BM) are in development.

4. Prognostication.

a. Radiation therapy group (RTOG) recursive partitioning analysis (RPA).

(1) Factors that influence prognosis include Karnofsky Performance Score (KPS), age, presence of extracranial metastases, and control of primary tumor. Patients can be categorized in three classes with median overall survival (OS) ranging from 2.3 (Class III) to 7.1 months (Class I).

b. Disease-specific graded prognostic assessment (DS-GPA).

(1) A histology-specific system that includes lung, breast, melanoma, renal, and gastrointestinal primaries. The factors that influence prognosis vary between

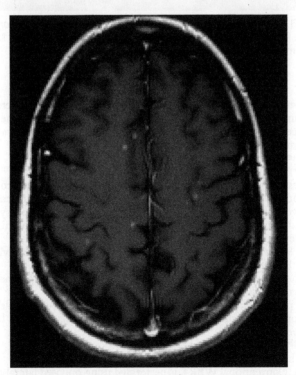

FIGURE 58.1 T1 postcontrast axial MRI. Numerous small enhancing lesions are noted bihemispherically in this non–small cell lung cancer patient with brain metastases. These lesions are noted predominantly at the gray–white interface.

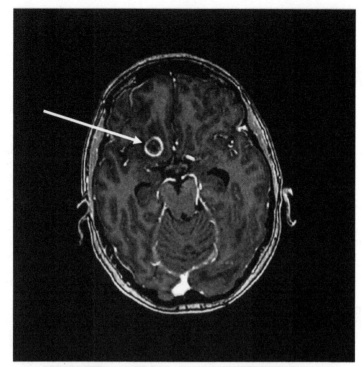

FIGURE 58.2 T1 postcontrast axial MRI. A larger ring-enhancing lesion (*arrow*) is noted in the inferior right frontal lobe in this patient with non–small cell lung cancer brain metastases. Peritumoral edema can be seen.

histologic groups and can include KPS, age, presence of extracranial metastases, number of brain metastases, and the molecular subtype of the tumor. Patients receive a summary score based on the addition of points for various prognostic factors. Median OS ranges between 2.79 and 25.30 months.

5. **Management.**
   a. **Surgery.**
      (1) Resection of a single brain metastasis followed by postoperative radiation has been shown to improve OS. The optimal surgical candidate has favorable prognostic factors, relatively well-controlled systemic disease, and reasonable systemic treatment options, as well as minimal surgical/anesthesia risk factors.
      (2) In larger symptomatic lesions there may be benefit from alleviating symptoms with surgical resection.
      (3) The role for surgical resection in the setting of multiple metastases and for recurrent disease is less clearly defined.
      (4) In patients with obstructive hydrocephalus an extra-ventricular drain, ventriculoperitoneal shunt, or third ventriculostomy may need to be performed to divert CSF flow.
   b. **Radiotherapy.**
      (1) Whole-brain radiation therapy (WBRT)
         (a) Conventional WBRT is performed using opposed lateral radiation beams. Although multiple fractionation schemes can be used, the most frequently employed is 30 Gy in 3 Gy fractions.
            1) The most frequently encountered acute toxicities are fatigue and alopecia. Some patients experience worsening of their focal neurologic deficits

because of progressive peritumoral edema. This can be diminished with the use of steroids. A small subset of patients develop acute encephalopathy.

    (b) Methods for limiting potential toxicity

        1) Hippocampal Avoidance WBRT (HA-WBRT). The use of an imaging-modulated radiation therapy plan administering a limited dose to the bilateral hippocampi has been evaluated and is undergoing additional investigation.

        2) Addition of neuroprotective agents such as memantine has demonstrated decreased rate of decline in performance on neurocognitive tests. This strategy is actively undergoing additional investigation.

    (c) Postoperative WBRT

        1) The randomized trials of surgical resection for single brain metastases all used postoperative WBRT. There has been a strong growing trend toward limited field radiation in the postoperative setting.

  (2) Stereotactic radiosurgery (SRS)

    (a) SRS describes the use of a large focal dose of radiation, typically administered in a single fraction. Its role in brain metastases has been extensively studied alone or in combination with surgery, WBRT, or systemic therapies.

    (b) Many would agree with a beneficial role for SRS in treating 1 to 4 brain metastases. It is less clear what the role is for SRS in the setting of >4 brain metastases. Other factors such as tumor histology, status of extra-CNS disease, and cumulative tumor volume may be of importance in defining the role for SRS. While the combination of SRS + WBRT provides more optimal local control it is not clear that it provides OS benefit.

c. Systemic therapies.

  (1) Systemic therapies for brain metastases currently do not have a role in the upfront setting. They are being investigated in clinical trials and they can be employed in select patients after progression post-standard of care.

  (2) As our understanding of the pathophysiology of disease advances the role for systemic therapies in the treatment and prophylaxis of brain metastases will likely evolve.

d. Symptom management.

  (1) Seizures.

    (a) The risk of seizures in patients with brain metastases is 20% to 80%. Factors such as tumor location (cortical/juxtacortical vs infratentorial, mesial temporal vs occipital) likely play a role in influencing incidence.

    (b) There are no formal guidelines recommending prophylactic antiepileptic drugs (AEDs).

    (c) When considering AEDs for the treatment of seizures in patients with brain metastases a number of factors in addition to efficacy should be considered. Absence of drug–drug interactions (lack of cytochrome P450 induction or inhibition) is preferred if possible. Cancer patients are often on other medications, including chemotherapies, the concentrations of which could be affected by cytochrome P450 metabolism. Lack of substantial hematologic or hepatic toxicities is also preferable, if possible. Additionally, the hematologic and hepatic toxicity of AEDs should be considered within the context of myelosuppressive/hepatotoxic chemotherapies. Finally, titration schedules should be considered in this patient population, which may be prone to frequent hospitalizations.

  (2) Cerebral edema and increased ICP.

    (a) Management of cerebral edema and increased ICP because of brain metastases is similar to the management because of other etiologies (see Chapter 63). It typically involves efforts to bring down ICP, often with the use of steroids or hyperosmolar agents such as mannitol.

B. Spinal metastases.

  1. Nomenclature. Numerous anatomic locations of metastases are at times lumped together as "spinal metastases." It is helpful to specify the specific anatomic localization (spinal cord parenchyma, CSF or dural disease affecting the cord, extradural disease affecting or potentially affecting the cord) as this influences clinical decision making. Often, "spinal

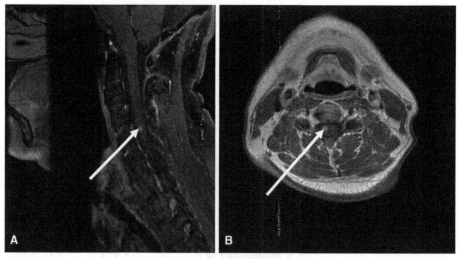

FIGURE 58.3 T1 postcontrast sagittal **(A)** and axial **(B)** MRI. These images demonstrate the less commonly encountered parenchymal spinal cord metastasis (arrow) in this patient with non–small cell lung cancer.

metastases" should be evaluated and managed emergently. Because of the potential for lesions at multiple levels, imaging of the entire spine is preferred in most cases.

2. Spinal cord metastases. The spinal cord is a relatively uncommon location for CNS metastases (Fig. 58.3A and B).
   a. Signs/Symptoms. Symptoms would localize to the level of the lesion and would have similarities to other etiologies injuring the cord at the equivalent level. As the metastases may grow without marked invasion of the parenchyma the severity of symptoms may be less pronounced than vascular or traumatic insults to the cord. Spinal cord metastases may also be associated with a syrinx above and/or below the lesion.
   b. Management. Data regarding optimal management are limited in comparison to brain metastases. Often concepts better studied in brain metastases are applied to spinal cord metastases. Steroids to diminish edema and the use of focal RT are the modalities that are likely the most frequently employed.
3. CSF and dural metastases (discussed further on) (Fig. 58.4A and B).
   a. Signs/Symptoms. Metastases involving the CSF and/or dura can cause direct injury to the spinal cord via compression and/or invasion.
   b. Management. Details regarding management of metastases in these anatomic locations will be discussed later. Unique to this location concern for cord compression often leads to the early administration of high-dose steroids to reduce edema within the cord.
4. Extradural metastases.
   a. Signs/Symptoms. Extradural metastases encompass metastases involving the vertebral bones and surrounding soft tissue. They can cause symptoms by compression of the cord, again with symptoms being associated with the level of the injury to the cord. There may be associated radicular pain if there is nerve root involvement or focal pain because of bony involvement. This may be exacerbated by percussion of the back.
   b. Management. There is randomized data to support the use of high-dose steroids (dexamethasone 10 to 96 mg) in symptomatic cord compression. Patients treated with high-dose steroids had a better ambulatory status at the completion of treatment and 6 months later. There is also data to support surgical decompression followed by RT over RT alone in patients with single symptomatic lesions. The surgical arm was superior on numerous outcome measures. However, the decision for surgical intervention should be made on a case-by-case basis.

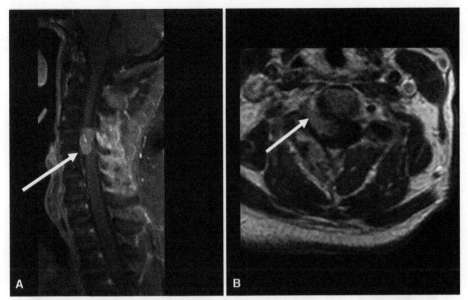

FIGURE 58.4 T1 postcontrast sagittal **(A)** and axial **(B)** MRI. An enhancing mass lesion in this patient with metastatic thyroid cancer is seen abutting the cervical spinal cord (*arrows*). It may be difficult to localize the lesion (cord vs. extraparenchymal) on the sagittal images, whereas the axial images more clearly demonstrate that this is an extradural lesion invading the spinal canal through the neural foramina.

C. **CSF metastases.**
   1. **Nomenclature.** A number of terms are used interchangeably to describe CSF metastases and include leptomeningeal metastases (LM) and leptomeningeal carcinomatosis (LC).
   2. **Epidemiology.**
     a. CSF involvement can be frequently seen with many hematologic malignancies. Breast cancer is the solid tumor with the highest incidence of LM.
   3. **Clinical presentation.**
     a. **Signs/Symptoms.**
       (1) Focal/localizable symptoms. Unlike with brain metastases, CSF metastases may manifest more commonly with cranial neuropathies and radiculopathies (including cauda equina syndrome). Often patients may have multifocal signs/symptoms, which are difficult to localize to a single lesion in the neuraxis. Patients may also develop seizures, although this is less frequently seen than in brain metastases.
       (2) Nonfocal/localizable symptoms. These are typically secondary to increased ICP and can consist of headaches (worse with lying flat and when first awakening in the morning), nausea, and vomiting. These are analogous to symptoms from increased ICP because of any etiology.
     b. **Imaging (Figs. 58.5, 58.6A and B).** Postcontrast CT or preferably MRI may demonstrate enhancement within the CSF. This can sometimes be seen as enhancement deep in the sulci or between the cerebellar folia. Spine imaging may also reveal enhancement, which may be diffuse or nodular. This may often be present on the surface of the cord or involving the nerve roots. The majority (75% to 90%) of patients with positive cytology will have abnormal MRI findings.
     c. **CSF studies.** Pathologic and cytologic evaluation of CSF is often a key component of the workup for CSF metastases. There are no other definitive biomarkers for diagnosis, prognosis, or prediction of response to therapy.
   4. **Prognostication.**
     a. The overall prognosis for patients with CSF metastases is poor. Survival is often measured in weeks to months. Clinical progression may be rapid. Patients with breast cancer as the underlying histology may fare best both with respect to the natural

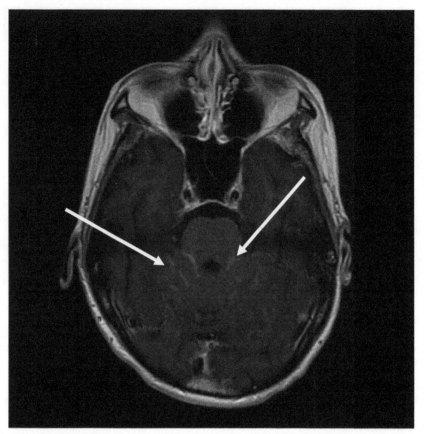

FIGURE 58.5 T1 postcontrast axial MRI. Enhancement between the cerebellar folia and adjacent to the brainstem can be noted bilaterally (*arrows*) in this patient with LC because of breast cancer. The posterior fossa is a typical location to radiographically detect evidence of LC. LC, leptomeningeal carcinomatosis.

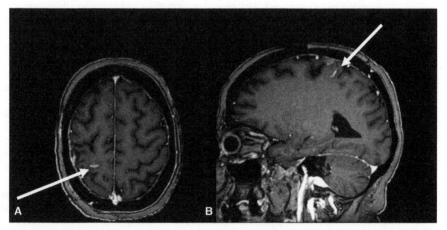

FIGURE 58.6 T1 postcontrast axial (A) and sagittal (B) MRI. Enhancement deep in the sulci is the only radiographic evidence of LC in this patient with breast cancer. Although this is a likely less often encountered radiographic picture in LC than posterior fossa enhancement, it is still relatively frequently seen.

history of the disease and response to therapy. Unlike with brain metastases, there are no formal widely employed prognostication systems. Performance status appears to be the most consistent predictor of outcome.

5. **Management.**
   a. Definitive evidence is lacking for an optimal management paradigm for LM. Often the decision making is made on an individualized basis. Do to the overall prognosis hospice is a reasonable management option to offer all patients with LM.
   b. **Radiation therapy.** The most frequently employed radiation regimen is WBRT. This can palliate symptoms and may prolong survival, but it does not address the entire CSF space. Craniospinal radiation, which does treat the entire CSF space, has limitations because of the significant toxicities that can be associated with it, particularly in this often very sick patient population. Additionally, the plan for craniospinal radiation may be further complicated by overlapping radiation fields from prior RT to extra-CNS areas of disease. Focal radiation to bulky disease is often also considered. This may palliate symptoms and has a higher likelihood of decreasing bulky tumor burden compared to systemic or intrathecal (IT) therapies.
   c. **Systemic therapies.** Most systemically administered therapies have not been extensively studied with respect to pharmacokinetics in the CSF. Of those that have, many do not reach adequate concentrations or have adequate therapeutic effects in the CSF. Although there are no data clearly establishing a role for systemic therapies in all patients with LM, responses or stability of disease have been noted in some patients. Often agents with good blood–brain barrier penetration such as lapatinib or temozolomide are considered.
   d. **IT therapies.** Evidence supports more favorable outcomes with administration of IT therapies through an intraventricular catheter such as an Ommaya reservoir as opposed to through lumbar punctures (LPs). The array of drugs available for safe administration into the CSF is limited.

D. **Dural metastases.**
   1. In about half of the patients with dural metastases, they are the only site of intracranial metastases.
   2. The most common solid tumors associated with dural metastases are prostate and breast primaries.
   3. No definitive management paradigm exists for dural metastases. Surgery, radiation, and systemic therapies may all be considered on a case-by-case basis.

Nonmetastatic Neurologic Complications of Cancer

A. Neurologic complications of cancer secondary to cancer not involving the nervous system.
   1. **Immune-mediated.**
      a. **Paraneoplastic syndromes.** These constitute a heterogeneous group of syndromes affecting the CNS, PNS, or both in the context of cancer. In approximately 2/3 of patients the onset of the paraneoplastic syndrome precedes the diagnosis of the underlying cancer. Establishment of the cancer diagnosis is necessary to appropriately treat the underlying neoplasm and to potentially improve the neurologic symptoms. A wide assortment of malignancies have been associated with paraneoplastic syndromes. The most commonly involved include small cell lung cancer (SCLC), teratomas, and thymomas. Oftentimes serum or CSF paraneoplastic antibodies are present. These antibodies can also be detected in immune-mediated non-neoplasm-related neurologic syndromes. Management of paraneoplastic syndromes includes treatment of the underlying cancer as well as possible immunomodulation. Numerous methods including high-dose steroids, intravenous immunoglobulin, plasma exchange, rituximab, cyclophosphamide, and mycophenolate mofetil have been used with varying degrees of success.
         (1) Associated with cell-surface antibodies. Pathogenic antibodies affecting structures on the cell surface include antibodies binding to N-methyl-D-aspartate (NMDA) receptors, α-amino-3-hydroxy-5-methyl-4-isoxazolepropionic acid (AMPA) receptors, voltage-gated potassium channels, calcium channels, and

acetylcholine receptors. Paraneoplastic syndromes associated with cell-surface antibodies are typically more responsive to treatment.

(a) Limbic encephalitis. Patients develop alteration in cognition, memory impairment, personality changes, and may demonstrate seizure activity. Symptoms may wax and wane in severity. This syndrome is most often seen in association with SCLC, germ cell tumors, and gynecologic malignancies. Antibodies to components of the VGKC, NMDA receptor, and AMPA receptor may be detected in the serum and/or CSF. These antibodies and this clinical syndrome can be found independent of an association with an underlying malignancy as well. When these antibodies are detected the patients may prove to be very responsive to treatment. When other antibodies such as anti-Hu (ANNA-1) are present, patients are much less responsive to treatment.

(b) Myasthenia gravis (MG). This is a syndrome of fatigable weakness. Extraocular muscles (EOM) as well as the larger proximal muscle groups are most often involved. This syndrome may or may not be associated with an underlying malignancy. Neurophysiologic studies demonstrate *decremental* response with repetitive stimulation. The tumor most often associated with this syndrome is thymoma. The majority of patients (in both paraneoplastic and nonparaneoplastic settings) are positive for antibodies to acetylcholine receptors on the postsynaptic neuromuscular junction (NMJ).

(c) Lambert–Eaton mysasthenic syndrome. This is a syndrome of weakness due to dysfunction of the presynaptic NMJ. It is less likely to involve the EOM compared to MG. Neurophysiologic studies demonstrate *incremental* response to repetitive stimulation. It is most often associated with SCLC. Patients are positive for VGCC antibodies.

(d) Paraneoplastic nerve hyperexcitability syndromes. Patients may develop motor and sensory symptoms including myokymia. They may also develop pain and dysautonomia. These are the result of antibodies targeting the PNS. Isaacs syndrome encompasses this constellation of symptoms. The addition of encephalopathy and sleep disturbance to the syndrome is classified as Morvan's syndrome. A range of malignancies can be associated with these syndromes. The most commonly associated antibodies are to components of the VGKC (Video 58.1).

(2) Associated with intracellular antibodies. These antineuronal antibodies (anti-Hu [ANNA-1], anti-Yo [PCA-1], anti-Ri [ANNA-2], amphiphysin, Ma2, CV2/CRMP5, and so on) are almost always associated with neoplasms. Syndromes associated with these intracellular antibodies are less likely to respond to treatment.

(a) Paraneoplastic cerebellar degeneration. Patients develop the subacute onset of ataxia. Cerebellar atrophy is seen on MRI over time. Breast cancer, gynecologic malignancies, SCLC, and Hodgkin's lymphoma are the most frequently associated cancers. The most frequently detected antibody is anti-Yo (PCA-1).

(b) Opsoclonus-myoclonus. This is a syndrome of irregular involuntary eye conjugate eye movements. Additionally, patients may have myoclonus and ataxia, overlapping somewhat with paraneoplastic cerebellar degeneration. This syndrome is often associated with neuroblastoma, and SCLC. This syndrome is most often associated with anti-Ri (ANNA-2) antibodies. Patients can experience rapid improvement with steroids.

(c) Paraneoplastic brainstem encephalitis. Patients develop subacute onset of signs and symptoms localizable to the brainstem. This can be seen with other nonparaneoplastic etiologies (autoimmune, infectious, and so on). When paraneoplastic in origin, this syndrome is associated with a range of autoantibodies (Hu, Ri, Ma2) and underlying malignancies including SCLC and gynecologic malignancies.

(d) Paraneoplastic parkinsonism (see Chapters 30 and 45). The clinical picture is similar to Parkinson's disease although the rapidity of symptom onset is quicker. Drug-induced parkinsonism because of antiemetics or antipsychotics should be ruled out before making this diagnosis. This is most often associated with Ma2 antibodies.

(e) Stiff-person syndrome. Patients develop sudden stiffening of the body or parts of the body. They may also develop severe dysautonomia including cardiac arrhythmias. Electroencephalography does *not* reveal any epileptiform activity. EMG, if performed during the muscle spasms, demonstrates continuous motor unit firing. It is most often associated with breast cancer. This syndrome is most often associated with GAD65 antibody (when *not* paraneoplastic) and anti-amphiphysin antibody (when paraneoplastic).

(f) Paraneoplastic chorea (see Chapters 28 and 45). Patients develop subacute onset of choreiform movements. They may also develop encephalopathy and ataxia. SCLC, thymoma, lymphoma, and testicular cancer are the most common underlying malignancies. This syndrome is most often associated with antibodies to CV2/CRMP5, less commonly with anti-Hu or anti-Yo.

(g) Paraneoplastic neuronopathy (see Chapter 51). Patients develop subacute sensory deficits and paresthesias. Motor function remains intact. The pattern of sensory symptoms is often patchy and does not correspond to specific peripheral nerves or nerve roots. It is most often associated with SCLC. The majority of patients are positive for anti-Hu (ANNA-1) antibodies.

(h) Paraneoplastic motor neuron disease. The clinical picture has overlap from idiopathic amyotrophic lateral sclerosis. It is most often associated with SCLC and the anti-Hu (ANNA-1) antibodies.

(i) Paraneoplastic myositis (see Chapter 52). Clinically patients can have syndromes consistent with dermatomyositis or polymyositis. These syndromes can be associated with an underlying neoplasm or may be nonparaneoplastic.

2. Vascular.
   a. Arterial.
      (1) Cancer patients may be on anticoagulation and in turn may be at slightly greater risk of CNS hemorrhagic events. They also may have had prior RT to extracranial blood vessels predisposing them to accelerated atherosclerosis. Depending on the location of said vessels this may increase their risk of stroke.
   b. Venous.
      (1) Venous sinus thrombosis. Patients with cancer are hypercoagulable and in turn at greater risk of venous clots. Although these most often clinically involve the veins of the lower extremities, they can occur anywhere, including the venous sinuses of the CNS. Venous sinus thrombosis typically requires anticoagulation to decrease the risk of venous infarctions.

B. Neurologic complications secondary to cancer treatment.
   1. Secondary to treatment of cancer involving the nervous system.
      a. Surgical complications.
         (1) The complications of surgery for CNS metastases are similar to complications of surgery for non-CNS metastases indications.
      b. Radiotherapy complications.
         (1) Involving the CNS
            (a) Acutely patients typically develop fatigue. They also develop alopecia in the area radiated.
            (b) Patients may develop subacute or delayed (years) areas of increased T2/FLAIR signal abnormality on MRI particularly in the white matter structures. This may be associated with cognitive symptoms including impairment of memory, processing speed, and executive functioning. HA-WBRT and systemic therapies to limit excitotoxicity (as discussed earlier) are methods being investigated to help minimize these symptoms.
            (c) Some patients develop radiation necrosis. Onset of this although variable most often occurs 6 to 12 months after RT. Radiographically heterogeneously enhancing lesions are seen. It may be difficult to differentiate radiation necrosis and progressive tumor. Noninvasive modalities such as PET and MRS can be used. Biopsy is sometimes needed to more firmly establish the etiology of radiographic changes. Symptoms from radiation necrosis may be self-limited. However, they may at times require treatment. Steroids are

typically the frontline therapy. There is randomized data to support benefit from the anti-VEGF antibody bevacizumab.

    (d) RT including the spinal cord in the field can lead to a delayed myelopathy. The risk of myelopathy is dose-dependent.

  (2) Involving the PNS

    (a) The most frequent RT-related injury to the PNS is likely plexopathy. Often, but not always, RT-related plexopathy is painless. Electromyography may demonstrate myokymic discharges, which are less often seen in plexopathy because of direct invasion of the plexus by tumor.

c. Systemic therapy complications.

  (1) As there are no specific systemic therapies definitively employed for the treatment of CNS metastases we will discuss the nervous system toxicities of systemic therapies in the following section (Section **B.2** under Nonmetastatic Neurologic Complications of Cancer).

d. IT therapies.

  (1) IT administration of drugs can be associated with an increased risk of infection (bacterial meningitis) as well as a chemical arachnoiditis, a pronounced inflammatory response with clinical features similar to a bacterial meningitis but typically lacking a fever. Bacterial meningitis is treated with antibiotics. Chemical arachnoiditis is treated with steroids.

  (2) If IT drugs are delivered through LP (as opposed to intraventricular reservoir) there is the potential risk of developing an epidural hematoma, particularly if platelet counts are low.

  (3) IT chemotherapy may also predispose patients to the development of leukoencephalopathy, a diffuse injury to the white matter tracts. The risk of this may be higher in specific subsets of patients (elderly, those who have received prior WBRT) as well as with specific agents (methotrexate).

2. Secondary to treatment of cancer not involving the nervous system.

  a. Systemic therapy complications.

    (1) Seizures

      (a) Some chemotherapies may increase the risk of seizures. Prophylactic AEDs are not recommended, however.

    (2) Cerebral edema

      (a) Some systemically administered chemotherapies such as cisplatin are thought to exacerbate cerebral edema. It is unclear what the exact mechanism of action for this is.

    (3) Encephalopathy

      (a) Many chemotherapies are associated with both acute and chronic encephalopathies. Agents such as ifosfamide are well known for their potential to cause acute encephalopathy. Chronic encephalopathy ("chemo brain") has been best studied in breast cancer. It is difficult to parcel out which specific agents contribute to this clinical picture.

    (4) Leukoencephalopathy

      (a) This describes a radiographic/histologic picture of diffuse white matter injury associated with encephalopathy. It can be a slow insidiously progressive process or it can progress quickly. It has been best described with the use of high-dose methotrexate most often in the setting of primary CNS lymphoma, but can occur with non-CNS tumors as well.

    (5) Cerebellar toxicity

      (a) The cerebellum is particularly sensitive to toxins. Agents such as high-dose cytarabine can cause acute cerebellar dysfunction. Others such as 5-fluorouracil may be associated with subacute development of symptomatology.

    (6) CNS infection (see Chapters 47 and 48)

      (a) Patients immune suppressed from systemic therapies are at greater risk for developing infections, including CNS infections.

    (7) Cerebrovascular complications

      (a) Bevacizumab. This monoclonal antibody targeting VEGF is used in the treatment of high-grade gliomas as well as other cancers. It is associated with an

increased risk of arterial and venous clotting events including stroke as well as increased risk of hemorrhage and posterior reversible encephalopathy syndrome.
(8) Neuropathy
    (a) Peripheral neuropathy is a common toxicity of a number of systemic therapies utilized to treat cancer.
        1) Agents that are associated with a high risk of treatment-related neuropathy include vinca alkaloids (vincristine), taxanes (paclitaxel, docetaxel), platinum agents (cisplatin, carboplatin, oxaliplatin), bortezomib
    (b) The most commonly encountered pattern is a symmetric length-dependent neuropathy. Neurophysiologic studies typically demonstrate a pattern of axonal (as opposed to demyelinating) injury. In addition to sensory and motor symptoms patients may have autonomic impairment, which can manifest with a variety of symptoms including constipation.
    (c) Patients with preexisting neuropathy or neuropathy risk factors are at greater risk of developing chemotherapy-related neuropathy.
    (d) There are no means to prophylax against or treat the underlying neuropathy so management is predominantly symptomatic.
    (e) Treatment-related neuropathy often improves slowly after treatment has been discontinued.

Key Points

- Nervous system complications of cancer can be divided into those directly caused by metastases to the nervous system and those which are nonmetastatic neurologic complications of cancer.
- Metastases can often affect the CNS and symptoms are based on the neuroanatomic localization.
- Brain metastases are the best studied of CNS metastases and in turn we have a clearer understanding of prognostication and management.
- Symptoms due to metastases affecting the spinal cord may respond to rapid therapeutic intervention.
- Metastases to the cerebrospinal fluid confer a poor prognosis, and while there exists a range of management options, in general efficacy is suboptimal.
- Nonmetastatic neurologic complication of cancer can either be because of indirect effects of the underlying malignancy or its treatment.
- Extra-CNS malignancy increases the risk of vascular events such as strokes as well as immune dysregulation leading to paraneoplastic syndromes with a myriad of clinical manifestations.
- Focal treatments of cancer such as surgery and radiation as well as systemic treatments of cancer can lead to CNS and PNS symptoms.

Recommended Readings

Eichler AF, Chung E, Kodack DP, et al. The biology of brain metastases-translation to new therapies. *Nat Rev Clin Oncol*. 2011;8(6):344–356.

Kak M, Nanda R, Ramsdale EE, et al. Treatment of leptomeningeal carcinomatosis: current challenges and future opportunities. *J Clin Neurosci*. 2015;22(4):632–637.

Khasraw M, Posner JB. Neurological complications of systemic cancer. *Lancet Neurol*. 2010;9(12):1214–1227.

Lin X, DeAngelis LM. Treatment of brain metastases. *J Clin Oncol*. 2015;33(30):3475–3484.

Lukas RV, Gabikian P, Garza M, et al. Treatment of brain metastases. *Oncology*. 2014;87(6):321–329.

Lukas RV, Lesniak MS, Salgia R. Brain metastases in non–small cell lung cancer: better outcomes through current therapies and utilization of molecularly targeted approaches. *CNS Oncol*. 2014;3(1):61–75.

Lukas RV, Mehta MP, Lesniak MS. Society for Neuro-Oncology 2014 annual meeting updates on central nervous system metastases. *Neurooncol Pract*. 2015;2(2):57–61.

Muldoon LL, Soussain C, Jahnke K, et al. Chemotherapy delivery issues in central nervous system malignancy: a reality check. *J Clin Oncol*. 2007;25(16):2295–2305.

Patchell RA, Tibbs PA, Regine WF, et al. Direct decompressive surgical resection in the treatment of spinal cord compression caused by metastatic cancer: a randomized trial. *Lancet*. 2005;366(9486):643–648.

Patchell RA, Tibbs PA, Walsh JW, et al. A randomized trial of surgery in the treatment of single metastases to the brain. *N Engl J Med*. 1990;322:494–500.

Rosenfeld MR, Dalmau J. Diagnosis and management of paraneoplastic neurologic disorders. *Curr Treat Options Oncol*. 2013;14(4):528–538.

Sperduto PW, Kased N, Roberge D, et al. Summary report on the graded prognostic assessment: an accurate and facile diagnosis-specific tool to estimate survival in patients with brain metastases. *J Clin Oncol*. 2012;30:419–425.

59 Neurotoxicology

Laura M. Tormoehlen and Daniel E. Rusyniak

Neurotoxins are compounds that are toxic, or potentially toxic, to the central nervous system (CNS) and/or peripheral nervous system (PNS). Capable of mimicking neurologic disorders, neurotoxins can be classified into one of three categories: (1) **Drugs** (prescription, over the counter, and illicit), (2) **Chemicals** (industrial, household, and abused agents), (3) **Environmental** (biologic agents and naturally occurring chemicals).

Establishing causation is paramount to the correct diagnosis and the treatment of any patient suspected of neurotoxic poisoning. The steps involved in determining if a neurotoxin is the causative agent are those established by Sir Austin Bradford Hill in differentiating association from causation in epidemiologic studies.

1. **Exposure.** Did an exposure occur? Requires quantifying the level of a toxin in biologic specimens (blood, urine, hair) or in the environment (air, water). In some cases, historical features alone may be adequate.
2. **Temporality.** Did symptoms begin concurrent with or after the exposure? A few toxins have long latent periods before symptoms develop but most cause symptoms shortly after the exposure.
3. **Dose–response.** Do persons receiving higher doses and/or longer exposures have more severe symptoms?
4. **Similarity to reported cases.** Are the symptoms similar to those previously reported?
5. **Improvement as exposure is eliminated.** Do symptoms improve when the exposure is eliminated or reduced? Most toxin-induced symptoms improve after cessation of exposure, although a period of worsening symptoms, or even permanent symptoms, can occur after exposure to a few toxins.
6. **Existence of animal model.** Do animal studies establish biologic feasibility? Animal studies can be helpful to predict toxicity in the absence of human studies; some toxins do not have animal models and some toxins have different effects in different animals.
7. **Other causes eliminated.** Are nontoxicologic causes excluded?

This overview is intended as a quick reference of those toxins clinicians are most likely to encounter. For more detailed work on the topic, see the recommended readings.

PERIPHERAL NERVOUS SYSTEM

A. Peripheral neuropathy. Toxic peripheral neuropathies typically present as acute or subacute, symmetric axonopathies first affecting the distal axons of the lower extremities.
   1. Heavy metals.
      a. Arsenic.
         (1) **Sources.** Ground and well water, seafood (organic arsenic, nontoxic), paints, fungicides, insecticides, pesticides, herbicides, wood preservatives, cotton desiccants, and as a homicidal agent.
         (2) **Route of exposure.** Ingestion is the most common, but absorption through skin, and inhalation can occur.
         (3) Acute toxicity (inorganic).
            (a) **Systemic signs.** Gastrointestinal (GI) (nausea, vomiting, abdominal pain, diarrhea) symptoms typically occur within 24 hours of exposure; if severe, symptoms can progress to hypovolemic shock, pancytopenia, and ventricular arrhythmias.
            (b) **Neurologic manifestations.** Within 2 weeks patients may develop a distal symmetric peripheral neuropathy presenting with burning and numbness

in the feet. In severe cases, patients may present with ascending weakness mimicking Guillain–Barré syndrome (GBS). Encephalopathy can also develop with severe poisoning.

(4) Chronic toxicity.

(a) Systemic signs. Hypertension, peripheral vascular disease, renal failure, hepatitis, keratoses of the palms and soles. Chronic exposure is associated with cancers of the skin, lung, liver, bladder, kidney, and colon.

(b) Neurologic manifestations: Peripheral neuropathy, stocking-glove distribution, sensory more than motor.

(5) Physical examination findings. Hyperpigmentation and keratosis develop on the palms and soles. Mees lines (transverse semilunar white bands across the nails) may be present in a minority of cases and can take as long as 40 days to develop.

(6) Mechanism of toxicity. Arsenic decreases ATP production by either binding sulfhydryl groups on enzymes involved in the Krebs cycle (trivalent arsenite) or by uncoupling oxidative phosphorylation (pentavalent arsenate).

(7) Diagnosis.

(a) Laboratory. The **24-hour urine** arsenic concentration is the gold reference standard for confirming recent exposures (<30 days): normal <100 μg/24 hours. False-positive results are common after seafood ingestion (from nontoxic organic arsenic) and necessitate repeating after abstaining from seafood. **Blood** testing (normal result <5 μg/L) is less reliable owing to short half-life of arsenic. **Hair** testing (normal <1 mg/kg dry weight) may be useful for chronic or remote exposures.

(b) Radiographs. May show radiopacities in the GI tract but this is unreliable.

(c) Nerve conduction studies (NCS). Severe acute exposure may cause conduction slowing characteristic of proximal demyelination (similar to acute inflammatory demyelinating polyradiculopathy), and distal, motor, and sensory axonopathy. In less severe, or chronic exposures, patients develop a distal, sensory more than motor axonopathy.

(d) Electrocardiography can show a prolonged QT interval with risk for Torsades des Pointes.

(8) Treatment.

(a) Removal of exposure

(b) If material is retained in the GI tract, consider either whole-bowel irrigation or use of cathartics.

(c) If clinical presentation is highly suggestive then begin chelation therapy before laboratory confirmation.

1) Dimercaptosuccinic acid (DMSA) is useful in the treatment of subacutely or chronically poisoned patients (10 mg/kg by mouth three times a day for 5 days then twice a day until the urinary arsenic level is less than 100 μg/L per 24 hours). Complications include transient increases in liver function tests.

2) British anti-lewisite (BAL) is useful in severe exposures when oral therapy cannot be given or the patient has an ileus. The dose is 3 to 5 mg/kg intramuscularly (IM) every 4 to 6 hours until urinary arsenic level is less than 100 μg/kg per 24 hours. Complications include pain over the injection site, hypertension, febrile reactions, and agitation.

3) Dimercaptoproprane-1-sulfonate is not approved in the United States but used in other countries (loading dose of 1,200 to 2,400 mg/day) in equal divided doses (100 to 200 mg 12 times daily) followed by maintenance of 100 mg orally two to four times a day.

(d) Red blood cell (RBC) and plasma exchange may be useful to remove components of RBC lysis and to further reduce arsenic levels in cases of intravascular hemolysis from arsine gas poisoning.

b. Lead.

(1) Sources. Lead-based paint (houses painted before 1978), soil, ceramic glaze, gun ranges, battery manufacturing, retained foreign bodies, ethnic folk remedies.

(2) Route of exposure. Ingestion or inhalation.

(3) **Systemic signs.** Abdominal pain, anorexia, constipation, anemia, nephropathy (Fanconi's syndrome), hypertension, and rarely gout.

(4) **Neurologic manifestations.**

(a) **CNS** signs are more common in children: encephalopathy, coma, visual perceptual defects, seizures and signs of increased intracranial pressure (bulging fontanel or papilledema).

(b) **PNS** signs are more common in chronically exposed adults and in persons with sickle cell disease: peripheral neuropathy manifesting as a motor axonopathy [arms > legs and extensors > flexors (causes foot or wrist drop)]. It can be symmetric or asymmetric.

(5) **Physical examination findings.** Bluish black lines around gums (Burton's lines) are rarely noted.

(6) **Mechanism of toxicity.** In children, lead affects many neurotransmitters by increasing the release of dopamine, acetylcholine, and γ-aminobutyric acid (GABA), and by blocking N-methyl-D-aspartate (NMDA) glutamate receptors. Disruption of intercellular junctions interferes with the blood–brain barrier causing capillary leakage and increasing pressure. In adults, lead causes Schwann cell destruction followed by demyelination and axonal destruction.

(7) **Diagnosis.**

(a) **Laboratory.** The gold standard for testing is **blood lead** levels. Normal result is <10 μg/dL. In **children** levels >10 μg/dL necessitate investigation and environmental lead reduction. Levels >45 μg/dL necessitate chelation. In **adults**, levels >40 μg/dL necessitate removal from work site. Levels >70 μg/dL with symptoms necessitate chelation. Complete blood count may show microcytic anemia with basophilic stippling.

(b) **Radiographs** may show lead lines (increased metaphyseal densities) in growth plates and retained radiopaque material in GI tract.

(c) **NCS** may show normal or decreased conduction velocity.

(8) **Treatment.**

(a) Remove from exposure.

(b) If material is retained in GI tract, consider either whole-bowel irrigation or cathartics.

(c) **Chelation therapy.**

1) **DMSA** may be used as the sole agent if patients are able to take oral medications (10 mg/kg by mouth three times a day for 5 days, then three times a day for 14 days), 1 week after cessation of therapy measure the lead level. Start for levels >45 μg/dL in children, or for symptomatic adults with levels >70 μg/dL. Continue until levels are <25 μg/dL in children or <30 μg/dL in adults.

2) **BAL** (3 to 5 mg/kg IM four times a day if unable to take orals).

3) **Ethylenediaminetetraacetic acid (EDTA)** [50 to 75 mg/kg every day by continuous intravenous (IV) infusion in combination with BAL]. Start 4 hours after initiation of BAL. Only use CaEDTA to avoid life-threatening hypocalcemia that can result from Na_2EDTA.

c. **Thallium.**

(1) **Sources.** Homicidal agent, rodenticides (no longer in United States), manufacturing of optic lenses and semiconductors.

(2) **Route of exposure.** Ingestion, dermal.

(3) **Systemic signs.** Constipation, myalgias and arthralgias, alopecia beginning approximately within 2 weeks of exposure.

(4) **Neurologic manifestations.** Within 1 week of exposure patients develop a rapidly progressive ascending, predominantly sensory, peripheral neuropathy (symptoms are dysesthesias and paresthesias of the feet, and less commonly the hands). Can see encephalopathy, insomnia and cranial neuropathies.

(5) **Physical examination findings.** Blackened hair roots (under low-power light microscopic), Mees' lines on fingernails (rarely).

(6) Mechanism of toxicity. Interferes with K^+-dependent processes resulting in a decrease in catabolism of carbohydrates and impaired ATP generation through oxidative phosphorylation, also inhibits sulfhydryl-containing enzymes.

(7) Diagnosis. 24-hour urine thallium concentration (normal <5 μg/specimen), hair thallium concentration (normal <20 ng/g), examination of darkened hair roots under light microscopy, and NCS show sensorimotor axonopathies with severity of abnormalities correlating with the severity of symptoms.

(8) Treatment. Prussian blue (3 g orally three times a day until urine concentrations <500 μg/specimen). If it cannot be obtained, multidose activated charcoal can be used until Prussian blue is available.

d. **Mercury.**

(1) Sources. There are three forms that differ in characteristic and toxicity:

   (a) Elemental mercury. Used in thermometers, barometers, thermostats, electronics, batteries, and dental amalgams.

   (b) Inorganic mercury salts. Found naturally as mercury (II) sulfide, mercuric chloride, mercuric oxide, mercuric sulfide, mercurous chloride, mercuric iodide, ammoniated mercury, and phenylmercuric salts. These compounds have been used in cosmetics and skin treatments. Most exposures come from old skin products and exposure to germicides, pesticides, and antiseptics.

   (c) Organic mercury. Used as preservatives and antiseptics, and previously common for industrial and medicinal purposes in the early twentieth century. Methyl mercury exposure occurs primarily through the consumption of predatory fish.

(2) Route of exposure. Elemental mercury exposure occurs by inhalation of the vapor or ingestion of the liquid. Ingestion is of little clinical consequence as mercury is poorly absorbed through intact GI mucosa. Ingestion of **inorganic mercury salts** results in the greatest absorption, but it may also be inhaled and dermally absorbed. **Organic mercury** exposure occurs primarily by ingestion and through dermal absorption.

(3) Systemic signs.

   (a) Elemental mercury. Acute toxicity presents within hours of a large inhalational exposure with GI upset, chills, weakness, cough, and dyspnea. Patients may progress to adult respiratory distress syndrome and renal failure. **Chronic toxicity** develops over weeks to months, depending on level of exposure, and presents with constipation, abdominal pain, poor appetite, dry mouth, headache, and muscle pains.

   (b) Inorganic mercury salts are corrosive to the GI mucosa causing oral pain, burning, nausea, vomiting, diarrhea, hematemesis, bloody stools, or abdominal discomfort with ingestions. Patients may develop acute tubular necrosis within 2 weeks exposure, and with chronic exposures patients can develop membranous glomerulonephritis and nephrotic syndrome.

   (c) Organic mercury. Patients may develop renal failure.

(4) Neurologic manifestations.

   (a) Elemental mercury. Chronic exposure can produce proximal weakness involving the pelvic and pectoral girdle. Patients can develop erethism (memory loss, drowsiness, lethargy, depression, and irritability). Patients also can suffer from incoordination, fine motor tremor of the hands, and a sensorimotor neuropathy without conduction slowing.

   (b) Inorganic mercury salts. Patients can develop erethism as above.

   (c) Organic mercury.

      1) PNS. Paresthesias of mouth and extremities occur as result of a predominantly sensory neuropathy.

      2) CNS. Damage occurs to gray matter of cerebral and cerebellar cortex, mainly affecting the temporal and occipital lobes. Patients present with concentric constriction of bilateral visual fields, ataxia, incoordination, tremor, dysarthria, and auditory impairment. In utero exposure may cause a cerebral palsy-like condition known as Minamata disease.

(5) Physical examination findings.

   (a) Elemental mercury. Oral findings include reddened, swollen gums, mucosal ulcerations, and tooth loss. Patients may display characteristics of acrodynia (sweating, hypertension, tachycardia, weakness, poor muscle tone, and an erythematous desquamating rash to the palms and soles). Symptoms associated with acrodynia may mimic pheochromocytoma (mercury elevates plasma and urinary catecholamine levels).

   (b) Inorganic mercury salts. Prolonged use can cause skin changes including hyperpigmentation most pronounced in skin folds of face and neck, swelling, and a vesicular or scaling rash. Patients can develop symptoms associated with acrodynia as described above.

   (c) Organic mercury. Mainly display abnormal neurologic exams as described in Section **A.1.d.(4).(c)** under Peripheral Nervous System.

(6) Mechanism of toxicity. All three forms combine with sulfhydryl groups on cell membranes and interfere with cellular processes.

(7) Diagnosis.

   (a) Elemental mercury. Clinical presentation, history of exposure, and elevated body burden of mercury. Because of a short half-life, blood levels have limited usefulness (concentrations are typically <10 μg/L). Twenty-four-hour urine levels are normally <20 μg/L of mercury.

   (b) Inorganic mercury salts. Twenty-four-hour urine levels are the gold standard.

   (c) Organic mercury. Best identified in blood or hair as 90% of methylmercury is bound to hemoglobin within the RBCs. Urinary mercury levels are unreliable because methylmercury is eliminated in bile. Normal whole blood values <0.006 mg/L. Diets rich in fish can increase levels to 0.200 mg/L or higher.

(8) Treatment.

   (a) Elemental mercury. Remove the patient from the source. As there is minimal toxicity from ingestion there is no role for GI decontamination. The usefulness of chelation therapy remains unclear. Suggested agents include **DMSA, dimercaprol,** and **D-penicillamine.** (See Section **A.1.a.(8).(c)** under Peripheral Nervous System for doses)

   (b) Inorganic mercury salts. Volume resuscitation and prompt chelation are critical to prevent renal injury. BAL is effective within 4 hours of ingestion but DMSA may be substituted if oral intake is tolerated. Hemodialysis is indicated in renal failure for elimination of dimercaprol–Hg complexes. See Section **A.1.a.(8).(c)** under Peripheral Nervous System for doses.

   (c) Organic mercury. Remove from the source. Chelation may be attempted although studies have not demonstrated appreciable improvement. BAL is not recommended because of increased CNS concentrations of mercury posttreatment.

e. Other metals.

   (1) Cisplatin. Used in chemotherapy, toxicity manifests as distal symmetric paresthesia that may not occur for months after treatment. NCS show sensory neuronopathy.

   (2) Gold salts. Used in rheumatoid arthritis, rarely associated with seizures and encephalopathy. Toxicity manifests as distal symmetric sensorimotor polyneuropathy.

   (3) Zinc. Sources include denture creams and vitamin supplements. Zinc toxicity results in copper deficiency by inhibiting dietary copper absorption. Copper deficiency is associated with anemia, neutropenia, and myeloneuropathy. Diagnosis is made by history and a complete blood count combined with serum and 24-hour urine copper and zinc levels. Treatment is removal of the zinc-containing product and copper supplementation.

   (4) Cobalt. Primary exposure source is cobalt-containing hip prosthesis. Chronic exposure can result in polycythemia, hypothyroidism, cardiomyopathy, and neurotoxicity (optic neuropathy, deafness, distal sensorimotor polyneuropathy). A blood level >7 μg/L should stimulate a referral for possible revision.

2. Solvents.

   a. N-hexane, methyl-n-butyl ketone, 2,5-hexandione.

   (1) Sources. Exist in industrial and household glues, varnish, cement, and ink.

   (2) Route of exposure. Inhalational, abused (huffing or bagging).

        (3) Systemic signs. Anorexia, weight loss, renal tubular acidosis (mixtures containing toluene).

        (4) Neurologic manifestations. Distal weakness, paresthesias, sensory loss, and areflexia. Progression of neuropathy may occur for weeks after exposure ends (coasting). NCS show motor more than sensory polyneuropathy with reduced sensory and motor amplitudes and prolonged motor conduction velocity.

        (5) Physical examination findings. Solvent odor on breath, absent Achilles reflexes.

        (6) Mechanism of toxicity. Impairs neurofilamentous transport.

        (7) Diagnosis.

           (a) Clinical history and physical examination findings

           (b) Sural nerve biopsy (axonal degeneration, demyelination, and paranodal axonal swelling with neurofilament accumulation)

           (c) Electromyography (denervation and decreased recruitment).

        (8) Treatment. Removal from the source results in improvement, although symptoms may progress for a time after exposure (coasting).

    b. 1-bromopropane.

        (1) Sources. Solvent that has replaced ozone-depleting agents. Used in dry-cleaning, as a metal degreaser, and in spray adhesives.

        (2) Route of exposure. Inhalational and dermal

        (3) Systemic signs. Confusion, nausea, headache

        (4) Neurologic manifestations. Central distal axonopathy with lower extremity paresthesias, decreased sensation, spastic paraparesis, proximal hyperreflexia, ataxic gait, and distal weakness.

        (5) Physical exam findings. Decreased vibration sense in stocking-glove distribution.

        (6) Mechanism of action. Unknown but may involve formation of S-propylcysteine protein adducts in the peripheral and CNS.

        (7) Diagnosis.

           (a) Clinical history and physical examination findings

           (b) Abnormal somatosensory evoked potentials

           (c) Laboratory evidence of bromide exposure: elevated serum chloride on basic chemistry or elevated serum (normal <10 mg/dL) bromide if measured

        (8) Treatment. Removal from the source may result in some improvement but permanent effects are possible.

    c. Other solvents.

        (1) Acrylamide. Sensorimotor neuropathy.

        (2) Carbon disulfide. Distal axonal neuropathy with axonal swellings, extrapyramidal signs, and psychosis.

        (3) Ethyl alcohol (chronic). Sensorimotor neuropathy effecting distal lower extremities first.

        (4) Ethylene oxide. Distal axonopathy.

        (5) Methyl-ethyl-ketone. Nontoxic alone, but synergistically promotes peripheral neuropathy from other solvents.

        (6) Methyl bromide. Both peripheral and pyramidal effects.

        (7) Styrene. Sensorimotor, demyelinating neuropathy.

        (8) Trichloroethylene. Cranial mononeuropathies.

    d. Organophosphates or carbamates.

        (1) Sources. Chemical warfare agents and pesticides.

        (2) Route of exposure. Ingestion, inhalation, and absorption through skin.

        (3) Systemic signs. Cholinergic excess secondary to stimulation of muscarinic receptors resulting in vomiting, diarrhea, lacrimation, salivation, diaphoresis, bronchospasm, bronchorrhea, miosis, bradycardia, or tachycardia (SLUDGE syndrome).

        (4) Neurologic manifestations.

           (a) CNS. Decreased responsiveness, seizures (rarely).

           (b) PNS.

               1) Acute. Excess acetylcholine causes depolarizing paralysis: fasciculations and cramping followed by flaccid paralysis.

               2) Intermediate syndrome. Proximal muscle weakness, including respiratory symptoms, beginning 1 to 4 days after cholinergic phase.

3) Organophosphate-induced delayed neurotoxicity. Occurs 1 to 4 weeks after organophosphate poisoning and manifests as symmetric, distal, predominantly motor polyneuropathy. NCS studies demonstrate denervation of affected muscles along with reduced amplitude and prolonged conduction velocity.

(5) Physical examination findings. Miosis, weakness, signs of cholinergic excess (acute exposure).

(6) Mechanism of toxicity. Acetylcholine excess through inhibition of acetylcholinesterase.

(7) Diagnosis.
  (a) History and physical examination findings
  (b) Plasma cholinesterase is less specific but has a rapid turnaround time (decrease in level by 50% of baseline or serial increasing levels after poisoning indicates exposure).
  (c) RBC cholinesterase is more specific but has a long turnaround time (decrease of 25% of baseline level indicates exposure).

(8) Treatment.
  (a) Remove from exposure and decontaminate the skin with soap and water.
  (b) Respiratory and cardiovascular support
  (c) Atropine initial dose of 2 mg IV and then double dose every 5 to 10 minutes until drying of respiratory secretions
  (d) Pralidoxime initial dose of 1.5 g IV over 30 minutes and then infusion of 500 mg/hour until resolution of muscle weakness
  (e) Diazepam 10 mg or **lorazepam** 2 mg IV for seizures with repetition of dosage as needed.

3. Gases.
  a. Nitrous oxide.
  (1) Sources. Anesthesic agent
  (2) Route of exposure. Inhalation.
  (3) Systemic signs. Signs similar to vitamin B_{12} (cobalamin) deficiency including fatigue, depression, psychosis, and glossitis.
  (4) Neurologic manifestations including sensorimotor **peripheral polyneuropathy** may result, in addition to **myelopathy** affecting the posterior and anterolateral columns of the cervicothoracic spinal cord. **Optic neuropathy** and **cognitive impairment** may also occur.
  (5) Physical examination findings. Megaloblastic anemia, ataxia, sensory loss, weakness, and Lhermitte's sign.
  (6) Mechanism of toxicity. Nitrous oxide disrupts methionine synthetase by oxidizing Cobalamin(I) to Cobalamin(II).
  (7) Diagnosis. Patients may have a normal cobalamin level. Elevated serum homocysteine and methylmalonic acid are useful for confirming the diagnosis (cobalamin is involved in their metabolism). Magnetic resonance imaging (MRI) of spinal cord may show increased signal intensity in the posterior and lateral columns on T2-weighted images. NCS show mainly sensorimotor axonopathy.
  (8) Treatment. Replace vitamin B_{12}: **cyanocobalamin** 1,000 to 2,000 mcg by mouth (P.O.) daily for 1 to 2 weeks followed by 100 mcg P.O. daily, or 1,000 mcg IM daily for 5 days, then 1,000 mcg IM weekly for 4 weeks, then 1,000 mcg IM every 1 to 3 months, or 1,500 mcg intranasally weekly for 3 to 4 weeks then 500 mcg intranasally weekly. Early intramuscular administration is preferred for patients with very low levels. Patients should slowly improve.
  b. Ethylene oxide. Chronic workplace exposure in industry or through the sterilization of hospital supplies can result in symmetric distal sensorimotor polyneuropathy.

4. Pharmaceuticals.
  a. Dapsone. Chronic use in dermatologic and rheumatologic disorders may result in a motor neuropathy characterized by weakness and atrophy affecting the upper extremities more than the lower. NCS show motor axonopathy. It may also cause anterior ischemic optic neuropathy or optic atrophy.

b. **Pyridoxine.** Sensory neuropathy can occur from either large acute doses or excessive long-term use. Permanent sensory neuropathy has been reported after massive doses (>50 g) over a short time. Recovery may occur after removal of the drug.

c. **Other pharmaceuticals** associated with peripheral neuropathy include amiodarone, colchicine, dideoxycytidine, hydralazine, isoniazid, metronidazole, nitrofurantoin, and thalidomide.

B. Toxins affecting ion channels.

1. Ciguatera poisoning.

a. Sources. Ingestion of reef fish (barracuda, sea bass, parrot fish, red snapper, grouper, amber jack, king fish, and sturgeon).

b. Systemic signs. Symptoms usually begin within 2 to 6 hours of ingestion and may include abdominal pain, vomiting and diarrhea, dysuria, and pruritus. Cardiovascular symptoms include arterial hypotension, bradycardia, or cardiac arrhythmias.

c. Neurologic manifestations. Headache, perioral paresthesias spreading centrifugally to hands and feet, hot–cold dysesthesia, and insomnia.

d. **Mechanism of toxicity** is from prolonged opening of sodium channels.

e. **Diagnosis** is based on the clinical symptoms and history. Samples of fish can be sent out for high-performance liquid chromatography and mass spectrometry to detect ciguatoxin.

f. Treatment. Supportive care, **mannitol** 1 g/kg IV over 30 minutes has been suggested as an effective treatment if given early; however, supporting studies are lacking. Complete recovery usually occurs within a few weeks, but fatigue and weakness may persist.

2. Tetrodotoxin poisoning.

a. Sources. Ingestion of puffer or globefish. Although processing of fugu (puffer fish fillets) is licensed, puffer fish poisoning accounts for more deaths than any other type of food poisoning in Japan.

b. Systemic signs. Vomiting, hypotension, respiratory arrest.

c. Neurologic manifestations. Paresthesia of the perioral region and extremities followed by paralysis of voluntary and respiratory muscles.

d. Mechanism of toxicity. Blockade of sodium channels.

e. Diagnosis. History of puffer fish ingestion and clinical features. NCS show complete conduction block effect on myelinated nerve fibers and sparing of axons.

f. Treatment. Supportive care.

3. Other toxins affecting ion channels. Grayanotoxin (rhododendron, sodium-channel opener), scorpion toxin (sodium-channel opener), saxitoxin (shellfish, sodium-channel blocker).

C. Toxins affecting neuromuscular junction.

1. Black widow spider venom.

a. Sources. Black widow spider (*Latrodectus mactans*).

b. Systemic signs. Hypertension, nausea, diaphoresis, restlessness.

c. Neurologic manifestations. Diffuse muscle spasms and rigidity.

d. Mechanism of toxicity. Increased release of neurotransmitters (e.g., acetylcholine, norepinephrine) followed by depletion of transmitter stores.

e. Diagnosis. History and clinical examination. Bite location may show a "target lesion" with a pale center surrounded by erythema.

f. Treatment. IV opioids for pain control and benzodiazepines for muscle relaxation. In severe cases, antivenin (equine-based antiserum) can be given, but carries a risk of anaphylaxis: Pretreatment with diphenhydramine and having epinephrine at the bedside is recommended.

2. Botulism.

a. Sources. Replicating *Clostridium botulinum*, and occasionally *Clostridium baratii* and *Clostridium butyricum*, produces distinctive botulinal neurotoxins (types A to G).

(1) **Food.** Ingestion of food contaminated with preformed toxin; often involves the consumption of improperly canned food.

(2) **Infant.** Ingestion of foods (honey) contaminated with *C. botulinum* spores.

(3) **Wounds.** Most commonly in IV drug users, infected with *C. botulinum*.

b. Systemic signs. Sore throat, dry mouth, vomiting, and diarrhea followed by abdominal distention and constipation.

c. **Neurologic manifestations.** Descending motor paralysis including ophthalmoplegia, dysphagia, mydriasis (in 50%), and skeletal and respiratory muscles. In infant botulism, babies have constipation followed by a subacute progression of bulbar and extremity weakness (within 4 to 5 days) manifested by inability to suck and swallow, weakened cry, ptosis, and hypotonia, which may progress to generalized flaccidity and respiratory compromise.

d. **Mechanism of toxicity** involves inhibition of presynaptic vesicles preventing the release of acetylcholine.

e. **Diagnosis.**

(1) **History and examination.** Difficult to differentiate from Miller Fisher variant of GBS, although ataxia, paresthesia, areflexia, and elevated cerebrospinal fluid (CSF) protein are more common in Miller Fisher syndrome. In infants, the differential diagnosis includes sepsis, viral syndrome, dehydration, diphtheria, cerebrovascular accident, hypothyroidism, hypermagnesemia, Lambert–Eaton myasthenic syndrome, myasthenia gravis, poliomyelitis, GBS, encephalitis, and meningitis.

(2) **Laboratory.** Confirmation of *C. botulinum* in serum, stool, gastric contents, wound culture, food specimens, or positive mouse bioassay.

(3) **NCS.** Facilitation on repetitive nerve stimulation (may be absent in severely affected patients on the ventilator).

f. **Treatment.**

(1) Supportive care and antibiotics for wound botulism. In infant botulism, respiratory decompensation is associated with administration of aminoglycoside antibiotics and neck flexion during positioning for lumbar puncture or imaging. Antibiotics are not indicated for infant botulism.

(2) **Botulinum (heptavalent) antiserum** for food and wound botulism. Obtained from the Centers for Disease Control and Prevention by the state health departments.

(3) For infant botulism, **human-derived IV botulinum immune globulin (BIG)** trials demonstrated safety and efficacy. BIG is now US Food and Drug Administration approved and is available only from the California Department of Health Services (24-hour telephone: 510-231-7600 or webpage http://www.infantbotulism.org/).

3. **Other toxins affecting the neuromuscular junction** include the venom of the funnel web spider (increases acetylcholine release), saliva from the *Ixodid* family of ticks (prevents acetylcholine release), hypermagnesemia (prevents acetylcholine release), venom from cobra, coral snake, mamba, and Mojave rattlesnakes (decreases nicotinic neurotransmission by various mechanisms).

D. **Myopathy.**

1. **Immobility.** Toxins that depress mental status or produce coma can result in extended periods of immobility compressing muscular compartments causing subsequent muscle breakdown and rhabdomyolysis. Examples include alcohol, barbiturates, benzodiazepines, and opioids.

2. **Excess activity.** Toxins, or activities, that result in skeletal energy consumption exceeding energy supply can cause rhabdomyolysis. This can be the direct effect of the drug or secondary to agitation. Examples include amphetamines, cocaine, phencyclidine (PCP), and anticholinergic drugs.

3. **Myotoxins.**

a. **Hypokalemia.** Drugs depleting total body potassium stores can cause muscle breakdown and rhabdomyolysis. Examples include toluene and amphotericin B (renal tubular acidosis), glycyrrhizinic acid in licorice (increases mineralocorticoid activity), and long-term use of diuretics.

b. **Metabolic poisons.** Compounds that interfere with the production of adenosine triphosphate can result in muscle breakdown and rhabdomyolysis. Examples include cyanide, hydrogen sulfide, salicylates, dinitrophenol, chlorophenoxy herbicides (2,4-D), and carbon monoxide.

c. **Direct-acting myotoxins.** Numerous agents exist that have direct toxic effects on muscles resulting in myopathy and rhabdomyolysis. Examples include ethanol, heroin, corticosteroids, antimalarials, 3-hydroxy-3-methyl-glutaryl-coenzyme A reductase inhibitors, colchicine, ingestion of Buffalo fish (Haff disease), and snake bites.

CENTRAL NERVOUS SYSTEM

A. Acute delirium.
   1. **Anticholinergic syndrome** occurs from blockade of central and peripheral muscarinic receptors.
      a. Sources. Pharmaceuticals: tricyclic antidepressants, antihistamines, antipsychotics, cyclobenzaprine, promethazine, benztropine, carbamazepine, amantadine, scopolamine. Plants: jimson weed, nightshades, mandrake.
      b. Systemic signs. Dry mouth, mydriasis, dry axilla, hypoactive bowel sounds, urinary retention, tachycardia, low-grade fever.
      c. Neurologic manifestations. Acute delirium with visual hallucinations, increased motor activity (e.g., picking at bed sheets), mumbling speech pattern.
      d. Treatment.
         (1) **Activated charcoal.** 1 g/kg by mouth if the patient is awake, not at risk of aspiration, and the ingestion is within 2 hours.
         (2) **Benzodiazepines.** Repeated IV doses for agitation and tachycardia.
         (3) **Butyrophenones** (haloperidol or droperidol) in addition to benzodiazepines for patients with severe agitation and acute psychosis (avoid in patients with a prolonged QT interval).
         (4) **Physostigmine.** May be useful as a diagnostic tool in differentiating anticholinergic syndrome from other neurologic causes (e.g., encephalitis). Because of its short half-life and potential complications, physostigmine is generally not recommended for treatment. The dosage is 1 to 2 mg slow IV push over 10 minutes. Complications such as seizures, cardiac dysrhythmia, and cholinergic crisis have been reported with use. Contraindicated in the care of patients with bradycardia, or known ingestions that increase the risk of seizures (e.g., tricyclic antidepressants).
         (5) **Supportive care.** IV hydration and serial measurement of creatine kinase (CK) for rhabdomyolysis.
   2. Sympathomimetic syndrome. Occurs from an increase in extracellular concentrations of central and peripheral monoamines.
      a. Sources. Pharmaceuticals: pseudoephedrine, phenylpropanolamine, methylphenidate, phentermine. Illicit drugs: cocaine, amphetamines, methamphetamine, methylenedioxymethamphetamine (MDMA), synthetic cathinones (bath salts), synthetic cannabinoids. Plants: ma huang.
      b. Systemic signs. Tachycardia, hypertension, diaphoresis, mydriasis, fever, chest pain, myocardial infarction, and ventricular dysrhythmia.
      c. Neurologic manifestations. Psychomotor agitation, seizures, mania, tactile hallucinations (formication), increased muscle tone, increased muscle stretch reflexes with clonus, impaired cognition and chronic psychiatric symptoms (e.g., psychosis), hyponatremia-induced cerebral edema, ischemic or hemorrhagic stroke.
      d. Treatment.
         (1) **Activated charcoal.** 1 g/kg by mouth if the patient is awake and is not at risk of aspiration and if ingestion is within 1 hour.
         (2) **Benzodiazepines.** Repeat IV doses for seizures, agitation, tachycardia, hypertension, and chest pain. Avoid use of β-blockers in cases presenting after acute ingestion secondary to unopposed α-stimulation and corresponding vasospasm.
         (3) **Butyrophenones** (haloperidol or droperidol) or atypical antipsychotics in addition to benzodiazepines for patients with severe agitation and acute psychosis.
         (4) **Supportive care.** IV hydration and serial measurement of CK for rhabdomyolysis. Active cooling of hyperthermic patients.
   3. Serotonin syndrome. Occurs from increase in extracellular concentrations of serotonin in the CNS. Typically occurs in patients taking more than one serotonergic agent or large ingestions of single agents.
      a. Sources. Pharmaceuticals: selective serotonin reuptake inhibitors, tricyclic antidepressants, monoamine oxidase inhibitors, meperidine, fentanyl, dextromethorphan, tramadol, trazodone, venlafaxine, amphetamines, linezolid, L-tryptophan, methylene blue,

bromocriptine, and lithium. Illicit drugs: cocaine, amphetamines, MDMA (ecstasy), synthetic cathinones (bath salts). Plants: St. John's wort.

b. **Systemic signs.** Tachycardia, hypertension, diaphoresis, mydriasis, hyperthermia.

c. **Neurologic manifestations.** Agitation, confusion, hallucinations, increased motor tone and activity (lower more than upper extremity), hyperreflexia with lower extremity clonus (Video 59.1).

d. **Treatment.**

(1) **Activated charcoal.** 1 g/kg by mouth if the patient is awake and is not at risk of aspiration and if ingestion is within 1 hour.

(2) **Benzodiazepines.** Repeated IV doses for agitation, tachycardia, and hypertension.

(3) **Cyproheptadine,** an antihistamine and 5-HT2a antagonist, can be given orally, 12 mg as first dose, then 8 mg every 6 hours. Some **atypical antipsychotics** (olanzapine) may also be beneficial secondary to 5-HT2a antagonism and parenteral administration. Avoid when possibility of neuroleptic malignant syndrome (NMS) exists.

(4) **Supportive care.** IV hydration and serial measurement of CK for rhabdomyolysis.

4. **Hallucinogens.**

a. **Sources.** Anticholinergic agents: see Section **A.1.a** under Central Nervous System. Illicit drugs: lysergic acid diethylamide, mescaline, PCP, ketamine, synthetic cannabinoids, phenethylamines (e.g., 25-I-NBOMe). Plants: morning glory, nutmeg, salvia. Mushrooms: *Amanita muscaria*, psilocybin mushrooms. Animals: bufotoxin from *Bufo* family of toads.

b. **Systemic signs.** Tachycardia, hypertension, diaphoresis, mydriasis.

c. **Neurologic manifestations.** Visual hallucinations, increased motor activity, hyperreflexia.

d. **Treatment.**

(1) **Activated charcoal.** 1 g/kg by mouth if the patient is awake and is not at risk of aspiration and if ingestion is within 1 hour.

(2) **Benzodiazepines.** Repeat IV doses as needed for agitation.

(3) **Butyrophenones** (haloperidol or droperidol) in addition to benzodiazepines for patients with severe agitation and acute psychosis.

(4) IV hydration and serial measurement of CK for rhabdomyolysis.

5. **GABA-agonist withdrawal syndromes** result in a hyperadrenergic state with symptoms similar to those of sympathomimetic syndrome.

a. **Benzodiazepines, barbiturates,** and **ethanol** can cause a life-threatening withdrawal syndrome characterized by a hyperadrenergic state (tachycardia, hypertension, diaphoresis, piloerection, fever), nausea, vomiting, diarrhea, altered mental status, hallucinations, and seizures. Management of acute symptoms involves repeated IV doses of benzodiazepines (high doses at times) followed by scheduled oral benzodiazepines for prevention.

b. **Baclofen** can cause a life-threatening withdrawal syndrome characterized by disorientation, hallucinations, fever, rebound spasticity, seizures, and coma. Treatment involves reinstituting oral or intrathecal baclofen and benzodiazepines.

c. *γ*-**Hydroxybutyrate (GHB).** Abrupt discontinuance of chronically abused GHB compounds results in a withdrawal syndrome similar to benzodiazepine and ethanol withdrawal. Treatment is with IV or oral benzodiazepines and supportive care.

6. **Wernicke encephalopathy.**

a. **At-risk populations** are persons with chronic alcoholism or patients with other thiamine deficiency states (e.g., hyperemesis gravidarum, anorexia nervosa, malignant tumor of the GI tract, pyloric stenosis, inappropriate parenteral nutrition, and in patients with gastric bypass surgery as early as 4 to 12 weeks postoperatively).

b. **Symptoms.** Characterized by altered mental status (global confusional state), ataxia, and ophthalmoplegia. Although classically diagnosed with the triad of mental confusion (66% of patients), staggering gait (51% of patients), and ocular abnormalities (40% of patients), Wernicke encephalopathy can occur in the absence of some or all of the symptoms.

c. **Diagnosis.** By clinical features and improvement with treatment. Laboratory assessments of thiamine deficiency include erythrocyte thiamine transketolase, the blood thiamine concentration, or urinary thiamine excretion (with or without a 5-mg thiamine load). Abnormal MRI findings are hyperintense signals in the dorsal medial thalamic nuclei, periaqueductal gray area, and the third and fourth ventricle. Mammillary bodies enhance acutely and demonstrate atrophy chronically. MRI has a sensitivity of 53% and a specificity of 93% for the diagnosis of Wernicke encephalopathy. Treatment should be primarily based on clinical suspicion.

   d. **Treatment.** IV thiamine (100 mg) and magnesium (2 g) followed by daily thiamine and multivitamin supplementation. Daily thiamine doses should be 50 to 100 mg for 7 to 14 days, then 10 mg/day until full recovery is achieved, followed by at least 1 to 2 mg/day.

   e. **Prognosis** is favorable for most patients, but residual neurologic effects, including Korsakoff psychosis, memory loss, ataxia, nystagmus, and neuropathy, may persist.

B. **Subacute encephalopathy.**

1. **Bismuth.** Long-term use of bismuth salts for ostomy odor or in the management of peptic ulcer disease can manifest as subacute progressive encephalopathy.

   a. **Symptoms.** Patients have symptoms of progressive dementia and delirium, ataxia, severe myoclonus, and in rare instances, seizures. Symptoms may not occur until after weeks or years of continued use. Other symptoms include dark stools and dark staining of the gums. This syndrome can be mistaken for Creutzfeldt–Jakob disease, Alzheimer's dementia, or other progressive forms of encephalopathy and can be fatal if not diagnosed.

   b. **Diagnosis.** In acute encephalopathy, the bismuth blood level is typically between 150 and 2,000 μg/100 mL instead of the normal 10 to 30 μg/100 mL. Head computed tomography (CT) may show increased attenuation in the basal ganglia and cerebral cortex.

   c. **Treatment.** Stop the drug and provide supportive care. The syndrome usually regresses in 3 to 12 weeks after cessation of bismuth.

2. **Lithium.** Chronic use or acute overdose of lithium salts can manifest as progressive encephalopathy. Impaired excretion (e.g., dehydration-induced renal insufficiency) and excessive intake of lithium are the usual causes of lithium intoxication.

   a. **Symptoms.** Patients come to medical attention with tremor, altered mental status, ataxia, myoclonus, and in rare instances, seizures. Other symptoms include nausea, vomiting, diabetes insipidus, hypothyroidism, mutism, and renal failure.

   b. **Diagnosis.** An elevated serum lithium level supports the diagnosis. Therapeutic levels of lithium range from 0.6 to 1.2 mEq/L. Toxic effects of lithium are generally related to serum levels, with mild to moderate severity seen with levels of 1.5 to 2.5 mEq/L, serious toxicity with levels of 2.5 to 3.0 mEq/L, and life-threatening toxicity with levels 3.0 to 4.0 mEq/L.

   c. **Treatment.** Patients with severe symptoms require urgent hemodialysis (impaired kidney function and a level >4.0 mEq/L or if demonstrating impaired consciousness, seizure, or life-threatening dysrhythmia). Dialysis clears extracellular lithium but the intracellular lithium may cause a rebound in the serum lithium concentrations after dialysis. IV saline should be given to rehydrate and avoid hyponatremia (excretion of sodium and lithium are related).

3. **Carbon monoxide (CO).** Patients with recent history of CO poisoning may have a syndrome known as **delayed neurologic sequelae,** occurring 2 to 40 days after exposure and recovery. The incidence of delayed neurologic sequelae increases with the duration of unconsciousness and age greater than 30.

   a. **Symptoms.** Manifested as altered mental status, personality changes, and memory loss. Patients may also have ataxia, seizures, urinary and fecal incontinence, parkinsonism, mutism, cortical blindness, and gait and motor disturbances. Physical examination findings may include hyperreflexia, frontal lobe release signs (glabellar reflex, palmar grasp), masked facies, and other parkinsonian features.

   b. **Diagnosis.** Neuropsychometric testing displays cognitive dysfunction. MRI findings may include bilateral globus pallidus infarcts (because of the acute hypoxia) and diffuse demyelination of subcortical white matter [because of delayed post-hypoxic leukoencephalopathy (DPHL)]. DPHL can also occur after exposure to other toxins that cause hypoxia (e.g., opioids).

c. **Treatment.** Supportive care. It is unclear whether treatment of acute CO poisoning influences the risk of delayed neurologic sequelae. The majority of patients will show some recovery.

4. **Aluminum.** Long-term use of aluminum phosphate binders, aluminum-contaminated dialysates, or medications containing aluminum (e.g., sucralfate) in the care of patients with renal failure can result in progressive encephalopathy. Patients come to medical attention with agitation, speech disorder, confusion, myoclonus, coma, and/or seizures. Aluminum exposure is also associated with osteomalacia and microcytic hypochromic anemia. Diagnosis is made by elevated aluminum level but if within normal limits and diagnosis is still suspected, bone biopsy may confirm the diagnosis. Treatment involves removal of sources of aluminum and for some patients chelation with deferoxamine.

5. **NMS.** Subacute encephalopathy associated with hyperthermia, rigidity with elevated CK, and autonomic instability in the setting of neuroleptic administration. Treatment is supportive care with external cooling and benzodiazepines as necessary. Consideration can also be given to bromocriptine and/or dantrolene for antidotal therapy. Care must be taken to differentiate NMS from serotonin syndrome (see Section **A.3** under Central Nervous System) as bromocriptine may worsen serotonin syndrome.

C. **Coma and CNS depression.** Many toxins causing CNS depression and coma can mimic brain death, including loss of brainstem reflexes. Many of these toxins have long half-lives, so clinical criteria of brain death do not apply.

1. **Sedative hypnotics.**
    a. **Sources.** Ethanol, benzodiazepines, barbiturates, central-acting muscle relaxants, chloral hydrate, buspirone, zolpidem, baclofen, clonidine, antihistamines, and numerous antidepressants and antipsychotics.
    b. **Systemic signs.** Pressure sores, arterial hypotension, bradycardia, hypothermia.
    c. **Neurologic manifestations.** Somnolence, coma, areflexia, nystagmus, amnesia. Coma from baclofen poisoning can be prolonged and profound with physical exam findings that can mimic brain death.
    d. **Treatment.** Supportive care, **activated charcoal** 1 g/kg by mouth if the patient is awake and is not at risk of aspiration and if ingestion is within 1 hour. The use of **flumazenil,** a benzodiazepine antagonist, is generally **not recommended** because of increased risk of seizures in habituated patients.

2. **Opioids, opiates.**
    a. **Sources.** Pharmaceuticals: hydrocodone, oxycodone, morphine, hydromorphone, oxymorphone, meperidine, fentanyl, methadone. Illicit drugs: Heroin, designer opioids.
    b. **Systemic signs.** Hypotension, bradycardia, bradypnea, pulmonary edema, track marks on skin, skin abscesses, decreased bowel sounds, cyanosis.
    c. **Neurologic manifestations.** Coma, miosis, deafness, areflexia, and seizures (meperidine). Seizures from meperidine are the result of elevated levels of normeperidine (a major metabolite of meperidine). Risk factors for normeperidine seizures are renal failure and chronic dosing. Naloxone (Narcan; Endo Pharmaceuticals, Chadds Ford, PA, USA) does not reverse meperidine- or propoxyphene-related seizures.
    d. **Treatment.** Supportive care, **Naloxone** 0.04 to 0.4 mg IV push followed by 0.04 to 0.4 mg every minute until reversal of respiratory depression or to a maximum of 8 mg. In habituated patients in whom immediate reversal is not warranted (not in cardiac or respiratory arrest) it is recommended to start with lower concentrations to avoid precipitating acute opioid withdrawal.

3. **GHB.**
    a. **Sources.** GHB (Xyrem), γ-butyrolactone, butanediol (used for mood enhancement, sleep induction, and by body builders for purported increased growth hormone release).
    b. **Systemic signs.** Bradycardia, hypotension, hypothermia, nystagmus, vomiting.
    c. **Neurologic manifestations.** Areflexic coma (typically short duration—less than 6 hours with rapid reversal), normal or miotic pupils, seizures.
    d. **Treatment.** Supportive care.

4. **Carbon monoxide.**
    a. **Sources.** Automotive exhaust, smoke inhalation, faulty heaters, external heating sources, propane- and gas-powered tools and vehicles.

    b. **Systemic signs.** Tachycardia, hypotension, chest pain, dyspnea, myocardial infarction, cardiac arrhythmia, flushed skin, pressure sores, nausea, vomiting.

    c. **Neurologic manifestations.** Headache, confusion, cognitive deficits, coma, seizures, stroke, parkinsonism, delayed neurologic sequelae (see Section **B.3** under Central Nervous System).

    d. **Diagnosis.** Carbon monoxide levels are indicative of exposure but are not reliable predictors of toxicity or symptoms. The normal result is <5% for nonsmokers and <10% for smokers.

    e. **Treatment.**

      (1) Removal from source of carbon monoxide

      (2) **100% oxygen** (via non-rebreather) for 6 to 12 hours for mild or moderate symptoms

      (3) Indications for **hyperbaric oxygen therapy** (although availability is limited):

        (a) Unconsciousness at the scene or hospital

        (b) Coma or persistent neurologic deficit or

        (c) Myocardial ischemia or ventricular dysrhythmia or

        (d) Hypotension or cardiovascular compromise or

        (e) Pregnancy with any of the above, levels >20%, or signs of fetal distress.

5. **Cocaine or stimulant washout syndrome** occurs among abusers of cocaine or other stimulants, the increased use of which decreases the level of CNS catecholamines resulting in depressed mental status, confusion, or coma (unresponsive to stimuli, including intubation). Patients may have dysconjugate gaze. Other physical examination findings, vital signs, and laboratory findings are generally normal. Symptoms may last for 8 to 24 hours, and treatment is supportive. This should always be a diagnosis of exclusion.

D. **Cerebellar disorders.**

1. **Toluene–solvent abuse syndrome.**

    a. **Sources.** Toluene-containing paint thinner, paint stripper, and glue.

    b. **Route of exposure.** Inhalational: huffing (inhaling soaked rags) or bagging (inhaling from bags containing solvent).

    c. **Systemic signs.** Abdominal pain, anorexia, weight loss, gastritis, possible renal tubular acidosis (hypokalemia and acidosis), rhabdomyolysis, hepatitis, solvent odor on breath.

    d. **Neurologic manifestations.** Tremor of the head and extremities, ataxia, staggering gait, cognitive deficits, personality changes, optic nerve atrophy, hearing loss, loss of smell, spasticity, and hyperreflexia.

    e. **Diagnosis.**

      (1) **Laboratory.** Elevated serum toluene levels and urine hippuric acid levels confirm exposure, but are not always detected.

      (2) **Imaging.** MRI of the brain often shows cerebellar and cerebral atrophy. Evidence of white matter disease can be seen with increased signal intensity on T2-weighted images in the periventricular, internal capsular, and brainstem pyramidal regions.

      (3) **Electrophysiologic studies.** Brainstem auditory evoked response testing may show sparing of early components and loss or decrement of the late components (waves III and IV). Abnormal pattern visual evoked cortical potentials and prolonged P100 peak latency may occur in patients with toxic optic neuropathy caused by toluene abuse.

    f. **Treatment.** Supportive care and addiction rehabilitation.

2. **Mercury poisoning** (see also Section **A.1.d** under Peripheral Nervous System). Poisoning with elemental mercury vapor or organic mercury (along with other symptoms described in Section **A.1.d** under Peripheral Nervous System) can result in cerebellar symptoms including ataxia and tremor with pathologic neuronal damage seen in visual cortex, cerebellar vermis and hemispheres, and postcentral cortex.

3. **Anticonvulsant drugs** including phenobarbital, phenytoin, and carbamazepine, in elevated concentration or acute overdose, manifest toxicity with predominantly ataxia, nystagmus, and CNS depression. Chronic use of phenytoin may also result in cerebellar atrophy.

4. **Ethanol.** Both acute intoxication and chronic abuse of ethanol can result in ataxia, tremor, and altered mental status. Wernicke encephalopathy should be considered when any

patient with chronic alcoholism has changes in mental status and ataxia not related to acute intoxication.

E. **Parkinsonism.**

1. **1-Methyl-4-phenyl-1,2,3,6-tetrahydropyridine (MPTP),** a byproduct in the production of a synthetic analog of meperidine, can cause acute parkinsonism in drug users, scientists, and pharmaceutical workers. Although not itself neurotoxic, MPTP is metabolized by monoamine oxidase to a compound (MPP+) that inhibits electron transport in dopaminergic neurons. This syndrome was characterized by the rapid (24 to 72 hours) development of end-stage parkinsonism with tremor, rigidity, bradykinesia, postural instability, masked facies, and decreased blink rate. Investigation of the mechanism of toxicity has led to the development of an animal model for Parkinson's disease.

2. **Manganese.** A parkinsonian-like illness has been described among miners or workers exposed to manganese oxide and among those who have ingested potassium permanganate, associated with methcathinone abuse. This syndrome is the result of degradation of the globus pallidus and striatum rather than the substantia nigra. It begins with a prodrome of nonspecific symptoms (insomnia, irritability, muscle weakness) and progresses to psychiatric manifestations (hallucinations, emotional lability, delusions) and finally to classic parkinsonian features of gait disturbance, masked facies, bradykinesia, rigidity, and less commonly tremor, which tends to be more postural or kinetic rather than resting. Patients with manganese-induced parkinsonism also experience dystonia consisting of facial grimacing and/or plantar flexion of the foot. These patients have little or no response to levodopa. Diagnosis is made by clinical history of significant exposure with associated physical exam and MRI findings. Fluorodopa positron emission tomography (PET) can help distinguish manganism (normal fluorodopa PET imaging) from Parkinson's disease.

3. **Neuroleptic drugs.** The use of neuroleptic agents, both typical and atypical, has been associated with the acute development of extrapyramidal side effects, most commonly parkinsonism. Patient's age and the duration and potency of neuroleptic treatment are risk factors for neuroleptic-induced parkinsonism. The presentation of neuroleptic-induced parkinsonism includes bradykinesia or akinesia, which may be associated with decreased arm swing, masked facies, drooling, decreased eye blinking, and soft, monotonous speech; tremor, that is most commonly a rhythmic, resting tremor; and rigidity of the extremities, neck, or trunk. Cessation of the neuroleptic typically results in resolution of symptoms within a few weeks. Patients can be treated with anticholinergics or dopaminergic agents although levodopa is not recommended because of insufficient efficacy and risk of exacerbating psychosis. Prolonged use of neuroleptics can result in tardive dyskinesia with choreiform movements of the face, tongue, and limbs. If recognized early, most symptoms of tardive dyskinesia resolve within 5 years.

4. **Mitochondrial toxins** (carbon monoxide, cyanide, hydrogen sulfide). Agents that inhibit the mitochondrial respiratory chain can cause development of bilateral globus pallidus infarction and subsequently a parkinsonian syndrome. This typically results from a combination of arterial hypotension and hypoxia in severe poisoning and can have neuropsychiatric manifestations or more classic parkinsonism.

F. **Seizures.** Toxins cause seizures by one of four mechanisms: (1) decrease in the seizure threshold of a patient with an underlying seizure disorder, (2) direct effects on the CNS, (3) withdrawal seizures, or (4) metabolic derangements. Most toxin-related seizures are generalized tonic–clonic. (If there is any suggestion of focal onset, then brain imaging is necessary.) Most patients with toxin-induced seizures can be treated with standard seizure algorithms, except that treatment is more often successful with benzodiazepines and barbiturates than with phenytoin.

1. **Stimulants** (see also Section A.2 under Central Nervous System).

   a. **Sources.** Cocaine, amphetamines, methamphetamine, PCP.

   b. **Mechanism of toxicity.** Secondary to increased extracellular levels of CNS catecholamines with subsequent excitation of the sympathetic nervous system. Can cause vasculitis, vasospasm, accelerated atherosclerosis, and increased risk of both ischemic and hemorrhagic stroke.

   c. **Treatment.**

      (1) **Diazepam** 10 mg or **lorazepam** 2 mg IV, repeat doses as needed, or

      (2) **Phenobarbital** 20 mg/kg IV at rate of 25 to 50 mg/minute for refractory seizures.

2. **Cholinergics** (see also Section A.3 under Peripheral Nervous System).
   a. Sources. Organophosphate and carbamate insecticides, chemical warfare agents.
   b. Mechanism of toxicity. Increased CNS concentration of acetylcholine with secondary release of glutamate.
   c. Treatment.
      (1) **Diazepam** 10 mg, **lorazepam** 2 mg IV, repeat doses as needed, or **phenobarbital** 20 mg/kg IV at rate of 25 to 50 mg/minute for refractory seizures.
      (2) **Atropine** 2 to 4 mg IV for signs of cholinergic excess.
      (3) **Pralidoxime** 1.5 g IV over 30 minutes for nicotinic symptoms.
3. **GABA antagonists.**
   a. Sources. Tricyclic antidepressants, phenothiazines, flumazenil, chlorinated hydrocarbons, hydrazines, cephalosporins, ciprofloxacin, imipenem, penicillins, isoniazid, steroids, clozapine, olanzapine. Plants: cicutoxin (water hemlock), picrotoxin (fish berries), and wormwood (absinthe).
   b. Mechanism of action. Direct or indirect inhibition of $GABA_A$ receptors or decreased synthesis of GABA through inhibition of either glutamic acid decarboxylase or pyridoxal kinase (e.g., isoniazid, hydrazines).
   c. Treatment.
      (1) **Diazepam** 10 mg, **lorazepam** 2 mg IV, repeat doses as needed, or **phenobarbital** 20 mg/kg IV at rate of 25 to 50 mg/minute for refractory seizures.
      (2) **Pyridoxine.** For isoniazid or hydrazine overdose. The amount of pyridoxine administered should be equivalent (gram for gram) to the estimated amount of isoniazid ingested. It can be given IV push to patients with severe symptoms or as an IV infusion. If an unknown amount of isoniazid has been ingested, 5 g IV can be given empirically.
4. **Glutamate agonists.**
   a. Sources. Domoic acid (shellfish), ibotenic acid (*A. muscaria* mushrooms), β-*N*-oxalylamino-L-alanine (BOAA found in legumes of the genus *Lathyrus*).
   b. Mechanism of action. Direct agonists at glutamate receptors (NMDA, α-amino-3-hydroxy-5-methyl-4-isoxazolepropionic acid).
   c. Other clinical features. Patients with lathyrism from BOAA have spastic paraplegia.
   d. Treatment.
      (1) **Diazepam** 10 mg or **lorazepam** 2 mg IV for seizures, repeat doses as needed or **phenobarbital** 20 mg/kg IV at a rate of 25 to 50 mg/minute for refractory seizures.
5. **Antihistamines.**
   a. Sources. First-generation (sedating) antihistamines (diphenhydramine, chlorpheniramine, brompheniramine).
   b. Mechanism of action. Central histamine-1 receptor antagonism.
   c. Other clinical features. See anticholinergic syndrome (Section **A.1** under Central Nervous System).
   d. Treatment.
      (1) **Diazepam** 10 mg or **lorazepam** 2 mg IV for seizures, repeat doses as needed, or **phenobarbital** 20 mg/kg IV at rate of 25 to 50 mg/minute for refractory seizures.
6. **Adenosine antagonists.**
   a. Sources. Theophylline, caffeine, theobromine, pentoxifylline, carbamazepine.
   b. Mechanism of action. Antagonism of presynaptic A1 receptors preventing inhibition of glutamatergic neurons, and A2 receptors causing cerebral vasoconstriction. Theophylline may decrease GABA levels by decreasing pyridoxal-5-phosphate levels.
   c. Other clinical features.
      (1) The manifestations of theophylline toxicity are similar to those of sympathomimetic syndrome (see Section **A.2** under Central Nervous System).
      (2) The manifestations of carbamazepine toxicity are similar to those of anticholinergic syndrome (see Section **A.1** under Central Nervous System).
   d. Treatment.
      (1) **Phenobarbital** 20 mg/kg IV at rate of 25 to 50 mg/minute for altered mental status, CNS agitation, theophylline levels greater than 100 μg/mL, or seizures additionally may use repeated doses of **diazepam** 10 mg or **lorazepam** 2 mg as needed. Avoid phenytoin and fosphenytoin.
      (2) **Hemodialysis** for theophylline or caffeine overdose with seizures.

7. **Withdrawal seizures.**
   a. **Sources.** Ethanol, benzodiazepines, barbiturates, baclofen.
   b. **Mechanism of action.** Prolonged use of GABA agonists results in decreased activity at GABA receptors and increased activity at glutamate receptors.
   c. **Other clinical features.** Delirium, hallucinations, tachycardia, arterial hypertension, fever, autonomic instability, and hypertonicity because of emergency of underlying tone (baclofen).
   d. **Treatment.**
      (1) **Diazepam** 10 mg or **lorazepam** 2 mg IV for seizures, repeat doses as needed, or **phenobarbital** 20 mg/kg IV at a rate of 25 to 50 mg/minute for refractory seizures.
      (2) For **baclofen** withdrawal oral baclofen should be restarted at the previous rate, or the baclofen pump should be refilled.

Key Points

Peripheral Nervous System

- Most peripheral neurotoxins cause a rapidly progressive symmetric distal axonopathy.
- Severe poisoning from arsenic or thallium can cause symptoms that mimic GBS.
- Chronic elemental or inorganic mercury exposure can cause symptoms that mimic pheochromocytoma.
- Chronic abuse of nitrous oxide or workplace exposure to 1-bromopropane can cause a myeloneuropathy syndrome.
- Botulism causes a descending paralysis that can mimic Miller Fisher variant of GBS.

Central Nervous System

- First-line treatment for toxin-induced agitated delirium, including anticholinergic, sympathomimetic, and serotonin syndromes, is benzodiazepines. High doses may be required.
- Toxin-induced seizures are best treated with GABA agonists, benzodiazepines followed by barbiturates if necessary. Supplementation with pyridoxine should be considered for refractory seizures that are not responding to GABA agonists.
- Wernicke encephalopathy should be considered in any patient with a history of alcohol use who presents with acute encephalopathy. Thiamine supplementation should be given empirically.
- CO poisoning can present with nonspecific symptoms and should be considered in patients whose symptoms are specific to one environment or who have family members or coworkers with similar symptoms. Identifying the source of the exposure is key for preventing further poisoning.
- Baclofen can cause prolonged, profound coma that may mimic the physical exam findings of brain death. Extreme caution should be used when considering a brain death examination in baclofen overdose.

Recommended Readings

Albin RL. Basal ganglia neurotoxins. *Neurol Clin.* 2000;18(3):665–680.

Bradberry SM, Wilkinson JM, Ferner RE. Systemic toxicity related to metal hip prostheses. *Clin Toxicol.* 2014;52(8):837–847.

Decker BS, Goldfarb DS, Dargan PI, et al. Extracorporeal treatment for lithium poisoning: Systematic review and recommendations from the EXTRIP workgroup. *Clin J Am Soc Nephrol.* 2015;10(5):875–887.

Dobbs MR. *Clinical Neurotoxicology: Syndromes, Substances, Environments.* Philadelphia, PA: Saunders Elsevier; 2009.

Hoffman RS, Howland MA, Lewin NA, et al, eds. *Goldfrank's Toxicologic Emergencies.* 10th ed. New York, NY: McGraw-Hill; 2014.

Ibrahim D, Froberg B, Wolf A, et al. Heavy metal poisoning: clinical presentations and pathophysiology. *Clin Lab Med.* 2006;26(1):67–97, viii.

Kao LW, Nanagas KA. Carbon monoxide poisoning. *Med Clin North Am.* 2005;89(6):1161–1194.

Kongsaengdao S, Samintarapanya K, Rusmeechan S, et al. Electrophysiological diagnosis and patterns of response to treatment of botulism with neuromuscular respiratory failure. *Muscle Nerve.* 2009;40(2):271–278.

London Z, Albers JW. Toxic neuropathies associated with pharmaceutic and industrial agents. *Neurol Clin.* 2007;25(1):257–276.

Majersik JJ, Caravati EM, Steffens JD. Severe neurotoxicity associated with exposure to the solvent 1-bromopropane (n-propyl bromide). *Clin Toxicol.* 2007;45(3):270–276.

O'Connor AD, Rusyniak DE, Bruno A. Cerebrovascular and cardiovascular complications of alcohol and sympathomimetic drug abuse. *Med Clin North Am.* 2005;89(6):1343–1358.

Rusyniak DE, Nanagas KA. Organophosphate poisoning. *Semin Neurol.* 2004;24(2):197–204.

Rusyniak DE, Sprague JE. Hyperthermic syndromes induced by toxins. *Clin Lab Med.* 2006;26(1):165–184, ix.

Spencer PS, Schaumburg HH, eds. *Experimental and Clinical Neurotoxicology.* 2nd ed. New York, NY: Oxford University Press; 2000.

Tormoehlen LM, Kumar N. Neurotoxicology: five new things. *Neurol Clin Pract.* 2015;2(4):301–310.

Walsh RJ, Amato AA. Toxic myopathies. *Neurol Clin.* 2005;23(2):397–428.

Wills B, Erickson T. Drug- and toxin-associated seizures. *Med Clin North Am.* 2005;89(6):1297–1321.

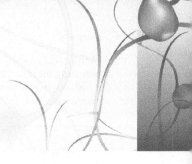

60 Sleep Disorders

Phyllis C. Zee and Alon Y. Avidan

Sleep disturbances are prevalent in the general population, but certain groups such as older adults, women, and patients with chronic comorbid medical, neurologic, and psychiatric disorders are at particular risk. Indeed, the most recent evidence points to a bidirectional relationship between health and sleep. Sleep problems influence health-related quality of life and may contribute to the development of, or exacerbate, medical and neurologic conditions. Patients who report disturbed sleep generally describe one or more of three types of problems—insomnia, excessive daytime sleepiness (EDS), and abnormal motor activities, complex behaviors, or disturbed sensations during sleep.

The 2014 revised international classification of sleep disorders: diagnostic and coding manual published by the American Academy of Sleep Medicine (AASM) (*ICSD-3*) lists five major categories of sleep disorders: insomnia—that is, disorder of initiating and maintaining sleep; sleep-related breathing disorders; hypersomnias—that is, disorders of excessive sleepiness; movement disorders; and circadian rhythm sleep–wake disorders (CRSWDs). To assist the clinician, in diagnosing and treating sleep disorders, a differential diagnosis-based classification adapted from the *ICSD-3* is used in this chapter.

INSOMNIA

Insomnia is characterized by persistent symptoms of difficulty with sleep initiation, duration, consolidation, or quality that occurs despite adequate opportunity and circumstances for sleep, and results in functional impairment. Insomnia is a chronic disorder (typically 3 months or more) that is made on the basis of a carefully detailed history. Insomnia is a 24-hour problem, so nighttime sleep difficulty must result in distress, impairment of function, health, and/or mood.

A. **Clinical course.** For the diagnosis of insomnia to be made, a patient has to have sleep difficulties that substantially affect daytime functioning and often have a learning or conditioning component that typically involves one or more of the following: daily worries about not being able to fall asleep or stay asleep accompanied by intense efforts to fall asleep each night; and somatized tension and anxiety associated with bedtime and the subject of sleep. The most difficult differential diagnosis is with generalized anxiety disorders in which anxiety is pervasive and involves most aspects of daily life rather than exclusively the inability to sleep. Differentiation from affective disorders, such as depression, also is important. Insomnia is a chronic inability to sleep, presumably associated with a predisposition for insomnia resulting from abnormality of the sleep–wake cycle, and autonomic activity or arousal system. Patients with this condition are a heterogeneous group. Most have a history of intermittent insomnia symptoms that are aggravated by precipitating factors such as stress and tension. Insomnia is often accompanied by other factors such as poor sleep hygiene, and psychiatric, neurologic and other medical disorders.

B. **Treatment and outcome.** Effective treatment begins with determining whether the chief problem is one of initiation, maintenance of sleep, early awakening, or a combination of these. The next step is to ascertain the severity of the problem by asking about the duration of insomnia, how often he/she experiences the problem, and how it affects their daytime functioning. Once the duration and severity have been established, it is important to identify precipitating and perpetuating factors such as poor sleep hygiene. Ask the patient about caffeine consumption; alcohol consumption; medications; medical, psychiatric, neurologic disorders; and symptoms of specific sleep disorders, such as sleep apnea, restless legs syndrome (RLS), and circadian rhythm disorders.

A multimodal individualized approach is indicated for most patients.

Optimizing the treatment of comorbid medical, neurologic, and psychiatric conditions, as well as identifying medications or behaviors that promote insomnia are essential first steps. A combined treatment approach involving good sleep hygiene, cognitive-behavioral therapy (CBT), and medications is most often employed. A 4- to 8-week program of sleep hygiene counseling, cognitive-behavioral modifications, and judicious use of hypnotics is recommended. If insomnia does not improve after this period of treatment, referral to a sleep specialist should be considered for further evaluation.

1. **Cognitive-behavioral therapy for insomnia (CBT-I).** The most widely used behavioral therapy program in the management of insomnia includes a combined program of sleep hygiene education, relaxation techniques, stimulus–control therapy, and sleep restriction therapy. Relaxation techniques may include progressive muscle relaxation, biofeedback, deep breathing, meditation, guided imagery, and other techniques to control cognitive arousal. These techniques are first taught during training sessions and then practiced daily for 20 to 30 minutes by the patient at home, usually around bedtime.

   A specific type of CBT-I is **stimulus–control therapy**, which is useful in the management of conditioned insomnia. This technique is an attempt to break the conditioning by teaching the patient to associate the bedroom with sleep behavior. The instructions for sleep hygiene and stimulus–control behavioral therapy are listed in Tables 60.1 and 60.2. Sleep restriction therapy involves curtailment of time in bed,

---

TABLE 60.1 Sleep Hygiene Instructions

Homeostatic drive for sleep

1. Avoid naps, except for a brief 10–15-min nap 8 hr after arising; check with your physician first, because in some sleep disorders naps can be beneficial.
2. Restrict sleep period to average number of hours you have actually slept per night in the preceding week. Quality of sleep is important. Too much time in bed can decrease quality on the subsequent night.
3. Get regular exercise every day, preferably 40 min in the afternoon. It is best to finish exercise at least 3 hr before bedtime.
4. Take a warm bath 90–120 min before bedtime to help lower body temperature.

Circadian factors

1. Keep a regular out-of-bed time (do not deviate more than 1 hr) 7 d/wk.
2. Do not expose yourself to bright light if you have to get up at night.
3. Expose yourself to bright light, either outdoor or artificial, during the day.

Drug effects

1. Do not smoke to get yourself back to sleep.
2. Do not smoke after 7:00 P.M.; give up smoking entirely.
3. Avoid caffeine and limit caffeine use to no more than three cups no later than 10:00 A.M.
4. Avoid alcoholic beverages after 7:00 P.M.

Arousal in sleep setting

1. Keep clock face turned away, and do not find out what time it is when you wake up at night.
2. Avoid strenuous exercise after 6:00 P.M.
3. Do not eat or drink heavily for 3 hr before bedtime. A light bedtime snack may help.
4. If you have trouble with regurgitation, be especially careful to avoid heavy meals and spices in the evening. You may have to raise the head of your bed.
5. Keep your room dark, quiet, well ventilated, and at a comfortable temperature.
6. Use a bedtime ritual. Reading before lights-out may be helpful if it is not occupationally related.
7. Do not try too hard to sleep; instead, concentrate on the pleasant feeling of relaxation.
8. Use stress management and relaxation techniques in the daytime.
9. Be sure your mattress pillow is of the right height and firmness.
10. Use the bedroom only for sleep; do not work or do other activities that lead to prolonged wakefulness.

TABLE 60.2 Stimulus–Control Behavioral Therapy

1. Go to bed only when sleepy. Stay up until you are really sleepy, then return to bed. If sleep still does not come easily, get out of bed again. The goal is to associate bed with falling asleep quickly.
2. Use the bed only for sleeping. Do not read, watch television, or eat in bed.
3. If unable to sleep, get up and move to another room.
4. Repeat the preceding step as often as necessary throughout the night.
5. Set the alarm and get up at the same time every morning, regardless of how much you slept during the night. This helps the body acquire a constant sleep–wake rhythm.
6. Do not nap during the day.

so that sleep efficiency (time asleep divided by time in bed) is 85% or greater. As sleep efficiency increases, time in bed is gradually lengthened. Shorter-duration behavioral interventions, and for patients who do not have access to formal face-to-face CBT-I training, Internet-based approaches are also available.

2. **Hypnotic drugs.** The most widely used prescription hypnotics are the benzodiazepine receptor agonists, which include benzodiazepines (BzRA) and the nonbenzodiazepine receptor agonist (non-BxRA) hypnotics, such as eszopiclone, zaleplon, and zolpidem. Traditionally, this class of medications was indicated for short-term use. More recently, with the recognition that insomnia is often chronic and with the availability of longer-term studies for up to a year, the short-term indication has been removed from the newly Food and Drug Administration (FDA)-approved hypnotics such as eszopiclone and zolpidem extended release (ER). Ramelteon, a melatonin receptor agonist; low-dose doxepin; and suvorexant, an orexin receptor antagonist, represent different classes of hypnotics with unique mechanisms of action that target the sleep/wake system.

The choice of hypnotic may depend on the timing of insomnia. For example, if the predominant difficulty is with sleep initiation, a fast-acting, short-half-life hypnotic may be preferable. If the problem is frequent awakenings during the night and sleep maintenance insomnia, a longer-acting hypnotic may be more effective. Most hypnotics approved by the FDA are indicated for the treatment of sleep-onset insomnia, whereas eszopiclone, zolpidem ER, low-dose doxepin, and suvorexant are also indicated for the treatment of sleep maintenance insomnia. In practice, sedating antidepressants, such as the tricyclic antidepressants and heterocyclics (trazodone), are frequently used off label for the treatment of insomnia. However, there is limited data regarding their efficacy or long-term safety for the treatment of insomnia that is not comorbid with depression. The exception is low-dose doxepin (3 to 6 mg), which is FDA approved for insomnia.

The most widely used prescription hypnotics and their properties are listed in Table 60.3. Although patients with chronic insomnia rarely become "great" sleepers after treatment, most can manage the perpetuating factors of insomnia by using sleep hygiene, cognitive-behavioral treatment, and, when indicated, hypnotics.

INSOMNIA ASSOCIATED WITH NEUROLOGIC, PSYCHIATRIC, AND MEDICAL DISORDERS

A. **Course.** Insomnia is often comorbid with neurologic and psychiatric conditions. Results of epidemiologic studies suggest that as many as 57% of persons with insomnia have a comorbid psychiatric condition or will have one within 1 year. The comorbid condition is usually a mood disorder, anxiety disorder, somatoform disorder, personality disorder, schizophrenia, pain syndrome, or substance abuse. Sleep in major depression is usually characterized by early morning awakening (2 to 4 hours after sleep onset), and frequent nocturnal awakening with inability to reinitiate sleep. Although depression and insomnia have a bidirectional relationship, insomnia often precedes the diagnosis of depression. The incidence of insomnia among patients with anxiety disorders is high. The typical symptoms are difficulty with sleep initiation and, to a lesser degree, nocturnal awakenings. Fatigue is common, but napping is unusual.

TABLE 60.3 FDA-Approved Hypnotics for the Management of Insomnia

Benzodiazepine Receptor Agonists (BzRA)

Agent	Dose (mg)	Onset of Action (min)	Half-Life (hr)	Active Metabolites
Triazolam (Halcion)	0.125–0.25 (0.125)	15–30	2–5	No
Temazepam (Restoril)	15–30 (7.5–15)	45–60	8–20	No
Estazolam (ProSom)	1–2 (0.5–1.0)	15–60	8–24	No
Flurazepam (Dalmane)	15–30 (7.5)	0.5–1 hr	47–100 including metabolites	Yes
Quazepam (Doral)	7.5–15 (7.5)	20–45	15–40 including metabolites	Yes

Nonbenzodiazepine Receptor Agonists (Nonbenzodiazepines)

Agent	Initiates Sleep	Maintains Sleep	Sleep with Limited Opportunity	Required Inactivity (hr)	Dose (mg)
Eszopiclone	√	√		8+	1, 2, 3[b]
Zaleplon	√		√	4	5, 10[b]
Zolpidem	√			7–8	5, 10[b]
ER	√	√		7–8	6.25, 12.5[b]
Zolpidem (sublingual)		√	√ (4 hr)[a]	4	1.75, 3.5
Zolpidem (oral spray)	√			4	5, 10[b]
Zolpidem (sublingual)	√			4	5, 10[b]
Doxepin		√		7–8	3, 6
Ramelteon	√			–	8
Suvorexant	√	√		7	5, 10, 15, 20

All have specific FDA indication for insomnia.
[a]Provided that 4 additional hours of sleep/time in bed are available.
[b]The reader is advised to check the most recent FDA warning about dose adjustments, specifically for women and patients >65 years.
Abbreviations: ER, extended release; FDA, Food and Drug Administration; SL, sublingual.

B. Treatment and outcome. Treatment should address the comorbid medical, neurologic, and psychiatric disorders as well as insomnia. For major depressive and anxiety disorders, this involves use of antidepressants or anxiolytics such as the selective serotonin reuptake inhibitors (SSRIs). An antidepressant with sedative properties is favored over a less-sedating one for patients with insomnia. Administration of the drug 30 minutes before bedtime also aids in promoting sleep.

Amitriptyline, trimipramine, doxepin, trazodone, and mirtazapine are the most sedating, whereas protriptyline and SSRIs such as fluoxetine and serotonin-norepinephrine reuptake inhibitors (SNRIs) have stimulating effects that may worsen insomnia and are best to be prescribed in the early part of the day. Antidepressants with anxiolytic properties are useful in the treatment of anxious, depressed patients and facilitate psychotherapeutic or pharmacologic treatment. Anticholinergic side effects of tricyclic antidepressants (cardiotoxicity, urinary retention, erectile dysfunction, and dry mouth) limit the usefulness of these agents, particularly in older patients.

Recent studies demonstrate that insomnia may persist despite adequate treatment of depression and that insomnia predicts future relapse of depression. Therefore, oftentimes, a parallel approach that combines treatment for both depression and insomnia is recommended. If the patient is refractory to treatment, a referral to a sleep specialist or psychiatrist is recommended for further evaluation of comorbid psychiatric or other underlying comorbid sleep disorders.

CIRCADIAN RHYTHM SLEEP DISORDERS

Circadian rhythms are generated by the internal neural clock located in the suprachiasmatic nucleus of the hypothalamus. Disruption of biologic timing, or the alignment between internal circadian rhythms with the external physical or social environment, results in circadian rhythm disorders that are most often associated with patients' reports of difficulty initiating and maintaining sleep, and excessive sleepiness. However, their impact extends beyond insomnia or hypersomnia to adverse health outcomes, impairments in social, occupational, and educational performance, and safety concerns.

CRSWDs are characterized by essentially normal total sleep time for age that is not synchronized with conventional environmental light–dark cycles and periods of sleep. Diagnosis requires specialized assessment, including use of a sleep diary for at least 7 days alone, or in combination with actigraphy when possible, physiologic markers of circadian timing such as core body temperature or melatonin onset. A careful history interview to elicit the appropriate major diagnostic criteria is key. CRSWDs include delayed sleep–wake phase disorder (DSWPD), advanced sleep–wake phase disorder (ASWPD), non-24-hour sleep–wake disorder (N24SWD), irregular sleep–wake rhythm disorder (ISWRD), shift work sleep–wake disorder, and jet lag disorder.

Effective treatment of CRSWDs typically requires a multifaceted approach to realign circadian rhythms with the use of timed bright light exposure and low-dose melatonin, together with cognitive-behavioral treatments that promote healthy sleep habits. The reader should be reminded that melatonin is not approved by the FDA for the treatment CRSDs, and one should also be aware of potential side effects such as headaches, vivid dreams, nausea, and cardiovascular effects.

A. DSWPD and ASWPD.

1. Clinical course.

DSWPD is characterized by a persistent inability to fall asleep until the early morning hours (typically between 1 and 3 A.M., and sometimes later) and profound difficulty waking up in the morning. If allowed, the patient would sleep until the late morning or early afternoon (10 A.M. to 2 P.M.). When the patient is forced to rise at 7 or 8 A.M., sleep is curtailed, and daytime sleepiness develops. Despite the daytime sleepiness, patients find that in the evening they become more alert and remain unable to fall asleep until the early morning hours. The prevalence rate is estimated to be between 1.7% (in the general population) and 7% (of those with insomnia complaints). Onset of this disorder typically occurs during adolescence or early adulthood.

ASWPD is characterized by early evening sleep onset, (typically at 7 to 9 P.M.), and early morning awakening (between 3 A.M. and 5 A.M.). Although DSWPD predominates at younger ages and ASWPD at older ages, both disorders can result in sleep problems throughout the life span. Because many features of the sleep of patients with depression resemble those of DSWPD or ASWPD, depression and other psychiatric disorders must be considered in the differential diagnosis.

2. Treatment and outcome.

a. **Chronotherapy** is a behavioral technique in which bedtime is systematically delayed (for DSWPD) or advanced (for ASWPD) in 2- to 3-hour increments each day until the desired sleep phase is achieved. The patient is then instructed to maintain the newly established bedtime rigidly. Although this approach works, it is an arduous procedure, and maintenance of the effect has been difficult.

b. Bright light therapy. Light intensity greater than 1,000 lux is considered bright. Appropriately timed bright light (white or blue/green enriched) exposure can reset the timing of circadian rhythms, and normalize circadian phase in DSWPD and ASWPD. Exposure to bright light in the early morning results in an advancement of circadian phase, whereas exposure to light in the evening delays circadian rhythms. For management of DSWPD, exposure to light is usually scheduled for 1 to 2 hours in the morning (close to the time of habitual awakening). For ASWPD, light exposure is recommended in the evening, approximately 2 to 4 hours before scheduled bedtime. Avoidance of bright light in the evening in DSWPD should also be encouraged. Despite high rates of success in achieving the desired sleep phase under immediate treatment, many patients do not continue the light regimen and have a relapse. Some patients are able to maintain a normalized phase without maintenance of light exposure for as long as several months, whereas others drift back toward the pretreatment phase within a few days.

   c. **Melatonin** has been shown to shift the phase of circadian rhythms in humans. Although not approved by the FDA, melatonin of 1 to 5 mg has been shown to be effective when taken in the early evening (5 to 6 hours before habitual falling asleep time) for patients with DSWPD.

B. **N24SWD.**

  1. Clinical course. Individuals with N24SWD typically have a longer than 24-hour circadian rhythm, similar to those living in temporal isolation. Because these patients are unable to achieve stable entrain to the external 24-hour physical, social, or activity cycles, sleep and wake periods progressively drift later each day. Diagnosis of N24SWD includes complaints of insomnia or excessive sleepiness associated with the misalignment between the endogenous circadian rhythm and the light–dark cycle. N24SWD is most common in blind people, but can occur in sighted persons. There is an overlap between severe DSWPD and N24SWD.

  2. Treatment and outcomes. Both behavioral and pharmacologic options are available for the treatment of non-24-hour sleep–wake rhythm disorder, depending on whether the patient is sighted or blind. For blind and sighted patients, planned sleep schedules and/or low-dose melatonin (0.5 to 3 mg) approximately 1 to 2 hours before habitual bedtime are recommended. Tasimelteon (20 mg), a melatonin receptor agonist, was recently approved by the FDA for the treatment of N24SWD. In sighted persons, the addition of timed exposure to bright light in the morning is also recommended.

C. **ISWRD.**

  1. Clinical course. ISWRD differs from the phase disorders in that there is a low amplitude to a complete loss of circadian rhythmicity, which results in the lack of a long, consolidated sleep period. Sleep is usually broken into three or more short sleep periods or naps during the course of 24 hours. Irregular sleep–wake patterns occur among patients with neurodevelopmental and neurodegenerative disorders, particularly in Alzheimer's disease and among other elderly persons in nursing homes.

  2. Treatment and outcomes. Management of irregular sleep–wake patterns and associated behavioral problems in this group of elderly and often cognitively impaired patients is a challenge. Treatment with sedative-hypnotics is prevalent in nursing homes. These medications have side effects that may not be well tolerated by older patients. The most promising is a multicomponent approach with structured physical and social activities and increasing light exposure during the day and optimizing the sleep environment by reducing noise and light at night.

    Studies have indicated that structured activity programs, increasing exposure to bright light and evening melatonin, may alleviate these sleep–wake and behavioral disorders. The effects of melatonin have been mixed, and a recent placebo-controlled multicenter study in Alzheimer's disease failed to demonstrate its effectiveness. Light therapy units are commercially available.

D. **Shift work disorder (SWD).**

  1. Clinical course. SWD is characterized by chronic symptoms of insomnia and excessive sleepiness that are due to unconventional work schedules, resulting in circadian misalignment. Typically, sleep is curtailed by 1 to 4 hours in patients with SWD, with most complaints associated with night and early morning work. Excessive sleepiness at work and commute poses important safety concerns.

  2. Treatment and outcomes. Clinical management of SWD is aimed at realigning circadian rhythms with the sleep and work schedules, as well as improving sleep, alertness, and safety. Nonpharmacologic treatments are basic to the management of SWD. Optimizing

the sleep environment, adherence to healthy sleep habits, and planned naps, when possible, should be encouraged for all patients.

   a. **Bright light therapy.** Timed bright light therapy and avoidance of light at the wrong time of the day can help accelerate and maintain entrainment to the shift schedule. For night workers, circadian rhythms need to be delayed, so that the highest sleep propensity occurs during the day, rather than at night. Intermittent bright light exposure (~20 minutes/hour blocks) and avoidance of bright light exposure in the morning during the commute to home (using driving safe sunglasses) have been shown to accelerate circadian adaptation to night shift.

   b. **Melatonin.** Studies on the effectiveness of melatonin for the treatment of SWD have been mixed. When taken at bedtime after the night shift, melatonin can improve daytime sleep, but may have limited effects on alertness at work. Other pharmaceuticals often used for the treatment of sleep disturbance and excessive sleepiness in shift workers include short-acting hypnotics for insomnia and FDA-approved stimulants such as modafinil and armodafinil for maintaining alertness. The required dose of these medications can vary among individuals and can be titrated. However, these approaches do not specifically address the issue of circadian misalignment, and thus should be used in concert with behavioral strategies as discussed above.

DISORDERS OF EXCESSIVE DAYTIME SLEEPINESS

Sleepiness severe enough to affect activities of daily living is estimated to be present among 30% of the population and is most commonly caused by self-imposed restriction of sleep. However, approximately 4% to 5% of the population has EDS as a result of a sleep disorder. Sleepiness is excessive and an indication of a sleep disorder when it occurs at undesirable times, such as while driving and during social activities. EDS can be divided into two types: extrinsic and intrinsic. Some extrinsic causes include environmental factors, drug dependency, sleep-disordered breathing, and movement disorders during sleep. The more common types of intrinsic hypersomnia usually associated with primary central nervous system (CNS) includes disorders such as narcolepsy and idiopathic hypersomnia (IH).

A. **Narcolepsy.**

   1. **Clinical features.** Narcolepsy is a syndrome characterized by a pentad of (i) severe unremitting excessive sleepiness (occurs in 100% of patients with narcolepsy), and is the sinequanone of the disorder, manifesting as sleep attacks; (ii) cataplexy (found in 60% to 70% of patients); (iii) sleep paralysis (SP) (impacting 25% to 50% of patients); (iv) hypnagogic hallucination and/or hypnopompic hallucination (HH) (in 20% to 40% of patients); and (v) disturbed nocturnal sleep (in 70% to 80% of patients). A description of these symptoms is provided in Table 60.4. Some patients will also have automatic behavior (20% to 40%), other comorbid primary sleep disorders such as restless leg syndrome, periodic leg movement disorder, rapid eye movement (REM)–sleep behavior disorder, and REM sleep without atonia (RSWA) (see Section H 1 b iii). All patients must have pathologic levels of daytime sleepiness. Cataplexy is defined by a sudden loss of skeletal muscle tone induced by strong emotional stimuli, typically laughter or joking, and is a pathognomonic feature for narcolepsy. Cataplexy is associated with a drop in H-reflex.

      Sleep apnea is noted in one-third of narcoleptic patients and may be related to the high body mass index (BMI) seen in narcolepsy patients, which could aggravate sleep attacks and is critical to screen for it, especially in patients whose sleepiness does not resolve with therapy or in overweight patients who snore.

   2. **Clinical course.** Narcolepsy is a manifestation of dissociation between wakefulness and sleep, particularly REM sleep. It is characterized by inability to maintain wakefulness during the day, but also by an inability to maintain sleep during the night. The onset usually occurs in adolescence or young adulthood, and men are affected more often than women. The prevalence of narcolepsy in the United States is estimated to be approximately 1 in 2,000 individuals, with most cases being sporadic. Studies have shown a strong genetic association between narcolepsy and the human leukocyte antigen (HLA) type DR2 and DQ1. A more sensitive marker for narcolepsy is the *HLA DQB1*0602* genotype, which appears to be correlated with both the frequency and severity of cataplexy.

TABLE 60.4 Narcolepsy Symptoms

Sleep attacks

Chronic and irresistible desire to fall asleep in inappropriate opportunities and at inappropriate places (i.e., while driving, playing, eating).

Cataplexy

Defined as a sudden loss of skeletal muscle tone universally preceded by a prodromal of strong emotional stimulus leading to a transient episode of muscle weakness. Typical emotions that trigger cataplexy include laughter and excitement or anger in more than 95% of the time. Episodes may be partial or complete and may manifest as momentarily head nodding, sagging of the jaw, buckling of the knees, with a duration of a few seconds to minutes. Consciousness is always preserved and neurologic examination reveals flaccidity of the muscles and absence or markedly reduced muscle stretch reflexes with decrease or absence of the H reflex and F responses. Cataplexy may occur months to years after the initial onset of sleepiness and sleep attacks, but it may be the initial manifestation, but may improve and sometimes disappear in older age.

Sleep paralysis (SP)

Episodes of paralysis of skeletal muscle tone occurring either during sleep or on awakening in the morning, and last from a few minutes to as long as 15–20 min. The patient experiences complete paralysis, is unable to move or speak, and is generally frightened, although he or she retains consciousness.

Hypnagogic and hypnopompic hallucinations

Found in 20%–40% of narcoleptic patients. Episodes occur during sleep onset (hypnagogic) or on awakening (hypnopompic) and generally appear months to years after the onset of sleep attacks. Hallucinations are most commonly vivid and visual (and often fear-inducing) but may also consist of auditory, vestibular, or somesthetic in nature. In 30% of patients, three of the four major manifestations of the narcoleptic tetrad (sleep attacks, cataplexy, SP, and hypnagogic hallucinations) occur together, and in about 10% of cases, all four major features occur together.

Disturbed night sleep

The paradox in narcolepsy is that while patients pathologically sleep during the day, as many as 70%–80% will experience significant disruption of their sleep.

Automatic behavior

Characterized by repeated performance of a single monotonous behavior such as driving or shopping without recollection, and speaking or writing in a meaningless manner. These occur in about 20%–40% of narcolepsy patients and are believed to originate from partial sleep episodes, frequent lapses, or microsleeps.

Abbreviations: HH, hypnopompic hallucination; SP, sleep paralysis.

The role of orexin [also known as hypocretin (Hcrt)] in narcolepsy is supported by the finding that Hcrt levels are abnormally low or undetectable in the cerebrospinal fluid of most narcoleptic patients. Values below 110 pg/mL are highly diagnostic for narcolepsy in the absence of severe brain pathology. The most consistent abnormalities were observed in the amygdala, where increased dopamine and metabolite levels were found.

The most plausible theory for the pathogenesis of narcolepsy–cataplexy syndrome suggests that the condition results from a depletion, either through degeneration or autoimmune disorder, of the Hcrt neurons, in patients who are at risk conferred by HLA-DQB1*0602 haplotype. New data reveal evidence of gliosis in the lateral hypothalamus, the location of the Hcrt neurons, prompting exploration for possible immune-related dysfunction in narcolepsy. Environmental triggers such as streptococcal infection and seasonal influenza, and more recent reports implicating the 2009 influenza pandemic A/H1N1 favor an immunologic mechanism for narcolepsy implicating a small epitope of H1N1, which resembles Hcrt and may be involved in molecular mimicry.

B. Classification of narcolepsy.

1. **Narcolepsy type 1 (NT-1) or Hcrt (orexin) deficiency syndrome.** (previously known as narcolepsy–cataplexy syndrome). Characterized by EDS for 3 months and at least one of the following:

   a. Cataplexy, and on Multiple Sleep Latency Test, a Mean Sleep Latency of <8 minutes and >2 sleep-onset rapid eye movement sleep periods (SOREMPs). One SOREMP may be on the preceding night's polysomnogram, OR

   b. CSF Hcrt-1 levels <110 pg/mL or one-third the baseline normal levels, and on multiple sleep latency testing (MSLT), MSL < 8 minutes > 2 SOREMPs (one SOREMP may be on the preceding night's polysomnogram)

2. **Narcolepsy type 2 (NT-2, with normal Hcrt levels)** (previously known as narcolepsy without cataplexy):

   Unlike NT-1, there is absence of cataplexy and Hcrt levels are normal. Positive polysomnography/multiple sleep latency test is met [(mean sleep latency of <8 minutes and ≥2 SOREMPs on the MSLT. A SOREMP (within 15 minutes of sleep onset) on the preceding nocturnal polysomnogram may replace one of the SOREMPs on the MSLT].

3. **Secondary narcolepsy.** Because of a known underlying CNS disorder, it is referred to as narcolepsy type 1 because of a medical condition (when Hcrt levels are low) or narcolepsy type 2 because of a medical condition (when Hcrt levels are normal).

   This condition is found in a number of key medical and neurologic conditions including abnormalities, genetic disorders associated such as Prader–Willi syndrome, structural lesions in the hypothalamic region, and inflammatory lesions such as multiple sclerosis and acute disseminated encephalomyelitis, midbrain tumors, vascular malformations, encephalitis, cerebral trauma, and paraneoplastic syndrome with anti-Ma2 antibodies and Niemann–Pick disease type C.

4. **Diagnosis.** In addition to the clinical history, nocturnal polysomnography (PSG) and MSLT are performed to establish a diagnosis of narcolepsy.

   a. Sleep studies.

   (1) **PSG.** A baseline sleep study is generally required for an accurate diagnosis of narcolepsy because of the spectrum of conditions that can cause excessive sleepiness. Most typically, the nocturnal PSG is required, followed by the MSLT. PSG features of narcolepsy include sleep disruption, repetitive awakenings, and decreased REM sleep latency. A SOREMP at night is highly predictive of narcolepsy and may be diagnostic of the condition along with the MSLT.

   (2) **The MSLT.** The MSLT during the day following the PSG is designed to determine a patient's propensity to fall asleep. As noted previously, the current criteria for narcolepsy include an MSL of ≤8 minutes and ≥2 SOREMPs, one of which may be a SOREM ≤15 minutes on the diagnostic polysomnogram.

   However, up to one-third of the general population may have an MSL of ≤8 minutes, so the finding of a short MSL alone, without any SOREMP, should be interpreted cautiously together with the clinical picture.

   Clinically, HLA-DQB1*0602 typing may be indicated when considering a CSF Hcrt measurement. Hcrt levels are generally normal if the patient is HLA-negative, unless the patient has a diencephalic lesion that explains the CNS hypersomnia (narcolepsy type 1 due to a medical condition).

5. **Treatment and outcome.** Treatment approaches to narcolepsy emphasize control of narcoleptic symptoms to allow optimal social and professional productivity by maintaining the patient's alertness throughout the day. Choice of treatment must take into account that narcolepsy is a lifelong disorder and that patients will have to take medications for many years. Clinicians are not unanimous in their approach to management of narcolepsy.

   a. The drugs commonly used to manage EDS and sleep attacks are the nonamphetamine stimulants (or wake-promoting agents) such as armodafinil and modafinil and CNS stimulants including methylphenidate and dextroamphetamine.

   Because of the frequent side effects of sympathomimetic stimulants, such as irritability, tachycardia, elevated blood pressure, and nocturnal sleep disturbance, methylphenidate and amphetamines are probably less preferred first-line treatment.

Armodafinil and modafinil have several advantages over other stimulants in that they have fewer cardiovascular side effects and longer half-lives and can therefore be taken once daily in the morning, and the prescription can be refilled.

Sodium oxybate is currently the only treatment approved for the management of both symptoms of hypersomnia and cataplexy in the setting of narcolepsy. Medications used in the management of EDS and the dosages are listed in Table 60.5. Drugs with norepinephrine-releasing properties have the greatest impact on sleepiness. However, evidence shows that even at the highest recommended doses, no drug is capable of returning a person with narcolepsy to a normal baseline level of alertness.

b. The management of abnormal REM intrusion phenomena such as cataplexy, SP, and hypnagogic hallucinations involves the use of sodium oxybate and tricyclic antidepressant medications. Sodium oxybate is currently approved for the management of cataplexy and daytime sleepiness in narcolepsy. Protriptyline and clomipramine have been used widely, often with good results. Other tricyclic medications, such as imipramine, desipramine, and amitriptyline, also are effective; however, anticholinergic side effects (particularly erectile dysfunction) limit the ability of many patients to tolerate these medications, particularly if high doses are needed to control cataplexy. Fluoxetine is somewhat less effective for cataplexy, but it has the advantage of being a mild stimulant (Table 60.5). An example of an initial regimen for narcolepsy among adults is provided in Table 60.6.

Status cataplecticus is an unusual state of repetitive cataplexy spells often following rapid withdrawal of anticataplectic treatment.

c. The third approach to the management of narcolepsy is to improve the nocturnal sleep of persons with narcolepsy. Improvement of nocturnal sleep not only decreases EDS but may also help address cataplexy. Nocturnal sleep disturbances may be related to periodic limb movement disorder of sleep (PLMDS), which frequently occur among patients with narcolepsy. They may, however, also be a complication of treatment with stimulants and tricyclic medications. Occasionally, management of PLMDS with dopamine agonist drug may be helpful.

d. Nonpharmacologic treatment. Scheduled short "power" naps and support therapy must be emphasized. Short naps of 15 to 20 minutes three times during the day help maintain alertness and have been shown to have a recuperative power in narcoleptic subjects.

(1) **Drug holiday.** In cases of tolerance, switching to a different class of medication or providing a drug holiday for 1 to 2 days can be useful.

(2) **Psychosocial considerations.** Patients with narcolepsy often experience social and professional difficulties owing to sleepiness and cataplexy. Narcolepsy can result in unemployment, academic difficulties, rejection by friends, and depression. For these reasons, it is important to encourage patients with narcolepsy to join support groups, like the Narcolepsy Network (http://www.narcolepsynetwork .org/), and to provide referral for psychotherapy when needed.

6. Side effects of stimulant medications. The amphetamine-like medications are typically associated with side effects such as hypertension, alterations in mood, and psychosis. Moreover, tolerance and, less frequently, addiction may be observed with drugs such as amphetamines. Interestingly, with high dosages of amphetamines (100 mg/day), a paradoxical effect of increased sleepiness may result. This paradoxical effect disappears with reduction of the daily dosage. Other common side effects include increased jitteriness, verbal aggressiveness, "racing thoughts," increased heart rate, tremor, and involuntary movements. The most commonly reported side effects of the nonamphetamine stimulants, armodafinil and modafinil, include headache, gastrointestinal (GI) irritability, and nausea. Both modafinil and armodafinil induce the hepatic cytochrome P45 and reduce the efficacy of hormonal methods of birth control. Women of childbearing age who take these agents should switch to another form of birth control. Side effects associated with sodium oxybate include disorientation in the middle of the night and morning grogginess, enuresis, and nausea at the time of initiating the medication and at higher doses.

TABLE 60.5 Medications Used to Treat CNS hypersomnias

Medication Name	Medication Class	Usual Daily Dose Range	Usual Starting Regimen	FDA Approval	FDA Pregnancy Category	Special Considerations
Amphetamine/ dextroamphetamine	Amphetamines	10–60 mg	10 mg daily	Yes	C	Black box warning—abuse
Dextroamphetamine		5–60 mg	5 mg b.i.d.	Yes	C	Same as above
Methamphetamine		5–60 mg	10 mg daily	No	C	Same as above
Methylphenidate	Amphetamine-like	10–60 mg	5 mg b.i.d.	Yes	C	Black box warning—Dependence
Mazindol		3–8 mg	2 mg b.i.d.	No	Unknown	
Pemoline		18.75–112.5 mg	37.5 mg daily	No	B	Not used because of liver toxicity
Modafinil	Nonamphetamine stimulants	100–400 mg	200 mg daily	Yes	C	Requires barrier contraception
Armodafinil		150–250 mg	150 mg daily	Yes	C	Requires barrier contraception
Sodium oxybate	Sedative-hypnotic	4.5–9 g	2.25 g × 2	Yes	C	Short half-life
Protriptyline	Tricyclic antidepressants	5–30 mg	5 mg daily	No	C	Black box warning—suicidality
Imipramine		25–150 mg	25 mg daily	No	D	Same as above
Clomipramine		25–125 mg	25 mg daily	No	C	Same as above
Fluoxetine	Serotonin specific reuptake inhibitors (SSRI)	10–40 mg	20 mg daily	No	C	Same as above
Selegiline	MAOI	5–10 mg	20 mg daily	No	C	
Venlafaxine	SNRI	75–225 mg	37.5 mg daily	No	C	Black box warning—suicidality
Atomoxetine	Norepinephrine reuptake inhibitors	40–80 mg	40 mg t.i.d.	No	C	Same as above
Bupropion	Norepinephrine-dopamine reuptake inhibitor	200–450 mg	100 mg b.i.d.	No	C	Same as above
Ritanserin	Type 2 serotonin (5-HT2) receptor antagonist	5–10 mg	5 mg daily	No	Unknown	

Abbreviations: b.i.d., twice a day; CNS, central nervous system; FDA, Food and Drug Administration; t.i.d., three times a day.
Adopted from Wise MS, Arand DL, Arger RR, et al. Treatment of narcolepsy and other hypersomnias of central origin. *Sleep.* 2007;1:30(12)1712–1727.

TABLE 60.6 Example of an Initial Treatment Plan for Narcolepsy in Adults

Behavioral therapy
Maintenance of regular sleep schedule and avoidance of sleep deprivation
Avoidance of heavy meals and alcohol intake
Regular timing of nocturnal sleep: 10:30 P.M.–7:00 A.M.
Naps. Strategically timed naps, if possible (e.g., 15 min at lunchtime and 15 min at 5:30 P.M.)

Medication
The effects of stimulant medications vary widely among patients. The dosing and timing of medications should be individualized to optimize performance. Additional doses, as needed, may be suggested for periods of anticipated sleepiness.
Armodafinil (150, 100, 200, or 250 mg daily upon awakening).
Modafinil: 200 mg/d (200 mg on awakening or 100 mg b.i.d.)
If difficulties persist: may increase modafinil to 400 mg/d
Methylphenidate: 5 mg (three or four tablets) or 20 mg SR in morning (on empty stomach)
If difficulties persist:
Methylphenidate (SR): 20 mg in morning, 5 mg after noon nap, 5 mg at 4:00 P.M.
If no response:
Dexedrine spansule (SR): 15 mg at awakening, 5 mg after noon nap, 5 mg at 3:30 or 4:00 P.M.
(or 15 mg at awakening and 15 mg after noon nap)

Abbreviation: b.i.d., twice a day.

C. **Hypersomnia other than narcolepsy.**
1. **Clinical course.** This group of disorders characterizes patients whose diagnosis does not meet that of narcolepsy but is associated with severe disabling hypersomnia without the associated cataplexy, which is unique with narcolepsy. The age at onset varies from adolescence to middle age. The symptoms are lifelong, with some potential for improvement if an associated condition is identified.
2. **Clinical features.** Patients report sleepiness throughout the day associated with prolonged naps, which, unlike narcolepsy, are not refreshing. Automatic behaviors and some features of REM sleep intrusion events (such as hypnogogic hallucinations) may occur during periods of drowsiness. These behaviors are often inappropriate, and patients usually do not have any recollection of these events. Patients have severe difficulty awakening in the morning.
3. **Examples of hypersomnia other than narcolepsy.**
   a. Idiopathic hypersomnia (IH) is characterized by greater than 3-month duration of EDS and an irrepressible need to sleep or daytime lapses into sleep in the absence, and after correction, of sleep deprivation.
   The onset of the disease is generally around the same age as narcolepsy (15 to 30 years). The sleep pattern, however, is different from that of narcolepsy. The patient generally sleeps for hours, but the sleep is not refreshing. Total 24-hour sleep time is typically 12 to 14 hours. The MSLT shows a mean sleep-onset latency of 8 minutes or less, and unlike narcolepsy, with *less* than two SOREMPs. Supportive features also include profound sleep inertia (aka sleep drunkenness, elucidated as prolonged difficulty waking up accompanied by irritability and repeated returns to sleep), dependence on others for awakening them, mental fatigability, and often prolonged (>60 minutes), unrefreshing naps. As part of the sleep drunkenness spectrum, some patients may have automatic behavior with amnesia for the events.
   The patient suffering from IH does not endorse a history of cataplexy, snoring, or repeating awakenings throughout the night. Physical examination uncovers no abnormal neurologic findings. This disabling and lifelong condition should be differentiated from other causes of EDS. REM intrusion phenomena such as SP and hypnagogic hallucinations may also be reported, but these are far less frequent than in narcolepsy and without clear association between IH and HLA. It is indeed very interesting that NT-1 may represent a completely separate and unique phenotype of hypersomnolence,

exemplified by HRCT deficiency and cataplexy in HLA-susceptible individuals, which is distinct from other central forms of hypersomnia such as NT-2 and IH.

   b. **Kleine–Levin syndrome (KLS aka recurrent hypersomnia, periodic hypersomnolence):** This is a very rare condition in which patients experience prolonged episodes of severe sleepiness separated by periods of normal alertness and function. The *ICSD-3* requires that there be at least two episodes of EDS lasting between 2 days and 5 weeks with periods of normalcy between episodes (normal alertness, cognition, and mood). KLS usually affects adolescent males, who also experience cognitive impairment, hyperphagia, megaphagia, and disinhibited behavior manifesting as hypersexuality. During the episodic sleep attacks, it is not uncommon for patients to sleep for 16 to 18 hours a day, eat voraciously while awake, and experience other behavioral disturbances during the episodes, including confusion, hallucinations, hyperorality, memory impairment, and polydipsia. The hypersomnia should not be better explained by another disorder, especially bipolar disorder.

D. **Hypersomnia caused by a medical condition.** *Hypersomnia may be* diagnosed when sleepiness is thought to be the direct result of a medical or neurologic condition, but the patient does not meet clinical or laboratory criteria for a diagnosis of narcolepsy. A variety of conditions may underlie this disorder, including associated neurologic disorders such as encephalitis, cerebrovascular accidents, brain tumor, head trauma, and Parkinson's disease. Common genetic conditions associated with sleepiness include Prader–Willi syndrome and myotonic dystrophy.

E. **Diagnosis.** The differential diagnosis includes narcolepsy and primary sleep disorders such as sleep-disordered breathing or periodic limb movement in sleep (PLMS), which may also be associated with significant daytime sleepiness. Therefore, the diagnosis is made by means of elimination of other causes of daytime sleepiness. Polysomnography should be performed to further assess these possibilities, and MSLT should be performed to document the level of objective daytime sleepiness.

   Mean sleep latencies are often less than 8 minutes but unlike narcolepsy, which is diagnosed electrographically when the MSL is <8 minutes and when two or more SOREMPs are present, the criteria for the latter must include less than two SOREMS and an equally short sleep latency.

F. **Treatment and outcome.** Because of multiple etiologic factors and the relative lack of understanding of the underlying pathophysiologic mechanism, treatment is symptomatic and the response is variable.

   Behavioral therapies and sleep hygiene instructions should be recommended but have only modest positive effect. The only medications that provide partial relief of excessive sleepiness are stimulant-like drugs. The most commonly suggested medications are armodafinil, modafinil, sodium oxybate, methylphenidate, and dextroamphetamine. Tricyclic antidepressants, selective SSRIs, clonidine, bromocriptine, amantadine, and methysergide have been used with varying success.

   Sometimes combinations of these drugs yield better control of sleepiness. Even with the highest recommended dose, complete control of daytime sleepiness is seldom achieved in this group of patients. Therefore, prescribing more than 400 mg of modafinil, more than 60 mg of methylphenidate, or 40 mg of dextroamphetamine does not provide significant additional symptomatic relief. The patient should be advised not to drive or engage in potentially dangerous activities that require high levels of alertness. Pemoline is not recommended because of its potential hepatotoxicity (see Table 60.5).

   Treatment for patients with KLS includes the amphetamine and nonamphetamine stimulants, and mood stabilizers such as lithium (probably most effective), valproic acid, and carbamazepine.

PARASOMNIAS

Parasomnias are a group of disorders that occur during sleep, are associated with abnormal wake-to-sleep transition, or abnormal arousal from sleep. These conditions with important consideration in neurology include REM sleep behavior disorder (RBD), sleepwalking (somnambulism), night terrors, nightmares, and confusional arousals. The ones that are most often encountered in adult clinical practice are discussed in this chapter.

A. **Non-REM parasomnias (aka disorders of arousal, DOA).** Examples include confusional arousals, sleepwalking (somnambulism), and sleep terrors (pavor nocturnus). They represent episodic arousals from non-REM sleep, typically slow-wave sleep, associated with amnestic behaviors.

1. **Clinical course.** The prevalence of sleepwalking and sleep terrors is estimated at approximately 6% of the population. These types of parasomnias are most frequent among children and often disappear by adolescence. These behaviors may be considered normal among children, but abnormal when they persist into adulthood, which may be related to sleep deprivation, underlying comorbid medical, sleep, or psychiatric conditions, and CNS-acting medications.

2. **Clinical features.** During these episodes, a variety of behaviors may occur ranging mild to severe: patients will exhibit a state of prolonged confusion with uttering irrelevant words (confusional arousals), sitting up, and getting up to walk (somnambulism/sleep walking), and may experience extreme autonomic sympathetic discharge culminating with screaming and sometimes aggression (sleep terrors). These episodes have the potential to become dangerous because patients may bump into walls and windows or fall down stairs. With all of these episodes, patients usually have only vague recollections of these events and are confused or agitated if awakened.

   a. **Unique subtypes.**

      (1) **Sleep sex (aka sexsomnias).** This is a variant of confusional arousals where patients experience automatic and inappropriate amnestic sexual behavior, out of character for the patient. It may be related to underlying untreated primary sleep disorders (i.e., sleep-disordered breathing, sleep deprivation).

      (2) **Sleep-related eating disorders.** The condition is a variant of sleepwalking and is common in younger women who are given a hypnotic agent. Episodes consist of recurrent episodes of involuntary eating and drinking during partial arousals from sleep without recollection/very partial recall. The eating behavior is sometimes unusual for the types of food items consumed (i.e., jam and cat food sandwich). The episodes may lead to weight gain and sometimes injury during food preparation. The condition can be either idiopathic, but occasionally in association with Willis–Ekbom Disease (WED) and use of CNS medications such as zolpidem.

3. **Diagnosis.** For adults, thorough evaluation of abnormal nocturnal behavior should be performed to differentiate non-REM parasomnias from other pathologic entities, particularly nocturnal seizures and REM parasomnias. The most common PSG findings are multiple abrupt arousals, arising predominantly from slow-wave sleep, but also from other stages of NREM sleep associated with the behavior, such as confusion, eating, walking, sympathetic hyperarousal. When ordering PSG in patients who may have parasomnia, it is important to arrange for the study to include expanded four-limb electromyographic (EMG) montage with high-definition video monometry, and ensure that the sleep laboratory is aware to ask patients about recollection of their spells, while ensuring that the monitoring environment is safe (monitoring bed is padded). Expanded EEG montage may also be utilized with nocturnal seizures on the differential diagnosis (especially for repetitive and stereotyped nocturnal spells) (Video 60.1).

4. **Treatment and outcome.** Therapy for non-REM parasomnias includes several approaches consisting of maximizing safety measures around the bedroom area (i.e., removal of sharp furniture, placing the mattress on the floor), preventive measures (avoidance of sleep deprivation, caffeine), psychological interventions, and when frequent/disruptive/severe, using medications (Table 60.7).

   a. **Preventive measures and psychological intervention.** Preventive measures are taken to avoid serious injury during episodes of sleepwalking. The patient should be advised to locate the bedroom on the ground floor, lock windows and doors, place door alarms, cover windows and glass doors with heavy draperies, and remove hazardous objects (sharps, knives, firearms) from the house.

      Comorbid sleep disorders such as sleep apnea and sleep deprivation should be addressed. Caffeine should be minimized. Although alcohol remains a known precipitant for some DOA, its specific role in provoking somnambulism is somewhat unclear/controversial.

TABLE 60.7 Treatment for Most Common Non-REM Parasomnias

	Treatment
Confusional arousal	Reassurance when benign in nature Avoid precipitants such as: • Sleep deprivation • Alcohol • CNS depressants Escitalopram (10 mg)—*for sexsomnia*
Somnambulism (sleep walking)	Safeguard the sleep environment and protect the patient Avoid precipitants: • Sleep deprivation • Lithium • Nonbenzodiazepine receptor agonists (i.e., zolpidem) Anticipatory awakenings Pharmacotherapy: Topirimate BzRA • Clonazepam (0.5–1 mg) • Diazepam (10 mg) • Triazolam (0.25 mg) Imipramine (50–300 mg)
Sleep terrors	Reassurance when benign in nature CBT Progressive muscle relaxation Biofeedback Hypnosis Psychotherapy Pharmacotherapy: • Paroxetine (20–40 mg) • Clonazepam (0.5–1 mg)

Abbreviations: BzRA, benzodiazepines; CNS, central nervous system; CBT, cognitive-behavioral therapy, REM, rapid eye movement.

Hypnosis and psychotherapy have also been used in the management of parasomnias. Hypnosis has been shown helpful, at least for a short time, to young adults. The need for psychotherapy depends on the association of psychological factors with the parasomnia. Psychotherapy has been used most widely to treat young adults for sleep terrors. Most cases of parasomnia increase in severity and frequency with psychological stress. Therefore, in addition to psychotherapy, relaxation programs, such as progressive muscle relaxation and biofeedback, may be beneficial. Anticipatory awakening has been reported as a treatment modality for sleepwalking and perhaps other DOA. The technique involves waking the patients between 15 and 30 minutes prior to the time of the typical episodes.

b. **Medications.** The BzRA—most commonly clonazepam, alprazolam, and diazepam—have been used. In the management of sleep terrors, tricyclic antidepressants (particularly imipramine) have been used either alone or in combination with BzRA to provide control of symptoms. In addition, several studies have shown that treatment with carbamazepine may be beneficial. An example of an initial therapeutic approach is to start with clonazepam (0.25 to 1 mg) approximately 30 minutes before bedtime. If the response is inadequate, the dose may be increased while balancing the side effects, which include confusion and daytime drowsiness. A secondary line of treatment includes initiation of low doses of tricyclic antidepressant drugs.

Results of management of non-REM parasomnias are poorly documented. However, the literature indicates that response to combinations of pharmacologic and nonpharmacologic therapies is generally good. After various lengths of time, as many as 70% of adult patients report improvement of the symptoms.

B. REM parasomnias.

This group consists of three important parasomnias, but one in particular, RBD, is of particular importance for neurologists.

1. RBDs.

a. Clinical course. REM sleep and dreaming is normally accompanied by skeletal muscle atonia. RBD is characterized by abnormal loss of REM-sleep atonia leading to excessive motor activation during sleep. Patients with this disorder most commonly experience vigorous and often aggressive dream behaviors that are accompanied by vivid dreams in which the patient is usually attacked by an intruder or animals. These behaviors may be quite violent and can result in serious injury to both patient and bed partner. Two specific RBD phenotypes may exist—a chronic form and an acute form. The chronic form usually occurs among older adults (>65 years of age) and is most common in male patients (having a 9:1 male-to-female predilection). It is encountered in association with alpha-synucleopathies such as Parkinson's disease and Parkinson's plus syndrome (multiple systems atrophy, Lewy body dementia). The acute form is usually associated with toxic–metabolic etiologic factors, most commonly, drug withdrawal states and antidepressant medications [i.e., antidepressants such as SSRI, SNRI, TCA, monoamine oxidase inhibitors (MAOIs)], various brainstem abnormalities, brainstem stroke, brainstem tumor, and demyelinating disease. The acute form is usually more common in younger (<50 years old) patients and does not have the gender predilection favoring males in the chronic form. Loss of REM EMG tone may also occur among patients taking medications that suppress REM sleep, such as tricyclic antidepressants and fluoxetine, and substances such as caffeine.

RBD may be idiopathic or secondary; however, it is currently believed that most patients most likely represent the secondary form and some have advocated replacing the term "idiopathic" with "cryptogenic" because of the high-degree phenoconversion to neurodegenerative diseases.

Besides the need to provide efficacious treatment for this potentially injurious REM parasomnia, the most important reason to properly diagnose this condition relates its strong prognostic utility as a predictor of neurodegeneration. RBD generally precedes the onset of the alpha-synucleinopathy by a few years to decades. Reviewing the underlying neurodegenerative disorders associated with RBD, 94% of recently reported cases were in the setting of alpha-synucleinopathies. The recent data on the rates of RBD phenoconversion to the emergence of a neurodegenerative disorder may exceed 90% over a 14-year observation period.

The differential diagnosis of RBD includes non-REM parasomnias, severe obstructive sleep apnea ("pseudo RBD"), and periodic movements of sleep, nocturnal seizures, and nocturnal rhythmic movements. It is important to recognize this condition and differentiate it from other nocturnal behaviors because RBD can be managed effectively.

Recent data demonstrate several potential markers of neurodegenerative diseases in idiopathic RBD (before the onset of dementia diagnosis) including impaired cognition, visuospatial dysfunction, impaired color vision, anosmia, and autonomic dysfunction, particularly orthostatic hypotension. Interestingly, for patients who have RBD but normal olfaction, the risk of developing a neurodegenerative disease over the next 5 years is approximately 15%. If anosmia is present, however, that risk increases dramatically to 65%.

b. Diagnosis. A diagnosis of RBD should be suspected in patients with a clinical history of recurrent dream-enactment behavior (DEB), but must be confirmed with polysomnography. The clinical evaluation should include a detailed interview of the patients, but equally, if not more important, the bed partner, as some patients are unable to adequately describe/recall the sleep-related events. One key question to ask the bed partner is "Have you ever seen the patient appear to "act out his or her dreams" (punched or flailed arms in the air, shouted, or screamed) while sleeping?"

As opposed to the DOA, a unique feature that may further differentiate RBD from other nocturnal spells is the timing of the episodes in the latter part of the night, where a greater REM occupies a larger percentage of the sleep cycle.

In patients who experience DEB, the diagnostic polysomnography is mandated for a definitive diagnosis to exclude DOA, nocturnal seizures, periodic limb movements, and sleep apnea ("pseudo RBD"). The presence of DEB by history/during the PSG along with evidence of RSWA is essential for diagnosis.

The ICSD diagnostic criteria for RBD require all of the following to be present:

i. Repeated episodes of sleep-related vocalization and/or complex motor behaviors
ii. The behaviors are documented by PSG during REM sleep or, based on clinical history of dream enactment, are presumed to occur during REM sleep.
iii. PSG recording confirms the presence of RSWA. The muscle augmentation may be based on recording from the limbs or chin EMG.
iv. The disturbance is not better explained by another sleep disorder, mental disorder, medication, or substance use.

c. **Treatment and outcome.** Management of RBD should begin with interventions that target environmental safety, and when appropriate proceed with pharmacologic therapy. When appropriate, disclosure of the risk for neurodegeneration should take place. The decision to treat and the specific treatment to select are based on a number of factors—frequency and severity of episodes and comorbidities such as sleep apnea.

(1) *Environmental safety* provides for the strongest level of evidence for managing RBD (level A evidence). Patients with frequent episodes of motor behavior should be advised to remove potentially dangerous objects from the bedroom, to pad hard and sharp surfaces/furniture around the bed, to cover windows with heavy draperies, and even to place the mattress on the floor, or to sleep in a sleeping bad, to avoid injury until pharmacotherapy is successful.

(2) The most commonly prescribed drug therapies include either clonazepam at a dosage of 0.25 to 2.0 mg, or melatonin at 3 to 12 mg at bedtime. If patients have significant OSA associated with RBD, they should be treated with positive pressure therapy because clonazepam may potentially exacerbate OSA, or be given melatonin instead. Clonazepam is effective in 90% of cases, and there is little evidence of abuse and infrequent in tolerance in this group of patients. Beneficial effects are observed within the first week of treatment. Typically, treatment with clonazepam results in control of vigorous, violent sleep behaviors, but mild to moderate limb movement. Discontinuation of treatment usually results in recurrence of symptoms.

Melatonin (3 mg titrated to clinical efficacy up to 12 mg q.h.s.) has been shown to be useful in improving DEB and has the added advantage of restoring muscle atonia. Melatonin may be advantageous over clonazepam because of its relative lack of sedation, cognitive impairment, and lack of respiratory suppression. When either melatonin or clonazepam fail to control the behavioral spells or disruptive hallucinations, both may be sued simultaneously, or the patient may be placed on a different therapy. Table 60.8 outlines the treatment options for RBD with the respective level of evidence based on a recent literature review. Both melatonin and clonazepam appear to have the strongest level of evidence in the management of this condition.

Although no specific treatment is available to prevent phenoconversion to neurodegenerative disease at present, RBD represents a unique opportunity to someday in the future provide a potential biomarker for selecting appropriate patients to be treated with neuroprotective agents to slow down or even prevent the conversion to neurodegeneration.

2. **Recurrent isolated SP.** Intrusion and persistence of muscle atonia of REM sleep into wakefulness is a central feature. Clinically, patients are unable to move or speak and experience a profound sense of impending doom and anxiety. As noted in the narcolepsy section, SP can occur as part of the classic narcolepsy pentrad, but in most individuals, SP is typically an isolated symptom and is specifically related to sleep deprivation. Specific treatment for SP is not needed in most patients as

TABLE 60.8 Treatment of RBD

	Dose	Level of Recommendation
Safety		Recommended
Clonazepam	0.25–2.0 mg q.h.s., usual recommended dose = 0.5–2.0 mg 30 min before bedtime	Suggested
Melatonin	3–12 mg q.h.s.	Suggested
Pramipexole	0.125 mg starting dose with effective dose ranging from 0.5 to 1.5 mg in the night	
Paroxetine	10–40 mg	May be considered
Donepezil	10–15 mg	May be considered
Rivastigmine	4.5–6 mg b.i.d.	May be considered
Temazepam	10 mg	May be considered
Alprazolam	1–3 mg	May be considered
Yi-Gan San	2.5 g t.i.d.	May be considered
Desipramine	50 mg q.h.s.	May be considered
Carbamazepine	500–1,500 mg q.d.	May be considered
Sodium oxybate	Unknown	May be considered

Abbreviations: b.i.d., twice a day; q.h.s., every night at bedtime; q.d., every day; RBD, REM sleep behavior disorder; t.i.d., 3 times a day.

avoidance of sleep deprivation is typically effective, and some patients with recurrent episodes unrelated to sleep loss may be managed with REM-suppressing therapy (such as SSRIs).

3. **Nightmare disorder.** The most prominent feature here consists of distressing visual imagery during REM sleep, with persistence into wakefulness. Unlike patients with sleep terrors, who are typically amnestic about event, those experiencing nightmares typically have good recollection of the episode, are able to detail their dream, but typically lack the abrupt and heightened autonomic hyperarousal and the episodes are not aggressive and lack motor activity.

Although specific pharmacotherapy of nightmares is usually not needed, patients with recurring and fearful nightmares may be managed with combined behavioral or psychotherapy and REM sleep-suppressant medications. Prazosin is helpful in reducing the severity and frequency of nightmares associated with posttraumatic stress disorder.

MOVEMENT DISORDERS OF SLEEP

A. **RLS and PLMDS.**

1. **Clinical course.** RLS, more appropriately referred to as WED (Willis-Ekbom disease), is characterized by a compulsive urge to move the lower, and occasionally in the upper, extremities, associated with irresistible movements of the extremities. The symptoms are often described by patients as creeping, crawling, and disagreeable sensations in the limbs, worse at rest (quiesogenic), and are relieved by movements such as stretching, rubbing, and walking. Lying down in bed and falling asleep is a major problem for patients with RLS. The need to move the lower extremities has a circadian predilection to be most severe at bedtime, and is often associated with sleep-initiation insomnia, which is often the most common reason for presentation. RLS must be differentiated from other conditions that could mimic RLS and clinically significant RLS is defined by symptoms leading to significant distress, sleep disturbance (insomnia/hypersomnia), or impairment of daily function.

Up to 80% of patients with RLS also have PLMS. However, PLMS can occur without RLS and has its own diagnostic category. Unlike RLS, which is a clinical diagnosis, PLMS is suspected when a patient or bed partner reports repeated leg kicks and is confirmed by periodic limb movements in the PSG. The typical PSG findings consist of stereotyped repetitive rhythmic movements. The leg movement must last for 0.5 to 10 seconds, and candidate leg movements are considered "periodic" if three or more occur with their onsets separated by 5 to 90 seconds. The leg movements consist of dorsiflexion of the foot, and occasionally may also involve the upper extremities. PLMS is usually more frequent during the first half of the night but can be present throughout sleep. Movements may be associated with sleep disruption. If numerous, the movements can result in nocturnal awakenings and EDS. The prevalence of PLMS increases with age, from 5% among those younger than 50 years to 44% among those 65 years and older. A PLM index is calculated by dividing the total number of periodic limb movements by the total sleep time (in hours), providing an average number of periodic limb movements per hour of sleep time. PLMS may be diagnosed if the patient has a PLM index greater than 15 per hour, in adults, or 5 per hour in children. PLMS is found out by PSG EMG, whereas an individual must report a sleep disturbance or a specific functional impairment that is causally related to the periodic limb movements, in which case the condition of termed PLMD. It is important to establish a cause-and-effect relationship between the insomnia or hypersomnia and the PLMS. The clinician should verify that other causes of insomnia (i.e., anxiety) or hypersomnia (i.e., narcolepsy, sleep apnea) are ruled out. PLMS is common but PLMD is believed to be less common in adults.

For most patients with RLS or PLMD, the cause is unknown and therefore termed **idiopathic.** In many cases, RLS is familial and has an autosomal-dominant inheritance with a significant genomewide association with a common variant in an intron of BTBD9 on chromosome 6p21.2, in addition to other gene variants (MEIS1, MAP2K5/LBXCOR, and PTPRD). Both RLS and PLMD are associated with anemia resulting from iron deficiency, particularly when the ferritin level is <45 mcg/L. Folic acid, vitamin B_{12} deficiency, neuropathy, myelopathy, rheumatoid arthritis, thyroid dysfunction, and uremia have also been shown to have an association. Results of studies suggest that RLS is associated with alteration in cerebrospinal fluid ferritin levels. Furthermore, PLMD may be induced or exacerbated by SSRIs and tricyclic antidepressants as well as by withdrawal from a variety of hypnotic agents. The existence of these conditions should be entertained in the differential diagnosis of PLMD so that patients receive the appropriate therapy. If these conditions are suspected, referral to the appropriate specialist is recommended.

2. **Treatment.** The four major classes of drugs that have been shown to be effective in the management of RLS are dopaminergic drugs, alpha-2-delta ($\alpha 2\delta$) ligands, BzRA, and opioids. Common medications used in the treatment of RLS are shown in Table 60.9.

   a. The first approach for patients with symptoms consistent with that of RLS is to draw a serum ferritin level. Patients with levels less than 45 mg/L should begin iron replacement therapy with iron sulfate along with vitamin C to improve absorption.

   b. When iron stores are normal, nonergotamine dopamine (D_2 D_3) agonists such as rotigotine, ropinirole, or pramipexole may be started. Two $\alpha 2\delta$ ligands, pregabalin and gabapentin enacarbi, have been shown to be effective in patients with primary moderate-to-severe RLS with painful symptoms and sleep disruption. Three dopamine agonists (rotigotine, ropinirole, and pramipexole) and one $\alpha 2\delta$ ligand, gabapentin enacarbi, are specifically FDA approved for the treatment of RLS. Major side effects include unpredictable sleep attacks, GI side effects, postural orthostatic hypotension, and, at higher doses, rare reports of impulse control behaviors (compulsive gambling). Patients on chronic dopamine therapy may experience augmentation, defined as a worsening of RLS symptoms earlier in the day with geographic spread to body parts other than the legs. Rebound may also occur and is characterized by a reappearance and worsening of symptoms as the effects of a medication wear off between doses.

   c. Historically carbidopa/levodopa (at a dose of 25 mg/100 mg q.h.s.) was initially widely used. However, its wide use is significantly limited because of the risk of rebound symptoms as well as frequent augmentation rates (up to 30%). It is better used in patients who require "on-demand" therapy of their RLS, such as when driving/flying long distances.

   d. The $\alpha 2\delta$ ligands, pregabalin and gabapentin enacarbi, of moderate-to-severe primary RLS in adults are not associated with impulse control behaviors or augmentation and

TABLE 60.9 Pharmacotherapy for RLS

Drug: Class (Generic/Brand)	Dose	Risks
Iron: Ferrous sulfate	325 mg b.i.d./t.i.d. Recommended for ferritin levels <45 mcg	GI side effects: constipation. Role in treatment under current investigation
Dopamine agonists		
Dopamine Agonists Pramipexole (Mirapex)[a] Ropinirole (Requip)[a]	0.125–0.5 mg, t.i.d Start low and increase slowly 0.25–2 mg b.i.d	Severe sleepiness, nausea reported in some cases Nausea, vomiting, sleep attacks, rare compulsive gambling
Rotigotine (Neupro)[a]	1, 2, or 3 mg q.d.	Allergic reactions, nausea, vomiting, sleep attacks, rare compulsive gambling
Dopamine Precursors Levodopa/Cardidopa (Sinemet)	25/200 mg: ½ tab–3 tabs 30 min before bedtime	Nausea, sleepiness, augmentation of daytime symptoms, insomnia, sleepiness, GI disturbances
$\alpha2\delta$ ligands: Gabapentin (Neurontin) Gabapentin enacarbil (Horizant)[a]	300–2,700 mg/d divided t.i.d. 600 mg/d taken with food at about 5:00 P.M.	Daytime sleepiness, nausea Somnolence/sedation and dizziness. May cause driving impairment
Benzodiazepines		
Clonazepam (Klonopin)	0.125–0.5 mg ½ hr before bedtime	Nausea, sedation, dizziness
Antihypertensives		
Clonidine: Catapres	0.1 mg b.i.d. May be helpful in patients with hypertension	Dry mouth, drowsiness, constipation, sedation, weakness, depression (1%), hypotension
Opioids		
Opioids: Darvocet (Darvoset-N) Darvon (Propoxyphene) Codeine	300 mg/d 65–135 mg at bedtime 30 mg	Nausea, vomiting, restlessness, constipation. Addiction, tolerance may be possible

[a]FDA-approved drugs for RLS as of October, 2016.
Abbreviations: BzRA, benzodiazepines; b.i.d., twice a day; GI, gastrointestinal; q.d., every day; RLS, restless legs syndrome; t.i.d., 3 times a day.

are effective when patients experience pain, anxiety, or insomnia as part of their RLS. Therapy, however, is sometimes limited by sedation, weight gain, and depression.

e. Several BzRA, including clonazepam, nitrazepam, lorazepam, and temazepam, have been found to improve the nocturnal sleep of patients with RLS and PLMS. Of these, clonazepam is the most widely used. The therapeutic action of clonazepam most likely results from its ability to decrease the number of arousals caused by leg movements. The usual starting dosage of clonazepam is 0.5 to 1.0 mg at bedtime for management of PLMS. Management of RLS may require additional doses to control symptoms during the day. Because BzRA are CNS depressants, they may aggravate sleep apnea, particularly among older persons.

f. Finally, opioids are highly effective in the management of RLS and PLMS. In severe cases refractory to other treatments, intermittent therapy with opioids provides good relief without evidence of augmentation.

SLEEP-DISORDERED BREATHING

The most commonly encountered types of abnormal nocturnal breathing are the sleep apnea and hypopnea. Sleep apnea is cessation of breathing for at least 10 seconds caused by obstruction of the upper airway (obstructive sleep apnea), loss of respiratory effort or rhythmicity (central apnea), or a combination of the two (mixed apnea). Hypopnea is a decrease in airflow, which can be obstructive or central in origin. Many patients with sleep apnea have combinations of the central and obstructive types, which suggest that the mechanisms of the different types of sleep apnea may overlap.

A. **Central sleep apnea (CSA).**

1. **Clinical course.** Patients with CSA constitute less than 10% of all patients with sleep apnea who undergo studies in sleep laboratories. Therefore, only a few studies have been reported, which limits knowledge of this disorder. Little information is available regarding the cardiovascular sequelae of CSA. The most common finding is sinus arrhythmia with bradycardia. Oxygen desaturation in patients with CSA tends to be generally mild to moderate compared with those with obstructive sleep apnea. Although the cause of CSA in most cases is unknown, it has been associated with certain diseases that should be considered in the differential diagnosis and management of this disorder. These diseases include central alveolar hypoventilation (Ondine's curse), obesity hypoventilation (Pickwickian) syndrome, congestive heart failure (Cheyne–Stokes breathing pattern), autonomic dysfunction (Shy–Drager syndrome, familial dysautonomia, and diabetes mellitus), neuromuscular disorders (muscular dystrophy, myasthenia gravis, and motor neuron disease), and brainstem lesions.

2. **Treatment** of patients with CSA is limited and not satisfactory. Studies regarding treatment usually have involved small numbers of patients, and very few have addressed the long-term efficacy of the proposed treatments.

   a. One approach is noninvasive nocturnal ventilation delivered by means of a nasal mask with a volume- or pressure-cycled ventilator. This approach is used to manage only the most severe cases of central alveolar hypoventilation or in the care of patients with neuromuscular disorders.

   b. Some patients with CSA have been shown to benefit from therapy with nasal continuous positive airway pressure (CPAP). This type of therapy is most beneficial to obese patients who also have signs of upper airway obstruction with predominantly central apnea. Nasal CPAP also has been shown effective in the treatment of patients with congestive heart failure in whom central apnea and periodic breathing are observed during sleep. Finally, oxygen therapy has been useful in managing central apnea.

   c. Adaptive seroventilation (ASV): ASV provides a relatively low baseline pressure and variable ventilatory support to establish a preset level of ventilation for each breath. If the patient's effort decreases, the ASV's inspiratory support increases to maintain a steady level of ventilation. This treatment is indicated in patients with CSA, but also OSA patients are refractory to standard CPAP. The term treatment-emergent sleep apnea (formerly known as "complex sleep apnea") refers to patients with OSA who develop CSA on initiation of CPAP. These patients with so-called treatment-emergent central apneas often experience spontaneous resolution of their disease with ongoing therapy.

      The reader needs to be aware that ASV is associated with an increased risk of cardiovascular mortality in the setting of symptomatic chronic heart failure with reduced ejection fraction (EF) [low EF ($\leq$45%)].

   d. For patients with medical or neurologic conditions known to be associated with CSA, the condition should be managed specifically and the central apnea reassessed. However, if the problem persists or if a cause is not found, several pharmacologic agents can be used. Acetazolamide, a carbonic anhydrase inhibitor, given at a dose of 250 mg four times a day, has been shown to improve CSA. The side effects associated with mild metabolic acidosis are usually well tolerated by this group of patients.

   e. Other medications, such as theophylline, naloxone, and medroxyprogesterone acetate, have been used with varying degrees of success. Because none of these medications has been studied systematically, more precise recommendations regarding their use are currently not available.

B. Obstructive sleep apnea (OSA).

1. **Clinical course.** The initial symptoms of OSA syndrome are loud snoring, excessive sleepiness, fatigue, morning headaches, memory problems, alterations in mood, and episodes of apnea witnessed by the bed partner. OSA is associated with considerable morbidity, including sleep fragmentation, daytime sleepiness that may lead to vehicular and industrial accidents, nocturnal hypoxemia, and cardiovascular as well as cerebrovascular sequelae (e.g., stroke, right heart failure, and hypertension). OSA is generally caused by upper airway obstruction resulting from obesity and skeletal and soft-tissue abnormalities. Examination of the nose and throat may indicate a possible cause. However, some patients with OSA may have normal findings at physical examination.

If OSA is suspected, PSG should be performed to ascertain the severity of the breathing disorder, which will determine the appropriate therapy. Some patients who have symptoms indistinguishable from those of OSA may have predominantly sleep hypopnea. Sleep hypopnea syndrome should be managed in the same manner as sleep apnea syndromes.

The apnea–hypopnea index (AHI) (number of respiratory events per hour of sleep) is used to measure sleep-disordered breathing. An index of 5 is generally accepted as the upper limit of the normal range. Patients who have milder indexes but whose respiratory events are accompanied by more significant oxygen desaturations and who have additional cardiovascular risk factors such as hypertension, history of heart disease, high cholesterol level, and cigarette smoking also should be treated.

In adults, a diagnosis of OSA is defined by either of the following:

a. AHI >5, in a patient with one or more of the following:
   (1) Sleepiness, nonrestorative sleep, fatigue, or insomnia symptoms
   (2) Waking up with breath holding, gasping, or choking
   (3) Habitual snoring, breathing interruptions, or both noted by a bed partner or other observer
   (4) Hypertension, mood disorder, cognitive dysfunction, coronary artery disease, stroke, congestive heart failure, atrial fibrillation, or type 2 diabetes mellitus
b. AHI >15, regardless of the presence of associated symptoms or comorbidities.

2. **Therapy.** The approach to management of obstructive sleep apnea and hypopnea syndromes involves both general measures and interventions that address specific abnormalities. For most patients, nasal CPAP is the most effective medical therapy for control of sleep apnea.

   a. **General measures** for identifying and addressing coexistent lifestyle issues that exacerbate OSA should be part of treatment of all patients. Although difficult to achieve, weight loss is an important factor in the treatment of obese persons with apnea. Sleep apnea generally improves with weight loss and may even be improved with weight loss of 40 to 50 pounds (18 to 23 kg). In addition to dietary control, this approach requires an exercise program and psychological counseling for long-lasting results. Unfortunately, results indicate that most patients regain the weight within 2 years. If sleep-disordered breathing is more prominent in the supine position, positional therapy to avoid sleep in the supine position is very useful. Alcohol, hypnotic drugs, and other CNS depressant drugs interfere with the arousal response that terminates apneic episodes. Therefore, patients should avoid alcohol use and should not take hypnotics or sedatives. If a specific cause for upper airway obstruction is found, an otorhinolaryngologic or maxillofacial evaluation is recommended for possible surgical intervention and trials of orthodontic devices, including tonsillectomy or adenoidectomy for enlarged tonsils or adenoids and correction of retrognathia or micrognathia. Results indicate that dental devices may be useful to those patients with mild-to-moderate sleep apnea with some degree of retrognathia or micrognathia. If chronic rhinitis is found, nasal steroid sprays may be beneficial.

   b. **Nasal CPAP.** If no specific cause of upper airway obstruction is found, nasal continuous positive airway pressure (CPAP) is the treatment of choice. This treatment is effective for most patients with obstructive apnea and hypopnea. The level of CPAP should be determined by means of titration of the therapeutic pressure in a sleep laboratory, respiratory data being obtained in all sleep stages. Nasal CPAP requires patency of the nasal airway. Therefore, this procedure may not be effective for patients with severe nasal obstruction. The most common causes of intolerance of nasal CPAP are nasal symptoms, dryness, discomfort from the mask, and social and psychological factors of having to use the mask during sleep (because of claustrophobia). Added humidification often alleviates dryness and associated nasal congestion. With higher pressures, bilevel positive airway pressure (BiPAP) may be a more comfortable alternative to CPAP. Most home-care companies provide both nasal CPAP and BiPAP services. If a patient with sleep apnea also has low baseline oxygen saturation during the day or during sleep, referral to an internist or pulmonologist is recommended. Although improvement of symptoms, including daytime sleepiness, may be observed within 1 or 2 days of treatment with nasal CPAP, maximal improvement may not occur for several weeks. Follow-up studies indicate that long-term compliance with nasal CPAP is a substantial problem for many patients not using CPAP throughout the night and on a daily basis. Compliance increases with close follow-up care. Follow-up visits should be scheduled 1 month after the start of CPAP and every 6 months thereafter.

The Centers for Medicare & Medicaid Services (CMS) has recently issued a memo that authorized payment for CPAP may take place only if formal PSG was performed and was diagnostic for OSA, and that CMS will pay for CPAP therapy for 3 months (and subsequently if OSA improves) for adults diagnosed with either PSG or with unattended home sleep-monitoring devices. The use of portable home monitoring devices may improve access to diagnosis and treatment of OSA.

However, these devices must be used as part of a comprehensive sleep evaluation program that includes access to board-certified sleep specialists, PSG facilities, and therapists experienced in fitting and troubleshooting CPAP devices.

c. **Oxygen therapy.** Oxygen has been previously reviewed for the treatment of OSA, but the data are quite limited, including limited population. An AASM practice parameter review from 2006 did not recommend oxygen as a primary treatment for OSA. In contrast, in some cases, oxygen may be utilized as a supplement to positive airway pressure therapy (PAP) in cases of refractory hypoxemia, chronic obstructive pulmonary disease overlapping with sleep apnea, and may, in some circumstances, be an option for individuals who fail or refuse all other OSA treatments and have significant nocturnal hypoxia associated with their sleep apnea.

d. **Oral appliances.** Custom-made oral appliances improve upper airway size, and prevent the collapse of the tongue and soft tissues in the back of the throat by supporting the jaw in a forward position, keeping the airway open during sleep. One specific type of an oral appliance, the mandibular repositioning appliance, covers the upper and lower teeth and holds the mandible in a relatively advanced position with respect to the resting position, improving the air space. Oral appliances may not be as efficacious as CPAP in treating sleep apnea, but are indicated for use in patients with mild-to-moderate OSA who do tolerate or respond to CPAP, or fail behavioral interventions to improve compliance. Oral appliances are appropriate for first-line therapy in patients with primary snoring who do not respond to weight-loss or positional therapy (refers to avoiding sleep in the supine position, which tends to worsens OSA). Patients with CSA, morbid obesity, poor dentition, and acute TMD derangement are not good candidates for oral appliances.

e. **Night shift.** A special device that is worn on the back of the neck, and vibrates when patients sleep on their back and slowly increases in intensity until a position change occurs. The therapy may be effective for treatment of positional OSA alone or in combination with other sleep apnea treatments such as CPAP.

f. **Winx sleep therapy system.** The device works by generating negative pressure in the oral cavity, which draws the soft palate and uvula forward, and stabilizes the tongue position, thus enlarging the upper airway.

g. **Expiratory positive airway pressure (or Provent Sleep Apnea Therapy).** During inhalation, the device opens, allowing patients to breathe in freely. However, during exhaling, the valve closes, increasing the pressure in the airway, allowing patients to keep the airways open until the next inhalation cycle.

h. **Somnoplasty.** Also known as temperature-controlled radio frequency, is a minimally invasive surgical technique that utilizes radiofrequency current to reduce tissue volume in a precise, targeted manner. Data demonstrate that the technique reduces snoring but is ineffective for sleep apnea.

i. **Uvulopalatopharyngoplasty (UPPP) with or without tonsillectomy.**
This technique enlarges the retropalatal upper airway by excising a portion of the posterior soft palate and uvula. Anatomy is the main predictor of success. While favorable anatomy for UPPP includes large tonsils and favorable tongue placement (small base of tongue), the technique may not resolve sleep apnea or protect patients from future development of OSA. It is estimated that these surgical approaches are effective for approximately 50% of the time for amelioration of sleep apnea but are more effective for snoring. Thus, patients may continue to have silent obstructive apnea after surgery.
A 2010 AASM's practice parameter on surgical treatment options for adult OSA patients reviewed the literature regarding the following specific surgical procedures: tracheostomy, maxillomandibular advancement, laser-assisted uvulopalatoplasty (LAUP), UPPP, RFA, and palatal implants.
Establishing a diagnosis of OSA and its severity by polysomnography prior to any surgical intervention was considered a standard recommendation by this position paper. In addition, in order that patients can make an informed decision regarding therapy, the standard proposed that all patients be advised of the anticipated success rates and potential complications, related to surgical intervention as compared to the alternative treatment options for their OSA (namely CPAP and oral appliances). If patients chose to have surgery, clinical follow-up including a nocturnal polysomnogram is a standard recommendation in order to demonstrate resolution of OSA as measures by the AHI, oxygen saturation, and sleep architecture. As for the specific surgical procedure, none, with the exception of LAUP, received more than a recommendation of option as an intervention for the management of OSA. The standard recommendation was not in favor of using LAUP as a treatment for OSA. A multidisciplinary approach is recommended to identify appropriate patients for surgical interventions.

j. **Bariatric surgery.** Gastric banding, sleeve gastrectomy, and gastric bypass surgery contribute to significant weight loss, resulting in improvements in OSA.

k. **Inspire upper airway stimulation.** An implanted system that senses breathing patterns and delivers mild stimulation to key airway muscles, by stimulating the hypoglossal nerve, which keeps the airway open during sleep.

l. **Drug therapy.** When nasal CPAP is not an option, patients with mild-to-moderate OSA may benefit from drug therapy. Protriptyline at a dosage of 10 mg at bedtime with upward adjustment depending on response and side effects may be an alternative treatment. Drug therapy is generally unsatisfactory for management of OSA. Recently, the FDA has approved the use of modafinil to improve wakefulness in patients who present with EDS associated with OSA if CPAP is used with adequate compliance and when total sleep time is adequate.

Key Points

- Sleep disturbances are very common in patients with neurologic disorders and may result in significant morbidity.
- Neurologists need to be aware of the major sleep disorders that may occur in their patients including chronic insomnia, sleep-disordered breathing such as obstructive sleep apnea, CNS hypersomnias including narcolepsy, circadian rhythm sleep disturbances, parasomnias such as RBD, and sleep-related movement disorders including RLS.
- Diagnosis is based on meticulous inventory of the clinical history, evaluation of the patients for problems such as snoring, apneic episodes, dream enactment, hypersomnolence, and urge to move the legs and an inability to initiate or maintain sleep.

- A detailed inventory of sleep patterns is an important step in the clinical interview, especially regarding bedtime habits and rituals that precede the typical sleep period and wake time, and daytime function.
- Questions reviewing the current medical and psychiatric problems, medications (with particular attention to activating and sedating drugs), social history, focusing on caffeine and alcohol ingestion as well as a family history for other first-degree relatives with similar complaints are very helpful.
- In some cases referral to a sleep laboratory for further evaluation with a nocturnal polysomnography (a sleep study) is indicated and may require the addition of additional EEG and EMG channels to evaluate for nocturnal seizures and parasomnias.
- RBD is increasingly recognized as a marker of an evolving neurodegenerative disease. It is very frequent in neurology practice, affecting up to two-thirds of patients with Parkinson's disease and may be confused with nocturnal seizures and parasomnia.

Recommended Readings

Allen R. Dopamine and iron in the pathophysiology of restless legs syndrome (RLS). *Sleep Med.* 2004;5:385–391.

Allen R, Becker PM, Bogan R, et al. Ropinirole decreases periodic leg movements and improves sleep parameters in patients with restless legs syndrome. *Sleep.* 2004;27:907–914.

American Academy of Sleep Medicine. *International Classification of Sleep Disorders, Revised: Diagnostic and Coding Manual.* 3rd ed. Darien, IL: American Academy of Sleep Medicine; 2014.

Aurora RN, Casey KR, Kristo D, et al. Practice parameters for the surgical modifications of the upper airway for obstructive sleep apnea in adults. *Sleep.* 2010;33(10):1408–1413.

Aurora RN, Zak RS, Maganti RK, et al. Best practice guide for the treatment of REM sleep behavior disorder (RBD). *J Clin Sleep Med.* 2010;6(1):85–95.

Avidan AY. Parasomnias and movement disorders of sleep. *Semin Neurol.* 2009;29(4):372–392.

Avidan AY, Kaplish N. The parasomnias: epidemiology, clinical features, and diagnostic approach. *Clin Chest Med.* 2010;31(2):353–370.

Avidan AY, Zee PC. *Handbook of Sleep Medicine.* 2nd ed. Philadelphia, PA: Wolters Kluwer Health; 2011.

Berry RB, Brooks R, Gamaldo CE, et al; for the American Academy of Sleep Medicine. *The AASM Manual for the Scoring of Sleep and Associated Events: Rules, Terminology and Technical Specifications*, Version 2.2. Darien, IL: American Academy of Sleep Medicine; 2015. http://www.aasmnet.org

Berry RB, Kryger MH, Massie CA. A novel nasal expiratory positive airway pressure (EPAP) device for the treatment of obstructive sleep apnea: a randomized controlled trial. *Sleep.* 2011;34(4):479–485.

Boeve BF, Molano JR, Ferman TJ, et al. Validation of the Mayo Sleep Questionnaire to screen for REM sleep behavior disorder in a community-based sample. *J Clin Sleep Med.* 2013;9:475.

Colrain IM, Black J, Siegel LC, et al. A multicenter evaluation of oral pressure therapy for the treatment of obstructive sleep apnea. *Sleep Med.* 2013;14:830–837.

Cowie MR, Woehrle H, Wegscheider K, et al. Adaptive servo-ventilation for central sleep apnea in systolic heart failure. *N Eng J Med.* 2015;373(12):1095–1105.

Dauvilliers Y, Siegel JM, Lopez R, et al. Cataplexy-clinical aspects, pathophysiology and management strategy. *Nat Rev Neurol.* 2014;10(7):386–395. doi:10.1038/nrneurol.2014.97.

Dodson ER, Zee PC. Therapeutics for circadian rhythm sleep disorders. *Sleep Med Clin.* 2010;5(4):701–715.

Earley CJ, Silber MH. Restless legs syndrome: understanding its consequences and the need for better treatment. *Sleep Med.* 2010;11(9):807–815.

Garcia-Borreguero D, Kohnen R, Silber MH, et al. The long-term treatment of restless legs syndrome/Willis-Ekbom disease: evidence-based guidelines and clinical consensus best practice guidance: a report from the International Restless Legs Syndrome Study Group. *Sleep Med.* 2013;14(7):675–684. doi:10.1016/j.sleep.2013.05.016.

Guilleminault C, Faull KF. Sleepiness in non-narcoleptic, nonsleep apneic EDS patients: the idiopathic CNS hypersomnolence. *Sleep.* 1982;5:S175–S181.

Harsora P, Kessmann J. Nonpharmacologic management of chronic insomnia. *Am Fam Physician.* 2009;79(2):125–130.

Holty JC, Guilleminault C. Surgical options for the treatment of obstructive sleep apnea. *Med Clin N Am.* 2010;94:479–515.

Iranzo A, Fernandez-Arcos A, Tolosa E, et al. Neurodegenerative disorder risk in idiopathic REM sleep behavior disorder: study in 174 patients. *PloS One.* 2014;9(2):e89741. doi:10.1371/journal.pone.0089741.

Kapur V, Maganti R, Owens J, et al; Standards of Practice Committee of the American Academy of Sleep Medicine. Practice parameters for the clinical evaluation and treatment of circadian rhythm sleep disorders. An American Academy of Sleep Medicine report. *Sleep.* 2007;30(11):1445–1459.

Kryger MH, Roth T, Dement WC. *Principles and Practice of Sleep Medicine.* 5th ed. Philadelphia, PA: Saunders; 2011.

Levendowski DJ, Seagraves S, Popovic D, et al. Assessment of a neck-based treatment and monitoring device for positional obstructive sleep apnea. *J Clin Sleep Med.* 2014;10(8):863–871.

Loube DI, Gay PC, Strohl KP, et al. Indications for positive airway pressure treatment of adult obstructive sleep apnea patients: consensus statement. *Chest.* 1999;115:863–866.

Manthena P, Zee PC. Neurobiology of circadian rhythm sleep disorders. *Curr Neurol Neurosci Rep.* 2006;6(2):163–168.

Mignot E. Narcolepsy: pharmacology, pathophysiology and genetics. In: Kryger M, Roth T, Dement WC, eds. *Principles and Practice of Sleep Medicine.* Philadelphia, PA: Elsevier Saunders; 2005:761–779.

Mitler M, Erman M, Hajdukovic R. The treatment of excessive somnolence with stimulant drugs. *Sleep.* 1993;16:203–206.

Morgenthaler TI, Kramer M, Alessi C, et al; American Academy of Sleep Medicine. Practice parameters for the psychological and behavioral treatment of insomnia: an update. An American Academy of Sleep Medicine report. *Sleep.* 2006;29(11):1415–1419.

Morgenthaler T; Kramer M; Alessi C et al. Practice parameters for the psychological and behavioral treatment of insomnia: an update. An American Academy of Sleep Medicine report. *Sleep.* 2006;29(11):1415–1419.

Neubauer DN, Flaherty KN. Chronic insomnia. *Semin Neurol.* 2009;29(4):340–353.

NIH State-of-the-Science Conference Statement on manifestations and management of chronic insomnia in adults. *NIH Consens State Sci Statements.* 2005;22(2):1–30.

Nishino S, Mignot E. Narcolepsy and cataplexy. In: Vinken PJ, Bruyn GW, eds. *Handbook of Clinical Neurology.* New York, NY: Elsevier B.V; 2011:783–814.

Overeem S, Mignot E, van Dijk JG, et al. Narcolepsy: clinical features, new pathophysiologic insights, and future perspectives. *J Clin Neurophysiol.* 2001;18(2):78–105.

Overeem S, Reading P. *Sleep Disorders in Neurology: A Practical Approach.* Chichester, West Sussex: Wiley-Blackwell; 2009.

Pack AI, Pien GW. Update on sleep and its disorders. *Annu Rev Med.* 2011;62:447–460.

Postuma RB, Bertrand JA, Gagnon JF, et al. Rapid eye movement sleep behavior disorder and risk of dementia in Parkinson's disease: a prospective study. *Mov Disord.* 2012;27(6):720–726.

Postuma RB, Gagnon JF, Montplaisir JY, et al. Olfaction and color vision identify impending neurodegeneration in rapid eye movement sleep behavior disorder. *Ann Neurol.* 2011;69(5):811–818.

Reid KJ, Chang AM, Zee PC. Circadian rhythm sleep disorders. *Med Clin North Am.* 2004;88(3):631–651.

Reid KJ, Zee PC. Circadian rhythm sleep disorders. In: Vinken PJ, Bruyn GW, eds. *Handbook of Clinical Neurology.* New York, NY: Elsevier B.V; 2011:963–977.

Riemann D, Perlis ML. The treatments of chronic insomnia: a review of benzodiazepine receptor agonists and psychological and behavioral therapies. *Sleep Med. Rev.* 2009;13(3):205–214.

Robinson A, Guilleminault C. Obstructive sleep apnea syndrome. In: Chokroverty S, ed. *Sleep Disorders Medicine: Basic Science, Technical Considerations, and Clinical Aspects.* 2nd ed. Boston, MA: Butterworth-Heineman; 1999:331–354.

Rubins JB, Kunisaki KM. Contemporary issues in the diagnosis and treatment of obstructive sleep apnea. *Postgrad Med.* 2008;120(2):46–52.

Schenck CH, Boeve BF, Mahowald MW. Delayed emergence of a parkinsonian disorder or dementia in 81% of older men initially diagnosed with idiopathic rapid eye movement sleep behavior disorder: a 16-year update on a previously reported series. *Sleep Med.* 2013;14(8):744–748. doi:10.1016/j.sleep.2012.10.009.

Silber MH, Becker PM, Earley C, et al; Medical Advisory Board of the Willis-Ekbom Disease F. Willis-Ekbom Disease Foundation revised consensus statement on the management of restless legs syndrome. *Mayo Clin Proc.* 2013;88(9):977–986. doi:10.1016/j.mayocp.2013.06.016.

Silber MH, Krahn LE, Morgenthaler TI. *Sleep Medicine in Clinical Practice.* 2nd ed. New York, NY: Informa Healthcare; 2010.

Strollo PJ, Soose RJ, Maurer JT, et al. Upper-airway stimulation for obstructive sleep apnea. *N Engl J Med.* 2014;370:139–149.

Sutherland K, Vanderveken O, Cistulli P. Oral appliance treatment for obstructive sleep apnea: an update. *J Clin Sleep Med.* 2014;10(2):215–227.

The National Institutes of Health Consensus Development Program. NIH state-of-the-science conference statement on manifestations and management of chronic insomnia in adults. *Sleep.* 2005;28:1049–1057.

Wise MS, Arand DL, Arger RR, et al. Treatment of narcolepsy and other hypersomnias of central origin. *Sleep.* 2007;30(12):1712–1727.

Zee PC, Goldstein CA. Treatment of shift work disorder and jet lag. *Curr Treat Options Neurol.* 2010;12(5):396–411.

61 Dizziness and Vertigo

Matthew L. Kircher and Sara Anderson-Kim

When investigating the source of dizziness in a patient, it is useful to organize potential etiologies into four groups. The four major causes of dizziness and vertigo are peripheral vestibular, central vestibular, medical, and unlocalized. True vertigo, particularly rotatory vertigo, is often because of a peripheral vestibular (inner ear) disorder. Presyncope and loss of consciousness are not associated with vertigo of peripheral origin and should direct the examiner to investigate other, often cardiovascular or central nervous system, causes. Common clinical scenarios illustrate the varied backgrounds from which a complaint of dizziness may arise, and these range in significance from benign annoyance to potentially life-threatening events.

Documentation of the impact of dizziness and vertigo on a patient's quality of life is essential in formulating a treatment plan. Treatment options are driven by the severity of disease and limitation in activities of daily living. Depending on the patient's job demands, symptoms may significantly impact their ability to work.

PERIPHERAL VESTIBULAR OR OTOLOGIC CAUSES OF VERTIGO

A. Benign paroxysmal positional vertigo.
1. **Clinical features.** Benign paroxysmal positional vertigo (BPPV) is characterized by vertigo triggered by changes in head position. BPPV is the most common cause of peripheral vertigo and results from stimulation of semicircular canal ampulla by loose otoconia dislodged from the utricle. The most common form of BPPV affects the posterior semicircular canal, and this section will focus on the diagnosis and treatment of posterior canal BPPV. The posterior semicircular canal lies in an inferior position within the labyrinth. With lying flat and to the affected side, otoconial debris will make its way into this canal and stimulate the vestibulo-ocular reflex thereby creating vertigo. Typically, the history is one of recurrent vertiginous episodes lasting not more than 1 minute and reproducible with repeated movement in the same direction. The dislodgement of otoconia or canaliths may occur after trauma or labyrinthitis, or even spontaneously. The Dix–Hallpike test is commonly employed to diagnose BPPV and identify the affected labyrinth **(see Chapter 16)**.
2. **Treatment.** Vestibular suppressant medications can lessen vertigo intensity but do not reduce the frequency of attacks. The mainstay of treatment is repositioning exercises to move the debris from the affected semicircular canal. Both office-based repositioning techniques and home exercises may be employed to accomplish this goal. If a patient has difficulty performing exercises owing to physical limitations or fear of inducing vertiginous symptoms, referring the patient to a trained physical therapist for repositioning is also a good option. Rarely, when positional vertigo is unresponsive to repositioning maneuvers, surgery may be considered.
   a. **Epley maneuver.** The Epley maneuver (**Video 61.1**) is a common technique used for canalith repositioning. It is most effectively used when the affected semicircular canal has been identified and can therefore be targeted for repositioning.
   (1) Technique (Fig. 61.1).
      (a) With the patient sitting upright, the head is turned 45 degrees to the offending side.
      (b) From this upright position with the head turned, the patient is reclined supine with slight neck extension; this position is held for at least 15 to 20 seconds while observing for nystagmus and/or inquiring about patient subjective dizziness.

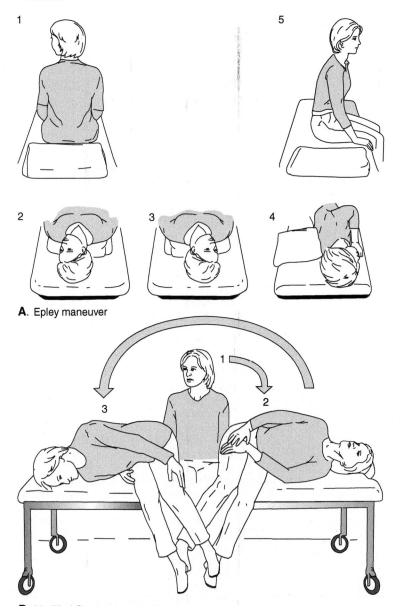

A. Epley maneuver

B. Modified Semont maneuver

FIGURE 61.1 Self-treatment of BPPV. **A:** Epley maneuver. **B:** Modified Semont maneuver. (From Radtke A, von Brevern M, Tiel-Wilck K, et al. Self-treatment of benign paroxysmal positional vertigo: semont maneuver vs Epley procedure. *Neurology*. 2004;63:150–152, with permission.).

(c) After nystagmus abates, the head is then slowly rotated away from the offending side, through midline, 90 degrees to the opposite side pausing again to monitor for generated nystagmus and to allow abatement.

(d) Keeping the head and neck in a fixed position relative to the body, the individual rolls onto their side, effectively rotating the head another 90 degrees away from the affected ear, completing a 180-degree rotation and pausing to allow nystagmus to abate.

    (e) After resolution of nystagmus and vertigo, the patient is returned to a seated position.

  b. Liberatory or Semont maneuver.

    (1) Technique (described for left-sided BPPV):

      (a) The patient sits upright on the edge of the bed with the head turned 45 degrees to the right.

      (b) The patient drops his/her head quickly to touch the left postauricular region to the bed while lying on the left trunk side and maintains this position for at least 30 seconds.

      (c) Keeping the head and neck in a fixed position relative to the body, the patient then swiftly rolls onto the right trunk side to touch the right side of the forehead down and maintains this position for at least 30 seconds.

      (d) The patient sits up again.

        These maneuvers should be performed multiple times per day as tolerated until symptoms abate.

  c. Surgery. Very rarely, repositioning techniques are ineffective, and in severe cases of refractory BPPV, surgery may be offered. Surgical options include semicircular canal plugging and vestibular neurectomy.

 3. Results. When applied to patients with BPPV, canalith repositioning is successful in relieving symptoms in up to 90% of patients. The techniques can be performed and taught by a wide range of clinicians. In those patients with recurrent symptoms, teaching the patient repositioning techniques will allow for self-treatment.

 4. Special circumstances. When BPPV is bilateral, treatment begins with the side that has a more robust nystagmus on Dix–Hallpike testing. Patients with severe disease may need pretreatment with 5 to 10 mg of diazepam 30 minutes before repositioning.

B. Vestibular neuritis and labyrinthitis.

 1. Clinical features. Vestibular neuritis and labyrinthitis are often discussed together because of their similar presenting feature of vertigo lasting for days to weeks, although labyrinthitis is associated with sensorineural hearing loss (SNHL), whereas vestibular neuritis is not. These conditions are typically self-limited and are generally attributed to a viral infection. During the acute phase of vestibular neuritis or labyrinthitis (acute vestibular syndrome), many patients present to the emergency department or urgent care concerned by the duration and intensity of their symptoms. Thorough assessment and, sometimes, imaging are necessary to rule out more serious cause of vertigo including vertebrobasilar stroke. After the acute phase, vestibular equilibrium gradually returns over the course of several weeks in most patients.

 2. Treatment. Using a combination of vestibular suppression, anti-inflammatory agents, antiemetics and vestibular rehabilitation, treatment aims to reduce the severity and duration of acute symptomatology while allowing for vestibular recovery.

  a. Vestibular suppression. Vestibular suppressants are generally grouped into three categories: benzodiazepines, antihistamines, and anticholinergics (Table 61.1). Benzodiazepines work through γ-aminobutyric acid (GABA) potentiation and subsequent inhibition of vestibular stimulation. Anticholinergics and antihistamines work to suppress vestibular input. These medications are generally well tolerated in low doses. However, it is important to realize that a high level of vestibular suppression may reduce central compensation and ultimately hinder recovery—"the brain can't fix what it can't see." Thus, it is wise to use vestibular suppressants in a limited fashion. Antiemetics are a fourth category of pharmacotherapy often used concurrently with vestibulosuppressants to target frequently associated nausea.

    (1) Antihistamines. Antihistamines, notably those of the histamine-1 antagonist group, are commonly used in the management of peripheral vertigo. They are believed to exert a vestibulosuppressant effect via a central anticholinergic mechanism. Meclizine is most commonly used, starting at small doses (12.5 to 25 mg two to three times daily) and titrating to effect. Its effect is limited, with

TABLE 61.1 Common Oral Medications for Treatment of Vertigo

Medication	Class	Dose
Clonazepam	Benzodiazepine	0.25–0.5 mg every 8 hr
Diazepam	Benzodiazepine	5–10 mg every 12 hr
Lorazepam	Benzodiazepine	1–2 mg every 8 hr
Dimenhydrinate	Antihistamine	50–100 mg every 4–6 hr not to exceed 400 mg daily
Diphenhydramine	Antihistamine	25–50 mg every 4–6 hr not to exceed 300 mg daily
Meclizine	Antihistamine	12.5–50 mg every 4–6 hr
Scopolamine	Anticholinergic	0.5 mg patch every 72 hr

adequate suppression typically lasting only 1 to 2 months. Promethazine is another antihistamine that also has antiemetic properties.

(2) **Anticholinergics.** Scopolamine is an anticholinergic medication commonly used in the prevention of motion sickness. It is not as valuable in the management of acquired vestibulopathy, but may be effective in the prophylaxis of motion sickness.

(3) **Benzodiazepines.** Benzodiazepines are a class of psychoactive drugs that work through central inhibitory GABA potentiation resulting in anxiolysis, sedation, and, in some cases, amnestic, anticonvulsant, and muscle relaxation effects. Lorazepam and diazepam are frequently used for their ability to prevent and mitigate attacks of dizziness and vertigo from a variety of etiologies. Diazepam at a low dose (5 to 10 mg) acts as a vestibulosuppressant and can be used for acute or chronic otologic dizziness. Care must be taken when utilizing benzodiazepines because of their increased potential for dependence and subsequent withdrawal symptoms on cessation of therapy.

(4) **Antiemetics** (Table 61.2). Antiemetics are used to relieve nausea and vomiting associated with vertigo. Prochlorperazine is a phenothiazine that exerts a strong antiemetic effect but also carries the risk of extrapyramidal side effects. Metoclopramide is a dopamine receptor antagonist and serotonin receptor antagonist/agonist with antiemetic and prokinetic properties. Ondansetron provides antiemesis via serotonin 5-HT$_3$ receptor antagonism.

b. **Corticosteroids/antivirals/antibiotics.** High-dose oral corticosteroids or intratympanic corticosteroids administered by an otolaryngologist may be effective in treating labyrinthitis-associated hearing loss. Prompt audiological evaluation and ENT referral are paramount because early initiation of corticosteroid therapy may improve hearing outcomes. Although most cases of labyrinthitis are believed to arise from viral infection, the addition of antiviral therapy to corticosteroids has not been shown to offer additional benefit. Antibiotics are of value in cases of bacterial or suppurative labyrinthitis; however, the decision to use antibiotics should be dictated by objective signs of infection.

c. **Vestibular rehabilitation.** Vestibular rehabilitation refers to physical therapy aimed at enhancing recovery from peripheral vestibulopathy. The exercises range from simple head-turning to increasingly more complex postural and ambulation challenges with and without head movement. Simple walking is a form of vestibular rehabilitation that

TABLE 61.2 Common Oral Medications for Treatment of Nausea

Medication	Dose
Metoclopramide	5–10 mg every 6 hr
Ondansetron	8 mg three times daily
Prochlorperazine	5–10 mg three to four times daily

can be recommended to patients with limited disequilibrium. The earlier vestibular rehabilitation takes place, the better the outcome, and patients should be titrated off vestibular suppressants to optimize vestibular challenge and recovery.

3. **Results.** Although there is some support for steroid use and vestibular rehabilitation enhancing vestibular recovery, randomized control trials are lacking. Fortunately, over 90% of patients with vestibular neuronitis or labyrinthitis will return to their presymptomatic baseline.

C. **Ménière's disease.**

1. **Clinical features.** Ménière's disease is characterized by the constellation of fluctuating SNHL, tinnitus, and vertigo. It is often associated with "aural fullness." Episodes are recurrent and typically last 20 minutes or longer. Over time, the involved peripheral vestibular system experiences a reduction in responsiveness or "burns out." It is a disease primarily of Caucasians, with a slight female bias and onset between 40 and 60 years of age. The histopathologic correlate is endolymphatic hydrops, the result of an overaccumulation of endolymph. One proposed pathophysiologic mechanism involves membranous labyrinth microruptures, allowing potassium-rich endolymph to mix with potassium-poor perilymph, thus disrupting biochemical gradients and neuronal conductivity.

2. **Treatments.** Treatment of Ménière's disease is focused on vertiginous symptom control, as tinnitus and hearing loss are less amenable to intervention. Medical therapy is used at the outset of treatment, with more invasive options reserved for symptoms refractory to conservative management.

   a. **Nonablative.**

   (1) **Acute.** As in labyrinthitis, antihistamines, anticholinergics, benzodiazepines, and antiemetics may be used to mitigate acute attacks of vertigo and nausea.

   (2) **Chronic.** Salt-restricted diet and diuretics are the mainstays of medical treatment. Their efficacy is believed to result from a reduction in endolymph. A combination of hydrochlorothiazide and triamterene is a commonly used regimen and can be titrated to effect. Also limiting alcohol, caffeine, and stress may be beneficial. Those patients with poor symptom control despite these measures may then be offered nonablative options such as intratympanic steroid injection or endolymphatic sac surgery (ESS). ESS is a hearing-preserving, nonvestibular-ablative endolymphatic sac decompressive procedure. The mechanisms by which it reduces vertigo are controversial.

   b. **Ablative.** For patients in whom conservative measures have failed, vestibular ablative options may be offered. Intratympanic gentamicin injection offers somewhat selective vestibular toxicity through a less invasive approach, but carries a significant risk of SNHL. Vestibular nerve section offers a high rate of vertigo control with minimal risk to hearing. Labyrinthectomy is a complete vestibular-ablative procedure well suited to patients with nonserviceable hearing.

3. **Results.** Diuretics have been shown to control vertigo and stabilize hearing in 50% to 70% of patients. In addition, the natural history of Meniere's disease allows for spontaneous remission of episodic vertigo in 60% to 80% of patients. For those few with refractory vertigo, intratympanic steroid and endolymphatic sac decompression are effective at controlling vertigo in approximately 80% of patients, while ablative procedures such as intratympanic gentamicin, vestibular neuronectomy, and labyrinthectomy can control vestibular symptoms in greater than 90% of patients.

D. **Perilymphatic fistula.**

1. **Clinical features.** Perilymphatic fistula is a controversial clinical entity. Theoretically it is characterized by the abnormal communication of perilymph between the labyrinth and the middle ear via the oval window, round window, or an aberrant pathway. It may result from barotrauma, penetrating middle-ear trauma, or stapedectomy or may occur spontaneously. The controversy in its diagnosis centers on the difficulty in identifying a microfistula intraoperatively and the lack of clear clinical criteria. It is described most often as vertigo with extreme pressure sensitivity that may be exacerbated by Valsalva maneuver and pneumatic otoscopy. It may also be associated with sudden or gradual hearing loss, thus mimicking Ménière's disease.

2. **Treatments.** Small fistulas may heal spontaneously with a short course of bed rest. In situations with stable hearing or when the clinical diagnosis is questioned, a trial of

vestibular rehabilitation may be attempted. When there is a clear temporal relationship between a predisposing insult (e.g., scuba diving, ear surgery, or penetrating middle ear trauma), surgery in the form of an exploratory tympanotomy may be undertaken to localize and patch the fistula with autogenous connective tissue. Postoperatively, a course of bed rest is undertaken to allow healing of the graft and efforts are made to minimize Valsalva coughing and straining.

3. Results. Bed rest is successful in many patients, and in cases where the fistula is evident, surgery can be very effective. Consideration of an alternate diagnosis such as superior semicircular canal dehiscence syndrome may be necessary in patients who undergo negative exploration.

E. Superior canal dehiscence syndrome.

1. Clinical features. Superior canal dehiscence syndrome (SCDS) is a sound- and pressure-induced vertigo caused by bony dehiscence of the superior semicircular canal. The characteristic torsional vertical nystagmus occurs in the plane of the affected canal with administration of sound and pressure changes. Patient complaints are variable and include autophony, sound-induced (Tullio's phenomenon) or pressure-induced vertigo, conductive hearing loss, and/or pulsatile tinnitus. Clinically, SCDS symptomatology overlaps with perilymphatic fistula and acquired horizontal canal dehiscence from cholesteatoma or chronic otitis media. However, history and physical examination direct clinical suspicion, and high-resolution computed tomography demonstrating superior canal dehiscence is diagnostic.

2. Treatments. Surgical plugging of the affected superior canal can be beneficial in patients with debilitating symptoms because of this disorder.

3. Results. Success rates of surgical plugging of superior canal dehiscence are reported to range from 50% to 90%.

F. Ototoxicity.

1. Clinical features. Ototoxicity may be associated with a number of medications and manifests as hearing loss, tinnitus and/or dizziness, and vertigo. Clinically significant ototoxicity is commonly associated with aminoglycosides and other antibiotics, platinum-based antineoplastic agents, salicylates, quinine, and loop diuretics. The aminoglycoside gentamicin is notably vestibulotoxic, and this property is selectively utilized when intratympanic injections are administered for vestibular ablation as previously mentioned. Cessation of ototoxic agent exposure will halt the continued insult, but recovery is variable and may be incomplete.

2. Treatments. Paramount to treatment is the avoidance of ototoxic medications whenever possible. Active treatment options are limited to vestibular rehabilitation and symptomatic supportive measures while central compensation and adaptation of the vestibulospinal and vestibulocervical reflexes occur.

3. Results. Although these compensatory mechanisms are of value, they are not typically sufficient in restoring complete function. Certainly prevention, if possible, is more effective than treatment in this condition.

G. Tumors involving the vestibulocochlear nerve.

1. Clinical features. Vestibular schwannoma is the most common lesion of the cerebellopontine angle (Fig. 61.2). These benign, slow-growing tumors can occupy the vestibular division of the eighth cranial nerve from the internal auditory canal to the cerebellopontine cistern. As the tumor enlarges, it can cause vestibulocochlear nerve dysfunction both from local compression as well as disruption of blood supply. Tumor progression is typically slow, allowing for contralateral vestibular and central compensation to mask vestibular loss. More commonly, unilateral hearing loss and tinnitus prompt patients to seek care. Advanced tumors may show signs of vestibulopathy and result in life-threatening hydrocephalus and brainstem compression.

2. Treatments. The slow-growing nature of vestibular schwannoma combined with varied clinical presentation requires that treatment options be tailored to each patient. Large tumors require surgical resection. Smaller tumors may be observed, because a certain percentage of tumors are quiescent. Growing tumors less than 2.5 cm may be considered for radiation treatment, which functions to arrest tumor growth in a large portion of patients. Microsurgical resection offers a chance for complete tumor resection with a

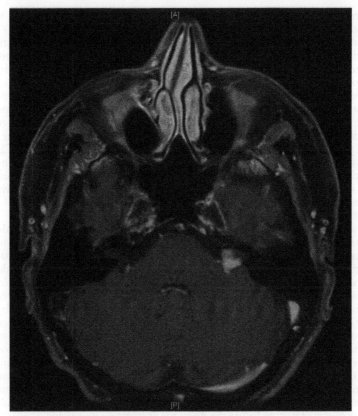

FIGURE 61.2 Left cerebellopontine angle vestibular schwannoma on contrast-enhanced T1-weighted axial MRI.

low rate of recurrence. Patient age, comorbidity, hearing status, and documentation of tumor growth must be considered in treatment planning.

3. **Results.** Success rates in the treatment of vestibular schwannoma must be weighed against the quiescent natural history of some tumors. Radiation therapy tumor control rates are reported to be greater than 95% in some series, although it is unknown what percentage of these tumors were growing. Outcomes for microsurgical control of vestibular schwannomas are comparable to radiotherapy. Hearing preservation is not always possible with surgery and is dependent on tumor size and location. However, hearing tends to decline in all vestibular schwannomas and it tends to decline in observed and radiated tumors at a similar rate, with hearing declining more rapidly in faster-growing tumors.

CENTRAL NEUROLOGIC CAUSES OF VERTIGO

A. Ischemia or infarction.
   1. **Clinical features.** Disruption of vertebrobasilar circulation to the brainstem, cerebellum, and peripheral vestibular system can cause dizziness and vertigo. The hallmark of this ischemia is the association of vertigo with other focal neurologic findings, particularly in a predictable anatomic distribution. Weakness, facial paresthesia, dysarthria, ataxia, diplopia, and visual disturbances are examples of symptoms that may also be present with transient ischemia or infarction of the brainstem. Because transient ischemia may

be responsible for episodic vertigo, it is important to recognize it as such to prevent potential stroke.

2. Treatments. General supportive measures and the use of antiplatelet and anticoagulant medications remain the cornerstones of medical therapy for the management of acute ischemic stroke. More importantly for the clinician evaluating episodic dizziness in the outpatient center is the recognition of signs of transient ischemic attacks (TIAs). Preceding TIAs are a risk factor for atherothrombotic brain infarction and should prompt evaluation of other vascular risk factors such as hypertension, diabetes mellitus, obesity, dyslipidemia, and smoking. Additionally, cardiac evaluation may be warranted in search of possible cardioembolic sources depending on presenting signs. Further discussion on the treatment and prevention of ischemic cerebrovascular disease is discussed elsewhere in **Chapter 40**.

3. Results. Appropriate lifestyle modifications and the addition of antithrombotic (antiplatelets or oral anticoagulants when indicated) therapy are effective in reducing the incidence of stroke and permanent deficit after stroke in at-risk individuals. No therapy is 100% effective.

B. Basilar migraine and migrainous vertigo.

1. Clinical features. Classically described as a condition of adolescent females, basilar migraine (see *ICHD-II*) can affect males and females of any age though it does have a female preponderance. It is characterized by an aura causing hemianopic visual changes, vertigo, ataxia, numbness, or dysarthria followed by a throbbing occipital headache often associated with nausea. Symptoms are self-limited, with the aura lasting from a few minutes to an hour and a headache of variable duration. Basilar migraine is considered a distinct clinical entity from migrainous vertigo, which is characterized by episodic vertigo, but without related neurologic symptoms and in some cases, even without headache. Because it is more difficult to diagnose without the associated symptoms, some question migrainous vertigo as a clinical entity. Diagnosis of migrainous vertigo relies on indirect evidence in the form of relationship of symptoms to migrainous triggers and response to antimigraine medications. In both cases, and particularly with vertibrobasilar migraine, there is overlap between migrainous symptoms and those of more serious cerebrovascular derangement, and a thorough evaluation should rule out other causes of vertigo before the diagnosis of migraine is applied.

2. Treatments. Multiple treatment regimens exist for migraine. Abortive medical therapy is directed at resolving the symptoms shortly after onset. Medications such as ergotamine and the triptans fall into this category. Patients whose symptoms are more frequent may be candidates for preventive medical therapy in the form of beta-blocking agents, tricyclic antidepressants, antiepileptic drugs (AEDs), and calcium-channel blockers. The treatment of migraine is discussed elsewhere in this text.

3. Results. With proper selection of medical therapy, the majority of migraine patients can achieve the goal of symptom prevention.

C. Multiple sclerosis (MS).

1. Clinical features. MS is often diagnosed in young adults. Vertigo can be an associated symptom of CNS dysfunction and may be followed some time later with isolated weakness or visual disturbance. Clinical diagnosis is confirmed with magnetic resonance imaging (MRI) and/or cerebrospinal fluid analysis.

2. Treatments. There are a number of immunomodulating agents used in the treatment of MS. These and other treatments are discussed in more detail elsewhere in Chapter 40.

3. Results. MS is a highly variable disease, and its effects on patients are myriad. Treatments are also varied with inconsistent results. The goal of appropriate therapy is to mitigate the severity of attacks while reducing their frequency.

D. Chiari malformations.

1. Clinical features. Symptoms suggestive of Chiari include headache, vertigo, ataxia, tinnitus, hearing loss, weakness, and numbness. Chiari malformations are often associated with downbeat nystagmus in the primary position.

2. Treatments. Conservative measures consisting of symptomatic control may be appropriate in certain patients. Those with progressive disease may require surgical decompression of the posterior fossa.

3. Results. Surgical decompression often relieves or at least halts the progression of brainstem compressive symptoms.

MEDICAL DIZZINESS

A. Postural hypotension.
  1. Clinical features. Postural hypotension is a classic finding in elderly patients and may result from any number of causes. Symptomatically it is described as lightheaded or presyncopal feeling when standing from sitting or lying. It can result from diminished cardiac output, antihypertensive medication with associated vasodilation or beta-blockade, dehydration, or autonomic insufficiency from underlying diabetic neuropathy, for example.
  2. Treatments. Most important in the treatment of postural hypotension is to recognize it as such. With this in mind, a systematic hemodynamic review must be undertaken. Modification of a current medication regimen is straightforward. Exercise and improved hydration can improve underlying cardiac decompensation, and elastic stockings may be of benefit in optimizing cardiac return.
  3. Results. Proper identification of hemodynamic insufficiency allows treatment modifications where able and is often successful at reducing the severity and frequency of postural hypotension.
B. Arrhythmia.
  1. Clinical features. Symptoms of cardiac arrhythmia frequently include palpitations with or without chest pain. They may be associated with presyncope or even loss of consciousness but are not typically associated with true vertigo. Diagnostic workup includes cardiac monitoring, particularly during an episode, to secure the diagnosis.
  2. Treatments. Cardiology referral is undertaken for evaluation and management of cardiac arrhythmia. Antiarrhythmic medications, pacemakers, and radiofrequency ablation of aberrant pathways of conduction may all be considered in treatment.
  3. Results. Appropriate treatment can be very effective in managing most cardiac arrhythmias.
C. Hypoglycemia.
  1. Clinical features. Metabolic derangements such as insulin-dependent diabetic hypoglycemia may be responsible for dysequilibrium but rarely true vertigo. Episodes of hypoglycemia and dysequilibrium may present acutely in patients who have used insulin for years.
  2. Treatments. Treatment of hypoglycemia is acutely directed at increasing the serum blood glucose level and may require tailoring the diabetic regimen to prevent future episodes.
  3. Results. Targeted treatment along with patient education is usually successful at resolving or decreasing the frequency of symptoms.
D. Medication-associated.
  1. Clinical features. Medications that mediate CNS effects, such as AEDs, benzodiazepines, and psychogenics, may cause primary effects and side effects that create a sensation of dysequilibrium. This dysequilibrium is distinct from postural hypotension that may arise from antihypertensive medications as described above.
  2. Treatments. Treatment is aimed at identifying, limiting, and/or removing the offending medication. Ideally, an alternative medication is found that offers a similar therapeutic profile.
  3. Results. Removing the offending medication will remove the associated symptoms, but as with most medications, treatment effect must be weighed against side-effect profile.
E. Infection.
  1. Clinical features. Infectious labyrinthitis occurring because of a number of viral, bacterial, and fungal agents may cause vertigo. Patient exposures, vaccination history, and associated signs and symptoms help to narrow the differential diagnosis.
  2. Treatments. Identification of the causative infectious agent allows effective treatment with antibiotics, antivirals, or other supportive measures. Administration of mumps, rubella, rubeola, and varicella-zoster vaccines is the best method to prevent viral inner ear infections. Hearing aid and cochlear implantation are audiologic rehabilitation options as well.
  3. Results. Results of treatment largely depend on the infectious etiology.

UNLOCALIZED VERTIGO

A. Psychogenic. Anxiety, depression, and personality disorder are common codiagnoses in patients complaining of dizziness. It is a bidirectional relationship in that severe organic vertigo can cause symptoms of depression and anxiety given the potential unpredictability of attacks. In addition, patients with primary psychiatric diagnoses may also identify dizziness as a complaint, described as an out-of-body experience, a sense of floating, or a racing sensation. It is important not to label a patient with a psychiatric diagnosis as having psychogenic dizziness until organic causes have been ruled out. Treatment should be directed at managing both organic and psychogenic factors simultaneously. SSRI medications and other antidepressants may be valuable in that role.

B. **Malingering.** Unfortunately, there are patients who misrepresent their symptoms for secondary gain. Objective testing, such as posturography, can be used to identify patients who may be falsely complaining of symptoms of dizziness.

C. **Postconcussive.** Concussions may be the result of mild to moderate traumatic brain injury (TBI) resulting in transient neurologic deficit with normal computed tomography imaging of the brain. Nausea, vomiting, headache, and dizziness may present acutely. Focal neurologic deficits typically resolve over weeks to months following mild to moderate TBI, but cognitive, psychological, and emotional dysfunction may persist in more severe injuries. Supportive measures and vestibular rehabilitation are utilized to speed vestibular recovery.

D. **Multifactorial.** Because balance is a multifactorial process maintained through visual, proprioceptive, and vestibular input, decline in one component may be masked through central compensation mechanisms. In some patients, however, particularly the elderly multiply comorbid patient, a decline in balance input may not be met with adequate central compensation and equilibrium will be difficult to reestablish. Peripheral neuropathy, poor vision, and multiple vestibulosuppressant medications are examples of factors contributing to dysequilibrium that should be addressed. Continued walking, with assistance if necessary, is often recommended in an effort to prevent further decompensation.

E. **Unknown.** Although thorough history, physical examination, and judicious ancillary testing are effective in identifying the cause of dizziness in most patients, there remain those few whose symptoms arise from an unidentifiable source. This can be frustrating for both clinician and patient, and requires the clinician to counsel the patient regarding reasonable expectations in achieving a mutually acceptable outcome.

Key Points

- Vertigo is a symptom for which numerous differential diagnoses must be examined. Peripheral vestibular, otologic, and central neurologic disorders as well as medical causes should be considered.
- True vertigo, particularly rotatory vertigo, is often because of a peripheral vestibular (inner ear) disorder.
- BPPV is the most common cause of peripheral vertigo. Repositioning exercises effectively treat the disorder by moving debris from the affected semicircular canal.
- Labyrinthitis and vestibular neuritis cause vertigo that lasts days to weeks. Both disorders are generally attributed to a viral infection.
- Ménière's disease is characterized by the constellation of fluctuating SNHL, tinnitus, and vertigo.
- When prescribing benzodiazepines, antihistamines, and anticholinergics, it is important to remember that a high level of vestibular suppression may reduce central compensation and ultimately hinder recovery.
- Peripheral neuropathy, poor vision, and multiple vestibulosuppressant medications should not be overlooked as factors contributing to disequilibrium.
- Diagnosis of migrainous vertigo is often made when there is a relationship between symptoms and exposure to migraine triggers. Many patients improve with diet changes and/or migraine medications.
- Vertigo associated with focal neurologic findings such as weakness, facial paresthesia, dysarthria, ataxia, diplopia, and/or visual disturbances suggests ischemia and potential for stroke.

Recommended Readings

Amarenco P. The spectrum of cerebellar infarctions. *Neurology.* 1991;41:973–979.

Brandt TH. Phobic postural vertigo. *Neurology.* 1996;46:1515–1519.

Chawla N, Olshaker JS. Diagnosis and management of dizziness and vertigo. *Med Clin North Am.* 2006;96:291–304.

Derebery MJ. The diagnosis and treatment of dizziness. *Med Clin North Am.* 1999;83:163–177.

Hain TC, Yacovino, D. Pharmacologic treatment of persons with dizziness. *Neurol Clin.* 2005;23:831–853.

Headache Classification Subcommittee of the International Headache Society. The International Classification of Headache Disorders: 2nd ed. *Cephalalgia.* 2004;24(suppl 1):9–160.

Lynn S, Pool A, Rose D, et al. Randomized trial of the canalith repositioning procedure. *Otolaryngol Head Neck Surg.* 1995;113:712–720.

Minor LB. Superior canal dehiscence syndrome. *Am J Otol.* 2000;21:9–19.

Radtke A, Von Brevern M, Tiel-Wilck K, et al. Self-treatment of benign paroxysmal positional vertigo: Semont maneuver vs Epley procedure. *Neurology.* 2004;63:150–152.

Solomon D. Distinguishing and treating causes of central vertigo. *Otolaryngol Clin North Am.* 2000;33(3):579–601.

Stangerup SE, Caye-Thomasen P, Tos M, et al. Change in hearing during 'wait and scan' management of patients with vestibular schwannoma. *J Laryngol Otol.* 2008;122(07):673–681.

Troost BT. Dizziness and vertigo. In: Bradley WG, Daroff RB, Fenichel GM, eds. *Neurology in Clinical Practice.* 4th ed. Boston, MA: Butterworth-Heineman; 2004:chap 18.

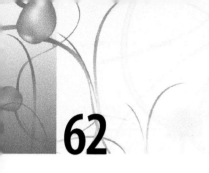

62

Neurologic Diseases in Pregnancy

Kathleen B. Digre and Michael W. Varner

In the United States, there are 4,000,000 live births per year. It is thus common to see neurologic conditions occur in association with pregnancy. Furthermore, the physiologic changes in pregnancy can mimic neurologic diseases and can affect the severity of neurologic signs and symptoms. Not only can neurologic conditions be affected by pregnancy, but also treatment frequently must be altered to accommodate a developing fetus. Finally, pregnancy-specific conditions can present with neurologic symptoms and signs. As unintended pregnancies occur frequently, every woman seen with neurologic conditions should be considered to have a prepregnancy visit with adequate counseling and excellent control of the condition before pregnancy. In general, optimum care of the mother will result in the best result for the baby (Video 62.1).

NORMAL PHYSIOLOGIC CHANGES IN PREGNANCY

A. Cardiovascular.
   1. Increase of 30% to 50% in cardiac output and blood volume with singleton pregnancy (70% with twins)
   2. Midpregnancy decrease in blood pressure by 5 to 10 mm Hg systolic and 10 to 15 mm Hg diastolic.
B. Pulmonary.
   1. Increase of 20% to 30% in minute volume.
   2. Increase in respiratory rate and partially compensated respiratory alkalosis.
C. Renal.
   1. Increase of 30% to 50% in renal blood flow.
   2. Decreased serum level of blood urea nitrogen and creatinine (because of increased renal clearance). Serum creatinine in mid-late pregnancy should be <1.0 mg%.
D. Gastrointestinal.
   1. Decreased motility as a result of progesterone-mediated decreases in smooth muscle activity.
   2. Elevated alkaline phosphatase level (placental). No pregnancy-associated changes in any other liver function tests.
   3. Increased cytochrome P-450 activity.
E. Hematologic.
   1. Decreased hematocrit (20% to 30% increase in red blood cell (RBC) volume, but 30% to 50% increase in blood volume).
   2. Increased white blood cell count; decreased platelet count.
F. Coagulation factors.
   1. Increased levels of plasminogen, fibrinogen, and factors VII, VIII, IX, and X.
   2. No change in factor V, antithrombin, or platelet adhesion.
   3. Thrombophilias (e.g., antiphospholipid antibodies, protein C and S deficiency, factor V Leiden) are more likely to produce thromboembolic complications.
G. Connective tissue. Thickening and fragmentation of reticular fibers with mild hyperplasia of smooth muscle cells.
H. Hormonal changes. Progressive increase in estrogens and progesterone until delivery.
I. Serum osmolality. Decreases from early in gestation, with resultant increase in extracellular fluid volume.

TABLE 62.1 Evaluating Neurologic Conditions in Pregnancy

Test	Risk to Mother	Risk to Fetus	Contraindications
MRI	None	None known	Metal, cardiac pacemaker, and otologic implant
MRI with gadolinium	None	None known	Same as above (risk category C)
CT	None	Minimal[a]	None
CT with contrast	None	Minimal[a]	Allergy to contrast medium
Angiography	Minimal in most	Minimal[a]	Allergy to contrast medium
LP	None	None	Incipient herniation or mass lesion
Ultrasonography	None	None	None
EEG	None	None	None
NCS/EMG	None	None	None
Tensilon test	Minimal	Minimal	Heart failure
Visual fields	None	None	None
Dilated eye examination	None	None with punctal occlusion	Incipient glaucoma
Fluorescein angiography	None	Minimal	Allergies, FDA risk category C

[a]Abdominal shielding.
Abbreviations: CT, computed tomography; EEG, electroencephalography; EMG, electromyography; FDA, Food and Drug Administration; LP, lumbar puncture; MRI, magnetic resonance imaging; NCS, nerve conduction studies.

J. **Neurologic.** Increase in pituitary size; slight decrease in brain volume that returns to baseline postpartum.
K. Evaluating neurologic conditions in pregnancy (Table 62.1).
L. US Food and Drug Administration (FDA) risk factor classification of drugs in pregnancy.
   1. **Class A.** Controlled studies show no risk to fetus in the first trimester; fetal harm is remote.
   2. **Class B.** No controlled studies have been completed, but there are no known risks.
   3. **Class C.** Studies on animals may show effects on fetuses, but no results of controlled studies are available. The drug can be used if the risk is justified.
   4. **Class D.** There are risks, but the drug may be used if serious disease or life-threatening conditions exist.
   5. **Class X.** Human and animal studies show risk. The risk of use outweighs any benefit.

SEIZURE DISORDERS IN PREGNANCY

A. **Frequency.** One percent of the population, about 500,000 women of childbearing age.
   1. In an unselected population, frequency is 7 to 8 per 1,000 deliveries. This is about 25,000 deliveries per year, or approximately one every 20 minutes.
   2. Some antiepileptic drugs (AEDs), particularly phenobarbital, phenytoin, and carbamazepine, lower the efficacy of some oral contraceptives in some individuals, making pregnancy more likely.
B. **Heredity.**
   1. About 2% to 5% of women have genetic susceptibility probability of vertical transmission if either parent has idiopathic epilepsy. Relatively higher if the parent is the mother; relatively lower if the parent is the father.
   2. No significant transmission if disease is acquired.
C. **Course of disease in pregnancy.**
   1. The best figures for disease activity during pregnancy include the following:
      a. Improved, 22%
      b. Exacerbated, 24% (most likely to occur in the first trimester)
      c. No change, 54%

2. Postulated mechanisms for changes in frequency during pregnancy include the following:
   a. Physiologic
      (1) Hormonal (estrogens decrease and progestins increase seizure threshold)
      (2) Metabolic (increased cytochrome P-450 activity)
   b. Sleep deprivation
   c. Noncompliance (e.g., fear of birth defects from taking medications)
   d. Pharmacokinetic changes in drug levels caused by: impaired absorption, increased volume of distribution, decreased albumin concentration, reduced plasma protein binding, and increased drug clearance
   e. Folate supplementation can reduce anticonvulsant levels
   f. Stress and anxiety decrease seizure threshold, making seizures more likely.
   g. Alcohol or other drug use makes seizures more likely.
3. Seizure frequency during pregnancy does not correlate with maternal age, seizure type, drug regimen, and seizure frequency in previous pregnancies.
4. Fetal risks with generalized convulsive seizure include the following:
   a. Physical injury from maternal abdominal trauma
   b. Hypoxic–ischemic injury because of maternal hypoxia

D. Therapeutic options.
   1. Pharmacologic.
      a. Be certain of the diagnosis, especially with new-onset seizures in pregnancy.
      b. Be familiar with and use the few drugs that are the most effective for the various types of seizures.
   2. **Surgery** in general should be addressed before or after pregnancy.
   3. General.
      a. Maintain good daily habits (regularly scheduled meals, adequate sleep, and minimize stress).
      b. Avoid alcohol and sedatives.
      c. Avoid hazardous situations.
      d. Avoid ketogenic diet.

E. Drug dosages, plasma levels, and clinical management.
   1. AED levels decline during pregnancy in almost all women. This does not necessarily equate with a need to increase dosage, unless seizures are not controlled.
      a. Free (non–protein-bound) drug level equates best with clinical status (seizure control and side effects) and should be obtained in pregnancies complicated by persistent or recurrent seizures or side effects.
      b. Total drug level (the usual laboratory result) sufficient if the patient has good clinical control.
      c. With the exception of valproic acid, the average decline in free levels is less than that for total levels.
   2. Frequency of measurement of levels.
      a. Ideally, preconceptional total and free levels should be obtained and optimized.
      b. Obtain non–protein-bound (free) levels every trimester (every 3 months), and again 4 weeks before term when seizure types do not interfere with activities of daily living and the epilepsy is well controlled.
      c. Obtain monthly free levels when uncontrolled seizures interfere with activities of daily living during the year before conception, previously controlled seizures recur during pregnancy, seizures are controlled but total drug levels decrease >50% on routine screens, troublesome or disabling side effects develop, and lack of compliance is suspected or confirmed.
      d. Always check levels postpartum and adjust dosage because levels often increase as the physiologic effects of pregnancy resolve within 10 to 15 days after delivery.
   3. Changing drug dosage.
      a. Reasons not to change dosage.
         (1) Total drug levels are declining in a woman with well-controlled seizures, unless there are >30% decline in free levels and a history of poor control.
         (2) A woman taking two or more AEDs discovers that she is pregnant (the time to change to monotherapy is before conception).

    b. **Reasons to change dosage.**
        (1) Increased numbers of tonic–clonic seizures
        (2) Complex partial or other seizure types that interfere with activities of daily life and the patient wants better control
        (3) Troublesome or disabling side effects
    c. Discontinuation of AED therapy should ideally be accomplished before conception but can be considered cautiously during pregnancy if a patient has been seizure-free for more than 2 years, has normal findings on neurologic examination, normal electroencephalographic findings, no structural brain disorder, and no history of prolonged convulsive seizures
4. AEDs used in pregnancy (Table 62.2); breast-feeding while taking AEDs does not appear to affect cognition.
5. Other drugs to add or consider for patients with epilepsy
    a. **Folic acid.**
        (1) Requirements may be further increased because of malabsorption, competitive metabolism, and increased hepatic metabolism.
        (2) Increased supplementation may precipitate seizures by lowering anticonvulsant levels.
        (3) Best advice is to maintain usual supplementation.
        (4) Compelling evidence links the folic acid antagonism properties of AEDs to relatively increased risk of fetal neural tube defects in women taking anticonvulsants during the first trimester (neural tube defects form, or do not form, 26 to 28 days after conception). *Women of reproductive potential should take continuous folic acid supplementation (400 mg/day) whether or not they are considering pregnancy.*
    b. Vitamin K should be administered (10 mg by mouth daily) to all pregnant women receiving AEDs beginning 4 weeks before expected delivery until birth to minimize the risk of neonatal hemorrhage. If a woman has not received vitamin K before delivery, consideration should be given to parenteral vitamin K administration.
    c. Vitamin D is not routinely supplemented.
6. Birth defects in infants of epileptic mothers
    a. Major birth defects in healthy pregnant women = 2% to 3%. In epileptic women on monotherapy = 3.2% to 7.8%. In epileptic women on polytherapy = 6.0% to 9.3%.
    b. Should be discussed with all epileptic women of reproductive age, irrespective of whether or not they are planning pregnancy (50% of pregnancies are unplanned)
    c. Other factors that may explain the increased incidence of anomalies in infants of epileptic mothers are as follows:
        (1) Increased incidence of anomalies in infants of epileptic mothers not taking AEDs. The only anomalies that are more common in phenytoin-exposed fetuses are hypertelorism and digital hypoplasia.
        (2) Increased incidence of characteristic malformations in infants of epileptic fathers, described as being intermediate between treated and untreated epileptic mothers
        (3) A specific metabolic defect (epoxide hydrolase deficiency) more common in persons with epilepsy may predispose to damage in some cases. Autosomal codominant and increased fetal anomalies
        (4) Epilepsy may represent an underlying genetic disease.
        (5) The defects may result from an AED-mediated relative folate deficiency. (Folate antagonists are known abortifacients and teratogens; see discussion above.)
7. **AED teratogenesis** should be discussed with all women with epilepsy of reproductive age, particularly because up to half of all pregnancies are unplanned.
    a. Fetal anticonvulsant syndrome occurs in 3% to 5% of epileptic women and can occur in association with use of any anticonvulsant medication. The relative risk is dose dependent. This syndrome is being seen with decreasing frequency as fewer women receive polytherapy and more receive monotherapy.
        (1) Craniofacial (cleft lip and palate) and digital dysmorphic changes
        (2) Growth deficiency
        (3) Microcephaly
        (4) Cardiac defects
        (5) Intellectual disability

TABLE 62.2 Medications Used in Epilepsy

Drug	Indication	Dosage	FDA Category	Side Effects	Breast-feeding[a]
Phenobarbital	Generalized seizures	1–2 mg/kg/d; 90–120 mg/d	D	Sedation	Potential toxicity
Phenytoin	Generalized seizures	4–5 mg/kg/d; 300–600 mg/d	D	Gingival hyperplasia and hirsutism	Compatible
Fosphenytoin	Status epilepticus	Maximum 100–150 mg	D	Infant risk possible PE/min IV	Compatible
Primidone	Generalized and partial complex seizures	500–2,000 mg/d in two or three divided doses	D	Fatigue, depression, nausea; folate deficiency	Potential toxicity
Carbamazepine	Generalized and, partial complex seizures	10–30 mg/kg/d divided t.i.d. or q.i.d.; maximum 1,600 mg/d	D	Diplopia, dizziness, neural tube defect headache, nausea	Compatible
Oxcarbazepine	Partial complex seizures	Initial: 600 mg/d divided b.i.d. Maintenance: 1,200 mg/d divided b.i.d.	C	Hyponatremia, rash	Probably compatible
Valproic acid, sodium valproate	Generalized and myoclonic seizures	15–60 mg/kg/d	D	1% neural tube defect	Compatible
Valproate IV	Status epilepticus, difficult to control	Loading dose of 20 mg/kg in 100 mL NS over 1 hr Maintenance: 15 mg/kg a day divided t.i.d.	D	Thrombocytopenia, injection-site erythema	Compatible seizures
Divalproex	Generalized seizure	15–60 mg/kg/d	X	Contraindicated in pregnancy	Compatible
Lamotrigine	Generalized seizures Adjunctive therapy	Starting dose: 25 mg b.i.d. slow start Maximum: 500 mg for partial seizures	C	Insomnia or drowsiness, rash, and nausea	Potential toxicity
Ethosuximide	Absence seizures	500–1,500 mg/d given as 1 or 2 doses	D	Nausea, vomiting, anorexia, agitation, and headache	Probably compatible
Felbamate	Partial onset with secondary generalization Mostly used in Lennox–Gastaut syndrome	300–400 mg t.i.d.	C	Aplastic anemia and liver failure	Potential toxicity
Gabapentin	Adjunctive for partial seizures	300–600 mg t.i.d.	C	Fatigue	Probably compatible
Pregabalin	Adjunct for partial seizures	75–150 mg divided dosage	C	Fatigue	Infant risk cannot be ruled out

Drug	Indication	Dosage	FDA Category	Side Effects	Breast-feeding[a]
Tiagabine	Partial and tonic–clonic seizures	30–50 mg/d divided doses	C	Dizziness and sedation	Probably compatible
Topiramate	Adjunctive, partial, and tonic–clonic seizures	12.5–25 mg/d with gradual increase to 6 mg/kg or 400 mg/d	D	Mental dullness, renal calculi; cleft palate	Potential toxicity
Zonisamide	Partial, generalized, or myoclonic seizures	Initial: 100–200 mg/d Maintenance: 400–800 mg/d divided b.i.d.	C	Hypersensitivity reaction and nephrolithiasis	Potential toxicity Probably compatible
Levetiracetam	Partial or generalized seizures	Initial: 1,000 mg/d divided b.i.d. Maintenance: 1,000–3,000 mg/d divided b.i.d.	C	Fatigue and weakness	Probably compatible
Trimethadione	Absence seizures	300–600 mg q.i.d.–t.i.d. (adult dosage)	X first trimester; D thereafter	Rash, sore throat, fever, drowsiness, fatigue, sunlight sensitivity	Probably compatible
Vigabratin	Adjunctive in treatment-resistant epilepsy, and refractory complex partial seizures	500 mg b.i.d.	C (D in Australia)	Watch vision; restricted use because of retinal toxicity	Possibly compatible
Lacosamide	Adjunctive in treatment of partial seizures	50 mg b.i.d. (Max dose 400 mg daily)	C	Blurred vision, imbalance, mood or behavioral changes, suicidal thoughts, syncope	Unknown
Perampanel	Adjunct partial and generalized seizures	8–12 mg bed time	C	Behavioral disorders and changes in mood, behavior or personality	Cannot rule out risk
Retigabine	Adjunct to partial seizures	100 mg three times daily	C	Retinal abnormalities and visual loss	Cannot rule out risk
Clobazam	Adjunct treatment Lennox–Gastaut seizure	10 mg initially and titrate slowly up to 20 mg divided doses	C	Somnolence	Compatible
Clonazepam, diazepam, lorazepam	Status epilepticus, adjunct	Check dosing for adults	D	Somnolence	Potential toxicity
Eslicarbazepine acetate	Partial seizure monotherapy or adjunct	400–800 mg	C		Cannot rule out risk

(continued)

TABLE 62.2 Medications Used in Epilepsy (*continued*)

Drug	Indication	Dosage	FDA Category	Side Effects	Breast-feeding[a]
Ezogabine	Partial seizures	100 mg initially maintenance 200–400 mg three times daily	C	Pigmentary changes in retina with long-term use, prolongation of QT interval; skin discoloration	Cannot rule out risk
Rufinamide	Lennox–Gastaut	400–800 mg	C	Can prolong QT interval	Risk cannot be ruled out

[a]Watch how infant does in all cases.
Abbreviations: b.i.d., twice a day; FDA, Food and Drug Administration; NS, normal saline solution; PE, pulmonary embolism; q.i.d., four times a day; t.i.d., three times a day.
Briggs GG, Freeman RK, Yaffe SJ. *Drugs in Pregnancy and Lactation*. 10th ed. Baltimore, MD: Lippincott Williams & Wilkins; 2015.
Micromedex 2.0, (electronic version). Greenwood Village, CO: Truven Health Analytics. Also available at: http://www.micromedexsolutions.com/. Accessed September 16, 2015.

    b. AEDs and neural tube defects.
       (1) Risk is 1% to 2% for valproic acid and slightly less for carbamazepine. It is <1% for other anticonvulsants. However, these risks are >0.1% population-wide risk in the United States.
       (2) The relative risk is dose related.
       (3) If the medications are necessary for seizure control, the patient should be offered maternal serum α-fetoprotein and ultrasound screening.
    c. Trimethadione is clearly teratogenic and is contraindicated in pregnancy.
  8. Breast-feeding.
    a. Most AEDs cross into breast milk, although at low levels; the higher the protein binding of the AED, the less that is passed into breast milk. Recent studies show no cognitive change in babies breast fed while mother takes AED.
    b. **Contraindications** to breast-feeding include poorly controlled maternal seizures and rapid somnolence on the part of an initially hungry infant, which suggests a drug effect.
F. Onset of seizures during pregnancy: differential diagnosis.
  1. Rule out eclampsia. The most common multisystem disease in late pregnancy is preeclampsia or eclampsia.
  2. **Cortical venous thrombosis,** especially late in pregnancy and in the immediate puerperium.
  3. **Tumors** are especially likely to manifest in the first trimester because this is when the pregnancy-associated increase in extracellular fluid begins. Meningioma tends to expand during pregnancy (response to the progressive increases in estrogen and progesterone).
  4. Intracranial hemorrhage.
  5. **Gestational epilepsy** is a diagnosis of exclusion and represents only a small fraction of all women who have initial seizures while pregnant.
  6. Drugs or toxins
G. Status epilepticus during pregnancy (follow guidelines for nonpregnant patients).
  1. Less than 1% of all pregnant epileptic women
  2. Not an indication for termination of pregnancy
  3. Management should follow standard treatment of status epilepticus. Hospitalize, securing the airway, intravenous (IV) access for normal saline solution and B vitamins, baseline laboratory studies including electrolytes, complete blood count, glucose, calcium, and arterial blood gases. Maternal and fetal vital signs, including electrocardiography (ECG) and fetal heart rate monitoring. In addition, administer the following:
    a. Glucose bolus (50 mL of D50)

b. Thiamine (100 mg intramuscularly or intravenously)

c. Begin lorazepam (0.1 mg/kg IV, not to exceed 2 mg/minute) or diazepam (5 to 15 mg IV in 5 mg boluses) and fosphenytoin (150 mg/minute) or phenytoin (10 to 20 mg/kg IV, not to exceed 50 mg/minute, with ECG and blood pressure monitoring, administered in non-glucose-containing fluids).

d. If seizures persist, intubate and begin either phenobarbital (20 to 25 mg/kg IV, not to exceed 100 mg/minute). Alternatives include midazolam, propofol, levetiracetam, or IV valproic acid (if absolutely necessary).

e. If seizures still persist, institute general anesthesia with halothane and neuromuscular junction blockade. (See Chapters 42 and 43.)

HEADACHE

A. The most common headache diagnoses are as follows:

1. **Migraine** (with or without aura) occurs in 10% to 20% of women of childbearing age. Unilateral or bilateral throbbing headaches associated with photophobia, phonophobia, nausea, or vomiting may be exacerbated by activity.

2. **Tension-type headache** is very common. Mild-moderate headache, without nausea and vomiting, may be relieved by activity.

B. Genetics of migraine. Migraine is more common in affected families. Hemiplegic migraine is autosomal dominant associated with three different gene loci affecting ionic channels; however, there are multiple polymorphisms associated with migraine.

C. Course of migraine in pregnancy.

1. The condition of most women with migraine improves when they are pregnant. This is especially true with menstrual migraine and migraine whose onset was at menarche. If migraines do not improve after the first trimester, it is likely to continue.

2. About 10% to 20% of headaches worsen or have the initial onset during pregnancy, usually in the first trimester. Many of these may be migraine aura without headache.

3. Migraineurs have no increased risk of complications during pregnancy, but headaches usually recur near term and in the puerperium.

4. Multiparous migraineurs may have an increase in headaches in the third trimester, whereas nulliparous women report less headache activity in pregnancy and the puerperium.

D. The **differential diagnosis** of headache or migraine occurring for the first time in pregnancy includes the following:

1. Severe preeclampsia/eclampsia—headache with hypertension should bring this diagnosis to the forefront.

2. Reversible cerebral vasoconstriction syndrome (RCVS)

3. Cerebral venous thrombosis

4. Stroke (carotid or vertebral artery dissection)

5. Intracranial hypertension [increased intracranial pressure (ICP)] or intracranial hypotension or hypovolemia

6. Intracranial hemorrhage

7. Brain tumor

8. Thrombocytopenia

E. Therapeutic options.

1. Nonmedication treatment.

   a. Adequate sleep, fluids, regular meals, and exercise

   b. Avoidance of dietary and environmental trigger factors

   c. Biofeedback, relaxation therapy, mindfulness, massage, physical therapy, and heat or ice packs

2. Acute medication treatment principles.

   a. Prevention of nausea (Table 62.3)

   b. Management of pain (Table 62.4)

   c. Sedation (Table 62.5)

3. Prophylactic treatment. In general, avoid daily medication for headaches, but if headaches are too severe or interfere excessively with life, daily treatment may be needed. In general, monotherapy should be attempted. The lowest dosage should be encouraged (Table 62.6).

TABLE 62.3 Acute Migraine Treatment in Pregnancy: Nausea Prevention

Drug	Dosage (mg)	FDA Schedule	Side Effects	Breast-feeding[a]
Promethazine	25–75 P.O., P.R.	C: trimester I B: trimester 2, 3	–	Probably compatible
Hydroxyzine	25–75 P.O., IM	C	Fatigue	Probably compatible
Prochlorperazine	10–25 P.O., P.R., IM, IV	C	Dystonic reaction	Potential toxicity
Trimethobenzamide	200–250 P.O., P.R.	C	–	Potential toxicity
Chlorpromazine	25 P.O., P.R., IM, IV	C	Dystonic reaction	Potential toxicity
Metoclopramide	5–10 IM, IV	B	Dystonic reaction	Probably compatible
Ondansetron	4 P.O., IV	B		Probably compatible

[a]Watch how infant does.
Abbreviations: FDA, Food and Drug Administration; IM, intramuscular; P.O., orally; P.R., rectally.
Source for classification, Briggs GG, Freeman RK, Yaffe SJ. *Drugs in Pregnancy and Lactation.* 10th ed. Baltimore, MD: Lippincott Williams & Wilkins; 2015.

TUMORS

A. Incidence.
 1. Probably 100 primary brain tumors per year nationwide
 2. Pregnancy does not increase the risk of brain tumors but does increase the likelihood of symptoms, primarily because of the decrease in serum osmolality.
 3. The types of tumors are identical to those observed in nonpregnant women of the same age, primarily glioma (32%), meningioma (29%), acoustic neuroma (15%), and others (24%).
 4. Metastatic tumors are relatively more common, with lung, breast, and gastrointestinal tract being the most common primary sites.
B. **Clinical features** include headache, nausea and vomiting, papilledema, focal deficits, or seizures.
C. **Diagnosis** is made by imaging: magnetic resonance imaging (MRI) with contrast enhancement (gadolinium) or computed tomography (CT) with contrast enhancement (Table 62.1).
D. Treatment.
 1. Surgery is the treatment of choice for most lesions. If the woman is clinically stable, meningiomas and low-grade malignant gliomas can be managed expectantly until after delivery. However, malignant tumors should be resected promptly.
 2. Dexamethasone (risk factor C)
  a. Dosage: 6 mg every 6 hours or 4 mg every 4 hours
  b. Problems: gastrointestinal; Cushingoid changes with prolonged use
 3. Mannitol (risk factor C) for acute brain swelling
E. Pituitary tumors.
 1. Course of disease.
  a. **Microadenoma** is rarely symptomatic (5%).
  b. **Macroadenoma** is symptomatic in 15% to 35% of cases.
 2. Serial **visual field evaluation** must be performed for macroadenoma.
 3. Treatment.
  a. Bromocriptine (risk factor B) or Cabergoline (risk factor B) may be taken throughout pregnancy if the tumor enlarges. (Caution is advised in breast-feeding.)
  b. If vision is threatened, surgical treatment is appropriate.

TABLE 62.4 Acute Migraine Treatment in Pregnancy: Pain Treatment

Drug	Dosage (mg)	FDA Schedule	Side Effects	Breast-feeding
Acetaminophen	350–500	B	–	Compatible
Aspirin	81 mg	C	Bleeding, diathesis, in utero closure of ductus arteriosus, oligohydramnios Risk first and third trimesters	Potential toxicity
Caffeine		B	–	Potential toxicity
Butalbital compounds		C	Possible neonatal withdrawal with heavy use	Potential toxicity
Isometheptene	Two at onset, then 1/hr to max 5/24 hr	C		Probably compatible
NSAIDs[a]				
Ibuprofen	200–800	B	Bleeding diathesis, oligohydramnios, in utero closure of ductus arteriosus	Compatible
Naproxen	200–500	B	Bleeding diathesis, oligohydramnios, closure of ductus arteriosus	Probably compatible
Ketorolac	Oral/IV	C		Probably compatible
Triptans				
Sumatriptan	25–100 P.O. 20 n.s. 4–6 s.c.	C	Contraindicated in coronary artery disease	Probably compatible
Zolmitriptan	2.5–5 P.O.	C	Contraindicated in coronary artery disease	Probably compatible
Naratriptan	1.25–2.5 P.O.	C	Contraindicated in coronary artery disease	Probably compatible
Rizatriptan	10 P.O.	C	Contraindicated in coronary artery disease	Probably compatible
Eletriptan	20–40	C	Contraindicated in coronary artery disease	Probably compatible
Almotriptan	12.5	C	Contraindicated in coronary artery disease	Probably compatible
Frovatriptan	2.5	C	Contraindicated in coronary artery disease	Probably compatible
Narcotic (use with antiemetic)				
Butorphanol	–	C	Respiratory depression, nausea	Probably compatible
Meperidine	50–100	B	Respiratory depression, nausea	Compatible
Ergotamine	Avoid	X	Possible abortifacient	Contraindicated

[a]Use in pregnancy should be restricted to <48 hr (>48 hr of consecutive therapy is associated with progressive risk of in utero closure of the ductus arteriosis, renal damage, and platelet dysfunction).
Abbreviations: NSAIDs, nonsteroidal anti-inflammatory drugs; n.s., nasal spray; P.O., orally; s.c., subcutaneously.
Source for FDA rating: Briggs GG, Freeman RK, Yaffe SJ. Drugs in Pregnancy and Lactation. 10th ed. Baltimore, MD: Lippincott Williams & Wilkins; 2015.

4. **Sheehan's syndrome** is pituitary infarction, frequently associated with tumor, placental abruption, or other causes of hemorrhagic shock.
   a. Manifests as inability to lactate, hypopituitarism, and hypothyroidism
   b. Treatment involves steroid and thyroid replacement.

TABLE 62.5 Acute Migraine Treatment in Pregnancy: Sedation

Drug	Dose	FDA Schedule	Side Effects	Breast-feeding[a]
Chloral hydrate	500–1,500	C	–	Probably compatible
Pentobarbital	–	D	Withdrawal	Potential toxicity
Hydroxyzine	25–75	C	–	Probably compatible
Meperidine (plus antiemetic)		B	–	Probably compatible
Diazepam	5–10	D	Lethargy	Potential toxicity
Lorazepam	–	D		Potential toxicity
Clonazepam	0.5–1.0	C–D	–	Potential toxicity
Chlorpromazine	25–50	C	Dystonic reaction; decreased pressure	Potential toxicity

[a]Watch infant.
Abbreviation: FDA, Food and Drug Administration.
Briggs GG, Freeman RK, Yaffe SJ. *Drugs in Pregnancy and Lactation*. 10th ed. Baltimore, MD: Lippincott Williams & Wilkins; 2015.

TABLE 62.6 Migraine Prophylaxis in Pregnancy

Drug	Dosage	FDA Schedule	Side Effects	Breast-feeding[a]
β-Blockers				
Propranolol	20–80	C	Possible IUGR[b], hypotension prematurity	Compatible
Nadolol	10–40	C	Possible IUGR	Compatible
Timolol	10–30	C	Possible IUGR	Compatible
Tricyclic antidepressants				
Amitriptyline in pregnancy	10–75	C	Limb deformities	Potential toxicity
Nortriptyline	10–75	C	–	Potential toxicity
Imipramine	10–75	D	–	Potential toxicity
Desipramine	10–75	C	–	Potential toxicity
Cyproheptadine	4 mg	B	Weight gain	Probably compatible
Calcium-channel blockers				
Verapamil	80–240	C	Constipation	Probably compatible
Nifedipine	10–30	C	Decreased blood pressure	Probably compatible
Amlodipine	2.5–5	C	–	Probably compatible
Anticonvulsant				
Gabapentin	100–300	C	Fatigue	Probably compatible
Topiramate	50–100 mg	D	Acidosis, weight loss; cleft palate	Potential toxicity
Valproate	500–1,000 mg	D	Weight gain, hair loss, neural tube defects	Potential toxicity
Other				
Onabotulinum toxin	As directed for chronic migraine	C	None known	Probably compatible
Magnesium	Up to 1 g daily	B	Diarrhea; used for women with preeclampsia	Probably compatible

[a]Watch infant.
[b]Contraindicated drugs: methysergide, valproic acid.
Abbreviations: FDA, Food and Drug Administration; IUGR, intrauterine growth retardation.

5. **Lymphocytic hypophysitis** mimics pituitary adenoma and suprasellar masses because it manifests as endocrinologic abnormalities, headaches, and a suprasellar mass at imaging. Lymphocytic hypophysitis occurs in pregnant and postpartum women. Biopsy is often needed to make the diagnosis. Steroid treatment with dexamethasone (category C) is often helpful.

PSEUDOTUMOR CEREBRI

Pseudotumor cerebri (idiopathic intracranial hypertension) is characterized by increased ICP not caused by an intracranial space-occupying lesion demonstrated at MRI or CT. Pregnancy does not cause pseudotumor cerebri. However, this disorder can occur in association with pregnancy. Pregnancy does not by itself cause visual loss. Pseudotumor cerebri does not cause miscarriage.

A. **Symptoms and signs.** Headache is the most common symptom (>90% of cases). Patients are otherwise alert and healthy. There are visual symptoms (transient visual obscurations) and auditory symptoms (whooshing noises). Signs include papilledema in almost all cases, and cranial nerve VI palsy. Most women are obese.

B. **Differential diagnosis of papilledema and no mass lesion in pregnancy.**
   1. Cerebral venous thrombosis (most important; most frequently needs to be excluded)
   2. Venous hypertension
   3. Meningitis
   4. Syphilis

C. **Evaluation** must include an imaging procedure (MRI and MR venography), cerebrospinal fluid (CSF) with opening pressure, and CSF constituents. Because the greatest threat to the patient is visual loss, visual acuity and visual field examinations must be performed frequently.

D. **Treatment options.**
   1. **Medical treatment.**
      a. Weight loss (restriction of weight gain is better than substantial weight loss)
      b. Frequent lumbar punctures (LPs)
         (1) Safe
         (2) Painful, often difficult
      c. Acetazolamide (500 to 2,000 mg) (risk C); can be continued in pregnancy; compatible with breast-feeding
      d. Furosemide (Lasix; Aventis, Bridgewater, NJ, USA) (risk C)
      e. Chlorthalidone (risk B); compatible with breast-feeding
   2. **Surgical treatment.**
      a. Optic nerve sheath decompression is the preferred procedure to save vision.
      b. Lumbar and ventriculo-peritoneal shunts can be difficult for pregnant patients because of displacement/compression from the enlarging uterus.

CEREBROVASCULAR DISEASE

A. Attributable risk of ischemic stroke or intracerebral hemorrhage in pregnancy or the puerperium is 8.1/100,000 pregnancies. The causes of stroke during pregnancy are listed in Table 62.7.
   1. Arterial stroke manifests as paresis but without altered consciousness or seizures; represents 90% of strokes *during pregnancy*.
   2. **Venous stroke** manifests as headache, seizures, increased ICP, and alteration of consciousness; represents 80% of strokes *during puerperium*.
   3. **Intracranial hemorrhage** characteristically manifests as sudden onset of headache, loss of consciousness, and accompanying neck stiffness and altered blood pressure.
   4. **Diagnosis.**
      a. CT and MRI (newer techniques of diffusion and perfusion may show early injury). Diffusion-weighted MR imaging and CT perfusion is very helpful.
      b. Angiography occasionally required (including CT angio, MR angio)
      c. Cardiac evaluation (transesophageal echocardiography—look also for right to left shunt)
      d. Appropriate laboratory studies. The factor V Leiden mutation is now thought to be associated with at least one half of all cases of venous thromboses among white

TABLE 62.7 Causes of Stroke in Pregnancy

Arterial occlusive disease
Thrombotic cause
  Atherosclerotic
  Cervicocephalic FMD
  Cervicocephalic arterial dissections
Embolic source
  Cardiac
    Peripartum cardiomyopathy
    Mitral valve prolapse
    Rheumatic heart disease
    Endocarditis (infective and nonbacterial)
    Paradoxical embolism
    Atrial fibrillation
    Amniotic or air embolism
Venous occlusive disease
  Infection
Drugs that can induce stroke
  Illicit drugs: cocaine, methamphetamine
  Other drugs: sympathomimetics: phenylpropanolamine; ergotamine, bromocriptine, isometheptene
Hypotensive disorders
  Watershed infarction
  Sheehan's pituitary necrosis
Hematologic disorders
  Lupus anticoagulant, Sneddon's syndrome
  Thrombotic thrombocytopenic purpura
  Sickle cell disease
  Antithrombin deficiency, protein C and protein S deficiencies
  Hyperhomocysteinemia
  Factor V Leiden mutation
  Prothrombin G20210A mutation
  MTHFR mutation
Arteritis and angiopathy
  SLE
  Infectious arteritis (syphilis, tuberculosis, meningococcal)
  Cerebral angiitis
  Takayasu's arteritis
  Postpartum cerebral angiopathy
  Cervicocephalic FMD and dissections
Intracerebral hemorrhage
  Eclampsia and hypertensive disorders
  Cerebral venous thrombosis
  Choriocarcinoma
  AVMs
  Vasculitis
  Infective endocarditis
  Moyamoya disease
  Tumors (primary and metastatic)
SAH
  Aneurysm (saccular, mycotic, traumatic, and so on)
  AVM (cerebral, spinal cord, and angiomas)
  Eclampsia
  Vasculitis
  Choriocarcinoma
  Cerebral venous thrombosis

Others
  Carotid cavernous fistula
  Dural vascular malformation
  Carotid and vertebrobasilar arterial dissection

Abbreviations: AVM, arteriovenous malformations; FMD, fibromuscular dysplasia; SAH, subarachnoid hemorrhage; SLE, systemic lupus erythematosus; MTHFR, methylene tetra hydrofolate reductase.
Modified from Digre KB, Varner MW, Skalabrin E, et al. Diagnosis and treatment of cerebrovascular disorders in pregnancy. In: Adams HP, eds. *Handbook of Cerebrovascular Diseases*. New York, NY: Marcel-Dekker; 2005:805–850.

women. Consider protein C or protein S deficiency (may be falsely depressed simply because of pregnancy), antithrombin, antiphospholipid antibodies, platelets, fibrinogen, and homocysteine levels. Vasculitic screen: ANA, ENA, ANCA. Toxicology screen if indicated

5. Treatment is directed at the underlying cause; treatment should be individualized.
   a. **Heparin,** unfractionated or low molecular weight, does not cross the placenta and can therefore be used safely during pregnancy. Low-molecular-weight heparin (risk category B) has been used. Safe for breast-feeding.
   b. **Warfarin** (risk category D; X in first trimester; compatible with breast-feeding) crosses the placenta and is contraindicated during pregnancy because of the embryopathy associated with use. Can be used for breast-feeding.
   c. **Low-dose aspirin** (81 mg/day) (risk category C) can be used safely in pregnancy when clinically indicated. Higher-dose aspirin is avoided. Other antithrombotic agents could be considered: Clopidogrel (risk category B) is an alternative to aspirin.
   d. Management of acute ischemic stroke with tissue plasminogen activator [e.g., Alteplase (FDA C)]; is not currently recommended although there are isolated case reports of benefit.
   e. Manage elevation of homocysteine levels with folate.

B. Cerebral venous thrombosis.
   1. Occurs primarily postpartum. The signs and symptoms include headache, seizures, hemiplegia, papilledema, and fluctuating obtundation and/or coma, especially in internal cerebral vein thrombosis.
   2. **Diagnosis** optimally with MRI and MR/CT venography; angiography, or venography is occasionally needed.
   3. Treatment.
      a. Correction of predisposing factors (infection and dehydration)
      b. Control of seizures
      c. Use of antiedema agents when appropriate
      d. Anticoagulation (see Sections **A.5.a.** to **c** under Cerebrovascular Disease)
   4. **Risk factors for cerebral venous thrombosis include** cesarean delivery, hypertension, infection other than pneumonia or influenza, drug abuse, especially cocaine, methamphetamines, and IV drug abuse.

C. **Postpartum cerebral angiopathy (also known as RCVS)** is a rare cause of a stroke-like syndrome characterized by seizure and focal neurologic deficits. Reversible cerebral vasoconstriction is found at angiography. Medications such as ergot alkaloids (e.g., ergonovine, bromocriptine, and ergotamine) and certain vasoconstrictive agents (isometheptene and sympathomimetic drugs) have been reported to cause the disorder. Treatment has been mainly supportive.

D. Hematologic disorders often manifest more frequently in pregnancy.
   1. Antiphospholipid antibody syndrome is associated with recurrent pregnancy loss, fetal growth restriction, and severe preeclampsia and eclampsia.
   2. Sickle cell disease
   3. Deficiencies of antithrombin, or protein C or S
   4. Thrombophilia, especially factor V Leiden mutation

E. Subarachnoid hemorrhage (SAH). Table 62.8 causes include:
   1. Intracranial aneurysm.
      a. Thought to be present in 1% of all women of reproductive age; more likely in older, parous women
      b. A significant contributor to maternal mortality

    c. Rupture probably equally likely throughout pregnancy

    d. Diagnosis requires CT and LP to look for RBCs, and angiography.

    e. Optimum outcomes with surgical correction

    f. Avoid nitroprusside because of its cyanide effect on the fetus. Hypertension can be controlled with verapamil or nimodipine.

    g. Vaginal delivery should be anticipated after successful clipping unless obstetric contraindications exist. If delivery occurs before clipping, cesarean section or forceps delivery with epidural anesthesia is indicated.

    h. Vasospasm can be managed with nimodipine (FDA C). Volume expansion must be monitored, because pregnant women are relatively more prone to pulmonary edema (decreased osmotic pressure).

    i. Outcome.

       (1) Grades 1 through 3: with expedited surgery, 95% successful outcome expected

       (2) Grade 4: 45% to 75% mortality

       (3) Fetal outcome: 27% mortality rate without surgery.

    j. Subsequent pregnancies after successful clipping have a good prognosis.

    k. Asymptomatic intracranial aneurysm should be evaluated on a case-by-case basis. When possible, these can be watched and treated after delivery (Video 62.2).

  2. Arteriovenous malformation (AVM)

    a. Characteristically occurs in younger women who have had fewer pregnancies.

    b. Diagnosis requires CT, LP, and angiography.

    c. The malformation should be corrected, if possible, surgically or with embolic therapy.

    d. Stereotactic radiation is not usually recommended during pregnancy.

    e. Delivery is vaginal with epidural anesthesia and low-outlet forceps.

F. Eclampsia, severe preeclampsia.

  1. Definition.

    a. Preeclampsia (new-onset hypertension and proteinuria beyond 20 weeks gestation) complicates 5% to 7% of pregnancies.

    b. Severe preeclampsia. One or more of the following is present: persistent blood pressures ≥160 mm Hg systolic and/or ≥110 mm Hg diastolic, 5 g proteinuria in 24 hours, oliguria (500 mL per 24 hours), elevated results of liver function tests, thrombocytopenia, persistent visual disturbances or headache, epigastric pain, pulmonary edema, or fetal growth restriction not explainable by other causes.

    c. Eclampsia. Seizures or coma in a woman with preeclampsia in whom no other explanation can be found.

    d. HELLP syndrome. A form of severe preeclampsia characterized by *h*emolysis, *e*levated results of *l*iver function tests, and *l*ow *p*latelet counts.

  2. Symptoms and physical findings.

    a. Headache, dizziness, scotomata, nausea, vomiting, and abdominal pain

    b. Generalized edema

    c. Funduscopic findings: segmental vasospasm, serous retinal detachment

    d. Neurologic finding: hyperreflexia; cortical blindness

    e. Bedside testing: visual acuity, Amsler grid for detection of scotomata

  3. CT and MRI findings.

    a. CT. Edema and hypodense lesions 75%, hemorrhage 9%

    b. MRI.

       (1) Severe preeclampsia. Deep white-matter signals on T2-weighted images

       (2) Eclampsia. Signals on T2-weighted images at gray matter–white matter junctions, particularly in the parietal–occipital areas; cortical edema, hemorrhage; images look similar to hypertensive encephalopathy or posterior reversible encephalopathy.

  4. Treatment.

    a. Delivery remains on the only definitive treatment and should be accomplished at such time as either the mother is better off not being pregnant anymore or when a baby can be expected to do as well, or better, in the nursery than in utero.

    b. Magnesium sulfate (FDA B; compatible with breast-feeding) is superior to IV diazepam and phenytoin in randomized controlled trials.

       (1) Administered in a 4 to 6 g loading dose followed by 2 g/hour intravenously.

      (2) Side effects include weakness, diplopia, ptosis, blurred vision, nausea, vomiting, and respiratory depression. *Use with caution in the care of patients with reduced renal clearance or neuromuscular diseases such as myasthenia gravis* (MG).

      (3) Neurologic findings of magnesium toxicity include diminished muscle stretch reflexes, ptosis and diminished accommodation, nausea, flushing, and respiratory depression.

    c. Blood pressure needs to be controlled to minimize risk of maternal vascular accidents (usually below 160 mm Hg systolic and 110 mm Hg diastolic) but kept high enough to adequately perfuse mother and fetus. The latter can be functionally assessed by maternal urine output and fetal heart rate monitoring.

    d. Control seizures with an AED such as diphenylhydantoin (fosphenytoin) only if $MgSO_4$ is unsuccessful.

    e. Manage cerebral edema or herniation with hyperventilation, steroids, or mannitol after delivery.

5. **Postpartum eclampsia** (one-third of eclamptic convulsions do not begin until after delivery, usually within 24 to 48 hours after delivery), usually defined as within 7 days of delivery. Late postpartum eclampsia can occur up to 10 to 14 days after delivery. Consider the possibility of stroke, venous thrombosis, or reversible angiopathy whenever the diagnosis of late postpartum eclampsia is being considered.

6. Outcome.
    a. The maternal mortality rate in the United States is 1% to 2%.
    b. The perinatal mortality rate is 13% to 30%.

7. Complications.
    a. Intracranial hemorrhage, frequently from uncontrolled hypertension
    b. Congestive heart failure, frequently from iatrogenic fluid overload
    c. Intrahepatic hemorrhage

MULTIPLE SCLEROSIS

A. Multiple sclerosis (MS) does not affect pregnancy per se, or vice versa. Although recent studies do show that there may be increased relapses postpartum, especially in the first 6 months postpartum (particularly in the relapsing–remitting form), pregnancy does not affect the rate of disability.

    1. Patients who have sphincter disturbances or paraplegia may experience increased difficulty during pregnancy.

    2. There is no evidence of vertical transmission of MS.

    3. MS does not occur more frequently in pregnancy.

B. Management of acute MS in pregnancy (Table 62.8).

    1. Semi-synthetic corticosteroids, most commonly methylprednisolone, are the mainstay for treatment of acute MS exacerbations during pregnancy (see Chapter 44).

    2. The interferons and copolymer are not yet recommended in pregnancy, although patients who were pregnant have used the medications without fetal harm.

    3. Avoid teriflunomide because it is currently labeled as an FDA Category X medication.

ROOT LESIONS AND PERIPHERAL NEUROPATHY

A. Lumbar disk.

    1. Signs and symptoms are the same as in nonpregnant patients.

    2. Generally treated nonoperatively. Consider surgery if there are bilateral symptoms or disturbances of sphincter function. Surgery during pregnancy is frequently associated with increased blood loss because of increased collateral flow.

B. Carpal tunnel syndrome.

    1. Often exacerbated during pregnancy because of increase in extracellular fluid.

    2. Pain and paresthesia are commonly worse at night and tend to be worse in the dominant hand.

    3. Symptoms usually respond to nocturnal wrist splinting and resolve within 3 months postpartum.

TABLE 62.8 Drugs Used in the Management of Multiple Sclerosis

Drug	Use in MS	FDA Schedule	Side Effects	Breast-feeding
IV Methylprednisolone	Acute exacerbations	C	Anxiety, gastrointestinal distress	Compatible
Interferon β-1a (Avonex) (Rebif)	Prevention of exacerbations (relapsing–remitting)	C	Fatigue, malaise, low fever	Probably compatible
Interferon β-1b (Betaseron) (Extavia)	Prevention of exacerbations (relapsing–remitting)	C	Fatigue, malaise	Probably compatible
Glatiramer acetate (Copaxone)	Prevention of exacerbations (relapsing–remitting)	B	Fatigue	Probably compatible
Methotrexate	Chronic progressive	X, do not use	–	Contraindicated
Azathioprine	Chronic progressive	D	–	Potential toxicity
Mitoxantrone (Novantrone)	Chronic progressive; progressive relapsing	D	Cardiac	Avoid
Natalizumab (Tysabri)	Relapsing–remitting	C	Spontaneous Abortions reported; also PML risk	Toxicity cannot be ruled out
Peginterferon Beta 1a (Extavia)	Relapsing–remitting	C		Risk cannot be ruled out
Dimethyl fumerate (Tecfidera)	Relapsing–remitting	C		Risk cannot be ruled out
Fingolimod (Gilyena)	Relapsing–remitting	C	Leukopenia	Toxicity cannot be ruled out
Intravenous immunoglobulin	Optic-spinal variants	C		Probably safe
Teriflunomide (Aubagio)	Relapsing–remitting	X	High incidence of malformations in animals; liver failure; women/men considering pregnancy should not use and if used, should have elimination period	Unknown
Alemtuzumab (Lemtrada)	Relapsing–remitting	C	Fatal autoimmune thrombocytopenia or kidney disorder	Cannot rule out risk
Symptomatic management of MS comorbidities				
Baclofen	Spasticity	B	–	Probably compatible
Amantadine	Fatigue	C	–	Potential toxicity
Modafinil (Provigil)	Fatigue	C		Potential toxicity

Abbreviations: FDA, Food and Drug Administration; MS, multiple sclerosis

From *Micromedex 2.0 (electronic version).* Greenwood Village, CO: Truven Health Analytics. Also available at: http://www.micromedexsolutions.com/. Accessed September 16, 2015.

C. **Bell's palsy.**
   1. Facial paresis of lower-motor neuron type when no other specific etiologic agent can be found. Signs and symptoms include abrupt onset, often with pain around the ear; feeling of facial stiffness and pulling to one side; difficulty closing the eye on the affected side; taste disturbances; and hyperacusis.
   2. Approximately three times more likely to occur during pregnancy, primarily in the third trimester or immediately postpartum
   3. Steroids are probably effective if given within the first 5 to 7 days (prednisone 1 mg/kg daily for 5 to 7 days). Surgery is ineffective.
D. **Other forms of cranial nerve palsy.**
   1. Cranial nerve IV: reported rarely to occur; mechanism similar to cranial nerve VII or VI palsy
   2. Cranial nerve VI: similar to above; usually resolve postpartum
E. **Meralgia paresthetica.**
   1. Causes numbness in the lateral aspect of the thigh
   2. Usually resolves within 3 months postpartum
F. **Sciatica and back pain.** Lumbosacral disk surgery should be reserved only for progressive atrophy or bowel or bladder dysfunction.
G. **Guillain–Barré syndrome.**
   1. Causes are not generally affected by pregnancy.
   2. Labor and delivery are otherwise normal.

MYASTHENIA GRAVIS

A. Variable weakness and fatigability of skeletal muscles resulting from defective neuromuscular transmission (reduced acetylcholine receptors in the neuromuscular junction)
B. Certain drugs should be avoided, including the following:
   1. **Ester anesthetics.** tetracaine (Pontocaine; Sanofi Winthrop, New York, NY, USA) and chloroprocaine (Nesacaine; AstraZeneca, Wilmington, DE, USA)
   2. Curare (and other nondepolarizing muscle relaxants)
   3. Halothane (Fluothane; Wyeth-Ayerst, Philadelphia, PA, USA)
   4. Aminoglycoside antibiotics
   5. Quinine and quinidine
   6. **Magnesium sulfate.** The antidote with MG is edrophonium (Tensilon; ICN, Costa Mesa, CA, USA), not calcium.
C. **Treatment.**
   1. **Antepartum.**
      a. Pregnancy per se does not affect the severity of preexisting disease.
      b. Perinatal mortality is increased because of increased risk of premature delivery as well as neonatal MG.
      c. Pharmacologic management of MG is not altered by pregnancy.
   2. **Intrapartum.**
      a. Oral medications should be discontinued at the onset of labor and the intramuscular equivalents continued until oral medications can again be ingested. Equipotent dosages are as follows:
         (1) Neostigmine 0.5 mg intravenously
         (2) Neostigmine 0.7 to 1.5 mg intramuscularly
         (3) Neostigmine 15 mg by mouth
         (4) Pyridostigmine 60 mg by mouth
      b. Analgesia and anesthesia for labor require the utmost caution because of the risks of respiratory depression and aspiration.
      c. Except for voluntary expulsive efforts in the second stage of labor, MG does not affect the progress of labor and is not an indication for cesarean section.
   3. **Postpartum.**
      a. Exacerbations are more likely to occur postpartum; tend to be sudden and severe in onset.
      b. Women with severe disease or whose babies have symptoms after nursing should not breast-feed.

c. Most women return to preconceptional oral dosage with modest increases in dose to allow for the additional stresses of early parenthood.
D. Neonatal myasthenia.
1. Occurs in 10% to 15% of cases
2. Results from transplacental transfer of maternal antibody against acetylcholine receptors.

MYOTONIC DYSTROPHY

A. Clinical characteristics.
1. Autosomal dominant; weakness and wasting in muscles of face, neck, and distal limbs; myotonia of hands and tongue
2. Variable age at onset. The condition sometimes is diagnosed in mothers only after an affected child is born (these pregnancies are frequently complicated by polyhydramnios that results from poor fetal swallowing).
3. Predisposition to cardiac arrhythmias
4. Treatment. There is none for the dystrophy. Severe myotonia: phenytoin (FDA C), quinine (FDA D), and procainamide (FDA D).
B. Effects on pregnancy.
1. Increased risk of spontaneous abortion
2. Increased risk of premature labor and polyhydramnios, particularly with fetal involvement
3. Normal first stage of labor
4. Normal response to oxytocin
5. Prolonged second stage of labor
C. **Labor management** includes outlet forceps, regional anesthesia; avoid succinylcholine (can cause hyperthermia); nonpolarizing agents are generally safe.

MOVEMENT DISORDERS

A. **Restless legs,** the most common movement disorder in pregnancy. Most cases respond to massage, flexion/extension leg exercises, and walking. Treat with iron or folate if any suggestion of concurrent deficiency.
B. Chorea Gravidarum.
1. Most commonly due to medications, toxins, or infections
2. May be the initial manifestation of another disorder (e.g., systemic lupus erythematosus, Sydenham's chorea)
3. Can be treated with low-dose haloperidol (FDA C)
C. **Parkinson's disease** in pregnancy is rare because the age at which most patients have the disease is past childbearing years. However, pregnancy has been successfully accomplished in patients with Parkinson's disease.
1. Pregnancy may adversely affect Parkinson's in that there may be exacerbations soon after pregnancy.
2. Drugs used in Parkinson's disease.
a. Levodopa (FDA C), MAO-B (selegiline, rasagiline—FDA C), dopamine agonists (pramipexole, ropinirole FDA C), and COMT inhibitor (entacapone FDA C).
b. Amantadine (FDA C) can increase the risk of complications and malformations.

Key Points

- Neurologic disorders are not rare in pregnancy, and all women seen, who are of childbearing age, should be considered to have a prepregnancy visit.
- Optimum control of the neurologic problem before pregnancy is ideal.
- The best outcome for the infant is optimal care of the woman in pregnancy.
- Use testing, including imaging, to determine the correct diagnosis.
- Use medications when necessary, keeping in mind the FDA drug classification.

Recommended Readings

Agarwal N, Guerra JC, Gala NB, et al. Current treatment options for cerebral arteriovenous malformations in pregnancy: a review of the literature. *World Neurosurg*. 2014;81(1):83–90.

Bove R, Alwan S, Friedman JM, et al. Management of multiple sclerosis during pregnancy and the reproductive years: a systematic review. *Obstet Gynecol*. 2014;124(6):1157–1168.

Briggs GG, Freeman RK, eds. *Drugs in Pregnancy and Lactation*. 10th ed. Philadelphia, PA: Lippincott Williams & Wilkins; 2014.

Bronby GM, Bell R, Claassen I, et al. Guidelines for the evaluation and management of status epilepticus. *Neurocrit Care*. 2012;17:3–23.

Bushnell C, Saposnik G. Evaluation and management of cerebral venous thrombosis. *Continuum (Minneap Minn)*. 2014;20(2 Cerebrovascular Disease):335–351.

Coyle PK. Multiple sclerosis in pregnancy. *Continuum (Minneap Minn)*. 2014;20(1 Neurology of Pregnancy):42–59.

Del Zotto E, Giossi A, Volonghi I, et al. Ischemic stroke during pregnancy and puerperium. *Stroke Res Treat*. 2011;2011:606780.

Digre KB. Headaches during pregnancy. *Clin Obstet Gynecol*. 2013;56(2):317–329.

Digre KB, Varner MW, Skalabrin E, et al. Diagnosis and treatment of cerebrovascular disorders in pregnancy. In: Adams HP, eds. *Handbook of Cerebrovascular Diseases*. New York, NY: Marcel-Dekker; 2005:805–850.

Falardeau J, Lobb BM, Golden S, et al. The use of acetazolamide during pregnancy in intracranial hypertension patients. *J Neuroophthalmol*. 2013;33:9–12.

Feske SK, Singhal AB. Cerebrovascular disorders complicating pregnancy. *Continuum (Minneap Minn)*. 2014;20(1 Neurology of Pregnancy):80–99.

Finkelsztein A, Brooks JB, Paschoal FM Jr, et al. What can we really tell women with multiple sclerosis regarding pregnancy? A systematic review and meta-analysis of the literature. *BJOG*. 2011;118:790–797.

Grear KE, Bushnell CD. Stroke and pregnancy: clinical presentation, evaluation, treatment, and epidemiology. *Clin Obstet Gynecol*. 2013;56:350–359.

Greving JP, Wermer MJ, Brown RD Jr, et al. Development of the PHASES score for prediction of risk of rupture of intracranial aneurysms: a pooled analysis of six prospective cohort studies. *Lancet Neurol*. 2014;13(1):59–66.

Guidon AC, Massey EW. Neuromuscular disorders in pregnancy. *Neurol Clin*. 2012;30(3):889–911.

Han IH. Pregnancy and spinal problems. *Curr Opin Obstet Gynecol*. 2010;22(6):477–481.

Harden CL, Hopp J, Ting TY, et al; American Academy of Neurology; American Epilepsy Society. Management issues for women with epilepsy-focus on pregnancy (an evidence-based review): I. Obstetrical complications and change in seizure frequency: report of the Quality Standards Subcommittee and Therapeutics and Technology Assessment Subcommittee of the American Academy of Neurology and the American Epilepsy Society. *Epilepsia*. 2009;50(5):1229–1236.

Harden CL, Meador KJ, Pennell PB, et al; American Academy of Neurology; American Epilepsy Society. Management issues for women with epilepsy-focus on pregnancy (an evidence-based review): II. Teratogenesis and perinatal outcomes: report of the Quality Standards Subcommittee and Therapeutics and Technology Subcommittee of the American Academy of Neurology and the American Epilepsy Society. *Epilepsia*. 2009;50(5):1237–1246.

Harden CL, Pennell PB, Koppel BS, et al.; American Academy of Neurology; American Epilepsy Society. Practice parameter update: management issues for women with epilepsy—focus on pregnancy (an evidence-based review): vitamin K, folic acid, blood levels, and breastfeeding: report of the Quality Standards Subcommittee and Therapeutics and Technology Assessment Subcommittee of the American Academy of Neurology and American Epilepsy Society. *Neurology*. 2009;73(2):142–149.

Hart LA, Sibai BM. Seizures in pregnancy: epilepsy, eclampsia, and stroke. *Semin Perinatol*. 2013;37(4):207–224.

Hutchinson S, Marmura MJ, Calhoun, A, et al. Epilepsy in pregnancy. *Clin Obstet Gynecol*. 2013;56:330–341.

Juvela S, Poussa K, Lehto H, et al. Natural history of unruptured intracranial aneurysms: a long-term follow-up study. *Stroke*. 2013;44(9):2414–2421.

Kesler A, Kuperminc M. Idiopathic intracranial hypertension and pregnancy. *Clin Obstet Gynecol*. 2013;56(2):389–396.

Kim YW, Neal D, Hoh BL. Cerebral aneurysms in pregnancy and delivery: pregnancy and delivery do not increase the risk of aneurysm rupture. *Neurosurgery*. 2013;72(2):143–149; discussion 150.

Klein A. Peripheral nerve disease in pregnancy. *Clin Obstet Gynecol*. 2013;56(2):382–388.

Liman TG, Bohner G, Heuschmann PU, et al. Clinical and radiological differences in posterior reversible encephalopathy syndrome between patients with preeclampsia-eclampsia and other predisposing diseases. *Eur J Neurol*. 2012;19(7):935–943.

Lynch JC, Gouvêa F, Emmerich JC, et al. Management strategy for brain tumor diagnosed during pregnancy. *Br J Neurosurg*. 2011;25(2):225–230.

MacGregor EA. Headache in pregnancy. *Continuum (Minneap Minn)*. 2014;20(1 Neurology of Pregnancy):128–124.

MacGregor EA. Migraine in pregnancy and lactation. *Neurol Sci*. 2014;35(suppl 1):61–64.

Marchenko A, Etwel F, Olutunfese O, et al. Pregnancy outcome following prenatal exposure to triptan medications: a meta-analysis. *Headache*. 2015;55(4):490–501.

Massey JM, De Jesus-Acosta C. Pregnancy and myasthenia gravis. *Continuum (Minneap Minn)*. 2014;20(1 Neurology of Pregnancy):115–127.

Molitch ME. Endocrinology in pregnancy: management of the pregnant patient with a prolactinoma. *Eur J Endocrinol*. 2015;172(5):R205–R213.

Picchietti DL, Hensley JG, Bainbridge JL, et al; International Restless Legs Syndrome Study Group (IRLSSG). Consensus clinical practice guidelines for the diagnosis and treatment of restless legs syndrome/Willis-Ekbom disease during pregnancy and lactation. *Sleep Med Rev*. 2015;22:64–77.

Razmara A, Bakhadirov K, Batra A, et al. Cerebrovascular complications of pregnancy and the postpartum period. *Curr Cardiol Rep*. 2014;16(10):532. doi:10.1007/211855-014-0532-1.

Signore C, Spong CY, Krotoski D, et al. Pregnancy in women with physical disabilities. *Obstet Gynecol*. 2011;117:935–947.

Varner M. Myasthenia gravis and pregnancy. *Clin Obstet Gynecol*. 2013;56:372–381.

Verheecke M, Halaska MJ, Lok CA, et al; ESGO Task Force 'Cancer in Pregnancy.' Primary brain tumors, meningiomas and brain metastases in pregnancy: report on 27 cases and review of literature. *Eur J Cancer*. 2014;50(8):1462–1471.

Wiese KM, Talkad A, Mathews M, et al. Intravenous recombinant tissue plasminogen activator in a pregnant woman with cardioembolic stroke. *Stroke*. 2006;37(8):2168–2169.

Winterbottom JB, Smyth RM, Jacoby A, et al. Preconception counseling for women with epilepsy to reduce adverse pregnancy outcome. *Cochrane Database Syst Rev*. 2008;(3):CD006645. doi:10.1002/14651858.CD006645.pub2.

Wlodarczyk BI, Palacios AM, George TM, et al. Antiepileptic drugs and pregnancy outcomes. *Am J Med Genet A*. 2012;158A:2071–2090.

63 The ABCs of Neurologic Emergencies

José Biller, Rochelle Sweis and Sean Ruland

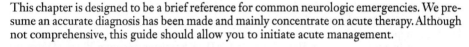

This chapter is designed to be a brief reference for common neurologic emergencies. We presume an accurate diagnosis has been made and mainly concentrate on acute therapy. Although not comprehensive, this guide should allow you to initiate acute management.

ELEVATED INTRACRANIAL PRESSURE

A. Maintain 30 degrees head-up in a neutral position with neck positioned midline to avoid jugular venous compression.
B. Correct factors exacerbating intracranial pressure (ICP).
   1. Hypercarbia
   2. Hypoxia
   3. Hyperthermia
   4. Acidemia
   5. Hypotension
C. Hyperventilate to $Paco_2$ 30 to 35 mm Hg as a temporizing measure.
   1. Implement emergently while awaiting surgical therapy.
   2. Prolonged use and $Paco_2$ below 25 mm Hg decrease cerebral blood flow (CBF) leading to ischemia.
   3. CBF decreases 4% for every 1 mm Hg decrement in $Paco_2$.
D. Mannitol (20% or 25% solution). 1 to 2 g/kg intravenously (IV) bolus followed by 0.25 to 1 g/kg every 4 to 6 hours, depending on ICP response. Monitor serum osmolality, osmolar gap, volume status, electrolytes, and renal function.
   1. Check serum osmolality, electrolytes, and osmolar gap prior to mannitol administration; hold mannitol if osmolar gap greater than 20 mOsm/L.
   2. Acute kidney injury is typically caused by decreased intravascular volume and not mannitol toxicity. Maintain euvolemia. Replace urine output using normal saline.
   3. Some authors recommend holding mannitol if serum osmolality is greater than 320 mOsm/L.
E. Consider hypertonic saline 3% solution 250 cc bolus or 23.4% solution 30 cc over 15 to 20 minutes.
   1. Target serum sodium 145 to 155 mEq/L.
   2. Hypertonic saline (3%) continuous infusion: start with 30 cc/hour and titrate up by 10 cc/hour until target reached.
   3. Avoid hypotonic solutions.
F. Indications for invasive ICP monitoring.
   1. Traumatic brain injury (TBI) with Glasgow Coma Scale (GCS) 8 or less and abnormal head computed tomography (CT)
   2. TBI with a normal head CT and two or more of the following: age over 40 years, posturing, or systolic blood pressure (BP) below 90 mm Hg.
   3. Place ventriculostomy catheter, which can also be therapeutic through cerebrospinal fluid (CSF) removal or an intraparenchymal probe.
   4. Maintain ICP below 20 mm Hg and cerebral perfusion pressure (CPP) above 50 mm Hg.
G. CSF diversion with ventriculostomy if obstructive hydrocephalus is present
H. Dexamethasone 10 mg IV once and then 4 to 6 mg IV every 6 hours if vasogenic edema is present
I. Sedation with propofol, benzodiazpeine, or opiates and paralysis if necessary

J. Barbiturate coma if hemodynamically can tolerate.
K. Hypothermia can lower cerebral metabolic rate (CMRO2) and ICP but has not improved outcome in two large multicenter randomized trials in adults with severe TBI.
L. Consider surgical decompression/evacuation for life-threatening intracranial hemorrhage. No outcome benefit for unilateral or bilateral craniectomy after diffuse TBI (see Chapter 40). Decompressive hemicraniectomy for malignant middle cerebral artery (MCA) infarction is discussed below (see section Malignant Cerebral Edema [Ischemic Stroke]).

COMA

A. Consider structural versus diffuse neuronal dysfunction versus psychogenic etiology.
B. Perform thorough general and neurologic examination.
C. ABCs. airway, breathing, and circulation.
D. Avoid hypotonic fluids.
E. Manage hypoglycemia with 50% glucose 50 cc IV. Administer thiamine 200 mg IV before glucose.
F. Consider empiric naloxone 0.4 to 2.0 mg IV if concern for opioid overdose.
G. Avoid flumazenil as it can precipitate benzodiazepine withdrawal and seizures in chronic users with life-threatening consequences.
H. Check arterial blood gas, electrolytes, renal function, liver enzymes, ammonia, complete blood count (CBC), urinalysis, blood and urine toxicology screens, human immunodeficiency virus (HIV), thyroid-stimulating hormone (TSH), troponin, and electrocardiography (ECG).
I. If focal neurologic signs, or history of head trauma, consider therapy for elevated ICP as above.
J. Emergent CT or magnetic resonance imaging (MRI) brain. If brainstem signs present, include CTA or MRA to assess for basilar artery occlusion.
K. Consider lumbar puncture (LP) for suspected subarachnoid hemorrhage (SAH) with normal findings on head CT or meningoencephalitis with addition of empiric IV antimicrobials if suspected (see Bacterial Meningitis).
L. Continuous EEG to assess for nonconvulsive seizures.

STATUS EPILEPTICUS

A. ABCs. Airway, breathing, and circulation.
B. Antiepileptic drug (AED) administration is more effective when given soon after seizure onset.
C. First line: benzodiazepine. Lorazepam 0.1 mg/kg IV at 1 mg/minute (maximum of 8 mg in adults), or midazolam 10 mg intramuscularly (IM) if no immediate IV access.
D. Second line. 5- to 30-minute trials needed. Options include:
   1. Valproate sodium.
     a. Loading. 20 to 40 mg/kg at 5 mg/kg/minute
     b. Maintenance. 4 to 6 mg/kg every 6 hour
   2. Levetiracetam.
     a. Loading. 1 to 6 g at 5 mg/kg/minute
     b. Maintenance. 500 to 1,500 mg IV or enteral every 12 hour
   3. Lacosamide.
     a. Loading. 200 to 400 mg over 15 to 30 minute
     b. Maintenance. 200 mg every 12 hour
   4. Fosphenytoin/phenytoin.
     a. Loading. 20 mg/kg IV at 150 mg/minute in adults
     b. Maintenance dose. 4 to 6 mg/kg/day IV or IM divided daily
     c. Check serum phenytoin level 1 hour after IV loading.
E. Third line. Continuous infusion therapy:
   1. Midazolam.
     a. Loading. 0.2 mg/kg over 5 minute
     b. Maintenance. 0.2 to 2 mg/kg/hour
   2. Propofol.
     a. Loading. 1 to 5 mg/kg over 5 to 10 minute
     b. Maintenance. Up to 4 mg/kg/hour if status persists and hemodynamics tolerate

c. Propofol usage above 4 mg/kg/hour for more than 48 hours has been associated with the propofol infusion syndrome, which can cause death.
3. Pentobarbital.
   a. Loading. 5 to 10 mg/kg slow infusion to avoid hypotension
   b. Maintenance dose. 0.5 to 5 mg/kg/hour
4. Ketamine.
   a. Loading. 1 to 3 mg/kg over 2 to 5 minute
   b. Maintenance. 0.5 to 10 mg/kg/hour
F. Endotracheal intubation and mechanical ventilator support
G. Peripheral or central venous access, IV fluids, and vasopressor support as needed
H. Avoid antihypertensive agents in the first 30 to 60 minutes of generalized convulsive status epilepticus as most patients are hypertensive.
I. Continuous EEG monitoring with goal of seizure cessation
J. CT or MRI brain
K. Consider thiamine 200 mg IV and 50% glucose 50 cc IV if hypoglycemia is suspected.
L. Manage medical complications including cerebral edema, hyperthermia, rhabdomyolysis, infections, venous thromboembolism (VTE), and pressure ulcers.
M. Treat etiology. LP if infectious, paraneoplastic, or autoimmune encephalitis suspected.

BACTERIAL MENINGITIS

A. Initiate empiric antibiotics immediately when suspected.
B. Manage elevated ICP if present.
C. Control seizures.
D. Manage complications including subdural empyema, cerebritis, brain abscess, ventriculitis, choroid plexitis, acute hydrocephalus, vasculitis, vasospasm, cerebral venous thrombosis, disseminated intravascular coagulation, shock, sodium abnormalities, and respiratory failure (Figs. 63.1 and 63.2A, B).
E. Initial antibiotic treatment for immunocompetent patients with community-acquired meningitis: ceftriaxone or cefotaxime *plus* vancomycin *plus* dexamethasone 10 mg IV once and then every 6 hours until CSF cultures and sensitivities are available to guide therapy. See Table 63.1 for antibiotic doses.
F. Consider ceftazidime, cefepime, or meropenem if *Pseudomonas* infection is suspected.
G. Consider ampicillin if *Listeria* infection is suspected, as in an immunocompromised host.
H. Consider doxycycline if *Rickettsia, Anaplasma, Ehrlichia*, or *Coxiella burnetii* is suspected.
I. Treat for 7 days regardless of organism but extend up to 4 weeks for *Listeria* meningitis or in immunocompromised patients.

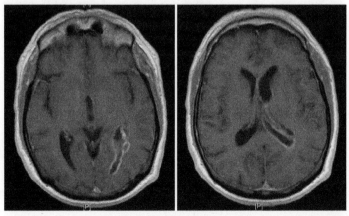

FIGURE 63.1 Axial T1-weighted MR images demonstrate diffuse abnormal enhancement extending along the ependymal surface of the left lateral ventricle and third ventricle consistent with ventriculitis/ependymitis in a 65-year-old man with *Streptococcus constellatus* meningitis.

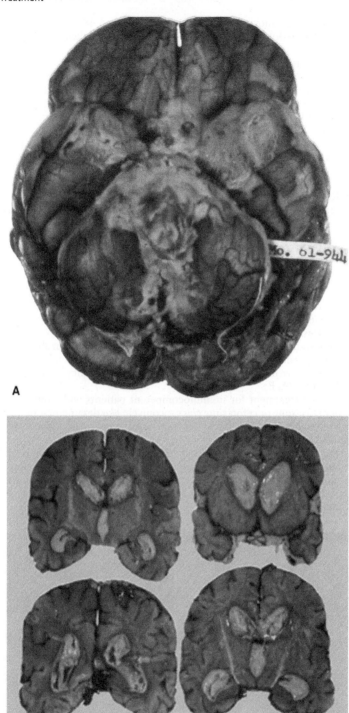

FIGURE 63.2 A: Gross image of pyogenic meningitis. **B:** Cross section of pyogenic ventriculitis. (See color plates.)

TABLE 63.1 Antibiotic Therapy for Bacterial Meningitis

	Total Daily Dose (Dosing Interval)	
Antibiotics	Adults	Children (Older than 2 mo)
Ceftriaxone	4 g (q12h–24h)	80–100 mg/kg (q12h–24h)
Cefotaxime	8–12 g (q4h–6h)	225–300 mg/kg (q6h–8h)
Vancomycin	30–45 mg/kg (q8h–12h)	40–60 mg/kg (q6h)
Ceftazadime	6 g (q8h)	150 mg/kg (q8h)
Ampicillin	12 g (q4h)	20–30 mg/kg (q8h)

J. Chemoprophylax household contacts and those with direct exposure to droplet secretions of patients with meningococcal and *Haemophilus influenzae* infection with rifampin 600 mg twice daily for 2 days.
K. Neuroimaging
L. Serum procalcitonin and C-reactive protein (CRP) can help differentiate bacterial from viral meningitis.

HERPES SIMPLEX ENCEPHALITIS

A. Most common cause of fatal sporadic encephalitis
B. Treatment. acyclovir IV 10 mg/kg every 8 hours for 14 to 21 days. Adjust dose for renal function and maintain adequate hydration to prevent crystal nephropathy.
C. Control seizures.
D. Neuroimaging
E. Predictors of poor outcome include age greater than 30 years, GCS less than 6, delayed initiation of acyclovir treatment more than 4 days after symptom onset
F. Untreated herpes simplex encephalitis has a 70% mortality rate (Fig. 63.3).

BRAIN ABSCESS

A. Classify according to suspected entry point of infection, which predicts microbial flora and guides empiric antimicrobial treatment.
  1. Most common source is direct or indirect seeding through emissary veins from paranasal sinus, middle ear, and teeth.
  2. Underlying pathology such as stroke or neoplasm can serve as a focus for abscess (Fig. 63.4).

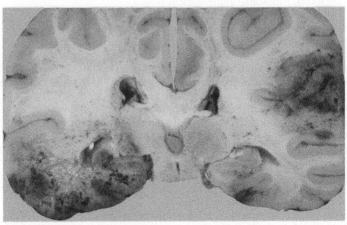

FIGURE 63.3 Cross section of the brain in a patient who had herpes simplex virus encephalitis. (See color plates.)

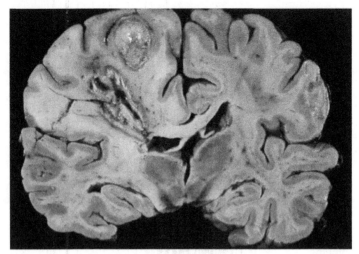

FIGURE 63.4 Cross section of the brain in a patient who had multiloculated cerebral abscesses. (See color plates.)

B. Gadolinium-enhanced MRI brain.
1. Allows for early recognition of cerebritis or abscess
2. Permits precise localization needed for surgical treatment
3. Serial MRI for treatment monitoring
4. Contrast-enhanced CT brain if MRI contraindicated

C. Antimicrobial treatment.
1. Antibiotics should not be withheld unless surgery is to be performed within several hours and no significant mass effect is present to preserve yield of positive cultures.
2. Community acquired. Third-generation cephalosporin: ceftriaxone (Table 63.1) (can also choose ceftazidime or cefotaxime) *plus* vancomycin (Table 63.1) *plus* metronidazole 500 mg every 6 hour in adults and 7.5 mg/kg every 8 hour in children.
3. Postoperative or posttraumatic. Meropenem or cefepime plus vancomycin.
4. Bone marrow transplant, stem cell transplant, solid organ transplant. Consider voriconazole and anti-toxoplasma therapy.
5. Nocardial abscess. Trimethoprim-sulfamethoxazole ± aspiration/excision.
6. Aspergillosis. Voriconazole
7. Mucormycosis. Liposomal amphotericin B
8. Coccidiomycosis. Fluconazole or itraconazole
9. Blastomycosis. Liposomal amphotericin B
10. Histoplasmosis: Liposomal amphotericin B × 3 months, then itraconazole × 12 months
11. Candidiasis. Combination IV liposomal amphotericin B *plus* oral flucytosine
12. Cryptococcus. Induction: combination liposomal amphotericin B *plus* flucytosine. Consolidation after 2 weeks: fluconazole 400 mg daily for 8 to 10 weeks for immunocompetent and 6 to 12 months for immunosuppressed patients
13. Actinomycosis. High-dose IV penicillin for 2 to 6 weeks, followed by P.O. amoxicillin, ampicillin, or penicillin for 6 to 12 months. Doxycycline, erythromycin, and clindamycin are also options.
14. Consider steroids for patients with significant mass effect due to vasogenic cerebral edema although there are no data supporting routine use.

D. Consider surgery for any abscess larger than 2.5 cm.
1. Aspiration is valuable for deep-seated abscesses. Excision allows for detection and treatment of extracranial communication.
2. Consider surgical treatment of primary infectious focus.

E. Treat complications including seizures, hyponatremia, obstructive hydrocephalus, ventriculitis, and cerebral edema.

CEREBRAL TOXOPLASMOSIS

A. High risk in HIV patients with CD4+ T cell counts less than 100 cells/μL or less than 200 cells/μL in the setting of concomitant opportunistic infection or malignancy

B. Treat with pyrimethamine 200 mg once then weight-based dosing.

C. **Less than 60 kg.** Pyrimethamine 50 mg P.O. daily *plus* sulfadiazine 1,000 mg P.O. q6h *plus* leucovorin 10 to 25 mg P.O. daily. Consider increasing to 50 mg daily or twice daily.

D. **Greater than 60 kg.** Pyrimethamine 75 mg P.O. daily plus sulfadiazine 1,500 mg P.O. q6h plus leucovorin 10 to 25 mg P.O. daily. Consider increasing to 50 mg daily or twice daily.

E. If patient is allergic to sulfa, consider clindamycin 600 mg IV or P.O. q6h.

F. Therapy duration: 6 weeks or longer if no clinical and radiologic improvement.

G. If no improvement after 10 to 14 days of therapy, consider alternative diagnosis.

SEPTIC CAVERNOUS SINUS THROMBOSIS

A. Etiology.
1. **Common.** Middle third facial infections and paranasal sinusitis
2. **Less common.** Otogenic, odontogenic, pharyngeal, and distant septic foci
3. Common organisms: *Staphylococcus aureus* (69%), *Streptococcus* (17%), *Pneumococcus* (5%), gram-negative species (5%), *Bacteroides* (2%), and *Fusobacterium* (2%)

B. **Clinical features.** Fever, tachycardia, hypotension, emesis, confusion, coma, chemosis, periorbital edema, ptosis, Horner's syndrome, ocular motility impairment, visual loss, papilledema, retinal vein dilatation, and pituitary insufficiency

C. Imaging.
1. CT brain provides bony details and air–soft tissue interface.
2. MRI brain has superior soft tissue resolution.

D. Treatment.
1. **Antimicrobial therapy.** Third-generation cephalosporin (ceftriaxone, ceftazidime, or cefotaxime), metronidazole, and vancomycin for at least 2 weeks.
2. Surgical treatment of nondraining primary infectious focus
3. Consider Ophthalmology and Otolaryngology consults.
4. Consider IV steroids for cranial nerve dysfunction or orbital inflammation after antimicrobial therapy initiated although evidence is limited.
5. Limited evidence regarding use of adjunctive anticoagulation
   a. Anticoagulation can be used safely in the absence of intracranial or systemic bleeding for patients deteriorating despite antimicrobial therapy.
   b. **Target.** twice baseline activated partial thromboplastin time (aPTT).
   c. **Duration.** 2 weeks to 3 months.

SUBDURAL EMPYEMA

A. Uncommon, suppurative, and loculated infection between the dura mater and the arachnoid; 95% intracranial and 5% spinal

B. Often unilateral and spreads rapidly throughout subdural space. Fatal if untreated

C. Etiology.
1. Paranasal sinusitis, meningitis, otitis media, mastoiditis, trauma, neurosurgical procedures, secondary infection of subdural hematoma (SDH) or hygroma, dental caries, and distant site infection (e.g., lungs) with hematogenous spread
2. Most common organisms.
   a. **Paranasal sinusitis.** Anaerobes, microaerophilic Streptococci.
   b. **Neurosurgical procedures.** *Pseudomonas aeruginosa* or *Staphylococcus epidermidis*.
   c. **Postoperative/posttraumatic.** *Staphylococcus aureus*.
   d. **Otitis media.** Streptococci species, *Pseudomonas aeruginosa*, *Bacteroides*.
   e. **Neonates.** *Enterobacteriaceae*, Group B streptococci, *Listeria monocytogenes*.
   f. **AIDS.** *Salmonella*.

D. **Clinical features.** Fever, seizures, headaches, vomiting, periorbital edema, sinusitis, meningismus, contralateral sensorimotor loss, mental status changes, stupor and coma.

E. Workup.
1. Gadolinium-enhanced MRI.
2. Contrast-enhanced CT if MRI contraindicated (lower sensitivity and specificity for intracranial subdural empyema compared to MRI)
3. LP. contraindicated if elevated ICP or spinal cord effacement present.
4. Erythrocyte sedimentation rate (ESR) and CRP.
F. Complications include seizures, cerebral infarction, cavernous sinus thrombosis, hydrocephalus, cerebral edema, and cranial/spinal osteomyelitis.
G. Treatment.
1. Empiric vancomycin *plus* third-generation cephalosporin (ceftriaxone, ceftazidime, cefotaxime) *plus* metronidazole
2. Early surgical drainage
3. Drainage of primary contiguous focus

ISCHEMIC STROKE: WITHIN 3 HOURS OF LAST KNOWN WELL

A. No intracranial hemorrhage on CT (Fig. 63.5; Video 63.1)
B. Age 18 years or older
C. IV tPA (alteplase) 0.9 mg/kg (maximum dose of 90 mg); 10% of total dose as bolus over 1 minute; and remainder infused over 60 minutes

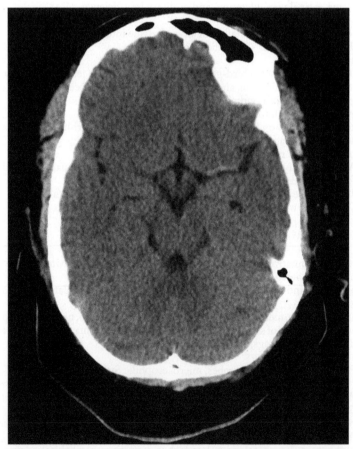

FIGURE 63.5 CT brain without contrast. Hyperdense left MCA sign in a patient presenting with nonfluent aphasia and right hemiplegia. CT, computed tomography; MCA, middle cerebral artery.

D. **Exclusion criteria.**
1. Stroke or serious head injury within 3 months
2. Frank hypodensity on CT more than 1/3 the MCA territory
3. Recent intracranial or intraspinal surgery
4. History of intracranial hemorrhage
5. Persistent systolic BP above 185 mm Hg or diastolic BP above 110 mm Hg despite reasonable attempts to reduce it
6. Intracranial neoplasm, arteriovenous malformation, or aneurysm
7. Symptoms suggestive of SAH
8. Active internal bleeding
9. Arterial puncture at a noncompressible site within 7 days
   a. Vitamin K antagonist or heparin used within 48 hours AND elevated aPTT, international normalized ratio (INR) above 1.7, or PT more than 15 seconds
   b. Other oral anticoagulant used within 48 hours
10. Platelet count below 100,000/μL
11. Blood glucose below 50 mg/dL
12. **Relative contraindications.**
    a. Recent surgery or major trauma within 14 days
    b. Pregnancy
    c. Gastrointestinal (GI) or urinary tract hemorrhage within 21 days
    d. Myocardial infarction within 3 months
    e. Rapidly improving or minor neurologic deficits likely to result in minimal or no deficit
E. No antithrombotic agents including VTE prophylaxis for 24 hours after IV tissue plasminogen activator (tPA)
F. Maintain BP below 180/105 mm Hg for 24 hours after IV tPA
G. Avoid IV enalaprilat as it increases risk of angiolingual edema associated with IV tPA.

ISCHEMIC STROKE 3 TO 4.5 HOURS FROM LAST KNOWN WELL

A. **Exclusion criteria.** In addition to above (Section **D** under Ischemic Stroke: Within 3 Hours of Last Known Well) exclusion criteria though not absolute, practitioners can consider the following exclusion criteria:
1. Age older than 80 years
2. National Institute of Health Stroke Scale (NIHSS) above 25
3. Combination of previous stroke and diabetes mellitus
4. Oral anticoagulant use regardless of INR values

ENDOVASCULAR INTERVENTION FOR ISCHEMIC STROKE UTILIZING MODERN STENT RETRIEVERS

1. **Inclusion criteria.**
   a. Prestroke modified Rankin Scale (mRS) score 0 to 1
   b. IV tPA administered within 4.5 hours
   c. Age 18 years or older
   d. Occlusion of internal carotid artery (ICA) terminus or proximal MCA (M1)
   e. NIHSS 6 or higher
   f. Alberta Stroke Program Early CT Score (ASPECTS) 6 or higher (endovascular treatment for ASPECTS less than 6 is uncertain)
   g. Groin puncture can be achieved within 6 hours of symptom onset
2. Effectiveness of endovascular treatment initiated beyond 6 hours is uncertain.
3. Endovascular treatment within 6 hours for anterior circulation occlusion is reasonable for patients with contraindications to IV tPA or those with occlusion of M2 or M3 portions of MCA, anterior cerebral arteries, vertebral arteries, or basilar artery.
4. Endovascular treatment is recommended over intra-arterial tPA within 6 hours.
5. Conscious sedation is preferred over general anesthesia if patient can protect airway.
6. CT brain should be completed prior to treatment and vascular imaging (CTA or MRA) is recommended. Benefits of perfusion imaging (CT/MRI) are uncertain.
7. Monitor patient in a neuroscience intensive care unit (NICU) after treatment.

ANGIOLINGUAL EDEMA ASSOCIATED WITH IV TPA ADMINISTRATION

A. Increased risk in patients on angiotensin-converting enzyme inhibitors (ACEIs)
B. Maintain airway.
  1. Endotracheal intubation may not be necessary if edema is limited to anterior tongue and lips.
  2. Edema involving larynx, palate, floor of mouth, or oropharynx with rapid progression (within 30 minutes) poses higher risk of requiring intubation.
  3. Awake fiberoptic intubation is optimal. Nasal-tracheal intubation may be required though poses risk of epistaxis post-tPA. Cricothyroidotomy is rarely needed and also problematic post-IV tPA.
C. Discontinue IV tPA infusion and hold ACEI.
D. Give IV methylprednisolone (IVMP) 125 mg, and diphenhydramine 50 mg IV.
E. Supportive care.

MALIGNANT CEREBRAL EDEMA

A. Associated factors include NIHSS above 20 (left hemispheric stroke) compared to above 15 (right hemispheric stroke), ICA terminus occlusion, impaired consciousness, headache, nausea/vomiting, leukocytosis, imaging 50% or greater MCA territory involvement on imaging, and additional involvement of ACA and PCA territories.
B. Decompressive hemicraniectomy within 48 hours after symptoms onset combined with best medical management in patients 18 to 60 years old with NIHSS 15 or higher, decreased level of consciousness, intact pupil reactivity, and at least 50% involvement of MCA territory on CT improves outcomes compared to best medical management alone.
  1. Fronto-temporo-parietal decompressive hemicraniectomy and durotomy at least 12 cm in diameter with extension to the floor of the middle cranial fossa with preservation of the superficial temporal artery and facial nerve branches.
  2. Mortality. 28% surgical versus 78% conservative.
  3. Functional outcome.
    a. mRS 1 to 4 at 12 months: 75% surgical versus 24% conservative.
    b. mRS 1 to 3 at 12 months: 43% surgical versus 21% conservative.
  4. Number needed to treat (NNT).
    a. mRS 0 to 4: 2
    b. mRS 0 to 3: 3
    c. Survival: 2
C. Decompressive hemicraniectomy within 48 hours in patients 61 to 82 years old increases survival and decreases severe disability.
  1. Mortality: 43% surgical versus 76% conservative
  2. Functional outcome.
    a. mRS 0 to 2: 0% surgical versus 0% conservative
    b. mRS 3 to 4: 38% surgical versus 16% conservative
  3. NNT.
    a. mRS 3 to 4: 4.5
    b. Survival: 3

MANAGEMENT OF INTRACRANIAL BLEEDING AFTER THROMBOLYTIC THERAPY

A. No evidence-based guidelines
B. Stop thrombolytic infusion.
C. CBC, PT/INR, aPTT, fibrinogen, and type and cross-match
D. STAT head CT
E. Cryoprecipitate (includes factor VIII): two adult doses infused over 10 to 30 minutes.
F. Platelets. One adult dose infused over 10 to 30 minutes.
G. Consider tranexamic acid. 1,000 mg IV infused over 10 minutes OR epsilon-aminocaproic acid 4-5 grams over 1 hour, followed by 1 gram IV until bleeding is controlled.
H. Consider hematology and neurosurgery consultations.
I. Supportive therapy including ICP, CPP, MAP, temperature, and glucose control.

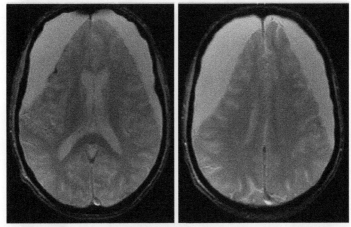

FIGURE 63.6 Axial gradient echo MRI shows large bilateral chronic SDHs. The right-sided SDH is slightly larger than the left. There is approximately 2 mm of right-to-left subfalcine shift. There is also evidence of previous hemorrhage along the lateral cortical surface of the right frontal lobe. The patient was an 83-year-old man with atrial fibrillation, on warfarin, who reported a subacute history of memory loss. INR on admission was 2.4. INR, international normalized ratio; MRI, magnetic resonance imaging; SDH, subdural hematoma.

MANAGEMENT OF INTRACRANIAL BLEEDING ASSOCIATED WITH WARFARIN

A. Discontinue warfarin (Figs. 63.6 and 63.7).
B. Vitamin K 10 mg slow IV injection
C. Four-factor (II, VII, IX, and X) prothrombin complex concentrate (PCC): 25 to 50 units per kg body weight based on INR *or* fresh frozen plasma 10 to 15 mL/kg
D. Rapid reversal is crucial.
E. Consider neurosurgery consultation.
F. Recombinant FVIIa not routinely recommended.

MANAGEMENT OF INTRACRANIAL BLEEDING ASSOCIATED WITH HEPARIN

A. Discontinue heparin.
B. Protamine sulfate. 1 mg/100 U of heparin administered in the preceding 4 hours infusion not to exceed 50 mg every 10 minutes. Adjust dose according to elapsed time from last heparin dose:
   1. 20 to 60 minutes. 0.5 to 0.75 mg/100 U of heparin.
   2. 60 to 120 minutes. 0.375 to 0.5 mg/100 U of heparin.
   3. More than 120 minutes. 0.25 to 0.375 mg/100 U of heparin.

MANAGEMENT OF INTRACRANIAL BLEEDING ASSOCIATED WITH NOVEL ORAL ANTICOAGULANTS

A. Stop novel oral anticoagulants (NOAC).
B. Check PT, INR, PTT, fibrinogen, and platelet count.
C. Treatment.
   1. Direct thrombin inhibitor (e.g., dabigatran). Four-factor PCC. Consider hemodialysis and activated charcoal if ingested within 2 hours. A fast acting antidote Idaruzizumab (Praxbind) has been recently approved by the US FDA.
   2. Anti-Xa agent (e.g., rivaroxaban, apixaban, edoxaban). Four-factor PCC. Consider activated charcoal within 3 hours for apixaban and edoxaban and up to 8 hours for rivaroxaban.
D. Other specific antidotes are currently in development.

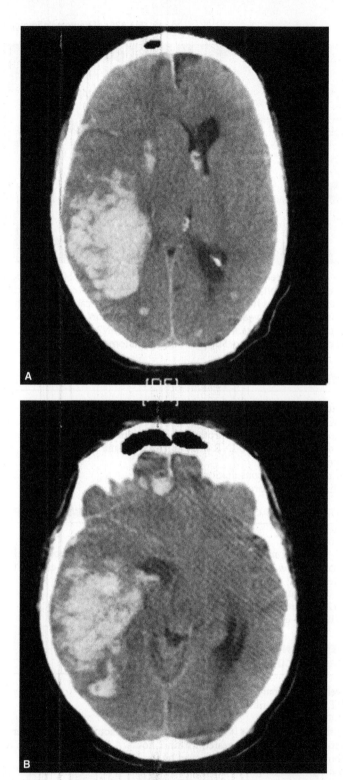

FIGURE 63.7 CT brain without contrast. Right temporo-parietal warfarin-related ICH with evidence of subfalcine and transtentorial herniation. CT, computed tomography; ICH, intracerebral hemorrhage.

SUBARACHNOID HEMORRHAGE

A. CT brain.
 1. Consider LP and MRI, if head CT is normal, depending on interval from onset.
 2. CT is more than 95% sensitive for SAH within 24 hours but rapidly decreases thereafter. CSF xanthochromia can take 12 hours to develop and distinguishing traumatic LP from SAH within 12 hours can be difficult.
 3. MRI is highly sensitive for subacute SAH and can reveal alternate diagnosis for thunderclap headache.
B. Neurosurgery and neuroendovascular consultation (clipping versus coiling)
C. Emergent CSF diversion with ventriculostomy if obstructive hydrocephalus present
 1. Vascular imaging with CTA or four-vessel catheter angiography followed by aneurysm treatment within 24 hours
  a. If renal insufficiency.
   (1) Normal saline 1 mL/kg/hour before and after angiography.
   (2) Consider acetylcysteine 600 mg enteral twice daily for 2 days.
D. Maintain normotension for unsecured aneurysm. Nicardipine and labetalol are preferred. Induced hypertension after aneurysm treatment may be necessary if delayed ischemic neurologic deficit develops.
E. Avoid hypotension and hypovolemia.
F. Enteral nimodipine 60 mg every 4 hours or 30 mg every 2 hours for 21 days if tolerated
G. Frequent neurologic assessments, analgesics, and stool softeners
H. AED if seizures occur.
I. Manage elevated ICP if present.
J. VTE prophylaxis.
 1. Pneumatic compression devices
 2. Consider SQ unfractionated heparin (UFH) 5,000 units every 8 or 12 hours, 24 hours after aneurysm secured.
K. Manage complications such as rebleeding, vasospasm, delayed cerebral ischemia, respiratory failure, cardiomyopathy, dysrhythmias, fevers, and hyponatremia.
 1. Antifibrinolytic therapy (epsilon aminocaproic acid or tranexamic acid) reduces risk of rebleeding but increases risk of cerebral ischemia and is reasonable if immediate aneurysm treatment not feasible.

CEREBELLAR HEMORRHAGE

A. ABCs. Airway, breathing, and circulation
B. Consider neurosurgery consultation (Figs. 63.8 and 63.9).
C. Emergent craniotomy with hematoma removal in patients with neurologic deterioration, brainstem compression, or obstructive hydrocephalus
D. Ventriculostomy placement for obstructive hydrocephalus may precipitate upward herniation. Recommend as an adjunct to surgical decompression.

INTRACEREBRAL HEMORRHAGE AND INTRAVENTRICULAR HEMORRHAGE

A. Intracerebral hemorrhage (ICH) represents 10% to 12% of all strokes.
B. Deep ICH (basal ganglia, thalamus, pons, and cerebellum) is commonly due to chronic hypertension.
C. Lobar ICH in elderly patients is commonly due to cerebral amyloid angiopathy.
D. ICH growth can occur within the first 6 hours.
E. Intraventricular hemorrhage (IVH) occurs in 40% of primary ICH and 15% of aneurysmal SAH (Fig. 63.10).
F. IVH with or without hydrocephalus is a predictor of poor outcome. Estimated 30-day mortality is 40% to 80%.
G. IVH can result in elevated ICP, decreased CPP, and if severe, herniation and death.
H. Intubate for depressed level of consciousness.

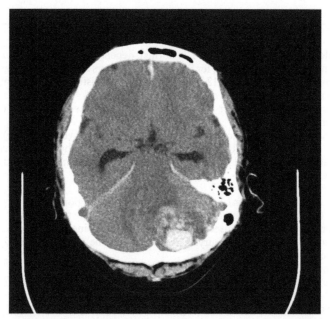

FIGURE 63.8 CT head without contrast demonstrates acute intraparenchymal hemorrhage of the left cerebellar hemisphere with effacement of the fourth ventricle and subsequent hydrocephalus of the third and lateral ventricles. The patient underwent placement of a right frontal ventriculostomy and a suboccipital craniectomy with bilateral decompression and removal of intracerebellar clot. CT, computed tomography.

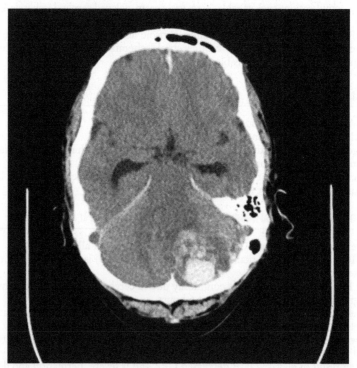

FIGURE 63.9 CT brain without contrast. Left cerebellar hemorrhage with mass effect and effacement of the fourth ventricle and resulting obstructive hydrocephalus. CT, computed tomography.

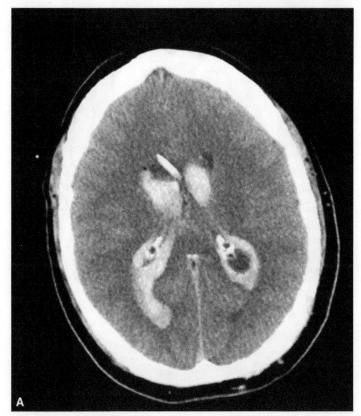

FIGURE 63.10 CT brain without contrast. Primary IVH with obstructive hydrocephalus. CT, computed tomography; IVH, intraventricular hemorrhage.

I. Ventriculostomy placement for patients with obstructive hydrocephalus. Check PT/INR, aPTT, and platelet count. Correct coagulopathy prior to ventriculostomy placement (see sections Malignant Cerebral Edema, Management of Intracranial Bleeding After Thrombolytic Therapy, and Management of Intracranial Bleeding with Warfin).

J. ICP control (see section Elevated Intracranial Pressure) if elevated despite CSF diversion

K. Consider additional brain (e.g., MRI) and vascular imaging to assess for bleeding source.

L. The efficacy of intraventricular tPA for clot lysis is uncertain but appears safe and may be reasonable in selected circumstances. Clinical trials are ongoing.
   1. Avoid in setting of unsecured aneurysms, vascular malformations, clotting disorders, hemorrhage instability, and within 48 hours of craniotomy.
   2. Consider if IVH involves greater than 30% of one of the lateral ventricles and/or the third or fourth ventricle and impaired consciousness.
   3. Dosing. 1 mg every 8 hours up to 12 doses or clearance of IVH from third and fourth ventricle.
   4. Administration. Withdraw CSF volume equivalent to volume of alteplase to be administered followed by 1 to 1.5 mL preservative-free saline flush.
   5. Clamp ventricular catheter for 2 hours. Unclamp if ICP rises above 25 mm Hg and drain 2 cc of CSF. Reclamp if ICP normalizes.

M. BP control. SBP below 140 mm Hg is safe and reasonable for ICH although no data support a target BP for isolated IVH.

N. Avoid hyperglycemia and hypoglycemia; treat fever; and initiate VTE prophylaxis within 48 hours of ICH/IVH stability.

O. AED for seizures. Prophylactic AED not recommended. Consider continuous EEG monitoring for patients with impaired consciousness out of proportion to anatomic injury.

P. Surgical evacuation for non-life-threatening ICH is not routinely recommended.

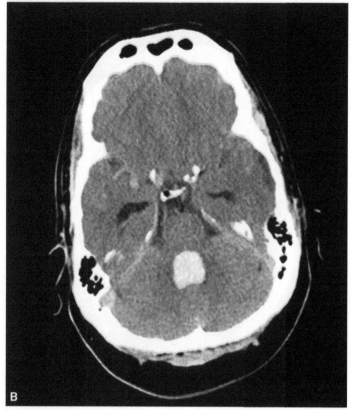

FIGURE 63.10 *(continued)*

METASTATIC EPIDURAL SPINAL CORD COMPRESSION

A. Emergent gadolinium-enhanced MRI of the spine
B. If MRI not feasible—CT myelography
C. Dexamethasone. Optimal dose uncertain. Boluses 16 to 100 mg IV have been used followed by 4 mg IV every 6 hours. Higher doses are not proven to be more effective and can lead to GI bleeding or perforation, psychosis, or sepsis.
D. Consider urgent radiation therapy within 24 hours.
E. Consider chemotherapy for chemosensitive tumors.
F. Consider surgical intervention.
   1. If worsening deficits during or following radiotherapy
   2. If radiation-resistant tumor
   3. If spinal instability, laminectomy is not recommended as it may destabilize spine.
G. Pain control with opioids
H. VTE prophylaxis
I. Bowel regimen.

SPINAL CORD INJURY

A. Central cord syndrome is the most common form of incomplete spinal cord injury (SCI).
   1. Traumatic hyperextension in patients with long-standing cervical spondylosis is the most frequent etiology (Fig. 63.11).

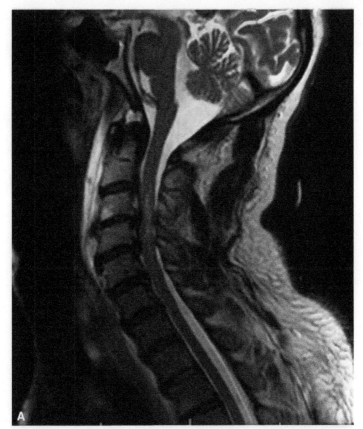

FIGURE 63.11 MRI cervical spine: T2-weighted sagittal image. C3–C4, C4–C5 disc herniations associated with underlying mild cervical canal stenosis causing spinal cord compression in a patient with central cord syndrome. MRI, magnetic resonance imaging.

    2. Other associations.
        a. Cervical spine fracture dislocations
        b. Congenital or acquired cervical canal stenosis
        c. Central spinal cord bleeding
    3. Disproportionate upper motor neuron pattern of weakness. Upper limbs are more affected than lower limbs.
    4. Muscle stretch reflexes are initially absent.
    5. Bladder dysfunction is common.
    6. Variable sensory loss below injury level
    7. Surgery is rarely indicated.
    8. Favorable prognosis in patients younger than 70 years without comorbidities
B. Other SCI. Transverse myelitis, Brown-Séquard (hemicord) syndrome, anterior spinal artery syndrome, posterior cord syndrome
C. Airway management for high cervical injury
D. Fluid resuscitation and vasopressor support with dopamine for neurogenic shock
E. Consider maintaining MAP above 85 mm Hg for the first 7 days.
F. Corticosteroids are not recommended by SCI guidelines.
    1. No class I or II evidence supporting clinical benefit of high-dose IVMP.
    2. High-dose IVMP associated with harmful side effects including wound infections, hyperglycemia, GI bleeding, myopathy, and increased mortality independent of injury severity

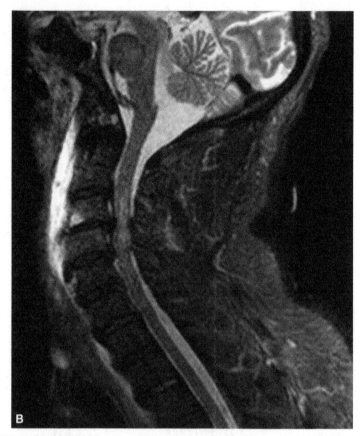

FIGURE 63.11 *(continued)*

G. Utility of hypothermia is uncertain.
H. Initiate VTE prophylaxis within 72 hours and continue for at least 3 months.
   1. Low-molecular-weight heparin
   2. Low-dose SQ UFH *plus* electrical stimulation or pneumatic compression boots
   3. Low-dose heparin or oral anticoagulation alone is not recommended (level II).
   4. Inferior vena cava filters are not recommended unless a patient has a contraindication to or fails pharmacologic prophylaxis.
   5. GI prophylaxis with proton-pump inhibitor or H2 blocker.

ACUTE CAUDA EQUINA SYNDROME

A. Emergent gadolinium-enhanced MRI lumbosacral spine
B. Bladder catheterization for urinary retention. Check serial post–void urinary residual if catheter has not been placed.
C. Analgesics, muscle relaxants (e.g., diazepam, baclofen)
D. Early surgical decompression within 24 hours
E. Radiation/chemotherapy for neoplastic etiologies
F. Intravenous steroids can be used for metastatic etiologies but otherwise have not been shown to improve outcome.
G. Physical and occupational therapy
H. Bowel regimen

SPINAL CORD DYSREFLEXIA

A. Occurs in up to 70% after SCI typically within 4 months and in those with injury above the sixth thoracic level. Commonly follows acute spinal shock.
B. Clinical features include SBP change by 20% or greater associated with change in pulse, sweating and piloerection above the injury level, facial flushing, headache, visual changes, anxiety, nausea, and nasal congestion. It can lead to posterior reversible encephalopathy syndrome, ICH, SAH, seizures, arrhythmia, pulmonary edema, retinal bleeding, coma, and death if untreated.
C. Nonpharmacologic management.
   1. Place patient in an upright position with legs lowered.
   2. Avoid constrictive garments or devices.
   3. Minimize precipitating stimuli including noxious stimuli below the injury level, bladder distention, bowel impaction, pressure ulcers, infection, urologic and endoscopic procedures, sympathomimetic agents, and sildenafil citrate.
D. Pharmacologic management if nonpharmacologic measures fail and SBP above 150 mm Hg. Utilize antihypertensive with rapid onset and short duration. Calcium-channel blockers, ACEIs, and nitrates are commonly used.

GUILLAIN–BARRÉ SYNDROME

A. Clinical features. Ascending areflexic weakness is common. Respiratory and bulbar muscles are frequently involved. Objective sensory loss is typically absent but lower extremity radicular distribution paresthesias/dysesthesias are commonly reported.
B. Workup.
   1. Nerve conduction studies including F waves
   2. CSF for albuminocytologic dissociation
C. Management.
   1. Endotracheal intubation if forced vital capacity (FVC) less than 15 mL/kg and/or negative inspiratory force (NIF) weaker than -25 cm H_2O
   2. Monitor for autonomic disturbances.
   3. Plasma exchange (PLEX) 200 to 250 mL/kg for 5 exchanges over 1 to 2 weeks *or* intravenous immunoglobulin (IVIG) 0.4 g/kg IV per day for 5 days.

MYASTHENIC CRISIS

A. Clinical features. Fatigable weakness. Ocular, bulbar, and respiratory muscles are frequently involved.
B. Workup.
   1. Neurophysiologic studies. Repetitive stimulation, single-fiber electromyography
   2. Serum acetylcholine receptor antibodies
   3. Edrophonium testing is not commonly performed for safety concerns.
C. Management.
   1. Closely monitor motor weakness, bulbar weakness, and respiration.
   2. Initiate noninvasive ventilation early. Intubate and mechanically ventilate when FVC is less than 15 mL/kg and/or NIF is < 25 cm H_2O or there is difficulty controlling secretions. Interpret VC and NIF with caution as poor oral seal on spirometer can adversely affect readings. Continuous end-tidal capnography may be useful.
   3. Assess for cholinergic signs and symptoms. Discontinue anticholinesterase if there is any concern for cholinergic toxicity.
   4. Avoid all drugs with anticholinergic properties.
   5. Manage concurrent infections.
   6. Administer PLEX every other day for 5 or more sessions depending on response *or* IVIG 0.4 g/kg IV daily for 5 days.
   7. Consider adjunctive immunosuppression.
   8. Monitor closely when initiating corticosteroids as early deterioration can occur. It is less of a concern if initiating concomitantly with PLEX or IVIG.

ACUTE DYSTONIC REACTION

A. Stop causative agent.
B. Diphenhydramine 50 mg IV.
C. Benztropine 2 mg IV.
D. Typically follow with oral anticholinergic agents such as benztropine 1 to 2 mg twice daily for 1 to 2 weeks, especially if due to long-acting dopamine receptor blocking agent.

NEUROLEPTIC MALIGNANT SYNDROME

A. Clinical features. Hyperthermia, rigidity, altered mental status, dysautonomia, elevated creatine kinase and transaminases and leukocytosis.
B. Management.
1. Immediately withdraw neuroleptics or dopamine-depleting agents or reinstitute previously withdrawn dopaminergic therapy.
2. Hydrate and maintain adequate urine flow.
3. Alkalinize urine if myoglobinuria is present.
4. Lower elevated body temperature.
5. Administer bromocriptine 2.5 to 5 mg four times daily. Increase dose until response occurs (maximum 50 mg daily).
6. Administer dantrolene 1 to 10 mg/kg daily in divided doses.
7. Other possible treatments include amantadine, levodopa, and carbamazepine.
8. If severe psychosis occurs during treatment, consider electroconvulsive therapy.

ACUTE SEROTONIN SYNDROME

A. Clinical features: Similar to neuroleptic malignant syndrome. Adventitial movements such as tremor, chorea, and myoclonus are common.
B. Management.
1. Discontinue serotonergic drugs.
2. Administer benzodiazepines—especially for agitation.
3. Administer cyproheptadine 12 to 32 mg daily. Consider initial dose in adults of 12 mg and maintenance dose of 8 mg every 6 hours.
4. Other possible treatments include propranolol, chlorpromazine, and methysergide (not available in the United States).
5. Monitor for seizures, arrhythmias, rhabdomyolysis, renal injury, hyperthermia, and coagulopathy.

GIANT CELL ARTERITIS (TEMPORAL ARTERITIS)

A. Clinical features. Unilateral or bilateral vision loss, jaw or tongue claudication, scalp tenderness, fever, and malaise.
B. Workup.
1. STAT ESR and CRP
2. Long-segment superficial temporal artery biopsy
C. Management. Initiate empiric oral prednisone 1 to 2 mg/kg daily or methylprednisolone 1 g IV daily for 3 days followed by oral prednisone 1 mg/kg daily, especially if there are visual symptoms or visual loss. Do not wait for biopsy confirmation to start treatment.

CENTRAL RETINAL ARTERY OCCLUSION

A. Four classifications.
1. Non-arteritic permanent central retinal artery occlusion (CRAO), which accounts for 2/3 of all CRAO
2. Non-arteritic transient CRAO, which accounts for 15% of all CRAO and has the best prognosis

3. Non-arteritic CRAO with cilioretinal sparing
4. Arteritic CRAO (e.g., giant cell arteritis), which accounts for <5% of all CRAO.

B. Management.
   1. No consensus.
   2. Treat hypertension, hyperglycemia, and hyperlipidemia. Avoid tobacco use.
   3. Pharmacologic treatment:
      a. Vasodilators. Pentoxyphylline, sublingual isosorbide dinitrite, hyperbaric oxygen, inhalation of carbogen, calcium-channel blockers, retrobulbar injection of papaverine or tolazoline, prostaglandin E1, CO_2 rebreathing, atropine, acetylcholine, lidocaine hydrochloride.
      b. Mannitol 1.5 to 2 g/ kg IV over 30 to 60 minutes
      c. Acetazolamide 250 to 500 mg IV four times daily for 24 hours
      d. IVMP
      e. Antiplatelet or anticoagulant agents
      f. Topical timolol 0.5% one eye drop in affected eye if elevated intraocular pressure
   4. Surgical treatment.
      a. Anterior chamber paracentesis
      b. Neodymium:yttrium-aluminum-garnet laser embolectomy
      c. Pars plana vitrectomy
   5. Ocular massage to dislodge embolus from central retinal artery
   6. Hemodilution
   7. Thrombolysis is not supported by randomized clinical trials.

WERNICKE'S ENCEPHALOPATHY

A. Thiamine deficiency state associated with chronic alcoholism, hyperemesis gravidarum, starvation, GI malignancies, pyloric stenosis, anorexia nervosa, inappropriate parenteral nutrition, digitalis intoxication, chronic hemodialysis, bariatric surgery, and thyrotoxicosis
B. Clinical features. acute confusion, ataxia, and ocular findings including nystagmus and gaze paresis.
C. Management.
   1. Administer thiamine 500 mg IV three times daily for 2 to 3 days. If there is partial response, continue 250 mg parenteral for 5 days.
   2. Avoid glucose without thiamine.

PITUITARY TUMOR APOPLEXY

A. Clinical features: Thunderclap headache, diplopia (cranial nerve III, IV, and VI palsies), decreased visual acuity, visual field defects (temporal or bitemporal hemianopsia), impaired consciousness, nausea/vomiting (Fig. 63.12A and B).
B. Precipitating and associated factors. Acute pituitary hemorrhage or infarct, head trauma, hypotension, anticoagulation, dopamine agonist use, pituitary dynamic testing thyrotropin-releasing hormone (TRH), corticotropin-releasing hormone (CRH), gonadotropin-releasing hormone (GNRH), insulin-induced hypoglycemia), history of hypertension or pituitary irradiation.
C. Workup. STAT MRI brain or pituitary CT scan if MRI cannot be performed.
D. Management.
   1. Hemodynamic resuscitation with fluids, vasopressors, and hydrocortisone 200 mg IV once followed by 50 mg IV four times daily or 100 mg IV thrice daily
   2. Endocrinology, neurosurgery, ophthalmology consultation
   3. Vascular imaging if concern for aneurysm
   4. Endocrine assessment. Serum electrolytes, renal function tests, PT (INR), aPTT, CBC, random cortisol, prolactin, free T4, TSH, Insulin-like growth factor 1 (IGF-1), IGF-1, growth hormone, luteinizing hormone, follicle-stimulating hormone, testosterone in men, estradiol in women
   5. Thyroid hormone replacement if deficient

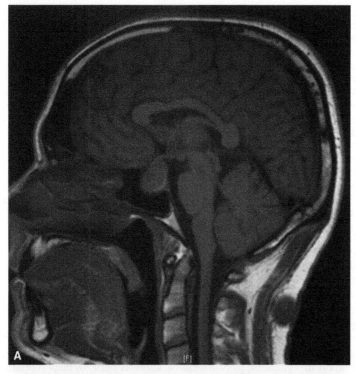

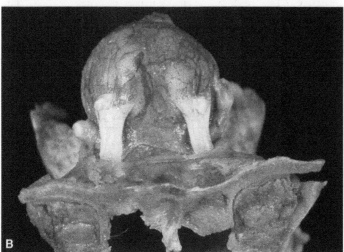

FIGURE 63.12 **A:** MRI brain demonstrating pituitary apoplexy. **B:** Pituitary apoplexy. MRI, magnetic resonance imaging. (See color plates.)

6. Indications for empiric steroids:
   a. Hemodynamic instability (see Pituitary Tumor Apoplexy)
   b. Altered consciousness
   c. Reduced visual acuity or severe visual defects
7. Urgent surgical trans-sphenoidal decompression for patients with severe neuro-opthalmologic symptoms if no contraindications. Surgery is optimal when performed within 7 days of onset.

8. Conservative management for patients with absent or mild neuro-opthalmologic symptoms including ocular palsies in the absence of visual field defects or visual acuity deficits, or early improvement of visual symptoms
9. Postoperative management.
   a. Check electrolytes, renal function, and plasma and urine osmolality if diabetes insipidus is suspected.
   b. Monitor for CSF leak, cortisol deficiency, visual loss, and meningitis.
10. Formal visual field testing when clinically stable.

POSTERIOR REVERSIBLE ENCEPHALOPATHY SYNDROME

A. Clinical features. Headache, visual changes, seizures, nausea/vomiting, and occasional sensorimotor deficits
B. Workup. MRI brain demonstrates posterior hemispheric white matter edema. Typically spares cortex. Can involve cerebellum and brainstem and occasionally frontal lobes. CT if MRI not feasible.
C. Management.
   1. Eliminate or treat precipitating causes such as hypertension, immunosuppressant medications, eclampsia, uremia, sepsis, and autoimmune disorders.
   2. Administer AED for seizures
   3. Treat hypertension. Do not decrease by more than 25% of presenting MAP within the first few hours.

Key Points

- This chapter is intended to serve as a uptodate quick reference guide to an audience composed of healthcare practitioners, including neurologists, neurosurgeons, critical care physicians, emergency medicine physicians, and nurses, involved in the care of neurologic and neurosurgical critically ill patients.
- Algorithms in accord with accepted evidence-based standards, highlighting concise and practical diagnostic testing and management strategies for a comprehensive index of neurologic and neurosurgical emergencies, are provided within this chapter.
- Radiologic images, histologic slides, and video highlighting different disease states discussed within this chapter are also provided, further contributing to a practitioner's rapid diagnosis and treatment of this patient population.

Recommended Readings

Agrawal A, Jake T, Pandit L, et al. A review of subdural empyema and its management. *Infect Dis Clin Pract.* 2007;15(3):149–153.

Aiyagari V, Ruland S, Gorelick PB. Chapter 40: Neurogenic hypertension including hypertension following stroke and with spinal cord injury. In: Floege J, Johnson R, Feehally J, eds. *Comprehensive Clinical Nephrology.* 5th ed. Philadelphia, PA: Saunders Publishing; 2015.

Aldrich, EM, Lee AW, Chen CS, et al. Local intraarterial fibrinolysis administered in aliquots for the treatment of central retinal artery occlusion: the Johns Hopkins Hospital experience. *Stroke.* 2008;39(6):1746–1750.

Bansal V, Ruland S, Aiyagari V. Chapter 2: Disorders of consciousness. In: Testai FD, Gorelick PB, eds. *Hankey's Clinical Neurology.* 2nd ed. Boca Raton, FL: CRC Press; 2014.

Beckham JD, Tyler KL. Initial management of acute bacterial meningitis in adults: summary of IDSA guidelines. *Rev Neurol Dis.* 2006;3(2):57–60.

Bhatia K, Jones NS. Septic cavernous sinus thrombosis secondary to sinusitis: are anticoagulants indicated? A review of the literature. *J Laryngol Otol.* 2002;116(9):667–676.

Biller J, Asconapé J, Kase CS, et al. Iatrogenic neurology. *Continuum.* 2001;7:1–224.

Biousse V, Calvetti O, Bruce BB, et al. Thrombolysis for central retinal artery occlusion. *J Neuroophthalmol.* 2007;27(3):215–230.

Bleck TP. Status epilepticus and the use of continuous EEG monitoring in the intensive care unit. *Continuum (Minneap Minn)*. 2012;18(3):560–578.

Bratton SL, Chesnut RM, Ghajar J, et al. Guidelines for the management of severe traumatic brain injury. *J Neurotrauma*. 2007;24:S1–S106.

Caroff SN, Campbell EC, Sullivan KA. Neuroleptic malignant syndrome in elderly patients. *Expert Rev Neurother*. 2007;7(4):423–431.

Chamberlain MC, Kornanik PA. Epidural spinal cord compression: a single institution's retrospective experience. *Neuro-oncology*. 2000;192:120–123.

Connolly ES, Rabinstein AA, Carhuapoma JR, et al. Guidelines for the management of aneurysmal subarachnoid hemorrhage a guideline for healthcare professionals from the American Heart Association/American Stroke Association. *Stroke*. 2012;43(6):1711–1737.

Cugati S, Varma DD, Chen CS, et al. Treatment options for central retinal artery occlusion. *Curr Treat Options Neurol*. 2013;15(1):63–77.

Dhall SS, Hadley MN, Aarabi B, et al. Deep venous thrombosis and thromboembolism in patients with cervical spinal cord injuries. *Neurosurgery*. 2013;72(suppl 2):244–254.

Dietrich U, Maschke M, Dorfler A, et al. MRI of intracranial toxoplasmosis after bone marrow transplantation. *Neuroradiology*. 2000;42(1):14–18.

Diringer MN, Zazulia AR. Osmotic therapy: fact and fiction. *Neurocrit Care*. 2004;1:219–233.

Dressler D, Benecke R. Diagnosis and management of acute movement disorders. *J Neurol*. 2005;252(11):1299–1306.

Edlow JA, Rabinstein A, Traub SJ, et al. Diagnosis of reversible causes of coma. *Lancet*. 2014;384(9959):2064–2076.

Enriquez A, Lip GY, Baranchuk A. Anticoagulation reversal in the era of the non-vitamin K oral anticoagulants. *Europace*. 2016;18(7):955–964.

Fugate JE, Kalimullah EA, Wijdicks EF. Angioedema after tPA: what neurointensivists should know. *Neurocrit Care*. 2012;16(3):440–443.

Fugate JE, Rabinstein AA. Posterior reversible encephalopathy syndrome: clinical and radiological manifestations, pathophysiology, and outstanding questions. *Lancet Neurol*. 2015;14(9):914–925.

Gardner A, Gardner E, Morley T. Cauda equina syndrome: a review of the current clinical and medico-legal position. *Eur Spine J*. 2011;20(5):690–697.

Greenlee JE. Subdural Empyema. *Curr Treat Options Neurol*. 2003;5(1):13–22.

Hattenbach LO, Kuhli-Hattenbach C, Scharrer I, et al. Intravenous thrombolysis with low-dose recombinant tissue plasminogen activator in central retinal artery occlusion. *Am J Ophthalmol*. 2008;146(5):700–706.

Hemphill JC, Greenberg SM, Anderson CS, et al. Guidelines for the management of spontaneous intracerebral hemorrhage a guideline for healthcare professionals from the American Heart Association/American Stroke Association. *Stroke*. 2015;46(7):2032–2060. doi:10.1161/STR-0000000000000069.

Hurlbert RJ, Hadley MN, Walters BC, et al. Pharmacological therapy for acute spinal cord injury. *Neurosurgery*. 2013;72(suppl 2):93–105.

Jauch EC, Saver JL, Adams HP Jr, et al. Guidelines for the early management of patients with acute ischemic stroke: a guideline for healthcare professionals from the American Heart Association/American Stroke Association. *Stroke*. 2015;44(3):870–947.

Johnson RT, Griffin JW, eds. *Current Therapy in Neurologic Disease*. 5th ed. St Louis, MO: Mosby; 1997.

Krassioukov A, Warburton DE, Teasell R, et al; Spinal Cord Injury Rehabilitation Evidence Research. A systematic review of the management of autonomic dysreflexia after spinal cord injury. *Arch Phys Med Rehabil*. 2009;90(4):682–695.

Lee EQ. Nervous system metastases from systemic cancer. *Continuum*. 2015;21(2 Neuro-oncology):415–428.

Lee GT, Antelo F, Mlikotic A. Cerebral toxoplasmosis. *Radiographics*. 2009;29(4):1200–1205.

Mathisen GE, Johnson JP. Brain abscess. *Clin Infect Dis*. 1997;25(4):763–779.

Munhoz RP, Scorr LM, Factor SA. Movement disorders emergencies. *Curr Opin Neurol*. 2015;28(4):406–412.

Nakagawa K, Smith WS (2011). Evaluation and management of increased intracranial pressure. *Continuum*. 2011;17(5 Neurologic Consultation in the Hospital):1077–1093.

Nawar RN, AbdelMannan D, Selman WR, et al. Pituitary tumor apoplexy: a review. *J Intensive Care Med*. 2008;23(2):75–90.

Noble J, Weizblit N, Baerlocher MO, et al. Intra-arterial thrombolysis for central retinal artery occlusion: a systematic review. *Br J Ophthalmol*. 2008;92(5):588–593.

Orjuela K, Ruland SD. Hypertensive encephalopathy and posterior reversible encephalopathy syndrome. In: Aiyagari V, Gorelick PB, eds. *Hypertension and Stroke: Pathophysiology and Management*. New York, NY: Humana Press; 2015.

Overturf G. Defining bacterial meningitis and other infections of the central nervous system. *Pediatr Crit Care Med*. 2005;6(3):S14–S18.

Pollack, Jr CV, Reilly PA, Eikelboom J, et al. Idarucizumab for Dabigatran Reversal. *N Engl J Med*. 2015;373:511–520.

Powers WJ, Derdeyn CP, Biller J, et al; American Heart Association Stroke. 2015 AHA/ASA Focused Update of the 2013 guidelines for the early management of patients with acute ischemic stroke regarding endovascular treatment: a guideline for healthcare professionals from the American Heart Association/American Stroke Association. *Stroke.* 2015;46:000–000. doi:10.1161/STR.0000000000000074.

Qureshi Al, Thurim S, Broderick JP, et al. Spontaneous intracerebral hemorrhage. *N Engl J Med.* 2001;344:1450–1460.

Rabinstein AA, Wijdicks E. *Tough Calls in Acute Neurology.* Boston, MA: Butterworth-Heinemann; 2004.

Radcliff KE, Kepler CK, Delasotta LA, et al. Current management review of thoracolumbar cord syndromes. *Spine J.* 2011;11(9):884–892.

Rajasekaran S, Vanderpump M, Baldeweg S, et al. UK guidelines for the management of pituitary apoplexy. *Clin Endocrinol.* 2011;74(1):9–20.

Robinson C, Ruland S. Chapter 16: Pitfalls in the diagnosis of subarachnoid hemorrhage. In: Biller J, Ferro J eds. *Common Pitfalls in Cerebrovascular Disease.* Cambridge, England; Cambridge Medicine Publishing; 2015.

Roos K, ed. *Central Nervous System Infectious Diseases and Therapy.* New York, NY: Marcel Dekker; 1997.

Ropper AH, ed. *Neurological and Neurosurgical Intensive Care.* 3rd ed. New York, NY: Raven Press; 1993.

Rosovsky RP, Crowther MA. What is the evidence for the off-label use of recombinant Factor VIIa (rFVIIa) in the acute reversal of warfarin? ASH evidence-based review 2008. *Hematology Am Soc Hematol Educ Program.* 2008:36–38. doi:10.1182/asheducation-2008.1.36.

Rossetti AO, Bleck TP. What's new in status epilepticus? *Intensive Care Med.* 2014;40(9):1359–1362.

Sarich TC, Seltzer JH, Berkowitz SD, et al. Novel oral anticoagulants and reversal agents: Considerations for clinical development. *Am Heart J.* 2015;169(6):751–757.

Sharma R, Mohandas K, Cooke RP. Intracranial abscesses: changes in epidemiology and management over five decades in Merseyside. *Infection.* 2009;37:39–43.

Silbergleit R, Durkalski V, Lowenstein D, et al. Intramuscular versus intravenous therapy for prehospital status epilepticus. *N Eng J Med.* 2012;366(7): 591–600.

Stochetti N, Maas AL, Chieregato A, et al. Hyperventilation in head injury: a review. *Chest.* 2005;127:1812–1827.

Temino VM, Peebles RS Jr. The spectrum and treatment of angioedema. *Am J Med.* 2008;121(4):282–286.

Thomson AD, Cook CC, Touguet R, et al. The Royal College of Physicians report on alcohol: guidelines for managing Wernicke's encephalopathy in the accident and Emergency Department. *Alcohol Alcohol.* 2002;37(6):513–521.

Treiman DM, Meyers PD, Walton NY, et al. A comparison of four treatments for generalized convulsive status epilepticus. Veterans Affairs Status Epilepticus Cooperative Study Group. *N Engl J Med.* 1998;339(12):792–798.

Wagner S, Schnippering H, Aschoff A, et al. Suboptimum hemicraniectomy as a cause of additional cerebral lesions in patients with malignant infarcts of the middle cerebral artery. *J Neurosurg.* 2001;94:693–696.

Wasterlain CG, Treiman DM, eds. *Status Epileptic Mechanisms and Management.* Cambridge, MA: MIT Press; 2006.

Wijdicks E, ed. *Neurologic Catastrophes in the Emergency Department.* Boston, MA: Butterworth-Heineman; 2000.

Index

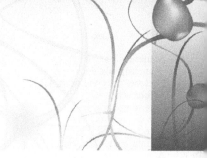

Page numbers with *f* refers to figures and *t* refers to tables.

Abnormal pupils
  anisocoria greater in darkness
    aberrant regeneration of oculomotor
      nerve, 130
    Horner's syndrome, 129–130
    physiologic anisocoria, 130–131
  light-near dissociation, 131
  mechanical anisocoria, 124, 125*f*
  pupil and eyelids, sympathetic
    innervation, 122*f*
  pupil size, 121, 123
  pupillary dilation, 121
  pupillary examination, 123
  pupillary light reflex, 121*f*, 123
  relative afferent pupillary defect, 123–124
  unilateral mydriasis, 124–129
    oculomotor (third cranial) nerve palsy, 125
    pharmacologic mydriasis, 128–129
    tonic pupil (Adie pupil), 125–128
Acephalgic migraine, 118
Acetazolamide, for central sleep apnea, 801
Acetylcholine, 1, 124, 593, 686
Acid maltase deficiency (Pompe's disease),
  681–682
Acoustic reflex thresholds (ARTs), 194
Acquired immunodeficiency syndrome (AIDS).
  See Neurologic complications in AIDS
Acrylamide, as peripheral nervous system
  toxin, 768
Acupuncture, migraine therapy, 697
Acute cauda equina syndrome, 856
Acute confusional state. *See* Confusion, acute
Acute delirium, and CNS toxins, 772–774
Acute disseminated encephalomyelitis
  (ADEM), 448
Acute dystonic reaction, 858
Acute inflammatory demyelinating neuropathy
  (GBS), 666, 670
Acute low back pain
  clinical manifestations and evaluation
    history, 250
    physical examination, 250
  diagnostic approach, 252
  differential diagnosis, 250
  etiology, 249
  serious causes of, 250*t*
  surgical referral, 256
  treatment, 254–255
Acute motor axonal neuropathy (AMAN), 342
Acute neurologic weakness
  acute disseminated encephalomyelitis, 448

Guillain–Barré syndrome, 447–448
  idiopathic transverse myelitis, 448
  infant botulism, 446–447
Acute serotonin syndrome, 858
Acute spinal cord injury, 651–654, 652*t*
Acute transient monocular visual loss (TMVL)
  approach to TMVL, 112
  clinical features, 111–112
  time course, 112
Acute transverse myelitis, 295
Acute vascular lesions
  arterial ischemic stroke, 449–450
  cerebral venous sinus thrombosis, 450
  intracranial hemorrhage., 449
Acyclovir, 610, 611, 633
Adenosine antagonists, 778
Advanced sleep–wake phase disorder (ASWPD),
  102–103, 785–786
AIDS. *See* Neurologic complications in AIDS
Alcoholic neuropathy, 668
Alemtuzumab (Lemtrada), for multiple
  sclerosis, 573
Algorithm
  acute, nontraumatic facial paralysis assessment
    algorithm, 166*f*
  for adult status epilepticus management, 456
  delayed, nontraumatic facial paralysis
    assessment algorithm, 167*f*
  for differential diagnosis of hypokinesia, 329*f*
  eight classical cortical aphasias, 33*f*
  for emergency evaluation of acute stroke, 394
Alpha coma, 413
Alprazolam (Xanax), for tremor, 585
Altered mental status/encephalopathy
  acute liver failure and neurologic sequelae, 452
  hypoxic ischemic encephalopathy, 451
  infectious meningitis and encephalitis,
    450–451
  methotrexate toxicity, 451
  posterior reversible encephalopathy
    syndrome, 451
Aluminum, 775
Alzheimer's disease, 17–19, 30
  aphasia, 30
  congophilic angiopathy, 496
  dementia, 17–19, 397
  end stages of, 464, 468
  and memory loss, 42–43
  sleep–wake disorder, 103
Amantadine (Symmetrel), for Parkinson's
  disease, 576
Amaurotic pupil, 109
American Academy of Sleep Medicine
  (AASM), 781

Amnesia
  anterograde, 44
  causes and conditions, 42t
  functional, 46
  posthypnotic, 46
  posttraumatic, 44
  retrograde, 44
  transient global, 46
Amyloid neuropathy, 671–672
Analgesics, migraine therapy, 698
Andersen's syndrome (or Andersen–Tawil
      syndrome), 677
Anesthesia dolorosa, 159
Angiolingual edema, 848
Anomic aphasia, 35
Anosognosia, dementia in, 602
Anoxia/ischemia, 45
Antalgic gait, 86
Anterior interosseous syndrome, 265
Anterior ischemic optic neuropathy (AION)
  arteritic AION, 114
  Leber's hereditary optic neuropathy, 114, 114f
  nonarteritic AION, 113, 113f
Anterograde amnesia (Learning defects), 44
Anterograde memory, 40–41
Antibiotics
  for bacterial meningitis, 843t
  for botulism, 771
  for vestibular neuronitis and labyrinthitis, 810
Anticholinergic syndrome, 772
Anticholinergics, for Parkinson's disease, 576–577
Anticoagulants, 484–488
Anticonvulsants, 776
  for central pain syndrome, 656
  for complex regional pain syndrome, 730
  for herpes encephalitis, 610–611
  and seizures, 66, 67
Antidepressants
  for chronic pain, 715, 716–717t
  for complex regional pain syndrome, 730
  migraine therapy, 701–702
Antidopaminergic agents, 2
Antiemetics
  migraine therapy, 700
  for vestibular neuronitis and labyrinthitis, 810
Antiepileptics
  for chronic pain, 715
  migraine therapy, 702
Antihistamines, 778
  for vestibular neuronitis and labyrinthitis,
      809–811
Antimicrobial therapy, for bacterial meningitis,
      605–606, 607–608t
Antimicrotubular myopathy, 683
Antiplatelet agents, 483–484
Antivirals
  for herpes encephalitis, 610
  for HIV, 621
  for vestibular neuronitis and labyrinthitis, 810
Anton syndrome, 119
Anxiety, in dementia, 595–596
Apathy, in dementia, 596
Aphasia, 29, 214
  anomic, 35

aprosodia, 35–36
Broca's, 33
clinical manifestations
  auditory comprehension impairment, 30
  nonfluency versus fluency, 30
  paraphasic errors, 30–31
  reading and writing, 31
  repetition impairment, 30
  word-finding difficulty (anomia), 31
conduction, 34
differential diagnosis
  mutism, 37
  thought disorders, 37
etiology, 30
evaluation, 31–32
extrasylvian 34
global, 34
mixed transcortical, 35
National Aphasia Association, 38
pathophysiology, 29
referral, 37–38
striatal-capsular, 35
syndromic diagnosis
  additional classical syndromes, 35–36
  aprosodia, 35–36
  extrasylvian, 34–35
  perisylvian, 33–34
  subcortical aphasia syndromes, 35
thalamic, 35
transcortical motor, 34
transcortical sensory, 34–35
Wernicke's, 33–34
Aphemia (apraxia of speech), 37
Aprosodia, 35–36
Aripiprazole, 13
  for tics, 582
Aristaless homeobox (ARX), 455
Arousal, 52
Arrhythmias, dizziness and vertigo in, 815
Arsenic as peripheral nervous system toxin,
      763–764
Arterial hypertension, 494–496
  emergency management, 506t
Arterial ischemic stroke (AIS), 449–450
Arteriography, 503–504
Ascending reticular activating system (ARAS), 52
Aseptic meningitis, 429, 624
ASPD. See Advanced sleep-wake phase disorder
      (ASWPD)
Aspirin, in stroke, 831
Ataxia
  acute, 440
  chronic nonprogressive, 440
  chronic progressive, 440
  diagnostic studies, 441
  evaluation, 441
  family history
    associated neurologic signs, 322–323
    autosomal-dominant ataxias, 321–322
    autosomal-recessive ataxias, 322
    brain MRI, 323–326, 324f, 325f
  Friedreich ataxia, 322
  history and examination, 318–321
  intermittent, 440

with oculomotor apraxia type 1 and 2, 322
  practical approach, 326
  rare genetic causes, 440–441
  telangiectasia, 322
Ataxic dysarthria, 37, 213
Ataxic gait, 84
Atenolol(Tenormin), for tremor, 585
Atonic seizures, 531
Attention deficit disorder (ADD), 582
Attention-deficit/hyperactivity disorder (ADHD), 432–433
Atypical facial pain, 157–158
Atypical odontalgia, 158
Auditory brainstem response (ABR), 195–196
Auditory steady-state responses (ASSR), 196
Auditory system, 190–191. *See also* Hearing loss
Autism Spectrum Screening Questionnaire (ASSQ), 438
Autonomic disorders
  alpha-synucleinopathies, 363
  differential diagnosis of MSA, 364t
  enteric ganglionitis, 365
  primary autonomic failure, 363–364
Autonomic dysreflexia, 655
Autonomic nervous system (ANS), 347
  blood pressure and heart rate responses, 351t
  clinical features of, 349t
  evaluation
    autonomic testing, 350–352
    electrophysiologic studies, 352
    history, 347
    physical examination, 347
    screening tests, 352
  selected autonomic disorders, 350t
Autonomic neuropathies, 364–365
Autonomic testing, 350–352
Autophagic myopathy, 683
Axillary freckling, 436f
Axonal neuropathy, 663
Azathioprine
  for inflammatory myopathy, 675
  for myasthenia gravis, 689

β-Adrenergic receptor antagonists
  migraine therapy, 701
  for tremor, 585
Baclofen withdrawal, 454
Bacterial meningitis, 605–609, 841–843
Balint's syndrome, 118–119
Barbiturates, migraine therapy, 700
Baroreflex pathways, 348f, 353t
Basilar migraine and migrainous vertigo, 814
Becker's muscular dystrophy, 679, 680
Behavioral therapy, for complex regional pain syndrome, 733
Bell's palsy, 162–163
  in pregnancy, 835
Benign occipital epilepsy, 511
Benign paroxysmal positional vertigo (BPPV), 807–809
Benzodiazepines, 6, 11, 13, 516, 525
  for anticholinergic syndrome, 744
  for epilepsies in children, 516, 525
  for epilepsy in adults, 555

for hallucinogens, 773
for restless legs syndrome, 800
for serotonin syndrome, 773
for spasticity in multiple sclerosis, 564
for status epilepticus, 547
for sympathomimetic syndrome, 772
for tardive dyskinesia, 583
for tremor, 585
for vestibular neuronitis and labyrinthitis, 810
Benztropine (Cogentin), for Parkinson's disease, 576
Bevacizumab, for high-grade gliomas, 739
Binocular visual loss, 116–117
Black widow spider venom, 770
Blink reflex, 143, 150
Botulinum toxin
  for chronic pain, 719
  for dystonia, 584
  injections, for tremor, 585
  for spasticity in multiple sclerosis, 564
Botulism, 342, 693–695, 770–771
  classic, 693–694
  infant, 694–695
  wound, 695
Brachial plexitis (Parsonage-Turner syndrome or neuralgic amyotrophy), 668
Brain abscess, 843–844
Brain attack, 473. *See also* Ischemic cerebrovascular disease
Brain death, 380. *See also* Coma
  assessments to declare, 382t
  coma and, 383
  corneal reflexes, 384
  ethical considerations, 387–388
  etiology, 380–381
  evaluation
    adult guidelines, 381
    apnea testing, 385, 386t
    confirmatory tests, 385–387
    neurologic examination, 384–385
    pediatric guidelines, 381–383
    prerequisites, 383–384
  metabolic parameters, 383
  neuroimaging, 383
  oculocephalic reflexes, 384
  oculovestibular reflexes, 384
  pathophysiology, 381
  pharmacologic interventions, 383
  physiologic parameters, 383–384
  practical problems, 388–389
  requirements, 386t
Brain edema, 482–483
Brain metastases, 750–753
Brain tumor, 221–222, 497–498. *See also* Central nervous system, tumors of
Brainstem auditory evoked potentials (BAEPs), for multiple sclerosis, 568
Branched-chain amino acids, for tardive dyskinesia, 583
Bright light therapy, for circadian rhythm sleep disorders (CRSD), 785–786, 787
Broca's aphasia, 29f, 33, 33f
1-bromopropane as peripheral nervous system toxin, 768

Brown–Séquard syndrome, 295
Bulbar motor neuron disease, 213f
Burning mouth syndrome, 160

Calcitonin gene-related peptide (CGRP)
    mechanism antagonists, migraine
    therapy, 703
Calcium-channel blockers
    for chronic pain, 718
    for complex regional pain syndrome, 731
    migraine therapy, 702
Cancer complications of nervous system,
    750–761
    brain metastases, 750–753, 751f, 752f
    cerebellar toxicity, 760
    cerebral edema, 760
    cerebrovascular complications, 760
    CNS infections, 760
    CSF metastases, 755–757, 756f
    defined, 750
    dural metastasis, 754, 755f, 757
    encephalopathy, 760
    extradural metastases, 754
    leptomeningeal metastasis, 755
    leukoencephalopathy, 760
    neuropathy, 761
    paraneoplastic syndromes, 757–759
    radiotherapy complications, 759–760
    seizures, 760
    spinal cord metastases, 754
    spinal metastases, 753–754, 753f
    surgical complications, 759
Candesartan, migraine therapy, 702
"CANOMAD" syndrome, 422
Capsaicin, for chronic pain, 719
Carbamazepine, 521
Carbon disulfide as peripheral nervous system
    toxin, 768
Carbon monoxide, 774–775, 775–776
Carcinomatous meningitis, 3, 11
Cardiac arrhythmias, 72
Cardiofacial syndrome, 166
Cardiovascular changes in pregnancy, 818
Carnitine-O-palmitoyltransferase II (CPT II)
    deficiency, 681t, 682
Carotid angioplasty and stenting
    (CAS), 488–489
Carotid endarterectomy (CEA), 488
Carotid sinus hypersensitivity, 72, 76
Catatonia, 6
Cauda equina syndrome, 296
Cefepime, 4–5, 10
Central auditory processing disorder, 198
Central cord syndrome, 657, 854–855
Central disorders of hypersomnolence. See
    Hypersomnolence, central disorders of
Central nervous system
    infections of, 605–615
        bacterial meningitis, 605–609
        cryptococcal meningitis, 612–613
        herpes encephalitis, 609–611
        herpes zoster (shingles), 611
        Lyme disease, 611–612
        neurocysticercosis, 614–615

    neurosyphilis in immunocompetent
        patients, 613
    tuberculous meningitis, 613
    lymphoma, 628–629
    toxins in, 772–779
    toxoplasmosis, 626–627
    tuberculosis, 633–635
    tumors of
        high-grade gliomas, 737–740
        low-grade gliomas, 740–742
        medulloblastoma, 746–748
        meningioma, 742–744
        primary CNS lymphomas (PCNSLs),
            745–746
Central pain syndrome, 655–656
Central pontine myelinolysis, 4
Central retinal artery occlusion, 858–859
Central sleep apnea (CSA), 801–802
Central vertigo, 173–174
Cerebellar disorders, and CNS toxins, 776–777
Cerebellar hemorrhage, 851
Cerebellar tremor, 304
Cerebral amyloid angiopathy, 496
Cerebral autoregulation, 482
Cerebral polyopia, 132
Cerebral toxoplasmosis, 845
Cerebral venous sinus thrombosis (CVST), 450
Cerebral venous thrombosis, in pregnancy, 831
Cerebrospinal fluid (CSF) metastases, 755–757
Cerebrovascular disease, in pregnancy,
    829–833, 830–831t. See also Ischemic
    cerebrovascular disease
Channelopathies, 676, 677t
Chemotherapy
    in low-grade gliomas, 742
    in medulloblastoma, 747–748
Chiari malformations, 174, 646
Childhood absence epilepsy, 63
Childhood Autism Rating Scale (CARS), 438
Chloride channel mutations, 677
Cholinergics, 778
Cholinesterase inhibitors (CEIs)
    for dementia, 593
    for myasthenia gravis, 687–688, 687t
Chorda tympanii, 162
Chorea, 581
    definition, 308
    differential diagnosis and evaluation
        adult-onset chorea, 311
        childhood-onset chorea, 311
    etiologic classification
        drug-induced chorea, 309
        genetic choreas, 308–309
        infectious chorea, 309
        metabolic or toxic encephalopathies, 309
        parainfectious and autoimmune
            disorders, 309
        structural basal ganglia lesions, 309
    hyperglycemic-induced hemichorea–
        hemiballismus, 310–311
    neuro-acanthocytosis, 310
    pathophysiology, 309
    PKAN, 310
    Sydenham's chorea, 310

Chorea gravidarum, in pregnancy, 836
Choreic gait, 85
Chronic and recurrent headache, 227, 441
 attributed to substances, 234–235
 Chiari I malformations, 234
 diagnostic studies, 230–231
 examination, 230
 history, 227–230
 Marfan or Ehler–Danlos syndromes, 234
 from nonvascular intracranial disorders,
  233–234
 posttraumatic headache, 231–232
 secondary to cerebrovascular disease, 232–233
 trigeminal autonomic cephalalgias, 237–238
 trigeminal neuralgia, 235
Chronic inflammatory demyelinating neuropathy,
  666–667
Chronic pain. *See* Pain, chronic
Chronic progressive external ophthalmoplegia
  (CPEO), 137
Chronotherapy, for circadian rhythm sleep
  disorders (CRSD), 785
Ciguatera poisoning, 770
Circadian rhythm sleep disorders (CRSD),
  785–787
 bright light therapy, 785–786, 787
 chronotherapy, 785
 course of, 785
 melatonin, 786, 787
 treatment and outcome, 785–786
Circadian rhythm sleep–wake disorders, 102–103
Cisplatin as peripheral nervous system toxin, 767
Classic botulism, 693–694
Clobazam, 523–524
Clonazepam, 523
 in epilepsy, 523
 for REM sleep behavior disorder (RBD), 795
 for tics, 582
 for tremor, 585
Clonidine
 for chronic pain, 719
 for complex regional pain syndrome, 731
 for tics, 582
Clopidogrel, 484
Clorazepate, 523
Clostridium botulinum, 693–695
Cluster headache, 221, 228, 238*t*. *See also*
  Headache
 preventive treatments, 706*t*, 707–708, 708*t*
 therapy and management, 706–709
Coagulation factors, 818
Cobalt as peripheral nervous system toxin, 767
Cocaine or stimulant washout syndrome, 776
Cognitive behavioral therapy, for insomnia,
  782–783, 782–783*t*
Cognitive enrichment, for dementia, 593
Cognitive neurorehabilitation, for dementia,
  593–594
Coma, 52, 840
 and arousal, 52
 ascending reticular activating system, 52
 CNS depression, 775–776
 differential diagnosis, 55–56
 etiology, 55

 evaluation, 52–55
 initial approach to patient, 56
 locked-in syndrome, 55
 management, 56–57
 patient with and without focal findings on
  neurologic examination, 57
 patient with fever or septic syndrome, 56–57
 patient with suspected hemorrhage, 56
 scales, 53*t*
 subarachnoid and cerebral hemorrhage, 52
 toxi-metabolic, 55
Comatose. *See* Coma
Comitant and incomitant, 133
Complex partial seizures of frontal lobe origin, 62
Complex regional pain syndrome, 724–734
 Budapest criteria for, 725*t*
 in children, 733
 clinical presentation, 724, 728–729
 course of, 728–729
 definition and types of, 724
 diagnosis of, 725–727
 differential diagnosis of, 725, 726*t*
 epidemiology of, 727
 interventional therapy, 731–732
 management of, 733
 pathophysiology of, 727–728
 pharmacologic therapy, 730–731
 quantitative sudomotor axon testing, 727
 stages of, 729
 treatment, 729–733, 734
Computed tomography (CT). *See also*
  Neuroimaging
 in acute confusional state, 11*f*, 396–397
 in acute headaches, 393–394
 in acute low back pain, 252
 in acute sensory loss, 299
 in acute stroke, 394
 in aphasia, 32
 in ataxia, 319
 of brain, 501–503, 502*f*, 503*f*
 in cervical spine injury, 392
 in closed head injury, 391–392
 in coma, 56
 in dementia, 17, 397
 in diplopia, 139
 in facial numbness, 150
 in facial weakness, 163, 166
 in gait disturbances, 88
 in headache, 222–223, 231
 in low back pain, 252, 402
 in lumbar disc disease with sciatica, 252
 in lumbar spinal stenosis, 252
 in memory impairment, 49
 in myelopathies, 403–404
 in neck pain, 240, 402
 in Parkinsonism, 373
 in penetrating head injury, 392
 in seizures, 63, 397–399, 398*f*
 in subacute headaches, 394
 in syncope, 78
 in UE pain and paresthesias, 263
 in vascular injury, 392
 in vision loss, 111, 401
COMT inhibitors, for Parkinson's disease, 579

Conduction aphasia, 34
Conductive hearing loss, 197
Confusion, acute, 1
    clinical manifestations, 7–10
    delirium (See Delirium)
    diagnostic testing, 10–12
    differential diagnosis, 6–7
    encephalopathy (See Encephalopathy)
    etiologies, 2–3t
        infections, 5
        metabolic, 3–4
        nutritional, 4
        structural, 3
        toxic, 4–5
    evaluation approach, 11f
    organized medical record review, 10
    pharmacologic management, 13
    prognosis, 13
Congenital facial paralysis, 166
Congenital myasthenia, 692
Connective tissue, changes in pregnancy, 818
Constipation, in Parkinson's disease, 579
Convergence and divergence, 133
Copper deficiency, 650
Cortical–subcortical neural system, 29
Corticosteroids
    cluster headache therapy, 708
    for complex regional pain syndrome, 730
    for myasthenia gravis, 688–689
    for neurocysticercosis, 614–615
    for primary CNS lymphoma, 745–746
    for vestibular neuronitis and labyrinthitis, 810
Cranial nerve palsy, in pregnancy, 835
Creutzfeldt-Jakob disease (CJD), 24–26, 118
Critical illness polyneuropathy, 668–669
Cryptococcal meningitis, 612–613, 625–626
Cubital tunnel syndrome, 265–266
Cyclophosphamide
    for inflammatory myopathy, 675
    for vasculitic neuropathy, 667
Cyclosporine
    for myasthenia gravis, 689–690
    for toxic myopathy, 682
Cysticercosis, in parasitic inflammatory
        myopathy, 676
Cysticidal therapy, for neurocysticercosis, 614
Cytomegalovirus (CMV), 630–632

Daily headache syndrome, 237
Dapsone, as peripheral nervous system toxin, 769
Declarative (explicit) memory, 41
Decompressive surgery, 489–490
Deep venous thrombosis, 654–655
Dejerine–Roussy syndrome, 295
Delayed sleep–wake phase disorder (DSWPD),
        102, 785–786
Delirium, 1
    hyperactive/hypoactive, 7
    management, 2, 13
    neurocognitive disorders and, 6
    pathophysiology, 1–2
Dementia, 588–602
    Alzheimer's disease, 17–19
    counseling and education, 601
    dementia with Lewy's bodies, 21

diagnostic criteria, 16–24
differential diagnosis, 26
early-onset, 601–602
epidemiology of, 15
etiology, 15, 16t
evaluation, 24–26
frontotemporal lobar degeneration, 21–24
mild cognitive impairment, 24
pathologic classification, 17t
psycho-pharmaceuticals in, 597–598
risk factors, 15
syndromic classification, 18t
treatment modalities
    cognitive remediation, 593–594
    disease modification, 588–593
    harm minimization, 600–601
    neuropsychiatric comorbidities, 594–600
vascular dementia, 19–21
Dementia with Lewy's bodies (DLB), 15–16, 21
Demyelinating disease, 149
Demyelinating lesions of spinal cord, 657
Demyelinating neuropathy, 663
Depression, 47
    in dementia, 594–595
    and spinal cord disorders, 655
    in stroke, 482
Dermatomyositis, 673, 674
Developmental delay
    ASD, 434
    cerebral palsy, 434
    disorders of white and grey matter, 435
    neurocutaneous disorders, 435–437
    progressive cognitive impairment, 435
    static encephalopathy, 433–434
Developmental disorders of spinal cord, 646–647
Dexamethasone, for bacterial meningitis, 605
Diabetic neuropathy, 669
Diagnostic and Statistical Manual of Mental
        Disorders (DSM-5), 1, 15, 42
Diastematomyelia, 646
Diffuse tongue atrophy and fasciculations, 213f
Dihydroergotamine (DHE), migraine therapy, 703
Dimethyl fumarate, for multiple sclerosis, 570, 572
Diplopia, 132, 429
    Bielschowsky's three-step test, 134
    chronic progressive external
        ophthalmoplegia, 137
    comitant and incomitant, 133
    convergence and divergence, 133
    cover–uncover test, 134
    ductions, 133
    esotropia, 133
    evaluation
        ancillary testing, 139
        clinical diagnosis, 138–139
        urgency of, 139–140
    examination
        head position and fixation, 133
        head tilt test, 134–135
        objective diplopia testing, 134
        other examination features, 135
        range of movement, 133
        subjective diplopia testing, 134
        testing saccades, 133–134
    exotropia, 133

giant cell arteritis, 138, 140
Graves' ophthalmopathy, 137
history, 132
hypertropia, 133
hypotropia, 133
increased intracranial pressure, 132
localization and etiologies
    brainstem, 135–136
    cranial nerves, 136–137
    extraocular muscles, 137–138
    orbit, 138
monocular *versus* binocular, 132
myasthenia, 137
neuromuscular junction disease, 137
orbital myositis, 137
orthophoria, 133
phoria, 133
sagging eye syndrome, 138
strabismus, 133
terminology, 133
treatment, 140
vasculopathic palsy, 136
versions, 133
Dipyridamole plus aspirin, 484
Discitis/osteomyelitis, 246–247
Disorders of arousal (DOA), 794–796, 795t
Distal symmetrical polyneuropathy, 670
Dix–Hallpike positional test, 179, 179f, 182
Dizziness and vertigo, 807–816
in arrhythmias, 815
audiologic testing, 180
basilar migraine and migrainous vertigo, 814
benign paroxysmal positional vertigo, 807–809
cervical vertigo, 174
chiari malformations, 174, 814
clinical manifestations, 175–176
diagnostic approach, 187
differential diagnosis, 182–187
Dix–Hallpike positional test, 179, 179f, 182
etiology of, 172t
    central vertigo, 173–174, 813–814
    medical vertigo, 174, 815
    otologic vertigo, 173, 807–813
    unlocalized vertigo, 174–175, 815–816
evaluation
    laboratory studies, 180–182
    patient history, 176–177
    physical examination, 177–180
examination procedures, 178t
head-shake test, 180
hypoglycemia, 815
in infection, 815
ischemia or infarction, 813–814
laboratory procedures, 181
medication-associated, 815
medications for treatment of vertigo, 810t
Ménière's disease, 185–186, 811
multiple sclerosis, 814
neck vibration test, 180
ototoxicity, 812
perilymphatic fistula, 811–812
postural hypotension, 815
referrals, 188
specific symptom complexes, 183t
superior canal dehiscence syndrome, 812

symptoms in patients with, 175t
treatment options, 809–810
tumors involving vestibulocochlear nerve,
    812–813
valsalva's test, 180
VEMP testing, 182
vertiginous migraine, 173
vestibular neuronitis and labyrinthitis, 809–811
vestibular testing, 181
Doose's syndrome, 514
Dopa-responsive dystonia (DYT5), 308
Dopamine, 1, 303, 373, 432, 576, 581, 594, 715
depleters, 583
receptor agonists, for Parkinson's disease, 577
Dopaminergic neurons, 1–2, 338, 777
Dravet's syndrome, 515
DSPD. *See* Delayed sleep-wake phase disorder
    (DSWPD)
Duchenne muscular dystrophy, 678–679, 680
Ductions, 133
Dural metastasis, 754, 755f, 757
Dysarthria, 36–37, 211
aphasia, 214
ataxic a, 213
clinical picture, 211
concomitant neurologic symptoms, 214
diagnostic evaluation, 214
differential diagnosis, 213–214
dysphonia, 214
evaluation of speech function, 214–215
flaccid, 211
hyperkinetic, 213
hypokinetic, 213
Lambert–Eaton myasthenic syndrome, 214
management, 215–216
mayo clinic classification, 212t
mixed, 212–213
spastic, 211–212
Dyschromatopsia, 563
Dysphagia
aspiration pneumonia, 204
clinical presentation, 203–204
common neurologic causes
    acute, 205
    chronic, 205–206
complications, 204–205
diagnostic evaluation, 206–208
fiberoptic endoscopic evaluation of
    swallowing, 208
main aspects of neurologic examination, 204t
normal swallowing, anatomy and physiology
    airway protection, 203
    central neurologic regulation, 203
    effects of normal aging, 203
    swallowing phases, 202
prognosis, 210
swallowing center, 203
symptoms and signs, 204t
treatment
    compensatory treatments, 208
    options, 209t
    rehabilitative treatments, 208–209
    surgical treatments, 209
    under investigation, 209
water swallowing test, 206

Dysphonia, 214
Dystonia, 584, 584t
  acquired dystonia, 307
  anti-N-methyl-d-aspartate receptor
    encephalitis, 308
  classification by age of onset, 305
  definition, 304–305
  dopa-responsive dystonia (DYT5), 308
  DYT6, 307
  etiologic classification, 305
  focal dystonia, 306–307
  myoclonus-dystonia (DYT11), 308
  Niemann–Pick type C, 308
  pathophysiology, 305
  phenomenologic classification, 305
  primary torsion dystonia, 305–306
  rapid-onset dystonia-parkinsonism (DYT12),
    308
  Wilson's disease, 307
Dystonic gait, 85
Dystrophinopathy, 678–679

Early-onset dementia, 601–602
EC/IC bypass surgery, 489
Eclampsia, in pregnancy, 831–832
Eculizumab, for myasthenia gravis, 690
Edrophonium test, for myasthenia gravis,
  685–686
EDS. See Excessive daytime sleepiness (EDS)
EEG. See Electroencephalography (EEG)
Electrical stimulation, for chronic pain, 720
Electroencephalogram (EEG), 10–11, 406
  abnormal activity
    altered states of consciousness, 412–414
    brain death, 414–415
    epilepsy, 407–412
  in acute sensory loss, 299
  in ADHD, 433
  alpha rhythm, 406
  in brain death, 385
  in coma, 55, 57
  in Creutzfeldt-Jakob's disease, 25
  in dementia, 25
  in dizziness and vertigo, 181
  in epilepsy (adults), 532
  in epilepsy (child), 510–511, 513–514
  epileptiform, 407
  findings in encephalopathic patients, 12t
  in headache, 231
  in hepatic encephalopathy, 412, 413f
  in hypokinesia, 334–335, 338
  in memory impairment, 50
  nerve conduction studies and, 415–422
  in neurocutaneous disorders, 438
  normal activity, 406–407, 407f
  in post cardiorespiratory arrest, 414f
  rhythms, 406
  in sleep disorders, 96, 100
  for status epilepticus, 526
  in syncope, 75, 78
Electromyography (EMG)
  for inflammatory myopathy, 674
  for myasthenia gravis, 686
Elevated intracranial pressure (ICP), 839–840

Emergencies. See Neurologic emergencies
Encephalopathy
  EEG findings in patients, 12t
  examination findings in patients, 8t
  hypertensive, 6
  metabolic, 3–4
  pathophysiology, 1–2
  treatment strategies, 12–13
Endocrine myopathy, 682
Entrapment neuropathies. See Lower extremity
  pain and paresthesias
Epilepsies in adults
  acute seizure cluster, 551
  and contraception, 554–555
  definitions and classifications of, 430–431
    of epilepsy or epileptic syndromes, 530–531
    of seizures, 530–532
  evaluation of, 532–533
  international classification of epileptic
    seizures, 59
  memory deficits in, 65
  and menstruation, 555
  in pregnancy, 551–555
  psychosocial problems, 558
  referrals
    epilepsy centers, 533, 558
    surgical treatment, 528
    vagal nerve stimulation (VNS), 527
  status epilepticus, 547–551
    in bacterial meningitis, 608–609
    cause of, 547–548
    definition of, 547
    drug therapy for, 549–550
    generalized convulsive status epilepticus
      (GCSE), 547
    management of, 558, 548t, 550–551
    prognosis of, 547
    refractory generalized convulsive status
      epilepticus (GCSE), 550
    types of, 547
  treatment of,
    AED discontinuation, 556–557
    antiepileptic drugs, 537–546
    first seizure, 546–547
    elderly and AEDs, 555–556
Epilepsies in children, 510–527
  classification of, 510–518
    generalized, 511–515
    localization- related (focal, partial), 510–511
    special syndromes, 517–518
    undetermined whether focal or generalized,
      515–517
  evaluation of, 518–519
    laboratory studies, 518–519
    physical examination, 518
    predisposing factors, 518
  in pregnancy, 819–825
  status epilepticus, 525–527
  treatment for, 519–527
    antiepileptic drugs (AEDs), 524
    indications for, 519
    medication withdrawal, 527
    psychosocial issues, 524
    single seizure, 519

surgery, 528
   vagal nerve stimulation, 527
Epley maneuver, for basilar migraine and
   migrainous vertigo, 807–809
Epworth sleepiness scale., 95f
Ergot alkaloids, migraine therapy, 699
Ergot derivatives, cluster headache therapy, 707
Esotropia, 133
Essential tremor (ET), 584–585
Ethanol poisoning, 776–777
Ethosuximide, 523
Ethyl alcohol as peripheral nervous system toxin,
   768
Ethylene oxide as peripheral nervous system
   toxin, 768, 769
Euthyroid Graves' disease, 139
Evoked potentials (EP), 422
   brainstem auditory, 424–425
   somatosensory, 426
   visual, 422–424
Excessive daytime sleepiness (EDS), 787–793
Exotropia, 133
Explicit memory, 41
Extradural metastases, 754
Extrapyramidal dysarthrias, 37
Extrasylvian aphasia, 34

Fabry's disease, 496
Facial numbness
   blink reflex, 143, 150
   causes of, 147–149
   classic clinical syndromes, 150–151
   demyelinating disease, 149
   diagnosis and management, 142
   history, 142
   leprosy and, 148
   localization, 144–147
   neuroanatomy of trigeminal nerve, 145f
   neurologic examination, 143–144
   numb cheek/chin syndrome, 151
   physical examination, 142
   sarcoidosis, 149
   syringobulbia, 149
   testing, 150
   treatment and referral, 150
Facial pain, 153
   anesthesia dolorosa, 159
   atypical facial pain, 157–158
   atypical odontalgia, 158
   burning mouth syndrome, 160
   causes, 158–160
   cluster headache, 156
   first bite syndrome, 158
   glossopharyngeal neuralgia, 155
   herpes zoster neuralgias, 155–156
   lower and oral pain, 158
   pearls for, 160
   persistent idiopathic facial pain, 157–158
   primary headache disorders, 156–157
   TMJ syndromes, 158
   trigeminal neuralgia, 153–154
   trigeminal trophic syndrome, 159
Facial weakness
   anatomy, 162–163

Bell's palsy, 162–163
blunt trauma, 165
cardiofacial syndrome, 166
clinical assessment, 163–164
congenital facial paralysis, 166
differential diagnosis, 164–170
Goldenhaar's syndromes, 166
House–Brackmann classification of facial
   function, 164t
Melkersson–Rosenthal syndrome, 165
Möbius syndrome, 166
Poland's syndromes, 166
Ramsay Hunt syndrome, 164–165
traumatic facial paralysis, 165f
Facioscapulohumeral muscular dystrophy,
   679, 681
Failed back syndrome, 283
   flat back syndrome, 286
   gate-control theory of pain, 286
   lumbar spondylosis, 285
   nonsurgical modalities, 285–286
   pain management, 286–287
   post-laminectomy spondylolisthesis, 287
   provocative diskography, 285
   pseudoarthrosis, 287
   radiographic evaluation, 288–289, 288f, 289f
   referrals, 289
   signs and symptoms
      claudication, 284
      flexion–extension radiographs, 285
      provocative diskography, 285
      radiculopathy, 284
      sharpy's fibers, 285
   somatic problems not related to spine, 285
   surgical management, 287–288
Familial amyloid neuropathy (FAP), 671
Familial temporal lobe epilepsy (FTLE), 60–61
Felbamate, 523
Femoral neuropathy, 273–275
Fingolimod, for multiple sclerosis, 572
First bite syndrome, 158
Flaccid dysarthria, 211
Flat back syndrome, 286
Flunarizine, migraine therapy, 702
Focal dystonia, 306–307
Focal motor seizures, 62
Folic acid deficiency, 649
Fosphenytoin, 516, 525
Foster Kennedy syndrome, 116
Fragile X tremor-ataxia syndrome
   (FXTAS), 586
Free radical scavengers, for complex regional
   pain syndrome, 734
Frenzel's goggles, 178–179
Friedreich ataxia, 322
Frontal lobe dementia, 43
Frontotemporal dementia, 43
Frontotemporal lobar degeneration (FTLD), 16,
   21–24
Fukuda stepping test, 88t
Functional amnesia, 46
Functional gait disorder, 373
Functional limb weakness/paralysis, 370–371
Functional movement disorders, 371–373

Functional neurologic disorders, 368
   classification, 368
   clinical manifestations and diagnostic
      approach, 370–375
   differential diagnosis, 376–377
   etiology and mechanism, 369–370, 369*f*
   evaluation, 375–376
   terminology, 368
   treatment and referral, 377–378
Functional/psychogenic gait, 86

Gabaergic agents, for chronic pain, 718
Gabapentin, migraine therapy, 702
Gait disturbance
   brainstem locomotor regions, 80–81
   classified
      high-level gait disorders, 85–86
      lower-level gait disorders, 83–84
      middle-level gait disorders, 84–85
      other gait disorders, 86
   clinical manifestations
      abnormal patterns of walking, 83–86
      features of normal walking, 81–83
      normal development of walking, 83
   cortical locomotor areas, 81
   criteria for diagnosis, 90
   diagnostic approach, 89
   differential diagnosis, 88–89
   etiology, 81
   evaluation, 86–88
   gait parameters, 83*t*
   inspection and examination, 87*t*
   neurologic causes, 89*t*
   pathophysiology, 80–81
   referral, 90–91
   spinal locomotor CPGs, 80
   supplementary motor area, 81
   vestibular evaluation, 88*t*
Gamma-aminobutyric acid (GABA)
      antagonists, 778
Gamma hydroxybutyrate (GHB), 775
Gases, PNS toxins, 769
Gastrointestinal changes in pregnancy, 818
Gastrointestinal dysfunction
   causes, 361
   esophageal, gastric, and intestinal
      dysfunction, 360
   evaluation, 361–362
   fecal incontinence, 361
   management of, *362*
   symptoms, 360
Gate-control theory of pain, 286
Generalized seizures, 530
Generalized tonic-clonic seizure (GTCS),
      64, 510
Germ cell therapy, 466
Giant cell arteritis (GCA), 138, 140, 858
Glasgow Coma Scale (GCS), 53*t*, 499
Glatiramer acetate, for multiple sclerosis, 570
Global aphasia, 34
Glossopharyngeal neuralgia, 155
Glutamate agonists, 778
Gold salts as peripheral nervous system toxin, 767
Goldenhaar's syndromes, 166

GON block
   cluster headache therapy, 707–708
   migraine therapy, 703
Gratification syndrome (masturbation), 443
Graves' ophthalmopathy, 137
Guanfacine, for tics, 582
Guillain-Barré syndrome (GBS), 211, 294, 447–
      448, 835, 857
Guyon's canal, 266

Hallpike's maneuver, 88*t*
Hallucinogens, 773
Haloperidol, for tics, 582
Hardy–Rand–Rittler pseudoisochromatic color
      plates, 109
Head computed tomography (CT), 231
Head size, abnormalities of, 444
Headache, 218
   arteriovenous malformations, 232
   associated with infection, 223
   chronic and recurrent, 227, 441
      attributed to substances, 234–235
      Chiari I malformations, 234
      diagnostic studies, 230–231
      examination, 230
      history, 227–230
      Marfan or Ehler–Danlos syndromes, 234
      from nonvascular intracranial disorders,
         233–234
      posttraumatic headache, 231–232
      secondary to cerebrovascular disease,
         232–233
      trigeminal autonomic cephalalgias, 237–238
      trigeminal neuralgia, 235
   cluster, 221, 228
   cyclic vomiting syndrome, 219
   evaluation, 442
   examination of patient, 224–225
   family history, 229–230
   ICHD-3 beta classification, 227*t*
   medication overuse headache, 235
   new daily persistent headache, 237
   orthostatic, 223
   pertinent history, 218–219
   postural orthostatic tachycardia syndrome,
      223–224
   in pregnancy, 825, 826–828*t*
   primary
      cluster headache, 221, 228, 238*t*
      hemicrania continua, 221
      migraine, 219, 235–236, 236*t*
      migraine with/without aura, 219–220
      tension-type headaches, 220–221, 227,
         236–237, 237*t*
   secondary
      brain tumors, 221–222
      due to increased intracranial pressure, 221
      exertional headaches, 222
      idiopathic intracranial hypertension, 222
      posttraumatic headache, 231–232
      red flags, 231*t*
      subdural hematoma, 222
   sentinel, 222
   sinusitis, 223

with stroke, 223
symptoms associated with, 218
tension-type headaches, 220–221, 227, 236–237, 442
thunderclap, 222
triggers or risk factors, 229
Hearing loss
assistive listening devices, 199
audiologic evaluation
audiogram, 192, 193f
pure-tone threshold audiometry, 192
range of hearing, 192
screening, 194
speech audiometry, 194
auditory neuropathy/dyssynchrony, 198
auditory system, anatomy and physiology
central auditory system, 191
external ear, 190
inner ear, 190–191
middle ear, 190
bone-anchored hearing aids, 199
central auditory processing disorder, 198
conductive hearing loss, 197–198
etiology, 190
hearing aid circuitry, 199
hearing aid styles, 199
management, 198–200
medical evaluation, 191–192
middle ear implantable hearing aids, 199
mixed hearing loss, 198
nonorganic, 190
otoscopic and otologic examination, 191
physiologic measures of hearing
auditory brainstem response, 195–196
auditory steady-state responses, 196
immittance audiometry, 194–195
otoacoustic emissions, 196–197
referral, 200
Rinne's test, 192
sensorineural hearing loss, 198
tuning fork tests, 191
Weber's test, 191
Heavy metals, PNS toxins, 763–767
Hematologic disorders in pregnancy, 831
Hemiballismus, 581
Hemifield slide, 116
Hemorrhagic cerebrovascular disease, 494
cause-specific treatment
saccular aneurysms, 508
vascular malformations, 507–508
causes
arterial hypertension, 494–496
bleeding disorders, 497
brain tumors, 497–498
cerebral amyloid angiopathy, 496
drug abuse, 497
of hemorrhagic stroke, 495t
moyamoya, 497
occult craniocerebral trauma, 494
other aneurysms, 496
saccular aneurysm, 496
vascular malformations, 496
vasculitis, 497
venous thrombosis, 497

diagnostic studies
arteriography, 503–504
cerebrospinal fluid examination, 503
computed tomography of brain, 501–503, 502f, 503f
MRI, 503
differential diagnosis
craniocerebral trauma, 500
ischemic stroke, 500
subarachnoid and primary intraventricular hemorrhage, 500–501
emergency management, 505t
manifestations
assessment of consciousness, 499–500
clinical presentation, 498
general examination, 498–499
neurologic examination, 500
treatment
general inpatient care, 507
general management, 505
halting continued bleeding, 505
increased ICP and brain edema, 505–506
prevention, 504
referral and admission, 505
surgical management, 506–507
treatment of arterial hypertension, 505
Heparin in stroke, 831
Herpes encephalitis, 609–611, 610f
Herpes simplex encephalitis, 45, 843
Herpes zoster (shingles), 148, 611
High-dose intravenous methotrexate, for primary CNS lymphoma (PCNSL), 746
High-grade gliomas (HGGs), 737–740
course of disease, 737
magnetic resonance imaging, 737–738, 738f
prognosis, 739–740
radiation therapy, 737–739
therapy for, 737–739
HIV. See Human immunodeficiency virus; Neurologic complications in AIDS
Holmes' tremor, 304
Hormonal changes in pregnancy, 818
Horner's syndrome, 129–130, 144
House–Brackmann classification of facial function, 164t
Human immunodeficiency virus (HIV). See also Neurologic complications in AIDS
distal sensory polyneuropathy, 622–624
HIV-associated neurocognitive disorder, 619–621, 620t
myelopathy, 622
myopathy, 622
neuropathy in, 670–671
Hunt–Hess Scale, 500t
Huntington's disease, 43
hyperkinetic movement disorders in, 581
Hyperextension-flexion injury (whiplash), 658–659
Hyperkalemic periodic paralysis, 677, 678
Hyperkinetic dysarthria, 213
Hyperkinetic movement disorders, 301, 301t, 581–586. See also Chorea; Dystonia; Myoclonus; Tics; Tremor

Hypersomnias, 791t, 792–793. *See also* Sleep
        disorders
    medical condition, result of, 793
    narcolepsy, 792–793
    recurrent hypersomnia, 793
Hypersomnolence, central disorders, 99–102
    associated with a psychiatric
        disorder, 102
    due to medical condition, 101–102
    due to medication or substance, 102
    idiopathic hypersomnia, 100–101
    insufficient sleep syndrome, 102
    Kleine–Levin Syndrome, 101
    narcolepsy (types 1 and 2), 99–100
Hypertropia, 133
Hypnosis, for chronic pain, 722
Hypnotic drugs, for sleep disorders, 783, 784t
Hypo-and hyperhidrosis, 362–363
Hypoglycemia, dizziness and vertigo in, 815
Hypokinesia, 328
    clinical findings of parkinsonism, 330–331
    diagnostic approach
        clinical, 337
        electrophysiology, 338
        general laboratory tests, 337
        genetic testing, 338
        neuropsychological testing, 338
        radiology, 337–338
        special diagnostic tests, 338
        therapeutic trial, 339
    differential diagnosis, 329f
        cerebrovascular disease, 334
        dementia syndromes, 336
        drug-induced parkinsonism, 333
        hemiatrophy–hemiparkinsonism, 334
        heredodegenerative diseases, 336–337
        IPD, 332–333
        normal pressure hydrocephalus, 333–334
        Parkinson-plus syndromes, 334–336
        toxins, 334
        Wilson's disease, 336
    evaluation of parkinsonism
        cognitive symptoms, 328–330
        direct motoric manifestations of
            parkinsonism, 328
        dysautonomia, 330
        family history, 330
        medication usage, 330
        psychiatric symptoms, 330
        response to medications, 328
        sleep disorders, 330
    neuroimaging, 332
    non-parkinsonian neurologic
        signs, 331–332
    referal, 339
Hypokinetic dysarthria, 213
Hypokinetic movement disorders, 575–580
Hypopigmented macule, 437f
Hypothyroid myopathy, 682
Hypotropia, 133
Hypoxic ischemic encephalopathy (HIE), 451
Hypsarrhythmia, 410

Iliohypogastric, ilioinguinal, and genitofemoral
        neuropathy, 279–280

Immune reconstitution inflammatory syndrome
        (IRIS), 636–637
Immunosuppressive therapy, for vasculitic
        neuropathy, 667–668
Implicit memory, 41
Inclusion body myositis (IBM), 673, 674
Infant botulism, 446–447, 694–695
Infarction
    dizziness and vertigo in, 813–814
    spinal cord, 650–651, 651f
Infection, dizziness and vertigo in, 815
Infectious–parainfectious neurologic diseases, 298
Inflammatory-demyelinating disease, 298
Inflammatory demyelinating polyneuropathy
        (IDP), 623–624
Inherited metabolic neurologic disorders,
        639–644
    classification of, 639–640
    diagnosis, 641–643
    incidence and prevalence of, 639
    large molecule disorders, 641, 642t
    prevention of, 643–644
    small molecule disorders, 640t
    treatment of, 643
Inherited polyneuropathies, neuropathy in, 671
Insomnia, 93–94, 781–785
    adjustment (acute) insomnia, 94
    associated disorders, 783–785
    behavioral insomnia of childhood, 95–96
    cognitive behavioral therapy, 782–783
    course of, 781
    due to drug or substance, 96
    due to medical condition, 96
    due to mental disorder, 95
    hypnotic drugs for, 783
    idiopathic insomnia, 95
    inadequate sleep hygiene, 95
    paradoxical insomnia, 94
    psychophysiologic insomnia, 94
    treatment and outcome of, 781–782
Interferons, for multiple sclerosis, 570
*International Classification of Sleep Disorders
        (ICSD)*, 93
Internuclear ophthalmoplegia, 563
Intracerebral hemorrhage, 851–853
Intracerebral Hemorrhage Scale, 500t
Intracranial aneurysm, in pregnancy, 831–832
Intracranial bleeding, 848–849
Intracranial hemorrhage, 449
    in pregnancy, 829
Intranasal capsaicin, cluster headache therapy, 709
Intranasal civamide, cluster headache therapy, 709
Intranasal lidocaine, cluster headache therapy, 707
Intravenous gamma globulin (IVIG)
    for acute inflammatory demyelinating
        neuropathy, 666
    for chronic inflammatory demyelinating
        neuropathy, 667
    for inflammatory myopathy, 675
Intravenous immunoglobulin (IVIG), for
        myasthenia gravis, 690
Intraventricular hemorrhage, 851–853
Irregular sleep–wake rhythm disorder (ISWRD),
        103, 786
Ischemia, dizziness and vertigo in, 813–814

Ischemic cerebrovascular disease, 473–475
  ischemic stroke, 475–479
  natural history and prognosis, 475–479
  prevention
    cigarette smoking, 479
    diabetes mellitus, 479
    excessive alcohol use, 480
    hyperlipidemia, 479–480
    hypertension, 479
    obesity and physical inactivity, 480
  surgical therapy
    carotid angioplasty and stenting, 488–489
    carotid endarterectomy, 488
    decompressive surgery, 489–490
    EC/IC bypass surgery, 489
  treatment
    anticoagulants, 484–488
    antiplatelet agents, 483–484
    brain edema, 482–483
    cerebral autoregulation, 482
    clopidogrel, 484
    depression, 482
    dipyridamole plus aspirin, 484
    electrolytic and metabolic disturbances, 481
    general measures, 480–482, 480f
    hemorrhagic transformation, 483
    pressure sores, 482
    rehabilitation, 483
    respiratory tract protection and infection,
      480–481
    seizures, 483
    urinary tract infections, 481
    venous thromboembolism, 481
Ischemic stroke, 500, 846–847
  from cardioembolism, 476
  from hemodynamic mechanisms, 476–477
  from hypercoagulable disorders, 477
  from large-artery atherosclerotic disease, 475
  from nonatherosclerotic vasculopathies, 477
  from small-vessel or penetrating artery disease
    (lacunes), 475–476
  of undetermined causation., 478–479
Ischemic–hemorrhagic neurologic disorders, 298

Jaundice, and coma, 53
Junctional syndrome, 113
Juvenile absence epilepsy, 63–64
Juvenile myoclonic epilepsy, 64

Ketamine, for chronic pain, 719
Kinetic perimetry, 111
Kleine–Levin syndrome (KLS), 793
Klonopin (clonazepam)
Korsakoff's syndrome, memory impairment in,
  41, 45

Lacosamide, 524
Lambert–Eaton myasthenic syndrome (LEMS),
  214, 417, 693
Lamotrigine, 522
Lance–Adams syndrome, 314
Landau–Kleffner syndrome, 438, 516
Large molecule disorders, 641, 642t
Lateral femoral cutaneous neuropathy
  clinical manifestations, 275

differential diagnosis, 275
  etiology, 275
  evaluation, 276
Lead as peripheral nervous system toxin, 764–765
Lennox–Gastaut syndrome, 64–65, 513
Leprosy, 148
Levetiracetam, 522
Levodopa, for Parkinson's disease, 577
Liberatory or Semont maneuver, for basilar
  migraine and migrainous vertigo, 809
Lidocaine, migraine therapy, 703
Limb-girdle muscular dystrophy, 679, 681
Lithium, 774
Lithium, cluster headache therapy, 709
Local anesthetics, for chronic pain, 718
Locked-in syndrome, 6t, 55
Long-term memory, 42, 47
Lorazepam, 525
  for status epilepticus, 608
Low back pain, acute
  clinical manifestations and evaluation
    history, 250
    physical examination, 250
  diagnostic approach, 252
  differential diagnosis, 250
  etiology, 249
  serious causes of, 250t
  surgical referral, 256
  treatment, 254–255
Low-grade gliomas (LGGs), 740–742
  course of disease, 740
  magnetic resonance imaging, 741f
  prognosis of, 742
  radiation therapy, 741–742
  therapy for, 741–742
Lower extremity pain and paresthesia, 272
  evaluation, 272–273
  miscellaneous neuropathies, 280–281
  piriformis syndrome, 276
  referrals, 281
  specific forms of mononeuropathy
    femoral and saphenous neuropathy, 273–275
    iliohypogastric, ilioinguinal, and
      genitofemoral neuropathy, 279–280
    lateral femoral cutaneous neuropathy,
      275–276
    medial and lateral plantar neuropathy, 279
    obturator neuropathy, 275
    peroneal neuropathy, 277–278
    sciatic neuropathy, 276–277
    tibial neuropathy, 278–279
LRP4 (low-density lipoprotein receptor-related
  protein 4), in myasthenia gravis, 686
Lumbar disc disease with sciatica
  clinical manifestations and evaluation
    history, 250
    physical examination, 251
  diagnostic approach, 252
  differential diagnosis, 251
  etiology, 249
  motor testing, 251
  sensory loss, 251
  straight-leg-raise testing, 251
  surgical referral, 256
  treatment, 255–256

Lumbar puncture, 427
  complications of, 429
  contraindications for, 428–429
  evaluation of results, 429–430
  and indications for CSF examination, 427–428
Lumbar spinal stenosis
  clinical manifestations and evaluation
    history, 250
    physical examination, 251
  diagnostic approach, 252, 253f
  differential diagnosis, 251–252
  etiology, 249–250
  surgical referral, 256
  treatment, 256
Lumbar spondylosis, 285
Lumbosacral plexopathy, 669
Lumbosacral spine, 254f
Lyme's disease, 611–612
  neuropathy in, 670
Lymphocytic hypophysitis, 829
Lysine acetylsalicylate, migraine therapy, 704

Macrocephaly, 444
Magnetic resonance angiography (MRA). See also
    Neuroimaging
  in dizziness and vertigo, 186
  in headache, 223, 393
  in impairment of ocular motility, 401
  in intermittent and chronic deficits, 395–396
  in pulsatile tinnitus, 399
  in vascular injury, 392
  in visual loss, 401
Magnetic resonance imaging (MRI). See also
    Neuroimaging
  in acute confusional state, 11f
  in acute sensory loss, 299
  in aphasia, 32
  of brain showing right vestibular
    schwannoma, 437f
  in dementia, 397
  in diplopia, 139
  in facial numbness, 150
  in facial weakness, 163, 166
  in gait disturbances, 88
  in low back pain, 252, 402–403
  in lumbar disc disease with sciatica, 252
  in lumbar spinal stenosis, 252
  in medulloblastoma, 747, 747f
  in meningioma, 743, 743f
  in multiple sclerosis, 566, 567t
  in myelopathies, 403–404
  in neck pain, 401–402
  for primary CNS lymphoma, 745–746, 745f
  in pulsatile tinnitus, 399
  in seizures, 397–399
  in syncope, 78
  in UE pain and paresthesias, 263
  in vertigo and ataxia, 400
  in vision loss, 111, 401
Magnetic resonance venography (MRV), 222
Major Neurocognitive Disorder.
    See Dementia
Malignant cerebral edema, 848
Manganese, 777

Mannitol, for increased intracranial pressure
    (ICP), 606
McArdle's disease, 682
Medial and lateral plantar neuropathy, 279
Medial longitudinal fasciculus (MLF), 563
Medical vertigo, 174
Medication overuse headache (MOH), 235
Medulloblastoma, 746–748
  course of disease, 746–747
  magnetic resonance imaging, 747f
  prognosis of, 748
  radiation therapy, 747–748
  therapy for, 747–748
Melatonin
  for circadian rhythm sleep disorders, 786, 787
  cluster headache therapy, 709
Melkersson–Rosenthal syndrome, 165
Memantine, for dementia, 593
Memory. See also Amnesia
  Alzheimer's disease, 42–43
  anoxia/ischemia, 45
  anterograde amnesia (learning defects), 44
  frontal lobe dementia, 43
  frontotemporal dementia, 43
  functional amnesia, 46
  hemispheric specialization of, 41t
  herpes simplex encephalitis, 45
  Huntington's disease, 43
  impairment of, 40–50
    clinical manifestations, 42–46
    depression, 47
    diagnostic criteria, 49
    differential diagnosis, 48–49
    evaluation, 46–48
    referral for, 49–50
    schizophrenia, 47
  Korsakoff's syndrome, 45
  neoplasms and, 45
  nonverbal memory tests, 47
  Parkinson's disease, 43
  Pick's disease, 43
  posthypnotic amnesia, 46
  posttraumatic amnesia, 44
  progressive supranuclear palsy, 43
  and psychiatric diseases, 47
  retrograde amnesia, 41, 44, 47
  subdivisions of, 40t
    anterograde, 40–41
    declarative (explicit) and nondeclarative
      (implicit), 41, 47
    long-term, 42, 47
    retrograde, 41, 44, 47
    short-term, 41
    verbal and nonverbal, 41
  transient global amnesia, 46
  vascular dementia, 44
  Wernicke–Korsakoff's syndrome, 45
  working, 40, 42
Mendelian mutations, 16
Meniere's disease, 185–186, 811
Meningioma, 742–744
  course of disease, 742–743
  prognosis of, 744
  therapy for, 743–744

Meralgia paresthetica, in pregnancy, 835
Mercury as peripheral nervous system toxin, 766–767
Mercury poisoning, 776
Mesial temporal sclerosis, 61
Mesial temporal system, 42
Metabolic myopathy, 681–682, 681t
Metabolic polyneuropathy, 668–669
Metastases
    brain, 750–753
    CSF, 755–757
    dural, 754, 757
    extradural, 754
    spinal, 753–754
    spinal cord, 754
Metastatic epidural spinal cord compression, 854
Methotrexate
    for inflammatory myopathy, 675
    for myasthenia gravis, 690
Methyl bromide as peripheral nervous system toxin, 768
Methyl-ethyl-ketone as peripheral nervous system toxin, 768
1-Methyl-4-phenyl-1,2,3,6-tetrahydropyridine (MPTP), 777
Methylphenidate, for tics, 582
Methysergide, cluster headache therapy, 709
Metronidazole, 4–5
Microcephaly, 444
Migraine, 219, 235–236, 236t, 441
    in pregnancy, 825, 826–828t
    preventive treatments for, 701t
Mild cognitive impairment (MCI), 16, 24
Mirtazapine, 581
Mitochondrial myopathies, 680, 681
Mitochondrial toxins, 777
Mixed dysarthria, 212–213
Mixed transcortical aphasia, 35
Möbius syndrome, 166
Modafinil, for tics, 582
Mononeuritis multiplex, 663
Mononeuropathy, 663
Motor disorders, 439–440
Movement disorders, 575–586. See also
        Hyperkinetic movement disorders;
        Hypokinetic movement disorders
    baclofen withdrawal, 454
    opsoclonus myoclonus syndrome, 454
    in pregnancy, 836
    sleep-related, 798–800 (See also Sleep
        disorders)
    status dystonicus, 455
Moyamoya, 497
Multiple sclerosis (MS), 561–573
    clinical features, 562–564, 563t
    course of, 568–569
    defined, 561
    diagnosis, 564–568, 565–567f
    dizziness and vertigo in, 814
    epidemiology of, 561–562
    pathogenesis of, 562
    in pregnancy, 573, 833, 834t
    therapy
        acute relapses, 569

disease-modifying therapies, 569–570
    for relapsing forms, 569–573, 571t
Multiple sleep latency testing (MSLT), 426–427, 789
Multiple systems atrophy (MSA), 72, 580
Muscle biopsy
    for inflammatory myopathy, 674
    for muscular dystrophy, 678
Muscle relaxants, for chronic pain, 718–719
Muscle weakness, acute, 340
    botulism, 342
    diagnostic approach, 344–345
    differential diagnosis
        acute anterior horn cell disease, 341
        acute intermittent porphyria, 342
        acute neuromuscular junction disorders, 342–343
        acute neuropathy, 342
        acute plexopathy, 341–342
        acute polyradiculoneuropathy, 341
        primary myopathy, 343–344
    diseases causing, 345t
    evaluation, 340–341
    laboratory studies, 344
    management, 345
    rhabdomyolysis, 343
    tick paralysis, 342
    West Nile Virus, 341
Muscular dystrophy, 678–681
    Becker's muscular dystrophy, 679, 680
    defined, 678
    Duchenne muscular dystrophy, 678–679, 680
    dystrophinopathy, 678–679
    facioscapulohumeral muscular dystrophy, 679, 681
    history and prognosis, 678–680
    limb-girdle muscular dystrophy, 679, 681
    mitochondrial myopathies, 680, 681
    myotonic dystrophy, 679–680, 681
    myotonic dystrophy type 2 or proximal
        myotonic myopathy, 680
    oculopharyngeal muscular dystrophy, 679, 681
    therapeutic approach, 680–681
    types of, 678
MuSK antibodies, in myasthenia gravis, 686
Mutism, 37
Myasthenia, 137
Myasthenia gravis (MG), 685–692
    associated autoimmune diseases, 685
    clinical features of, 685
    congenital myasthenia, 692
    definition and causes of, 685
    diagnosis, 685–686
        ACh receptor antibodies, 686
        edrophonium test, 685–686
        EMG testing, 686
        LRP4, 686
        MuSK antibodies, 686
    in pregnancy, 835–836
    prognosis of, 686–687
    transient neonatal myasthenia, 692
    treatment, 687–692
        alternative immunosuppressive drug
            therapy, 689–690

Myasthenia gravis (MG) (*continued*)
cholinesterase inhibitors, 687–688, 687*t*
corticosteroids, 688–689
drugs to avoid in, 691
high dose intravenous immunoglobulin, 690
management guidelines, 690–691
plasma exchange, 690
specific therapy guidelines, 691–692
thymectomy, 688
Myasthenic crisis, 446–447, 691, 691*t*, 857
Mycophenylate mofetil
for inflammatory myopathy, 675
for myasthenia gravis, 689
Myoclonic astatic epilepsy (MAE), 514
Myoclonic seizures, 530
Myoclonus, 10, 582, 583*t*
brainstem myoclonus, 313
cortical myoclonus, 313
definition, 312
epilepsia partialis continua, 313
etiologic classification, 312
Lance–Adams syndrome, 314
opsoclonus-myoclonus syndrome, 312
palatal myoclonus, 314
Parkinsonian disorders, 313
pathophysiology, 312–313
propriospinal myoclonus, 313
Myoclonus-dystonia (DYT11), 308
Myopathies. *See also* Muscular dystrophy
defined, 673
idiopathic inflammatory, 673–676
diagnosis, 674
history and prognosis, 673–674
therapy, 674–676
metabolic, 681–682, 681*t*
acid maltase deficiency (Pompe's disease),
681–682, 681*t*
carnitine-O-palmitoyltransferase II (CPT
II) deficiency, 681*t*, 682
McArdle's disease, 681*t*, 682
parasitic inflammatory, 676
periodic paralyses, 676–678
channelopathies, 676, 677*t*
history and prognosis, 676–677
prevention and therapeutic approach,
677–678
toxic, 682–683
antimicrotubular, 683
autophagic, 683
endocrine, 682
hypothyroid, 682
steroid, 683
thyrotoxic, 682
toxic necrotizing, 682
viral inflammatory, 676
Myotonia congenita, 578, 677
Myotonic dystrophy, 679–680, 681
in pregnancy, 836
Myotonic dystrophy type 2, 680

N-hexane, methyl-*n*-butyl ketone,
2,5-hexandione as peripheral nervous
system toxin, 767–768
Nadolol, for tremor, 585

Narcolepsy, 787–790. *See also* Sleep disorders
classification of, 789
clinical features, 787
course of, 787–789
defined, 787
diagnosis of, 789
drugs for, 791–792*t*
symptoms of, 788*t*
treatment and outcome of, 789–790
Natalizumab, for multiple sclerosis, 572–573
National Aphasia Association, 38
NCSE. *See* Nonconvulsive status epilepticus
(NCSE)
Neck pain
with arm pain from bone spurs, 243
etiology, 244
evaluation, 244
referral, 244–245
with arm pain from soft cervical disk bulges/
herniations (radiculopathy)
anatomy, 242
etiology, 242
evaluation, 242–243
referral, 243
of arthritic origin (nontraumatic)
etiology, 241
evaluation, 241
referral, 241
due to metastatic cancer of cervical spine, 246
miscellaneous
discitis/osteomyelitis, 246–247
rheumatoid arthritis, 246, 248*f*
motor strength classification, 242*t*
Nurick classification, 244*t*
posttraumatic, 240*t*
scans and X-rays, 246, 274*f*
tumors and, 246, 274*f*
without arm pain (traumatic)
etiology, 240
evaluation, 240
medication, 240
referral, 240–241
soft collar, 240
time-off from work, 240–241
Nervous system. *See* Cancer complications of
nervous system; Central nervous system;
Peripheral nervous system
Neurocysticercosis, 614–615
Neurogenic orthostatic (postural) hypotension,
352–354
Neuroimaging
in altered level of consciousness, 396–397
in back pain, 402–403
in cerebral ischemia
acute stroke, 394
dural sinus and cortical vein thrombosis,
395
intermittent and chronic deficits, 395–396
in chemosis and proptosis, 401
in dementia, 397
in headache
acute, 393–394
chronic, 394
subacute, 394

in hearing loss, 399
in impairment of ocular motility, 401
in myelopathies, 403–404, 403*f*, 404*f*
in neck pain and cervical radiculopathy,
  401–402, 401*f*
in nonpulsatile tinnitus, 399
in pulsatile tinnitus, 399
in seizures
  known seizure disorder, 397
  new-onset adult, 397
  pediatric, 397–399
in trauma
  cervical spine injury, 392
  closed head injury, 391–392
  penetrating head injury, 392
  vascular injury, 392
in vertigo and ataxia, 400
in visual loss, 401
Neuroleptic malignant syndrome (NMS), 4, 858
Neuroleptics, 777
  for tardive dyskinesia, 583
Neurologic changes in pregnancy, 818
Neurologic complications in AIDS, 617–637
  conditions attributed to HIV infection,
    619–624
    aseptic meningitis, 624
    HIV-associated neurocognitive disorder,
      619–621, 620*t*
    HIV distal sensory polyneuropathy,
      622–624
    HIV myelopathy, 622
    HIV myopathy, 624
    inflammatory demyelinating
      polyneuropathy, 623–624
  entities causing, 618–619*t*
  general considerations, 617
  highly active antiretroviral therapy, 617
  opportunistic illnesses, 624–637
    CNS lymphoma, 628–629
    CNS toxoplasmosis, 626–627
    CNS tuberculosis, 633–635
    cryptococcal meningitis, 625–626
    cytomegalovirus, 630–632
    immune reconstitution inflammatory
      syndrome, 636–637
    neurosyphilis, 635–636
    progressive multifocal leukoencephalopathy,
      629–630
    varicella-zoster virus, 632–633
Neurologic conditions in pregnancy, 819, 819*t*
Neurologic emergencies, 839–861
  acute cauda equina syndrome, 856
  acute dystonic reaction, 858
  acute serotonin syndrome, 858
  angiolingual edema, 848
  bacterial meningitis, 841–843
  brain abscess, 843–844
  central cord syndrome, 854–855
  central retinal artery occlusion, 858–859
  cerebellar hemorrhage, 851
  cerebral toxoplasmosis, 845
  coma, 840
  elevated intracranial pressure, 839–840
  giant cell arteritis (temporal arteritis), 858

Guillain-Barré's syndrome, 857
herpes simplex encephalitis, 843
intracerebral hemorrhage, 851–853
  associated with heparin, 849
  associated with warfarin, 849
  in thrombolytic therapy, 848
intracranial bleeding, 848–849
intraventricular hemorrhage, 851–853
ischemic stroke, 846–847
malignant cerebral edema, 848
metastatic epidural spinal cord
  compression, 854
myasthenic crisis, 857
neuroleptic malignant syndrome, 858
pituitary tumor apoplexy, 859–861
posterior reversible encephalopathy
  syndrome, 861
septic cavernous sinus thrombosis, 845
spinal cord injury, 854–856
status epilepticus, 840–841
subarachnoid hemorrhage, 851
subdural empyema, 845–846
Wernicke's encephalopathy, 859
Neurology, ethical issues
  approaches to
    brain death, 463–464
    chronic pain, 469
    neurogenetic diseases, 466–467
    research in neurology, 468
    static or progressive disorders with impaired
      cognition, 467–468
    static or progressive disorders with intact
      cognition, 467
    vegetative state, 464–465
  background and implications, 459–460
  case method approach, 462
  case studies, 470–471
  ethical decision making in general, 462–463
  ethical theories
    criteria of adequate theory, 460
    types, 460–461
  interface with law, 469
  medical profession and drug industry, 469–470
  referrals, 470
  in 21st century, 459
Neurology, pediatric
  acute neurologic weakness
    acute disseminated encephalomyelitis, 448
    Guillain–Barré syndrome, 447–448
    idiopathic transverse myelitis, 448
    infant botulism, 446–447
  acute vascular lesions
    arterial ischemic stroke, 449–450
    cerebral venous sinus thrombosis, 450
    intracranial hemorrhage, 449
  altered mental status/encephalopathy
    acute liver failure and neurologic
      sequelae, 452
    hypoxic ischemic encephalopathy, 451
    infectious meningitis and encephalitis,
      450–451
    methotrexate toxicity, 451
    posterior reversible encephalopathy
      syndrome, 451

Neurology, pediatric (*continued*)
  epilepsy, 455–456
  movement disorders
    baclofen withdrawal, 454
    opsoclonus myoclonus syndrome, 454
    status dystonicus, 455
Neuromuscular junction disorders, 685–695. *See
    also* Myasthenia gravis
  botulism, 693–695
  Lambert–Eaton myasthenic syndrome, 693
Neuronopathy, 663
Neuropathic pain, 713
Neuropathy, peripheral, 663–672
  definition and terms, 663
  diagnosis and management of specific
      conditions, 666–668
    acute inflammatory demyelinating
        neuropathy, 666
    brachial plexitis (Parsonage-Turner
        syndrome or neuralgic amyotrophy), 668
    chronic inflammatory demyelinating
        neuropathy, 666–667
    vasculitic neuropathy, 667–668
  management based on symptoms, 663–666
    cramping, 665
    pain, 663–665
    paresthesia, 665
    sensory loss, 665
    unstable balance, 665–666
    weakness, 665
  medication-induced, 669–670
  new developments in, 671–672
    amyloid neuropathy, 671–672
    small fiber neuropathy, 671
  polyneuropathies due to infections, 670–671
    human immunodeficiency virus, 670–671
    inherited, 671
    Lyme's disease, 670
  toxic or metabolic, 668–669
    alcoholic neuropathy, 668
    critical illness polyneuropathy, 668–669
    diabetic neuropathy, 669
Neurophysiologic electrodiagnostic studies, 406
Neurosyphilis, 613, 635–636
Neurotoxins, 763–779
  causation in, 763
  central nervous system toxins, 772–779
    acute delirium, 772–774
    cerebellar disorders, 776–777
    coma and CNS depression, 775–776
    Parkinsonism, 777
    seizures, 777–779
    subacute encephalopathy, 774–775
  classification and definition of, 763
  myotoxins, 771
  peripheral nervous system toxins, 763–771
    gases, 769
    heavy metals, 763–767
    pharmaceuticals, 769–771
    solvents, 767–769
  toxins affecting ion channels, 770
  toxins affecting neuromuscular junction, 770
New daily persistent headache (NDPH), 237
Nightmare disorder, 798

Nitrous oxide as peripheral nervous system
    toxin, 769
NMDA receptor antagonists, for complex
    regional pain syndrome, 734
NMDA-receptor antibody encephalitis, 581
Non-24-hour sleep–wake isorder (N24SWD),
    103, 786
Non-REM parasomnias, 794–796, 795*t*
Nonconvulsive status epilepticus (NCSE),
    5, 9–10
Nondeclarative (implicit) memory, 41, 47
Nonepileptic paroxysmal disorders, 443
Nonorganic visual loss, 119–120
Nonsteroidal anti-inflammatory drugs (NSAIDs)
    for chronic pain, 713–714
    for complex regional pain syndrome, 730
    migraine therapy, 698–699
Normocephaly, 444
NSAIDs. *See* Nonsteroidal anti-inflammatory
    drugs
Numb cheek/chin syndrome, 151
Numb chin syndrome, 294
Nurick scale, 245
Nutraceuticals, migraine therapy, 703
Nystagmus, 88*t*

Obsessive–compulsive behavior, 582
Obstructive sleep apnea (OSA), 802–804
  expiratory positive airway pressure, 803
  nasal CPAP, 802–803
  night shift, 803
  oral appliances, 803
  oxygen therapy, 803
  somnoplasty, 804
  surgery, 804
  uvulopalatopharyngoplasty for, 804
  winx sleep therapy system, 803
Obturator neuropathy, 275
Occipital lobe seizures, 63
Occipital nerve stimulation, migraine
    therapy, 704
Occult craniocerebral trauma, 494
Occupational therapy, for chronic pain, 720
Ocular bobbing, 55
Ocular coherence tomography (OCT), for
    multiple sclerosis, 568
Oculomotor (third cranial) nerve palsy, 125
Oculopharyngeal muscular dystrophy, 679, 681
Ohtahara's syndrome, 515
Olanzapine, for tics, 582
Onabotulinum toxin A, migraine therapy, 702–703
Onionskin sensory loss, 146*f*
Ophthalmoscopy, 109
Opioids, 775
    for chronic pain, 714–715, 714*t*
    for complex regional pain syndrome, 731
    migraine therapy, 700
Opsoclonus myoclonus syndrome (OMS),
    312, 454
Optic neuritis, 563
Orbital myositis, 137
Organophosphates or carbamates as peripheral
    nervous system toxin, 768–769
Orthophoria, 133

Orthostatic headache, 223
Orthostatic hypotension
   nonpharmacologic treatment, 355t
   pharmacologic treatment, 356t
Otoacoustic emissions, 196–197
Otologic vertigo, 173
Otosclerosis, 198
Ototoxicity, 812
Oxcarbazepine, 521
Oxygen inhalation, cluster headache therapy,
   706–707

Pain, chronic, 713–722
   defined, 713
   management of, 713–722
   medications for, 713–720
   neuropathic, 713
   nonpharmacologic treatments for, 720–722
   somatic, 713
   visceral, 713
Paraneoplastic syndromes, cancer and, 757–759
Parasitic inflammatory myopathy, 676
Parasomnias, 793–798. See also Sleep disorders
   defined, 793
   non-REM, 794–796
   NREM-related, 103–104
   REM, 104, 796–798
Paretic dysarthria, 36
Parietal lobe seizures, 63
Parkinsonian disorders, 313
Parkinsonian gait, 85
Parkinsonian tremor, 303
Parkinsonism, and CNS toxins, 777
Parkinson's disease, 43, 575–580, 576t
   hypokinetic movement disorders in, 575–580
   in pregnancy, 836
Parkinson's disease dementia (PDD), 21
Paroxysmal infant shuddering, 443
Parsonage-Turner syndrome or neuralgic
   amyotrophy, 668
Partial (focal) seizures, 530
Partial myelitis, 563
Partial seizures, 59, 61–63
   complex partial seizures of frontal
      lobeorigin, 62
   focal motor seizures, 62
   occipital lobe seizures, 63
   parietal lobe seizures, 63
   supplementary motor seizures, 62
   temporal lobe seizures, 61
PCNSL. See Primary CNS lymphoma
PCOM. See Posterior communicating artery
   (PCOM)
Pediatric neurology
   acute neurologic weakness
      acute disseminated encephalomyelitis, 448
      Guillain–Barré syndrome, 447–448
      idiopathic transverse myelitis, 448
      infant botulism, 446–447
   acute vascular lesions
      arterial ischemic stroke, 449–450
      cerebral venous sinus thrombosis, 450
      intracranial hemorrhage, 449
   altered mental status/encephalopathy
      acute liver failure and neurologic
         sequelae, 452
      hypoxic ischemic encephalopathy, 451
      infectious meningitis and encephalitis,
         450–451
      methotrexate toxicity, 451
      posterior reversible encephalopathy
         syndrome, 451
   epilepsy, 455–456
   movement disorders
      baclofen withdrawal, 454
      opsoclonus myoclonus syndrome, 454
      status dystonicus, 455
Penicillamine, for Wilson's disease, 586
Pentobarbital, for increased intracranial pressure
   (ICP), 607
Perampanel, 524
Perilymphatic fistula, 811–812
Periodic hypersomnolence, 793
Periodic lateralized epileptiform discharges
   (PLEDs), 61
Periodic paralyses, 676–678
Periodic paralysis secondary, 677
Peripheral nerve stimulation, migraine therapy,
   704–705
Peripheral nervous system (PNS), toxins in,
   763–771
Peripheral neuropathy, 663. See Neuropathy,
   peripheral
Perisylvian language zone, 29f, 30–31,
   34–35
Peroneal neuropathy
   clinical manifestations, 277–278
   differential diagnosis, 278
   etiology, 277
   evaluation, 278
Persistent idiopathic facial pain, 157–158
Pharmaceuticals, PNS toxins, 769–771
Phenobarbital, 516, 521
Phenytoin, 538
   for status epilepticus, 608
Phenytoin, 521
Phoria, 133
Physical therapy
   for chronic pain, 720
   for complex regional pain syndrome, 732
   for Duchenne muscular dystrophy, 680
Physiologic tremor, 302
Pick's disease, 43
Pimozide, for tics, 582
Piriformis syndrome, 276
Pituitary tumor apoplexy, 859–861
Pituitary tumors, in pregnancy, 826–829
Plain radiography, for complex regional pain
   syndrome, 725
Plasma exchange (PLEX)
   for acute inflammatory demyelinating
      neuropathy, 666
   for chronic inflammatory demyelinating
      neuropathy, 667
   for myasthenia gravis, 690
Platybasia, 647
Pleocytosis, 429
Plexopathy and plexitis, 663

PNS disorders, UE pain and paresthesias
  brachial plexopathy
    idiopathic brachial, 269
    neurogenic TOS, 269
    in patients with malignancy, 269–270
  mononeuropathy
    axillary nerve, 267
    dorsal scapular nerve, 268
    median nerve, 264–265
    musculocutaneous nerve, 267–268
    radial nerve, 266–267
    suprascapular nerve, 268
    ulnar nerve, 265–266
Poland's syndromes, 166
Polymyalgia rheumatica (PMR), 673, 674
Polymyositis, 673, 674
Polyneuropathy, 663
Polyradiculitis, 671
Polyradiculoneuropathy, 663
Polyradiculopathy, 663
Polysomnography (PSG), 426, 789
Pompe's disease, 681–682
Post-laminectomy spondylolisthesis, 287
Postconcussion syndrome, 445
Posterior communicating artery (PCOM), 9
Posterior reversible encephalopathy syndrome
      (PRES), 4, 6, 12–13, 118, 451, 861
Posthypnotic amnesia, 46
Postpartum cerebral angiopathy, in
      pregnancy, 831
Postpartum eclampsia, in pregnancy, 833
Posttraumatic amnesia, 44
Posttraumatic headache, 231–232
Posttraumatic neck pain, 240t
Postural hypotension, dizziness and vertigo in, 815
Postural orthostatic tachycardia syndrome
      (POTS), 223–224, 354. See also POTS
POTS, 78, 223, 350–351t, 354
Prednisone, for inflammatory myopathy, 674–675
Preeclampsia, in pregnancy, 831–832
Pregnancy
  cerebrovascular disease, 829–833
  chorea gravidarum, 836
  epilepsy in, 819–825
  headache in, 825, 826–828t
  movement disorders in, 836
  multiple sclerosis, 833, 834t
  myasthenia gravis, 835–836
  myotonic dystrophy, 836
  neurologic conditions in, 819, 819t
  neurologic diseases in, 818–836
  pseudotumor cerebri, 829
  root lesions and peripheral neuropathy, 833, 835
PRES. See Posterior reversible encephalopathy
      syndrome (PRES)
Presbyopia, 108
Pressure sores, 482, 654
Primary CNS lymphoma (PCNSL), 745–746
  course of disease, 745
  high-dose intravenous methotrexate, 746
  magnetic resonance imaging, 745–746, 745f
  prognosis, 746
  radiation therapy, 746
  therapy for, 745–746

Primary hypokalemic periodic paralysis, 676,
      677–678
Primary progressive aphasia (PPA), 30
Primidone, for tremor, 585
Progressive multifocal leukoencephalopathy
      (PML), 629–630
Progressive supranuclear palsy (PSP), 43, 580
Pronator teres syndrome, 265
Propranolol, for tremor, 585
Proximal myotonic myopathy, 680
Pseudo-Foster Kennedy syndrome, 116
Pseudoarthrosis, 287
Pseudosyncope, 73
Pseudotumor cerebri, in pregnancy, 829
Psychogenic seizures, 66
Pulfrich phenomenon, 563
Pulmonary changes in pregnancy, 818
Pupils, abnormal
  anisocoria greater in darkness
    aberrant regeneration of oculomotor nerve,
        130
    Horner's syndrome, 129–130
    physiologic anisocoria, 130–131
  light-near dissociation, 131
  mechanical anisocoria, 124, 125f
  pupil and eyelids, sympathetic
        innervation, 122f
  pupil size, 121, 123
  pupillary dilation, 121
  pupillary examination, 123
  pupillary light reflex, 121f, 123
  relative afferent pupillary defect, 123–124
  unilateral mydriasis, 124–129
    oculomotor (third cranial) nerve palsy, 125
    pharmacologic mydriasis, 128–129
    tonic pupil (Adie pupil), 125–128
Pyridoxine, 516
Pyridoxine as peripheral nervous system
      toxin, 770

Quantitative sudomotor axon testing (QSART),
      for complex regional pain syndrome, 727
Quetiapine, for Parkinson's disease, 578

Radiation therapy
  in meningioma, 744
  for primary CNS lymphoma (PCNSL), 746
Radiculopathy, 663
Ramsay Hunt syndrome, 164–165
Rapid-onset dystonia-parkinsonism
      (DYT12), 308
Rasagiline, for Parkinson's disease, 575
Recurrent and nonrecurrent seizures, 59
Recurrent hypersomnia, 793
Reflex syncope, 355
Relative afferent pupillary defect (RAPD), 109,
      112–113
REM parasomnias, 796–798, 798t
Renal changes in pregnancy, 818
Reserpine, for tardive dyskinesia, 583
Respiratory tract protection and infection,
      480–481
Retinal nerve fiber layer (RNFL), 114f
Retrograde memory, 41, 44, 47

Reversible cerebral vasoconstriction syndrome (RCVS), 223
Reye's syndrome, viral inflammatory myopathy in, 676
Rheumatoid arthritis, 246, 248f
Rifampin, for meningococcal meningitis, 609
Rinne's test, 192
Risperidone, for tics, 582
Rituximab
  for inflammatory myopathy, 676
  for myasthenia gravis, 690
  for primary CNS lymphoma, 746
Root lesions and peripheral neuropathy, in pregnancy, 833, 835
Rufinamide, 523

Saccular aneurysm, 496, 508
Sagging eye syndrome (SES), 138
Sandifer's syndrome, 443
SANTE trial, 67
Saphenous neuropathy, 273–275
Sarcoidosis, 149
Schizophrenia, 47
Sciatic neuropathy
  clinical manifestations, 276
  differential diagnosis, 277
  etiology, 276
  evaluation, 277
Sciatica and back pain, in pregnancy, 835
Secondary hypokalemic periodic paralysis, 677
Sedative hypnotics, 775
Seizures, 59–68. See also Epilepsy
  in acute confusional state, 3, 3t
  and anticonvulsants, 66
  aura in, 66
  in bacterial meningitis, 608–609
  clinical manifestations of, 61–65
  and CNS toxins, 777–779
  comprehensive epilepsy center, 67
  in dementia, 26
  diagnostic approach for, 66–67
  differential diagnosis of, 66
  dizziness and vertigo in, 172t, 173
  etiology of, 59–60
  evaluation of, 65–66
  familial temporal lobe epilepsy, 60–61
  generalized tonic–clonic, 64, 483
  international classification, 59
  Lennox–Gastaut syndrome, 64–65
  neuroimaging for, 397–399, 398f
  partial, 59, 61–63
    complex partial seizures of frontal lobe origin, 62
    focal motor seizures, 62
    occipital lobe seizures, 63
    parietal lobe seizures, 63
    supplementary motor seizures, 62
    temporal lobe seizures, 61
  in pregnancy, 819–825
  primary (idiopathic) generalized epilepsy, 63–64
    childhood absence epilepsy, 63
    generalized tonic-clonic seizures, 64
    generalized tonic-clonic status epilepticus, 64
    juvenile absence epilepsy, 63–64
    juvenile myoclonic epilepsy, 64
  psychogenic, 66
  recurrent and nonrecurrent, 59
  referral of, 67–68
  secondary (symptomatic) generalized epilepsy, 64
    Lennox-Gastaut's syndrome, 64–65
    West's syndrome, 64
  sleep disorders and, 66–67
  and syncope, 66
  typical features, 74t
  West's syndrome, 64
Selegiline, for Parkinson's disease, 575
Sensorimotor polyneuropathy, 669
Sensorineural hearing loss, 198
Sensory loss, acute, 291
  acute transverse myelitis, 295
  albuminocytologic dissociation, 299
  anosognosia, 295
  brachial plexus, 296
  Brown–Séquard syndrome, 295
  cauda equina syndrome, 296
  clinical aspects in area of trunk, 295–298
  clinical manifestations
    examination of sensory modalities, 291–292
    functional sensory loss, 292
    negative sensory symptoms, 292
    positive sensory symptoms, 292
  Dejerine–Roussy syndrome, 295
  diagnostic approaches
    blood work, 299
    brain evaluation, 299
    examination of cerebrospinal fluid, 299–300
    nerve biopsy, 299
    PNS evaluation, 298–299
    spinal cord evaluation, 299
  etiology, 298
  Guillain–Barré syndrome, 294
  hemibody sensory disturbance, 294
  infectious–parainfectious neurologic diseases, 298
  inflammatory-demyelinating disease, 298
  ischemic–hemorrhagic neurologic disorders, 298
  localization of pathologic processes
    brachial and lumbosacral plexus, 293
    cortex, 293
    cranial nerve and brainstem, 293
    nerve roots, 292
    peripheral nerves, 292
    sensory receptors, 292
    spinal cord, 293
  lumbosacral plexus, 296
  numb chin syndrome, 294
  "onionskin-like" sensation, 294
  over scalp and neck, 294–295
  referrals, 300
  sensory disturbance in face, 293–294
  sensory useless hand syndrome, 295
  syringobulbia, 294
  Tolosa–Hunt syndrome, 294
  traumatic–compressive lesions, 298
Sensory useless hand syndrome, 295

Sentinel headaches, 222
Septic cavernous sinus thrombosis, 845
Serotonin syndrome, 4, 5t, 9, 772–773
Serum osmolality in pregnancy, 818
Sexsomnias, 794
Sexual dysfunction
  erectile dysfunction, 357–358
  laboratory testing, 357
  lifestyle changes, 357
  pathophysiology, 356–357
  somatosensory stimulation, 357
Shagreen patch, 438f
Sharpy's fibers, 285
Sheehan's syndrome, 827
Shift work sleep–wake disorder, 103, 786–787
Short-term memory, 41
Sickle cell anemia, 148
Sinusitis, 223
Sleep disorders, 781–804
  advanced sleep–wake phase disorder, 102–103
  central disorders of hypersomnolence, 99–102
    associated with a psychiatric disorder, 102
    due to medical condition, 101–102
    due to medication or substance, 102
    idiopathic hypersomnia, 100–101
    insufficient sleep syndrome, 102
    Kleine–Levin Syndrome, 101
    narcolepsy (types 1 and 2), 99–100
  circadian rhythm sleep–wake disorders , 102–
      103, 785–787
    bright light therapy, 785–786, 787
    chronotherapy, 785
    course of, 785
    melatonin, 786, 787
    treatment and outcome, 785–786
  definition and categories of, 781
  delayed sleep–wake phase disorder, 102
  in dementia, 596
  Epworth sleepiness scale, 95f
  excessive daytime sleepiness, 787–793
    defined, 787
    narcolepsy (See also Narcolepsy)
  general approach
    sleep history, 93
    subjective measure scales, 93
    wake history, 93
  hypersomnias, 792–793
    medical condition, result of, 793
    narcolepsy, 792–793
    recurrent hypersomnia, 793
  insomnia, 93–94
    adjustment (acute) insomnia, 94
    behavioral insomnia of childhood, 95–96
    due to drug or substance, 96
    due to medical condition, 96
    due to mental disorder, 95
    idiopathic insomnia, 95
    inadequate sleep hygiene, 95
    paradoxical insomnia, 94
    psychophysiologic insomnia, 94
  insomnia, 781–785
    associated disorders, 783–785
    cognitive behavioral therapy, 782–783
    course of, 781

hypnotic drugs for, 783
  treatment and outcome of, 781–782
investigational tools and options, 105
irregular sleep–wake rhythm disorder, 103
maintenance of wakefulness test, 105
movement disorders, 798–800
  periodic limb movement disorder, 798–800
  restless legs syndrome, 798–800, 800t
non-24-hour sleep–wake rhythm disorder, 103
parasomnias, 793–798
  defined, 793
  non-REM, 103–104, 794–796
  REM, 104, 796–798
shift work disorder, 103
sleep-disordered breathing, 801–804
  central sleep apnea, 801–802
  obstructive sleep apnea, 802–804
sleep-related breathing disorders
  CSA syndromes, 97–98
  obstructive sleep apnea, 96–97
  sleep-related hypoventilation disorders,
      98–99
sleep-related movement disorders
  periodic limb movement disorder, 104–105
  restless legs syndrome, 104
Sleep-related breathing disorders (SRBDs)
  CSA syndromes, 97–98
  hypoventilation disorders, 98–99
  obstructive sleep apnea, 96–97
Sleep-related eating disorders, 794
Sleep-related movement disorders
  periodic limb movement disorder, 104–105
  RLS, 104
Sleep sex, 794
Sleep terrors, 104
Sleepwalking, 104
Small fiber neuropathy, 671
Small molecule disorders, 640t
Solvents, PNS toxins, 767–769
Somatic pain, 713
Somatosensory evoked potentials (SSEPs), for
      multiple sclerosis, 568
Sotalol, for tremor, 585
Spasmus nutans, 443
Spastic dysarthria, 36, 211–212
Spastic gait, 84
Spasticity, in spinal cord disorders, 659–661
Speech awareness threshold (SAT), 194
Speech recognition threshold (SRT), 194
Speech–language pathologist (SLP), 214
SPG stimulation, migraine therapy, 704–705
Spina bifida occulta, 646
Spinal cord disorders, 646–661
  acute spinal cord injury, 651–654, 652–653t
  central cord syndrome, 657
  demyelinating lesions of spinal cord, 657
  developmental disorders, 646–647
  hyperextension-flexion injury (whiplash),
      658–659
  infarctions, 650–651, 651f
  sequelae of spinal cord injuries, 654–656
  spasticity in, ,659–661, 659–660t
  spinal epidural abscesses, 656–657
  vascular malformation of spinal cord, 650

vitamin deficiencies, 647–650
Spinal cord injury, 854–856
Spinal cord metastases, 754
Spinal cord stimulation
    for chronic pain, 720
    for complex regional pain syndrome, 731–732
Spinal epidural abscesses, 656–657
Spinal metastases, 753–754
Status cataplecticus, 790
Status dystonicus, 455
Status epilepticus, 608–609, 840–841
Steppage gait, 83
Stereocilia, 191
Steroid myopathy, 683
Stilbamidine, 148
Stimulants, 777
Stimulus–control behavioral therapy, for
    insomnia, 782, 783t
Strabismus, 133
Styrene as peripheral nervous system toxin, 768
Subacute encephalopathy, and CNS toxins,
    774–775
Subarachnoid hemorrhage (SAH), 501t, 851
    in pregnancy, 831–832
Subcutaneous octreotide, cluster headache
    therapy, 707
Subdural empyema, 845–846
Sundowning, 7
Superior canal dehiscence syndrome, 812
Supplementary motor seizures, 62
Supraorbital neurostimulation, migraine
    therapy, 704
Surgery
    for basilar migraine and migrainous vertigo, 809
    for cluster headache, 710
    for high-grade gliomas, 738
    for low-grade gliomas, 741
    for medulloblastoma, 747
    in meningioma, 744
    for Parkinson's disease, 579–580
    thymectomy for myasthenia gravis, 688
    for tremor, 585
Surgical sympathectomy, for complex regional
    pain syndrome, 732
Sydenham's chorea, 310
Sympathetic block, for complex regional pain
    syndrome, 726
Sympathetic ganglion blocks, for complex
    regional pain syndrome, 731
Sympathomimetic syndrome, 772
Syncope, 66, 70–78
    and carotid sinus hypersensitivity, 72, 76
    etiology
        cardiac arrhythmias, 72
        cerebrovascular, 72–73
        neurally mediated syncope, 70–72
        orthostatic hypotension/intolerance
            syndromes, 72
        pseudosyncope, 73
        structural heart disease, 72
    evaluation
        blood laboratory testing, 77
        comorbid conditions, 75
        device interrogation, 78

echocardiography, 77
electrocardiography, 76–77
electrophysiologic testing, 77
events leading to syncope, 74–75
patient history, 74–75
physical examination, 76
postsyncopal events, 75
prodromal signs and symptoms, 75
radiographic studies/MRI, 78
stress testing or coronary angiography, 77
tilt-table testing, 77–78
    management, 78
    typical features, 74t
    of unknown origin, 73
Syringobulbia, 149
Syringomyelia, 647

Tacrolimus
    for myasthenia gravis, 690
    for toxic myopathy, 682
Tardive akathisia, 316
Tardive dyskinesia, 582–583
Tardive dystonia, 316, 583
Tardive syndromes
    definition, 316
    drugs to cause, 316
    risk factors, 316
Temporal lobe seizures, 61
Temporomandibular joint (TMJ)
    syndromes, 158
Tension-type headache, 220–221, 227, 236–237.
    See also Headache
    in pregnancy, 825, 826t
    therapy, 705–706
Teriflunomide, for multiple sclerosis, 572
Tethering of spinal cord, 646
Tetrabenazine(Xenazine), 581
    for tardive dyskinesia, 583
Tetrathiomolybdate, for Wilson's disease, 586
Tetrodotoxin poisoning, 770
Thallium as peripheral nervous system toxin,
    765–766
Thermal testing, for complex regional pain
    syndrome, 726
Thiothixene, for tics, 582
Thoracic radiculopathy, 669
Thunderclap headache, 222
Thyrotoxic myopathy, 682
Thyrotoxic periodic paralysis, 677, 678
Tibial neuropathy, 278–279
Tick paralysis, 342
Tics, 582
    definition, 314
    etiologic classification, 315
    pathophysiology, 315
    phenomenologic classification, 314
    Tourette's syndrome, 315
Timolol, for tremor, 585
TLOC (Transient loss of consciousness), 70, 73
Tolosa–Hunt syndrome, 294
Toluene–solvent abuse syndrome, 776
Tonic pupil (Adie pupil), 125–128
Tonic seizures, 531
Tonic–clonic seizures, 531

Topiramate, 522
  cluster headache therapy, 709
  migraine therapy, 702
  for tremor, 585
Tourette's syndrome (TS), 315, 582
Toxi-metabolic coma, 55
Toxic myopathy, 682–683
  antimicrotubular, 683
  autophagic, 683
  endocrine, 682
  hypothyroid, 682
  steroid, 683
  thyrotoxic, 682
  toxic necrotizing, 682
Toxic necrotizing myopathy, 682
Toxic polyneuropathy, 668–669
Toxoplasmosis, in parasitic inflammatory
    myopathy, 676
Transcortical motor aphasia, 34
Transcortical sensory aphasia, 34–35
Transcranial magnetic stimulation, migraine
    therapy, 705
Transcutaneous electrical nerve stimulation
    (TENS), 241
Transient global amnesia, 46
Transient ischemic attacks (TIAs), 71–72,
    111–112, 172, 175, 220, 532
  stroke and, 173t, 473
Transient loss of consciousness (TLOC), 70, 73
Transient neonatal myasthenia, 692
Transmagnetic stimulation, for chronic pain, 720
Traumatic brain injury (TBI), 231
Traumatic facial paralysis, 165f
Tremor, 584–586, 585t
  cerebellar tremor, 304
  definition, 301
  essential tremor, 303
  etiologic classification, 302
  Holmes' tremor, 304
  Parkinsonian tremor, 303
  pathophysiology, 302
  phenomenologic classification
    action tremor, 302
    rest tremor, 301–302
  physiologic tremor, 302
Trichinosis, in parasitic inflammatory
    myopathy, 676
Trichloroethylene as peripheral nervous system
    toxin, 768
Tricyclic antidepressants (TCAs), migraine
    therapy, 701–702
Trientine, for Wilson's disease, 586
Trifluoperazine, for tics, 582
Trigeminal neuralgia, 153–154, 235
Trigeminal trophic syndrome, 159
Trihexyphenidyl, for Parkinson's disease, 576
Triple-phase bone scan, for complex regional
    pain syndrome, 725–726
Triptans
  cluster headache therapy, 707
  migraine therapy, 699–700
Trivalent botulinum antitoxin, for classic
    botulism, 694
Tuberculous meningitis, 613

Tumors. See also Central nervous system,
    tumors of
  compressing the eighth cranial nerve in
    otologic vertigo, 172t, 173
  facial numbness in, 147
  involving vestibulocochlear nerve, 812–813
  in pregnancy, 826–829
Tuning fork tests, 191
Tympanometry, 194, 195f

Uhthoff phenomenon, 563
Unlocalized vertigo, 174–175, 815–816
Unresponsive wakefulness syndrome, 55
Upper extremity (UE) pain and paresthesias
  anterior interosseous syndrome, 265
  cubital tunnel syndrome, 265–266
  diagnostic approach, 263–264
  differential diagnosis, 258, 259t
  etiology, 258, 259t
  evaluation, 258–263
  Guyon's canal, 266
  motor vehicle accident, 260
  MSK disorders, 270
  muscle inspection, 261
  muscle strength ratings, 261–262
  muscle tone and, 262
  PNS disorders, brachial plexopathy
    idiopathic brachial plexopathy, 269
    neurogenic TOS, 269
    in patients with malignancy, 269–270
  PNS disorders, mononeuropathy
    axillary nerve, 267
    dorsal scapular nerve, 268
    median nerve, 264–265
    musculocutaneous nerve, 267–268
    radial nerve, 266–267
    suprascapular nerve, 268
    ulnar nerve, 265–266
  pronator teres syndrome, 265
  referral, 271
  symptoms
    motor, 259–260
    sensory, 258–259
  systemic illnesses, 261
Urinary bladder dysfunction, 358
  anatomy, 358
  clinical evaluation
    examination, 359
    history, 359
    urodynamic investigations, 359
  clinical presentations
    urinary incontinence, 360
    neurogenic bladder dysfunction, 359t
    treatment, 360
Urinary frequency medications, in multiple
    systems atrophy (MSA), 580
Urinary tract infections (UTI), 10, 13, 481
UTI. See Urinary tract infection (UTI)

Vagal nerve stimulation, migraine therapy, 705
Vagus nerve stimulation (VNS), 533
Valproate, migraine therapy, 702, 704
Valproic acid, 522
Varicella-zoster virus (VZV), 632–633

Vascular dementia, 16, 44, 19–21
Vascular malformation of spinal cord, 650
Vasculitic neuropathy, 667–668
Vasculopathic palsy, 136
Venlafaxine, migraine therapy, 702
Venous thromboembolism, 481
Venous thrombosis, 497
Verapamil, cluster headache therapy, 708–709
Verapamil, migraine therapy, 702
Verbal and nonverbal memory, 41
Versions, 133
Vertiginous migraine, 173
Vestibular neuronitis and labyrinthitis, 809–811
Vestibular rehabilitation, for vestibular neuronitis
    and labyrinthitis, 810–811
Vigabatrin, 523
Viral inflammatory myopathy, 676
Visceral pain, 713
Vision loss
    acute transient monocular visual loss, 111–112
    AION
        arteritic AION, 114
        Leber's hereditary optic neuropathy,
            114, 114f
        nonarteritic AION, 113, 113f
    Balint's syndrome, 118–119
    binocular visual loss due to optic chiasm
        dysfunction, 116–117
    clinical examination
        color vision testing, 109
        confrontation visual fields, 109
        electrophysiologic testing, 111
        neuroimaging, 111
        ophthalmoscopy, 109
        pupils, 109
        visual acuity, 108–109
        visual field testing, 109–111
    electroretinography, 111
    Foster Kennedy syndrome, 116
    hemifield slide, 116
    history, 108
    homonymous hemianopia, 117–118
    Humphrey visual fields, 110f
    nonorganic visual loss, 119–120
    ophthalmoscopy, 109
    persistent monocular visual loss
        acute/subacute clinical syndromes, 113–114
        chronic monocular visual loss from optic
            neuropathy, 114–115

posterior reversible encephalopathy
    syndrome, 118
presbyopia, 108
prosopagnosia, 119
pseudo-Foster Kennedy syndrome, 116
sudden binocular vision loss, 116
vision disturbances related to higher cognitive
    dysfunction, 118–119
visual evoked potentials, 111
Visual evoked potentials (VEPs), for multiple
    sclerosis, 568
Visual hallucinations and psychosis, in
    Parkinson's disease, 579
Vitamin B12 (cobalamin) deficiency, 647–649
Vitamin deficiencies, 647–650
Vitamin E deficiency, 649–650

Waddling and Trendelenburg gaits, 83–84
Warfarin, in stroke, 831
Weber's test, 191
Wechsler Memory Scale, fourth edition
    (WMS-IV), 47
Wernicke encephalopathy, 773–774
Wernicke–Korsakoff's syndrome, 45
Wernicke's aphasia, 29f, 33–34, 33f
Wernicke's encephalopathy, 4, 859
West Nile virus (WNV), 341
West's syndrome, 64
Whiplash (hyperextension-flexion injury),
    658–659
Wilson's disease, 307, 586
Withdrawal seizures, 779
Working memory, 40, 42, 47
Wound botulism, 695

X-linked dystrophinopathy, 678

Zelapar (Valeant), for Parkinson's
    disease, 575
Zidovudine (AZT) for HIV, 621
Zinc as peripheral nervous system toxin, 767
Ziprasidone (Geodon), 582
Zolmitriptan, 699
Zonisamide, 523
    for chronic pain, 718
    in epilepsy, 523, 542, 543
    for tremor, 585
Zydis selegiline (Zelapar), for Parkinson's
    disease, 575